615.
7

ROW

Clinical Pharmacokinetics and Pharmacodynamics

CONCEPTS AND APPLICATIONS

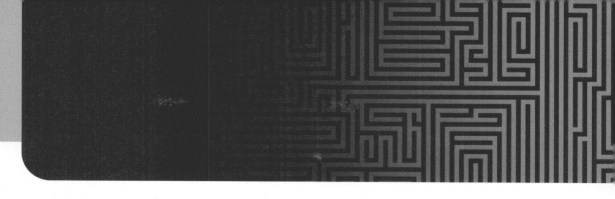

FOURTH EDITION

Clinical Pharmacokinetics and Pharmacodynamics

Concepts and Applications

Malcolm Rowland, DSc, PhD

Professor Emeritus
School of Pharmacy and
    Pharmaceutical Sciences
University of Manchester
Manchester, United Kingdom

Thomas N. Tozer, PharmD, PhD

Professor Emeritus
School of Pharmacy and
    Pharmaceutical Sciences
University of California, San Francisco
Adjunct Professor of Pharmacology
Skaggs School of Pharmacy and
    Pharmaceutical Sciences
University of California San Diego

With Online Simulations by
Hartmut Derendorf, PhD
Distinguished Professor
Guenther Hochhaus, PhD
Associate Professor
Department of Pharmaceutics
University of Florida
Gainesville, Florida

Wolters Kluwer | Lippincott Williams & Wilkins
Health

Philadelphia • Baltimore • New York • London
Buenos Aires • Hong Kong • Sydney • Tokyo

Acquisitions Editor: David B. Troy
Product Manager: Matt Hauber
Marketing Manager: Allison Powell
Designer: Doug Smock
Compositor: Maryland Composition Inc./ASI

Fourth Edition

Library of Congress Cataloging-in-Publication Data

Rowland, Malcolm.
   Clinical pharmacokinetics and pharmacodynamics : concepts and applications / Malcolm Rowland and Thomas N. Tozer. —4th ed.
     p. ; cm.
   Rev. ed. of: Clinical pharmacokinetics. 1995.
   ISBN 978-0-7817-5009-7
   1. Pharmacokinetics. 2. Chemotherapy. I. Tozer, Thomas N. II. Rowland, Malcolm. Clinical pharmacokinetics. III. Title.
   [DNLM: 1. Pharmacokinetics. 2. Drug Therapy. QV 38 R883c 2009]
   RM301.5.R68 2009
   615′.7—dc22

                                                      2009028928

To Dawn and Margaret
for their continual love, patience, and tolerance.

MALCOLM ROWLAND

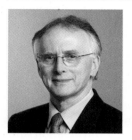

Malcolm Rowland is Professor Emeritus and former Dean (1998–2001), School of Pharmacy and Pharmaceutical Sciences, University of Manchester, and Adjunct Professor, School of Pharmacy, University of California, San Francisco. He was President of the European Federation of Pharmaceutical Sciences (1996–2000) and Vice-President, International Pharmaceutical Federation (FIP; 2001–2008), the organization that represents and serves pharmacy and pharmaceutical sciences around the globe. He received his pharmacy degree and PhD from the University of London, and was on faculty at the School of Pharmacy, University of California, San Francisco (1967–1975).

Dr. Rowland, together with Dr. Thomas Tozer, authored the introductory textbook, *Introduction to Pharmacokinetics and Pharmacodynamics: The Quantitative Basis of Drug Therapy*. He has authored over 300 scientific articles and chapters. His research interest is primarily in physiologically-based pharmacokinetics and its application to drug development and clinical use. In particular, he has pioneered the concept and application of clearance and developed approaches to the prediction of pharmacokinetics of drugs from a combination of physicochemical properties and in vitro information. He was an editor of the Journal of Pharmacokinetics and Pharmacodynamics (1973–2006), the premier journal dedicated to the subject, and has established workshops for teaching both basic- and advanced-level pharmacokinetics. He is an advisor to the pharmaceutical industry and sits on various scientific advisory boards.

Dr. Rowland has been awarded honorary doctorate degrees from the University of Poitiers (France) and Uppsala University (Sweden) as well as Honorary Membership of the Royal College of Physicians (London). He received various awards including the Distinguished Investigator Award of the American College of Clinical Pharmacology (ACCP, 2007) and the Millennial Pharmaceutical Scientist Award (FIP BPS, 2000). He has been made a fellow of the Academy of Medical Sciences, ACCP (Hon), American Association of Pharmaceutical Scientists, the Royal Pharmaceutical Society of Great Britain, and the Institute of Mathematics.

THOMAS N. TOZER

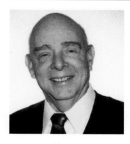

Dr. Tozer, Professor Emeritus of Biopharmaceutical Sciences and Pharmaceutical Chemistry, School of Pharmacy, University of California, San Francisco, received his BS, PharmD, and PhD degrees from the University of California, San Francisco. He is currently an Adjunct Professor of Pharmacology at the University of California, San Diego, where he teaches biopharmaceutics and clinical pharmacokinetics at the Skaggs School of Pharmacy and Pharmaceutical Sciences. After a 2-year postdoctoral fellowship in the laboratory of Dr. B. B. Brodie, National Institutes of Health,

Bethesda, Maryland, he joined the Faculty of the School of Pharmacy in San Francisco in 1965. Although now in emeritus status, he continues to teach courses and workshops in pharmacokinetics/pharmacodynamics and clinical pharmacokinetics at several institutions in the United States and Europe.

Dr. Tozer, together with Dr. Malcolm Rowland, authored *Clinical Pharmacokinetics: Concepts and Applications*, the title of the first three editions of this textbook. He has published more than 155 scientific papers on a variety of research topics with emphasis on the development and application of kinetic concepts in drug therapy. Dr. Tozer's research before retirement was focused in four areas: colon-specific drug delivery, toxicokinetics, kinetics of potential contrast agents for magnetic resonance imaging, and nonlinear pharmacokinetics. Other research included determination of drug disposition in disease states, particularly end-state renal disease. Emphasis here was placed on evaluating and predicting when and how drug administration to renal disease patients should be altered.

Dr. Tozer was a corecipient of the 2000 Meritorious Manuscript Award, American Association of Pharmaceutical Scientists, and was a Visiting Professor (1996–1999) at the University of Manchester, Manchester, England. He is a Fellow of the American Association of Pharmaceutical Scientists and has served as a consultant to the Food and Drug Administration and to many pharmaceutical companies.

PREFACE

Much has happened in the field of our textbook since the last edition was published in 1995. First, in recognition that there was a readership that sought a less in-depth textbook we wrote a companion, entitled *Introduction to Pharmacokinetics and Pharmacodynamics: The Quantitative Basis of Drug Therapy*; it was published in 2006. While emphasizing pharmacokinetics, the widening to include pharmacodynamics as an integral part of this introductory text reflected the increasing body of knowledge linking the two elements that explain the relationship between drug administration and response. We have continued this trend of integrating pharmacodynamics with pharmacokinetics in the current text, which is reflected in the title. Second, in addition to an expanding knowledge of pharmacodynamics, there has been an explosion in our understanding at the molecular and mechanistic levels of all the processes controlling the pharmacokinetics of drugs. The availability of the introductory text has therefore allowed us the opportunity to expand in this current edition on these new insights for those readers wishing to gain a greater in-depth understanding of the subject. This has required some enlargement over previous editions, but every attempt has been made to limit the size of the book.

As in our previous three editions, we are committed to developing and applying the concepts to explain and improve the therapeutic use of drugs. As such, we continue to have students and practitioners in pharmacy, medicine, pharmacology, and allied professions in mind as our readers. Accordingly, although the principles have wide application, emphasis continues to be at the clinical level. We recognize, however, that pharmacokinetics and pharmacodynamics are cornerstones in the industrial design, selection, and development of new drugs, and so believe that this textbook is of equal value to scientists engaged in all aspects of the pharmaceutical industry, as well as those working in regulatory agencies evaluating drug applications.

In addition to more detailed consideration of the basic principles compared to the introductory text, the current textbook expands greatly on why individuals vary in their response to drugs, which is central to personalizing drug therapy. Furthermore, there is an increase in the number of thought-provoking problems at the end of each chapter, with answers provided in the last appendix. While maintaining the overall structure and organization, there are also significant improvements over the third edition. In particular, we have incorporated advances in our understanding of the role of enzymes and transporters in pharmacokinetics, and of genetics in both pharmacokinetics and pharmacodynamics. As briefly mentioned above, we have greatly expanded on pharmacodynamics, which was a single chapter in the specialized topic section of the last edition, and have integrated it throughout the book. We have also incorporated Turnover Concepts and Dialysis, which were also previously specialized topics, into the body of the book, recognizing that these are fundamental to the subject. We have also added two new chapters. One deals with protein drugs, reflecting the rapid increase in recent years in the number of such medicines that have become a part of the armamentarium of modern therapeutics. The second concerns the prediction of human pharmacokinetics from in vitro and preclinical data, and subsequent simulation of likely kinetics in patients under a wide variety of clinical conditions and situations, which can improve the chances of selecting compounds that have desirable pharmacokinetic characteristics in planning clinical drug trials and in ensuring their subsequent optimal use.

We have also updated all chapters and replaced many of the examples and case histories with more modern ones, while providing many new problems with answers. To help approach these problems, we have provided at the end of each chapter a summary of key relationships. In addition, Drs. Hartmut Derendorf and Guenther Hochhaus, University of Florida, have prepared web-based simulations of many of the concepts presented throughout the book. The simulations allow the reader to explore the influence of changes in parameter values in both pharmacokinetics and pharmacodynamics on drug concentration and response with time following drug administration. Finally, to conform to the quality of all new figures, of which there are many, we have redrawn or improved the figures retained from previous editions.

ACKNOWLEDGMENTS

As with all previous editions, we wish to thank the many students, as well as participants of various workshops that we have taught, and colleagues for helping us shape the fourth edition. Their enthusiasm, commitment, and appreciation continue to be a source of immense satisfaction to us. We would also like to thank in particular Joe Balthasar for critiquing the protein drug chapter and Amin Rostami for assistance in the simulation of pharmacokinetic profiles in virtual patient populations.

It is now 30 years since the first edition of our textbook was published. Throughout this period, we have been enormously gratified by the wide and varied readership around the world, sometimes in the most unexpected of places. Our wish has always been to contribute to the improved design and more rational use of medicines. We hope that this fourth edition helps further this aspiration.

Malcolm Rowland, Manchester, UK
Thomas N. Tozer, San Francisco, California

TABLE OF CONTENTS

Preface   ix
Nonproprietary and Brand Names of Drugs in Text and Illustrations   xiii
Definition of Symbols   xix

SECTION I   BASIC CONSIDERATIONS

1 Therapeutic Relevance 3
2 Fundamental Concepts and Terminology 17

SECTION II   EXPOSURE AND RESPONSE AFTER A SINGLE DOSE

3 Kinetics Following an Intravenous Bolus Dose 49
4 Membranes and Distribution 73
5 Elimination 111
6 Kinetics Following an Extravascular Dose 159
7 Absorption 183
8 Response Following a Single Dose 217

SECTION III   THERAPEUTIC REGIMENS

9   Therapeutic Window 245
10 Constant-Rate Input 259
11 Multiple-Dose Regimens 293

SECTION IV   INDIVIDUALIZATION

12 Variability 333
13 Genetics 357
14 Age, Weight, and Gender 373
15 Disease 403
16 Nonlinearities 445
17 Drug Interactions 483
18 Initiating and Managing Therapy 527

SECTION V SUPPLEMENTAL TOPICS

19 Distribution Kinetics 561

20 Metabolites and Drug Response 603

21 Protein Drugs 633

22 Prediction and Refinement of Human Kinetics from In Vitro, Preclinical, and Early Clinical Data 663

APPENDICES

A. Assessment of *AUC* 687

B. Ionization and the pH Partition Hypothesis 691

C. Distribution of Drugs Extensively Bound to Plasma Proteins 695

D. Plasma-to-Blood Concentration Ratio 703

E. Well-stirred Model of Hepatic Clearance 705

F. Absorption Kinetics 709

G. Wagner-Nelson Method 713

H. Mean Residence Time 717

I. Amount of Drug in Body on Accumulation to Plateau 723

J. Answers to Study Problems 727

Index   819

NONPROPRIETARY AND BRAND NAMES OF DRUGS IN TEXT AND ILLUSTRATIONS

(For those drugs available only by brand name at time of manuscript submission, the brand name is provided.)

Abacavir	Ziagen	Asparaginase	Elspar
Abatacept		Aspirin	
Abciximab	ReoPro	Astemizole	
Acenocoumarol		Atenolol	
Acetaminophen		Atorvastatin	Lipitor
Acetazolamide		Azathioprine	
Acetylsalicylic acid		Azelastine	
Acyclovir		Azithromycin	
Adalimumab	Humira		
Adefovir		Bacitracin	
Agalsidase		Barbital	
Albendazole	Albenza	Basiliximab	Simulect
Albuterol		Benzylpenicillin	
Aldesleukin		Bethanechol	
Alefacept	Amevive	Chloride	
Alemtuzumab	Campath	Bevacizumab	Avastin
Alendronate sodium	Fosamax	Bivalirudin	Angiomax
Alfentanil		Bosentan	Tracleer
Alglucosidase alfa	Myozyme	Budesonide	Pulmicort
Allopurinol			Respules® and
Alprazolam			Entocort EC
Alprenolol		Bufurolol	
Alteplase		Bumetanide	
Amikacin		Buprenorphine	
Amiloride		Bupropion	
Aminosalicylic acid		Buspirone	
Amiodarone		Busulfan	
Amitriptyline			
Amoxicillin		Caffeine	
Ampicillin		Calcitonin-salmon	Miacalcin
Amprenavir	Agenerase	Capromab pendetide	ProstaScint Kit
Amrinone		Captopril	
Anakinra	Kineret	Carbamazepine	
Anidulafungin		Carbenicillin	
Antipyrine		Carmustine	
Antihemophilic		Cefamandole	
Factor (VIII)		Cefazolin	
Antithrombin III		Cefepime	
Aprepitant	Emend	Cefonicid	
Aprotinin		Ceforanide	
Ascorbic acid		Cefotaxime	

Cefprozil		Daclizumab	Zenapax
Cefsulodin		Dapsone	
Ceftazidime		Darifenacin	
Ceftizoxime		Debrisoquine	
Ceftriaxone		Delavirdine mesylate	Rescriptor
Cefuroxime		Denileukin diftitox	Ontak
Celecoxib	Celebrex	Desflurane	Suprane
Cephalexin	Keflex	Desipramine	
Cephalothin		Desirudin	Iprivask
Cephradine		Desloratadine	Clarinex
Cerivastatin	Baycol	Desmopressin acetate	DDAVP
Cetirizine		Dextroamphetamine	
Cetuximab	Erbitux	Dextromethorphan	
Chlordiazepoxide		Diazepam	
Chloroquine	Aralen	Diclofenac	
Chlorothiazide		Dicloxacillin	
Chlorpheniramine		Dicumarol	
Chlorpromazine		Didanosine	
Chlorzoxazone		Diethylcarbamazepine	
Cholestyramine		Diflunisal	
Chorionic gonadotropin		Digitoxin	
		Digoxin	
Cidofovir		Digoxin immune Fab	Digibind
Cilastatin	Primaxin	Diltiazem	
Cimetidine		Diphenhydramine	
Ciprofibrate		Dipyridamole	
Ciprofloxacin		Disopyramide	
Cisapride		Dobutamine	
Citalopram	Celexa	Dolasetron mesylate	Anzemet
Cladribine		Donepezil	Aricept
Clarithromycin		Dornase alfa	Pulmozyme
Clavulanate		Doxepin	
Clobazam		Doxorubicin	
Clofibric acid		Doxycycline	
Clonazepam		Draflazine	
Clonidine		Dronabinol	Marinol
Clopidogrel	Plavix	Droperidol	
Clotting Factor VIIa		Dutasteride	Avodart
Clotting Factor IX			
Cloxacillin		Efalizumab	Raptiva
Clozapine		Efavirenz	
Cocaine		Enalapril	
Codeine		Encainide	
Collagenase		Enfuvirtide	Fuzeon
Cortisol		Enoxacin	
Cosyntropin		Epinephrine	
Crotalidae immune Fab		Epipodophyllotoxin	
		Epoetin alfa	Epogen
Curare		Eptifibatide	Integrilin
Cyclophosphamide		Ergonovine	
Cyclosporine		Erythromycin	
Cytarabine	DepoCyt Injection	Esmolol	
		Estradiol	

Etanercept	Enbrel	Halothane	
Ethambutol		Heparin	
Ethchlorvynol		Hepatitis B immune globulin	
Ethinyl estradiol		Heptabarbital	
Etonogestrel	NuvaRing (combined with ethinyl estradiol)	Hirudin	
		Hydralazine	
		Hydrocortisone	
		Hydroxyzine	
Ezetimibe	Zetia (also combined with simvastatin [Vytorin®])		
		Ibandronate	
		Ibuprofen	
		Imiglucerase	Cerezyme
		Imipenem	Primaxin
		Imipramine	
Felbamate	Famvir	Imirestat	
Felodipine		Indinavir	Crixivan
Fenoldopam		Indocyanine green	
Fentanyl		Indomethacin	
Fexofenadine	Allegra	Infliximab	Remicade
Fibrinolysin		Insulin	
Filgrastim	Neupogen	Insulin glargine	Lantus
Flecainide		Interferon alfacon-1	Infergen
Flesinoxan			
Fluconazole		Interferon Alpha-2b (pegylated)	Pegintron
Flumazenil	Romazicon		
Fluorouracil		Interferon Beta-1a	Rebif
Fluoxetine		Interleukin-11 (Oprelvekin)	Neumega
Flurazepam			
Flurbiprofen		Intravenous gamma globulin	Gammagard
Fluvastatin			
Fluvoxamine		Irbesartan	Avalide, Avapro
Fosamprenavir	Lexiva	Irinotecan	Camptosar
Furosemide		Isoflurane	
		Isoniazid	
Gabapentin		Isosorbide dinitrate	
Ganciclovir	Cytovene	Itraconazole	
Gemcitabine	Gemzar		
Gemtuzumab ozogamicin	Mylotarg	Ketamine	
		Ketoconazole	
Gentamicin		Ketoprofen	
Gladase		Ketorolac	
Glibenclamide			
Glyburide		Labetalol	
Glipizide		Lansoprazole	
Glucagon		Laronidase	
Gonadotropin-releasing hormone		Leflunomide	Arava
		Lepirudin	Refludan
Goserelin	Zoladex	Leucovorin	
Griseofulvin		Leuprolide acetate	
Growth hormone		Levodopa	
		Levofloxacin	
Halazepam		Levonorgestrel	
Haloperidol		Lidocaine	

Lithium		Norelgestromin	Ortho Evra
Lomefloxacin			(combined
Lomustine			with ethinyl
Loperamide			estradiol)
Lopinavir	Kaletra	Norepinephrine	
	(combined	Norfloxacin	
	with ritonavir)	Normal immune	
Lorazepam		globulin	
Losartan	Hyzaar	Nortriptyline	
Lovastatin			
Lymphocyte		Octreotide	
anti-thymocyte		Olsalazine	
immune globulin		Omalizumab	Xolair
		Omeprazole	
Maprotiline		Ondansetron	
Mefloquine	Arima	Orlistat	Xenical
Meloxicam		Otenzapad	
Memantine		Oxacillin	
Menotropins	Menopur	Oxaliplatin	
Meperidine		Oxazepam	
Mercaptopurine		Oxycodone	
Mesalamine		Oxytocin	
Metformin			
Methamphetamine		Paclitaxel	
Methotrexate		Palivizumab	Synagis
Methyldopa		Pamidronate	Aredia
Methylphenidate		Pancuronium	
Methylprednisolone		Panitumumab	Vectibix
Metoprolol tartrate		Para-aminohippuric	
Metronidazole		acid	
Mibefradil		Pancrelipase	
Midazolam		Pantoprazole	
Minocycline		Papain	
Minoxidil		Paroxetine	
Misonidazole		Pegvisomant	
Misoprostol		Penciclovir	Denavir
Montelukast	Singulair	Penicillin G	
Morphine		Pentagastrin	
Moxalactam		Pentazocine	Talwin®
Muromomab-CD3			(combined
			with
Naloxone			naloxone)
Naproxen		Pentobarbital	
Nelfinavir mesylate	Viracept	Pentoxyphylline	
Neomycin		Pertussis immune	
Nesiritide		globulin	
Niacin		Phenelzine	
Nicardipine		Phenobarbital	
Nicotine		Phenprocoumon	
Nicoumalone		Phenylbutazone	
Nifedipine		Phenytoin	
Nitrazepam		Pimozide	
Nitroglycerin		Piperacillin	

Piroxicam	
Pivampicillin	
Polymyxin	
B Sulfate	
Pravastatin	
Prazepam	
Prednisolone	
Prednisone	
Primaquine	
Primidone	
Probenecid	
Procainamide	
Procarbazine	
Progesterone	
Proguanil	
Promazine	
Propafenone	
Propantheline	
Propofol	
Propranolol	
Propylthiouracil	
Protriptyline	
Pyridostigmine	
Quinacrine	
Quinidine sulfate	
Rabies immune globulin	
Ranibizumab	Lucentis
Ranitidine	
Rasburicase	Elitek
Remifentanil	Ultiva
Rho(D) immune globulin	
Rifampin	
Ritonavir	Norvir
Rituximab	Rituxan, Mabthera
Rivastigmine	Exelon
Rolipram	
Rosiglitazone	Avandia
Rosuvastatin	Crestor
Salicylic acid	
Saquinavir mesylate	Invirase
Saruplase	
Scopolamine	
Sermorelin	
Sertraline	
Sevoflurane	Ultane
Sildenafil citrate	Viagra
Simvastatin	

Sirolimus	Rapamune
Somatropin	
Sparteine	
St. John's Wort	
Streptomycin	
Succinylcholine	
Sucralfate	
Sufentanil	
Sulfamethazine	
Sulfasalazine	
Sulfinpyrazone	
Sulindac	
Sumatriptan	
Tacrolimus	
Tamoxifen	
Tamsulosin	Flomax
Taxol	
Teicoplanin	
Telithromycin	Ketek
Tenecteplase	TNKase
Terazosin	
Terbutaline	
Terfenadine	
Teriparatide	Forteo
Testosterone	
Tetanus immune globulin	
Theophylline	
Thioguanine	
Thiopental	
Thyroxine	
Ticlopidine	Ticlid
Timolol maleate	
Tipranavir	
Tirofiban	Aggrastat
Tissue-type plasminogen activator (t-PA)	
Tobramycin	
Tolbutamide	
Tolmetin	
Tolterodine tartrate	Detrol
Tositumomab	Bexxar
Trandolapril	Mavik
Trastuzumab	Herceptin
Triazolam	
Trimipramine	Surmontil
Troleandomycin	
Tubocurarine	
Urokinase	

Vaccinia immune globulin	
Valganciclovir	Valcyte
Valproic acid	
Valsartan	Diovan
Vancomycin	
Varicella-zoster immune globulin	Varivax
Vasopressin	
Venlafaxine	Effexor
Verapamil hydrochloride	

Vinblastine		
Vincristine		
Viomycin		
Vitamin C		
Voriconazole		
Warfarin		
Zafirlukast	Accolate	
Zidovudine		
Zileuton	Zyflo	
Zoledronic acid	Reclast, Zometa	

(Typical units are shown)

A	Amount of drug in body, mg or μmol.
Aa	Amount of drug at absorption site remaining to be absorbed, mg or μmol.
$A_{av,ss}$	Average amount of drug in body during a dosing interval at steady state, mg or μmol.
Ae	Cumulative amount of drug excreted in the urine, mg or μmol.
Ae_∞	Cumulative amount of drug excreted in the urine after a single dose to time infinity, mg or μmol.
A_{inf}	Amount of drug in body during a constant-rate infusion, mg or μmol.
$A(m)$	Amount of metabolite in the body, mg or μmol.
A_{min}	The minimum amount of drug in body required to obtain a predetermined level of response, mg or μmol.
$A_{max,N}; A_{min,N}$	Maximum and minimum amounts of drug in body after the Nth dose of fixed size and given at a fixed dosing interval, mg or μmol.
$A_{N,t}$	Amount of drug in body at time t after the Nth dose, mg or μmol.
A_{ss}	Amount of drug in body at steady state during constant-rate administration, mg or μmol.
$A_{max,ss}; A_{min,ss}$	Maximum and minimum amounts of drug in body during a dosing interval at steady state on administering a fixed dose at a fixed dosing interval, mg or μmol.
AUC	Area under the plasma drug concentration-time curve. Total area from time 0 to infinity is implied unless the local context indicates a specific time interval (e.g., a dosing interval), mg-hr/L or μM-hr.
AUC_b	Area under the blood concentration-time curve, mg-hr/L or μM-hr.
$AUC(m)$	Area under the plasma metabolite concentration-time curve, mg-hr/L or μM-hr.
AUC_{ss}	Area under the plasma concentration-time curve within a dosing interval at steady state, mg-hr/L or μM-hr.
$AUMC$	Total area under the first moment-time curve, mg-hr^2/L or μM-hr^2.
BMI	Body mass index, kg/m^2.
BSA	Body surface area, m^2.
C	Concentration of drug in plasma (or reservoir), mg/L or μM.
C_{50}	Concentration giving one-half the maximum effect, mg/L or μM.
$C(0)$	Initial plasma concentration obtained by extrapolation to time zero, after an intravenous bolus dose, mg/L or μM.
C_A	Drug concentration in arterial blood, mg/L or μM.

$C_{av,ss}$ — Average drug concentration in plasma during a dosing interval at steady state on administering a fixed dose at equal dosing intervals, mg/L or μM.

C_{inf} — Concentration of drug in plasma during a constant-rate infusion, mg/L or mM.

C_b — Concentration of drug in blood, mg/L or μM.

CL — Total clearance of drug from plasma, L/hr or mL/min.

CL_b — Total clearance of drug from blood, L/hr or mL/min.

$CL_{b,H}$ — Hepatic clearance of drug from blood, L/hr or mL/min.

CL_{cr} — Renal clearance of creatinine, mL/min or L/hr.

CL_D — Clearance by dialysis procedure, L/hr or mL/min.

CL_H — Hepatic clearance of drug from plasma, L/hr or mL/min.

CL_{int} — Intrinsic clearance of drug in organ of elimination (well-stirred model), L/hr or mL/min.

CL_R — Renal clearance of drug from plasma, L/hr or mL/min.

CLu — Clearance of unbound drug, L/hr or mL/min.

C_{lower}, C_{upper} — Lower and upper bounds of the therapeutic window of plasma concentrations, mg/L or μM.

C_{max} — Highest drug concentration observed in plasma after administration of an extravascular dose, mg/L or μM.

$C_{max,ss}, C_{min,ss}$ — Maximum and minimum concentrations of drug in plasma at steady state on administering a fixed dose at equal dosing intervals, mg/L or μM.

$C(m)$ — Concentration of a metabolite in plasma, mg/L or μM.

$C(m)_{ss}$ — Concentration of a metabolite in plasma at steady state during a constant-rate infusion of a drug, mg/L or μM.

C_{min} — Concentration of drug in plasma required to give the minimum effect, mg/L or μM.

C_{out} — Concentration leaving the extractor in the reservoir model, mg/L or μM.

C_{ss} — Concentration of drug in plasma at steady state during constant-rate administration, mg/L or μM.

C_T — Average concentration of drug in tissues outside plasma, mg/L or μM.

Cu — Unbound drug concentration in plasma, mg/L or μM.

Cu_H — Unbound drug concentration within hepatocytes, mg/L or μM.

C_V — Concentration of drug in venous blood, mg/L or μM.

D_L — Loading (or priming) dose, mg.

D_M — Maintenance dose given every dosing interval, mg

$D_{M,max}$ — Largest maintenance dose that will keep systemic exposure within the therapeutic window, mg.

E — Extraction ratio, no units.

In pharmacodynamics, E means "effect," which may be either clinically desirable or adverse. Units are those of response measured.

E_H — Hepatic extraction ratio, no units.

E_{max} — Maximum effect, units of response measurement.

E_R — Renal extraction ratio, no units.

F	Bioavailability of drug, no units.
f_D	Fraction of total elimination occuring by dialysis, no units.
fe	Fraction of drug systemically available that is excreted unchanged in urine, no units.
F_{ev}	Bioavailability of drug after extravascular administration, no units.
FEV_1	Forced expiratory volume in one second, L.
F_F	Fraction of an oral dose that enters the gut wall, no units.
F_G	Fraction of drug entering the gut that passes on to the portal circulation, no units.
F_H	Fraction of drug entering the liver that escapes elimination on single passage through the organ, no units.
fm	Fraction of drug systemically available that is converted to a metabolite, no units.
Fm	Fraction of administered dose of drug that enters the general circulation as a metabolite, no units.
F_R	Fraction of filtered and secreted drug reabsorbed in the renal tubule, no units.
fu	Ratio of unbound and total drug concentrations in plasma, no units.
fu_b	Ratio of unbound and whole blood concentrations available for binding, no units.
fu_P	Ratio of unbound and total sites on a plasma protein, no units.
fu_R	Apparent fraction unbound in intracellular fluids, no units.
fu_T	Ratio of unbound and total drug concentrations in tissues (outside plasma), no units.
γ	Steepness of concentration–response relationship, no units.
GFR	Glomerular filtration rate, mL/min or L/hr.
k	Elimination rate constant, hr^{-1}.
ka	Absorption rate constant, hr^{-1}.
Ka	Association equilibrium constant, L/mol.
Kd	Dissociation constant for saturable binding, mg/L.
K_I	Inhibition equilibrium constant, mg/L or μM.
Km	Michaelis-Menten constant, mg/L or μM.
K_p	Equilibrium distribution ratio of drug between tissue and plasma, no units.
$K_{p,b}$	Equilibrium distribution ratio of drug between tissue and blood, no units.
K_T	Constant for saturable transport model, mg/L.
k_t	Fractional turnover rate, hr^{-1}.
k_T	Fractional rate at which drug leaves a tissue, hr^{-1}.
λ_1, λ_2	Exponential coefficients, hr^{-1}
m	Slope of the relationship between response and the log of the plasma concentration (between 20 and 80% of maximum response), units of the response.
MRT	Mean residence time of a drug molecule within the body, hr.
n	A unitless number.
N	Number of doses, no units.

P	Permeability coefficient, cm/sec.
P_T	Total concentration of binding protein in plasma, mM.
Q	Blood flow, L/min or L/hr.
Q_H	Hepatic blood flow (portal vein plus hepatic artery), L/min or L/hr.
Q_R	Renal blood flow, L/min or L/hr.
R_{ac}	Accumulation ratio (index), no units.
R_d	Ratio of unbound clearance of an individual patient with renal function impairment to that of a typical patient, no units.
RF	Renal function in an individual patient as a fraction of renal function in a typical patient, no units.
R_{inf}	Rate of constant intravenous infusion, mg/hr.
R_{syn}	Rate of synthesis or input of a substance into the body, mg/hr or μg/hr
R_t	Turnover rate, mg/hr.
SA	Surface area, m^2.
τ	Dosing interval, hr.
t_{max}	Maximum dosing interval to remain within the limits of C_{lower} and C_{upper}, hr.
t	Time, hr.
t_D	Duration of response, hr
t_{inf}	Duration of a constant-rate infusion, hr.
Tm	Maximum rate of drug transport, mg/hr.
t_{max}	Time at which the highest drug concentration occurs after administration of an extravascular dose, min or hr.
t_t	Turnover time, hr.
$t_{1/2}$	Elimination half-life, hr.
$t_{1/2,a}$	Half-life of systemic absorption, hr.
V	Volume of distribution (apparent) based on drug concentration in plasma, L.
V_1	Initial dilution space or volume of central compartment in a two-compartment model, L.
V_b	Volume of distribution (apparent) based on drug concentration in whole blood, L.
V_B	Blood volume, L.
Vm	Maximum rate of metabolism by a given enzymatic reaction, mg/hr or μmol/hr.
$V(m)$	Volume of distribution (apparent) of a metabolite based on its plasma concentration, L.
V_P	Plasma volume, L.
V_R	Aqueous volume of intracellular fluids, L.
V_{ss}	Volume of distribution (apparent) under steady state conditions based on drug concentration in plasma, L.
V_T	Physiologic volume outside plasma into which drug appears to distribute, L.
Vu	Unbound volume of distribution, L.
W	Body weight, kg.

Basic Considerations

Therapeutic Relevance

CLINICAL SETTING

Those patients who suffer from chronic ailments such as diabetes and epilepsy may have to take drugs every day for the rest of their lives. At the other extreme are those who take a single dose of a drug to relieve an occasional headache. The duration of drug therapy is usually between these extremes. The manner in which a drug is taken is called a **dosage regimen**. Both the duration of drug therapy and the dosage regimen depend on the therapeutic objective, which may be the cure, the mitigation, or the prevention of disease or conditions suffered by patients. Because all drugs exhibit some undesirable effects, such as drowsiness, dryness of the mouth, gastrointestinal irritation, nausea, and hypotension, successful drug therapy is achieved by optimally balancing the desirable and the undesirable effects. To achieve optimal therapy, the appropriate "drug of choice" must first be selected. This decision implies an accurate diagnosis of the disease or condition, a knowledge of the clinical state of the patient, and a sound understanding of the pharmacotherapeutic management of the disease. Then the questions of, how much? how often? and how long? must be answered.

The question, how much? recognizes that the magnitudes of the therapeutic and adverse responses are functions of the size of dose given. To paraphrase the 16th-century physician Paracelsus, "all drugs are poisons, it is just a matter of dose." For example, 25 mg of aspirin does little to alleviate a headache; a dose closer to 300 to 600 mg is needed, with little ill effect. However, 10 g taken all at once can be fatal, especially in young children. The question, how often? recognizes the importance of time, in that the magnitude of the effect eventually declines with time following a single dose of drug. The question, how long? recognizes that some conditions are of limited duration, while a cost (in terms of side effects, toxicity, economics) is incurred with continuous drug administration. In practice, these questions cannot be completely divorced from one another. For example, the convenience of giving a larger dose less frequently may be more than offset by an increased incidence of toxicity.

What determines the therapeutic dose of a drug and its manner and frequency of administration, as well as the events experienced over time by patients on taking the recommended dosage regimens, constitutes the body of this book. It aims to demonstrate that there are concepts common to all drugs and that, equipped with these concepts, not only can many of the otherwise confusing events following drug administration be rationalized, but also the key questions surrounding the very basis of dosage regimens can be understood. The intended result is a better and safer use of drugs for the treatment or amelioration of diseases or conditions suffered by patients. Bear in mind, for example, that still today, some 5% of patients admitted into hospital are there because of the inappropriate use of drugs, much of which is avoidable.

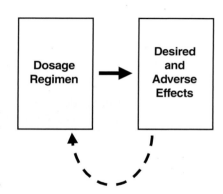

FIGURE 1-1. An empirical approach to the design of a dosage regimen. The effects, both desired and adverse, are monitored after the administration of a dosage regimen of a drug and used to further refine and optimize the regimen through feedback (*dashed line*).

It is possible, and indeed it was a common past practice, to establish the dosage regimen of a drug through trial and error by adjusting such factors as the dose and interval between doses and observing the effects produced as depicted in Fig. 1-1. A reasonable regimen might eventually be established but not without some patients experiencing excessive adverse effects and others ineffective therapy. Certainly, this was the procedure followed to establish that digoxin needed to be given at doses between 0.125 mg and 0.25 mg only once a day for the treatment of congestive cardiac failure, whereas morphine sulfate needed to be administered at doses between 10 mg and 50 mg up to 6 times a day to adequately relieve the chronic severe pain experienced by patients suffering from terminal cancer. However, this empirical approach not only fails to explain the reason for this difference in the regimens of digoxin and morphine but also contributes little, if anything, toward establishing the principles underlying effective dosage regimens of other drugs. That is, our basic understanding of drugs has not been increased.

INPUT–RESPONSE PHASES

Progress has only been forthcoming by realizing that concentrations at active sites, rather than dose administered, drive responses, and that to achieve and maintain a response, it is necessary to ensure the generation of the appropriate exposure–time profile of drug within the body, which in turn requires an understanding of the factors controlling this exposure profile. These ideas are summarized in Fig. 1-2, where now the input–response relationship (which often runs under the restrictive title "dose–response," as not only dose is altered) is divided into two parts, a **pharmacokinetic phase** and a **pharmacodynamic phase** both with roots derived from the Greek word *pharmacon*, meaning a drug, or interestingly, a poison. The pharmacokinetic phase covers the relationship between drug input, which comprises such adjustable factors as dose, dosage form, frequency and route of administration, and the concentration achieved *with time*. The pharmacodynamic phase

FIGURE 1-2. A rational approach to the design of a dosage regimen. The pharmacokinetics and pharmacodynamics of the drug are first defined. Then, responses to the drug, coupled with pharmacokinetic information, are used as a feedback (*dashed lines*) to modify the dosage regimen to achieve optimal therapy. For some drugs, active metabolites formed in the body may also need to be taken into account.

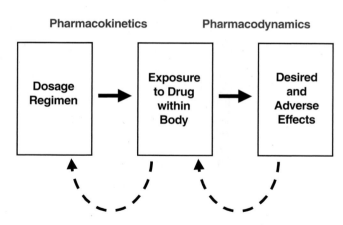

covers the relationship between concentration and both the desired and adverse effects produced *with time*. In simple terms, **pharmacokinetics** may be viewed as how the body handles the drug, and **pharmacodynamics** as how the drug affects the body. Sometimes, the metabolites of drugs formed within the body have activity and also need to be taken into account when relating drug administration to response.

Several other basic ideas have helped to place drug administration on a more rational footing. The first, and partially alluded to above, is that the intensity or likelihood of effect increases with increasing exposure to the drug, but only to some limiting, or maximum value, above which the response can go no higher, regardless of how high the exposure. Second, drugs act on different parts of the body, and the maximum effect produced by one drug may be very different from that of another, even though the measured response is the same. For example, both aspirin and morphine relieve pain, but whereas aspirin may relieve mild pain, it cannot relieve the severe pain experienced by patients with severe trauma or cancer even when given in massive doses. Here, morphine, or another opioid analgesic, is the drug of choice. Third, which follows in part from the second idea, is the realization that drugs produce a multiplicity of effects, some desired and others undesired, which when coupled with the first idea, has the following implication. Too low an exposure results in an inadequate desired response, whereas too high an exposure increases the likelihood and intensity of adverse effects. Expressed differently, there exists an optimal range of exposures between these extremes, the **therapeutic window**, shown schematically in Fig. 1-3. For some drugs, the therapeutic window is narrow, and therefore the margin of safety is small. For others, it is wide. Although the appropriate concentration should be that at the site of action, rarely it is accessible; instead, the concentration is generally measured at an alternative and more accessible site, the plasma.

Armed with these simple ideas, it is now possible to explain the reason for the difference in the dosing frequency between digoxin and morphine. Both drugs have a relatively

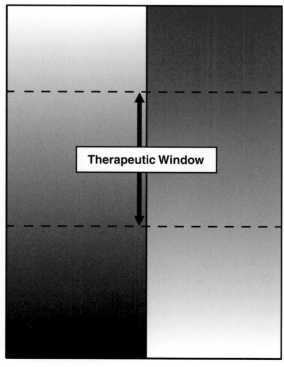

FIGURE 1-3. At higher concentrations or higher rates of administration on chronic dosing, the probability of achieving a therapeutic response increases (from gray to white), but so does the probability of adverse effects (toward increasing redness). A window of opportunity, called the "therapeutic window," exists, however, within which the therapeutic response can be attained without an undue incidence of adverse effects.

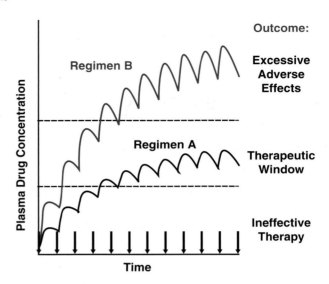

FIGURE 1-4. When a drug is given in a fixed dose and at fixed time intervals (denoted by the arrows), it accumulates within the body until a plateau is reached. With regimen A, therapeutic success is achieved although not initially. With regimen B, the therapeutic objective is achieved more quickly, but the drug concentration is ultimately too high, resulting in excessive adverse effects.

narrow therapeutic window, but whereas morphine is eliminated very rapidly from the body, so that it must be given frequently to maintain an adequate concentration to ensure relief of pain without excessive adverse effects, such as respiratory depression, digoxin is relatively stable and so with little lost each day, once daily administration suffices. These principles also help to explain an added feature of digoxin. Given daily, digoxin was either ineffective acutely or eventually produced unacceptable toxicity when a dosing rate sufficiently high to be effective acutely was maintained. Because it is eliminated slowly with little lost each day, it accumulates appreciably with repeated daily administration, as depicted schematically in Fig. 1-4. At low daily doses, the initial concentration is too low to be effective but eventually, it rises to within the therapeutic window. Increasing the daily dose brings the concentration within the therapeutic window earlier, but with the concentration still rising, eventually the concentration becomes too high, and unacceptable toxicity ensues. However, what was needed was rapid achievement and subsequent maintenance of adequate digoxin concentrations without undue adverse effects. The answer was to give several small doses within the first day, commonly known collectively as a *digitalizing dose*, to rapidly achieve therapeutic concentrations followed by small daily doses to maintain the concentration within the therapeutic window. The lesson to be learned from the case of digoxin and indeed most drugs is that only through an understanding of the temporal events that occur after the drug's administration can meaningful decisions be made regarding its optimal use.

The issue of time delays between drug administration and response is not confined to pharmacokinetics but extends to pharmacodynamics too. Part of such delays is a result of the time required for drug to distribute to the target site, which is often in a cell within a tissue or organ, such as the brain. This is certainly the case with digoxin, where the peak effect on the heart occurs several hours after observing the peak exposure in plasma. Part is also a result of delays within the affected system within the body, as readily seen with the oral anticoagulant warfarin, used as a prophylaxis in the prevention of deep vein thrombosis and other thromboembolic complications. Even though the drug is rapidly absorbed, yielding high, early concentrations throughout the body, as seen in Fig. 1-5, the peak effect, in terms of prolongation of the clotting time, occurs approximately 2 days after a dose of warfarin. Clearly, it is important to take this lag in response into account when deciding how much to adjust dose to achieve and maintain a given therapeutic response. Failing to do so and attempting to adjust dosage based, for example, on the response seen after 1 day, before the full effect develops, increases the danger of overdosing the patient, with serious potential consequences, such as internal hemorrhage, with this low margin-of-safety drug.

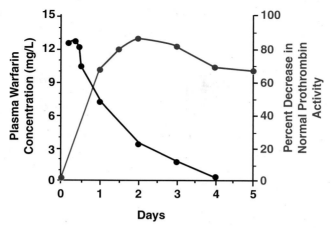

FIGURE 1-5. The sluggish response in the plasma prothrombin complex activity (colored line), which determines the degree of coagulability of blood, is clearly evident following administration of the oral anticoagulant warfarin. Although the absorption of this drug into the body is rapid, with a peak concentration seen within the first few hours, for the first 2 days after giving a single oral 1.5 mg/kg dose of sodium warfarin, response (defined as the percent decrease in the normal complex activity) steadily increases reaching a peak after 2 days. Thereafter, the response declines slowly as absorbed drug is eliminated from the body. The data points are the averages of five male volunteers. (From: Nagashima R, O'Reilly RA, Levy G. Kinetics of pharmacologic effects in man: The anticoagulant action of warfarin. Clin Pharmacol Ther 1969;10:22–35.)

Another example of a time delay in pharmacodynamics concerns an adverse effect, a safety issue, seen in Fig. 1-6 after a single intravenous dose of the anticancer drug paclitaxel. A common and clinically significant toxicity of many anticancer drugs is leukopenia, an abnormal fall in the number of leukocytes in blood. Leukocytes are important in the immunological defense of the body and if the leukocyte counts fall too far, it places the patient at severe risk. Most clinical focus therefore is on the lowest leukocyte count after chemotherapy treatment, but the time course of the fall in count and return to baseline is also important. Despite paclitaxel being eliminated from the body within

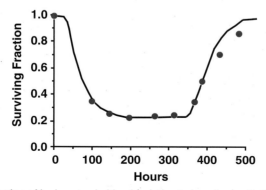

FIGURE 1-6. The fraction of leukocytes in blood (relative to baseline) with time in a patient receiving a single intravenous dose of paclitaxel. Notice the sluggish return of the leukocyte count to the baseline value. The continuous line is the best line fit of a model of the production and destruction of leukocytes to the data, with paclitaxel inhibiting mature cell production. (From: Minami H, Sasaki Y, Saijo N, et al. Indirect-response model for the time course of leukopenia with anticancer drugs. Clin Pharmacol Ther 1998;64:511–521.)

2 days, the changes in the fraction of leukocytes in blood is extremely sluggish, taking over a week to reach the lowest count and only returning to the baseline value 3 weeks after drug administration. Leukocytes in blood reflect the balance between production and destruction. The direct inhibitory effect of paclitaxel is upstream on progenitor cells within the bone marrow thereby reducing the production of mature leukocytes. Fewer mature leukocytes feed into the vascular pool so that the pool size declines, but a long time is needed to produce a sufficient number of mature leukocytes to again restore the normal blood pool.

As mentioned, an interesting feature of many drugs is that they exhibit different effects with plasma concentration. An unusual but telling example is seen with clonidine. Originally developed as a nasal decongestant, when evaluated for this indication, some subjects became faint, because of a then unexpected hypotensive effect. Today, the therapeutic use of this drug is as an antihypertensive. However, further investigation showed that it was possible to produce not only a hypotensive effect but also hypertension, depending on the plasma concentration. Clonidine acts on two classes of receptor, one causing a lowering of blood pressure and the other an elevation in blood pressure. At low concentrations achieved with therapeutic doses, the lowering effect on blood pressure predominates, but at high concentrations, as might well be achieved during an overdose, the hypertensive effect predominates, although this effect will subside and the hypotensive effect will again predominate as the systemic exposure falls. For some other drugs, such as warfarin, the mechanism of action is the same for producing desired and adverse effects. Warfarin's almost singular action is anticoagulation, yet this effect is defined as therapeutic when the concentration is such as to minimize the risk of development of an embolism and as adverse at higher concentrations at which the risk of internal hemorrhage becomes high, associated with excessive anticoagulation. The lesson is clear. Understanding the specific concentration–response time relationships helps in the management and optimal use of drugs.

VARIABILITY IN DRUG RESPONSE

If we were all alike, there would only be one dose strength and regimen of a drug needed for the entire patient population. But we are not alike; indeed, we often exhibit great interindividual variability in response to drugs. This is generally not so important for drugs with wide therapeutic windows, because patients can tolerate a wide range of exposures for similar degrees of benefit, particularly when the dose employed ensures that the maximum beneficial effect is experienced by essentially all patients, in which case a single dose of drug, the "one-dose-for-all" idea, suffices. Although some patients may still not respond to therapy because they lack the putative receptor on which the drug acts, a rare individual may experience a hypersensitivity reaction, such as an acute allergic episode. Clearly, the drug is contraindicated in the last two types of patient. The problem of variability becomes particularly acute for drugs with an intermediate or narrow therapeutic window, of which there are many, including the immunosuppressive agent cyclosporine, used to prevent organ rejection following transplantation, and the antiepileptic drug, phenytoin (Fig. 1-7), in addition to the examples of morphine and digoxin mentioned previously. For these drugs, the solution is the availability of an array of dose strengths, with titration of each patient to the required dosage.

Variability in the response among patients to phenytoin and many other drugs is primarily pharmacokinetic in origin. In other cases, pharmacodynamics is the major cause of variability in response, as shown, for example, in Fig. 1-8 by the wide range in plasma concentrations of the oral anticoagulant warfarin needed to maintain a similar degree of anticoagulation in patients.

The causes of variability in dose response are manifold and include the patient's age, weight, degree of obesity, type and degree of severity of disease, other drugs concurrently administered, and environmental factors. Another important and pervasive one is genetics.

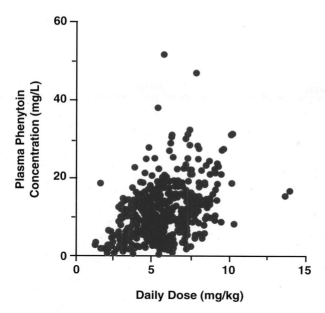

FIGURE 1-7. Although the average plasma concentration of phenytoin on chronic dosing tends to increase with the dosing rate, there is large variation in the individual values. (From: Lund, L. Effects of phenytoin in patients with epilepsy in relation to its concentration in plasma. In Davies DS, Prichard BNC, eds. Biological Effects of Drugs in Relation to Their Plasma Concentration. London and Basingstoke: Macmillan, 1973:227–238.)

This was known for many years, in that when evaluated, there were only minor differences in the pharmacokinetics and response to drugs between identical twins even when they lived apart and in different social environments, compared with the often experienced wide differences in response within the patient population. The importance of genetics was also known from familial studies and studies in different ethnic groups. One example, arising during World War II, which occurred when the fighting spread to tropical regions where malaria was rife, was the observation that approximately 10% of African American soldiers, but few white ones, developed acute hemolytic anemia when given a typical dose of the antimalarial drug primaquine. Subsequent investigations showed that this sensitivity to primaquine and some other chemically related antimalarial drugs was a result of an inherited deficiency among many African Americans of an important enzyme, glucose-6-phosphate dehydrogenase (G6PD), residing in red blood cells and a component responsible for their

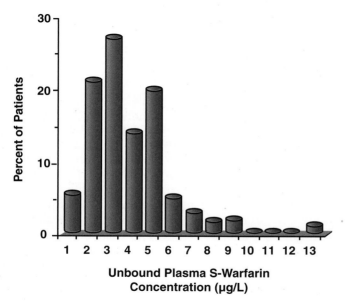

FIGURE 1-8. There is considerable interindividual pharmacodynamic variability in response to the oral anticoagulant warfarin as demonstrated by the substantial spread in the unbound concentration of the active S-isomer associated with a similar degree of anticoagulation in a group of 97 patients on maintenance therapy. (From: Scordo MG, Pengo V, Spina E, et al. Influence of CYP2C9 and CYP2C19 genetic polymorphisms of warfarin maintenance dose and metabolic clearance. Clin Pharmacol Ther 2002;72:702–710.)

integrity. Further checking found that G6PD is located on chromosome X, and that more than 400 million people carry one of the many different variants of 6GDP, which places them at risk to hemolysis when exposed to certain drugs. Returning to warfarin, much of the variability in pharmacodynamics has been traced to mutant variations in the gene that produces a protein that regulates the level of vitamin K epoxide reductase in the liver. Warfarin acts by lowering the concentration of reduced vitamin K by decreasing its regeneration from the inactive vitamin K epoxide pool in the vitamin K cycle, through inhibition of vitamin K epoxide reductase. Vitamin K is an essential cofactor for the synthesis of the vitamin K-dependent clotting factors that control the degree of coagulation.

Another example of the importance of genetics is the one that was experienced with the drug debrisoquine, a now defunct antihypertensive drug. In most patients, this proved to be an effective and relatively safe drug, but in about 8% of whites, even a modest dose caused a major hypotensive crisis which, because it was then unpredictable, in that there was no ability to predict who would manifest this severe adverse effect, resulted in the drug being withdrawn. With progress in deciphering the human genome, or more accurately human genomes, as we all are different in a myriad of ways, we are beginning to understand the molecular basis for genetic differences. In the case of the debrisoquine-induced crisis, the cause was eventually traced to the presence within this minority white group of defective variants of a cytochrome-metabolizing enzyme located within the liver, cytochrome P4502D6, which is almost exclusively responsible for metabolism of this drug and many others. Normally, debrisoquine is rapidly eliminated from the body, but with an inability to readily remove this drug in this minority group, usual doses of debrisoquine produce excessively high concentrations within the body and excessive effect. Today, the importance of genetics is becoming clearer, and the possibility of using genomic information to both predict and individualize therapy for various medicines is on the horizon.

Drug–drug interactions are another major source of variability in drug response. Many patients, particularly the elderly, are on multiple drug therapy, often administered to treat several concomitant conditions or diseases. The potential of one or more of these drugs affecting the pharmacokinetics or pharmacodynamics of one of the others is therefore ever present. Occasionally, the interaction is sufficiently severe as to contraindicate the combination or, on rare occasions, when not recognized at the time, has been fatal. For example, death in some patients taking the usually safe antihistamine terfenadine was traced to torsade de pointes, a rare heart condition, induced by the presence of extremely high exposures of this antihistamine caused by coadministration of the oral antifungal agent ketoconazole. The mechanism, poorly understood at the time, involves strong inhibition by ketoconazole of the enzyme predominantly responsible for the elimination of terfenadine. Indeed, because there are so many strong inhibitors of this enzyme, and the risk of the interaction is so severe, the decision was taken to withdraw terfenadine from the market. Fortunately, in most cases, the interaction is not so severe and the risk is minimized by adjusting the dose of the affected drug when it needs to be coadministered with the interacting one. In making the adjustment, use is made of the fact that such interactions are graded, with the intensity of the interaction varying with the concentration of the interacting drug, and hence with dose and time, in a known manner.

To make a point, many of the examples mentioned previously are at the extreme. Usually, the therapeutic situation is less stark or of lesser concern. This is often because drugs are metabolized by several enzymes, so that genetic variation, or inhibition, of any one of them, has only a partial effect on overall elimination. Also, as mentioned, for many drugs, the therapeutic window is quite wide, so that a wide variation in exposure among patients, or within the same patient, does not manifest in any appreciable variation in drug response. Still, there are many exceptions, so it is important to deal with each drug on a case specific basis. Nonetheless, the principles briefly enumerated here and stressed throughout this book hold and help to rationalize and optimize drug therapy.

ADHERENCE

If only patients adhered to the prescribed dosage regimen of their medicines, we would at least have some idea whether a failure to respond or an excessive response can be attributed to the drug itself. However, the problem of nonadherence, or what is commonly called noncompliance, is, to some extent, part and parcel of human behavior. There are those patients who are compulsive in taking their medicines as instructed, but many others are much less reliable, missing doses or times of dosing or even stopping taking them before the full course of treatment is complete, referred to as lack of persistence of treatment. This is clearly evident from the data displayed in Fig. 1-9, which show that, in a cohort of patients prescribed once daily antihypertensive medication, approximately 50% had discontinued therapy 1 year from the start of treatment, despite the

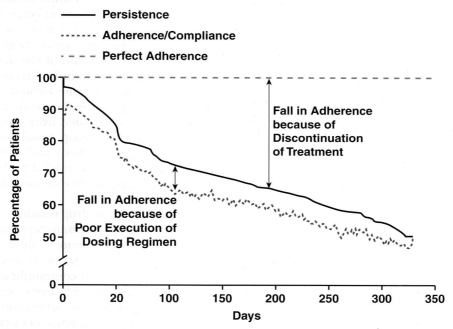

FIGURE 1-9. Nonadherence to prescribed medication is a major source of variability in drug therapy. Shown is the gradual but persistent decrease in adherence in the percent of patients prescribed various once-a-day antihypertensive therapies because of discontinuation of treatment, such that by toward the end of the first year, only 50% of the patients prescribed the treatment for an indefinite duration continue to take the prescribed medication. The initial 3% drop in adherence is a result of some patients never even starting the medication. The data were obtained using an electronic monitoring device that detects and logs each time the container with the medication is opened. (From: Vrijens B, Vincze G, Kistanto P, et al. Adherence to prescribed antihypertensive drug treatments: longitudinal study of electronically compiled dosing histories. BMJ 2008;17:1114–1117.)

intention that such treatment be "for life." Reasons for nonadherence are manifold. Patients either feel better and decide that there is no point in taking the drug any longer, are just not convinced of the benefits, or experience some adverse effect, which they had not anticipated or feel that they cannot tolerate, and decide that this adverse effect is worse than the condition for which they are being treated. The result is that we need to broaden the scheme depicted in Fig. 1-2 to include this issue of adherence, as shown in Fig. 1-10, if we wish to relate drug response to prescribed regimens in the real world. In the past, reliance was placed on what the patient said about their adherence to the

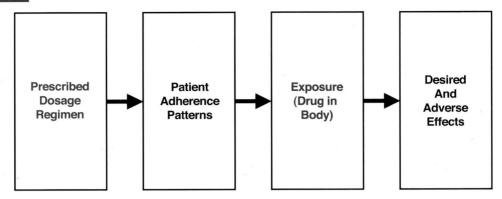

FIGURE 1-10.   To adequately relate prescribed dosage regimens of drugs to response outcomes in patients in the real world of clinical practice, it is necessary to insert the adherence pattern of drug usage between the prescribed regimen and systemic exposure.

prescribed dosage, but it has become clear, based on much more objective evidence using electronic monitoring devices that record, for example, each time a bottle of tablets is opened (which was the method used to obtain the data in Fig. 1-9), if proof is needed, that many patients are untruthful about their adherence pattern. However, for some drugs, a certain degree of nonadherence is tolerable without major therapeutic consequences, for some others, close adherence to the prescribed regimen is vital to the success of therapy. The latter is particularly true in the case of drugs used in the treatment of many infections, such as those caused by the human immunodeficiency virus (HIV; the cause of acquired immune deficiency syndrome [AIDS]) and tuberculosis. Failure to be almost fully compliant, which ensures an adequate exposure to the medication at all times, can lead to the emergence of resistant strains, with fatal consequences, including those to whom the infection spreads. But being fully compliant is often very demanding on the patient, particularly those suffering from AIDS, who are often receiving a combination of many drugs taken several times a day and sometimes at different times of the day. Some argue that we would not be in the situation that we are today—that is, the emergence of resistant microorganisms (such as methicillin-resistant *Staphylococcus aureus,* which has caused so many deaths in hospitals, where this organism is increasingly prevalent)—if we had ensured full adherence to the regimens of the existing armament of antibiotics for the full duration of treatment.

THE INDUSTRIAL PERSPECTIVE

The industrial process of discovering new therapeutic targets and identifying and selecting potentially useful drugs against them, together with their subsequent evaluation, development, and registration, depicted schematically in Fig. 1-11, is a long, complex, costly, and uncertain process, taking on average 10 to 12 years between inception of the idea and the marketing of a new medicine. In many cases, many tens of thousands of compounds are evaluated before a successful one emerges. Although the process appears to be unidirectional, from discovery to registration of a medicine with the regulatory authorities, in reality, there is a continuous feedback at every stage of the process to improve understanding and help identify the best possible compound and its most appropriate use. Increasingly, with progress in a wide variety of different fields, including molecular biology, genomics, systems biology, medicinal chemistry, material science, and computational and modeling tools, the process is becoming more predictive, although some empiricism prevails as there is much about many diseases and conditions that is still not well understood.

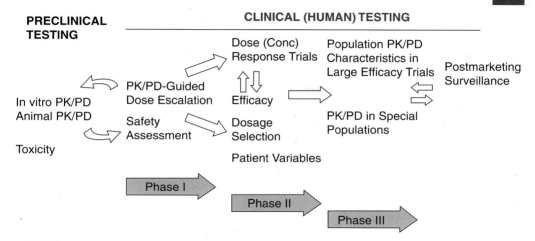

FIGURE 1-11.   The development and subsequent marketing of a drug. The preclinical data helps to identify promising compounds and to suggest useful doses for testing in humans. Phases I, II, and III of human assessment generally correspond to the first administration to humans, early evaluation in selected patients, and the larger trials, respectively. Pharmacokinetic (PK) and pharmacodynamic (PD) data gathered during all phases of drug development help to efficiently define safe and effective dosage regimens for optimal individual use. Postmarketing surveillance, particularly for safety, helps to refine the PK/PD information.

Awareness of the benefits of understanding pharmacokinetics and concentration–response relationships has led in recent years to the extensive application of such information by the pharmaceutical industry to the design, selection, and development of drugs. For example, a potent compound found to be poorly and unreliably absorbed and intended for oral administration may be shelved in favor of a somewhat less potent but more extensively and reliably absorbed compound. Also, many of the basic processes controlling both pharmacokinetics and response are similar across mammalian species such that data can be extrapolated from animals to predict quantitatively the likely behavior in humans, while increasingly in vitro systems, using human or human-expressed materials, and early and sensitive measures of the biological action in vivo, are being employed to further aid in the prediction. This quantitative framework improves the chances of selecting not only the most promising compounds but also the likely correct range of safe doses to first test in humans. Incorporation of both pharmacokinetic and pharmacodynamic elements with these early phase I studies, usually in healthy subjects, together with assessment of any acute side effects produced, helps to define candidate dosage forms and regimens for evaluation in phase II studies conducted in a small number of patients, to test whether the drug will be effective for the intended clinical indication, commonly known as the "proof-of-concept" stage. These phase I and II learning studies, which provide important mechanistic information as well as identifying and quantifying the magnitude and causes of variability in pharmacokinetics and pharmacodynamics, are also aimed at defining the most likely safe and efficacious dosage regimens for use in the subsequent larger confirmatory phase III clinical trials, often involving many thousands of patients. Ultimately, some compounds prove to be of sufficient therapeutic benefit and safety to be approved for a particular clinical indication by drug regulatory authorities. Even then, the drug undergoes virtually continuous postmarketing surveillance and study through its life time of use, to further refine its pharmacotherapeutic profile. Occasionally, this may lead to a change in the recommended therapeutic dose range, sometimes greater and sometimes lower than that originally indicated or, even more rarely, removal of the drug from the market.

ORGANIZATION OF BOOK

The problems and issues encountered in assuring optimal drug therapy, discussed earlier, are expanded on in the balance of the book. Both pharmacokinetics and pharmacodynamics are covered, although there is a more in-depth consideration of pharmacokinetics. This, in part, is because the underlying pharmacokinetic concepts apply to all drugs, whereas many pharmacodynamic issues are specific to a particular system of the body, such as one in the brain, the liver, or the cardiovascular system. In addition, there is an increasing understanding of mechanisms controlling the pharmacokinetics of drugs, be they small or large molecules, whereas, probably because of the greater complexity of many systems of the body, the mechanisms and quantitative features of many pharmacodynamic processes have yet to be elucidated.

The book is divided into five sections. Section I examines the therapeutic relevance of the subject of the book and the basic concepts involved in relating exposure to drug input and response to systemic exposure. Section II deals with the physiologic and anatomic features governing the pharmacokinetic and pharmacodynamic events following administration of a single dose of drug. Section III covers the principles used to achieve and maintain drug response with time. Constant rate of input by intravenous infusion or specific devices and repeated fixed dose regimens are emphasized. Section IV examines sources of variability and how to adjust drug administration in the individual to accommodate the omnipresent variability, whereas Section V the last section, as the title implies, deals with several additional issues, namely distribution kinetics, metabolite kinetics, protein drugs, and prediction of human pharmacokinetics, that the reader may find helpful in providing a more rounded understanding on the subject. In addition, Appendices A through I are included as supplements to various aspects introduced in Sections II and III, and are applied in the subsequent two sections.

This book deals with the quantitative principles underlying drug therapy and how events evolve over time following drug administration. With an emphasis on quantitation, a certain amount of mathematics is inevitable, if one is to be able to grasp the concepts and understand their application. However, every effort has been made to back the principles with both graphical illustrations and examples where these principles are applied to drugs in clinical practice. In addition, appendices have been provided for those wishing to know more about the basis of some of the material contained in the body of the book. In common with many aspects of mathematics, symbols are employed as a form of shorthand notation to denote common terms, for ease of reading and presentation. Each of these symbols is defined the first time it is used. In addition, a list of all common symbols with their definitions and units, where appropriate, are provided immediately after the preface. Symbols used only in a limited context may not be included.

A word on generic and brand names of drugs is warranted. During the patent life of a compound, a drug is registered worldwide not only by its generic name but also under the innovator company's brand name, which may vary from country to country, although today, global branding is common. In practice, a drug is marketed as a formulation, such as a tablet or capsule, aimed at ensuring not only the optimal quality and performance of the drug but also its acceptability to patients, and it is this product (or series of products containing the active compound) that carries the brand name. Once the patent has expired, however, other companies may produce versions that are sufficiently similar so that they may be considered interchangeable with the original product. In such cases, the products are known as generic products. Throughout this book the policy has been to use the generic name of the active principle as the default when describing a drug product. However, it is recognized that during its patent life, the product is the only one available and is usually referred to by its brand name, which is familiar to both clinician and patient alike. For example, the brand name of the chemical sildenafil is Viagra but when asked, few would know the generic name of this widely used drug. Accordingly, for drugs still under patent, we have provided the brand name at its first mention in the book. A list of all generic and currently patented drugs (at the time of publishing this book) is provided immediately after the "Definition of Symbols."

To aid in the learning of the material, at the beginning of each of Chapters 2 through 22 is a list of objectives, which should be thought of as points that you might reasonably be expected to answer after you have completed each chapter. Also, as an aid to answering quantitative problems, a list of key relationships is at the end of each chapter, with the exception of the first and last chapters. In addition, key words and phrases are emboldened within the text where they are first introduced.

Finally, to aid in the learning of the material, at the beginning of each of the 21 subsequent chapters is a list of objectives which should be thought of as points that you might reasonably be expected to answer after you have completed each chapter. In addition, for those wishing to practice problem solving and/or to examine the basic models used in pharmacokinetics and pharmacodynamics, two different kinds of additional exercises are available. First, study problems are given at the end of Chapters 2 to 21. Answers to these problems are given in Appendix J. Some problems require the plotting of data on graph paper. To this end, blank graph paper (linear and semilogarithmic, identified as Regular Graph Paper, 2-Cycle Semilogarithmic Graph Paper, 3-Cycle Semilogarithmic Graph Paper, and Log-log Graph Paper) can be downloaded from the website given below. Alternatively, a software program like Excel, can be used to prepare such plots. Second, for quantitatively visualizing the behavior of changes in parameter values of selected pharmacokinetic and pharmacodynamic models, interactive online simulations, prepared by Drs. Hartmut Derendorf and Guenther Hochhaus, School of Pharmacy, University of Florida, are available on the companion web site: http://thePoint.lww.com/Rowland4e.

2

Fundamental Concepts and Terminology

OBJECTIVES

The reader will be able to:

- Define the following terms: agonist, all-or-none response, antagonist, baseline, bioavailability, biomarker, clinical response, compartment, cumulative frequency, disease progression, disposition, distribution, elimination, endogenous, enterohepatic cycling, excretion, exogenous, extravascular administration, first-pass loss, fractional turnover rate, full agonist, full antagonist, graded response, intestinal absorption, intravascular administration, local administration, maximum effect, metabolic interconversion, metabolism, metabolites, parenteral administration, partial agonist, partial antagonist, pharmacokinetic–pharmacodynamic (PK/PD) modeling, placebo, pool size, potency, prodrug, quantal response, safety biomarker, specificity, steepness factor, surrogate endpoint, systemic absorption, turnover, turnover rate, turnover time, up-or-down regulation.

- Discuss the limitations to interpretation of pharmacokinetic data imposed by assays that fail to distinguish between compounds administered (e.g., R- and S-isomers) or between drug and metabolite.

- Show the general contribution of mass balance concepts to drug absorption and drug and metabolite disposition.

- Explain why plasma drug concentration can serve as a useful correlate of response.

- Briefly discuss issues involved in the assessment of drug effect.

- Describe, with examples, how the intensity of a graded response changes with concentration at the site of action.

- Describe the parameters of the model that often characterize the relationship between a graded response and plasma concentration.

- Describe how a quantal response is related to plasma concentration.

- Discuss the relative value of potency, maximum effect, and specificity in drug therapy.

- Briefly discuss how the condition being treated influences the relative importance of the features of the exposure–time profile after a single oral dose.

This chapter introduces input–exposure (pharmacokinetics) and exposure–response (pharmacodynamic) relationships and defines the terms commonly used in these areas. Concepts in these areas play many key roles, as listed in Table 2-1, in the development and use of medicinal agents. The chapter begins with a definition of systemic exposure and consideration of basic models and methods for evaluating it.

TABLE 2-1	**Applications of Pharmacokinetics and Pharmacodynamics in Drug Therapy**

- To relate temporal patterns of response (efficacy, harm) to drug administration following acute and chronic dosing.
- To help provide a rational basis for drug design, drug selection, and dosage regimen design.
- To aid in the design of protocols to evaluate events in vivo and in subsequent interpretation of the data obtained.
- To help evaluate quantitatively drug product performance in vivo and to establish appropriate in vitro dissolution specifications to help ensure maintenance of the quality of the manufacturing process.
- To provide a means for rationally initiating and individualizing drug administration in patients.

Before considering the subject of exposure, a distinction must be made between those drugs that act locally and those that act systemically. Locally acting drugs are administered at the local site where they are needed. Examples of products intended for **local administration** are eye drops, nasal sprays, intravaginal creams, and topical preparations for treating skin diseases. This chapter, and indeed much of the book, emphasizes those drugs that act within the blood or that must be delivered to the site of action by the circulatory system. In general terms, we say such drugs act **systemically**.

PHARMACOKINETICS

SYSTEMIC EXPOSURE

Needless to say, the response produced by a systemically acting drug is related, in one way or another, to the amount entering the body and its duration there. While responses can be observed, often noninvasively, such as monitoring blood pressure, drug within the body, which causes the change in blood pressure in the first place, is usually monitored invasively. To understand the relationship between the administration of drugs and the responses produced, we need to follow the events occurring within the body with time. A key to doing so is to measure the body's internal exposure to the drug. Here, our options are limited. It is rare when we can measure drug directly at the site of action, such as the brain or heart. Rather, we turn to more accessible sites to assess the systemic exposure to the drug.

Sites of Measurement.   Various sites of exposure assessment are used, including plasma, serum, whole blood, breath, milk, saliva, and urine. The first three fluids (plasma, serum, and blood) are obtained by invasive techniques. The differences among plasma, serum, and whole blood drug concentrations are shown in Table 2-2. Breath, milk, saliva, and urine are obtained noninvasively. Drug concentrations at these sites reflect the concentrations in plasma, blood, or serum.

The two fluids most commonly sampled are blood and urine. Drug within blood generally equilibrates rapidly with drug in blood cells and on plasma proteins. Accordingly, any of the fluids (whole blood, plasma, or serum) can be used to reflect the systemic time course of drug. In practice, plasma is preferred over whole blood primarily because components in blood cause interference in many assay techniques. Plasma and serum usually yield equivalent drug concentrations, but plasma is considered easier to prepare, as blood must be allowed to clot to obtain serum. During this process, hemolysis can occur, producing a concentration that is neither that of drug in plasma or blood, or causing interference in the assay.

Unbound Drug Concentration.   A comment is in order at this stage with respect to the binding of drugs to plasma proteins. The total plasma (or serum) concentration includes

TABLE 2-2	Differences Among Plasma, Serum, and Whole Blood Drug Concentrations

Fluid	Comment
Plasma	Whole blood is centrifuged after adding an anticoagulant, such as heparin or citric acid. Cells are precipitated. The supernatant fluid, plasma, contains proteins that often bind drugs. The concentration in plasma comprises bound and unbound drug.
Serum	Whole blood is centrifuged after the blood has been clotted. Cells and material forming the clot, including fibrinogen and its clotted form, fibrin, are removed. Binding of most drugs to fibrinogen and fibrin is insignificant. Although the protein composition of serum is slightly different from that of plasma, the drug concentrations in serum and plasma are virtually identical.
Whole Blood	Whole blood contains red blood cells, white blood cells, platelets, and various plasma proteins. An anticoagulant is commonly added and during analysis, the drug is commonly extracted into an organic phase often after denaturing the plasma proteins. The blood drug concentration represents an average over the total sample. Concentrations in the various cell fractions and in plasma may be very different.

both unbound and bound drug. Drug distribution and elimination, as well as pharmacodynamic responses, are dependent on the unbound concentration. It is only the unbound drug that passes through cell membranes to reach sites of storage, metabolism, or activity. Because the ratio of unbound to total drug, **fraction unbound**, usually does not change, it makes little difference whether total or unbound drug is measured. However, in those conditions in which binding is altered, such as the presence of another drug that displaces the drug of interest from its binding protein, renal disease, hepatic disease, surgery, severe burns, and pregnancy, measurement of the unbound concentration becomes important.

Exposure–Time Profile. The systemic exposure–time profile is a function of the rate and extent of drug input, distribution, and elimination. Figure 2-1 shows the salient features of the systemic exposure–time profile after ingesting a single oral dose. The highest concentration is called the maximum concentration, C_{max}, or maximum systemic exposure. The time of its occurrence is called the time of maximum concentration, t_{max}, or time of maximum exposure. Both C_{max} and t_{max} depend on how quickly the drug enters

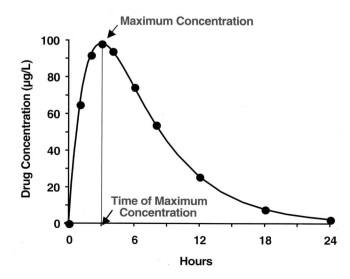

FIGURE 2-1. Drug concentration–time curve following a single oral dose showing the maximum systemic exposure (C_{max}) and the time of its occurrence (t_{max}). The concentration could represent drug in whole blood, plasma, or serum.

into and is eliminated from the body. The area under the concentration–time curve over all time, abbreviated as *AUC*, is a measure of the total systemic exposure to the drug. The concentration profile before the peak is a function of how quickly the drug enters the systemic circulation; after the peak, it is a function of how quickly the drug is eliminated.

The measured peak concentration (peak systemic exposure) of the example in Fig. 2-1 is 96 µg/L and the peak time is 3.0 hr. To get the *AUC*, the concentration must be integrated with respect to time. One common way to accomplish this is by approximating the areas between measurements as trapezoids and summing up the areas of the successive trapezoids (see Appendix A for further details).

Period of Observation. A basic kinetic principle is to make observations within the time frame of interest. An atomic physicist measures atomic events that occur within microseconds or nanoseconds. A geologist, on the other hand, may be studying plate tectonics, which occur on the scale of hundreds of thousands to millions of years. To appreciate the events, both of these individuals must make their observations consistent with the time frame of the kinetic events.

The same principles apply to drugs. Sometimes, drugs have a very short sojourn within the body. Following an intravenous (i.v.) bolus dose of such drugs, most of the dose may leave the body within minutes to hours. Other drugs remain in the body for days, weeks, months, and in a few instances, years. The period of measurement of systemic exposure must then be tailored to the kinetics of the specific drug of interest.

CHEMICAL PURITY AND ANALYTIC SPECIFICITY

A general statement needs to be made about the chemical purity of prescribed medicines and the specificity of chemical assays.

Over the years, a major thrust of the pharmaceutical industry has been to produce therapeutic agents and products that are not only as safe and effective as possible, but well characterized to ensure reproducible qualities. The majority of administered drug products today are therefore prepared with essentially pure drugs and, coupled with specific analytic techniques for their determination in biologic fluids, definitive information about their pharmacokinetics is gained. However, a large number of drug substances are not single chemical entities but rather mixtures. This particularly applies to stereoisomers and proteins. The most common stereoisomers found together in medicines are optical isomers, or compounds for which their structures are mirror images; the drug substance is often a racemate, a 50:50 mixture of the R- and S-isomers. Some drug substances contain geometric isomers (e.g., *cis* and *trans*) and still others, especially proteins of high molecular weight derived from natural products or through fermentation, may be a mixture of structurally related, but chemically distinct, compounds. Each chemical entity within the drug product can have a different pharmacologic, toxicologic, and/or pharmacokinetic profile. Sometimes these differences are small and inconsequential, other times the differences can be therapeutically important. For example, dextroamphetamine (S-isomer) is a potent central nervous stimulant, whereas the R-isomer is almost devoid of such activity. Sometimes the exposure–time profiles of the enantiomers are very different when given orally in racemic form, as shown in Fig. 2-2 for acenocoumarol, an oral anticoagulant, and methylphenidate, used to treat hyperactivity in children (reasons for the differences are explained in the "Study Problems" of Chapter 6). Despite the occasional occurrence of such striking differences in pharmacokinetics or pharmacodynamics, historically, many chemical assays have not distinguished between stereoisomers. Obviously, under these circumstances, attempting to quantify the various processes and to relate plasma concentration to response has many problems with no simple solution. Notwithstanding these problems, specific information about each chemical entity should be sought whenever possible. To avoid these problems,

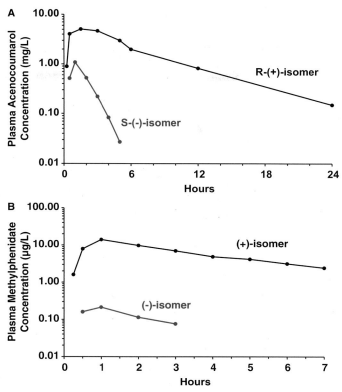

FIGURE 2-2. **A.** The exposure–time profiles of the R-(+) and S-(−) isomers of acenocoumarol, an agent used in some countries, differ strikingly after oral administration of 20 mg of a 50/50 racemic mixture to a subject. (From: Gill TS, Hopkins KJ, Rowland M. Stereospecific assay of acenocoumarol: application to pharmacokinetic studies in man. Br J Clin Pharmac 1988;25:591–598.) **B.** The peak and total systemic exposures to the (−) isomer of methylphenidate (colored) is negligible compared to the (+) isomer (black) following the oral administration of 30 mg of a racemic mixture of the two isomers, the common form of the drug. (From: Aoyama T, Kotaki H, Sasaki T, et al. Nonlinear kinetics of threo-methylphenidate enantiomers in a patient with narcolepsy and in healthy volunteers. Eur J Clin Pharmacol 1993;44:79–84.)

stereospecific assays are now more commonly used to measure individual isomers, and stereoisomers are being developed and marketed as single chemical entities, such as S-naproxyn, a nonsteroidal anti-inflammatory agent, and tamsulosin (R-isomer: Flomax), an α-adrenergic blocking agent used to treat benign prostatic hyperplasia. In contrast, many new protein and polypeptide drugs are being introduced that may, in many instances, lack high purity. Furthermore, these latter substances are often measured by assays that lack chemical specificity.

Some medicinal products contain several active compounds, an example being the combination of a thiazide diuretic and a β-blocker to lower blood pressure, each acting by a different mechanism. Specific assays are therefore needed to follow the pharmacokinetics of each compound. Herbal preparations contain a myriad of compounds, some of which may well be active. However, given the variable composition of such preparations and the uncertainty as to what might contribute to any observed effect, attempting to characterize the input–exposure relationships for many herbal products is highly problematic.

An added concern exists following drug administration, namely, the formation of **metabolites**, compounds formed from the drug usually by enzymatic reactions. To be of value, an analytic procedure must distinguish between drug and metabolite(s), many of which have very different pharmacokinetic and pharmacodynamic properties compared to the parent compound. Today, most assays have this desired specificity, except for many of those used to measure protein and polypeptide drugs.

A potential problem exists when using radiolabeled drugs to determine the fate of drug and related materials following drug administration. Incorporation of one or more radionuclides, usually ^{14}C and ^{3}H, into the molecular structure allows for simple and ready detection within a complex biologic milieu, but not necessarily of the administered drug. Complete recovery of all of a radiolabeled dose in urine, following oral drug administration, is useful in identifying the ultimate location of drug-related material but may provide little to no kinetic information about the drug itself. Consider, for example, a case in which the entire dose of an orally administered drug is destroyed in the gastrointestinal tract, yet degradation products enter the body and are ultimately excreted into the urine. Full recovery of radioactivity may suggest that the drug is completely available systemically when, in fact, none is. A basic lesson is learned here: Distinguish carefully between drug and metabolite(s). Each chemical entity must be considered separately for kinetic data to be meaningful.

ACTIVE METABOLITES AND PRODRUGS

Metabolites are sometimes thought of as weakly active or inactive end-products. For many drugs this is the case, but for many others it is not. Sometimes, the compound administered is an inactive **prodrug** that must be metabolized to the active compound. A prodrug is often developed intentionally to overcome an inherent problem with the active drug, such as poor or highly variable oral absorption. Examples of prodrugs include dolasetron mesylate (Anzemet), used to prevent chemotherapy-induced nausea and vomiting, famciclovir (Famvir), an antiviral agent, and most of the angiotensin-converting enzyme inhibitors, used to lower blood pressure. Many drugs have metabolites that augment the activity of the administered compound, as is the case with sildenafil (Viagra), an agent used to treat erectile dysfunction. Some drugs form metabolites that produce other effects. For example, acyl glucuronides of a number of drugs (polar esters of the drug formed by its conjugation with glucuronic acid), including several nonsteroidal anti-inflammatory agents, react with some proteins and have been implicated in a wide range of adverse effects, including hypersensitivity reactions and cellular toxicity. Metabolites may also, by inhibiting drug metabolism, prolong or enhance drug response, or when acting to increase drug metabolism, shorten or diminish drug response. Delavirdine mesylate (Rescriptor), a reverse transcriptase inhibitor of the human immunodeficiency virus type 1 (HIV-1), is an example of the former.

Drug (or prodrug) and metabolites often have very different systemic exposure–time profiles, as shown in Fig. 2-3 for aspirin and its primary metabolite, salicylic acid. It is well to remember that therapeutic or adverse effects may reside with either the compound administered or with one or more of the metabolites. Differences in their exposure–time profiles can, therefore, have a major impact on drug response. This topic is expanded on in Chapter 20, *Metabolites and Drug Response.*

ANATOMIC AND PHYSIOLOGIC CONSIDERATIONS

As previously stated, measurement of a drug in the body is usually limited to plasma and occasionally, blood. Nonetheless, the information obtained at these sites has proven to be very useful. Such usefulness can be explained by anatomic and physiologic features that affect a drug's sojourn within the body following its administration.

Blood is the most logical site for measurement of drug in the body. Blood receives drug from the site of administration and carries it to all the organs, including those in which the drug acts and those in which it is eliminated. This movement of drug is depicted schematically in Fig. 2-4 (page 24).

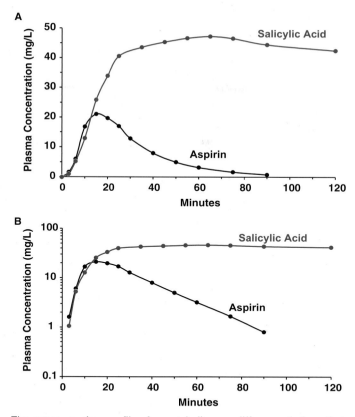

FIGURE 2-3. The exposure–time profile of a metabolite can differ greatly from that of the administered drug, as shown for salicylic acid (colored) and aspirin (black) on linear **(A)** and semilogarithmic **(B)** plots following the oral ingestion of 650 mg of aspirin. Consideration of the exposure–time profiles of metabolite(s) becomes particularly important therapeutically when the metabolite contributes to the therapeutic response or is associated with adverse events. When aspirin is given for its anticlotting activity, all the therapeutic activity lies with the drug, but when given for anti-inflammatory or antipyretic effects, most of the activity lies with the metabolite. (From: Rowland M, Riegelman S, Harris PA, Sholkoff SD. Absorption kinetics of aspirin in man following oral administration of an aqueous solution. J Pharm Sci 1972;61:379–385.)

Sites of Administration. There are several sites at which drugs are commonly administered. These sites may be classified as either intravascular or extravascular. **Intravascular** administration refers to the placement of a drug directly into the blood (i.e., either intravenously or intra-arterially).

Extravascular modes of administration include the buccal (between the cheek and the gums), intradermal, intramuscular, oral, pulmonary (inhalation), subcutaneous (into fat under the skin), rectal, and sublingual (under the tongue) routes, as listed in Table 2-3. Whether given through the alimentary canal (food canal or gastrointestinal tract) or any other extravascular route, an additional step, absorption, is required for drug to reach the systemic site of measurement relative to that required after intravascular administration.

Another term often used is **parenteral administration**. This refers to administration *apart from the intestines.* Today, the term is generally restricted to those routes of administration in which drug is injected through a needle. Thus, parenteral administration includes intramuscular, intravascular, and subcutaneous routes. Although the use of other routes, such as skin patches or nasal sprays (for systemic delivery), are strictly forms of parenteral administration, this term is not used for them.

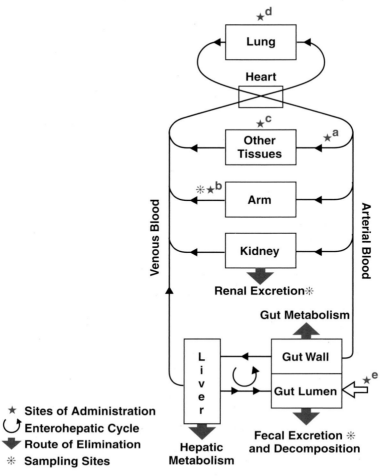

FIGURE 2-4.   Once absorbed from any of the many sites of administration, drug is conveyed by blood to all sites within the body including the eliminating organs and site(s) of action. Sites of administration include: *a*, artery; *b*, peripheral vein; *c*, muscle and subcutaneous tissue; *d*, lung; and *e*, gastrointestinal tract, the open arrow. When given intravenously into an arm vein, the contralateral arm should then be used for sampling. The movement of virtually any drug can be traced from site of administration to site(s) of elimination.

TABLE 2-3	Extravascular Routes of Administration for Systemic Drug Delivery*

Via Alimentary Canal

| Buccal | Rectal |
| Oral | Sublingual |

Other Routes

Inhalation	Subcutaneous
Intramuscular	Transdermal
Intranasal	

*Routes such as intra-articular, intrathecal, intravaginal, ocular, and subdural are usually used to achieve a local effect.

Drug may also be administered regionally (e.g., into the pleural or peritoneal cavities or into the cerebrospinal fluid). Regional administration also includes intra-arterial injection into the vessel leading to a tissue to be treated (e.g., a cancerous tumor). It is a potential means of gaining a selective therapeutic advantage. This advantage, in comparison with other routes of administration, comes about by increasing drug exposure locally, where it is needed, and decreasing or producing little or no change in exposure throughout the rest of the body, where it is not wanted.

Events After Entering Systemically. Once entered systemically, a drug is distributed to the various organs of the body by the blood. Distribution is influenced by organ blood flow, organ size, binding of drug within blood and in tissues, and transport across tissue membranes.

The two principal organs of elimination, the liver and the kidneys, are shown separately in Fig. 2-4. The kidneys are the primary organs for excretion of the chemically unaltered or unchanged drug. The liver is the usual organ for drug metabolism; however, the kidneys, the intestinal tissues, and other organs can also play an important metabolic role for certain drugs. The metabolites so formed are either further metabolized or excreted unchanged, or both. The liver may also secrete unchanged drug into the bile. The lungs are, or may be, an important route for eliminating volatile substances, for example, gaseous anesthetics. Another potential route of elimination (not shown) is lactation. Although generally an insignificant route of elimination in the mother, drug in the milk may be consumed in sufficient quantity to affect a suckling infant.

Drugs are rarely given alone as the pure substance. They are formulated into a product that is convenient for the patient and optimizes the drug's performance when administered. For example, tablets and capsules permit a fixed dose to be easily administered orally. The formulation of the product may result in rapid release of the active drug, or its release may be modified to diminish fluctuation in systemic exposure between doses or to allow less frequent dosing.

MODELS FOR DRUG ABSORPTION AND DISPOSITION

A model is useful to summarize data and facilitate extrapolation and prediction after drug administration. The complexities of human anatomy and physiology would appear to make it difficult, if not impossible, to model how the body handles a drug. Perhaps surprisingly then, it is a simple pharmacokinetic model, depicted in Fig. 2-5, which has proved useful in many applications and is emphasized throughout much of this book.

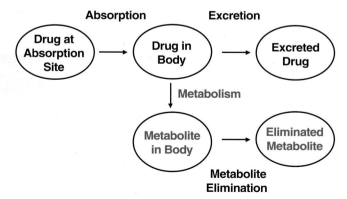

FIGURE 2-5. A drug is simultaneously absorbed into the body and eliminated from it, by excretion and metabolism. The processes of absorption, excretion, and metabolism are indicated with arrows and the compartments with ovals. The compartments represent different locations and different chemical species (color = metabolite). Metabolite elimination may occur by further metabolism or excretion.

The boxes in Fig. 2-5 represent **compartments** that logically fall into two classes: transfer and chemical. The site of administration, the body, and excreta are clearly different places. Each place may be referred to as a location or transfer compartment. In contrast, metabolism involves a chemical conversion; drug and metabolite in the body are clearly in compartments that differ chemically, but not by location. The same principle applies to excreted drug and metabolite.

The model is based on amounts of drug and metabolite. However, they can only be directly measured in urine and feces. The total amount of drug metabolized includes metabolites in, as well as eliminated from, the body. The amount in the body is usually determined from measurement of the blood or plasma concentration. Estimates of drug in the absorption compartment are also usually made indirectly from either blood or urine data. Drug at the absorption site includes that which is never absorbed, for example, drug that is ultimately decomposed in the gastrointestinal tract or lost in the feces after oral administration.

The model is readily visualized from mass balance considerations. The dose is accounted for at any one time by the molar amount of substance in each of the compartments:

$$Dose = \frac{Amount\ at}{Absorption\ Site} + \frac{Amount}{in\ Body} + \frac{Amount}{Excreted} + \frac{Amount}{Metabolized} \qquad 2\text{-}1$$

The mass balance of drug and related material with time is shown in Fig. 2-6. Because the sum of the molar amounts of drug in transfer and chemical compartments is equal to the dose, the sum of the rates of change of the drug in these compartments must be equal to zero so that:

$$\frac{Rate\ of\ Change}{of\ Drug\ in\ Body} = \frac{Rate\ of}{Absorption} - \left[\frac{Rate\ of}{Excretion} + \frac{Rate\ of}{Metabolism} \right] \qquad 2\text{-}2$$

The relationships expressed in Eqs. 2-1 and 2-2 apply under all circumstances, regardless of the nature of the absorption and elimination processes. They are particularly useful in developing more complex models for quantifying drug absorption and disposition. **Pharmacokinetics** is the quantitation of the time course of a drug and its metabolites in the body and the development of appropriate models to describe observations and predict outcomes in other situations.

Examples of other common models used in pharmacokinetics are shown in Fig. 2-7. One form (A) is the use of equations, which may consist of either integrated or differential equations, or both. Physiologic models (B) are also common, such as those depicting

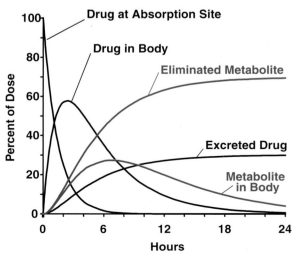

FIGURE 2-6. Time course of drug and metabolite in each of the compartments shown in Fig. 2-5. The amount in each compartment is expressed as a percentage of the dose administered. In this example, all the dose is absorbed. At any time, the sum of the molar amounts in the five compartments equals the dose.

A. Equations, e.g.,

<u>Integrated</u>   <u>Differential</u>

$$C = C(0)e^{-kt} \qquad \frac{dA}{dt} = ka \cdot Aa - k \cdot A$$

B. Physiologic Models

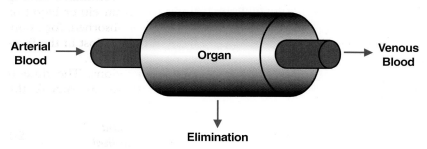

Arterial Blood → Organ → Venous Blood

Elimination

C. Compartmental Models

1. One-compartment (Body) Model

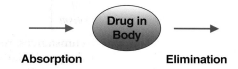

Absorption   Drug in Body   Elimination

2. Two-compartment (Body) Model

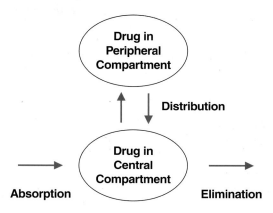

Drug in Peripheral Compartment

Distribution

Absorption   Drug in Central Compartment   Elimination

FIGURE 2-7. Several kinds of models are used in pharmacokinetics. **A.** Differential and integral eqs. can be one way of modeling the kinetic behavior of drugs in the body. **B.** Symbolic models are also used. An example is a physiologic model, in which the degree of complexity varies with the intended use of the model. When the multiple organs of the body are included, and are arranged anatomically, as in Fig. 2-4, a full physiologically based model is obtained. **C.** An additional kind of model is one in which drug distribution within the body is approximated by compartments, which are kinetically defined. One-compartment and two-compartment models, the ones used most commonly for characterizing drug in the body, are shown.

movement of a drug through a tissue or organ of elimination. Figure 2-4 is such a physiologic model of drug absorption and disposition in the whole body. The disposition of a drug is often simulated using compartmental models (C) for drug distribution within the body. Shown are one- and two-compartment models. The two-compartment model, in which drug distributes from a central compartment, of which the plasma is a part, to a peripheral compartment, which is generally viewed as the tissues, is a very common one.

DEFINITIONS OF PHARMACOKINETIC TERMS

The processes of absorption, distribution, metabolism, and excretion (ADME) are schematically shown in Fig. 2-8. They are defined below, but their meanings are truly apparent only within the context of experimental observations.

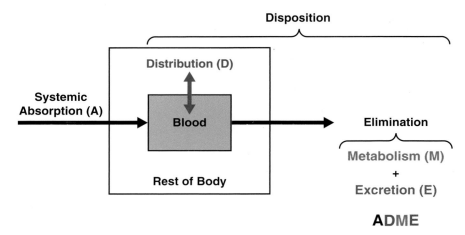

FIGURE 2-8. The terms absorption (systemic), distribution, metabolism, and excretion (ADME) used in pharmacokinetics are schematically defined relative to the process of moving from the site of administration into the body (large box), absorption, moving between locations within the body, distribution, or moving out of the body, elimination. All of the processes are defined relative to the site of measurement, usually plasma. Disposition refers to the combined processes of distribution and elimination. Compounds are eliminated from the body by both excretion (irreversible loss of unchanged drug) and metabolism (conversion to another chemical entity).

Systemic Absorption. **Systemic absorption** is defined as the process by which unchanged drug proceeds from site of administration to site of measurement within the body, usually plasma in an arm vein. To illustrate why systemic absorption is defined this way, consider the events depicted in Fig. 2-9 as a drug, given orally, moves from the site of administration (mouth) to the general systemic circulation.

There are several possible sites of loss along the way. One site is the gastrointestinal lumen where decomposition may occur. Suppose, however, that a drug survives destruction in the lumen, only to be completely metabolized by enzymes as it passes through the membranes of the gastrointestinal tract. One would ask, Is the drug absorbed? Even though the drug leaves the gastrointestinal tract, it would not be detected in the general circulation. Hence, the drug is not absorbed systemically. Taking this argument one step further: Is the drug absorbed if all of the orally administered drug were to pass through the membranes of the gastrointestinal tract into the portal vein only to be metabolized completely on passing through the liver? If one were to sample the portal blood entering the liver, the answer would be positive. If, however, blood or plasma in an arm vein is the site of measurement, then, because no drug would be detected, the answer would be negative. Indeed, loss at any site prior to the site of measurement contributes to a decrease in systemic absorption. The gastrointestinal tissues and the liver, in particular, are often

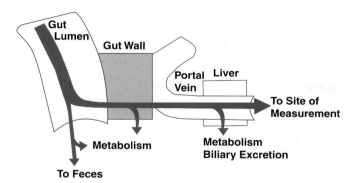

FIGURE 2-9. A drug, given as a solid, encounters several barriers and sites of loss in its sequential movement through gastrointestinal tissues and the liver. Incomplete dissolution or metabolism in the gut lumen or by enzymes in the gut wall is a cause of incomplete input into the systemic circulation. Removal of drug as it first passes through the liver may further reduce systemic input.

sites of loss. The requirement for an orally administered drug to pass through these tissues, prior to reaching the site of measurement, interconnects the extent of systemic absorption and elimination. This loss of drug during its first passage through these tissues is **first-pass loss**. Drugs that show extensive first-pass loss may require much larger oral than i.v. doses to achieve the same therapeutic effect.

The movement of drug across the intestinal epithelium is often called absorption, or more precisely, **intestinal absorption**. But it is extremely difficult to measure in practice. As mentioned, assessment of intestinal absorption would require measurement of drug in the portal vein draining the intestine, a very invasive procedure. Moreover, in itself, intestinally absorbed drug is only of interest clinically if the drug acts directly on or within the liver. In most cases, and specifically the ones of primary focus in this book, drugs act systemically and, to that extent, intestinal absorption is only one component of **systemic absorption** (hereafter often simply called **absorption**).

Absorption is not restricted to oral administration. The term applies as well following intramuscular, subcutaneous, and all other extravascular routes of administration. Monitoring intact drug in plasma offers a useful means of assessing the entry of drug into the systemic circulation.

The term **bioavailability** is commonly applied to both rate and extent of drug input into the systemic circulation. Throughout the book, unless qualified otherwise, this term is limited to denoting the extent of drug input and is defined as the fraction, or percent, of the administered dose systemically absorbed intact.

Disposition. As absorption and elimination of drugs are interrelated for physiologic and anatomic reasons, so too are distribution and elimination. Once absorbed systemically, a drug is delivered simultaneously by blood to all tissues, including organs of elimination. Distinguishing between elimination and distribution as a cause for a decline in concentration in plasma is therefore often difficult. Disposition is the term used to embrace both processes. Disposition may be defined as all the kinetic processes that occur to a drug subsequent to its systemic absorption. By definition, the components of disposition are distribution and elimination.

Distribution. **Distribution** is the process of reversible transfer of a drug to and from the site of measurement and the peripheral tissues. An example is distribution between blood and muscle. The pathway for return of drug need not be the same as that leaving the circulation. For example, drug may be secreted in the bile, stored in and released from the gallbladder, transit into the small intestine, and be reabsorbed there back into the circulation. By doing so, the drug completes a cycle, the **enterohepatic cycle**, a component of distribution (see Fig. 2-10). The situation is analogous to one in which water is pumped from one reservoir into another, only to drain back into the original one.

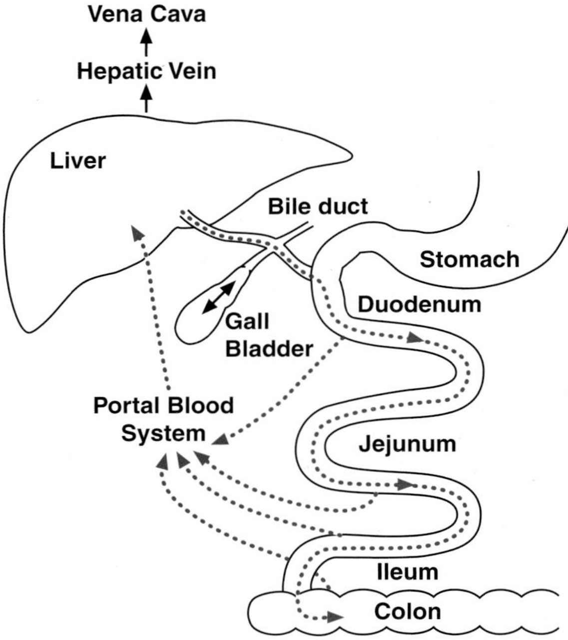

FIGURE 2-10. Drugs sometimes are excreted from the liver into the bile and stored in the gall bladder. On emptying the gall bladder, particularly when induced by food, drug passes into the lumen of the small intestine, where it may be absorbed into a mesenteric vein draining the small intestine and colon, and conveyed by blood back to the liver via the portal vein. The drug has then completed a cycle, the enterohepatic cycle, as shown in color.

Elimination. **Elimination** is the irreversible loss of drug from the site of measurement. Elimination occurs by two processes, excretion and metabolism. **Excretion** is the irreversible loss of chemically unchanged compound. **Metabolism** is the conversion of one chemical species to another. Occasionally, metabolites are converted back to the drug. As with enterohepatic cycling, this **metabolic interconversion** becomes a route of elimination only to the extent that the metabolite is excreted or otherwise irreversibly lost from the body.

BILIARY SECRETION AND FECAL EXCRETION

When a compound fails, partially or completely, to be reabsorbed from the gastrointestinal tract after biliary secretion, it is excreted from the body via the feces or decomposed in the intestines. For example, the hydroxylated metabolites of zafirlukast (Accolate), an antiasthmatic drug, are quantitatively excreted in the feces.

PHARMACODYNAMICS

Drugs produce a therapeutic effect when there is an adequate exposure profile at the target site. Often the target is distant from the site of application, a common example being that of antidepressant drugs taken orally. For these drugs, exposure at the target site within the brain occurs via delivery of drug by the systemic circulation. And, as drug concentration cannot be or is rarely measured within the brain, or indeed at any other site of action within the body, measurement of systemic drug exposure offers a generally useful substitute for exposure at the active site. Although the potential role of metabolites should always be kept in mind, the subsequent discussion is based on the assumption that it is the administered compound that drives the response.

Drugs interact with components within the body to produce a response. These components are commonly proteins, such as enzymes or receptors, or they may be a gene or DNA itself. Drugs can produce their effects by causing **up-or-down regulation** of a protein responsible for the drug's effect by increasing or decreasing its concentration. They can also modulate an endogenous system. Drugs that act on receptors are said to be either

agonists or **antagonists** depending on whether they increase or diminish the functional response of the receptor. When they produce the maximum possible effect, they are said to be **full agonists** or **full antagonists**. Compounds that fail to achieve the full effect, even at very high concentrations, are said to be **partial agonists** or **partial antagonists**. Some drugs, such as the estrogens, are agonists at one range of concentrations and antagonists at another.

In this chapter, we primarily consider the relationship between systemic exposure and response, that is, the **pharmacodynamics** of the drug. In subsequent chapters, we integrate pharmacokinetics with response over time, in which case we speak of **PK/PD modeling** in the sense that we are linking a model of the pharmacokinetics with a model of the pharmacodynamics of a drug to obtain a complete picture of the relationship between drug administration and response over time.

Response is an all-embracing term applied to a wide variety of measurements. It may be one that reflects the effect of a drug at a particular moment in time; it may be an observation that integrates past effects, as in the case of the increase in daily urinary sodium excretion and urine volume produced by the diuretic furosemide.

CLASSIFICATION OF RESPONSE

There are various ways to classify response. Clinically, the most important is whether the effect produced is desired or harmful. However, this classification gives little insight into the mechanisms involved. For example, for some drugs the adverse effect is simply an extension of the desired effect and is entirely predictable from its pharmacology. An example is the oral anticoagulant warfarin. It is used clinically to reduce the risk of developing an embolism by decreasing the tendency of blood to clot, whereas the adverse and potentially fatal effect is internal hemorrhage caused by excessive anticoagulation. In many other cases, the adverse effect occurs via a completely different and often more unpredictable mechanism, such as the hepatic or cardiac toxicity caused by some antibiotics.

Another form of classification is whether the measured effect is a **clinical response**, a **surrogate endpoint**, or a **biomarker**. Clinical responses may be divided into subjective and objective measures. Subjective ones are those that the patients themselves assess, such as a feeling of well-being, a sense of nausea, and a greater sense of mobility, which collectively form part of a global measure of "quality of life." Examples of objective ones are an increase in survival time, stroke prevention, or prevention of bone fracture. However, although these objective measures are clearly therapeutically relevant, the need for another measure arises in many cases because the clinical response may not be fully manifested for many years, and a more immediate measure is sought to guide therapy or simply to know that an effect is being produced. An example is the use of antihypertensive agents to reduce the risk of morbidity of several sequelae of prolonged hypertension, such as blindness and renal failure, and premature mortality. These outcomes are evident only after many years of prolonged treatment. A more rapid, ready, and simple measure of effect, which correlates with the clinical outcome and which can be used to guide therapy, is the lowering of blood pressure in a hypertensive patient to values within the normotensive range. And because lowering of blood pressure has been shown through many large long-term studies to correlate with the clinical effect, it is called a surrogate (or substitute) endpoint, in this case, one which is on the causal pathway to the clinical effect.

The last category of response is the biomarker, which broadly may be considered within the context of pharmacodynamics as any measurable effect produced by a drug. The term is usually applied to situations in which the measure has some diagnostic or prognostic value. It may be a change in a laboratory test, such as blood glucose when evaluating antidiabetic drug therapy, a change in a physiologic test, such as the response time in a simulated driving test when evaluating an antidepressant with concern about possible changes in motor reflex, or it may be the binding of a positron-emitting labeled drug to a specific brain receptor determined using positron emission tomography, a noninvasive technique that measures externally the location and quantity of the labeled compound within the brain. These are examples of biomarkers that are intended to relate in some way to the desired action of the drug. Others, called **safety biomarkers**, are general measures not specifically related to the drug and are used to monitor for potential adverse effects. Examples are liver function tests, white cell count, erythrocyte sedimentation rate, and fecal blood loss. Drugs often produce multiple effects; the biomarker may therefore not be at all related to the clinical effect of the drug. In this sense, all pharmacodynamic responses are biomarkers unless they are either accepted as the clinical response, which is rarely the case, or they have been shown through rigorous evaluation to predict clinical response, in which case they are classified as surrogate endpoints. Clearly, biomarkers are most likely to serve as surrogate endpoints if they are on the causal pathway between drug action and clinical response.

The majority of drugs used clinically act reversibly in that the effect is reversed on reducing concentration at the site of action. An exception is the class of anticancer drugs known as alkylating agents, such as busulfan. These compounds covalently, and hence irreversibly, bind to DNA causing death of proliferating cells, taking advantage of the fact that cancer cells proliferate more rapidly than most healthy cells within the body.

Many responses produced are **graded**, so called because the magnitude of the response can be scaled or graded within an individual. An example of a graded response, shown in Fig. 2-11, is anesthesia produced by ketamine given intravenously. The intensity of the response varies continuously with the drug concentration in plasma. Many other pharmacologic and adverse responses do not occur on a continuous basis; these are known as **quantal** or **all-or-none** responses. One example is the suppression of a cardiac

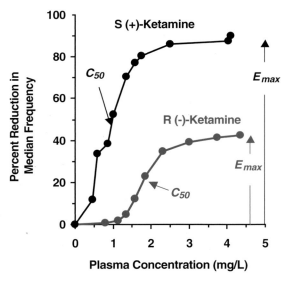

FIGURE 2-11.   Changes in the electroencephalographic median frequency were followed to quantify the anesthetic effect of R($-$)-ketamine and S($+$)-ketamine in a subject who received an i.v. infusion of these two optical isomers on separate occasions. Shown is the percent reduction in the median frequencies versus plasma concentration. Although characteristic S-shaped, or sigmoidal, curves are seen with both compounds, they differ in both maximum effect achieved, E_{max}, and concentration needed to produce 50% of E_{max}, the C_{50}. These relationships may be considered direct ones as no significant time delay was found between response and concentration. (From: Schuttler, J, Stoeckel H, Schweilden H, Lauvan PM. Hypnotic drugs. In: Stoeckel H, ed. Quantitation, modeling and control in anaesthesia. New York: Thieme; 1985, pp. 196–210.)

arrhythmia. The arrhythmia is either suppressed or not. Another obvious but extreme example of an adverse all-or-none event is death.

An effect of drug treatment may be assessed relatively frequently during the course of treatment, such as the almost daily monitoring of blood glucose in a diabetic patient receiving insulin treatment, or it may be assessed at some defined time, such as the percent of cancer patients surviving after 5 years following drug treatment.

ASSESSMENT OF DRUG RESPONSE

Most drugs do not occur naturally within the body, so that when they are found in plasma, we can be confident that they have been administered. Exceptions are those drugs that are normally produced within the body, that is, **endogenous compounds**, such as insulin. There is always a basal plasma concentration of insulin, a protein secreted by the pancreas, and a correction is needed in its measured concentration if we wish to characterize the kinetics of externally, or **exogenously**, administered insulin.

In contrast to drug concentration, a **baseline** almost always exists when attempting to assess drug effect. For example, antihypertensive drugs act by lowering blood pressure in hypertensive patients. Hence, the drug effect is the difference between the high baseline blood pressure in such a patient and the blood pressure when the patient is on antihypertensive therapy. For many drugs, there is an additional factor to consider—**the placebo effect**. A placebo effect is a deviation from the baseline value produced when the patient takes or receives what has all the appearances of drug treatment but lacks the active principle. This may take the form of giving the patient a tablet that looks and tastes identical to the one containing the drug. Thus, in general, when attempting to assess response following drug administration, we can write

$$\frac{Measured}{Response} = \frac{Drug}{Response} + \frac{Placebo}{Response} + Baseline \qquad \text{2-3}$$

An additional issue is that not only do drug responses vary with time following drug administration but commonly, so do both the placebo effect and the baseline. Hence, separating out and characterizing the true drug effect with time requires careful attention to these other factors. This is equally true when assessing both the desired and adverse effects of the drug. Several examples are considered to illustrate these points.

Figure 2-12 shows forced expiratory volume in 1 second (FEV_1; the volume exhaled during the first second of a forced expiration started from the level of total lung capacity), a common measure of respiratory function, with time following the oral administration of placebo and 10-mg montelukast (Singulair), a specific leukotriene receptor antagonist that improves respiratory function. Notice both the appreciable placebo response and also the positive effect of montelukast seen as the difference in FEV_1 between the two treatments, which is sustained over the 24-hr period of study. In this study, and commonly, there is no specific and independent assessment of the normal changes in baseline over time; these are subsumed in the assessment following drug treatment and placebo, and assumed to be independent of treatment.

Sometimes the baseline is relatively stable over the period of assessment of drug effect. Other times, and indeed commonly, it is not. Many physiologic processes undergo rhythmic changes with time. For some, the period of the cycle approximates a day (a so-called circadian rhythm), such as seen with the hormone cortisol. For others, the period is much shorter or much longer than 1 day, sometimes being as long as 1 month, such as with hormones associated with the estrous cycle. Correcting for the variable baseline is then more difficult. Returning to Fig. 2-12, we see that following placebo FEV_1 first increases with time and then wanes (with a time course relatively similar to that observed following drug administration), although this is not always the case. However, without independent baseline data, it is not possible to know how much of the temporal change in FEV_1 is caused by a change in the baseline function, and how much to the placebo.

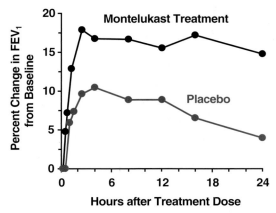

FIGURE 2-12. Changes in FEV_1 (forced expiratory volume in 1 second), a measure of respiratory function, with time following administration of a single dose of a placebo (colored circle) or montelukast (10 mg; black circle), a specific leukotriene receptor antagonist. Notice both the appreciable placebo difference in FEV_1 between the two treatments, which is sustained over the 24-hr period, and also the positive effect of montelukast seen as the difference in FEV_1 between the two treatments, which is sustained over the 24-hr period of study. (From: Dockhorn RJ, Baumgartner RA, Leff JA, et al. Comparison of the effects of intravenous and oral montelukast on airway function: a double blind, placebo controlled, three period, crossover study in asthmatic patients. Thorax 2000;55:260–265.)

Placebo effects can be quite subtle even when using what are thought to be objective assessments, such as loss of weight. They are commonly extensive when assessing subjective effects, such as a feeling of well-being or depression, or a sense of nausea or dizziness. Indeed, the interaction between the mind and various physiologic processes can be quite strong. Because placebo effects can be clinically significant, double blind placebo controlled trials, in which neither the clinician nor the patient know whether placebo or active treatment has been given, are usually employed to assess drug effects.

Occasionally, it is not appropriate to use a placebo arm for a study. This can occur when the drug is tested for a disease or condition in which there is a standard treatment, although perhaps not highly effective, already available. It may be unethical to use a placebo group, especially if the current treatment prevents some deaths, reduces intense pain or discomfort, or has any other effect of which a patient should not be deprived. In this case, the new treatment might then be compared with the standard treatment, instead of a placebo. Whether a placebo or standard treatment is given, ethics again enters the picture if there is evidence that the new treatment, for example, a new antimicrobial agent, is much more effective than the standard treatment. For example, there may be a considerable reduction in the number of deaths or a prolongation of life. Here, the code for the double blinding may need to be broken before the end of the study so that all patients can benefit from the new treatment.

As mentioned previously, the clinical benefit of many drugs requires that drug treatment be continued for many months or years. During this time, the baseline itself often changes, reflecting the natural course of the disease or condition. Consider, for example, the data in Fig. 2-13 showing the change in average muscle strength in a group of boys with Duchenne dystrophy, a degenerating muscle disease associated with a gene defect. The aim of the study was to assess the potential benefit of the corticosteroid prednisone. The study was randomized and double blinded. Patients were assigned to one of three treatments: placebo, 0.3 mg/kg prednisone, or 0.75 mg/kg prednisone in the form of one capsule daily, with the study period extending over 6 months. These data showed several interesting points. First, at best, the placebo appeared to produce

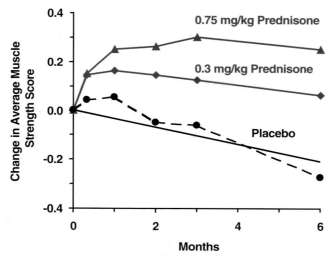

FIGURE 2-13. Mean changes in the score for average muscle strength in placebo (black circle, dashed line) and prednisone-treated groups (colored diamond, 0.3 mg/kg daily; colored triangle, 0.75 mg/kg daily) of patients suffering with Duchenne dystrophy after the initiation of treatments. The solid continuous straight line represents the average natural course of the changes observed in a group of 177 such patients who received no treatment. (From: Griggs RC, Moxley RT, Mendell JR, et al. Predisone in Duchenne dystrophy. Arch Neurol 1991;44:383–388.)

an initial slight benefit when judged against the natural progression of the disease, but it was not significant. Second, prednisone had a dose-dependent positive effect. For patients receiving 0.3 mg/kg prednisone daily, muscle strength increased to a maximum by the end of the first month of treatment and then declined in parallel with the natural course of the disease, indicating that there is no further benefit gained with this dose of drug. A similar pattern was seen in the patient group receiving the 0.75 mg/kg daily dose, except that the improvement was greater and continued over approximately 3 months of treatment, before declining once again in parallel with the natural history of the disease. From these findings, we can conclude that prednisone provides relief of the symptoms but does not alter the course of the underlying disease.

Figure 2-14 schematically generalizes the distinction between symptomatic relief and cure against the background of the natural course of a physiologic function. A characteristic of physiologic functions is that they tend to decline with advancing age beyond around 20 years. The rate of decline varies for different functions but is commonly around 1% per year (see also Chapter 12, *Variability*). Many chronic diseases accelerate this rate of decline, as it occurs for example in patients with chronic renal disease or Alzheimer's disease. As discussed previously, prednisone provides symptomatic improvement by treating the symptoms of a disease but not the underlying disease itself. Alternatively, a drug may arrest the **disease progression**, thereby stabilizing the function, such that the measured function subsequently declines at the normal physiologic rate. A drug is curative if it restores the function in the patient back to within the normal range expected of an otherwise healthy person. For example, some drugs cure certain cancers in that such patients no longer exhibit the signs of the disease and go on to live a normal life span. This is an example of a long-term cure. An example of a short-term cure is the abolition of a severe "stress" headache, which fails to return. Obviously, there are many shades of effectiveness between symptomatic relief and long-term cure.

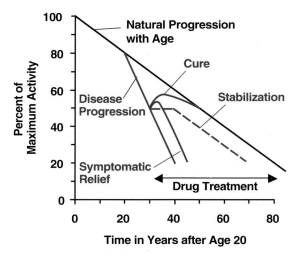

FIGURE 2-14. Schematic diagram illustrating various scenarios of effectiveness of a drug in the treatment of patients suffering from a disease that causes a faster rate of decline of a measured function than seen in otherwise healthy subjects. Treatment is symptomatic if after a period of initial benefit, the measured function returns to a rate of decline seen in patients not receiving treatment. Treatment is stabilizing if it arrests the disease, returning the rate of function decline to that in otherwise healthy subjects; it may also temporarily stop further deterioration of function. Cure is achieved if the drug treatment returns the patient to the trend line for normal physiologic function with age. Drug effectiveness can, of course, lie anywhere between these various extremes.

RELATING RESPONSE TO EXPOSURE

Because sites of action lie mostly outside the vasculature, delays often exist between plasma concentration and the response produced. Such delays can obscure underlying relationships between concentration and response. One potential solution is to measure concentration at the site of action. Although this may be possible in an isolated tissue system, it is rarely practical in humans. Apart from ethical and technical issues that often arise, many responses observed in vivo represent an integration of multiple effects at numerous sites within the body. Another approach is to develop a model that incorporates the time course of drug movement between plasma and site of action, thereby predicting "effect site" concentrations that can then be related to response. Yet, another approach is to relate plasma concentration to response under conditions whereby a constant concentration is maintained using a constant rate of drug input, which obviates consideration of the time course of distribution. Whatever the approach adopted, the resulting concentration–response relationships for most drugs have features in common.

Graded Response. Response increases with concentration at low concentrations and tends to approach a maximum at high values. Such an effect is seen for the anesthetic ketamine, as illustrated in Fig. 2-11. R(−)-ketamine and S(+)-ketamine are optical isomers which, as the racemate (50:50 mixture of the isomers), constitute the commercially available i.v. anesthetic agent, ketamine. Although both compounds have an anesthetic effect, they clearly differ from each other. Not only is the maximum response (E_{max}) with R(−)-ketamine less than that with S(+)-ketamine, but the plasma concentration required to produce 50% of E_{max}, referred to as the C_{50} value, is also greater (1.8 mg/L versus 0.7 mg/L). Although the reason for the differences is unclear, these observations stress the importance that stereochemistry can have in drug response, and that drugs acting on even the same receptor do not necessarily produce the same maximal response.

An equation to describe the response E associated with the types of observations seen in Fig. 2-11 for ketamine is

$$E = \frac{E_{max} \cdot C^{\gamma}}{C_{50}^{\gamma} + C^{\gamma}}$$

2-4

where E_{max} and C_{50} are as defined above and γ is a **steepness factor** that accommodates for the steepness of the curve around the C_{50} value. The intensity of response is usually a change in a measurement from its basal value expressed as either an absolute difference, or a percent change. Examples are an increase in blood pressure and a decrease in blood glucose, expressed as a percent of the baseline. One should always keep in mind that unbound drug drives response, and therefore the unbound concentration should be used when relating response to systemic exposure, particularly when plasma protein binding varies.

Although empirical, Eq. 2-4 has found wide application. Certainly, it has the right properties; when $C = 0$, E is zero, and when C greatly exceeds C_{50} response approaches E_{max}. Figure 2-15A shows the influence of γ on the shape of the concentration–response relationship. The larger the value of γ, the greater is the change in response with concentration around the C_{50} value. For example, if $\gamma = 1$ then, by appropriate substitution into Eq. 2-2, the concentrations corresponding to 20% and 80% of maximal response are 0.25 and 4 times C_{50}, respectively, a 16-fold range. Whereas, if $\gamma = 2$, the corresponding concentrations are 0.5 and 2 times C_{50}, only a fourfold range. Using the percent decrease in heart rate during a standard exercise as a measure of response to the β-adrenergic blocking agent propranolol, the average value of γ is close to 1 (Fig. 2-15A). Generally, the value of γ lies between 1 and 3. Occasionally, it is much greater, in which case the effect appears almost as an all-or-none response, because the range of concentrations associated with minimal and maximal responses becomes so narrow.

A common form of representing concentration–response data is a plot of the intensity of response against the *logarithm* of concentration. Figure 2-15B shows this transformation of the curves in Fig. 2-15A. This transformation is popular because it expands the

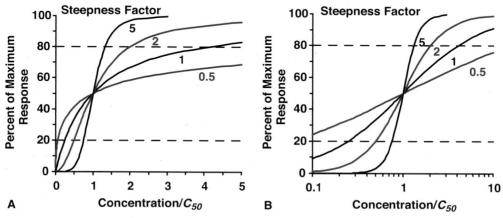

FIGURE 2-15. Linear (**A**) and semilogarithmic (**B**) concentration–response plots, predicted according to Eq. 4, for four hypothetical drugs that have different values of the steepness factor, γ. At low concentrations the effect increases almost linearly with concentration (**A**), when $\gamma = 1$, approaching a maximal value at high concentrations. The greater the value of γ, the steeper is the change in response around the C_{50} value. Between 20% and 80% of maximal effect, the response appears to be proportional to the logarithm of the concentration (**B**) for all values of γ. Concentrations are expressed relative to C_{50}.

initial part of the curve, where response is changing markedly with a small change in concentration, and contracts the latter part, where a large change in concentration produces only a slight change in response. It also shows that between approximately 20% and 80% of the maximum value, response appears to be proportional to the logarithm of concentration regardless of the value of the steepness factor, γ. This relationship occurs with propranolol within the range of unbound concentrations of 1 and 10 μg/L, as shown in Fig. 2-16B after transformation of the data in Fig. 2-16A.

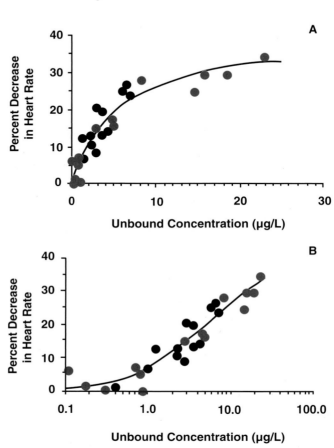

FIGURE 2-16. **A.** Response, measured by the percent decrease in exercise-induced tachycardia, to propranolol increases with the unbound concentration of the drug in plasma. **B.** The same data as in **A**, except now concentration is plotted on a logarithmic scale. The data points represent measurements after single and multiple (daily) oral doses of two 80-mg tablets of propranolol (●) or a 160-mg modified-release capsule (colored) in an individual subject. The solid line is the fit of Eq. 2-4 to the data. The response appears to follow the Hill eq. with a γ of 1, an E_{max} of 40%, and a C_{50} of 5.3 μg/L. (From: Lalonde RL, Straka RJ, Pieper JA, et al. Propranolol pharmacodynamic modeling using unbound and total concentrations in healthy volunteers. J Pharmacokinet Biopharm 1987;15:569–582.)

The greatest response produced clinically for some drugs may be less than that pharmacologically possible. For example, for a drug stimulating heart rate, the entire cardiovascular system may deteriorate, and the patient may die long before the heart rate approaches its maximum value. Other adverse effects of the drug or metabolite(s) may further limit the maximally tolerated concentration in vivo. As a general rule, it is more difficult to define the E_{max} of an agonist than it is of an antagonist. For an antagonist, such as a neuromuscular blocking agent used to prevent muscle movement during surgery, the maximum possible effect is easy to identify; it is the absence of a measurable response. That is, total muscle paralysis. For an agonist, it is not always certain how great the response produced can be.

Quantal Response. All the preceding examples are graded responses. Unlike a graded response, a quantal response, being all-or-none and hence discontinuous, cannot be correlated continuously with concentration. Instead, the overall response is evaluated from the **cumulative frequency** or likelihood of the event with concentration. This is illustrated in Fig. 2-17 by a plot of cumulative frequency of satisfactory control in patients receiving the

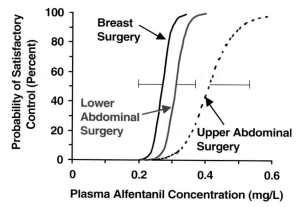

FIGURE 2-17. The relationship between the cumulative frequency in satisfactory response versus the mean arterial concentration obtained for alfentanil, an opioid analgesic, during the intraoperative period in each of three surgical groups of patients receiving nitrous oxide anesthesia. Notice, for any group, the narrow range of alfentanil concentrations between that which just begins to produce a satisfactory response in some patients to that which produces a satisfactory response in all patients. Notice also that the concentration needed to produce 50% satisfactory response is in the order: breast (0.27) < lower abdomen (0.31) < upper abdomen (0.42). (From: Ausems ME, Hug CC, Stanski DR, Burm AGL. Plasma concentrations of alfentanil required to supplement nitrous oxide anesthesia for general surgery. Anesthesiology 1986;65:362–373. Reproduced by permission of J.B. Lippincott.)

opioid analgesic alfentanil to supplement nitrous oxide anesthesia during surgery. In such cases, the C_{50} refers to the concentration that produces the predetermined response in 50% of the patients, and the shape of the cumulative probability–concentration curve is determined by the distribution of values in the patient population. Figure 2-17 also shows that the concentration needed to produce an effect may vary with the specific application. In this case, the mean C_{50} values for the three surgical procedures were in the order, upper abdominal > lower abdominal > breast. In common with other opioids, the cumulative frequency of the response–concentration curve is very steep in all three groups.

Sometimes, a limit is set on a graded response below which an effect is said not to occur clinically. For example, a potentially toxic effect of antihypertensive therapy is an excessive lowering of blood pressure. The lowering of blood pressure produced by antihypertensive agents is a graded response, but hypotensive toxicity is said to occur only if blood pressure falls to too low a value. Here the clinical endpoint is all-or-none, but the pharmacologic response is graded. Another common example is the division clinically of pain relief (a therapeutic response) or pain itself (an adverse response) into mild, moderate, or full for drugs acting reversibly on pain receptors. Again, the clinical endpoints are quantal, but the pharmacologic response is graded.

Desirable Characteristics. There is a tendency to think that the most important pharmacodynamic characteristic of a drug is its **potency**, expressed by its C_{50} value. The lower the C_{50}, the greater is the potency of the compound. Certainly, it is important as it often leads to the need for only a small dose of drug to produce an effect, but there are several other factors that are also, if not more, important. One is the **specificity** of the drug, that is, a greater production of desired relative to undesired effects. One way of increasing potency is to increase lipophilicity, for example, by adding lipophilic groups onto the molecule that increase binding to the target site. However, this approach also tends to increase its nonspecific binding to many other sites within the body, which may result in either an increase or a decrease in its overall specificity.

Another very important factor is the **maximum effect** of the drug. That is, the greatest possible effect, E_{max}, that can be achieved with the compound. Returning to the example of ketamine, it is apparent that however high we increase the concentration of R(−)-ketamine, we can never achieve the same maximum response as can be achieved with the S(+)-isomer. Clearly, if the desired therapeutic response demands that the effect be greater than can be achieved with R(−)-ketamine, then no matter how potent this compound, it would be of little therapeutic value when given alone. The last important pharmacodynamic factor for a graded response is the steepness factor, γ. If it is very high, it may be difficult to manage the use of the drug as only a small shift in concentration around the C_{50} causes the response to change from zero to full effect, and vice versa. In contrast, if the value of γ is very small, then large changes in drug concentration are needed to cause the response to change significantly, particularly beyond the C_{50} value. Clearly, a value between these two extremes is desirable.

DOSE–TIME–RESPONSE RELATIONSHIPS

So far, relationships between dose and measures of drug exposure and between response and exposure have been explored. In clinical practice, decisions have to be made as to the dosage regimen to employ to ensure optimal benefit within the confines of the conditions in which the patient receives a drug. This is a complex decision involving consideration of many factors including not only the pharmacokinetics and pharmacodynamics of the drug, but also the nature of the disease being treated, as well as a host of patient factors, both clinical and social. Some of these aspects are considered in the remainder of the book. However, at this point some broad issues, centered on exposure–response relationships, are worth considering.

Drugs are given to achieve therapeutic objectives; the practical question is how best to do so? One approach is to examine the pharmacokinetics of a drug. Figure 2-18 contains typical plots of plasma drug concentration with time following oral administration of a single dose. One may then ask: What feature of the exposure profile is most important in the context of the desired therapeutic objective? In Fig. 2-18A are displayed the concentration–time profiles for two drugs achieving the same maximum concentration (C_{max}) and the same time to reach C_{max} (t_{max}) but differing in the kinetics of decline in their concentrations beyond the peak. For some drugs intended to be given chronically, it is only important to maintain the plasma concentration above a defined minimum, below which

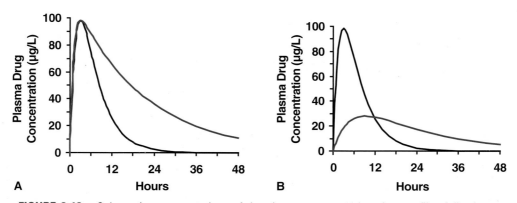

FIGURE 2-18. Schematic representations of the plasma concentration–time profiles following a single oral dose. **A.** For two drugs that produce similar peak concentrations and time to peak, but one (colored line) declines more slowly than the other thereby creating a greater total exposure (*AUC*) and higher concentrations at later times. **B.** For a drug that produces the same total *AUC* when given on two occasions, but on one of these occasions (colored line) the peak concentration is lower and later due to a slowing of absorption.

minimal if any clinical benefit is derived, even though a pharmacologic response may be measurable at still lower concentrations. Then a distinct advantage exists for the drug with the slower decline in exposure, as the duration of clinical effect is clearly longer. For other drugs, however, such as ones taken for the relief of a headache, the critical factor is the rapid achievement of an adequate concentration, after which maintenance of exposure becomes less important. Then C_{max} and t_{max} become the important determinants of efficacy, in which case there may be little difference between the two drugs in Fig. 2-18A. However, there may be benefit in having a rapid fall in plasma concentration if prolonged exposure to the drug leads to an increased risk of adverse effects. Now consider the kinetic events depicted in Fig. 2-18B in which total exposure (AUC) is the same for a drug but input is slower in one case than the other, leading to a slower decline in concentration. A slowed input may be a disadvantage if response is related directly to concentration as C_{max} would be lower and t_{max} would occur later, with the possibility of failing to achieve a sufficiently adequate clinical response. Speed of input would however be of limited importance if the clinical benefit for the drug were determined by the total exposure (total AUC) rather than a particular concentration. These simple scenarios clearly demonstrate that the relative therapeutic importance of different parts of the exposure–time profile of a drug depends on the clinical application and the nature of the exposure–response relationship.

TURNOVER CONCEPTS IN DRUG RESPONSE

Frequently, the response one measures does not directly reflect the actual effect of the drug. This occurs because the measured effect relates to the concentration of an endogenous substance within the body, and the direct effect is to either increase or decrease its rate of formation or elimination. The response is then often delayed, which can be explained by the turnover of the endogenous substance or system. Examples are oral anticoagulants, which lower the plasma concentrations of certain clotting factors by inhibiting their synthesis; antihyperlipidemics, which lower the input of cholesterol and other related substances; uricosuric agents, which lower the plasma concentration of uric acid by increasing its renal clearance; and epoetin alfa, which stimulates red blood cell production. Accordingly, to be able to relate sensibly the pharmacokinetics of a drug to its pharmacologic effect when an endogenous compound or system is involved or to interpret the concentration of an endogenous compound or state of the system to assess body function, the kinetics of the endogenous compound or system must be understood.

The concentrations of many body constituents remain fairly constant with time. They are said to be at steady state. This does not mean, however, that they are in a static state. Indeed, they are often being replaced, or synthesized and eliminated, at a rapid rate; they are said to be "turning over." The concept of **turnover** can be applied to plasma proteins, enzymes, hormones, electrolytes, water, and in fact, to virtually every endogenously formed substance and system within the body.

Turnover implies that an endogenous substance or system is at steady state. Thus, the rate of renewal equals the rate of elimination. This rate, the **turnover rate**, does not fully convey the speed of the process. To do that, the turnover rate must be related to the amount of substance or constituent present, frequently called the **pool size**. The ratio of the turnover rate, R_t, to the pool size, A_{ss}, is called the **fractional turnover rate**, k_t, that is,

$$k_t = \frac{R_t}{A_{ss}} \qquad \text{2-5}$$

A second useful parameter for measuring turnover is **turnover time**, t_t. It is the time required to input the amount in the pool. This is not the time to fully renew the substance, as complete renewal actually requires an infinite period of time, because newly entering substance continuously mixes with that already in the pool. Turnover time can be readily defined, however, by the time required to bring into the pool the amount that is in it, therefore,

$$t_t = \frac{A_{ss}}{R_t}$$ 2-6

Consequently, the relationship between turnover time and fractional turnover rate is

$$t_t = \frac{1}{k_t}$$ 2-7

The input may be either synthetic or involve a transfer of substance into the pool from elsewhere, or both. A good example is total body water, which is both imbibed and synthesized by catabolism of foodstuffs. Figure 2-19 schematically shows the turnover of water in the body. From the values given in the figure and Eqs. 5 to 7, the following average turnover values for water are obtained:

Turnover rate = 2.5 L (or kg)/day
Fractional turnover rate = 0.06 day^{-1} (or 6%/day)
Turnover time = 17 days

Although the turnover rate (2.5 kg/day) is a large value, the actual turnover of body water is quite slow as reflected by the fractional turnover rate (6%/day) or turnover time (17 days). Clearly, both of these parameters characterize turnover better than turnover rate alone.

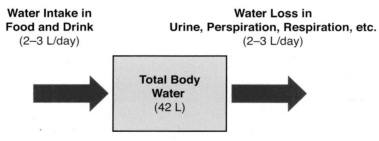

FIGURE 2-19. The turnover of total body water.

The input or output may involve several pathways. For body water, urinary and fecal excretion, perspiration, and respiration are the major routes of loss. In a hot, dry desert climate, the last two pathways, especially perspiration, may increase dramatically. Intake must then be increased to compensate for increased loss. The pool size remains essentially constant, although turnover rate may be increased to 21 L/day under these extreme conditions. In this situation, fractional turnover rate and turnover time of water become 0.5 day^{-1} and 2 days, respectively. The pool size of many body constituents, including water, is kept constant by feedback control mechanisms that maintain homeostasis.

In contrast to water, the pool size, rather than fractional turnover rate or turnover time, of many other constituents in the body change when the renewal rate is altered. This results in a change in the concentration or amount of the substance in the system. One example is that of cholesterol, which is both synthesized within the body and input from food. Some antihyperlipidemic drugs are given to decrease cholesterol input from food, such as ezetimibe (Zetia); others, such as simvastatin (Zocor), are given to decrease the synthesis of the substance. The combination of the two kinds of agents is used as well (Vytorin, ezetimibe + simvastatin). Another example is that of filgrastim (Neupogen), a granulocyte-colony stimulating factor, which increases the white blood cell count by increasing the production of white blood cells. In both examples, there is an altered turnover rate and pool size.

Armed with the fundamental concepts and terminology of pharmacokinetics and pharmacodynamics, we now focus our attention on the next section, *Exposure and Response after a Single Dose,* for a more in-depth consideration of these concepts when a single i.v. or extravascular dose is administered. This is followed by Section III, *Therapeutic Regimens,* in which the concepts are extended to the more common situations of continuous or repetitive administration of drugs.

KEY RELATIONSHIPS

$$Dose = \frac{Amount\ at}{Absorption\ Site} + \frac{Amount}{in\ Body} + \frac{Amount}{Excreted} + \frac{Amount}{Metabolized}$$

$$\frac{Rate\ of\ Change}{of\ Drug\ in\ Body} = \frac{Rate\ of}{Absorption} - \left[\frac{Rate\ of}{Excretion} + \frac{Rate\ of}{Metabolism} \right]$$

$$\frac{Measured}{Response} = \frac{Drug}{Response} + \frac{Placebo}{Response} + Baseline$$

$$E = \frac{E_{max} \cdot C^{\gamma}}{C_{50}{}^{\gamma} + C^{\gamma}}$$

$$k_t = \frac{R_t}{A_{ss}}$$

$$t_t = \frac{1}{k_t}$$

STUDY PROBLEMS

(Answers to Study Problems are in Appendix J.)

1. Define the terms listed in the first objective at the beginning of this chapter.

2. Would you expect the concentration of a drug in **whole blood** or **plasma** to be greater, or are they about the same in each of the following situations? *Circle your answer.* Except in situation d., the unbound drug concentration is the same in plasma water and cellular fluids.

   a. There is extensive binding to plasma proteins, but not within or to blood cells.

   WHOLE BLOOD   SAME   PLASMA

   b. There is extensive binding to blood cell components, but no binding to plasma proteins.

   WHOLE BLOOD   SAME   PLASMA

   c. There is no binding to plasma proteins or blood cell components.

   WHOLE BLOOD   SAME   PLASMA

   d. There is no binding to plasma proteins or blood cells, and the drug is unable to cross the membranes of blood cells.

   WHOLE BLOOD   SAME   PLASMA

3. a. Briefly state why an analytical method that does not distinguish between R- and S-isomers can lead to problems in the interpretation of plasma data following administration of a racemic mixture.

b. Do you think that first-pass metabolism can explain the observed differences (Fig. 2-2B) in the concentration–time profiles of the methylphenidate optical isomers?

4. Identify which one or more of the following statements below is/are correct after a single oral dose. For any incorrect ones, state the reason why or supply a qualification.

a. A 100% recovery of unchanged drug in urine indicates that the drug is completely absorbed systemically and not metabolized.

b. The maximum amount of drug in the body occurs when the rate of absorption and rate of elimination are equal.

c. The rate of change of amount of drug in the body equals the rate of elimination at all times after drug absorption is complete.

d. A drug is labeled with a radioactive atom. Complete recovery of all the dose of radioactivity in urine implies that the drug is completely absorbed systemically.

e. A drug is completely recovered (100%) as a glucuronide in the feces. Fecal excretion is therefore the route of elimination of this drug.

f. The rate of change of drug in the body approaches the rate of absorption at the peak time.

5. State why enterohepatic cycling contributes to the elimination of a drug from the body only when it is incomplete.

6. Comment on the accuracy of the following statements:

a. For a graded response, the C_{50} is the steady-state plasma drug concentration that produces 50% of the maximum response.

b. For responses less than 20% of the maximum, the response is directly proportional to drug concentration only when γ of the Hill equation equals one.

c. Hysteresis in a response versus plasma drug concentration curve cannot be observed after i.v. administration of a bolus dose of drug.

d. Measuring a placebo effect is necessary under all conditions.

7. The data in Fig. 2-20 were obtained in a human subject with AF-DX116, an experimental cardioselective muscarinic agent at the time of the publication of the article. In parallel with measurement of heart rate, blood samples were drawn and centrifuged for measurement of the plasma concentration of the drug.

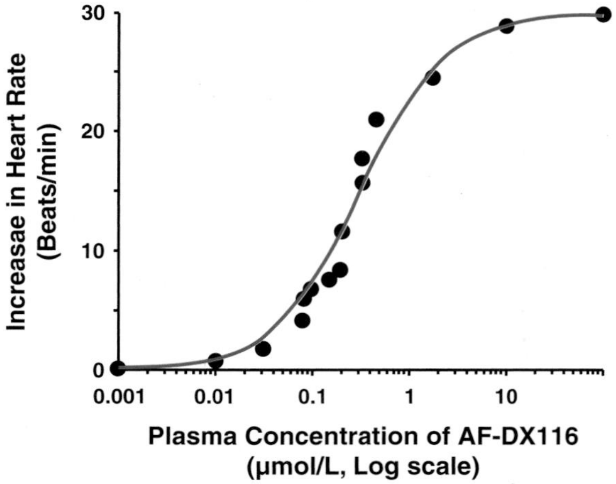

FIGURE 2-20. Pharmacodynamic data for an experimental drug. (From: Schute B, Valz-Zang C, Mutschler E, et al. AF-DX116, a cardioselective muscarinic antagonist in humans: pharmacodynamic and pharmacokinetic properties. Clin Pharmacol Ther 1991;50:372–378.)

a. Is this a graded or a quantal response?

b. The data in the figure show the increase in heart rate as a function of the logarithm of the plasma drug concentration. Estimate the approximate values for E_{max}, C_{50}, and γ of the Hill equation (Eq. 2-4) for the line shown.

8. The concentration–response relationship for a drug that produces a graded response is characterized by a C_{50} of 10 mg/L and a γ value of 2.5. To be effective, the response to the drug must be kept between 20% and 80% of the maximal value. Calculate the range of concentrations that are needed to achieve this objective. Equilibrium of drug at the site of action with drug in plasma is essentially instantaneous.

9. Figure 2-21 is a plot of the cumulative incidence of hepatic toxicity (taken to be greater than a threefold increase in serum alanine aminotransferase [ALT], a measure of inflammation of the liver) and the total AUC of a drug in the patient population. Corresponding plots against the maximum plasma concentration, or concentration at any particular time after administration of the drug, failed to show as significant a relationship as seen with AUC.

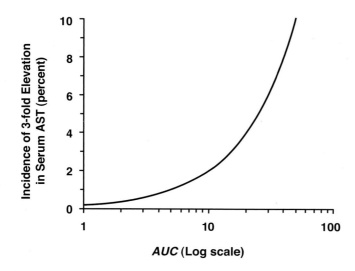

FIGURE 2-21. Incidence of hepatic toxicity (expressed as percent of the patient population) against the AUC of a drug.

a. Is the measured effect graded or quantal? Explain how you come to your conclusion.

b. Why might hepatic toxicity be better correlated with AUC than any particular concentration of the drug?

10. Given that the total amount of albumin in the body is 350 g and that its turnover time is 16 days, calculate:

a. The amount of albumin formed per day.

b. The fractional turnover rate of albumin.

Exposure and Response after a Single Dose

3

Kinetics Following an Intravenous Bolus Dose

OBJECTIVES

The reader will be able to:

- Define the meaning of the following terms: clearance, compartmental model, disposition kinetics, distribution phase, elimination half-life, elimination phase, elimination rate constant, extraction ratio, extravasation, first-order process, fraction excreted unchanged, fraction in plasma unbound, fractional rate of elimination, glomerular filtration rate, half-life, hepatic clearance, loglinear decline, mean residence time, monoexponential equation, renal clearance, terminal phase, tissue distribution half-life, volume of distribution.

- Estimate from plasma and urine data following an intravenous (i.v.) dose of a drug:
  - Total clearance, half-life, elimination rate constant, and volume of distribution.
  - Fraction excreted unchanged and renal clearance.

- Calculate the concentration of drug in the plasma and the amount of drug in the body with time following an i.v. dose, given values for the pertinent pharmacokinetic parameters.

- Ascertain the relative contribution of the renal and hepatic routes to total elimination from their respective clearance values.

- Describe the impact of distribution kinetics on the interpretation of plasma concentration–time data following i.v. bolus administration.

- Determine the mean residence time of a drug when plasma concentration–time data after a single bolus dose are provided.

- Explain the statement, "Half-life and elimination rate constant depend upon clearance and volume of distribution, and not vice versa."

A dministering a drug intravascularly ensures that the entire dose enters the systemic circulation. By rapid injection, elevated concentrations of drug can be promptly achieved; by continuous infusion at a controlled rate, a constant concentration, and often response, can be maintained. With no other route of administration can plasma concentration be as promptly and efficiently controlled. Of the two intravascular routes, the i.v one is the most frequently employed. Intra-arterial administration, which has greater inherent manipulative dangers, is reserved for situations in which drug localization in a specific organ or tissue is desired. It is achieved by inputting drug into the artery directly supplying the target tissue.

The disposition characteristics of a drug are defined by analyzing the temporal changes of drug in plasma and urine following i.v. administration. How this information is obtained following rapid injection of a drug, as well as how the underlying processes control the profile, form the basis of this chapter, Chapter 4, *Membranes and Distribution,* and Chapter 5, *Elimination.* These are followed by chapters dealing with the kinetic events following an extravascular dose and the physiologic processes governing drug absorption. The final chapter in this section of the book deals with the time course of drug response after administering a single dose. The concepts laid down in this section provide a foundation for making rational decisions in therapeutics, the subject of subsequent sections.

APPRECIATION OF KINETIC CONCEPTS

Toward the end of Chapter 2, we considered the impact that various shapes of the exposure-time profile following an oral dose may have on the clinical utility of a drug. Figures 3-1 and 3-2 provide a similar set of exposure–time profiles except that the drugs are now given as an i.v. bolus. Notice that following the same dose, the two drugs displayed in Fig. 3-1 have the same initial concentration but different slopes of decline, whereas those displayed in Fig. 3-2 have different initial concentrations but similar slopes of decline. The reasons for these differences are now explored.

Several methods are employed for graphically displaying plasma concentration–time data. One common method that has been mostly employed in the preceding chapters and shown on the left-hand side of Figs. 3-1 and 3-2 is to plot concentration against time on regular (Cartesian) graph paper. Depicted in this way, the plasma concentration is seen to fall in a curvilinear manner. Another method of display is a plot of the same data on semilogarithmic paper (right-hand graphs in Figs. 3-1 and 3-2). The time scale is the same as before, but now, the ordinate (concentration) scale is logarithmic. Notice now that all the profiles decline linearly and, being straight lines, make it easier in many ways to predict the concentration at any time. But why do we get a linear decline when plotting the data on a semilogarithmic scale (commonly referred to as a **loglinear decline**), and what determines the large differences seen in the profiles for the various drugs?

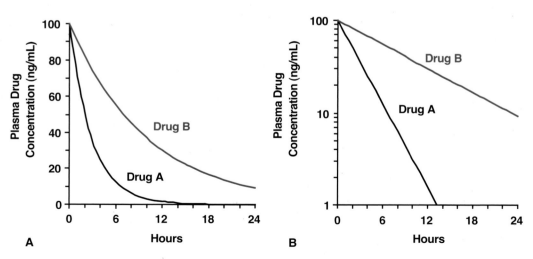

FIGURE 3-1. Drugs A (*black line*) and B (*colored line*) show the same initial (peak) exposure but have different half-lives and total exposure–time profiles (*AUC*). **A.** Regular (Cartesian) plot. **B.** Semilogarithmic plot. Doses of both drugs are the same.

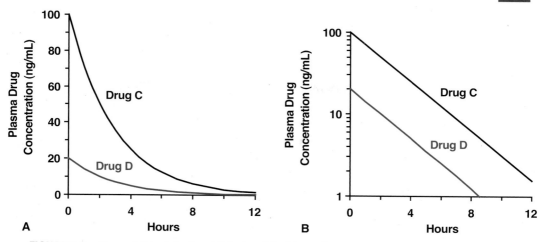

FIGURE 3-2. Drugs C (black line) and D (colored line) have the same half-life but have different initial concentrations and total exposure–time profiles. **A.** Regular (Cartesian) plot. **B.** Semilogarithmic plot. Doses of both drugs are the same.

VOLUME OF DISTRIBUTION AND CLEARANCE

To start answering these questions, consider the simple scheme depicted in Fig. 3-3. Here, drug is placed into a well-stirred reservoir, representing the body, whose contents are recycled by a pump through an extractor, which can be thought of as the liver or kidneys, that removes drug. The drug concentrations in the reservoir, *C*, and that coming out of the extractor, C_{out}, can be measured. The initial concentration in the reservoir, *C(0)*, depends on the amount introduced, *Dose*, and the volume of the container, *V*. Therefore,

$$C(0) = \frac{Dose}{V} \qquad\qquad 3\text{-}1$$

Fluid passes through the extractor at a flow rate, *Q*. With the concentration of drug entering the extractor being the same as that in the reservoir, *C*, it follows that the rate of presentation to the extractor is then $Q \cdot C$. Of the drug entering the extractor, a fraction, *E*, is extracted (by elimination processes) never to return to the reservoir. The correspon-

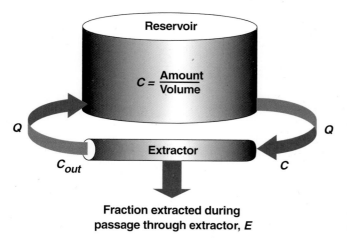

$$C = \frac{Amount}{Volume}$$

Reservoir

Extractor

C_{out} *C*

Q   *Q*

Fraction extracted during passage through extractor, *E*

FIGURE 3-3. Schematic diagram of a perfused organ system. Drug is placed into a well-stirred reservoir, volume V, from which fluid perfuses an extractor at flow rate *Q*. The rate of extraction can be expressed as a fraction *E* of the rate of presentation, $Q \cdot C$. The rate that escaping drug returns to the reservoir is $Q \cdot C_{out}$. For modeling purposes, the amount of drug in the extractor is negligible compared to the amount of drug contained in the reservoir.

ding rate of drug leaving the extractor and returning to the reservoir is therefore $Q \cdot C_{out}$. The rate of elimination (or rate of extraction) is then:

$$Rate\ of\ elimination = Q \cdot C \cdot E = Q(C - C_{out}) \qquad 3\text{-}2$$

from which it follows that the **extraction ratio**, **E**, of the drug by the extractor is given by

$$E = \frac{Rate\ of\ elimination}{Rate\ of\ presentation} = \frac{Q \cdot (C - C_{out})}{Q \cdot C} = \frac{(C - C_{out})}{C} \qquad 3\text{-}3$$

Thus, we see that the extraction ratio can be determined experimentally by measuring the concentrations entering and leaving the extractor and by normalizing the difference by the entering concentration.

Conceptually, it is useful to relate the rate of elimination to the measured concentration entering the extractor, which is the same as that in the reservoir. This parameter is called **clearance**, **CL.** Therefore,

$$Rate\ of\ elimination = CL \cdot C \qquad 3\text{-}4$$

Note that the units of clearance are those of flow (e.g., mL/min or L/hr). This follows because rate of elimination is expressed in units of mass per unit time, such as μg/min or mg/hr, and concentration is expressed in units of mass per unit volume, such as μg/L or mg/L. An important relationship is also obtained by comparing the equalities in Eqs. 3-2 and 3-4, yielding

$$CL = Q \cdot E \qquad 3\text{-}5$$

This equation provides a physical interpretation of clearance. Namely, clearance is the volume of the fluid presented to the eliminating organ (extractor) that is effectively, completely cleared of drug per unit time. For example, if $Q = 1$ L/min and $E = 0.5$, then effectively 0.5 L of the fluid entering the extractor from the reservoir is completely cleared of drug each minute. Also, it is seen that even for a perfect extractor ($E = 1$) the clearance of drug is limited in its upper value to Q, the flow rate to the extractor. Under these circumstances, we say that the clearance of the drug is sensitive to flow rate, the limiting factor in delivering drug to the extractor.

Two very useful parameters in pharmacokinetics have now been introduced, **volume of distribution** (volume of the reservoir in this example) and **clearance** (the parameter relating rate of elimination to the concentration in the systemic circulation [reservoir]). The first parameter predicts the concentration for a given amount in the body (reservoir). The second provides an estimate of the rate of elimination at any concentration.

FIRST-ORDER ELIMINATION

The remaining question is: How quickly does drug decline from the reservoir? This is answered by considering the rate of elimination ($CL \cdot C$) relative to the amount present in the reservoir (A), a ratio commonly referred to as the **fractional rate of elimination**, **k**

$$k = \frac{Rate\ of\ elimination}{Amount\ in\ the\ reservoir} = \frac{CL \cdot C}{A} = \frac{CL \cdot C}{V \cdot C} \qquad 3\text{-}6$$

or

$$k = \frac{CL}{V} \qquad 3\text{-}7$$

This important relationship shows that k depends on clearance and the volume of the reservoir, two independent parameters. Note also that the units of k are reciprocal time. For example, if the clearance of the drug is 1 L/hr and the volume of the reservoir is 10 L, then $k = 0.1\ hr^{-1}$ or, expressed as a percentage, 10% per hour. That is, 10% of that in the reservoir is eliminated each hour. When expressing k, it is helpful to choose time units so that the value of k is much less than 1. For example, if instead of hours, we had

TABLE 3-1	Amount Remaining in the Reservoir over a 5-Hr Period after Introduction of a 100-mg Dose of a Drug with an Elimination Rate Constant of 0.1 hr^{-1}

Time Interval (h)	Amount Lost during Interval (mg)	Amount Remaining in Reservoir at the End of the Interval (mg)^a
0	—	100
0–1	10	90.0
1–2	9	81.0
2–3	8.1	72.9
3–4	7.3	65.6
4–5	6.56	59.04

^{a}If the time unit of k had been made smaller than hours the amount lost, and hence remaining in the reservoir, with time would be slightly different because in this calculation the assumption is made that the loss occurs at the initial rate throughout the interval, when in reality it falls exponentially. In the limiting case, the fraction remaining at time t is $e^{-k \cdot t}$ (Eq. 3-17), which in the above example is 60.63% at 5 hr.

chosen days as the unit of time, then the value of clearance would be 24 L/day, and therefore $k = 2.4$ day^{-1}, implying that the fractional rate of elimination is 240% per day, a number which is clearly misleading.

To further appreciate the meaning of k, consider the data in Table 3-1, which shows the loss of drug in the reservoir with time, when $k = 0.1$ hr^{-1}. Starting with 100 mg, in 1 hr, 10% has been eliminated, so that 90 mg remains. In the next hour, 10% of 90 mg, or 9 mg, is eliminated, leaving 81 mg remaining at 2 hrs, and so on. Although this method illustrates the application of k in determining the time course of drug elimination, and hence drug remaining in the body, it is rather laborious and has some error associated with it. A simpler and more accurate way of calculating these values at any time is used (see "Fraction of Dose Remaining" later in this chapter).

Considering further the rate of elimination, there are two ways of determining it experimentally. One method mentioned previously is to measure the rates entering and leaving the organ. The other method is to determine the rate of loss of drug from the reservoir, since the only reason for the loss from the system is elimination in the extractor. Hence, by reference to Eq. 3-6

$$\textit{Rate of elimination} = -\frac{dA}{dt} = k \cdot A \qquad 3\text{-}8$$

where $-dA$ is the small amount of drug lost (hence the negative sign) from the reservoir during a small interval of time dt. Processes, such as those represented by Eq. 3-8, in which the rate of the process is directly proportional to the amount present, are known as **first-order processes**, in that the rate varies in direct proportion with the amount there raised to the power of one ($A^1 = A$). For this reason, the parameter k is frequently called the **first-order elimination rate constant**. Then, substituting $A = V \cdot C$ on both sides of Eq. 3-8, and dividing by V gives

$$-\frac{dC}{dt} = k \cdot C \qquad 3\text{-}9$$

which, on integration, yields

$$C = C(0) \cdot e^{-k \cdot t} \qquad 3\text{-}10$$

where e is the natural base with a value of 2.71828 . . . Equation 3-10 is known as a **monoexponential equation**, in that it involves a single exponential term. Examination of this equation shows that it has the right properties. At time zero, $e^{-k \cdot t} = e^{-0} = 1$, so that $C = C(0)$ and, as time approaches infinity, $e^{-k \cdot t}$ approaches zero and so therefore does concentration. Equation 10 describes the curvilinear plots in Figs. 3-1 and 3-2. To see why such curves become linear when concentration is plotted on a logarithmic scale, take the logarithms of both sides of Eq. 3-10.

$$ln\ C = ln\ C(0) - k \cdot t \tag{3-11}$$

where ln is the natural logarithm. Thus, we see from Eq. 3-11 that $ln\ C$ is a linear function of time with a slope of $-k$, as indeed observed in Figs. 3-1 and 3-2. Moreover, the slope of the line determines how fast the concentration declines, which in turn is governed by V and CL, independent parameters. The larger the elimination rate constant k the more rapid is drug elimination.

HALF-LIFE

Commonly, the kinetics of drugs is characterized by a **half-life** ($t_{1/2}$), the time for the concentration (and amount in the reservoir) to fall by one half, rather than by an elimination rate constant. These two parameters are of course interrelated. This is seen from Eq. 3-10. In one half-life, $C = 0.5 \times C(0)$, therefore

$$0.5 \times C(0) = C(0) \cdot e^{-k \cdot t_{1/2}} \tag{3-12}$$

or

$$e^{-k \cdot t_{1/2}} = 0.5 \tag{3-13}$$

which, on inverting and taking logarithms on both sides, gives

$$t_{1/2} = \frac{ln\ 2}{k} \tag{3-14}$$

Further, given that $ln\ 2 = 0.693$,

$$t_{1/2} = \frac{0.693}{k} \tag{3-15}$$

or, on substituting k by CL/V, leads to another important relationship, namely,

$$t_{1/2} = \frac{0.693 \cdot V}{CL} \tag{3-16}$$

From Eq. 3-16, it should be evident that half-life is controlled by V and CL, and not vice versa.

To appreciate the application of Eq. 3-16, consider creatinine, a product of muscle catabolism and used as a measure of renal function. For a typical 70-kg, 60-year-old patient, creatinine has a clearance of 4.5 L/hr (75 mL/min) and is evenly distributed throughout the 42 L of total body water. As expected by calculation using Eq. 3-16, its half-life is 6.5 hr. Inulin, a polysaccharide also used to assess renal function, has the same clearance as creatinine in such a patient, but a half-life of only 2.5 hr. This is a consequence of inulin being restricted to the 16 L of extracellular body water (i.e., its "reservoir" size is smaller than that of creatinine).

FRACTION OF DOSE REMAINING

Another view of the kinetics of drug elimination may be gained by examining how the fraction of the dose remaining in the reservoir ($A/Dose$) varies with time. By reference to Eq. 3-10 and multiplying both sides by V

$$\frac{Fraction\ of\ dose}{remaining} = \frac{A}{Dose} = e^{-k \cdot t} \tag{3-17}$$

Sometimes, it is useful to express time relative to half-life. The benefit in doing so is seen by letting n be the number of half-lives elapsed after a bolus dose ($n = t/t_{1/2}$). Then, as $k = 0.693/t_{1/2}$, one obtains

$$\frac{Fraction\ of\ dose}{remaining} = e^{-0.693n} \tag{3-18}$$

Since $e^{-0.693} = 1/2$, it follows that

$$Fraction\ of\ dose\atop remaining = \left(\frac{1}{2}\right)^n \qquad\qquad 3\text{-}19$$

Thus, one half or 50% of the dose remains after 1 half-life, and one fourth ($\frac{1}{2} \times \frac{1}{2}$) or 25% remains after 2 half-lives, and so on. Satisfy yourself that by 4 half-lives, only 6.25% of the dose remains to be eliminated. You might also prove to yourself that 10% remains at 3.32 half-lives.

If one uses 99% lost (1% remaining) as a point when the drug is considered to have been for all practical purposes eliminated, then 6.64 half-lives is the time. For a drug with a 9-min half-life, this is close to 60 min, whereas for a drug with a 9-day half-life, the corresponding time is 2 months.

CLEARANCE, AREA, AND VOLUME OF DISTRIBUTION

We are now in a position to fully explain the different curves seen in Figs. 3-1 and 3-2, which were simulated applying the simple scheme in Fig. 3-3. Drugs A and B in Fig. 3-1A have the same initial (peak) concentration following administration of the same dose. Therefore, they must have the same volume of distribution, V, which follows from Eq. 3-1. However, Drug A has a shorter half-life, and hence a larger value of k, from which we conclude that, since $k = CL/V$, it must have a higher clearance. The lower total exposure (area under the curve [AUC]) seen with Drug A follows from its higher clearance. This is seen from Eq. 3-4, repeated here,

$$Rate\ of\ elimination = CL \cdot C$$

By rearranging this equation, it can be seen that during a small interval of time dt

$$Amount\ eliminated\ in\ interval\ dt = CL \cdot C \cdot dt \qquad\qquad 3\text{-}20$$

where the product $C \cdot dt$ is the corresponding small area under the concentration–time curve within the time interval dt. For example, if the clearance of a drug is 0.1 L/min and the AUC between 60 and 61 min is 0.1 mg-min/L, then the amount of drug eliminated in that minute is 0.01 mg. The total amount of drug eventually eliminated, which for an i.v. bolus equals the dose administered, is assessed by adding up or integrating the amounts eliminated in each time interval, from time zero to time infinity, and therefore,

$$Dose = CL \cdot AUC \qquad\qquad 3\text{-}21$$

or, rearranging,

$$CL = \frac{Dose}{AUC} \qquad\qquad 3\text{-}22$$

where AUC is the total exposure. Thus, returning to the drugs depicted in Fig. 3-1, since the clearance of Drug A is higher, its AUC must be lower than that of Drug B for a given dose. Several additional points are worth noting. First, because clearance, calculated using Eq. 3-22, relates to total elimination of all drug from the body, irrespective of how eliminated, it is sometimes called **total clearance**. Second, in practice, once AUC is known, clearance is readily calculated. Indeed, if this is the only parameter of interest, there is no need to know either the half-life or volume of distribution to calculate clearance. Third, Eq. 3-22 is independent of the shape of the concentration–time profile. The critical factor is to obtain a good estimate of AUC (see Appendix A, *Assessment of AUC*). Lastly, it follows from Eqs. 3-7 and 3-22 that volume of distribution is given by

$$V = \frac{CL}{k} = \frac{Dose}{AUC \cdot k} \qquad\qquad 3\text{-}23$$

That is, once clearance and k (or half-life) are known, V can be calculated.

Now consider the two drugs, C and D, in Fig. 3-2 in which, once again, the same dose of drug was administered. From the regular plot, it is apparent that as the initial concentration of Drug C is higher, it has a smaller V. And, as the total exposure (AUC) of Drug C is the greater, it has the lower clearance. However, from the semilogarithmic plot, it is apparent that, as the slopes of the two lines are parallel, they must have the same value of the elimination rate constant, k (Eq. 3-11), and hence the same value of half-life (Eq. 3-15). These equalities can only arise because the ratio CL/V is the same for both drugs. The lesson is clear. The important determinants of the kinetics of a drug following an i.v. bolus dose are clearance and volume of distribution. These parameters determine the resultant kinetic process, reflected by the secondary parameters, k and $t_{1/2}$.

MEAN RESIDENCE TIME

Another view of the events occurring following drug administration is to consider how long molecules stay in the body, their **residence times**, before being eliminated. Molecules eliminated soon after administration have short residence times, whereas those eliminated later have longer ones. The average time molecules stay in body is known as the **mean residence time**, MRT. The MRT can be calculated in the following manner.

A measure of the number of molecules in the body is the amount there; the number and the amount are directly related to each other by Avogadro number, which for all compounds is the same, 6.022×10^{23} molecules per mole of compound. On giving a bolus dose, initially all the molecules are in the body, the dose; thereafter the number of molecules, and hence the amount, falls. The MRT is therefore obtained by simply summing, or integrating, the number of residing molecules over all times and dividing by the total number of molecules, the dose. Thus,

$$MRT = \frac{\int_0^\infty A \cdot dt}{Dose} \qquad 3\text{-}24$$

So, returning to the reservoir model, the amount in the body with time is $Dose \cdot e^{-k \cdot t}$ (Eq. 3-17), which on substitution into Eq. 3-24 and integration yields

$$MRT = \frac{1}{k} \qquad 3\text{-}25$$

Thus, we see that MRT is simply the reciprocal of the elimination rate constant. For example, when $k = 0.1\ hr^{-1}$, $MRT = 10$ hr. That is, when the fractional elimination rate of a compound is 0.1 per hour, on average drug molecules stay in the body for 10 hr. MRT is further explored in Chapter 19, *Distribution Kinetics*.

A CASE STUDY

In reality, the body is more complex than depicted in the simple reservoir model. The body comprises many different types of tissues and organs. The eliminating organs, such as the liver and kidneys, are much more complex than a simple extractor. To gain a better appreciation regarding how drugs are handled by the body, consider the data in Fig. 3-4 showing the decline in the mean plasma concentration of midazolam displayed in both regular and semilogarithmic plots, following an 8.35-mg i.v. bolus dose of midazolam hydrochloride (equivalent to 7.5-mg midazolam base) of this hypnotic sedative and anxiolytic drug in a group of subjects with an average weight of 79 kg. We would obviously have preferred to consider each individual separately, but as is commonly the case, mean data are usually provided in published literature. However, for our purpose, let us assume that the data are those of an individual.

As expected, the decline in concentration displayed on the regular plot (Fig. 3-4A) is curvilinear. However, contrary to the expectation of the simple reservoir model, the decline in the semilogarithmic plot (Fig. 3-4B) is clearly biphasic, rather than monoexponential, with the concentration falling very rapidly for about 1 hr. Thereafter, the decline is slower and linear. The early phase is commonly called the **distribution phase** and the latter, the **terminal** or **elimination phase**.

A

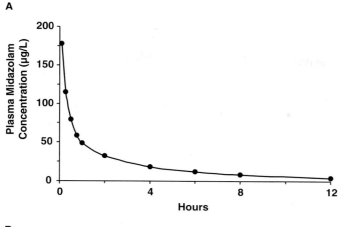

B

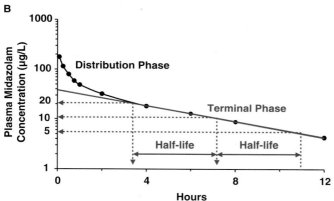

FIGURE 3-4. **A.** Plasma concentration of midazolam with time in an individual after an 8.35-mg i.v. bolus dose of midazolam hydrochloride (7.5 mg of the base) in a healthy adult. **B.** The data in A are redisplayed as a semilogarithmic plot. Note the short distribution phase. (From: Pentikäinen PJ, Välisalmi L, Himberg JJ, Crevoisier C. Pharmacokinetics of midazolam following i.v. and oral administration in patients with chronic liver disease and in healthy subjects. J Clin Pharmacol 1989;29:272–277.)

DISTRIBUTION PHASE

The distribution phase is called such because distribution into tissues primarily determines the early rapid decline in plasma concentration. For midazolam, distribution is rapid and occurs significantly even by the time of the first measurement in Fig. 3-4, 5 min. This must be so because the amount of midazolam in plasma at this time is only 0.61 mg. This value is calculated by multiplying the highest plasma concentration, 180 μg/L (0.18 mg/L), by the physical volume of plasma expected in an average 79-kg adult, 3.4 L (the standard value is 0.043 L/kg). The majority, 6.9 mg or 92% of the total 7.5-mg dose of midazolam base, must have already left the plasma and been distributed into other tissues, which together with plasma comprise the **initial dilution space**. Among these tissues are the liver and the kidneys, which also eliminate drug from the body. However, although some drug is eliminated during the early moments, the fraction of the administered dose eliminated during the distribution phase is less than 50% for midazolam and much less so for many other drugs. This statement is based on exposure considerations and is discussed more fully later in this chapter. Nonetheless, because both distribution and elimination are occurring simultaneously, it is appropriate to apply the term **disposition kinetics** when characterizing the entire plasma concentration–time profile following an i.v. bolus dose.

TERMINAL PHASE

During the distribution phase, changes in the concentration of drug in plasma reflect primarily movement of drug within, rather than loss from, the body. However, with time, distribution equilibrium of drug in tissue with that in plasma is established in more and more tissues, and eventually changes in plasma concentration reflect a proportional change in the concentrations of drug in all other tissues and, hence, in the amount of drug in the body. During this proportionality phase, the body acts kinetically as a single container or compartment, much like in the reservoir model. Because decline of the plasma concentration is now associated solely with elimination of drug from the body, this phase is often called the **elimination phase**, and parameters associated with it, such as k and $t_{1/2}$, are often called the **elimination rate constant** and **elimination half-life**.

Elimination Half-Life The elimination half-life is the time over which the plasma concentration, as well as the amount of the drug in the body, falls by one half. The half-life of midazolam determined by the time to fall, for example, from 20 to 10 µg/L, is 3.8 hr (Fig. 3-4B). This is the same time that it takes for the concentration to fall from 10 to 5 µg/L, or by half anywhere along the terminal decline. In other words, the elimination half-life of midazolam is independent of the amount of drug in the body. It follows, therefore, that less drug is eliminated in each succeeding half-life. Initially, there are 7.5 mg of midazolam in the body. After 1 half-life (3.8 hr), assuming that distribution equilibrium was virtually spontaneous throughout this period, 3.75 mg remains in the body. After 2 half-lives (7.6 hr), 1.88 mg remains, and after 3 half-lives (11.4 hr), 0.94 mg remains. In practice, the drug may be regarded as having been eliminated (99%) by 6.64 half-lives (25 hr, or approximately 1 day).

Once the half-life is known, the elimination rate constant, k, and the mean residence time in the body, *MRT*, can be readily calculated from Eqs. 3-15 and 3-25. These are 0.182 hr^{-1} and 5.5 hr, respectively. Midazolam clearly is removed relatively quickly from the body.

Clearance This parameter is obtained by calculating total exposure, since $CL = Dose/AUC$. For midazolam total AUC is 287 µg-hr/L (0.287 mg-hr/L), and so $CL = 7.5$ mg/0.287 mg-hr/L, or 26 L/hr, or 43 mL/min. That is, 26 L of plasma are effectively cleared completely of drug each hour.

Volume of Distribution The concentration in plasma achieved after distribution is complete is a function of dose, the extent of distribution of drug into tissues, and the amount eliminated while distributing. This extent of distribution can be determined by relating the concentration obtained with a known amount of drug in the body. This is analogous to the determination of the volume of the reservoir in Fig. 3-3 by dividing the amount of compound added to it by the resultant concentration, after thorough mixing. The volume measured is, in effect, a dilution space but, unlike the reservoir, this volume is not a physical space but rather an apparent one.

The apparent volume into which a drug distributes in the body at equilibrium is called the **(apparent) volume of distribution**. Plasma, rather than blood, is usually measured. Consequently, the volume of distribution, V, is the volume of plasma at the drug concentration, C, required to account for the entire amount of drug in the body, A.

$$V = \frac{A}{C}$$

$$\text{Volume of distribution} \quad \frac{\text{Amount of drug in body}}{\text{Plasma drug concentration}}$$

3-26

Volume of distribution is useful in estimating the dose required to achieve a given plasma concentration or, conversely, in estimating amount of drug in the body when the plasma concentration is known.

Calculation of volume of distribution requires that distribution equilibrium be achieved between drug in tissues and that in plasma. The amount of drug in the body is known immediately after an i.v. bolus; it is the dose administered. However, distribution equilibrium has not yet been achieved, so, unlike the reservoir model, we cannot use, with any confidence, the concentration obtained by extrapolating to zero time to obtain an estimate of *V.* To overcome this problem, use is made of a previously derived important relationship $k = CL/V$, which on rearrangement gives

$$V = \frac{CL}{k} \qquad \qquad 3\text{-}27$$

or, since $k = 0.693/t_{1/2}$ and the reciprocal of 0.693 is 1.44,

$$V = 1.44 \cdot CL \cdot t_{1/2} \qquad \qquad 3\text{-}28$$

So, although half-life is known, we need an estimate of clearance to estimate *V.* Substituting $CL = 26$ L/hr and $t_{1/2} = 3.8$ hr into Eq. 3-28 gives a value for the volume of distribution of midazolam of 142 L.

Volume of distribution is a direct measure of the extent of distribution. It rarely, however, corresponds to a real volume, such as for a 70-kg adult, plasma volume (3 L), extracellular water (16 L), or total body water (42 L). Drugs distribute to various tissues and fluids of the body. Furthermore, binding to tissue components may be so great that the volume of distribution is many times the total body size.

To appreciate the effect of tissue binding, consider the distribution of 100 mg of a drug in a 1-L system composed of water and 10 g of activated charcoal, onto which 99% of the drug is adsorbed. After the charcoal has settled, the concentration of drug in the aqueous phase is 1 mg/L; thus, 100 L of the aqueous phase, a volume 100-times greater than that of the entire system, is required to account for the entire amount in the system.

CLEARANCE AND ELIMINATION

Knowing clearance allows calculation of rate of elimination for any plasma concentration. Using Eq. 3-4, since $CL = 26$ L/hr, the rate of elimination of midazolam from the body is 0.26 mg/hr at a plasma concentration of 0.01 mg/L (10 µg/L). One can also calculate the amount eliminated during any time interval, as illustrated in Fig. 3-5. Thus, it follows from Eq. 3-20 that multiplying the area between any two times, for example from time 0 to time t [$AUC(0, t)$], by clearance gives the amount of drug that has been eliminated up to that time.

Alternatively, when the area is expressed as a fraction of the total *AUC,* one obtains the fraction of the dose eliminated. The fraction of the total area beyond a given time is a measure of the fraction of dose remaining to be eliminated. For example, in the case of midazolam, by 2 hr, the area is 48% of the total *AUC,* and hence 48% of the administered 7.5-mg dose, or 3.6 mg, has been eliminated from the body and 3.9 mg has yet to be eliminated.

DISTRIBUTION AND ELIMINATION: COMPETING PROCESSES

Previously, it was stated that relatively little midazolam is eliminated before attainment of distribution equilibrium. Or to be more precise, relatively little more has been eliminated than expected had distribution equilibrium occurred instantaneously. This conclusion is

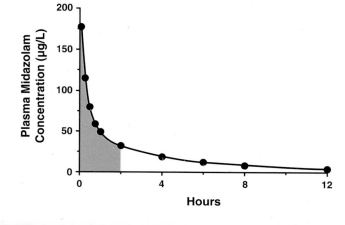

FIGURE 3-5. A linear plot of the same plasma concentration–time data for midazolam as displayed in Fig. 3-4A. The area up to 2 hr is 48% of the total *AUC* indicating that 48% of the dose administered has been eliminated by then. The area beyond 2 hr represents the 52% of the administered drug remaining to be eliminated.

based on the finding that the area under the concentration–time profile during the distribution phase (up to about 2 hr, see Fig. 3-4B) represents less than 50% of the total *AUC*, and hence less than 50% of the total amount eliminated. One would expect 30% to have been eliminated anyway during the 2-hr interval (2/3.8 of one half-life). This occurs because the speed of tissue distribution of this, and of many other drugs, is faster than that

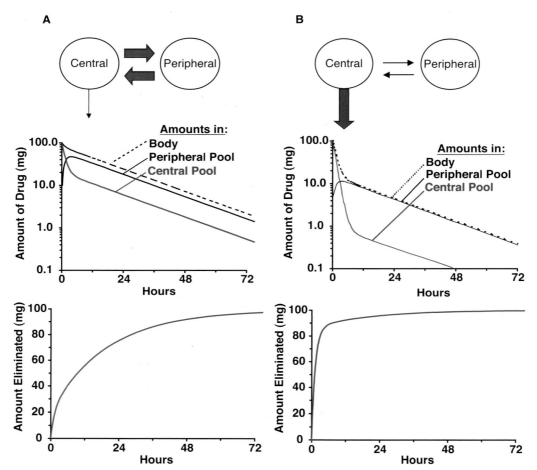

FIGURE 3-6. The events occurring within the body after a 100-mg i.v. bolus dose are the result of interplay between the kinetics of distribution and elimination. Distribution is depicted here as an exchange of drug between a central pool, comprising blood and rapidly equilibrating tissues, including the eliminating organs, liver and kidneys, and a pool containing the more slowly equilibrating tissues, such as muscle and fat. Because of distribution kinetics, a biexponential decline is seen in the semilogarithmic plot of drug in the central pool (and hence plasma). Two scenarios are considered. The first (left-hand set of panels, **A**) is one in which distribution is much faster than elimination, shown by large arrows for distribution and a small one for elimination. Distribution occurs so rapidly that little drug is lost before distribution equilibrium is achieved, when drug in the slowly equilibrating pool parallels that in the central pool, as is clearly evident in the semilogarithmic plot of events with time. Most drug elimination occurs during the terminal phase of the drug; this is seen in the linear plot of percent of dose eliminated with time. In the second scenario (right-hand set of panels, **B**), distribution (small arrows) is much slower than elimination (large arrow). Then, although, because of distribution kinetics, a biexponential decline from the central pool is still evident, most of the drug has been eliminated before distribution equilibration has been achieved. Then the phase associated with the majority of elimination is the first phase, and not the terminal exponential phase, which reflects redistribution from the slowly equilibrating tissues.

of elimination. These competing events, distribution and elimination, which determine the disposition kinetics of a drug, are shown schematically in Fig. 3-6. Here, the body is portrayed as a **compartmental model**, comprising two body pools, or compartments, with exchange of drug between them and with elimination from the first, often called central, pool. One can think of the blood, liver, kidneys, and other organs into which drug equilibrates rapidly as being part of this central pool where elimination and input of drug occurs, and the more slowly equilibrating tissues, such as muscle and fat, as being part of the other pool. The size of each arrow represents the speed of the process; the larger the arrow the faster the process. Two scenarios are depicted. The first, and most common, depicted in Fig. 3-6A, is one in which distribution is much faster than elimination. Displayed is a semilogarithmic plot of the fraction of an i.v. bolus dose within each of the pools, as well as the sum of the two (total fraction remaining in the body), as a function of time. Notice that, as with diazepam, a biphasic curve is seen and that little drug is eliminated from the body before distribution equilibrium is achieved; thereafter, during the terminal phase, drug in the two pools is in equilibrium, and the only reason for the subsequent decline is elimination from the body. The decline of drug in plasma then reflects changes in the amount of drug in the body.

Next consider the situation, albeit less common, depicted in Fig. 3-6B. Here, distribution of drug between the two pools is slow, and elimination from the central pool is rapid. Once again, a biphasic curve is seen. Also, during the terminal phase, at which time distribution equilibrium has been achieved between the two pools, the only reason for decline is again elimination of drug from the body and events in plasma reflect changes in the rest of the body. But there the similarity ends. Now, most of the drug has been eliminated from the body *before distribution equilibrium is achieved,* so there is little drug left to be eliminated during the terminal phase. An example of this latter situation is shown in Fig. 3-7 for the aminoglycoside antibiotic, gentamicin. This is a large polar compound

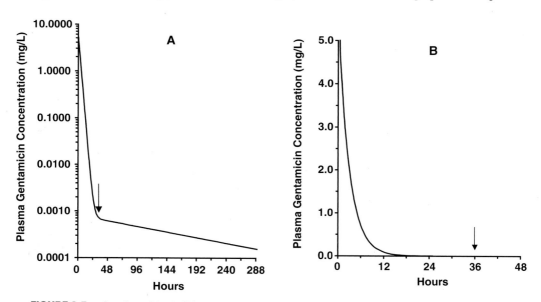

FIGURE 3-7. Semilogarithmic **(A)** and linear **(B)** plots of the decline in the mean plasma concentration of gentamicin following an i.v. bolus dose of 1 mg/kg to a group of 10 healthy men. Notice that, although a biexponential decline is seen in the semilogarithmic plot with the terminal phase reached by 36 hr (indicated by the arrow), based on analysis of the linear plot, essentially all the area, and hence elimination, has occurred before reaching the terminal phase. This is a consequence of elimination occurring much faster than tissue distribution. (From: Adelman M, Evans E, Schentag JJ. Two-compartment comparison of gentamicin and tobramycin in normal volunteers. Antimicrob Agents Chemother 1982;22:800–804.)

that is rapidly cleared from the body via the kidneys, but which permeates very slowly into many cells of the body. Over 95% of an i.v. dose of this antibiotic is eliminated into the urine before distribution equilibrium has occurred. Hence, with respect to elimination, it is the first phase and not the terminal phase that predominates. In conclusion, assigning the terminal phase as the elimination phase of a drug is generally reasonable, and unless mentioned otherwise, is assumed to be the case for the rest of this book. However, keep in mind, there are always exceptions.

PATHWAYS OF ELIMINATION

Some drugs are totally excreted unchanged in urine. Others are extensively metabolized, usually within the liver. Knowing the relative proportions eliminated by each pathway is important as it helps to predict the sensitivity of clearance of a given drug in patients with diseases of these organs or who are concurrently receiving other drugs that affect these pathways, particularly metabolism. Of the two, renal excretion is much the easier to quantify, achieved by collecting unchanged drug in urine; there is no comparable method for determining the rate of hepatic metabolism.

RENAL CLEARANCE

Central to this analysis of urinary excretion is the concept of *renal clearance*. Analogous to total clearance, renal clearance (CL_R) is defined as the proportionality term between urinary excretion rate and plasma concentration:

$$Rate\ of\ excretion = CL_R \cdot C \qquad 3\text{-}29$$

with units of flow, usually mL/min or L/hr.

Practical problems arise, however, in estimating renal clearance. Urine is collected over a finite period (e.g., 4 hr, during which time the plasma concentration is changing continuously. Shortening the collection period reduces the change in plasma concentration but increases the uncertainty in the estimate of excretion rate owing to incomplete bladder emptying. This is especially true for urine collection intervals of less than 30 min. Lengthening the collection interval, to avoid the problem of incomplete emptying, requires a modified approach for the estimation of renal clearance. This approach is analogous to that taken with total clearance. By rearranging Eq. 3-29, during a very small interval of time, dt,

$$Amount\ excreted = CL_R \cdot C \cdot dt \qquad 3\text{-}30$$

where $C \cdot dt$ is the corresponding small area under the plasma drug concentration–time curve. The urine collection interval (denoted by Δt) is composed of many such very small increments of time, and the amount of drug excreted in a collection interval is the sum of the amounts excreted in each of these small increments of time, that is,

$$Amount\ excreted\ in\ collection\ interval = CL_R \cdot [AUC\ within\ interval] \qquad 3\text{-}31$$

The problem in calculating renal clearance therefore rests with estimating the *AUC* within the time interval of urine collection (see Appendix A). The average plasma drug concentration during the collection interval is given by (*AUC* within interval)/Δt. This average plasma concentration is neither the value at the beginning or at the end of the collection time but is the value at some intermediate point. When the plasma concentration changes linearly with time, the average concentration occurs at the midpoint of the collection interval. Because the plasma concentration of drug is in fact changing exponentially with time, the assumption of linear change is reasonable only when loss during the interval is small relative to the amount in the body. In practice, the interval should be less than an elimination half-life. This method of calculating renal clearance is useful when addressing questions of change in this parameter with time or urine pH (further examined in Chapter 5, *Elimination*).

Integrating Eq. 3-30 over all time intervals, from zero to infinity, one obtains the useful relationship

$$Renal\ clearance = \frac{Total\ amount\ excreted\ unchanged}{AUC} \qquad 3\text{-}32$$

where AUC is the total area under the plasma drug concentration–time curve. To apply Eq. 3-32, care must be taken to ensure that all urine is collected and for a sufficient period of time to gain a good estimate of the total amount excreted unchanged. In practice, the period of time must be at least 6 elimination half-lives of the drug. Thus, if the half-life of a drug is in the order of a few hours, no practical difficulties exist in ensuring urine collections taken over an adequate period of time. Severe difficulties with compliance in urine collection occur, however, for drugs such as the antimalarial mefloquine, with a half-life of about 3 weeks, since all urine excreted over a period of at least 4 months must be collected. In this case, because of practical problems to ensure complete urine collection, renal clearance is usually determined over a shorter time interval, applying Eq. 3-31.

RENAL EXCRETION AS A FRACTION OF TOTAL ELIMINATION

The **fraction excreted unchanged** of an i.v. dose, fe, is an important pharmacokinetic parameter. It is a quantitative measure of the contribution of renal excretion to overall drug elimination. Knowing fe aids in establishing appropriate modifications in the usual dosage regimen of a drug for patients with diminished renal function. Among drugs, the value of fe in patients with normal renal function lies between 0 and 1.0. When fe is low (<0.3), which is common for many highly lipophilic drugs that are extensively metabolized, excretion is a minor pathway of drug elimination. Occasionally, as in the case of gentamicin and the β-adrenergic blocking agent atenolol, used to lower blood pressure, renal excretion is virtually the sole route of elimination, in which case the value of fe approaches 1.0. By definition, the complement, $1 - fe$, is the fraction of the i.v. dose that is eliminated by other mechanisms, usually hepatic metabolism.

An estimate of fe is most readily obtained from cumulative urinary excretion data following i.v. administration, since by definition,

$$fe = \frac{Total\ amount\ excreted\ unchanged}{Dose} \qquad 3\text{-}33$$

In practice, care should be taken to ensure all urine is collected and over a sufficient period of time to obtain a good estimate of total amount excreted unchanged.

Substituting Eq. 3-33 for fe and Eq. 3-21 for CL into Eq. 3-32 indicates that CL_R can be estimated directly from the relationship

$$CL_R = fe \cdot CL \qquad 3\text{-}34$$

Thus, fe may also be defined and estimated as the ratio of renal and total clearances. This approach is particularly useful in those situations in which total urine collection is not possible.

ESTIMATION OF PHARMACOKINETIC PARAMETERS

To appreciate how the pharmacokinetic parameters defining disposition are estimated, consider the plasma and urine data in Table 3-2 obtained following an i.v. bolus dose of 100 mg of a drug.

PLASMA DATA ALONE

From the table, the plasma concentration is seen to drop progressively with time, but only after the data are plotted semilogarithmically (Fig. 3-8), when a polyphasic decline is still seen, is there clear evidence of distribution kinetics. Initially, concentration falls rapidly until after about 2 hr, when distribution equilibrium has been achieved, after

TABLE 3-2   Plasma and Urine Data Obtained Following an Intravenous 100-mg Bolus Dose

Observation							
Plasma Data		**Urine Data**			**Treatment of Data**		
Time (hr)	**Concentration (mg/L)**	**Time interval of collection (hr)**	**Volume of urine (mL)**	**Concentration of unchanged drug (μg/ml)**	**AUC within interval (mg-hr/L)**	**Amount excreted within interval (mg)**	**Cumulative amount excreted (Ae, mg)**
0.25	3.0						
0.5	2.8						
0.75	2.4						
1	2.2						
1.5	2.0						
2	1.8						
4	1.4						
6	1.2						
8	1.1						
12	0.9	0–12	907	13.3	17.4	12.06	12.06
24	0.55	12–24	950	7.05	8.7	6.70	18.76
30	0.45						
36	0.36	24–36	1232	3.35	5.43	4.13	22.89
48	0.23	36–48	784	3.32	3.54	2.60	25.49
60	0.15						
72	0.10	48–72	1430	1.91	3.78	2.73	28.22

which time it falls monoexponentially, the terminal phase. Only then can the elimination half-life and associated rate constant be readily determined. The half-life, taken as the time for the concentration to fall in half (e.g., from 1.2 to 0.6 mg/L or 0.6 to 0.3 mg/L), is 18 hr, so that k is 0.038 hr^{-1}, and therefore the MRT is 26.3 hr. Clearance is determined by dividing dose (100 mg) by AUC. The total AUC, estimated using the trapezoidal rule (Appendix A, *Assessment of AUC*), is 41.48 mg-hr/L. Accordingly, clearance is 2.41 L/hr. Volume of distribution, estimated from CL/k (Eq. 3-23), is therefore 63.4 L. Lastly, for this drug one can be sure that little has been eliminated before distribution equilibrium is reached. This is readily seen by calculating the area above the line when the terminal slope in Fig. 3-8 is extrapolated back to zero time. This area comprises only 7% of the total AUC. That is, only 7% of the dose has been eliminated during the attainment of distribution equilibrium above that expected from the terminal half-life.

PLASMA AND URINE DATA

The cumulative amount excreted unchanged up to 72 hr is 28.2 mg. During this period, 4 half-lives have elapsed, and based on half-life considerations (Eq. 3-19), 93.75% of the ultimate amount will have been excreted. Hence, a reasonable estimate of the total amount excreted unchanged (Ae_∞) is 28.2/0.973 or 30 mg, so that the fraction of the dose excreted unchanged, fe, is 30 mg/100 mg, or 0.30.

Both plasma and urine data are required to estimate renal clearance. This parameter can be obtained from the slope of a plot of the amount excreted within a collection interval against AUC within the same time interval (Fig. 3-9). The straight line implies that

A

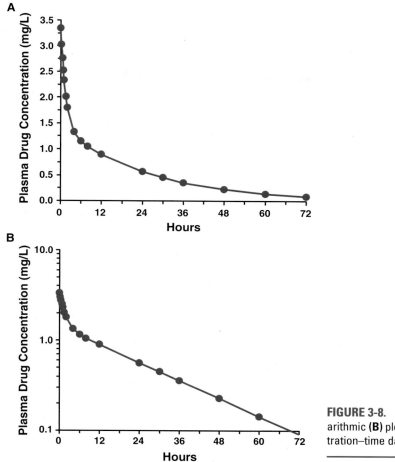

B

FIGURE 3-8. Regular **(A)** and semilogarithmic **(B)** plots of the plasma concentration–time data given in Table 3-2.

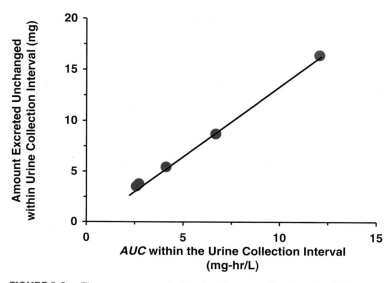

FIGURE 3-9. The amount excreted is directly proportional to the *AUC* measured over the urine collection interval. Renal clearance is given by the slope of the line. (Data from Table 3-2.)

renal clearance is constant and independent of plasma concentration over the range covered. The slope of the line indicates that the renal clearance of this drug is 0.74 L/hr. Essentially the same value is obtained by multiplying total clearance (2.5 L/hr) by fe (0.30) (cf., Eq. 3-34).

A QUESTION OF PRECISION

Had you plotted the same data and calculated the pharmacokinetic parameters by visual inspection, you may have obtained answers that differ from those given. This is not unusual and will occur in many cases when you check your answers to the problems at the end of each chapter against those given in Appendix J. The reason lies in differences in where you draw your line through the data, after they have been plotted, and in rounding-off numbers. All measurements have errors associated with analytic methods, conditions of storage, and handling of samples prior to analysis, leading to some uncertainty in knowing the true curve.

Also, had the study just considered been repeated subsequently in the same individual, the estimated half-life may have been 16.5 or 19.1 hr instead of 18 hr. For almost all clinical situations, this degree of within individual variation is acceptable. To reflect the acceptable 5% to 10% variation, most answers here and throughout the remainder of the book are usually given to no more than two or three significant places.

In this chapter, many symbols have been defined, as it is the first time that they are used. These symbols are reused repeatedly throughout the book. To avoid continually redefining them in every chapter and to facilitate reference to them, the "Definitions of Symbols" appear in a table just before Chapter 1. Some infrequently used symbols that occur only within one chapter are defined there and may not be included in the table.

MEASUREMENT FLUID

Strictly speaking, when referring to concentration, one should use the terminology *concentration of drug in plasma* (or *whole blood*, or *plasma water*, as appropriate). For expediency, in much of this chapter and throughout the rest of the book, this phrase is often shortened to *plasma* (or *blood*) *drug concentration*. Indeed, this is sometimes even further shortened to *plasma concentration* (or *blood concentration*) in many contexts in which concentration of a drug is understood. Similarly, the phrase *amount in body* refers to the amount of drug in the body, unless otherwise stated.

USE OF COMPUTERS

Today, computers are used to analyze pharmacokinetic and pharmacodynamic data and make predictions. Implicit in the approach is the application of a model. Based on statistical criteria, the parameter values giving the best fit of the parameters of the appropriate equation or model to the experimental data are obtained. This approach not only provides the best estimate of the parameters but also one's confidence in them. Furthermore, application of the same computer program to a set of data results in the same answers independent of the operator. This consistency cannot be achieved by fitting graphical data by eye. Moreover, unlike an exponential equation, there are many situations in pharmacokinetics and particularly pharmacodynamics that require equations that cannot be linearized. Obtaining a best fit by eye then becomes virtually impossible. This limitation does not arise using a computer. Nonetheless, a great deal is learned by displaying data graphically. One gains a feeling for the quality of the data and the equation or model that is most likely to describe them appropriately. Ultimately, the suitability of a model can be judged by how well predictions match observations at all times. Because of the great benefits to learning pharmacokinetics and pharmacodynamics gained by plotting data and interpreting graphical representations, this element is incorporated throughout the book and emphasized in study problems and simulation exercises.

CHANGE IN DOSE

An adjustment in dose is often necessary to achieve optimal drug therapy. The kinetic consequences of adjustment are made more readily when the values of the pharmacokinetic parameters of a drug do not vary with dose or with concentration. For example, the *AUC* is expected to double when the single i.v. dose of 50 mg is doubled to 100 mg, because clearance is unchanged. There are, however, many reasons for a change in a parameter value (e.g., *CL*, with dose). These are dealt with in Chapter 16, *Nonlinearities*. Throughout the majority of the book, however, pharmacokinetic parameters are assumed not to change with either dose or time.

KEY RELATIONSHIPS

$$E = \frac{(C - C_{out})}{C}$$

$$Rate\ of\ elimination = CL \cdot C$$

$$CL = Q \cdot E$$

$$k = \frac{CL}{V}$$

$$Rate\ of\ elimination = -\frac{dA}{dt} = k \cdot A$$

$$C = C(0) \cdot e^{-k \cdot t}$$

$$ln\ C = ln\ C(0) - k \cdot t$$

$$t_{1/2} = \frac{0.693}{k}$$

$$t_{1/2} = \frac{0.693 \cdot V}{CL}$$

$$\frac{Fraction\ of}{dose\ remaining} = e^{-k \cdot t} = \left(\frac{1}{2}\right)^{n}$$

$$Dose = CL \cdot AUC$$

$$V = \frac{A}{C}$$

$$V = 1.44 \cdot CL \cdot t_{1/2}$$

$$MRT = \frac{1}{k}$$

$$fe = \frac{Total\ drug\ excreted\ unchanged}{Dose}$$

$$Renal\ clearance = fe \cdot CL$$

$$CL_R = \frac{Rate\ of\ excretion}{Plasma\ concentration}$$

$$Renal\ clearance = \frac{Total\ amount\ excreted\ unchanged}{AUC}$$

STUDY PROBLEMS

(Answers to Study Problems are in Appendix J.)

1. Define the following terms: clearance, compartmental model, disposition kinetics, elimination half-life, elimination rate constant, extraction ratio, first-order process, fraction excreted unchanged, fraction in plasma unbound, fractional rate of elimination, half-life, mean residence time, monoexponential equation, renal clearance, terminal phase, volume of distribution.

2. Given that the disposition kinetics of a drug is described by a one-compartment model, which of the following statements is (are) correct? The half-life of a drug following therapeutic doses in humans is 4 hr, therefore,

   a. The elimination rate constant of this drug is 0.173 hr^{-1}.
   b. It takes 16 hr for 87.5% of an i.v. bolus dose to be eliminated.
   c. It takes twice as long to eliminate 37.5 mg following a 50 mg bolus dose as it does to eliminate 50 mg following a 100-mg dose.
   d. Complete urine collection up to 12 hr is needed to provide a good estimate of the ultimate amount of drug excreted unchanged.
   e. The fraction of the administered dose eliminated by a given time is independent of the size of the dose.

3. For a drug exhibiting one-compartment disposition kinetics, calculate the following:

   a. The fraction of an i.v. dose remaining in the body at 3 hr, when the half-life is 6 hr.
   b. The half-life of a drug, when 18% of the dose remains in the body 4 hr after an i.v. bolus dose.

4. The average values of clearance and volume of distribution of valproic acid, an antiepileptic drug, in the adult patient population are 0.5 L/hr and 9 L, respectively.

   a. Calculate the rate of elimination of valproic acid when the plasma concentration is 30 mg/L.
   b. Calculate the half-life of valproic acid.
   c. What is the amount of valproic acid in the body at distribution equilibrium when the plasma concentration is 60 mg/L?
   d. What is the expected plasma concentration 12 hr after an i.v. 700-mg dose of valproic acid (administered as the equivalent amount of the sodium salt)?

5. A drug that displays one-compartment disposition kinetics is administered as a 100-mg single bolus dose. Depicted in Fig. 3-10A is the plasma concentrations of drug observed initially (10 mg/L) and 10 hr later (2.5 mg/L). Depicted in Fig. 3-10B is the cumulative urinary excretion of unchanged drug at 48 hr (60 mg). Complete the figures by drawing continuous lines that depict the fall of drug concentration in plasma and the accumulation of drug in urine with time.

6. From 0 to 3 hr after a 50-mg i.v. bolus dose of drug, the *AUC* is 5.1 mg-hr/L. The total *AUC* is 22.4 mg-hr/L and the cumulative amount excreted unchanged, Ae_{∞}, is 11 mg.

   a. Determine the amount of drug remaining in the body at 3 hrs as a percent of the administered dose.
   b. Calculate total clearance.

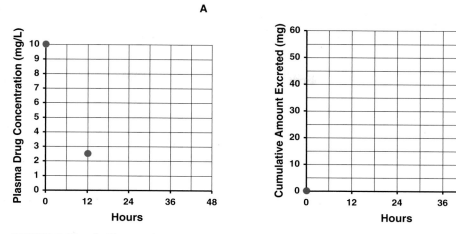

FIGURE 3-10. **A.** Plasma drug concentration-time profile. **B.** Cumulative amount excreted unchanged with time. Only two points are shown in each graph.

c. Calculate the renal clearance of the drug.

d. What is the fraction of the dose that is eliminated by renal excretion?

7. When 100 mg of a drug was given as an i.v. bolus, the following plasma concentration–time relationship (C in mg/L and t in hours) was observed,

$$C = 7.14e^{-0.051t}$$

Calculate:

a. Volume of distribution.

b. Elimination half-life.

c. Total AUC.

d. Total clearance.

e. The plasma concentration 70 min after a 250-mg i.v. bolus dose.

8. A 10-mg dose of diazepam is injected intravenously into a patient with status epilepticus. The half-life and volume of distribution of the drug are 48 hr and 80 L, respectively, in the patient. Calculate your expectation for each of the following:

a. The elimination rate constant.

b. The plasma diazepam concentration 12 hr after giving the dose.

c. The fraction of the dose remaining in the body 48 hr after the dose is given.

d. The clearance of diazepam.

e. The initial rate of elimination when the entire dose is in the body.

f. The AUC.

g. The amount of drug in the body 1 week after giving the dose.

9. The data given in Table 3-3 are the plasma concentrations of cocaine as a function of time after i.v. administration of 33 mg cocaine hydrochloride to a subject. (Molecular weight of cocaine hydrochloride = 340 g/mol; molecular weight of cocaine = 303 g/mol.) (Adapted from Chow MJ, Ambre JJ, Ruo TI, et al. Kinetics of cocaine distribution, elimination, and chronotropic effects. Clin Pharmacol Ther 1985;38:318–324.)

a. Prepare a semilogarithmic plot of plasma concentration versus time. Graph paper is available online at the companion web site: http//thePoint.lww.com/Rowland4e. Regular Graph Paper, 2-Cycle Semilogarithmic Graph Paper, 3-Cycle Semilogarithmic Graph Paper, and Log-log Graph Paper are available. You may prefer to plot the data using Excel or some other software program.

b. Estimate the half-life.

TABLE 3-3	Plasma Concentrations of Cocaine with Time After a Single Intravenous Dose of 33-mg Cocaine Hydrochloride						
Time (hr)	0.16	0.5	1.0	1.5	2.0	2.5	3.0
Concentration (μg/L)	170	122	74	45	28	17	10

c. Estimate the total *AUC* of cocaine by integration of the exponential equation and by use of the trapezoidal rule (Appendix A, *Assessment of AUC*). Comment on any differences between these two estimates.

d. Calculate the clearance of cocaine.

e. Given that the body weight of the subject is 75 kg, calculate the volume of distribution of cocaine in L/kg.

10. Figure 3-11 shows a semilogarithmic plot of the plasma concentration–time profile of theophylline following a 500-mg i.v. bolus dose in a 70-kg patient. Notice that the decline is biexponential, with the break in the curve at around 30 min. Theophylline is 40% bound in plasma and freely passes across membranes and distributes into all body water spaces. It is also extensively metabolized with only 10% of the dose excreted in the urine unchanged.

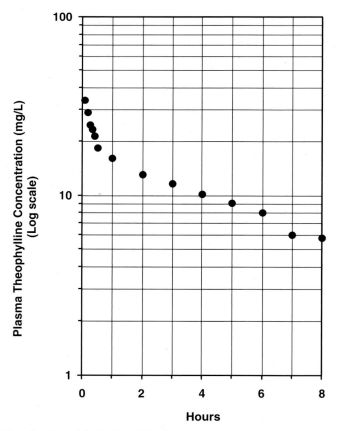

FIGURE 3-11. Semilogarithmic plot of the plasma concentration–time profile of theophylline following a 500-mg i.v. bolus dose in a 70-kg patient. (From: Mitenko PA, Ogilvie RI. Pharmacokinetics of intravenous theophylline. Clin Pharmacol Ther 1973;14:509–513.)

a. The total area under the plasma-concentration time profile of theophylline is 125 mg-hr/L. Calculate the total clearance of theophylline.
b. Is it appropriate to call the initial decline phase up to about 30 min the distribution phase knowing that the *AUC* of theophylline up to that time is 13.1 mg-hr/L?
c. The plasma concentration at the first sampling time of 5 min is 33 mg/L. What percent of the dose has left the plasma by then and to where does the drug primarily go?
d. Calculate the renal clearance of theophylline.
e. From the plot, estimate the half-life of theophylline.
f. Estimate the volume of distribution of theophylline.

4

Membranes and Distribution

OBJECTIVES

The reader will be able to:

- Define the following terms: hydrophilic, hydrophobic, lipophilic, lipophobic, active transport, paracellular transport, passive facilitated transport, permeability, transcellular transport, and transporter.
- List two examples of transporters involved in systemic absorption after oral administration and three involved in the distribution of drugs into and out of tissues, including eliminating organs.
- Define the following terms:
  a. Perfusion limitation in distribution
  b. Permeability limitation in distribution
  c. Tissue-to-blood equilibrium distribution ratio
  d. Fraction unbound
  e. Plasma protein binding
- Distinguish between perfusion rate-limited and permeability rate-limited passage of drugs through membranes.
- Describe the role of pH in the movement of drugs through membranes.
- Describe the consequences of the reversible nature of movement of drugs through membranes.
- Determine the plasma concentration, the amount of drug in the body, and the apparent volume of distribution at distribution equilibrium when any two of these values are known.
- Describe the effects of perfusion limitation, permeability limitation, and the tissue-to-blood equilibrium distribution ratio on the time required for drug to distribute into and out of tissues.
- Ascertain whether, for a given amount of drug in the body at distribution equilibrium, the unbound plasma concentration is likely to be sensitive to variation in plasma protein binding when the volume of distribution is known.
- From knowledge of the volume of distribution and the fraction unbound for a drug bound only to albumin in plasma, calculate the fraction of drug in the body at equilibrium that is:
  a. Unbound
  b. In the extracellular fluids
  c. Outside the extracellular fluids
  d. Bound to plasma proteins
  e. Bound to plasma proteins in the extracellular fluids
  f. Bound intracellularly (in or on tissue cells)
- Anticipate the effect of altered plasma protein binding on the half-life of a drug, bound to albumin and with a volume of distribution less than 15 L.

I n the last chapter, emphasis was placed on general input–exposure relationships after a single intravenous (i.v.) bolus. We now examine the role and function of membranes primarily in the context of determinants of drug distribution, but the principles apply as well to drug elimination (Chapter 5, *Elimination*) and drug absorption (Chapter 7, *Absorption*). Drugs must also pass through membranes to reach the site of action.

This chapter also explores the process of distribution itself and its role in clinical pharmacokinetics from a physiologic point of view. The chapter begins with kinetic considerations and ends with equilibrium concepts involved in drug distribution, the reversible transfer of drug from one location to another within the body.

Before examining membranes as a determinant of drug absorption and disposition, a few terms commonly applied to the physicochemical properties of drugs need to be defined. **Hydrophilic** and **hydrophobic** are adjectives that refer to water (hydro-) loving (-philic) and fearing (-phobic) properties. Similarly, **lipophilic** and **lipophobic** are adjectives that relate to lipid (lipo-) loving and fearing properties. In general, the terms hydrophilic and lipophobic are interchangeable. When referring to substances, both these terms imply that the substances are soluble in water, but very poorly soluble in nonpolar lipids. Similarly, the terms lipophilic and hydrophobic are interchangeable and refer to substances that are soluble in lipids, but very poorly soluble in water. A common measure of lipophilicity of a substance is its partitioning between n-octanol (an organic solvent with hydrogen bonding properties aimed at mimicking the physicochemical properties of tissue membranes) and water. The higher the **partition coefficient**, ratio of drug concentrations at equilibrium (approximated by the ratio of solubilities) in the two phases, the greater is the lipophilicity. Many drugs contain both hydrophobic and hydrophilic groups and vary in their solubilities in water and n-octanol. Some compounds, such as alcohol, are readily soluble in both water and n-octanol or other lipid-like solvents. Others, such as digoxin, are poorly soluble in both water and lipids. Thus, both solubility and partition coefficient are important in drug absorption and disposition.

MEMBRANES

Movement through membranes is known as **drug transport**, a term that is often used more specifically to describe the processes and transport systems (transporters) that facilitate movement across membranes. Understanding how physicochemical, anatomic, and physiologic factors determine the rapidity of drug transport is a prerequisite to an appreciation of factors controlling the pharmacokinetics and pharmacodynamics of drugs.

Cellular membranes are composed of an inner, predominantly lipoidal, matrix covered on each surface by either a continuous layer or a lattice of protein (Fig. 4-1, upper section of drawing). The hydrophobic portions of the lipid molecules are oriented toward the center of the membrane and the outer hydrophilic regions face the surrounding aqueous environment. For some drugs, facilitative mechanisms are embedded in the protein lattice. Narrow aqueous-filled channels exist between some cells (e.g., in most blood capillary membranes, the glomerulus of the kidney, and intestinal epithelia).

The transport of drugs is often viewed as movement across a series of membranes and spaces, which, in aggregate, serve as a "functional" macroscopic unit. The cells and interstitial spaces that lie between the intestinal lumen and the capillary blood and the structures between the sinusoidal space and the bile canaliculi in the liver, as well as the skin (see Fig. 4-1), are examples. Each of the interposing cellular membranes and spaces impede drug transport to varying degrees, and any one of them can be the slowest step, rate-controlling the overall transport process. In the skin, the stratum corneum is the major site of impedance. In the small intestine, it is the apical side of the epithelial cells, that is, the side facing the lumen. These complexities of structure make accurate extrapolation of the quantitative features of drug transport from one membrane to another difficult.

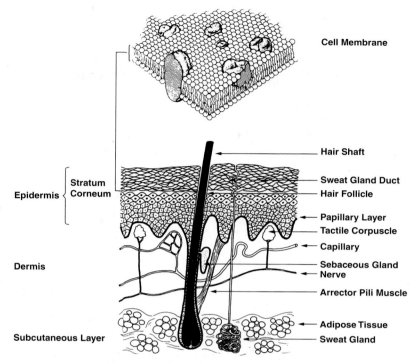

Cell Membrane

Hair Shaft

Sweat Gland Duct

Hair Follicle

Papillary Layer

Tactile Corpuscle

Capillary

Sebaceous Gland

Nerve

Arrector Pili Muscle

Adipose Tissue

Sweat Gland

Stratum Corneum

Epidermis

Dermis

Subcutaneous Layer

FIGURE 4-1. Functional membranes vary enormously in structure and thickness. They can be as thin as a single-cell membrane of approximately 1×10^{-6} cm thickness (*top*), to as thick as the multicellular barrier of the skin. This multicellular barrier extends from the stratum corneum to the upper part of the papillary layer of the dermis, adjacent to the capillaries of the microcirculation; a distance of approximately 2×10^{-2} cm (*bottom*). The cell membrane comprises a bimolecular leaflet, with a lipid interior and a polar exterior, dispersed through which are globular proteins, depicted as large solid irregular shaped bodies. (From: Singer SJ, Nicolson GL. The fluid mosaic model of the structure of cell membranes. Science 1972;175:720. Copyright 1982 by the AAAS; skin was kindly drawn by Mandy North.)

Nonetheless, much can be gained by considering the general qualitative features governing drug transport across these "functional" membranes.

TRANSPORT PROCESSES

Drug transport can broadly be divided into **transcellular** and **paracellular** processes, as shown in Fig. 4-2. Transcellular movement, which involves the passage of drug through cells, is the most common route of drug transport. Some drugs, however, are too polar to pass across the lipoidal cell membrane and for them only the paracellular pathway, between the cells, is generally available. Other drugs move across some cell membranes by facilitative mechanisms.

PROTEIN BINDING

Before considering the determinants of the permeability of drug itself, a comment needs to be made about protein binding. Many drugs bind to plasma proteins and tissue components (discussed later in this chapter). Such binding is generally reversible and usually so rapid that equilibrium is established within milliseconds. In such cases, the associated (bound) and dissociated (unbound) forms of the drug can be assumed to be at equilibrium at all times and under virtually all circumstances. Only **unbound** drug is capable of

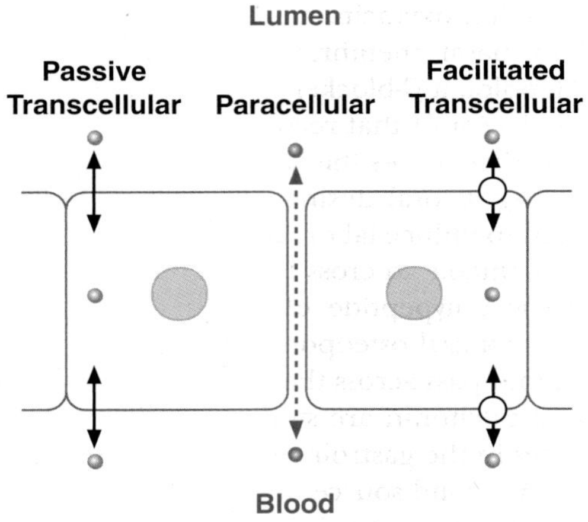

FIGURE 4-2. Movement of drugs across membranes occurs by paracellular and transcellular pathways. Paracellular movement (*dashed colored arrow*) of drug (●) is influenced by the tightness of the intercellular junctions. The transcellular pathways can be divided into two categories: those in which the passage is by simple diffusion (*solid arrows*) and those in which facilitative mechanisms (*arrows with a circle*) are involved.

diffusing through cell membranes. Proteins, and hence protein-bound drugs, are much too large to do so. Hence, the unbound concentration, not the total concentration, is the driving force for drug transport across a cell membrane.

DIFFUSION

One process by which drugs pass through membranes is **diffusion**, the natural tendency for molecules to move down a concentration gradient. Movement results from the kinetic energy of the molecules, and because no work is expended by the system, the process is known as **passive diffusion**.

To appreciate the properties of passive diffusion across a membrane, consider a simple system in which a membrane separates two well-stirred aqueous compartments. The driving force for drug transfer is the difference between the unbound concentrations in compartment 1, Cu_1, and compartment 2, Cu_2. The net rate of transport is:

$$Net\ rate\ of\ transport = \underset{\text{Permeability}}{P} \cdot \underset{\substack{\text{Surface}\\\text{area}}}{SA} \cdot \underset{\substack{\text{Concentration}\\\text{difference}}}{(Cu_1 - Cu_2)} \qquad 4\text{-}1$$

The importance of the surface area of the membrane is readily apparent. For example, doubling the surface area doubles the probability of collision with the membrane and thereby increases the penetration rate twofold. Some drugs readily pass through a membrane, others do not. This difference in ease of penetration is quantitatively expressed in terms of the **permeability**, P. Note that the product $P \cdot SA$ has the units typical of flow, volume/time (cm^3/min). With SA, *surface area involved*, having units of cm^2, it is apparent that permeability has units of velocity, distance/time (cm/min).

Drug Properties Determining Permeability. Three major molecular properties affecting, and sometimes limiting, the passage of a drug across a given membrane are size, lipophilicity, and charge (or degree of ionization). These properties, together with the nature of the membrane and the medium on either side, determine the overall speed of movement of a compound across the membrane.

Molecular size has only a small impact on diffusion of substances in water. However, molecular size has a major impact on movement through membranes. This sensitivity to size is because of the relative rigidity of cell membranes, which sterically impedes drug movement. For some membranes, water-soluble materials cannot move through cells; instead, they move paracellularly through narrow channels between cells. Here, molecular size is the primary determinant of transport. To appreciate the impact of molecular size on paracellular transport, consider the passage of three water-soluble drugs, atenolol, oxytocin, and calcitonin-salmon across two membranes, the relatively loosely knit nasal membranes and the relatively tightly knit gastrointestinal membranes. Atenolol, a β-blocker used in the treatment of hypertension, is a small stable molecule (246 g/mol) that readily passes across the nasal membranes and is even reasonably well absorbed across the gastrointestinal membranes, with an oral bioavailability of 50%, facilitating its oral dosing. Oxytocin, a moderately sized cyclic nanopeptide (1007 g/mol) used to induce labor, also rapidly crosses nasal membranes paracellularly but is almost totally unable to cross the gastrointestinal membranes. Whereas calcitonin-salmon, a synthetic polypeptide of 32 amino acids (3432 g/mol) used in the treatment of postmenopausal osteoporosis, is so large that it is only 3% absorbed from a nasal spray and cannot pass across the intestinal epithelium. Furthermore, most nasally applied oxytocin and calcitonin are swallowed and undergo extensive degradation (digestion) by peptidases in the gastrointestinal tract, so that these drugs are not orally administered.

A second source of variation is lipophilicity. Generally, the more lipophilic the molecule the greater is its permeability but, as mentioned, size is also important. Small lipid-soluble, un-ionized drugs tend to traverse lipid membranes transcellularly with ease. This tendency and the effect of molecular size are shown in Fig. 4-3 for transdermal passage of various uncharged molecules. Notice, as mentioned above, as size increases permeability drops sharply. For example, for only a doubling of molecular weight (MW) from 400 to 800 g/mol for molecules with the same lipophilicity, permeability decreases by a factor of almost 2.5 log units, or 300-fold.

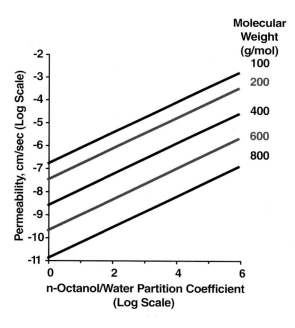

FIGURE 4-3. Permeability across skin as a function of molecular size and lipophilicity of neutral molecules. Lipophilicity is expressed as the n-octanol/water partition coefficient. Each line represents substances of the same molecular weight but different lipophilicity. Note, to offset the effect of reducing permeability on doubling of molecular weight, from 400 to 800 g/mol, lipophilicity has to increase by 4 log units, from 2 to 6, equivalent to a 10,000-fold increase in the partition coefficient. (From: Potts RO, Guy RH. Predicting skin permeability. Pharm Res 1992;9:633–669. Reproduced with permission of Plenum Publishing Corporation.)

The importance of lipophilicity and molecular size is also supported by observations of the movement of various drugs into the central nervous system (CNS), as shown in Fig. 4-4. The brain and spinal chord are protected from exposure to various substances. The protective mechanism was observed many years ago when various hydrophilic dyes, injected intravenously into animals, stained most tissues of the body, but not the CNS, which appeared to exclude them. Thus, the concept of high impedance to the movement of these substances into brain arose, namely, the **blood-brain barrier**. The barrier exists because of very tight junctions between the endothelial capillary cells as well as the presence of glial processes surrounding the capillaries highly resistant to polar substances.

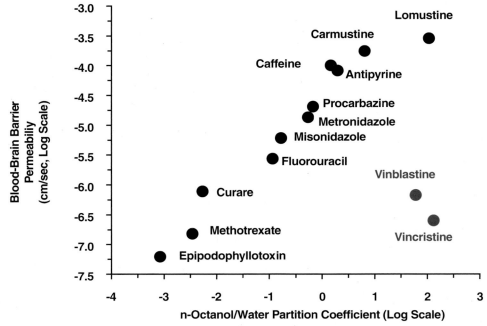

FIGURE 4-4. Relationship between permeability of a drug across the blood-brain barrier and its n-octanol/water partition coefficient. Generally, permeability increases progressively with increasing lipophilicity, but not always. For compounds such as vinblastine and vincristine (*colored*) the permeability is lower than expected, due in large part to their being substrates for the efflux transporter, P-glycoprotein. Both axes are logarithmic. (From: Greig N. Drug delivery to the brain by blood-brain barrier circumvention and drug modification. In: Neuwelt E, ed. Implication of the Blood-Brain Barrier and Its Manipulation. Vol. 1. Basic Science Aspects; 1989:311–367.)

Figure 4-4 clearly shows that lipophilicity, as measured by the n-octanol/water partition coefficient, is a major determinant of the transport of drugs across the blood-brain barrier. The two major exceptions, the anticancer drugs vinblastine and vincristine, are moderately large molecules (molecular masses of 814 and 824 g/mol) and as stated above, size is also a major determinant of passage across membranes. The drugs are also substrates of efflux transporters.

Charge is the third major constraint to transmembrane passage. Again, there is considerable variation in the impedance of different membranes to charged molecules, but the effect of charge is, with a few exceptions (e.g., those involving paracellular transport across the blood capillary membranes and renal glomerulus), always large. The larger and more hydrophilic a molecule, the slower is its movement across membranes. Movement is slowed even more if the molecule is also charged. Some drugs are only partially charged (or ionized) at physiologic pH. Therefore, the degree of ionization is also important in determining movement across membranes.

Most drugs are weak acids or weak bases and exist in solution as an equilibrium between un-ionized and ionized forms. Increased total concentration of drug on the side of a membrane where pH favors greater ionization of drug has led to the **pH partition hypothesis**. According to this hypothesis, only un-ionized nonpolar drug penetrates the membrane, and at equilibrium, the concentrations of the un-ionized species are equal on both sides, but the total concentrations may be very different because of the differences in degree of ionization, as shown in Fig. 4-5. The topic of ionization and the pH partition hypothesis is expanded upon in Appendix B, *Ionization and the pH Partition Hypothesis.*

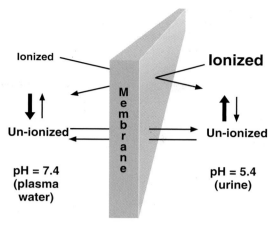

FIGURE 4-5. When a drug is a weak acid or weak base, its total concentration on one side of a lipophilic membrane may be very different from that on the other at equilibrium, if the pH values of the two aqueous phases are different. One mechanism producing this concentration difference is the pH partition hypothesis, which states that only the un-ionized form can cross the membrane and that the total concentration on each side at equilibrium depends on the degree of ionization. The side with greater ionization has the higher total concentration. For weak bases, the example shown, the total concentration is greater on the side with the lower pH; the opposite applies to weak acids. The relative concentrations of un-ionized and ionized drug on both sides of the membrane are shown by the font sizes. The weak base has a pKa of 6.4.

Most evidence supporting the pH partition hypothesis stems from studies of gastrointestinal absorption, renal excretion, and gastric secretion of drugs, all anatomical locations where pH is highly variable. The pH of gastric fluid varies between 1.5 and 7.0; that of intestinal fluids varies between 6.2 and 7.5, whereas urine pH varies between 5.0 and 7.5. Elsewhere in the body, changes in pH tend to be much smaller and to show less deviation from the pH of blood, 7.4. An exception is the acidic (pH 5) lysosomal region within cells where digestion of intracellular material takes place.

Despite its general appeal, the pH partition hypothesis fails to explain certain observations. Some small quaternary ammonium compounds (e.g., bethanechol chloride), which are always ionized, are absorbed and elicit systemic effects when given orally. Movement of these compounds through the gastrointestinal membranes occurs, although at a slow and unpredictable rate. Part of this movement is paracellular, but for many compounds, influx and efflux transporters are involved. For these reasons, quantitative prediction of the influence of pH on the movement of drugs across a membrane, based solely on the pH partition hypothesis, is often inaccurate.

Membrane Characteristics. Although molecular size, lipophilicity, and charge are generally key determinants of transmembrane passage of compounds, properties of the membrane are important as well. Some membranes, such as the renal glomerulus and blood capillaries of most tissues, are highly permeable to molecules up to 5000 g/mol in size with little effect of charge or lipophilicity. In these cases, drug transfer occurs paracellularly by movement through large fenestrations (windows) in the membrane. Movement of water through the membranes (a convective process) tends to augment the transport in the direction of flow. Table 4-1 lists membranes in general ascending order with regard to the influence of size (up to 5000 g/mol), lipophilicity, and charge on drug transport.

Another determinant of permeability is membrane thickness, the distance a molecule has to traverse from the site of interest (e.g., an absorption surface) to a blood capillary. The shorter the distance, the higher is the permeability. This distance can vary from

TABLE 4-1   **Properties of Different Membranes**

Blood capillaries (except in testes, placenta, and most of the central nervous system) Renal glomerulus	Transport through membranes is basically independent of lipophilicity, charge, and molecular size (up to ~5000 g/mol). For larger molecules, charge is also important, with negatively charged molecules showing lower permeability.
Nasal mucosa Buccal mucosa Gastrointestinal tract Lung	Transport affected by lipophilicity, charge, and molecular size. Nasal mucosa generally more porous than gastrointestinal tract.
Hepatocyte Renal tubule Blood-brain barrier	Transport highly dependent on lipophilicity, charge, and molecular size.

about 0.005 to 0.01 μm (for cell membranes) to several millimeters (at some skin sites; see Fig. 4-1, lower part of figure).

Drug transport continues toward equilibrium, a condition in which the concentrations of the diffusing (generally unbound and uncharged) species are the same in the aqueous phases on both sides of the membrane. Movement of drug between these phases still continues at equilibrium, but the net flux is zero. Equilibrium is achieved more rapidly with highly permeable drugs, and when there is a large surface area of contact with the membrane, that is when the $P \cdot SA$ product is high (see Eq. 4-1).

Initially, when drug is placed on one side of the membrane, it follows from Eq. 4-1 that rate of drug transport is directly proportional to concentration (Fig. 4-6). For example, rate of transport is increased twofold when concentration of drug is doubled. Stated differently, each molecule diffuses independently of the other, and there is no upper limit to the rate of transport, unless the drug alters the nature of the membrane. Both absence of competition between molecules and lack of an upper limit to the rate of transport are characteristics of passive diffusion.

FIGURE 4-6. Initial rate of drug transport is plotted against the concentration of drug placed on one side of a membrane. With passive diffusion, the rate of transport increases linearly with concentration. With carrier-mediated transport, the rate of transport approaches a limiting value at high concentrations, the transport maximum.

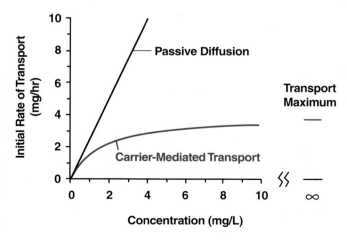

CARRIER-MEDIATED TRANSPORT

Although many drugs are passively transported through cells, for many others the transport is facilitated, that is, the transport across the membrane is faster than expected from their physicochemical properties. Figure 4-7 shows several types of facilitated transport. The first example is **passive facilitated diffusion** in which movement is facilitated by a

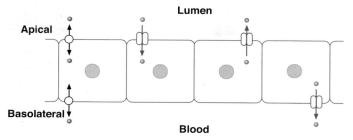

FIGURE 4-7. The intestinal epithelium, which exemplifies the general transport properties of membranes, forms a selective barrier against the entry of drugs into blood. Movement into (influx) and out of (efflux) the epithelial cells occurs by facilitative mechanisms, involving equilibrating transporters (bidirectional passive transport at either or both the apical and basolateral membranes) and concentrating transporters (*in color*). Concentrating transporters require energy and may involve influx, in which case the drug concentrates in the cell, or efflux, in which case drug is kept out of the cell.

transporter, or transport system, which aids in speeding up the bidirectional process but does not change the condition at equilibrium. Such transporters are sometimes known as **equilibrating transporters**.

Passive facilitated diffusion is exemplified by the gastrointestinal absorption and transmembrane passage into and out of tissue cells of many nucleosides and nucleobases. It is a passive process; the nucleosides and nucleobases move down a concentration gradient without expenditure of energy and, at equilibrium, the unbound concentrations across the membrane are equal. At high plasma drug concentrations, however, the rate of transport reaches a limiting value or **transport maximum**. This is a characteristic of facilitated transport processes, as shown in Fig. 4-6. Furthermore, in common with other carrier-mediated systems, passive facilitated transport is reasonably specific and is inhibited by other competing substrates of the same carrier. Drugs, so handled, include cytarabine, used to treat hairy cell leukemia, and gemcitabine, used in treating pancreatic cancer.

Additional types of facilitated transport, shown in Fig. 4-7 for intestinal transport, require energy and are capable of moving drug against an opposing concentration gradient. They are adenosine triphosphate (ATP) dependent and are examples of **active** transport systems, sometimes known as **concentrating transporters**. The direction of net movement may be either into the cell (**influx** transporter) or out of the cell (**efflux** transporter) and may occur on either the apical (lumen) or basolateral (blood) side of the membrane. Intracellular metabolizing enzymes may convert the drug to another substance before they both reach the blood. Apical efflux transporters and intracellular enzymes may, by concerted action, materially reduce systemic absorption, particularly for some drugs given orally.

Efflux transporters also play a major role in removing metabolic end products and xenobiotic (foreign) substances from cells and organs. Our awareness of the therapeutic importance of efflux transporters was heightened when certain tumor cells were observed to be resistant to specific anticancer drugs. A transporter appeared to exclude many drugs from the cell; it was called the multiple drug-resistant receptor (MDR1). A specific glycoprotein, which resides in the cell membrane and is called *permeability* glycoprotein, or **P-glycoprotein** (170,000 g/mol), was found to be responsible. This ATP-dependent transporter is located in many organs and tissues. It plays a major role in the hepatic secretion into bile of many drugs, the renal secretion of many others, and the rate and extent of absorption of some drugs from the gastrointestinal tract. Many other drug transporters have since been identified. Examples of hepatic and renal transporters and their substrates are listed in Table 4-2. The location of these and other transporters

TABLE 4-2 **Human Liver and Kidney Transporters Important in Drug Disposition**

Gene Symbol	Protein Name	Full Protein Name	Representative Substrates
Influx transporters			
SLC22A1	OCT1	Organic cation transporter 1	Metformin, oxaliplatin
SLC22A2	OCT2	Organic cation transporter 2	Metformin, amantadine
SLC22A4	OCTN1	Novel organic cation transporter 1	Gabapentin
SLC22A5	OCTN2	Novel organic cation transporter 2	Carnitine
SLC22A6	OAT1	Organic anion transporter 1	Adefovir, tenofovir
SLC22A7	OAT2	Organic anion transporter 2	Ganciclovir, allopurinol
SLC22A8	OAT3	Organic anion transporter 3	Cimetidine, cefotaxime
SLC22A11	OAT4	Organic anion transporter 4	Bumetanide, ketoprofen
SLC22A12	URAT1	Urate anion exchanger 1	Uric acid, oxypurinol
SLCO1A2	OATP1A2	Organic anion transporting polypeptide A	Methotrexate, fexofenadine
SLCO1B1	OATP1B1	Organic anion transporting polypeptide C	Pravastatin, repaglinide
SLCO1B3	OATP1B3	Organic anion transporting polypeptide B	Digoxin, paclitaxel
SLCO2B1	OATOP2B1	Organic anion transporting polypeptide B	Atorvastatin benzylpenicillin
SLC47A1	MATE1	Multidrug and toxin extrusion 1	Cimetidine, metformin
SLC47A2	MATE2-K	Multidrug and toxin extrusion 2	Cimetidine, metformin
Efflux transporters			
ABCB1	P-gp	P-glycoprotein	Etoposide, imatinib
ABCB11	BSEP	Bile salt export pump	Paclitaxel
ABCC1	MRP1	Multidrug resistance-associated protein 1	Methotrexate
ABCC2	MRP2	Multidrug resistance-associated protein 2	Doxorubicin, cisplatin
ABCC3	MRP3	Multidrug resistance-associated protein 3	Etoposide, methotrexate
ABCC4	MRP4	Multidrug resistance-associated protein 4	Methotrexate
ABCC6	MRP6	Multidrug resistance-associated protein 6	Anthracyclines
ABCG2	BCRP	Breast cancer resistance protein	Mitoxantrone, doxorubicin

From: Cropp CD, Yee SW, Giacomini KM. Genetic variation in drug transporters in ethnic populations. Clin Pharmacol Ther 2008;84:412–416.

and the processes in which they are involved in drug absorption and disposition are shown schematically in Fig. 4-8.

The CNS exemplifies, perhaps to the greatest extent, the consequences of the presence of carrier-mediated transport on drug distribution. The apparent lack of movement of many drugs across the blood-brain barrier is explained not only by the lipoidal nature of the barrier and the virtual absence of paracellular spaces, but also by the presence of efflux transporters. Many of these efflux transporters, P-glycoprotein being the most important identified so far, have the potential to keep the unbound concentration in the CNS relatively low compared to that in plasma, even at equilibrium.

To appreciate whether a transporter is likely to influence the relative concentration of drug on either side of a membrane, consider Fig. 4-9, which schematically shows three transport processes in brain. The dashed arrow is passive diffusion; the open arrow is passive facilitated diffusion, and the solid arrow is one involving an active efflux process.

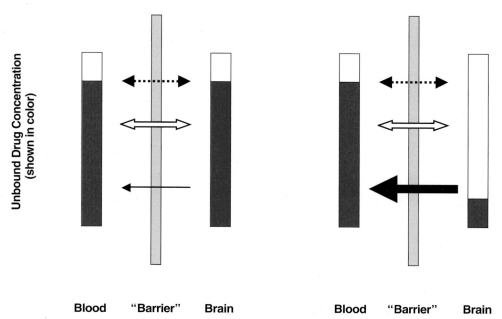

Key	Process	Example Transporter
A	Intestinal Uptake	OATPs
B	Intestinal Efflux	MDR1*, BCRP
C	Hepatic Uptake	OATPs
D	Hepatic Efflux	MRP3
E	Biliary Secretion	MDR1, MRP2
F	Renal Uptake	OAT3
G	Renal Secretion	MDR1, MRP2
H	Renal Reabsorption	SVCT1
I	Brain Uptake	LAT1
J	Brain Efflux	MDR1, BCRP

*Commonly called P-glycoprotein

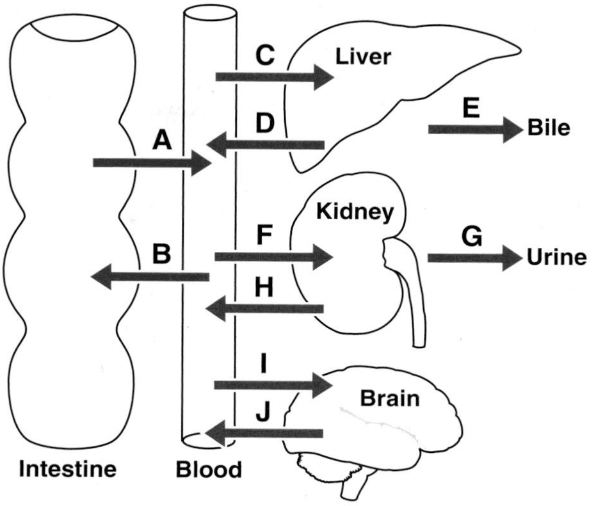

FIGURE 4-8. Selected transporters involved in intestinal absorption and in disposition of drugs within the liver, kidney, and brain. The names of these transporters and their general transport function within each of these tissues are identified.

FIGURE 4-9. Substances enter the brain by simple diffusion (*dashed arrow*) and facilitated diffusion (*open arrow*). Even when active efflux transporters (*solid arrow*) are also present, the equilibrium ratio of unbound concentrations, brain to blood, can be close to one if the passive processes are inherently faster than the efflux transport (*on left*) or close to zero if the opposite is true (*on right*). For substances whose physicochemical properties (small in size, lipophilic, no charge) make them diffuse quickly, equilibrium tends to be rapidly achieved with left-hand condition prevailing.

In Fig. 4-9A, the passive processes are fast and active efflux transport is relatively slow or absent. As a consequence, at equilibrium, the unbound concentration in brain is virtually the same as that in plasma. In Fig. 4-9B, the passive processes are slow compared to the efflux process so that the unbound concentration within the brain always remains low compared to that in blood. The apparent lack of entry into the CNS is shown in Fig. 4-10 for indinavir (Crixivan), a moderately large compound (MW = 712 g/mol) used for treating human immunodeficiency virus (HIV) infections.

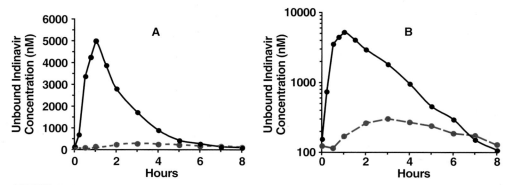

FIGURE 4-10. The mean steady-state unbound concentration–time profile of the HIV protease inhibitor indinavir in cerebrospinal fluid (*colored*) and plasma (*black*) over dosing interval during chronic oral administration of 800 mg every 8 hr in 8 symptom-free adults with HIV type 1 infection. **A.** Linear plot. **B.** Semilogarithmic plot. Note the much lower average unbound indinavir concentration in cerebrospinal fluid than in plasma. Also note that the unbound cerebrospinal fluid concentration peaks much later than does that of plasma and has a greatly reduced fluctuation. These observations are consequences of slow passive diffusion and efficient efflux, resulting in a slow and incomplete movement of drug into the cerebrospinal fluid. (From: Haas DW, Stone J, Clough LA, et al. Steady-state pharmacokinetics of indinavir in cerebrospinal fluid and plasma among adults with human immunodeficiency virus type 1 infection. Clin Pharmacol Ther 2000;68:367–374.)

Antihistamines further demonstrate the importance of drug transport and lipophilicity in drug action. Unlike the "first generation" antihistamines (e.g., chlorpheniramine, diphenhydramine, and hydroxyzine), which caused drowsiness, the "second generation" antihistamines (e.g., azelastine [Astelin], cetirizine [Zyrtec], fexofenadine [Allegra], and desloratadine [Clarinex]) are essentially devoid of sedative properties, not because they interact at a different receptor, or have a stimulating effect, but rather because they poorly penetrate the blood-brain barrier. This poor penetration is a consequence of their being good substrates for the efflux transporter, P-glycoprotein, as well as their being more hydrophilic than the "first generation" compounds.

REVERSIBLE NATURE OF TRANSPORT

It is important to remember that drug transport across membranes is generally bidirectional. One tends, for example, to think of the transport between gastrointestinal lumen and mesenteric blood as unidirectional, resulting in drug absorption. Normally, with very high initial concentrations of drug in the gastrointestinal lumen following oral administration, relative to the unbound drug concentration in mesenteric blood, the net rate of transport is indeed toward the systemic circulation. However, important applications can be made of transport in the opposite direction. For example, repeated oral administration of the adsorbent, activated charcoal, or the ion-exchange resin cholestyramine can hasten removal from the body of drugs such as digoxin, phenobarbital, and the

TABLE 4-3	Time to Reduce the Plasma Concentration of the Active Metabolite of the Prodrug, Leflunomide, by 50% in the Presence and Absence of Activated Charcoal Treatment*

	No Charcoal Treatment	**With Charcoal Treatment†**
Time for plasma concentration to drop in half.	14–18 days	1–2 days

*Suspension of activated charcoal was given (orally or via nasogastric tube) in a dose of 50 g every 6 hr.
†From: Rozman B. Clinical pharmacokinetics of leflunomide. Clin Pharmacokinet 2002;41:421–430.

active immunomodulatory metabolite of the prodrug leflunomide (Arava), in cases of overdose. Data for the leflunomide metabolite are given in Table 4-3. Because of repeated administration of charcoal and extensive adsorption of the drug to charcoal, the lumen of the gastrointestinal tract acts as a sink. The systemically circulating metabolite is removed both directly from blood via the intestinal membranes and by preventing its reabsorption after biliary secretion. In general, to optimize removal it is important to maintain distribution of adsorbent along the entire gastrointestinal tract by administering it repeatedly. Even with proper distribution of the adsorbent, the overall rate of transfer into the intestinal lumen depends on the permeability of the functional membranes along the length of the gut, as well as on blood flow to these various sites. When elimination primarily occurs by biliary excretion, as with the leflunomide metabolite, then it may be particularly important for the adsorbent to be in the duodenum in sufficient amounts to substantially adsorb drug when the gall bladder empties (i.e., after eating). Also of importance is how much loss occurs by the adsorbent treatment relative to that by the body's own ability to eliminate the drug.

Adsorbents, such as charcoal and cholestyramine, are also administered (often by a nasogastric tube) to decrease the rate and extent of absorption of drugs and other substances after their oral intake in cases of acute overdose. One key to the success of these procedures is to administer the adsorbent while much of the substance still resides in the stomach, to prevent or slow its subsequent intestinal absorption. Even if most of the dose has been systemically absorbed, the adsorbent may still help remove the substance from the systemic circulation by the processes discussed in the previous paragraph.

RATE OF DISTRIBUTION TO TISSUES

Although it may have great viewer impact on TV and films to portray a person succumbing instantly to the deadly effects of an ingested drug or poison acting on the heart, brain, or respiratory center, reality is very different. Even if systemic absorption were instantaneous, which of course it is not, tissue distribution also takes time; it occurs at various rates and to various extents, as illustrated by the experimental data in Fig. 4-11. Several factors determine the distribution pattern of a drug with time. Included are delivery of drug to tissues by blood, ability to cross tissue membranes, binding within blood and tissues, and partitioning into fat. Tissue uptake from blood, commonly called **extravasation**, continues toward equilibrium of the diffusible form of the drug between tissue and blood perfusing it.

Distribution can be rate-limited by either **perfusion** (a delivery limitation) or **permeability** (ease of crossing a membrane). A **perfusion-rate limitation** prevails when the tissue membranes present essentially no barrier to distribution. As expected, this condition is likely to be met by small lipophilic drugs diffusing across most membranes of the body and, by almost all drugs, except macromolecules diffusing across loosely knit membranes, such as capillary walls of muscle and subcutaneous tissue (see also Chapter 6, *Kinetics Following an Extravascular Dose*, and Chapter 21, *Protein Drugs*).

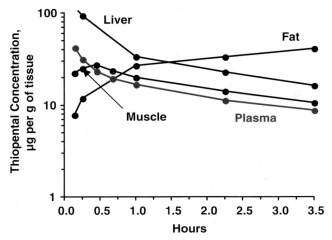

FIGURE 4-11. Semilogarithmic plot of the concentration (µg per g of tissue) of thiopental, a lipophilic drug, in various tissues and plasma (*colored line*) following an i.v. bolus dose of 25 mg/kg to dog. Note the early rise and fall of thiopental in a well-perfused tissue (liver), the slower rise in muscle, a poorly perfused tissue, and still slower rise in adipose, a poorly perfused tissue with a high affinity for thiopental. After 3 hr, much of the drug remaining in the body is in adipose tissue. (From: Brodie BB, Bernstein E, Mark LC. The role of body fat in limiting the duration of action of thiopental. J Pharmacol Exp Ther 1952;105:421–426. Copyright Williams & Wilkins.)

PERFUSION RATE LIMITATION

Blood, perfusing tissues, delivers and removes substances. Accordingly, viewing any tissue as a whole, the movement of drug through membranes cannot be separated from perfusion considerations. When movement through a membrane readily occurs, the slowest or rate-limiting step in the entire process becomes perfusion, not permeability, as shown in Fig. 4-12. The initial rate of movement of drug into the tissue is determined by the rate of its delivery, which depends on blood flow.

Perfusion is usually expressed in units of milliliters of blood per minute per gram of tissue. As seen in Table 4-4 (page 88), the perfusion rate of tissues varies from approximately 10 mL/min per g of tissue for lungs down to values of only 0.025 mL/min per g of tissue for fat or resting muscle. All other factors remaining equal, well-perfused tissues take up a drug much more rapidly than do poorly perfused tissues. Moreover, as the subsequent analysis shows, there is a direct correlation between tissue perfusion rate and the time required to distribute a drug to a tissue.

Figure 4-13 (page 88) shows blood perfusing a tissue in which distribution is perfusion rate-limited and no elimination occurs. The rate of presentation to the tissue is the product of blood flow, Q, and arterial blood concentration, C_A, that is,

$$Rate\ of\ presentation = Q \cdot C_A \qquad 4\text{-}2$$

The net rate of **extravasation**, movement from blood into the tissues, is the difference between rates of presentation and leaving, $Q \cdot C_V$, where C_V is the emergent venous blood concentration. Therefore,

$$Rate\ of\ extravasation = Q \cdot (C_A - C_V) \qquad 4\text{-}3$$

The maximum initial rate of uptake is the rate of presentation, $Q \cdot C_A$. Further, with no effective impedance to movement into the tissue, blood and tissue can be viewed kinetically as one compartment, with the concentration in emergent venous blood (C_V) in equilibrium with that in the tissue, C_T.

At any time, therefore,

$$Amount\ in\ tissue = V_T \cdot C_T = V_T \cdot Kp_b \cdot C_V \qquad 4\text{-}4$$

A. Perfusion-Rate Limitation

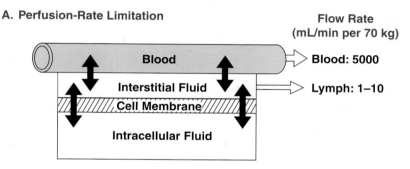

B. Permeability-Rate Limitation

1. *At Cell Membrane*

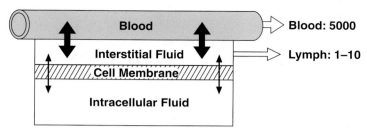

2. *At Both Capillary and Cell Membranes*

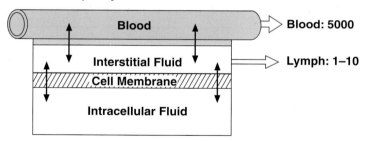

FIGURE 4-12. The limiting step controlling rate of movement of drug across membranes, from blood to tissue or the converse, varies. **A.** If membranes offer no resistance (noted by large arrows), drug in the blood leaving the tissue is in virtual equilibrium with that within the interstitial fluids and cells; blood and tissue may be viewed as one compartment. Here, movement of drug is rate-limited by blood flow. **B.** A permeability-rate limitation exists if membrane permeability to drug movement becomes low (noted by small arrows); movement into such tissues is both slow and insensitive to changes in perfusion. Also, equilibrium is not achieved between cells and blood by the time the blood leaves the tissue; blood and tissue cells must now be viewed as separate drug compartments. For some tissues (i.e., muscle, kidneys, heart), the permeability limitation is at the cell membrane **(B1)**. For others (e.g., the central nervous system and testes), an additional permeability limitation occurs at the capillary membrane **(B2)**. Interstitial fluid also flows into the lymphatic system. Although low, 1–10 mL/min per 70 kg, compared to a blood flow of 5000 mL/min per 70 kg, lymph flow plays a major role in keeping the concentration of slowly diffusing molecules, especially proteins, low in the interstitial fluid, relative to that in blood. The lymphatic pathway is also important for the systemic absorption of macromolecules after intramuscular and subcutaneous administration (see Chapter 21, *Protein Drugs*). These large molecules move through the capillary membranes so slowly that, by default, they mostly reach the systemic blood by moving through the lymphatic vessels, which in turn empty into the systemic blood via the vena cava. For macromolecules, then, the heavy arrows in the lower graph become very thin ones and movement into lymph predominates.

TABLE 4-4   **Blood Flow, Perfusion Rate, and Relative Size of Different Organs and Tissues Under Basal Conditions in a Standard 70-kg Young Healthy Adult**

Organ*	Percent of Body Weight	Blood Flow (ml/min)	Percent of Cardiac Output	Perfusion Rate (mL/min per g of tissue)
1. Adrenal glands	0.03	25	0.2	1.2
2. Blood	7	(5000)*	(100)	-
3. Bone	16	250	5	0.02
4. Brain	2.0	700	14	0.5
5. Adipose	15†	200	4	0.025
6. Heart	0.4	200	4	0.6
7. Kidneys	0.5	1100	22	4.0
8. Liver	2.3	1350	27	0.8
Portal	1.7 (Gut)	(1050)	(21)	-
Arterial	-	(300)	(6)	-
9. Lungs	1.6	5000	100	10.0
10. Muscle (inactive)	43	750	15	0.025
11. Skin (cool weather)	11	300	6	0.04
12. Spleen	0.3	77	1.5	0.4
13. Thyroid gland	0.03	50	1	2.4
Total Body	100	5000	100	0.071

*Some organs (e.g., stomach, intestines, spleen, and pancreas) are not included.
†Includes fat within organs. Because 75–80 kg is more typical of body weight today, a better estimate of this value in an average person is closer to 20%.
From: Guyton AC. Textbook of Medical Physiology. 7th ed. Philadelphia: WB Saunders; 1986:230; Lentner C, ed., Geigy Scientific Tables, vol. 1. Edison, NJ: Ciba-Geigy; 1981; and Davies B, Morris T: Physiological parameters in laboratory animals and humans. Pharm Res 1993;10:1093–1095.

where V_T is the tissue volume and Kp_b is the tissue-to-blood equilibrium distribution ratio (C_T/C_V). Furthermore, the fractional rate of leaving the tissue, k_T, is given by

$$k_T = \frac{Rate\ of\ leaving}{Amount\ in\ tissue} = \frac{Q \cdot C_V}{V_T \cdot Kp_b \cdot C_V} = \frac{Q/V_T}{Kp_b} \qquad 4\text{-}5$$

where Q/V_T is the perfusion rate of the tissue. The parameter k_T, the **distribution rate constant**, with units of reciprocal time, may be regarded as a measure of how rapidly drug would

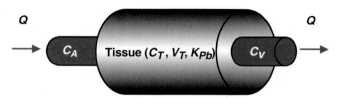

FIGURE 4-13.   Drug is presented to a tissue at an arterial concentration of C_A and at a rate equal to the product of blood flow, Q, and C_A. The drug leaves the tissue at a venous concentration, C_V, and at a rate equal to $Q \cdot C_V$. The tissue concentration, C_T, increases when the rate of presentation exceeds the rate of leaving in the venous blood, and the converse. The amount of drug in the tissue is the product of V_T, the volume of the tissue, and the tissue drug concentration. The ratio of C_T to C_V at equilibrium is Kp_b.

leave the tissue if the arterial concentration were suddenly to drop to zero. It is analogous to the elimination rate constant for loss of drug from the whole body and, like elimination, the kinetics of tissue distribution can be characterized by a **tissue distribution half-life** for which

$$Distribution\ half\text{-}life = 0.693 \cdot \frac{Kp_b}{Q/V_T} \qquad 4\text{-}6$$

Thus, drug leaves slowly from tissues that have a high affinity ($K_{P,b}$) for it and that are poorly perfused.

Suppose now, that the arterial blood concentration is maintained constant with time. Then tissue uptake continues, but at a decreasing rate as tissue concentration rises, until equilibrium is achieved, when the net rate of uptake is zero, $C_V = C_A$ and $C_T = K_{P,b} \cdot C_A$. This situation is analogous to events occurring during a constant-rate infusion of drug into the body (Chapter 10, *Constant-Rate Input*), with the equation defining the rise of tissue concentration to its plateau being given by

$$Tissue\ concentration = K_{P,b} \cdot C_A \cdot (1 - e^{-k_T \cdot t}) \qquad 4\text{-}7$$

Thus, the approach to plateau is determined solely by the tissue distribution half-life. In one half-life, the tissue concentration is 50% of its plateau value; in two half-lives, it is 75%; at 3.32 half-lives, it is 90%; and so on.

To appreciate the foregoing, consider the events depicted in Fig. 4-14. Shown are plots of concentration in various tissues with time during the maintenance of a constant

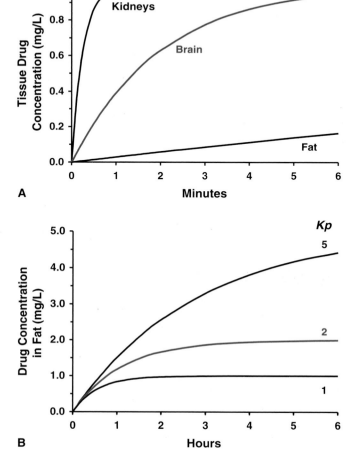

FIGURE 4-14. When distribution is perfusion rate-limited, the time to reach distribution equilibrium in tissue, when the arterial blood concentration is constant (1 mg/L), depends on the perfusion rate and the tissue-to-plasma distribution equilibrium ratio. **A.** Concentrations with time in kidney, brain, and fat tissues with different perfusion rates for a drug with a $Kp_b = 1$ in all three tissues. **B.** Concentrations with time in fat of three drugs with Kp_b values of 1, 2, and 5, respectively. Note the difference in time scales of **A** (minute) and **B** (hour).

arterial blood concentration of 1 mg/L. First consider panel A in which the $K_{P,b}$ values of a drug in kidneys, brain, and adipose tissue are the same and equal to one. Given that the perfusion rates to these tissues are 4, 0.5, and 0.03 mL/min per g of tissue, respectively (Table 4-4), it follows that the corresponding half-lives for distribution are 0.17, 1.4, and 23 min. Thus, by 1 min (more than four half-lives), drug in the kidneys has reached equilibrium with that in blood, while it takes closer to 5 and 75 min (>3.32 half-lives) for 90% of equilibrium to be reached in brain and fat, tissues of lower perfusion. Next, consider panel B, in which events in adipose tissue are shown for drugs with different $K_{P,b}$ values, namely 1, 2, and 5. Here the corresponding half-lives are 23, 46, and 115 min. Now, not only is the time taken for drug in tissue to reach equilibrium different, but so are the equilibrium tissue concentrations.

These simple examples illustrate two basic principles. Namely, both the approach toward equilibrium in, and the loss of drug from, a tissue take longer the poorer the perfusion and the greater the partitioning of drug into a tissue. The latter is contrary to what one might intuitively anticipate. However, the greater the tendency to concentrate in a tissue, the longer it takes to deliver to that tissue the amount needed to reach distribution equilibrium and the longer it takes to redistribute drug out of that tissue. Stated differently, an increased affinity for a tissue accentuates an existing limitation imposed by perfusion.

A **perfusion limitation** is exemplified in Fig. 4-15 for the passage of selected hydrophilic substances across the jejunal membranes of a rat, from lumen to perfusing blood. The blood acts as a sink by carrying drug away from the absorption site to the other tissues of the body. Tritiated water (MW = 18 g/mol) moves freely through the membrane, and its rate of passage increases with increasing perfusion. The passage of

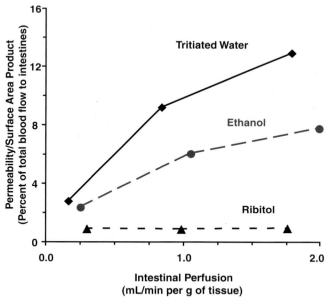

FIGURE 4-15. The rate of passage of a substance across the jejunum of a rat was determined by measuring its rate of appearance in intestinal venous blood. The passage is perfusion rate-limited when, like tritiated water and many small lipophilic compounds, the molecule freely permeates the membrane. With poorly permeable substances, like the polar molecule ribitol and many polar antibiotics, the passage is limited by transmembrane permeability, not by perfusion. The permeability only approaches about 15% of total blood flow to the intestines because only 15% of the intestinal blood flow perfuses the region of the intestines where absorption occurs. (From: Winne D, Remischovsky J. Intestinal blood flow and absorption of non-dissociable substances. J Pharm Pharmacol 1970;22:640–641.)

ethanol (MW = 46 g/mol) is similarly mostly perfusion rate-limited, as is the passage of many small lipophilic molecules across the intestinal epithelium (not shown) and many other membranes.

PERMEABILITY-RATE LIMITATION

As cell membrane resistance to drug transport increases, the rate limitation moves from one of perfusion to one of permeability. The problem now lies in penetrating the membrane, not in delivering drug to, or removing it from, the tissue. As mentioned previously, this increase in resistance may arise for the same drug crossing membranes of increasing thickness; for example, the multiple cell layers of the skin epidermis are less permeable to a drug than the single cell layer of the capillary epithelium. For the same membrane, as previously discussed, resistance increases with increasing size and polarity of the molecule. Thus, transport across the jejunum is slower for the pentose sugar ribitol (MW = 152 g/mol) and many other large polar compounds than for ethanol or water, which results in decreased sensitivity to changes in perfusion (see Fig. 4-15).

A permeability-rate limitation arises particularly for polar drugs diffusing across tightly knit lipoidal membranes, as demonstrated in Fig. 4-16 for the passage of compounds into the cerebrospinal fluid. In this study, the concentration of each drug was measured in cerebrospinal fluid, relative to that in plasma water (unbound), with time following attainment and maintenance of a constant plasma concentration. Differences in ease of entry are a function of both lipid-to-water partition coefficient and degree of ionization, suggesting that only the un-ionized drug penetrates brain. For example, the lipophilicity (expressed by the n-octanol/water partition coefficient) of salicylic acid and pentobarbital are similar, yet the time required to reach distribution equilibrium is far shorter for pentobarbital than for salicylic acid because, being

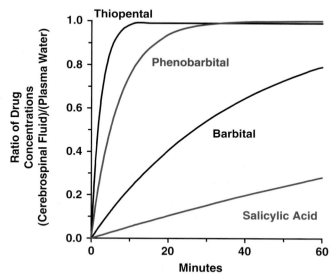

FIGURE 4-16. Equilibration of drug in the cerebrospinal fluid with that in plasma is often permeability rate-limited. The ratio of drug concentrations (cerebrospinal fluid/unbound drug in plasma) is shown for various drugs in the dog. The plasma concentration was kept relatively constant throughout the study. Notice that when a permeability rate limitation occurs the time to achieve equilibrium is longer than that when uptake is perfusion rate limited, as occurs with the lipophilic thiopental. (From: Brodie BB, Kurz H, Schanker LS. The importance of dissociation constant and lipid-solubility in influencing the passage of drugs into the cerebrospinal fluid. J Pharmacol Exp Ther 1960;130:20–25. Copyright 1960, The Williams & Wilkins Co., Baltimore.)

the weaker acid (pKa 8.1 versus 3.0 for salicylic acid), a greater fraction of pentobarbital is un-ionized in both plasma and cerebrospinal fluid, pH 7.4.

With large differences in perfusion and permeability of various tissues, it would appear to be impossible to predict tissue distribution of a drug. However, either of these two factors may limit the rate of extravasation, thereby simplifying the situation and allowing some conclusion to be drawn. Consider, for example, the following question: "Why, on measuring total tissue concentration, does the i.v. anesthetic propofol enter the brain much more rapidly that it does muscle tissue; yet for penicillin, the opposite is true?" The explanation lies in both the physicochemical properties of these drugs and the anatomical features of these tissues.

Propofol is a nonpolar, lipophilic, very weak acid (pKa = 11) that is insignificantly ionized at plasma pH (7.4). As such, its entry into both brain and muscle occurs readily and is perfusion rate-limited. Since perfusion of the brain, average of 0.5 mL/min per g of tissue, is much greater than that of muscle, 0.025 mL/min per g of tissue, entry of propofol into the brain is the more rapid process and explains its use in rapidly inducing anesthesia.

Penicillin G, a relatively large polar compound, does not readily pass through cell membranes. The faster rate of entry of penicillin into muscle than into brain arises from the greater porosity of blood capillaries in muscle than in brain. As depicted in Fig. 4-12B1, for many tissues (e.g., muscle and subcutaneous tissue), capillary membranes are very porous and have little influence on the entry of drugs of usual MW (100–400 g/mol), and even larger molecules up to 3000 g/mol, into the interstitial fluids between cells, regardless of the drug's physicochemical properties. There may well be a permeability limitation at the tissue cell membrane, but in terms of measurement of drug in the *whole* tissue, there would appear to be minimal impedance to entry of either ionized or polar compounds, or both, into muscle. Other tissues, for example, much of the CNS, anatomically have a permeability limitation at the capillary level that impedes movement of drug into the tissue as a whole, as observed with penicillin. Efflux transporters play a key role here as well. As mentioned previously, the general observation, especially with several polar organic dyes, led to the concept of the blood-brain barrier.

For large macromolecules (>5000 g/mol), especially charged or polar ones, movement across the capillary membrane is slow (permeability rate-limited). As a consequence, molecules that do move from blood to the interstitial space tend to primarily return via the lymphatic system, which drains interstitial fluid from virtually all tissues. The lymphatic route is then faster than return via the capillaries. The average flow of interstitial fluid into the lymph capillaries within the body is about 10 mL/min, whereas the rate of return of lymph to the blood is about 1 mL/min. The difference is accounted for by reabsorption of water from the lymphatic vessels and lymph nodes. As shown in Fig. 4-12, the flow of interstitial fluid into lymph capillaries and the return of lymph to the blood are very much slower than the flow of blood to and from the body's tissues (about 5000 mL/min). Nevertheless, the lymphatic system plays a major role in keeping the concentration of such large molecules lower in the interstitial fluids than in plasma. It is also important in determining the rate and extent of systemic absorption of macromolecules following their intramuscular or subcutaneous administration, a topic covered in Chapter 21, *Protein Drugs*.

The effect of a high equilibrium distribution ratio (Kp_b) on the time to achieve distribution equilibrium, discussed previously for a perfusion-rate limitation, applies equally well to a permeability-rate limitation. A permeability-rate limitation simply decreases the rate of entry and hence increases the time to reach distribution equilibrium *over that of perfusion*. Where the equilibrium lies is independent, however, of which process is rate-limiting.

If the arterial concentration is maintained long enough, the unbound concentration in tissue becomes the same as that in plasma. Sometimes, however, this equality is not ob-

TABLE 4-5	Distribution of Albumin in the Standard Young, Healthy Adult	
Organ	**Amount (g/70-kg person)**	**Concentration (g/kg)**
Intravascular		
Plasma	140	43
Blood cells	0	0
Extravascular		
Muscle	50	2.3
Skin	40	7.7
Liver	2	1.4
Gut	8	5
Other tissues	110	3
Total	210	
Total body	350	8.3*

*Amount (g) per total body water (42 L).
From: Peters T. Serum albumin. In: Putnam FW, ed. The plasma proteins. 2nd ed., vol. 1. New York: Academic Press; 1975:162.

served. Reasons for lack of equality include maintenance of sink conditions by intracellular metabolism, active transport, bulk flow of interstitial fluids through both lymphatic channels and ducts, and pH gradients across cell membranes. Inequality in unbound concentration is frequently observed in the cerebrospinal fluid relative to plasma for large polar molecules (e.g., many antibiotics). One likely explanation here is that fluid formation is sufficiently fast relative to diffusion that the resulting concentration, even at steady state, remains below that of the diffusible unbound drug in plasma. An example is that of the distribution of albumin in the body (Table 4-5). Albumin slowly diffuses across the endothelial linings of the capillaries. The bulk flow of water in the interstitial fluids and lymphatic vessels provides a means of removing albumin from the tissues. The resulting interstitial concentration is well below that of plasma. Albumin also diffuses into the cerebrospinal fluid, but the rate process is so slow compared to that of production of the fluid that the albumin concentration is very low. When there is a breakdown in the blood–cerebrospinal-fluid barrier, as occurs for example in meningitis, the albumin concentration in the cerebrospinal fluid increases as a result of an increased permeability to this protein.

EXTENT OF DISTRIBUTION

Multiple equilibria occur within plasma where drug can bind to various proteins, examples of which are listed in Table 4-6. Acidic drugs commonly bind to albumin, the most abundant plasma protein. Basic drugs often bind to α_1-acid glycoprotein, and neutral lipophilic compounds associate with lipoproteins. Proteins, such as γ-globulin, transcortin, fibrinogen, sex hormone-binding globulin, and thyroid-binding globulin, bind specific compounds. Many large protein drugs also have specific protein carriers. Commonly, more than one plasma protein is involved. Tissue distribution can also involve multiple equilibria. Ionized basic compounds, for example, form ion pairs with the abundant acidic phospholipids in tissues. Their un-ionized forms may also partition into adipose tissue.

TABLE 4-6	Representative Proteins to Which Drugs Generally and Specifically Bind in Plasma		
Protein	Molecular Weight (g/mol)	Normal Concentrations g/L	μm
General			
Albumin	67,000	35–50	500–700
α_1.Acid glycoprotein	42,000	0.4–1.0	9–23
Lipoproteins	200,000–2,400,000	Variable	
Specific			
Cortisol binding globulin (transcortin)	53,000	0.03–0.07	0.6–1.4
Sex-hormone binding globulin	90,000	0.0036	0.04

APPARENT VOLUME OF DISTRIBUTION

The concentration in plasma achieved after distribution throughout the body is complete is a result of the dose administered and the extent of tissue distribution. At equilibrium, the extent of distribution is defined by an apparent volume of distribution (V):

$$V = \frac{Amount\ in\ body\ at\ equilibrium}{Plasma\ drug\ concentration} = \frac{A}{C} \qquad 4\text{-}8$$

This parameter is useful in relating amount in body to plasma concentration, and the converse. Volumes of distribution vary widely, with illustrative values (Fig. 4-17) ranging

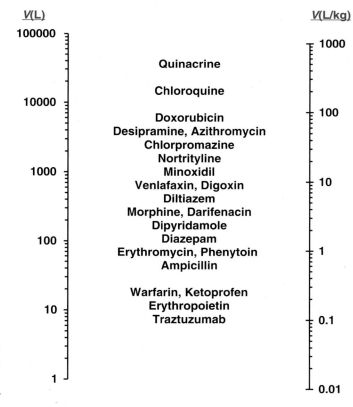

FIGURE 4-17. The apparent volume into which drugs distribute varies widely.

from 3 to 40,000 L, a value far in excess of total body size. Knowing plasma volume, V_P, and volume of distribution, V, the fraction of drug in body within and outside plasma can be estimated. The amount in plasma is $V_P \cdot C$; the amount in the body is $V \cdot C$. Therefore,

$$\textit{Fraction of drug in body within plasma} = \frac{V_P}{V} \qquad \text{4-9}$$

It is evident that the larger the volume of distribution, the smaller is the fraction in plasma. For example, for a drug with a volume of distribution of 100 L, only 3% resides in plasma. The remaining fraction, given by

$$\textit{Fraction outside plasma} = \frac{(V - V_P)}{V} \qquad \text{4-10}$$

includes drug in the blood cells. For the example considered above, 97% is outside plasma. Although this fraction can be readily determined, the specific tissues into which the drug distributes outside plasma cannot.

The reason why the volume of distribution is an apparent volume and why its value differs among drugs may be appreciated by considering the simple model shown in Fig. 4-18. In this model, drug in the body is entirely accounted for in plasma, of volume V_P, and one tissue compartment, of volume V_T. At distribution equilibrium, the amount of drug in each compartment can be expressed in terms of plasma concentration, C, volumes of the two compartments, and the tissue-to-plasma equilibrium distribution ratio, K_p, as follows:

$$A = V_P \cdot C + V_T \cdot K_P \cdot C \qquad \text{4-11}$$

$$\begin{matrix} \text{Amount} & \text{Amount} & \text{Amount} \\ \text{in body} & \text{in plasma} & \text{in tissue} \end{matrix}$$

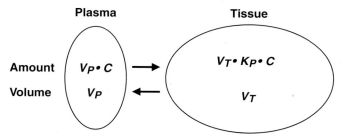

FIGURE 4-18.   The effect of tissue binding on volume of distribution is illustrated by a drug that distributes between plasma and a tissue. The physiologic volumes are V_P and V_T, respectively. At equilibrium, the amount of drug in each location depends on the equilibrium distribution (partition) ratio, Kp, the plasma and tissue volumes, and the plasma concentration.

And because $A = V \cdot C$ (Eq. 4-8), it follows, on dividing the equation above by C, that

$$V = V_P + V_T \cdot K_P \qquad \text{4-12}$$

The product $V_T \cdot K_P$ is the apparent volume of a tissue viewed from measurement of drug in plasma. Thus, by expanding the model to embrace all individual tissues of the body, it is seen that the volume of distribution of a drug is the volume of plasma plus the sum of the apparent volumes of distribution of each tissue, namely,

$$V = V_P + V_{T_1} \cdot K_{P_1} + V_{T_2} \cdot K_{P_2} \cdots \cdots \qquad \text{4-13}$$

For some tissues the value of K_P is large, which explains why the sum of the volume of distribution terms $(V_{T_i} \cdot K_{P_i})$ of some drugs can be much greater than total body size. Adipose tissue, for example, occupies approximately 20% of body volume. If the K_P value in adipose tissue is 5, then this tissue alone has an apparent volume of distribution equal to that of total body volume.

The volume of distribution of a specific drug can vary widely among patients. The reasons for such differences are now explored. Before doing so, however, a general point is considered.

BINDING WITHIN BLOOD

Within blood, drug can bind to many components including blood cells and plasma proteins. As a consequence of binding, the concentration of drug in whole blood (C_b), in plasma (C), and unbound in plasma water (Cu) can differ greatly, as discussed in Chapter 2, *Fundamental Concepts and Terminology*. For ease of chemical analysis, plasma is the most common fluid analyzed. In many respects, this choice is unfortunate. One of the primary goals of measuring concentration is to relate the measurement to pharmacologic response and toxicity. However, only unbound drug can pass through most cell membranes, the protein-bound form being too large. Accordingly, the unbound drug concentration is undoubtedly more closely related to the activity of the drug than is the total plasma concentration. Yet unbound concentration is only occasionally measured, primarily because the methods for doing so are often tedious, lack accuracy and precision, and are costly. Nonetheless, it is helpful to define an unbound volume of distribution, Vu,

$$Vu = \frac{Amount\ in\ body\ at\ equilibrium}{Unbound\ plasma\ concentration} = \frac{A}{Cu} \qquad 4\text{-}14$$

which permits the amount of drug in the body to be related to the unbound drug concentration.

Sometimes, whole blood concentration is measured, especially when extraction concepts are considered (see Chapter 5, *Elimination*). Once again, an appropriate volume term, V_b, can be defined. Namely,

$$V_b = \frac{Amount\ in\ body\ at\ equilibrium}{Unbound\ plasma\ concentration} = \frac{A}{C_b} \qquad 4\text{-}15$$

As the amount of drug in body is independent of the site of measurement, it follows from Eqs. 4-8, 4-14, and 4-15 that

$$V \cdot C = Vu \cdot Cu = V_b \cdot C_b \qquad 4\text{-}16$$

The values of these volume terms can differ markedly for a given drug. The term most often quoted in the literature is based on measurement of drug in plasma (i.e., V). Examples of drugs with differing values of V are given in Fig. 4-17, whereas examples of differing values of V, V_b, and Vu for a few selected drugs are listed in Table 4-7. Note that all the volumes are nearly the same for caffeine, which does not bind appreciably either in plasma or tissues. Also note that some drugs (e.g., amitriptyline, maprotiline, mibefradil, and propofol) have very large unbound volumes of distribution, in large part a consequence of being highly bound in tissues, as discussed below.

PLASMA PROTEIN BINDING

The principal concern with plasma protein binding is related to its variability within and among patients in various therapeutic settings. The degree of binding is frequently expressed as the bound-to-total concentration ratio. This ratio has limiting values of 0 and 1.0. Drugs with values greater than 0.9 are said to be extensively bound.

As stated previously, unbound, rather than bound, concentration is more important in therapeutics. Therefore, the fraction of drug in plasma unbound, fu, is

$$fu = \frac{Cu}{C} \qquad 4\text{-}17$$

The fraction unbound is of greater utility than fraction bound. Obviously, only if fu is constant is total plasma concentration a good measure of changes in unbound drug con-

TABLE 4-7 Distributional Properties of Selected Drugs

Drug	Class*	Volume of Distribution V (L/70 kg)	Volume of Distribution Based on Concentration in Whole Blood V_b (L/70 kg)	Volume of Distribution Based on Unbound Concentration in Plasma Vu (L/70 kg)	Ratio of Plasma and Whole Blood Concentrations C/C_b	Fraction Unbound in Plasma fu	Fraction Unbound in Tissues[†] fu_T
Amitriptyline	B	581	676	10,375	1.16	0.056	0.0038
Caffeine	N	47	45	67	0.96	0.7	0.62
Fluvastatin	A	29	16	3722	0.54	0.0079	0.012
Ibuprofen	A	7	13	1148	1.82	0.0061	0.059
Maprotiline	B	3010	1771	25,083	0.56	0.12	0.0016
Metoprolol	B	242	212	269	0.88	0.90	0.147
Mibefradil	B	213	333	28,373	1.2	0.0075	0.134
Propofol	N	340	272	12,150	1.2	0.25	0.0032

*Class: A = acidic drug, B = basic drug, N = neutral compound throughout physiologic pH range.
[†]Calculated using a rearrangement of Eq. 4-25 and letting V_P = 3 L and V_T = 39 L.
From: Rodgers T, Rowland M. Mechanistic approaches to volume of distribution predictions: understanding the processes. Pharm Res 2007;24:918–933.

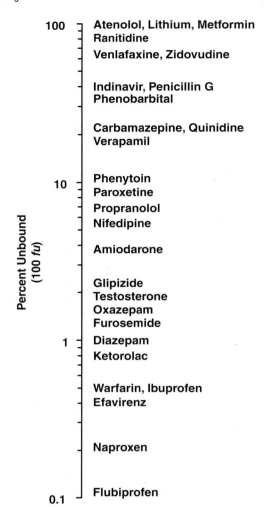

FIGURE 4-19. The percent of drug in plasma unbound varies widely among drugs.

centration. Approximate values of *fu* usually associated with therapy for representative drugs are shown in Fig. 4-19.

Binding is a function of the affinity of the protein for the drug. The affinity is characterized by an association constant, K_a. Because the number of binding sites on a protein is limited, binding also depends on the molar concentrations of both drug and protein. For a single binding site on the protein, the association is simply summarized by the following reaction:

$$Drug + Protein \rightleftharpoons Drug\text{–}protein\ Complex$$

Equilibrium may lie either to the right or to the left. High affinity, of course, implies that equilibrium lies far to the right. This is a relative statement, however, as the greater the protein concentration for a given drug concentration, the greater the bound drug concentration and the converse. From mass law considerations, the equilibrium is expressed in terms of the concentrations of unbound drug, *Cu*, unoccupied protein, *P*, and bound drug, C_{bd}, thus,

$$Ka = \frac{C_{bd}}{Cu \cdot P} \qquad\qquad 4\text{-}18$$

The unoccupied protein concentration, *P*, depends on the total protein concentration, P_t. These two concentrations are related by $fu_p = P/P_t$, where fu_p is the fraction

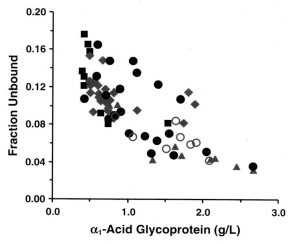

FIGURE 4-20. The fraction unbound of propranolol varies with the plasma concentration of α_1-acid glycoprotein, its binding protein, in 78 patients with various diseases (renal, ●; arthritis, ○; Crohn's disease, ▲; cirrhosis, ■) and in healthy volunteers (◆). In all cases, the protein is not saturated; the molar concentration of propranolol is below that of α_1-acid glycoprotein. (From: Tozer TN. Implications of altered plasma protein binding in disease states. In: Benet LZ, Massoud N, Gambertoglio JG, eds. Pharmacokinetic Basis for Drug Treatment. New York: Raven Press; 1983:173–193. Original data from Piafsky KM, Borgá O, Odar-Cederlöf I, et al. Increased plasma protein binding of propranolol and chlorpromazine mediated by disease-induced elevations of plasma α_1-acid glycoprotein. N Engl J Med 1978;299:1435–1439. Reproduced with permission of Raven Press.)

of the total number of binding sites unoccupied. Furthermore, the unbound concentration is $fu \cdot C$ and the bound concentration is $(1 - fu) \cdot C$. Appropriately substituting into Eq. 4-18, it therefore follows upon rearrangement that

$$fu = \frac{1}{(1 + Ka \cdot fu_p \cdot P_t)} \qquad 4\text{-}19$$

From this relationship, the value of fu is seen to depend on the total protein concentration, as illustrated in Fig. 4-20 for the binding of propranolol to α_1-acid glycoprotein in plasma. Often the binding site is not saturated at therapeutic concentrations, so that fu_p remains close to 1.0, and fu is given by $1/(1 + K_a \cdot P_t)$. If also fu is small (<0.1), Eq. 4-19 is approximately $1/(K_a \cdot P_t)$. By taking the ratio of this equation for normal and altered conditions, the value of fu (fu') when the concentration of binding protein is altered (P_t') is,

$$fu' = \frac{P_t}{P_t'} \cdot fu \qquad 4\text{-}20$$

Consider, for example, the change in fu expected for ibuprofen ($fu = 0.005$), a drug bound primarily to albumin, when the albumin concentration is decreased from 43 g/L to 28 g/L, a condition that can arise in alcoholic cirrhosis. The fraction unbound is expected to increase to 0.0077, a 54% increase.

Usually, as previously stated, only a small fraction of the available sites on binding proteins is occupied ($fu_p \approx 1$) at the therapeutic concentrations of most drugs; the fraction unbound is then relatively constant at a given protein concentration and independent of drug concentration. Occasionally, therapeutic concentrations are sufficiently high so that most of the available binding sites are occupied. Then both fu and fu_p are concentration-dependent (see Chapter 16, *Nonlinearities*).

In subsequent chapters, it will be helpful to remember that pharmacologic activity relates to the unbound concentration. Plasma protein binding, then, is often only of interest because the total plasma concentration is measured. The total plasma concentration depends on both the extent of protein binding and the unbound concentration, that is,

$$C = \frac{Cu}{fu} \qquad 4\text{-}21$$

When conceptualizing dependency and functionality, this equation should not be rearranged.

TISSUE DISTRIBUTION

The tissue-to-plasma equilibrium distribution ratio, K_p, can be large or small whether or not a drug is bound to plasma proteins. Two kinds of processes, binding to tissue components and transport (uptake and efflux transporters), are involved in determining the ratio.

Tissue Binding. The fraction of drug in body located in plasma can depend on its binding to both plasma and tissue components, as shown schematically in Fig. 4-18 (page 95). A drug may have a great affinity for plasma proteins, but may still be located primarily in tissue if the tissue has an affinity even greater than that of plasma (see data for mibefradil in Table 4-7). Unlike plasma binding, binding of a drug to tissue components cannot readily be measured. The tissue would have to be disrupted, with a resulting loss of its integrity. Even so, tissue binding is important in drug distribution.

Tissue binding may be inferred from measurement of drug binding in plasma. Consider, for example, the following mass–balance relationship,

$$\underset{\substack{\text{Amount} \\ \text{in body}}}{V \cdot C} \quad = \quad \underset{\substack{\text{Amount} \\ \text{in plasma}}}{V_P \cdot C} \quad + \quad \underset{\substack{\text{Amount} \\ \text{outside plasma}}}{V_{TW} \cdot C_{TW}} \qquad 4\text{-}22$$

in which V_{TW} is the aqueous volume outside of plasma into which the drug distributes, and C_{TW} is the corresponding total drug concentration required to account for the mass of drug in tissue. Dividing by C,

$$\underset{\substack{\text{Apparent volume} \\ \text{of distribution}}}{V} \quad = \quad \underset{\substack{\text{Volume of} \\ \text{plasma}}}{V_P} \quad + \quad \underset{\substack{\text{Apparent} \\ \text{volume of tissue}}}{V_{TW} \cdot \frac{C_{TW}}{C}} \qquad 4\text{-}23$$

Recall that $fu = Cu/C$. Similarly, for the tissue, $fu_T = Cu_T/C_{TW}$. Given that distribution equilibrium is achieved when the unbound concentrations in plasma, Cu, and in tissues, Cu_T, are equal, that is, concentrating transporters are not involved, then

$$\frac{C_{TW}}{C} = \frac{fu}{fu_T} \qquad 4\text{-}24$$

which, on substituting into Eq. 4-22, yields

$$V = V_P + V_{TW} \cdot \frac{fu}{fu_T} \qquad 4\text{-}25$$

From this relationship, it is seen that the apparent volume of distribution increases when fu is increased and decreases when fu_T is increased. Note that in Eq. 4-25, fu_T is the average value across all tissues into which drug distributes, and that to change appreciably, the affected tissues must represent the dominant ones, such as muscle, influencing V.

Clearly, a change in binding within brain alone, which comprises just 2% of the total body weight (Table 4-4), is unlikely to be reflected noticeably within plasma.

By comparing Eqs. 4-25 and 4-12, it is seen that $Kp \approx fu/fu_T$. That is, K_P is a measure of the relative binding of a drug between plasma and tissue. However, although equivalent, the advantage of Eq. 4-25 over Eq. 4-12 is that it allows for the interpretation of drug distribution among drugs, as well as when binding is altered for a specific compound. To appreciate this interpretation, first consider the statement made earlier that the volumes of distribution of basic drugs are much larger than those of acidic ones. The difference cannot be ascribed to differences in plasma binding. Examination of the data in Fig. 4-17 shows that there is no clear pattern in the fraction unbound in plasma between these two classes of compounds. For example, fu is 0.02 to 0.04 for furosemide and amiodarone, an acidic and a basic drug, respectively; yet the former has a volume of distribution of 10 L and the latter 7000 L. Therefore, the difference between acidic and basic drugs must lie in the much higher tissue binding of bases (lower fu_T). Next, consider the data for propranolol in Fig. 4-21, which shows large differences in V among different subjects. The linear relationship between V and fu not only indicates, from Eq. 4-25, that V_T/fu_T is relatively constant, (and, as the body-water content does not vary much among individuals, hence tissue binding is constant) but also that differences in binding of propranolol in plasma among subjects account for most of the variation observed in its volume of distribution.

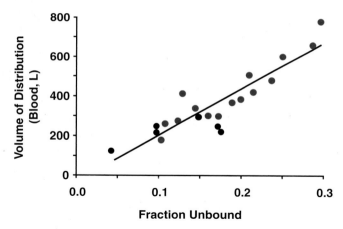

FIGURE 4-21. The volume of distribution of (+)-propranolol varies with the fraction unbound in plasma. The observation was made in 6 control subjects (●) and in 15 patients (●) with chronic hepatic disease after an i.v. 40-mg bolus dose of (+)-propranolol. (From: Branch RA, Jones J, Read AE. A study of factors influencing drug disposition in chronic liver disease, using the model drug (+)-propranolol. Br J Clin Pharmacol 1976;3:243–249.)

The equilibrium distribution ratio (K_P, concentration in tissue/concentration in plasma) varies from one tissue to another. For basic drugs, K_P appears to vary with the tissue concentration of acidic phospholipids, a primary site to which basic drugs have an affinity in the tissue (Fig. 4-22). This is undoubtedly a major contributor to the observation that bases have volumes of distribution that are much larger than those of acids.

Transporters. Uptake transporters can concentrate drug in tissues and efflux transporters can effectively keep drugs out. A useful model is derived from the schematic of Fig. 4-7 (page 81). The rate of transport into a cell is the permeability-surface area product times Cu, $P_{uptake} \cdot A \cdot Cu$, whereas that for efflux from the cell is $P_{efflux} \cdot A \cdot Cu_T$, where Cu_T is the unbound intracellular concentration. At steady state, the net movement into

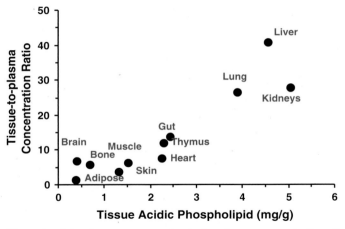

FIGURE 4-22. The ratio of the tissue concentration to the plasma concentration, K_P, of metoprolol varies with the acidic phospholipid content of tissues in the rat, suggesting that this is a primary determinant of the drug's tissue distribution. (From: Rodgers T, Leahy D, Rowland M. Tissue distribution of basic drugs: accounting for enantiomeric, compound and regional differences amongst beta-blocking drugs in rat. J Pharm Sci 2005;94:1237–1248.)

the cell is zero, therefore, the unbound concentration within the cell relative to that outside the cell is:

$$\frac{Cu_T}{Cu} = \frac{P_{uptake}}{P_{efflux}}$$

4-26

When, because of active uptake, P_{uptake} is greater than P_{efflux}, then $Cu_T > Cu$, and the converse when active efflux predominates. Recall that $Cu = fu \cdot C$ and $Cu_T = fu_T \cdot C_T$, so that

$$\frac{C_T}{C} = \frac{fu}{fu_T} \cdot \frac{Cu_T}{Cu}$$

4-27

Combining Eqs. 4-26 and 4-27, therefore, yields

$$\frac{C_T}{C} = \frac{fu}{fu_T} \cdot \frac{P_{uptake}}{P_{efflux}}$$

4-28

which on substitution into Eq. 4-25 gives

$$V = V_P + V_{TW} \cdot \frac{fu}{fu_T} \cdot \frac{P_{uptake}}{P_{efflux}}$$

4-29

As with fu_T, both P_{uptake} and P_{efflux} reflect global events in some tissues throughout the body, and are relatively insensitive to events occurring in some tissues because of limited distribution or small size, such as brain, that contribute little to the volume of distribution of the drug. Furthermore, note that if permeability is passive, $P_{uptake} = P_{efflux} = P_{passive}$, Eq. 4-29 reduces to Eq. 4-25.

The relationships expressed in Eq. 4-29 explains why, because of plasma and tissue binding and transport processes, V rarely corresponds to a defined physiologic space, such as plasma volume (3 L), extracellular water (16 L), or total body water (42 L). Even if V corresponds to the value of a physiologic space, one cannot conclude unambiguously that the drug distributes only into that physical volume. Binding of drugs in both plasma and specific tissues complicates the situation and often prevents making any conclusion about the actual volume into which the drug distributes. An exception would occur when drug is restricted to plasma; the volumes of distribution, apparent and real, are then the same, about 3 L in an adult. This last situation is expected for small MW drugs that are highly bound to plasma proteins but not bound in the tissues. However, this apparent volume cannot be an equilibrium value, because plasma proteins themselves equilibrate slowly between plasma and other extracellular fluids. The apparent volume of plasma proteins, about 7.5 L for albumin, is perhaps a better estimate of the minimum value for such drugs.

For drugs of high MW (greater than approximately 70,000 g/mol), extravascular distribution is very slow to nonexistent. For such drugs, the volume of distribution then tends to approach that of plasma, 3 L. For example, for adalimumab (Humira), a recombinant human monoclonal antibody (MW = 142,000 g/mol) used to treat patients suffering from moderate to severe active rheumatoid arthritis, V is about 5 to 6 L.

For very polar drugs that are bound in neither tissues nor plasma, the volume of distribution varies between the extracellular fluid volume (16 L) and the total body water (42 L), depending on the degree to which the drug gains access to the intracellular fluids. Examples of compounds that distribute in total body water, and which do not appreciably bind within plasma and tissues, are caffeine and alcohol, both small molecules that pass freely through membranes. The volume of distribution of these two compounds is about 40 L.

SMALL VOLUME OF DISTRIBUTION

MODEL

The model expressed by Eq. 4-25 is conceptually useful, but it does not take into account that plasma proteins distribute throughout extracellular fluids, as shown for albumin in Table 4-5 (page 93). A model is therefore needed to distinguish, in tissues, between binding to plasma protein and binding to other constituents. This need is particularly great for drugs that bind to a plasma protein and that have small (<15 L) volumes of distribution. Much of the drug in the body is then bound to the plasma protein and any change in binding or in the distribution of the protein can substantially influence the distribution of unbound drug within the body. A model to describe such distribution is derived in Appendix C, *Distribution of Drugs Extensively Bound to Plasma Proteins.*

For a drug bound to albumin, the approximate relationship between V and binding to albumin and other sites is

$$V = 7.5 + \left(7.5 + \frac{V_R}{fu_R} \right) \cdot fu \qquad 4\text{-}30$$

where fu is the fraction unbound, V_R is the aqueous volume of the intracellular fluids into which drug distributes (total available volume = 27 L), and fu_R is the apparent fraction unbound in the intracellular fluids. The virtue of this model is that it provides a means of analyzing the distribution of both drug and the plasma protein to which it binds. Representative drugs with volumes of distribution less than 15 L and to which this model is specifically applicable are given in Table 4-8. The drugs are either weak acids or macromolecules. As previously stated, basic drugs tend to have much greater tissue binding than acidic drugs. Consequently, basic drugs do not have a small volume of distribution. Large macromolecules, because of their size and hydrophilic nature, tend to be restricted, in large part, to plasma.

To illustrate the utility of the proposed model, consider the data in Fig. 4-23. Shown is a linear relationship between V and fu for a series of cephalosporins. This dependence might have been explained by the general model, $V = V_P + V_{TW} \cdot fu/fu_T$, assuming fu_T does not vary among the cephalosporins. A major problem would have been noticed here, however. The observed volume intercept when fu approaches zero is 7 L, a value much larger than the plasma volume, V_P, of 3 L. The observations are much better ex-

TABLE 4-8	Representative Drugs With Volumes of Distribution of 15 L or Less*		

Small Molecules (MW <500 g/mol)*

Acetylsalicylic acid	Cefotaxime	Dobutamine	Piroxicam
Bumetanide	Ceftriaxone	Dicloxacillin	Probenecid
Carbenicillin	Cefuroxime	Diflunisal	Salicylic acid
Cefamandole	Chlorothiazide	Ibuprofen	Tolbutamide
Cefazolin	Clofibric acid	Ketoprofen	Tolmetin
Cefonicid	Cloxacillin	Naproxen	Valproic acid
Ceforanide	Diclofenac	Piperacillin	Warfarin

Macromolecules (MW >10,000 g/mol)

Adalimumab (148,000)[†]	Denileukin diftitox (58,000)	Etanercept (150,000)	Rasburicase (34,000)
Anakinra (17,300)	Epoetin alfa (30,400)	Infliximab (149,100)	Somatropin (22,000)

*Binding to albumin is known or assumed.
[†]Approximate molecular size in grams per mol.

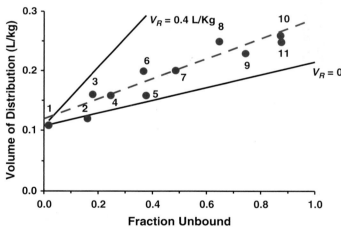

FIGURE 4-23. The volumes of distribution of a series of cephalosporin antibiotics increase with the fraction unbound to plasma proteins. The slope of the line of best fit (*colored*) lies between the expected relationships for drugs that do not enter tissue cells, $V_R = 0$, and those that do, $V_R = 28$ L or 0.4 L/kg (Eq. 4-25), but do not bind to cellular components ($fu_R = 1$). The cephalosporins shown are: 1 = cefonicid, 2 = cefazolin, 3 = ceforanide, 4 = cefamandole, 5 = cefotaxitin, 6 = cephalothin, 7 = moxalactam, 8 = cefotaxime, 9 = ceftazidime, 10 = cephalexin, and 11 = cephradine. (From: Dudley MN, Nightingale CH. Effects of protein upon activity of cephalosporins: New beta-lactam antibiotics: A review from chemistry to clinical efficacy of the new cephalosporins. Neu HC, ed. Philadelphia: Francis Clark Wood Institute for the History of Medicine, College of Physicians of Philadelphia; 1982:227–239.)

plained by the proposed model. The discrepancy between the two models lies in the distribution of the plasma protein. The proposed model suggests that albumin is the major binding protein for these antibiotics in that those cephalosporins that are tightly bound have distribution characteristics in common with albumin.

The volumes of distribution of the cephalosporins at higher fractions unbound, however, indicate that the drugs must partially enter cells or be bound to some extravascular structures. The extent of this distribution outside the extracellular fluids, on average, must be relatively small in that by extrapolation to $fu = 1$, corresponding to a cephalosporin with no binding to plasma albumin, the volume is 20 L (0.29 L/kg), a value greater than the extracellular volume, about 16 L, but considerably less than total body water (42 L).

The unbound volumes of distribution within the series of cephalosporins (Fig. 4-24) in contrast to the total volume of distribution (see Fig. 4-23), dramatically decrease as the fraction unbound increases. For those cephalosporins that are highly bound (low fu), the binding protein effectively ties up the drug. The consequence of plasma protein binding here is that a much larger amount of drug must be in the body to give the same antimicrobial effect for those drugs with the same minimum inhibitory unbound concentration.

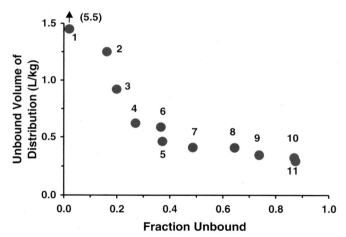

FIGURE 4-24. The unbound volumes of distribution of the same cephalosporins shown in Fig. 4-23 decrease dramatically with an increase in the fraction unbound. For those cephalosporins with unbound volumes much greater than the extracellular space ($V_E = 0.22$ L/kg) or the total body water (0.6 L/kg), binding to plasma proteins clearly reduces the concentration of the active form for a given dose.

LOCATION IN BODY

The fractions of drug in the body that are in plasma (bound and unbound), in or outside extracellular fluids, and bound in plasma or throughout extracellular fluids can be useful pieces of information, particularly with those conditions, examples listed in Table 4-9, in which there are changes in the distribution of plasma proteins. Relationships to calculate these fractions are given in Table 4-10. Their derivations are given in Appendix C, *Distribution of Drugs Extensively Bound to Plasma Proteins.*

When the apparent volume of distribution of a drug is large (>50 L), Eq. 4-25 approximately reduces to

$$V \approx V_R \cdot \frac{fu}{fu_R}$$

TABLE 4-9	Examples of Conditions in Which the Plasma Concentration of the Two Major Plasma Proteins to Which Drugs Bind Are Altered	
Plasma Protein	**Condition**	**Change in Concentration of Plasma Protein**
Albumin	Hepatic	Decrease
	Burns	Decrease
	Nephrotic syndrome	Decrease
	End-stage renal disease	Decrease
	Pregnancy	Decrease
α_1-**Acid glycoprotein**	Myocardial infarction	Increase
	Surgery	Increase
	Crohn's disease	Increase
	Trauma	Increase
	Rheumatoid arthritis	Increase

TABLE 4-10	Approximate Relationships for Analyzing Distribution of a Drug That Binds to Albumin and Distributes Throughout Total Body Water
Fraction of Drug in Body That is:	**Relationships***
In plasma	$\dfrac{V}{3}$
Outside plasma	$\dfrac{V-3}{V}$
Unbound in body water	$\dfrac{42 \cdot fu}{V}$
Unbound in extracellular fluids	$\dfrac{15 \cdot fu}{V}$
In extracellular fluids	$\dfrac{7.5(1 + fu)}{V}$
Outside extracellular fluids	$\dfrac{V - 7.5(1 + fu)}{V}$
Bound to proteins in plasma	$\dfrac{3(1 - fu)}{V}$
Bound to extracellular proteins	$\dfrac{7.5(1 - fu)}{V}$
Bound outside the extracellular fluids (in tissues)	$\dfrac{V - 25 \cdot fu - 75}{V}$

*Derivations are given in Appendix C, *Distribution of Drugs Extensively Bound to Plasma Proteins.*

which is virtually the same as that predicted by Eq. 4-25. The major practical application of Eq. 4-26, however, is for drugs with small volumes of distribution, that is, with values approaching 7.5 L/70 kg (0.11 L/kg) for a drug bound to albumin.

ALTERED BINDING AND LOADING DOSE

Loading doses are sometimes given to rapidly achieve a therapeutic response, putatively by rapidly producing a desired unbound concentration (Chapter 11, *Multiple-Dose Regimens*). With variations in both plasma and tissue binding, the question arises whether or not the loading dose needs to be adjusted.

For many drugs, volume of distribution is greater than 50 L, that is, much greater than the apparent volume of the binding protein, implying that only a small fraction of drug in body resides on the plasma protein. Therefore, ignoring the first two terms in Eq. 4-25 and realizing that $fu \cdot C = Cu$, it follows that

$$\text{Amount in body} = \frac{V_R}{fu_R} \cdot Cu$$

This equation indicates that Cu is independent of plasma binding, and thus, no adjustment in loading dose in a patient is needed. The total plasma concentration does, of course, change with altered plasma binding, but this is of no therapeutic consequence with respect to loading dose requirements. If, however, tissue binding (fu_R) were to change, so would the initial value(s) of Cu (and C), necessitating a decision to change the loading dose.

We will subsequently examine (Chapter 5, *Elimination*) the physiologic concepts underlying the elimination of drugs from the body and integrate the kinetic principles following a single i.v. dose with these concepts.

KEY RELATIONSHIPS

$$\text{Net rate of transport} = \underset{\substack{\text{Permeability}}}{P} \cdot \underset{\substack{\text{Surface} \\ \text{area}}}{SA} \cdot \underset{\substack{\text{Concentration} \\ \text{difference}}}{(Cu_1 - Cu_2)}$$

$$\text{Distribution half-life} = 0.693 \cdot \frac{Kp_b}{Q/V_T}$$

$$V = \frac{\text{Amount in body at equilibrium}}{\text{Plasma drug concentration}} = \frac{A}{C}$$

$$V = V_P + V_{T_1} \cdot K_{P_1} + V_{T_2} \cdot K_{P_2} \cdots$$

$$\text{Fraction of drug in body within plasma} = \frac{V_P}{V}$$

$$\text{Fraction outside plasma} = \frac{V - V_P}{V}$$

$$V \cdot C = Vu \cdot Cu = V_b \cdot C_b$$

$$fu = \frac{Cu}{C}$$

$$fu = \frac{1}{(1 + Ka \cdot fu_p \cdot P_t)}$$

$$V = V_P + V_{TW} \cdot \frac{fu}{fu_T}$$

$$Kp = \frac{C_T}{C} = \frac{fu}{fu_T} \cdot \frac{Cu_T}{Cu}$$

$$V = V_P + V_{TW} \cdot \frac{fu}{fu_T} \cdot \frac{P_{uptake}}{P_{efflux}}$$

$$V = 7.5 + (7.5 + \frac{V_R}{fu_R}) \cdot fu$$

STUDY PROBLEMS

(Answers to Study Problems are in Appendix J.)

1. Define the following terms related to:
   a. *Movement across membranes*
      Active transport, extravasation, paracellular transport, passive facilitated transport, permeability, transcellular transport, and transporter.
   b. *Drug distribution*
      Apparent volume of distribution, fraction unbound, tissue-to-blood equilibrium distribution ratio, and perfusion-rate and permeability-rate limitations in drug distribution.

2. Briefly state the meaning of the following physicochemical properties and how they are commonly assessed: hydrophilic, hydrophobic, lipophilic, and lipophobic.

3. How accurate are each of the following statements?
   a. When distribution is perfusion-rate limited, the ratio of tissue-to-blood concentrations across a capillary membrane is virtually one at all times.
   b. When the surface area of a membrane is doubled, so is its permeability.
   c. Passive diffusion across a membrane stops when the unbound concentrations on both sides are the same.
   d. Carrier-mediated transport is one in which energy is needed to transfer drug across a membrane.
   e. Protein binding in the aqueous phases diminishes the permeability of membranes.

4. The volume of distribution of paroxetine (Paxil), a psychotropic drug, is about 300 L. The fraction unbound in plasma is 0.06.
   a. The plasma concentration when 30 mg of drug is in the body would therefore be _____ mg/L.
   b. The amount of drug in the body when the plasma concentration is 0.2 mg/L is _____ mg.
   c. The percentage of drug in the body that is:
      (1) In plasma is _____.
      (2) Outside plasma is _____.

5. State how transporters are involved in the systemic absorption, distribution, and elimination of drugs, and give an example of each.

6. For each of the following statements, indicate whether it is true or false. If false or ambiguous, provide an explanation for why it is so.

   a. The difference between equilibrating and concentration transporters is that drug only reaches equilibrium across a membrane in the case of the former kind of transporter.

   b. When the initial rate of distribution of a drug into a tissue fails to increase with an increase in the rate of blood perfusing it, the distribution to that tissue is said to be *permeability rate-limited.*

   c. All other factors being the same, absorption from solution within a given region of the small intestine where the pH is 6.4 is expected to be faster for a weak acid with a pKa of 10.0 than for a weak base with a pKa of 10.0.

7. Explain how ingestion of activated charcoal can be used to both *reduce* the oral absorption of a drug, if the charcoal is given concurrently with the drug or soon thereafter, and *remove* drug from systemic circulation after drug absorption is complete.

8. Molecular size is an important determinant of permeability. Figure 4-3 summarizes the results of skin penetration for various un-ionized compounds. Using the figure, describe the effect of doubling MW on the permeability for a series of compounds of equal lipophilicity (e.g., n-octanol/water partition coefficients on log scale are all equal to 2).

9. Using the information in Table 4-11, calculate the time required for the amounts in each of the tissues listed to reach 50% of the equilibrium value for a drug with perfusion rate-limited distribution when the arterial blood concentration is kept constant with time. Rank the times and the corresponding tissues.

TABLE 4-11	Equilibrium Distribution Ratio and Perfusion Rate of a Drug in Selected Organs	
Organ	**Equilibrium Distribution Ratio**	**Perfusion Rate (mL/min per g of tissue)**
Heart	3	0.6
Kidneys	4	4
Liver	15	0.8
Lungs	1	10
Skin	12	0.024

10. The volume of distribution of a drug (MW = 351 g/mol) in a 70-kg subject is observed to be 8 L. Indicate which one (or more) of the following statements is (are) consistent with this observation. The drug is:

    a. Highly bound to plasma proteins.
    b. Bound to components outside plasma and is highly bound to proteins in plasma.
    c. Not bound to plasma proteins.

11. Ganeval et al. studied the pharmacokinetics of warfarin in 11 patients with the nephrotic syndrome. Table 4-12 illustrates the differences in warfarin kinetics in the two populations. No data on differences in body weight between the two groups were given. For the purposes of this problem, both groups averaged 70 kg.

    a. Given a fraction unbound of 0.005 in the control group, estimate the value expected in the nephrotic group.

TABLE 4-12	Mean Pharmacokinetic Parameters and Serum Albumin Concentrations in 11 Control and 11 Nephrotic Patients After Oral Administration (8 mg) of Warfarin	
Parameters	**Control Group**	**Nephrotic Patients**
V (L)	9.4 ± 2.7	13.7 ± 6.6
CL (L/hr)	0.20 ± 0.07	0.58 ± 0.26
$t_{1/2}$ (hr)	36 ± 14	18 ± 11
Serum albumin (g/L)	43 ± 5	12.5 ± 6.5

From: Ganeval D, Fischer AM, Barre J, et al. Pharmacokinetics of warfarin in the nephrotic syndrome and effect on vitamin K-dependent clotting factors. Clin Nephrol 1986;25:75–80.

b. Warfarin has a small volume of distribution. Calculate the expected volume of distribution in the patients with the nephrotic syndrome if fu is increased to the value calculated in "a." Does it agree with the observed value? Hint: determine the value of fu_R in the control group, and assume it is the same in the nephrotic patients.

c. Had the half-life data not been given, could you have predicted the observed shortening of the value in nephrotic patients? This condition usually suggests induction of metabolism.

12. Briefly comment on the validity of each of the following statements.

a. The equilibrium distribution ratio for a drug between liver (1.6 L in size) and plasma (3 L) is 50; therefore, its volume of distribution must be at least 75 L in a man weighing 70 kg.

b. A drug that essentially reaches distribution equilibrium within 30 min, yet whose volume of distribution in a 70-kg man is 200 L, must distribute primarily into highly perfused organs.

Elimination

OBJECTIVES

The reader will be able to:

- Define the meaning of the following terms: extraction ratio, glomerular filtration rate, hepatic acinus, hepatic sinusoids, hepatocellular activity, microsomal enzymes, nephron, perfusion, perfusion rate-limited elimination, phase I and phase II reactions, plasma-to-blood concentration ratio, primary metabolic pathways, prodrug, secondary metabolic pathways, sequential reactions, sinusoids (hepatic).

- Define the following using both words and equations: biliary clearance, blood clearance, clearance, enterohepatic cycle, filtration clearance, intrinsic clearance, intrinsic metabolic clearance, intrinsic excretory clearance, hepatic clearance, renal clearance, secretion clearance, and unbound clearance.

- Calculate the extraction ratio across an eliminating organ given blood clearance and blood flow to that organ.

- Define glomerular filtration, tubular secretion, and tubular reabsorption.

- State the average values of hepatic blood flow, renal blood flow, and glomerular filtration rate.

- Ascertain from the value of its extraction ratio whether the clearance of a drug by an organ is sensitive to perfusion or cellular activity and plasma protein binding.

- Describe where filtration, secretion, and reabsorption of drugs occur within the nephron.

- Given renal clearance and plasma protein binding data, determine if a drug is predominantly reabsorbed from or secreted into the renal tubule.

- Anticipate those drugs for which a change in urine pH may alter the value of their renal clearance and the direction of the alteration.

- Anticipate those drugs for which a change in urine flow may alter the value of their renal clearance and the direction of the alteration.

- Ascertain the relative contribution of the renal and hepatic routes to total elimination from their respective clearance values.

- Describe the role that biliary secretion can play in drug disposition.

- Determine the biliary clearance of a drug from its bile-to-plasma concentration ratio and the bile flow.

- Explain the statement, "Half-life and elimination rate constant depend on clearance and volume of distribution, and not vice versa."

- List examples of physiologic variables that may alter the primary pharmacokinetic disposition parameters: hepatic clearance, renal clearance, and volume of distribution.

- Given plasma (or blood) concentration versus time data in normal and altered states following an intravenous (i.v.) bolus dose, determine the changes that have occurred in the primary and secondary pharmacokinetic parameters and list the possible physiologic mechanism(s) involved.
- Predict and graphically demonstrate the effects of an alteration in plasma protein or tissue binding, organ perfusion, or cellular eliminating activity on the time course of drug in plasma following an i.v. bolus dose when the appropriate primary pharmacokinetic parameters of the drug are known.

T his chapter is concerned with elimination processes and particularly with the concept of clearance. In Chapter 3, *Kinetics Following an Intravenous Bolus Dose*, the method of quantifying clearance following a single i.v. bolus dose was presented. Here, its physiologic meaning is given. The chapter ends with integration of kinetic and physiologic concepts applied to the events following an i.v. bolus dose.

PROCESSES OF ELIMINATION

The clearance of drugs varies widely. Before answering the question as to why this is so, a few words are in order about processes of elimination and about clearance in general, with particular emphasis on relatively small drug molecules, generally less than 1200 g/mol. Larger molecules, such as polypeptides and proteins are dealt with in Chapter 21, *Protein Drugs*.

Elimination occurs by excretion and metabolism. Some drugs are excreted via the bile. Others, particularly volatile substances, are excreted in the breath. For most drugs, however, excretion occurs predominantly via the kidneys. Some drugs are eliminated almost entirely by urinary excretion, but these are relatively few. Rather, metabolism is the major mechanism for elimination of drugs from the body as shown in Fig. 5-1 for the top 200 prescribed drugs, and for most of these drugs, metabolism occurs predominantly in the liver. Occasionally, however, a drug is extensively metabolized in one or more other tissues, such as the kidneys, lungs, blood, and gastrointestinal wall.

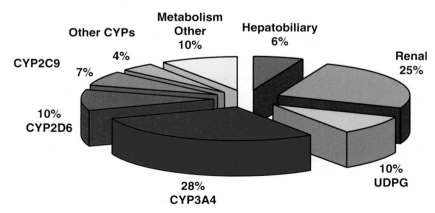

FIGURE 5-1. Relative importance of route and mechanism of elimination of the top 200 prescribed drugs. The segments of the pie in color refer to phase I metabolic reactions. The remaining segments refer to either phase II conjugative reactions or excretory processes within the liver and kidney. (From: Williams JA, Hyland R, Jones BC, et al. Drug-drug interactions for the UDP-glucuronsyltransferase substrates: a pharmacokinetic explanation for typically observed low exposure [*AUCi/AUC*] ratios. Drug Metab Dispos 2004;32:1201–1208.)

The most common metabolic reactions are oxidation, reduction, hydrolysis, and conjugation. Conjugation reactions include glucuronidation (conjugation with glucuronic acid), sulfation, and acetylation. Frequently, a drug simultaneously undergoes metabolism by several competing (**primary**) pathways. The fraction going to each metabolite depends on the relative rates of each of the parallel pathways. Metabolites may undergo further (**secondary**) metabolism. For example, oxidation, reduction, and hydrolysis are often followed by a conjugation reaction. These reactions occur in series or are said to be **sequential**. Because they often occur first, oxidation, reduction, and hydrolysis are commonly referred to as **phase I reactions**, and conjugations as **phase II reactions**. Some drugs, however, only undergo primary elimination via phase II reactions.

Table 5-1 illustrates patterns of biotransformation (metabolism) of representative drugs. The pathways of metabolism are classified by chemical alteration. Several of the transformations occur in the endoplasmic reticulum of cells of the liver and certain other tissues; others occur in the cytosol or on the surface of the hepatocyte. On homogenizing these tissues, the endoplasmic reticulum of cells is disrupted with the formation of small vesicles called **microsomes**. For this reason, metabolizing enzymes of the endoplasmic reticulum are called **microsomal enzymes**. Drug metabolism, therefore, may be classified as microsomal and nonmicrosomal.

TABLE 5-1	Patterns of Biotransformation* of Representative Drugs[†]

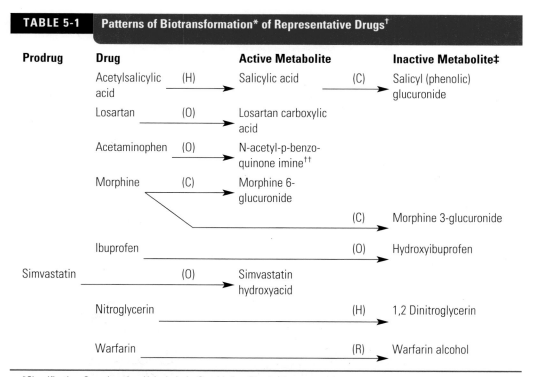

Prodrug	Drug		Active Metabolite		Inactive Metabolite[‡]
	Acetylsalicylic acid	(H)	Salicylic acid	(C)	Salicyl (phenolic) glucuronide
	Losartan	(O)	Losartan carboxylic acid		
	Acetaminophen	(O)	N-acetyl-p-benzo-quinone imine[††]		
	Morphine	(C)	Morphine 6-glucuronide		
				(C)	Morphine 3-glucuronide
	Ibuprofen			(O)	Hydroxyibuprofen
Simvastatin		(O)	Simvastatin hydroxyacid		
	Nitroglycerin			(H)	1,2 Dinitroglycerin
	Warfarin			(R)	Warfarin alcohol

*Classification: C, conjugation; H, hydrolysis; O, oxidation; R, reduction.
[†]For some drugs, only representative pathways are indicated.
[‡]Inactive at concentrations obtained following the therapeutic administration of the parent drug.
[††]Cause of hepatotoxicity, and sometimes death, in cases of acetaminophen overdose.

The major enzymes responsible for the oxidation and reduction of many drugs belong to the superfamily of cytochrome P450 enzymes. This superfamily, which comprises many enzymes, is divided in humans into three major distinct families, designated CY(cytochrome)P(450)1, 2, and 3, each further divided into subfamilies, A through E. Arabic numerals are used to refer to individual enzymes (gene products) within each subfamily. The enzymes of this family display a relatively high degree of structural specificity; a drug

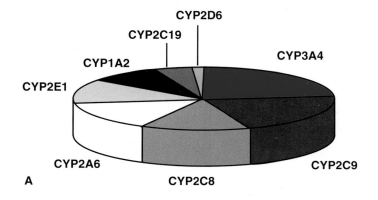

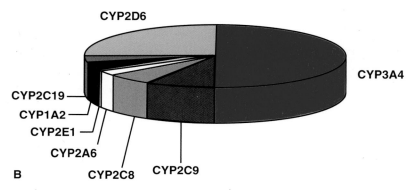

FIGURE 5-2. **A.** Relative abundance of the major hepatic P450 cytochromes in human liver. **B.** Relative contribution of the major hepatic P450 cytochromes in the P450-mediated clearance of 403 marketed drugs in the United States and Europe. (From: Clarke SE, Jones BC. Hepatic cytochromes P450 and their role in metabolism-based drug-drug interactions. In: Rodriguez AD, ed. Drug-drug Interaction. New York: Marcel Dekker, 2002:55–88.)

is often a good substrate for one enzyme but not another. Figure 5-2 displays the major P450 enzymes by abundance and by relevance to drug metabolism. The most abundant, CYP3A, metabolizes many drugs of relatively diverse structure and size and, unlike many of the other P450 enzymes, is found in the intestinal wall as well as in the liver. The abundance of a particular cytochrome in the liver does not necessarily reflect its importance to drug metabolism. For example, although comprising only approximately 2% of the total CYP content, CYP2D6 is involved to the overall extent of 25% of the clearance of prescribed drugs, and particularly basic ones. Many acidic drugs are metabolized preferentially by CYP2C9 and CYP2C19. Examples of substrates for various CYP enzymes are shown in Fig. 5-3. There is also a superfamily of UDP-glucuronosyltransferases (UGTs), responsible for formation of glucuronides of some drugs and many of their metabolites. Glucuronidation is the major pathway of elimination of some drugs and endogenous compounds, such as irinotecan, estradiol, etoposide, and bilirubin, which are primarily substrates of UGT1A1, and zidovudine, which is a substrate of UGT2B7.

The consequences of drug metabolism are manifold. Biotransformation provides a mechanism for ridding the body of undesirable foreign compounds and drugs; it also pro-

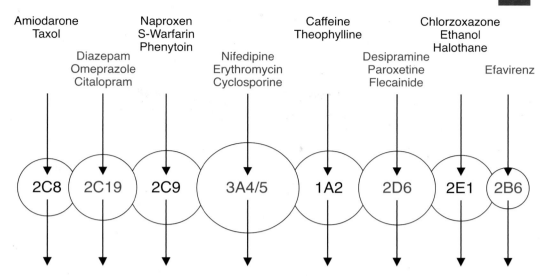

FIGURE 5-3. Graphic representation of the different forms of human cytochrome-P450 enzyme (*circles*) with different but often overlapping substrate specificities. The arrows indicate the single metabolic pathways. Representative substrates are listed above each enzyme.

vides a means of producing active compounds. Numerous examples are now recognized in which the administered drug is really an inactive **prodrug**, which is converted into a pharmacologically active species. Sometimes, one or more metabolites have a pharmacologic profile similar to the parent drug; others have a different profile, and some are responsible for adverse effects. The duration and intensity of the responses to a drug relate to the time courses of all active substances in the body. The pharmacokinetics of active metabolites, as well as that of the compound administered, is therefore of therapeutic concern. The kinetics of metabolites after drug administration is presented in Chapter 20, *Metabolites and Drug Response*. The administered drug and its elimination processes are emphasized in all subsequent chapters through Chapter 19, *Distribution Kinetics*.

CLEARANCE IN GENERAL

Of the concepts in pharmacokinetics, **clearance** has the greatest potential for clinical applications. It is also the most useful parameter for the evaluation of an elimination mechanism.

Recall from Chapter 3, *Kinetics Following an Intravenous Bolus Dose*, clearance is defined as the proportionality factor that relates rate of drug elimination to the plasma (drug) concentration. That is,

$$Rate\ of\ elimination = CL \cdot C \qquad\qquad 5\text{-}1$$

Alternatively, clearance may be viewed from the loss of drug across an organ of elimination. This approach has several advantages, particularly, in predicting and in evaluating the effects of changes in blood flow, plasma protein binding, enzyme activity, or secretory activity on the elimination of a drug, as will be seen. Figure 5-4 summarizes the various ways of viewing mass balance across an eliminating organ. In this scheme, drug in the eliminating organ is assumed to have reached distribution equilibrium; thus, the sole reason for any difference between the arterial and venous concentrations is elimination. For all but the earliest moments, this assumption is reasonable for the kidneys and the liver, which are among the most highly perfused and hence most rapidly equilibrating organs in the body.

1. Mass Balance

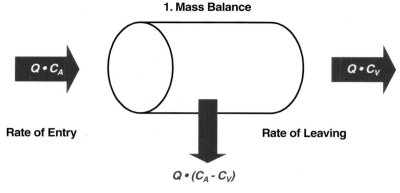

2. Mass Balance Normalized to Rate of Entry

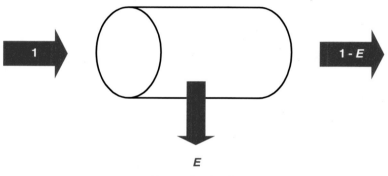

3. Mass Balance Normalized to Entering Concentration

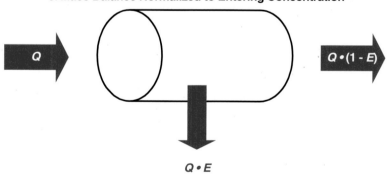

FIGURE 5-4. The extraction of a drug by an eliminating organ under steady-state conditions may be considered from the fundamental concepts of mass balance. **1.** The extraction of drug may be accounted for from its rates in and out of the organ. **2.** Normalizing to the rate of entry provides a means of determining the fraction extracted, the extraction ratio, E. **3.** Normalizing to the entering concentration allows one to account for the drug in terms of blood clearance, CL_b, and blood flow, Q. C_A and C_V are the blood concentrations entering and leaving the organ, respectively.

Before proceeding further, however, a point of distinction needs to be made between these two ways of viewing clearance. In the first, clearance is simply a proportionality term. The second is derived from mass–balance considerations, by relating the rate of extraction to the rate of presentation to the eliminating organ. In the reservoir model used in Chapter 3, *Kinetics Following an Intravenous Bolus Dose*, to introduce this concept, the fluid perfusing the eliminating organ (the extractor) is water, containing drug (see Fig. 3-3). In vivo, the fluid presented to the liver and kidneys is whole blood, and the rate of presentation of drug to the kidneys, for example, is $Q_R \cdot C_A$, where Q_R and C_A are renal blood flow and the concentration in the arterial blood perfusing the kidneys, respectively. So, when the extraction ratio, E_R, approaches one, everything in the incoming blood (both in the blood cells and plasma) is cleared of drug, not just that in plasma. For this reason, when calculating organ extraction ratio, *it is important to relate renal blood clearance (CL_b) to renal blood flow and not plasma clearance to plasma flow.* For the kidneys then,

$$CL_{b,R} \quad = \quad Q_R \quad \cdot \quad E_R \qquad\qquad 5\text{-}2$$

Renal	Renal	Renal
blood	blood	extraction
clearance	flow	ratio

And for the liver,

$$CL_{b,H} \quad = \quad Q_H \quad \cdot \quad E_H \qquad\qquad 5\text{-}3$$

Hepatic	Hepatic	Hepatic
blood	blood	extraction
clearance	flow	ratio

From these relationships, it is apparent that blood clearance cannot be of any value. If the extraction ratio approaches 1.0, then blood clearance approaches a maximum, organ blood flow. For the kidneys and liver, the average blood flows in an adult are 1.1 and 1.35 L/min (Table 4-4), respectively.

Before considering clearance of drug by specific organs, several comments are in order.

DESCRIPTION OF CLEARANCE BY ORGAN, PROCESS, OR SITE OF MEASUREMENT

Clearance can be described in terms of the eliminating organ (e.g., hepatic clearance, renal clearance, or pulmonary clearance). It can also be described by the difference between renal excretion and elimination by all other processes (e.g., renal clearance and extrarenal clearance). How an organ clears the blood of drug may also be described by the nature of the elimination process (e.g., metabolic clearance or excretory clearance). Furthermore, the clearance value depends on the reference fluid. Thus, to be specific, the clearance of a drug eliminated (e.g., by metabolism in the liver), using plasma concentration measurements would then be hepatic metabolic plasma clearance. Similarly, "clearance by excretion of drug in the kidneys" would be renal excretory plasma clearance. In practice, the term *plasma* is dropped, because plasma is the common site of measurement. In addition, one often drops *metabolic* or *excretory* when describing clearance by the liver and kidneys, respectively, because these processes generally occur in these respective organs. However, metabolism does occur in the kidneys, and excretion (into bile) does occur in the liver. Therefore, the assumptions underlying the clearance nomenclature for a specific drug should always be questioned.

PLASMA VERSUS BLOOD CLEARANCE

Because plasma is the most commonly measured fluid, plasma clearance is much more frequently reported than blood clearance. For many applications in pharmacokinetics, all that is needed is a proportionality term, in which case it matters little which clearance value for a drug is used. As seen above, the exception is if one wishes to estimate extraction ratio, then, one needs to convert plasma clearance to blood clearance. This conversion is readily accomplished by experimentally determining the **plasma-to-blood concentration ratio** (C/C_b), most often by preparing a known concentration in whole blood, centrifuging, and determining the resulting concentration in the plasma. This ratio generally ranges from 0.3 to 2, although it can be very much lower for drugs that associate extensively with blood cells. This concentration ratio is a function of the hematocrit and of the binding of drug to both plasma proteins and blood cell components. The relationship is derived in Appendix D, *Plasma-to-Blood Concentration Ratio*. When binding to blood cells is extensive, the plasma-to-blood ratio may be much less than 1.0 with the lower limit approaching zero. In contrast, strong binding to plasma proteins produces a ratio greater than 1.0 ($1/[1 - \text{hematocrit}]$), with an upper limit close to 2 when drug is restricted to plasma. Some relatively polar drugs, such as antibiotics, do not partition onto, or enter, blood cells and for these, likewise, drug is restricted to plasma.

Because, by definition, the product of clearance and concentration is equal to the rate of elimination, which is independent of what fluid is measured, it follows that:

$$Rate\ of\ elimination = CL \cdot C = CL_b \cdot C_b = CLu \cdot Cu \qquad 5\text{-}4$$

where CLu is the **unbound clearance**, that is, the clearance with reference to unbound drug in plasma water, which therapeutically is the important concentration driving response.

Equation 5-4 allows one to calculate one clearance from another, given the appropriate ratio. For example, **blood clearance**, CL_b, is given by

$$CL_b = CL \cdot \left(\frac{C}{C_b}\right) \qquad 5\text{-}5$$

Similarly, unbound clearance is given by

$$CLu = \frac{CL}{fu} \qquad 5\text{-}6$$

For example, if the plasma clearance of a drug, by default simply called clearance, is 1.3 L/min and the drug is extensively eliminated by hepatic metabolism, there is a potential danger in believing that it has a high extraction ratio. However, knowing that the plasma-to-blood concentration ratio is 0.1 indicates that blood clearance is only 0.13 L/min, much lower than hepatic blood flow, 1.35 L/min. Hence, this drug is one of low-extraction ratio, and clinically, the implications are very different, as discussed below.

ADDITIVITY OF CLEARANCE

The clearance of a drug by one organ adds to the clearance by another. This is a consequence of the anatomy of the circulatory system. Consider, for example, a drug that is eliminated by both renal excretion and hepatic metabolism. Then

$$\frac{Rate\ of}{elimination} = \frac{Rate\ of}{renal\ excretion} + \frac{Rate\ of}{hepatic\ metabolism} \qquad 5\text{-}7$$

Dividing the rate of removal associated with each process by the incoming drug concentration (blood or plasma), which for both organs is the same (C), gives the clearance associated with that process:

$$\frac{\dfrac{Rate\ of}{elimination}}{C} = \frac{\dfrac{Rate\ of}{renal\ excretion}}{C} + \frac{\dfrac{Rate\ of}{hepatic\ metabolism}}{C} \qquad 5\text{-}8$$

Analogous to total clearance, renal clearance (CL_R) is defined as the proportionality term between urinary excretion rate of unchanged drug and plasma concentration.

Similarly, hepatic clearance (CL_H) is the proportionality term between rate of hepatic metabolism and plasma concentration. Therefore,

$$\underset{\substack{\text{Total} \\ \text{clearance}}}{CL} = \underset{\substack{\text{Renal} \\ \text{clearance}}}{CL_R} + \underset{\substack{\text{Hepatic} \\ \text{clearance}}}{CL_H} \qquad \text{5-9}$$

Recall from Chapter 3, *Kinetics Following an Intravenous Bolus Dose*, that total clearance is determined from the total exposure (*AUC*) following an i.v. dose (see Eq. 3-21) and that renal clearance can be determined from the fraction excreted unchanged and total clearance (see Eq. 3-34). In contrast, rate and extent of metabolism can rarely be measured directly, but by taking advantage of the additivity of clearance, hepatic clearance is readily estimated as the difference between total and renal clearance, that is, $CL_H = (1 - fe) \cdot CL$.

One exception to the simple additivity of clearance is pulmonary clearance. This is caused in part by the blood supply to the lungs being in series, rather than in parallel, with other organs of elimination and in part to the total cardiac output passing through the lungs before reaching the site of measurement, usually blood in a peripheral vein. The concentration measured in the systemic circulation reflects that leaving, rather than entering, the lungs. The use of this concentration to calculate clearance is inconsistent with its definition. If the pulmonary extraction ratio is high, clearance values calculated in the usual manner may even exceed cardiac output, making interpretation problematic.

Clearances of drugs by the liver and the kidneys are now examined. Each organ has special anatomic and physiologic features that require its separate consideration.

HEPATIC CLEARANCE

As with other organs of elimination, the removal of drug by the liver may be considered from mass–balance relationships, as shown in Eq. 5-3. For the liver, Q_H is the sum of two blood flows, the hepatic portal venous flow, draining the gastrointestinal tract, and the hepatic arterial blood flow, with average values of 1050 and 300 mL/min, respectively. Also, elimination can be by metabolism, secretion into the bile, or both.

PERFUSION, PROTEIN BINDING, AND HEPATOCELLULAR ACTIVITY

The following principles, relating changes in clearance and extraction ratio to alterations in perfusion, plasma protein binding, or inherent elimination characteristics, apply in general to all organs of elimination.

The clearances of drugs vary widely owing to differences in organ perfusion, plasma protein binding, and inherent elimination characteristics within cells, involving metabolism and secretion. Changes in perfusion can occur in disease and during exercise. One drug can compete for the binding sites of another, thereby increasing the fraction unbound of the affected drug. The cellular activity, controlling the elimination processes, is sometimes affected by disease and by other drugs taken by a patient. Although the following principles, relating changes in clearance and extraction ratio, are exemplified here with hepatic extraction, they apply in general to all organs of elimination.

The functional anatomical unit of the liver is the **acinus**. The most abundant cell type comprising the acinus is the hepatocyte, where most drug elimination occurs. Another cell type, the Kupffer cell, which is part of the reticuloendothelial scavenger system, appears to be primarily involved in removing large protein drugs. Cells in the acinus are arranged broadly into three zones. Cells in zone 1 are closest to incoming arterioles and venules and are the first to receive drugs and nutrients from the incoming blood. Cells in zone 3, which appear to be richer in CYP450 and hydrolytic enzymes, are farthest from the distributing vessels and closest to the vessels draining the central vein and bile cannaliculae. Cells in zone 2 have functional and morphological characteristics intermediate between those of zones 1 and 3. The capillaries of the liver are termed **sinusoids**, comprising a discontinuous layer of fenestrated endothelial cells. The fenestrae (or windows) are about 100 nm in diameter, allowing ready exchange of materials, even as large as albumin, between the plasma in the sinusoids and the interstitial fluid, within the space of Disse, bathing the hepatocytes.

At least six processes, as shown in Fig. 5-5, may affect the ability of the liver to extract and eliminate drug from blood. In addition to perfusion, there is binding within the perfusing blood, to cells and proteins, and permeation or transport of unbound drug into the cell, where subsequent elimination occurs, via metabolism or secretion into the bile, or both. The scheme in Fig. 5-5 would appear to be such a complex interplay of

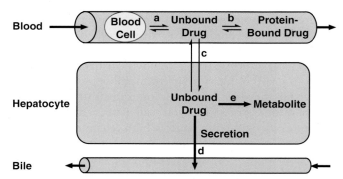

FIGURE 5-5.   Drug in blood is bound to blood cells (process *a*) and to plasma proteins (process *b*); however, it is the unbound drug that permeates (process *c*) into the hepatocyte. Within the hepatocyte, unbound drug is subjected to secretion into bile (process *d*) or to metabolism (process *e*). The formed metabolite leaves the hepatocyte via blood or bile, or is subjected to further metabolism. Any one of these five processes, or perfusion, can be the slowest, or rate-limiting, step in the overall process of drug elimination within the liver. Formed metabolite can be either further metabolized, returned to blood, or secreted into bile.

processes as to preclude any ready conclusion about how any one of these factors may influence clearance. Fortunately, the task becomes relatively simple by dividing drugs into whether they are of high ($E_H > 0.7$), low ($E_H < 0.3$), or intermediate extraction within the liver, as has been done for representative drugs eliminated primarily by either hepatic or renal routes in Table 5-2. However, before addressing the specific issues of perfusion and protein binding, we need to bring forward the concept of **intrinsic clearance**.

Intrinsic Clearance.   Although clearance is measured from observations in plasma or blood, elimination only occurs because a drug is a substrate for one or more of the eliminating mechanisms within the cell. In all cases, the externally observed rate of elimination is therefore a measure of, and indeed, equal to the rate of elimination occurring within the cell. This rate is dependent on the intracellular unbound concentration, Cu_H, to which the metabolic enzymes and excretory transporters are exposed. Because, by definition, clearance is simply the proportionality constant between rate of elimination and concentration, it therefore follows that

$$Rate\ of\ elimination = CL \cdot C = CL_{int} \cdot Cu_H \qquad\qquad 5\text{-}10$$

where CL_{int} is the **intrinsic clearance** of the drug, so called because it is a measure of the **intrinsic hepatocellular** eliminating activity, separated from other external factors, such as blood flow and plasma protein binding. Many drugs are substrates for more than one enzyme or eliminating transporter, so that analogous to the partitioning of hepatic clearance into hepatic metabolic and excretory (biliary) clearances, hepatic intrinsic clearance

TABLE 5-2	Hepatic and Renal Extraction Ratios of Representative Drugs

	Extraction Ratio		
	Low **(<0.3)**	**Intermediate** **(0.3–0.7)**	**High** **(>0.7)**
Hepatic Extraction*	Carbamazepine	Aspirin	Alprenolol
	Diazepam	Codeine	Cocaine
	Ibuprofen	Cyclosporine	Meperidine
	Nitrazepam	Ondansetrone	Morphine
	Paroxetine	Nifedipine	Nicotine
	Salicylic acid	Nortriptyline	Nitroglycerin
	Valproic acid		Propoxyphene
	Warfarin		Verapamil
Renal Extraction*	Amoxicillin	Acyclovir	Metformin
	Atenolol	Benzylpenicillin	p-Aminohippuric acid[†]
	Cefazolin	Cimetidine	Penciclovir
	Digoxin	Cephalothin	
	Furosemide	Ciprofloxacin	
	Gentamicin	Ranitidine	
	Methotrexate		
	Pamidronate		

*At least 30% of drug eliminated by pathway.
[†]Used as a diagnostic to measure renal plasma flow.

is equal to the sum of the intrinsic metabolic ($CL_{int,m}$) and excretory ($CL_{int,ex}$) clearances associated with each of the primary processes. That is,

$$\text{Hepatic intrinsic clearance, } CL_{int} = \sum CL_{int,m} + \sum CL_{int,ex} \qquad 5\text{-}11$$

where the symbol $\sum$ denotes summation.

Perfusion. When the hepatic extraction ratio of a drug approaches 1.0 ($E_H > 0.7$), its hepatic blood clearance approaches hepatic blood flow. The drug must clearly have had sufficient time on its passage through the liver to partition out of the blood cells, dissociate from the plasma proteins, pass through the hepatic membranes, and be either metabolized by an enzyme or transported into the bile, or both. To maintain the sink conditions necessary to promote the continuous entry of more drug into the cell to be eliminated, as depicted in Fig. 5-6A, drug must obviously have a high hepatocellular uptake permeability and be an excellent substrate for the elimination processes within the hepatic cells. In this condition, with blood clearance approaching its maximum value, hepatic blood flow, *elimination becomes rate-limited by perfusion* and not by the speed of any of the other processes depicted in Fig. 5-5. *Clearance is then sensitive to changes in blood flow but relatively insensitive to changes in, for example, plasma protein binding or hepatocellular eliminating activity.* Furthermore, for a given systemic concentration, changes in blood flow are expected to produce corresponding changes in rate of elimination, but the extraction ratio is virtually unaffected.

In contrast to high extraction, elimination of a drug with a low extraction ratio (approaching zero) must be rate-limited somewhere else in the overall scheme other than

FIGURE 5-6. A,B. Exchange of drug between plasma and hepatocyte and its removal from this cell involves unbound drug (*Cu*). When the extraction is high (*E_H* >0.7), *Case A*, essentially all the drug is removed from blood on entering the liver (entering concentration, *C_{in}*), whether bound to blood cells or plasma proteins. Clearance is then rate-limited by perfusion. In contrast, when the extraction ratio is low (*E_H* <0.3), *Case B*, little drug is removed (exiting concentration, *C_{out}* approaches *C_{in}*), and any one of the many processes (other than perfusion) can rate limit drug elimination. Generally, it is because the drug is a poor substrate for the hepatic enzymes or biliary transporters. Occasionally, it is cell membrane permeability. Clearance is then governed by hepatocellular activity and fraction unbound in plasma. Arrows denote mass flow of drug; the thicker the arrow the greater the speed of mass transfer occurring via the associated process.

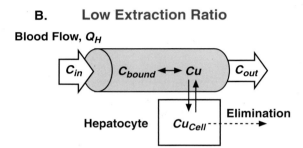

A. High Extraction Ratio

Blood Flow, *Q_H*

B. Low Extraction Ratio

Blood Flow, *Q_H*

perfusion (see Fig. 5-5). The most common reason is that the drug is a poor substrate for the elimination process, usually metabolism. Occasionally, for polar drugs of insufficient lipophilicity to permeate readily into the cell, elimination is rate-limited by membrane permeability. Whatever the cause of the limitation, drug concentration in arterial and venous blood, entering and leaving the liver, are virtually identical when the extraction ratio is low (Fig. 5-6B). Therefore, changes in blood flow should produce virtually no change in the drug concentration within the organ, in rate of elimination, or by definition in clearance. From Eq. 5-3, however, it is seen that the hepatic extraction ratio varies inversely with blood flow when clearance is constant. These expectations regarding perfusion for drugs of high and low extraction ratios are illustrated in Fig. 5-7.

A word of caution is needed here. Although mass–balance principles state that changes in blood flow are not expected to alter the clearance of drugs of low extraction ratio, there are physiologic mechanisms that may secondarily produce such an effect. Examples are the presence of homeostatic control mechanisms and a perfusion-limited supply of cofactors such as oxygen or sulfate needed in the metabolism of a drug.

Plasma Protein Binding. For a drug with a *high extraction ratio*, the liver is clearly capable of removing all the drug presented to it in spite of binding to blood cells and to plasma proteins. Rate of elimination then depends on total concentration in blood. Certainly, a decrease in binding aids in removing a drug; but in this case, it is essentially all removed anyway. Therefore, neither extraction ratio nor clearance is materially affected by changes in binding, and certainly not within the normally less than threefold range in fraction unbound seen for a drug in clinical practice.

For a drug with a *low extraction ratio*, clearance depends on plasma protein binding because only unbound drug penetrates membranes and is available for elimination and because the drop in drug concentration across the liver is small. The unbound concentration in plasma leaving the liver is almost identical to that entering the liver, *Cu*. The unbound concentration throughout the blood vessels within the liver therefore is then virtually the same, and again equal to *Cu*. And, as equilibrium is reached when the unbound concentrations within and outside the cell are equal for drugs able to readily permeate the hepatocyte, it follows that unbound concentration in the cell, *Cu_H*, equals *Cu*.

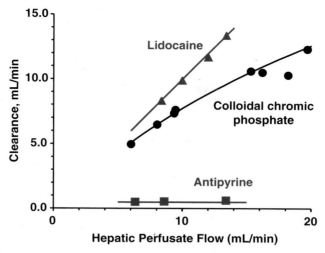

FIGURE 5-7. Composite data showing that the sensitivity of the clearance of a compound to changes in blood flow varies. When extraction ratio is low, as occurs with antipyrine, clearance is low and independent of blood flow. Clearance varies in direct proportion to flow rate for lidocaine, a drug with an extraction ratio close to 1.0. Between these extremes is colloidal chromic phosphate, the clearance of which moves away from a perfusion-rate limitation at higher flows. All data, obtained in an isolated, perfused rat liver, have been normalized to a 10-g liver. The lines are drawn by eye. (From: Antipyrine and lidocaine: Pang KS, Rowland M. Hepatic clearance of drugs. II. Experimental evidence for the acceptance of the "well-stirred" model over the "parallel tube" model using lidocaine in the perfused rat liver in situ preparation. J Pharmacokinet Biopharm 1977;5:655–680; Colloidal chromic phosphate: Brauer RW, Leong GF, McElroy RF Jr, Holloway RJ: Circulatory pathways in the rat liver as revealed by ^{32}P chromic phosphate colloid uptake in the isolated, perfused liver preparation. Am J Physiol 1956;184:593–598.)

Then, the rate of drug elimination in the liver is directly related to the concentration of drug unbound in the incoming, systemically delivered plasma. Accordingly, substituting Cu for Cu_H in Eq. 5-10, yields

$$Rate\ of\ elimination = CL_{int} \cdot Cu$$

| | Intrinsic clearance | Unbound Concentration | 5-12 |

Expressing the rate of hepatic elimination relative to the plasma concentration, it is apparent, therefore, that the hepatic plasma clearance varies in direct proportion with changes in the fraction unbound in plasma.

$$Hepatic\ clearance = CL_{int} \cdot fu \qquad 5\text{-}13$$

Intrinsic clearance   Fraction in plasma unbound

For example, if fu varies twofold, so does hepatic clearance; intrinsic clearance remains unchanged.

Notice from the equalities of Eqs. 5-4 and 5-13 that when the extraction ratio is low, $CLu \approx CL_{int}$. However, this is clearly not the case when extraction ratio is high. For example, if clearance of a drug approaches blood flow, then by substitution into Eq. 5-6 $CLu = Q_H/fu$. Hence, CLu varies reciprocally with fu, a parameter quite independent of CL_{int}.

The data in Fig. 5-8 obtained in the isolated perfused liver illustrate the points made above. In this system, protein binding can be readily altered by changing the

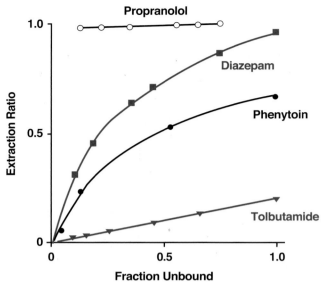

FIGURE 5-8. Composite mean data, obtained in an isolated, perfused rat liver, showing that the sensitivity of hepatic extraction ratio to changes in fraction of drug unbound varies. Extraction ratio is proportional to fraction unbound only when the extraction ratio is low, as observed over the entire range of binding for tolbutamide but only over a limited range for diazepam and phenytoin. When the extraction ratio is high, as occurs with phenytoin and diazepam at low binding ($fu > 0.5$) and with propranolol at all degrees of binding studied, extraction ratio is relatively insensitive to changes in fraction unbound. Notice that in this preparation, in which the fraction unbound is varied over a wide range by modifying the concentration of albumin, the binding protein, a drug such as diazepam can be changed from one of high to one of low extraction. The solid lines are drawn by eye. (From: Phenytoin: Shand DG, Cotham RH, Wilkinson GR. Perfusion-limited effects of plasma drug binding on hepatic extraction. Life Sci 1976;19:125–130; Diazepam: Rowland M, Leitch D, Fleming G, Smith B. Protein binding and hepatic clearance: discrimination between models of hepatic clearance with diazepam, a drug of high intrinsic clearance, in the isolated, perfused rat liver preparation. J Pharmacokinet Biopharm 1984;12:129–147; Tolbutamide: Schary WL, Rowland M. Protein binding and hepatic clearance: studies with tolbutamide, a drug of low intrinsic clearance, in the isolated, perfused rat liver preparation. J Pharmacokinet Biopharm 1983;11:225–243; Propranolol: Jones DB, Ching MS, Smallwood RA, Morgan DJ. A carrier-protein receptor is not a prerequisite for avid hepatic elimination of highly bound compounds: a study of propranolol elimination by the isolated, perfused rat liver. Hepatology 1985;5:590–593.)

concentration of the binding protein in the blood perfusing the liver, and perfusion can be held constant. Consider first tolbutamide, a drug of low extraction even in the absence of binding ($fu = 1.0$). As expected, the extraction ratio (and clearance) of tolbutamide is directly proportional to fu.

The observations with diazepam are illuminating. The extraction ratio (and clearance) changes from a value close to 1.0 (in the absence of binding, $fu = 1.0$) to one close to zero on decreasing the fraction unbound (increasing the extent of binding). Clearly, protein binding can limit extraction if binding is high enough. However, this situation is nonphysiologic in that the fraction unbound is varied between 1.0 and 0.05, a 20-fold change. In practice, a threefold change in fu would be considered particularly large for a drug bound to albumin, although larger changes are seen for drugs bound to other plasma proteins, such as α_1-acid glycoprotein. Under these more restricted conditions, the expected relationship between clearance and fu holds. Thus, for diazepam, in the region where extraction ratio is low (low fu), clearance is directly proportional to fu. At the other extreme, in the region where the extraction ratio is high, clearance varies little with a moderate change in fu. Finally, for the even more highly extracted drug propranolol, changes in binding produce no perceptible change in clearance, or extraction ratio, over a very wide range of *fu* values.

Hepatocellular Eliminating Activity. The influence of changing the activity of the elimination process within the liver cell may perhaps be most easily visualized by examining Fig. 5-9, which shows changes in extraction ratio and clearance as a function of hepatocellular (intrinsic) activity. When E_H is low, because the limitation is intrinsic activity, any change in this activity (e.g., caused by induction or inhibition by another drug) is directly reflected by a change in the extraction ratio, and hence, clearance. Equation 5-13 then applies. In contrast, when eliminating activity is very high, both E_H and clearance approach their limiting values, of one and blood flow, respectively. Then, both parameters are relatively insensitive to even large changes in eliminating activity.

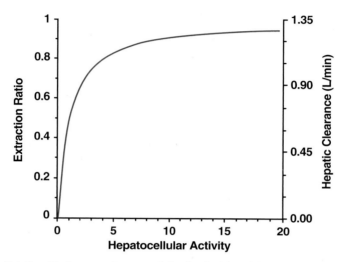

FIGURE 5-9. Relationship between hepatocellular (intrinsic) activity, hepatic extraction ratio and hepatic clearance, for an assumed hepatic blood flow of 1.35 L/min expected based on the well-stirred model. When hepatocellular activity is low, extraction ratio and clearance increase in almost direct proportion to hepatocellular activity. However, as hepatocellular activity increases, extraction ratio approaches the limiting value of 1, and clearance approaches the limiting value of hepatic blood flow. In this upper limiting region, large changes in hepatocellular activity produce minimal changes in clearance. Hepatocellular activity is the parameter that relates rate of hepatic elimination to the unbound concentration in the hepatocyte.

Finally, there are some drugs that have intermediate extraction ratios, such as codeine and nortriptyline (see Table 5-2). The clearance of these compounds is sensitive to all the above-mentioned factors, but not to the same extent as expected at the extremes of extraction ratio.

A MEMORY AID

The general principles just discussed can be difficult to remember. Models of hepatic elimination have been developed to quantify changes in clearance when perfusion, plasma protein binding, and enzyme activity are altered. One of these models, the **well-stirred model**, in which instantaneous and complete mixing is assumed to occur within the liver, is particularly attractive because it can readily be used to summarize these principles (see Appendix E, *Well-Stirred Model of Hepatic Clearance*). Even though it may not be quantitatively accurate, the model allows one to predict those situations in which either clearance or extraction ratio is affected and the expected direction of change. It is used, for example, to generate the curve in Fig. 5-9.

The well-stirred model states that

$$CL_{b,H} = Q_H \cdot E_H = Q_H \cdot \left[\frac{fu_b \cdot CL_{int}}{Q_H + fu_b \cdot CL_{int}} \right] \qquad 5\text{-}14$$

where Q_H is the hepatic blood flow; CL_{int} is the intrinsic clearance, and fu_b is the ratio of unbound concentration in plasma (Cu) to whole blood (C_b) concentration. The term fu_b can readily be estimated from fu if the ratio C/C_b is known, as $Cu = fu \cdot C = fu_b \cdot C_b$; then $fu_b = fu \times plasma/blood\ concentration\ ratio$. From Eq. 5-14, it follows that the hepatic extraction ratio is

$$E_H = \left[\frac{fu_b \cdot CL_{int}}{Q_H + fu_b \cdot CL_{int}} \right] \qquad 5\text{-}15$$

These last two equations have the desired properties at the limits. When E_H approaches 1.0 (the perfusion rate-limited elimination case), a condition that arises because $fu_b \cdot CL_{int}$ is much greater than Q_H, clearance approaches Q_H (Eq. 5-14). Changes in CL_{int} and fu_b here are not expected to influence $CL_{b,H}$ or E_H much. Conversely, when E_H is small, Q_H must be much greater than $fu_b \cdot CL_{int}$. Now E_H and $CL_{b,H}$ are approximated by $fu_b \cdot CL_{int}/Q_H$ and $fu_b \cdot CL_{int}$, respectively; the value of the extraction ratio depends on all three factors, whereas clearance depends only on fu_b and CL_{int}.

Equation 5-15 offers an explanation on why the extraction ratios of most drugs appear to be either low ($E_H < 0.3$) or high ($E_H > 0.7$). Suppose, for example, that the hepatocellular activity (intrinsic clearance) varied evenly from 0.01 to 100 L/min among a large group of compounds (i.e., more than a 10,000-fold range) and that none is bound within blood ($fu_b = 1.0$). Then substitution of these values into Eq. 5-15 shows that only those few drugs with an intrinsic clearance in the narrow range of $0.43 \cdot Q_H$ to $2.3 \cdot Q_H$ have an intermediate extraction ratio (i.e., with values between 0.3 and 0.7).

Strictly, as whole blood delivers drug to the liver, the fraction unbound in Eqs. 5-14 and 5-15 should refer to that in blood, not plasma. The exception are those compounds, such as large polar molecules and protein drugs, many of which are restricted within blood to plasma, because they cannot permeate blood cells. For didactic purposes, however, here and throughout the remainder of the book, unless otherwise stated, where Eqs. 5-14 and 5-15 are applied, as a first approximation, fu and fu_b can be thought of as equivalent. This a reasonable approximation for the majority of drugs in that the ratio of plasma-to-blood concentrations does not differ by more than a factor of two. A major discrepancy occurs, however, when the plasma-to-blood concentration ratio is much smaller than 1, and due correction would then need to be made.

SOME COMPLEXITIES

There are several factors that render the situation more complex than indicated so far. Two of these are considered. The first is permeability and the second is the relative location of enzymes and transporters.

Permeability. So far, it has been assumed that drugs readily pass into the hepatocyte. This is true for many, particularly lipophilic, drugs. However, for larger molecules (molecular weight greater than approximately 600 g/mol) or more polar ones, membrane permeability is often low. This general dependence of hepatocellular uptake permeability on lipophilicity is clearly seen in Fig. 5-10. Shown is the relationship between the permeability-surface area product ($P \cdot SA$) across the basolateral (sinusoidal) membrane (between base of the hepatocyte and blood) of a series of compounds with different lipophilicities. For small highly lipophilic compounds, such as diclofenac and diazepam, the $P \cdot SA$ well exceeds blood flow to the liver, indicating that the rate-limiting step in drug uptake is blood flow. However, as lipophilicity declines so does $P \cdot SA$, and for more polar compounds such as the antibiotic cefodizime, and the angiotensin-converting enzyme

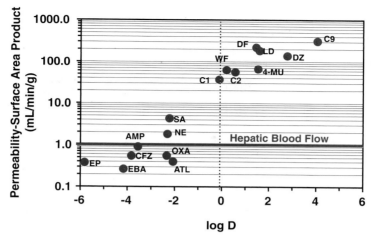

FIGURE 5-10. Relationship between the uptake permeability-surface area product in the isolated perfused rat liver and the logarithm of the n-octanol:water partition coefficient at pH 7.4 (logD), a measure of lipophilicity at plasma physiologic pH, of a series of compounds. Note, the lower the lipophilicity of the compound the lower is its permeability, and for some sufficiently hydrophillic compounds uptake moves toward permeability rate-limited when the permeability-surface area product is considerably less than hepatic blood flow (*colored horizontal line*), whereas for the more lipophilic compounds, blood flow and not permeability becomes the rate-limiting step controlling the kinetics of distribution. AMP ampicillin; ATL, atenolol; C1, 5-methyl-5-ethylbarbituric acid; C2, barbital; C9, 5-n-nonyl-5-ethylbarbituric acid; CFZ cefodizime; DZ, diazepam; DF, diclofenac; EBA, 5-ethylbarbituric acid; EP, enalaprilat; LD, lidocaine; 4-MU, 4-methylumbelliferone; NE, norepinephrine; OXA, oxacillin; SA, salicylic acid; WF, warfarin. (From: Chou C, McLachlan AJ, Rowland M. Membrane permeability and lipophilicity in the isolated perfused rat liver: 5-ethyl barbituric acid and other compounds. J Pharmacol Exp Ther 1995;275:933–940.)

(ACE) inhibitor enalaprilat, it is less than blood flow, and then uptake becomes permeability rate-limited. Occasionally, as appears to be the case with the pravastatin, rosuvastatin (Crestor), and valsartan (Diovan) uptake permeability is so low as to rate limit the overall elimination of drug by the liver. Such drugs then have a low extraction ratio and clearance. Furthermore, under these circumstances, the important component determining clearance is basolateral membrane permeability rather than metabolic activity or biliary secretion (see Appendix E, *Well-stirred Model of Hepatic Clearance*).

Location of Transporters. Recall from Chapter 4, *Membranes and Distribution*, many drugs are substrates for one or more of the hepatic transporters, which are located on either the basolateral (between blood and interior of hepatic cell) membrane upfield of the enzymes or apical (between the cell interior and bile cannaliculae) membrane of the hepatocyte, downfield of the enzymes. On the basolateral membrane, some transporters are involved in transporting drug into the hepatocytes (such as OATP1B1) and others in effluxing drug out of the cell back into the perfusing blood. Consequently, any change in transporter activity can potentially influence observed clearance. Normally, as mentioned above, permeability of the basolateral membrane is so high as not to limit intracellular access, in which case, the main determinants of clearance are the activities of the intracellular enzymes and apical transporters (such as P-glycoprotein and multidrug resistance protein 2) secreting drug into bile. However, occasionally uptake is, or becomes, the slowest process. Then changes in these basolaterally located transporters, caused for example by disease, genetics, competing drugs, or endogenous compounds, will affect the observed clearance of the compound, but not the relative fractions eliminated by hepatic metabolism and biliary secretion.

BILIARY EXCRETION AND ENTEROHEPATIC CYCLING

Small molecular weight drugs are found in bile, whereas protein drugs tend to be excluded. Drug in bile enters the small intestine via the common bile duct after storage in the gallbladder. In the small intestine, it may be reabsorbed to complete an **enterohepatic cycle**. Drug may also be metabolized in the liver (e.g., to a glucuronide). The glucuronide is then secreted into the intestine, where the β-glucuronidase enzymes of the resident flora may hydrolyze it back to the drug, which is then reabsorbed. Enterohepatic cycling of drugs directly and indirectly through a metabolite is represented schematically in Fig. 5-11. Recall from Chapter 2, *Fundamental Concepts and Terminology*, that enterohepatic cycling is a component of distribution, not elimination.

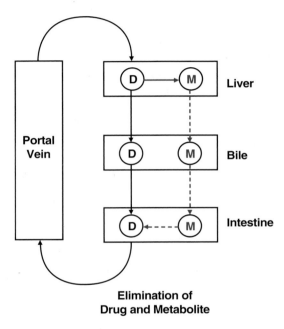

FIGURE 5-11. When a drug (*D*) is absorbed from intestine, excreted in bile, and reabsorbed from intestine, it has undergone enterohepatic cycling (*black arrows*), a component of distribution. Similarly, when a drug is converted to a metabolite (*M*) that is secreted in bile, converted back to drug in the intestine (*colored arrows*), and drug is reabsorbed, the drug has also undergone enterohepatic cycling, in this case, indirectly through a metabolite.

Elimination of Drug and Metabolite

Any drug in bile not reabsorbed, either directly or indirectly via a metabolite, is excreted from the body via the feces. For some drugs, this is the major route of elimination following i.v. administration. The efficiency of biliary excretion can be expressed by biliary clearance.

$$Biliary\ clearance = \frac{(Bile\ flow) \cdot (Concentration\ in\ bile)}{Concentration\ in\ plasma} \qquad 5\text{-}16$$

Bile production in the liver has a relatively steady flow of 0.5 to 0.8 mL/min. Thus, for a drug with a concentration in the bile equal to or less than that in plasma, biliary clearance is very low. A drug that concentrates in the bile, however, may have a relatively high biliary clearance. The bile-to-plasma concentration ratio can approach 1000, when the drug is a very good substrate for one or more of the apical efflux transporters. Therefore, biliary clearances of 500 mL/min or higher can be achieved. Eventually, of course, biliary clearance is limited by hepatic perfusion.

Bile is not a product of filtration, but rather of secretion of bile acids and other solutes. The pH of bile averages about 7.4. The biliary transport of drugs, however, is similar to active secretion in the kidneys in that it may be saturated and competitively inhibited. This topic is further discussed in Chapter 16, *Nonlinearities*.

A few generalizations can be made regarding the characteristics of a drug needed to ensure high biliary clearance. First, the drug must be actively secreted, as occurs extensively for the relatively hydrophilic statin, pravastatin; separate secretory mechanisms exist for acids, bases, and un-ionized compounds. Second, it must be polar, and, last, its molecular weight must exceed 350 g/mol. The latter two requirements may be a consequence of the apparent porous as well as lipophilic nature of bile cannaliculae. Both nonpolar and small molecules may be reabsorbed. These arguments do not aid in predicting the nature and specificity of the secretory mechanisms, but they do aid in predicting the likelihood of a high biliary clearance. For example, glucuronide conjugates of drugs are polar, ionized, pKa about 3, and have molecular weights exceeding 350 g/mol. They are often extensively cleared into bile.

RENAL CLEARANCE

Drugs vary widely in their renal clearance (see Table 5-2). Although the general principles governing renal clearance are the same as for the liver, the mechanisms involved and the relative importance of each differs.

THE NEPHRON: ANATOMY AND FUNCTION

The basic anatomic unit of renal function is the nephron (Fig. 5-12). Basic components are the glomerulus, proximal tubule, loop of Henle, distal tubule, and collecting tubule. The glomerulus receives blood first and filters about 120 mL of plasma water each minute. The filtrate passes down the tubule. Most of the water is reabsorbed, resulting in a urine flow of only 1–2 mL/min. On leaving the glomerulus, the same blood

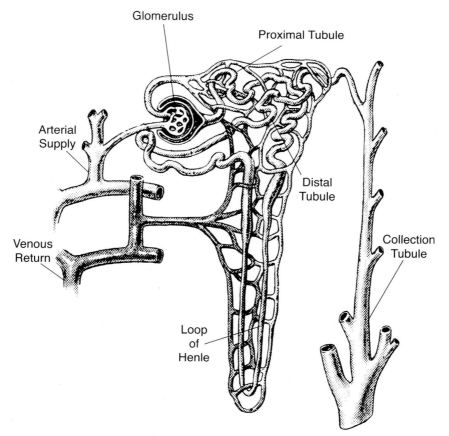

FIGURE 5-12. The functional nephron, an anatomic view. (From: Smith HW. The Kidney: Structure and Function in Health and Disease. New York: Oxford University Press; 1951.)

perfuses both proximal and distal portions of the tubule through a series of interconnecting channels.

Appearance of drug in the urine is the net result of filtration, secretion, and reabsorption. The first two processes add drug to the lumen in the proximal part of the nephron; the last process involves the movement of drug from the lumen back into the bloodstream. The excretion rate is, therefore,

$$Rate\ of\ excretion = (1-F_R)\left[\begin{array}{c} Rate\ of \\ filtration \end{array} + \begin{array}{c} Rate\ of \\ secretion \end{array}\right] \qquad 5\text{-}17$$

where F_R is the fraction reabsorbed from the lumen. A schematic representation of these processes and their approximate location in the nephron are given in Fig. 5-13. Dividing throughout by plasma concentration, therefore leads to

$$CL_R = \dfrac{\begin{array}{c} Rate\ of \\ excretion \end{array}}{C} = (1-F_R)\left[\dfrac{\begin{array}{c} Rate\ of \\ filtration \end{array}}{C} + \dfrac{\begin{array}{c} Rate\ of \\ secretion \end{array}}{C}\right] \qquad 5\text{-}18$$

$$= (1-F_R)[CL_f + CL_S]$$

where CL_f and CL_S are the filtration and secretion clearances, respectively. Let us look at each process in turn.

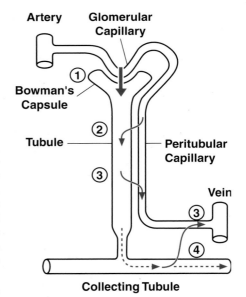

FIGURE 5-13. Schematic representation of the functional unit of the kidney, the nephron. Drug enters the kidney via the renal artery and leaves partly in the exiting renal vein and partly in urine. Urinary excretion (**4**) is the net effect of glomerular filtration of unbound drug (**1**) and tubular secretion (**2**), processes adding drug into the proximal part of the lumen of the tubule, and tubular reabsorption of drug from the lumen and collecting tubule back into the perfusing blood (**3**).

Glomerular Filtration. Approximately 20% to 25% of cardiac output, or 1.1 L of blood per minute, goes to the kidneys. Of this volume, about 10% is filtered at the glomerulus by the hydraulic pressure exerted by the arterial blood. As a general rule, only unbound drug in plasma water (concentration Cu) is filtered; protein-bound drug is too large to pass through the fenestrations in the glomerulus.

The rate at which plasma water is filtered, 120 mL/min in a 70-kg, 20-year-old man, is conventionally called the **glomerular filtration rate**, *GFR*. Therefore,

$$Rate\ of\ filtration = GFR \cdot Cu \qquad 5\text{-}19$$

Recall that fu is the ratio of the unbound to total plasma drug concentration; therefore,

$$Rate\ of\ filtration = fu \cdot GFR \cdot C \qquad 5\text{-}20$$

If a drug is only filtered and all filtered drug is excreted into the urine, then the rate of urinary excretion is the rate of filtration and its renal clearance is its filtration clearance, CL_f. Because renal clearance, CL_R, by definition, is

$$CL_R = \frac{Rate\ of\ urinary\ excretion}{Plasma\ concentration} \qquad \text{5-21}$$

it follows that for such a drug, its renal clearance is $fu \cdot GFR$. The extraction ratio of such a drug is low. For example, even if the drug is totally unbound in blood ($Cu = C_b$), the extraction ratio is still only 0.11. This follows because

$$Extraction\ ratio = \frac{Rate\ of\ extraction}{Rate\ of\ presentation} = \frac{GFR \cdot Cu}{Q_R \cdot C_b} = \frac{120\ mL/min}{1100\ mL/min} = 0.11$$

Creatinine, an endogenously produced compound, is neither bound to plasma proteins nor secreted, and the entire filtered load is excreted into the urine. Accordingly, its renal clearance is a measure of GFR. Under normal conditions, GFR is relatively stable and insensitive to changes in renal blood flow.

Active Secretion. Filtration always occurs but, as shown above, renal extraction of a drug by this mechanism alone is low, especially if drug is highly bound in plasma. Secretion, active transport from blood to lumen of nephron, facilitates extraction. Mechanisms exist for secreting many acids (anions) and bases (cations), and even some large neutral drugs, such as digoxin. The secretory processes are located predominantly in the proximal tubule, on both the basolateral and apical membranes, with sequential uptake and efflux facilitating renal secretion. Although active, these transport systems appear to lack a high degree of specificity, as demonstrated by the wide variety of substances transported by them. As expected, however, substances transported by the same system can compete with each other, and, in doing so, may affect their renal clearances.

Secretion is inferred when rate of excretion ($CL_R \cdot C$) exceeds the rate of filtration ($fu \cdot GFR \cdot C$). Stated differently, secretion is apparent when $CL_R > fu \cdot GFR$. Some reabsorption may still occur, but it must be less than secretion.

Protein Binding and Perfusion. The influence of protein binding on secretion depends on the efficiency of the secretion process and on the contact time at the secretory sites. These conclusions are similar to those drawn for hepatic elimination. Blood resides at the proximal tubular secretory sites for approximately 30 sec. When a drug is secreted, but poorly, this contact time is insufficient to transport much drug into the lumen, and accordingly, the drop in drug concentration across the region is small. Then, the unbound concentration at the secretion site is almost identical to the unbound concentration in plasma, Cu. Because the rate of secretion depends on the unbound drug concentration, or $fu \cdot C$, it follows that clearance resulting from secretion, CL_S, obtained by dividing rate of secretion by C, is directly proportional to fu. As variation in renal blood flow does not cause any change in the plasma drug concentration, no change in renal clearance with perfusion is expected under these circumstances. Furthermore, the sum of clearances associated with filtration ($fu \cdot GFR$) and secretion, must also be directly proportional to fu. Obviously, the extraction ratio of such a drug is low. Figure 5-14 supports these predictions for furosemide in an isolated rat kidney preparation. Furosemide is secreted and is bound to albumin. In this preparation, the fraction unbound could be varied over a wide range.

Some drugs are such excellent substrates for the secretory system that they are virtually completely removed from blood perfusing the kidneys within the time they are in contact with the active transport site, even when they are bound to plasma proteins or located in blood cells. In such cases, evidently dissociation of the drug–protein complex and movement of drug out of the blood cells is sufficiently rapid so as not to limit the

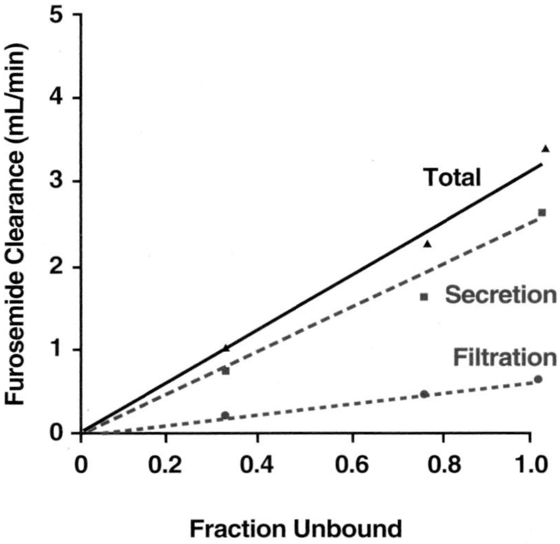

FIGURE 5-14. Contribution of glomerular filtration (●) and tubular secretion (■) to the total renal clearance (▲) of furosemide at different values of fraction unbound. (From: Hall S. Doctoral dissertation, University of Manchester, 1985.)

secretory process. Para-aminohippuric acid (PAH) is handled in this manner and is not reabsorbed. Accordingly, the extraction ratio of PAH is close to 1.0, and hence its renal blood clearance is a measure of renal blood flow, the clinical use of this compound. Obviously, under these circumstances, clearance is perfusion rate-limited. Examples of drugs with various renal extraction ratios are listed in Table 5-2. Although many drug conjugates have high renal extraction ratios, because of a combination of being good substrates for the renal uptake and secretion processes and minimal tubular reabsorption caused by their being hydrophilic, it is rare that drugs in general are highly extracted in the kidneys. This is in contrast to the liver for which a substantial proportion of drugs show high extraction. Also, because it affects oral bioavailability, hepatic extraction is very important in therapeutics, given that most drugs are taken orally.

Tubular Reabsorption. Reabsorption is the third factor controlling the renal handling of drugs. Reabsorption must occur if the renal clearance is less than the calculated clearance by filtration ($CL_R < fu \cdot GFR$). Some secretion may still occur, but it must be less than reabsorption. Reabsorption varies from being almost absent to being virtually complete. Active reabsorption occurs for many vital endogenous compounds, including vitamins, electrolytes, glucose, and amino acids. However, for most exogenous compounds, reabsorption occurs by a passive process. The degree of reabsorption depends on the properties of the drug (e.g., its lipophicity and state of ionization). As with many membranes throughout the body, the lipoidal membranes of the cells that form the tubule act as a barrier to water-soluble and ionized substances. Thus, lipophilic molecules tend to be extensively reabsorbed, whereas polar molecules, such as many conjugates, do not. Reabsorption also depends on physiologic variables such as urine flow and urine pH.

Reabsorption occurs all along the nephron, associated with the reabsorption of water filtered at the glomerulus. The majority, 80% to 90%, of the filtered water is reabsorbed in the proximal tubule. Most of the remainder is reabsorbed in the distal tubule and collecting tubules, where urine flow is controlled. If no water is reabsorbed in the distal tubule, urine flow is about 15 to 20 mL/min. Normally, however, water is so extensively reabsorbed that urine flow is only 1 to 2 mL/min or lower.

Consequently, with water reabsorption, drugs concentrate in the filtrate. In fact, if a drug were neither reabsorbed (generally polar) nor secreted, with approximately 99% water reabsorption, the concentration in the urine would be about 100 times as great as that unbound in plasma. Thus, reabsorption of water favors the reabsorption of a drug.

Urine flow and protein binding. Urine flow can only have a substantial effect on renal clearance if a drug is mostly reabsorbed. Certainly, the effect is most dramatic when reabsorption approaches equilibrium.

As only unbound drug diffuses through membranes, equilibrium is reached when the concentration in urine and that unbound in plasma, Cu, are equal. Consequently, since

$$CL_R = \frac{Urine\ flow \cdot Urine\ concentration}{Plasma\ concentration} \qquad 5\text{-}22$$

and since $Cu = fu \cdot C$, it follows that

$$Renal\ clearance = fu \cdot Urine\ flow \qquad 5\text{-}23$$

This last relationship is a simple test of how close reabsorption of un-ionized drug is to equilibrium. A drug may have a renal clearance below this value if it is actively reabsorbed. Moreover, if drug is highly bound to plasma proteins, renal clearance (and extraction ratio) would be extremely low because urine flow is normally only 1 to 2 mL/min. Note also that renal clearance is directly proportional to fu, when urine flow is constant.

Ethyl alcohol is an example of a compound that is not significantly bound to plasma proteins and is reabsorbed to the extent that its concentration in urine is virtually the same as that in the plasma regardless of urine flow. Consequently, it follows from Eqs. 5-22 and 5-23 that renal clearance of alcohol is approximately equal to urine flow and, therefore, urine-flow dependent.

Urine pH. For weak acids and weak bases, urine pH is an additional factor affecting reabsorption. The extremes of urine pH are 5.0 and 7.5 under forced acidification and alkalinization, respectively. These extremes contrast with the narrow range of plasma pH, 7.3 to 7.5. On the average, urine pH is close to 6.3. Thus, a large pH gradient may exist between plasma and urine.

Urine pH is altered by diet, drugs, and the clinical state of a patient. It also varies during the day. Respiratory and metabolic acidosis produces acidification, and respiratory and metabolic alkalosis produces alkalinization of urine. When metabolic acidosis is of renal origin, for example, renal tubular acidosis, the urine is alkaline. Drugs that substantially inhibit carbonic anhydrase, such as acetazolamide, produce alkaline urine.

Equilibrium Considerations. Renal clearances of several weak acids and bases, listed in Table 5-3, were calculated using Eq. 5-23. The urine-to-plasma concentration ratio was calculated using the Henderson-Hasselbalch equation (Appendix B, *Ionization and the pH*

TABLE 5-3	Calculated Renal Clearances (mL/min) of Selected Nonpolar Weak Acids and Weak Bases at Various Values of Urine pH under Equilibrium Conditions*		
Drug	**Nature**	**pKa**	**Urine pH**
			4.4	**6.4**	**7.9**
A	**Acid**	2.4	0.001	0.1	3
B		6.4	0.1	0.2	3
C		10.4	1.0	1.0	1.0
D	**Base**	2.4	1.0	1.0	1.0
E		6.4	90	2	0.9
F		10.4	1000	10	0.3

*Conditions: no binding of drug to plasma proteins; $fu = 1$, urine flow of 1 mL/min; plasma pH 7.4.

Partition Hypothesis), given that these compounds do not bind to plasma proteins, that equilibrium is achieved between un-ionized drug in urine and plasma, and that the ionized form is not diffusible. It appears that the renal clearance of some acids, pKa less than 6.0, can be much less than urine flow (1 mL/min), whereas that of any base cannot, because urine pH is never much higher than plasma pH.

An interesting observation may be made about weak bases. At low urine pH, renal clearance, by calculation, approaches renal blood flow, which usually suggests active secretion. It is unlikely, however, that such a high clearance value can be obtained by passive diffusion—for three reasons. First, the fraction of renal blood flow that reaches the end of the distal tubule and collecting tubule, where the major change in pH occurs, is small. Second, the calculation of renal clearance in Table 5-3 is based on the ratio of urine concentration to plasma concentration leaving, rather than entering, the kidneys. The venous concentration here is less than that entering the kidneys, particularly when the extraction ratio of the drug is high—a perfusion rate-limited condition. Third, the high values of calculated clearance apply to those bases, which, at blood pH, tend to be almost completely ionized; thus, the rate of movement through the membranes, which depends on the concentration of un-ionized drug, is reduced. A similar argument applies to weak acids. Accordingly, a renal clearance value greater than $fu \cdot GFR$ for either an acid or a base at normal urine pH probably suggests active secretion.

A Rate Process in Reality. The foregoing discussion was based primarily on equilibrium concepts, but tubular reabsorption of drug may not approach equilibrium, as there is only a finite time available as drug passes down the distal tubules where most of the reabsorption occurs. In reality, then, reabsorption should be considered more from a kinetic rather than equilibrium point of view, as is true for absorption of drugs from the gastrointestinal tract (Chapter 7, *Absorption*).

The rate at which reabsorption occurs depends on the ability of the un-ionized drug to diffuse across membranes, its polarity, and the fractions un-ionized in the lumen and plasma. The percentages un-ionized for the same drugs listed in Table 5-3 are given in Table 5-4. The calculation is based on the Henderson-Hasselbalch equation (Appendix B, *Ionization and the pH Partition Hypothesis*).

TABLE 5-4	Percent of Unionized of Selected Weaks Acids and Weal Bases at Various Values of Urine pH*			
Drug	**Nature**	**pKa**	**Urine pH**		
			4.4	**6.4**	**7.9**
A	Acid	2.4	1.0	0.01	0.0003
B		6.4	99	50	3
C		10.4	100	100	99.7
D	Base	2.4	99	100	100
E		6.4	1.0	50	97
F		10.4	0.0001	0.01	0.3

*Same drugs as in Table 5-3.

Weak Bases. The effect of urine pH on the cumulative amount of unchanged methamphetamine (pKa 10) that is excreted in the urine is shown in Fig. 5-15. After 16 hr, about 16% of the dose is excreted unchanged when the urine pH is not controlled, average pH = 6.3. On sustained alkalinizing of urine (e.g., by chronic ingestion of sodium bicarbonate), only 1% to 2% of the dose is in the urine, whereas sustained acidification by

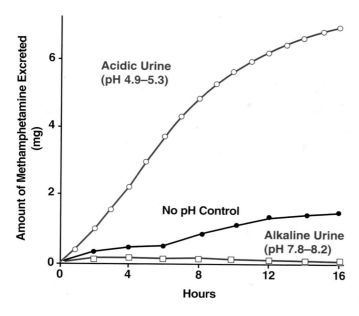

FIGURE 5-15. Mean cumulative urinary excretion of methamphetamine (11 mg, orally) in man varies with the urine pH. (From: Beckett AH, Rowland M. Urinary excretion kinetics of methylamphetamine in man. Nature 1965;206:1260–1261.)

repetitively ingesting ammonium chloride results in 70% to 80% recovery in the urine. Clearly, for this drug, urine pH is important in determining the contribution of renal to total elimination; and hence, it strongly influences total clearance and half-life. Under conditions of no pH control, urine pH varies throughout the day, and the excretion of methamphetamine fluctuates accordingly. The explanation for these observations is contained in Tables 5-3 and 5-4. At low urine pH, both equilibrium and kinetic considerations favor high renal clearance of a basic drug of pKa 10. In particular, the percent un-ionized, and hence the un-ionized concentration in the renal tubule, is so small that there is little opportunity for reabsorption within the time that the drug resides in the nephron. At high urine pH, with a greater percent of drug un-ionized in the tubule, both equilibrium and rate considerations favor reabsorption. *Drugs that show these substantial changes in renal clearance are said to be pH sensitive.*

The effect of urine pH on the reabsorption of basic drugs, in general, can be summarized as follows:

1. A basic drug that is polar in its un-ionized form is not reabsorbed, regardless of its degree of ionization in the urine, unless actively transported. The hydrophilic aminoglycoside gentamicin is an example; its renal clearance approximates that of GFR and is independent of urine pH.
2. A very weakly basic nonpolar drug, whose pKa is around 7.0 or below, such as diazepam, is extensively reabsorbed, and renal clearance is accordingly very low, at all values of urine pH because virtually 100% is un-ionized regardless of urine pH. Furthermore, equilibrium favors reabsorption.
3. For a basic nonpolar drug with a *pKa value between 7.0 and 12,* the extent of reabsorption may vary from negligible to almost complete (equilibration) with changes in urine pH. The renal clearance of such a drug (e.g., methamphetamine) can therefore vary markedly with urine pH, being higher at lower pH values. Basic drugs with a pKa >12 would be expected to be minimally reabsorbed being essentially completely ionized at all values of urine pH.

Weak Acids. The principles developed for weak bases also apply to weak acids. However, for acids, an increase in pH causes more ionization, not less. Consequently, acids are reabsorbed less and have larger renal clearances at higher urine pH.

Again, the effect of pKa on reabsorption is seen by inspecting Tables 5-3 and 5-4. An acid with a pKa value of 2.0 or less (e.g., chromoglycic acid) is so completely ionized at all urine pH values that it is simply not reabsorbed; its renal clearance is generally high and insensitive to pH. At the other extreme, a very weak acid with a pKa value above 8.0, such as phenytoin, is mostly un-ionized throughout the range of urine pH; its renal clearance is always low and insensitive to pH. Only for a nonpolar acid whose pKa *lies between 3.0 and 7.5* might renal clearance be pH sensitive. Note in Table 5-3 that for all nonpolar acids equilibrium favors reabsorption.

Data supporting the expected urine pH sensitivity in renal clearance of nonpolar weak acids with a pKa between 3 and 7.5 and nonpolar weak bases with a pKa between 6 and 12 are provided by salicylic acid, pKa 3 (Fig. 5-16), and the anthelmintic diethylcarbamazine, pKa 10 (Table 5-5), respectively.

Weak acids and bases that show pH-sensitive reabsorption also generally show flow-rate dependence. Again, however, the degree to which renal clearance is changed by urine flow depends on the extent of reabsorption. If 50% of that filtered and secreted is reabsorbed at normal urine flow, 50% is excreted. Increased urine flow decreases reabsorption toward zero, but renal clearance cannot be increased by more than a factor

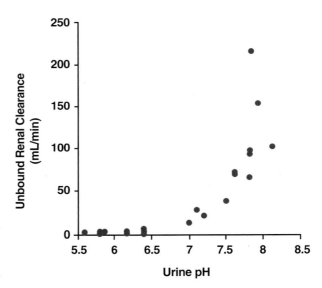

FIGURE 5-16. The unbound renal clearance of salicylic acid increases dramatically with an increase in urine pH above 6.5. (From: Smith PK, Gleason HL, Stall CG, Ogorzalek S. Studies on the pharmacology of salicylates. J Pharmacol Exp Ther 1946; 87:237–255.)

TABLE 5-5	Sensitivity of Diethylcarbamazine Renal Clearance to Change in Urine pH
Urine pH	**Renal Clearance (L/hr)**
Not controlled (~6.3)*	8.6
Acidic, <5.5	38.0
Alkaline, >7.0	1.0

*Typical pH of urine.
From: Edwards G, Breckenridge AM, Adjepon-Yamoah KK, et al. The effect of variations in urinary pH on the pharmacokinetics of diethylcarbamazine. Brit J Clin Pharmacol 1981;12:807–812.

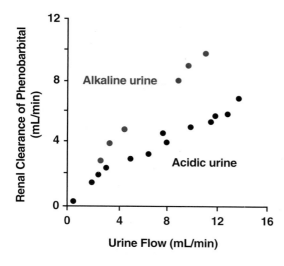

FIGURE 5-17. Renal clearance of phenobarbital varies with urine flow in man. It is also a function of urine pH: without alkalinization (*black circles*), with alkalinization (*colored circles*). (From: Linton AL, Luke RG, Briggs JD. Methods of forced diuresis and its application in barbiturate poisoning. Lancet 1967;290:377–390.)

of 2. Figure 5-17 shows how the renal clearance of phenobarbital (pKa 7.2) varies with urine flow. As expected, the renal clearance of this drug is pH sensitive as well as urine flow-rate dependent.

Forced Diuresis and Urine pH Control. Increased urine flow by forced intake of fluids and, in some cases, the coadministration of mannitol or another diuretic, can increase the excretion of some drugs. More rapid elimination is, of course, desirable for the purpose of detoxifying a patient who is overdosed. Several criteria must be met for forced diuresis to be of value:

1. Renal excretion under conditions of forced diuresis must be or become the major route of drug elimination. Increasing the renal clearance of a drug 10-fold, for example, does little to hasten drug elimination from the body if renal clearance normally is only 1% of total clearance. Although renal excretion may be a relatively modest pathway of elimination at therapeutic doses, it may become the major route of elimination during drug overdose if the metabolic pathways become saturated.
2. The compound must normally be extensively reabsorbed in the renal tubule.
3. If the reabsorption is pH sensitive, both forced diuresis and pH control may be of value. This applies if forced diuresis or pH control alone only partially prevents reabsorption.

The last point bears further discussion. Suppose that, on alkalinizing the urine, the reabsorption of a weak acid is decreased from 90% to 10% of that filtered and secreted. The addition of forced diuresis will be of little additional value; the excretion rate can only be increased by a further 10%. The converse applies to the use of pH control when forced diuresis almost completely prevents reabsorption.

RENAL METABOLISM

Emphasis so far has been on the kidney as an excretory organ. Yet, this organ contains various enzymes capable of hydrolysis, oxidation, and conjugation of drugs. Often, however, this is a minor route of metabolism, but not always. Direct evidence of the involvement of the kidney in drug metabolism is normally difficult to obtain. Evidence is usually most clearly discerned when studying handling of drug in patients with renal impairment, an aspect explored in greater detail in Chapter 15, *Disease*, and in

Chapter 21, *Protein Drugs*. It is in such patients that the impact of renal metabolism is greatest.

DEPENDENCE OF ELIMINATION KINETICS ON CLEARANCE AND DISTRIBUTION

The physiology of the body dictates that several pharmacokinetic parameters are related to and dependent on one another. Perhaps the most fundamental dependency in clinical pharmacokinetics is that of half-life on (total) clearance and volume of distribution. This dependency is derived as follows.

HALF-LIFE IN PLASMA

Recall from Chapter 3, *Kinetics Following an Intravenous Bolus Dose*, that the elimination rate constant (i.e., fractional rate of drug elimination) at distribution equilibrium, k, is related to total clearance, CL, and volume of distribution, V, by the expression

$$k = \frac{Rate\ of\ elimination}{Amount\ in\ body} = \frac{CL}{V} \qquad 5\text{-}24$$

Because clearance is the volume of plasma cleared of drug per unit of time and V is the volume that drug appears to occupy at a concentration equal to that in plasma, it is apparent from Eq. 5-24 that fractional rate of drug elimination can be thought of as the fraction of the volume of distribution from which drug is removed per unit time. Furthermore, recall that half-life, $t_{1/2}$, is related to k, or to V and CL through the expressions

$$t_{1/2} = \frac{0.693}{k} = \frac{0.693 \cdot V}{CL} \qquad 5\text{-}25$$

To appreciate the dependence of half-life on clearance and volume of distribution, consider a drug that undergoes complete enterohepatic cycling yet distributes to bile and subsequently to the intestines in significant amounts as a result of slow intestinal reabsorption. The consequence of biliary obstruction would be a decreased volume of distribution, but no change in total clearance, and therefore a shorter half-life. On the other hand, if there is no enterohepatic cycling, the bile and the intestines are not part of the volume of distribution. Biliary obstruction, by decreasing clearance without affecting distribution, would then cause the half-life to increase.

Figure 5-18 illustrates half-lives of drugs with various combinations of clearance and volume of distribution. One striking feature is the enormous range of values for both of these parameters, with volume of distribution ranging 2000-fold, from 3 to 7000 L, and clearance ranging from 0.01 to close to 100 L/hr, a 10,000-fold range. Another striking feature is the large number of drugs with similar half-lives (e.g., 20 to 50 hr), comprising different combinations of clearance and volume of distribution. Note also, when clearance is low and volume of distribution is large, the half-life can be weeks or months. There is a paucity of drug examples with these characteristics. A small volume (4–10 L/70 kg) and a very low clearance (<0.1 L/hr) is common for a particular class of therapeutic agents, the monoclonal antibodies (see Chapter 21, *Protein Drugs*). Three examples are given in Fig. 5-18, namely, daclizumab, infliximab, and adalimumab.

The relative lack of very long-life drugs is not surprising, because drug accumulation would be extensive and occur slowly on daily dosing for prolonged periods. Furthermore, detoxification of a patient who exhibits toxicity while on such a drug would generally be slow, without intervention with a rescue procedure, such as the administration of activated charcoal (see Chapter 4, *Membranes and Distribution*) or hemodialysis (see Chapter 15, *Disease*).

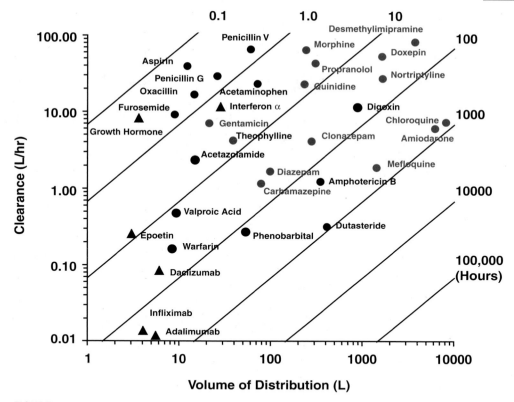

FIGURE 5-18. Clearance (ordinate) and volume of distribution (abscissa) of selected acidic (●, digoxin is neutral) and basic (●), as well as protein (▲), drugs varies widely. The diagonal lines show the combination of clearance and volume with the same half-lives (in hours). Note that drugs with very low clearance and very large volumes (lower right-hand quadrant of graph) are uncommon; their half-lives are often too long for these drugs to be used practically in drug therapy. Note also that protein drugs have volumes of distribution close to plasma volume, and that basic compounds tend to have larger volumes of distribution than acids. Digoxin is a neutral compound, whereas amphotericin B is both an acid and a base.

HALF-LIFE IN BLOOD AND PLASMA WATER

The interrelationships expressed in Eqs. 5-24 and 5-25 are just as readily derived from clearance and volume parameters based on measurements of drug in blood (CL_b, V_b) or in plasma water (CLu, Vu). Thus, recall

$$Rate\ of\ elimination = CL \cdot C = CL_b \cdot C_b = CLu \cdot Cu$$

and, at distribution equilibrium

$$Amount\ in\ body = V \cdot C = V_b \cdot C_b = Vu \cdot Cu$$

Note that each clearance or volume term can be related to the other using the definitions $fu = Cu/C$ and $fu_b = Cu/C_b$. For example, $CL = fu \cdot CLu$. Dividing each clearance term by the respective volume term gives

$$k = \frac{CL}{V} = \frac{CL_b}{V_b} = \frac{CL_u}{V_u} \tag{5-26}$$

and on substituting Eq. 5-24 into Eq. 5-23, it follows that

$$t_{1/2} = \frac{0.693\ V}{CL} = \frac{0.693\ V_b}{CL_b} = \frac{0.693\ V_u}{CL_u} \tag{5-27}$$

Thus, the value of the elimination rate constant, k, or the half-life, $t_{1/2}$, is independent of the site of measurement in blood.

The clearance parameter based on measurement of drug in blood is useful in considerations of drug extraction in the eliminating organs. Volume and clearance parameters based on the unbound drug concentration are particularly useful in therapeutics, because it is the unbound drug that is thought to relate most closely to the effects of a drug. Both sets of parameters are of value in anticipating and evaluating the pharmacokinetic and therapeutic consequences of alterations in protein binding, blood flow, and other physiologic variables. In practice, plasma drug concentrations are usually measured, but the application of the volume and clearance parameters so obtained is limited. We now illustrate the benefits of integrating physiologic concepts with kinetics.

INTEGRATION OF KINETIC AND PHYSIOLOGIC CONCEPTS

Reference is frequently made to *the* half-life or *the* clearance of a drug, as if there were only one value for each parameter. The pharmacokinetic parameters of a drug can, and do however, change—with disease, with concomitant drug therapy, and even within the same individual with time. An ability to assign likely physiologic and pathologic mechanisms to these observed changes in the kinetics of a drug is important, as is the prediction of the kinetic consequences of an alteration in a physiologic variable. Both approaches are taken in this last part of the chapter with respect to events following an i.v. bolus (i.e., disposition kinetics) to integrate and practice the physiologic and pharmacokinetic concepts learned to this point. No attempt is made to examine situations involving all possible changes of physiologic variables because the theoretical possibilities are too numerous. In subsequent chapters, especially in Chapter 6, *Kinetics Following an Extravascular Dose*, Chapter 10, *Constant-Rate Input*, Chapter 11, *Multiple-Dose Regimens*, Chapter 15, *Disease*, Chapter 16, *Nonlinearities*, and Chapter 17, *Drug Interactions*, additional examples that demonstrate and require integration of physiologic and kinetic concepts are given.

Frequently, conditions that produce a change in one physiologic parameter cause changes in others as well. For example, renal disease appears not only to decrease the renal clearance of digoxin, but to reduce its tissue distribution and extrarenal clearance as well (see Chapter 15, *Disease*). The interaction of quinidine and digoxin is another example. Similar to renal disease, quinidine decreases tissue distribution and both renal and extrarenal clearances of digoxin. Thus, neither of these situations is a good example of the kinetic consequences of any *one* of the alterations that occur. Yet, these kinds of observations occur frequently. The first step in analyzing such situations is to examine the expectations for an alteration in each physiologic variable involved. The overall picture is then gained by integrating these expectations.

INTERRELATIONSHIPS AMONG PHARMACOKINETIC PARAMETERS AND PHYSIOLOGIC VARIABLES

A summary of the interrelationships among pharmacokinetic parameters and physiologic variables is appropriate here.

Primary Parameters and Physiologic Variables. The processes affecting disposition depend on many physiologic variables. Distribution is influenced by binding to both plasma proteins and tissue components and by body composition. Renal excretion may depend on secretion (active transport), urine pH, and urine flow. Hepatic elimination depends on enzyme and biliary activity, binding within blood, and blood flow. Each of these physiologic variables is affected by numerous factors. Thus, for example, exercise affects tissue blood flow, food affects intestinal blood flow, urine flow depends on fluid intake and water loss, and diseases and drugs produce many effects.

The disposition kinetics of a drug can be described with reference to systemic concentration by relatively few parameters. Recall extent of distribution can be characterized by the volume of distribution, and elimination can be characterized by hepatic and renal clearances. Each of these parameters may be directly affected by changes in physiologic variables. Because of this direct relationship, these parameters are referred to in this book as **primary pharmacokinetic parameters**. It is recognized, however, that each of these parameters is controlled by many other cellular and molecular events.

Secondary Pharmacokinetic Parameters and Derived Values. Half-life, elimination rate constant, and fraction excreted unchanged in urine are examples of *secondary pharmacokinetic parameters*, in that their values depend on those of the primary pharmacokinetic parameters. Furthermore, there are several observations, such as area under the curve (*AUC*), that depend not only on the primary pharmacokinetic parameters but also on dose administered. These dependencies are summarized briefly in Table 5-6.

TABLE 5-6	Dependence of Secondary Pharmacokinetic Parameters and Observations on Primary Pharmacokinetic Parameters
Secondary Pharmacokinetic Parameters	**Equations**
Elimination half-life	0.693 · Volume of distribution/Clearance
Elimination rate constant	Clearance/(Volume of distribution)
Fraction excreted unchanged	(Renal clearance)/(Total clearance)
Observations	
Area under curve (i.v.)	Dose/Clearance
C_{max}	Dose/Volume of distribution
Amount excreted unchanged	Dose · (Renal clearance)/(Total clearance)

The equations in Table 5-6 plus a few previous equations provide the basic relationships for interpreting and predicting alterations in kinetic behavior. Particularly useful is the memory aid of Eqs. 5-14 and 5-15, namely

$$CL_{b,H} = Q_H \cdot \left[\frac{fu_b \cdot CL_{int}}{Q_H + fu_b \cdot CL_{int}} \right]$$

and

$$E_H = \left[\frac{fu_b \cdot CL_{int}}{Q_H + fu_b \cdot CL_{int}} \right]$$

Volume of distribution depends on binding to both plasma proteins and tissue constituents. For a drug with a large volume (>50 L) and whose distribution is not materially affected by transporters,

$$V \approx V_R \cdot \frac{fu}{fu_R}$$

whereas for a low molecular weight (<500 g/mol) drug with a small volume of distribution (<0.2 L/kg), which are generally acidic drugs, *V* tends to be independent of changes in *fu* (Chapter 4, *Membranes and Distribution*).

The subsequent examples are analyzed using these relationships. They exemplify alterations in intrinsic hepatocellular activity (induction and inhibition), hepatic blood flow, active tubular secretion, and plasma protein binding.

Induction of Metabolism. Some drugs induce the metabolism of others by increasing the rate of synthesis of the enzyme(s) involved. The kinetic and therapeutic consequences depend on whether the affected drug initially has a low or a high extraction ratio in the eliminating organ in which induction occurs.

Low extraction ratio. Figure 5-19 demonstrates the kinetic effect of induction of metabolism of the opioid analgesic alfentanil by the antitubercular agent rifampin. Alfentanil is almost exclusively metabolized in the liver; a negligible fraction is excreted in urine unchanged. Rifampin induces the metabolism of CYP3A4, the primary enzyme responsible for alfentanil metabolism.

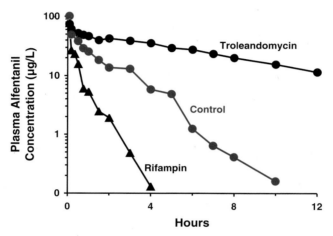

FIGURE 5-19.   The influence of altered hepatocellular enzymatic (CYP3A4) activity on the disposition kinetics of the opioid analgesic alfentanil. Semilogarithmic plot of the mean plasma alfentanil concentration–time profiles administered as a single i.v. bolus dose (20 μg/kg) to a group of male subjects, alone (●), following administration of the enzyme inducer rifampin (▲) and the enzyme inhibitor troleandomycin (●) on separate occasions. Rifampin (600 mg, orally) was taken for five consecutive mornings before alfentanil administration, whereas troleandomycin (500 mg, orally) was taken 2 hr before, and then 12, 24, and 36 hr following the dose of alfentanil. Notice that compared with the control, rifampin increases and troleandomycin reduces the clearance of alfentanil, a drug with a low extraction ratio, with reciprocal changes in half-life. (From: Kharasch ED, Russell M, Mautz D, et al. The role of cytochrome P450 3A4 in alfentanil clearance: Implications for interindividual variability in disposition and perioperative drug interactions. Anesthesiology 1997;87:36–50.)

The data in Fig. 5-19 support alfentanil having a low hepatic extraction ratio. This conclusion is based on the calculation of clearance. Thus, during the control phase clearance, obtained by dividing dose (20 μg/kg) by *AUC* (63 μg-hr/L), is 0.32 L/hr per kilogram. The plasma-to-blood concentration ratio is close to 1, so that blood clearance is considerably lower than hepatic blood flow, 81 L/hr/70 kg or 1.2 L/hr per kilogram, with an estimated hepatic extraction ratio of 0.27. In the presence of rifampin, the *AUC* of alfentanil is clearly decreased compared with that of the control value, reflecting a higher clearance. This observation is consistent with induction of hepatic enzymes; the clearance of a drug of low hepatic extraction ratio is expected to be sensitive to changes in hepatocellular enzymatic activity. The data suggest no effect of rifampin on alfentanil distribution. The estimated volumes of distribution are 0.37 and 0.44 L/kg during the control and rifampin phases, respectively. These values are probably not significantly different. Finally, half-life reflects reciprocally the increase in clearance, as it decreases with rifampin treatment.

High extraction ratio. Induction of metabolism of a drug with a high hepatic extraction ratio has kinetic consequences very different from those of a drug with a low hepatic extraction ratio, as illustrated in Fig. 5-20. Pretreatment with the enzyme inducer pentobarbital has little effect on the pharmacokinetics of alprenolol after its i.v. administration. At first glance, this observation appears to be inconsistent with enzyme induction. Knowing that this drug is eliminated almost exclusively by metabolism in the liver, with only traces found in urine, and on calculating (from dose and *AUC* and knowing that the plasma-to-blood concentration is 1.3) a blood clearance of 1.2 L/min in this individual, the explanation is clear.

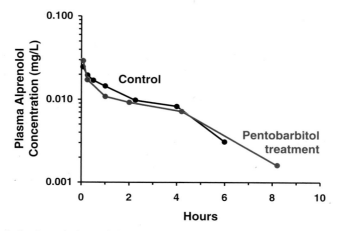

FIGURE 5-20. Induction of alprenolol metabolism by pentobarbital treatment produces minimal change in the plasma concentration with time when given as a 5-mg i.v. bolus. Alprenolol was administered before (*black lines*: ●) and 10 days into (*colored lines*: ●) a pentobarbital regimen of 100 mg at bedtime. Despite in vitro evidence that pentobarbital induces drug metabolism, there is no material change in the disposition kinetics of alprenolol following pentobarbital treatment because the clearance of alprenolol, a drug with a high hepatic extraction ratio, is limited by blood flow, which is unaltered by pentobarbital treatment. (From: Alván G, Piafsky K, Lind M, von Bahr C. Effect of pentobarbital on the disposition of alprenolol. Clin Pharmacol Ther 1977;22:316–321.)

The hepatic extraction ratio of alprenolol is inherently high; its clearance approaches hepatic blood flow, approximately 1.35 L/min, even before induction. Because clearance is therefore perfusion rate-limited, and relatively insensitive to changes in intrinsic metabolic clearance associated with enzyme induction, and there is no evidence in humans that pentobarbital alters hepatic blood flow, there is only a modest increase in clearance with pentobarbital administration. Calculation shows that the increase in hepatic extraction ratio, and hence clearance, is only about 20% (from 0.78–0.94), which is difficult to detect in practice. Furthermore, the lack of change in terminal half-life after induction indicates that pentobarbital has no effect on the volume of distribution of alprenolol. In the absence of any auxiliary information, one might well have concluded that no induction had occurred. Two additional pieces of information demonstrate, however, that induction by pentobarbital occurs. One is a body of in vitro data, showing clear evidence of induction of the enzymes responsible for the metabolism of alprenolol by pentobarbital. The other, discussed at greater depth in Chapter 7, *Absorption,* is reduction in the oral bioavailability of alprenolol, from 22% to 6%, after coadministration with pentobarbital.

Metabolic Inhibition. Examples of drugs that inhibit the metabolism of other drugs are given in Chapter 17, *Drug Interactions.* Reduced metabolism can also be a consequence of hepatic disease (Chapter 15, *Disease*), dietary deficiencies (Chapter 12, *Variability*), and other conditions. Whatever the cause of decreased metabolic activity, the kinetic consequences depend on the hepatic extraction ratio of the drug.

Low extraction ratio. The effect of decreasing hepatocellular activity for a drug of low hepatic extraction ratio is illustrated by data of the effect of the macrolide antibiotic troleandomycin on alfentanil. Recall, alfentanil is primarily eliminated by CYP3A4-catalyzed metabolism, and troleandomycin is a potent inhibitor of this enzyme.

The concentration–time profile of the alfenanil after a 20 µg/kg i.v. bolus dose is clearly very different from that following troleandomycin administration (Fig. 5-19), with *AUC* increased and half-life substantially prolonged. Specifically, mean clearance and half-life values were 0.32 L/kg and 1.0 hr in the absence and 0.066 L/kg and 10.5 hr in the presence of troleandomycin. The effect of decreased hepatocellular activity is clear for a drug with a low extraction ratio; clearance decreases and half-life increases.

High extraction ratio. The kinetic consequences of inhibition of metabolism of a drug with a high hepatic extraction ratio are illustrated by the coadministration of the antifungal agent, itraconazole, and the analgesic opioid fentanyl (Fig. 5-21). That, unlike alfentanil, fentanyl is a drug of high hepatic extraction ratio is deduced from its blood clearance, 1.5 L/hr per kilogram (estimated by dividing the i.v. dose by the corresponding *AUC* and knowing that the plasma-to-blood concentration is 1), is in the same order as hepatic blood flow, and from the knowledge that fentanyl is eliminated almost exclusively by hepatic metabolism.

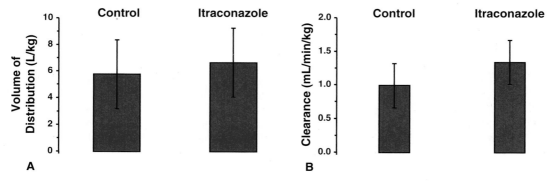

FIGURE 5-21. **A,B.** Neither volume of distribution or clearance of the opioid analgesic fentanyl following an i.v. bolus dose (3 µg/kg) is influenced by the coadministration of itraconazole (200 mg orally for 4 days prior to fentanyl administration), despite its known inhibition of CYP3A4, the enzyme primarily responsible for the metabolism of fentanyl. The explanation lies in the very high hepatic clearance of fentanyl for which clearance is blood flow limited, even in the presence of this dosage of itraconazole. (From: Palkama VJ, Neuvonen PJ, Olkkola KT. The CYP 3A4 inhibitor itraconazole has no effect on the pharmacokinetics of i.v. fentanyl. Br J Anaesth 1998;81:598–600.)

Notice, there is no significant change in the clearance of fentanyl, despite knowing that this opioid, like alfentanil, is eliminated almost exclusively by hepatic metabolism via CYP3A4, and that in vitro itraconazole has been clearly shown to be a reasonably strong inhibitor of CYP3A4. The explanation lies in the clearance of fentanyl being perfusion rate-limited under control conditions, with calculations based on the well-stirred model showing that the intrinsic hepatocellular clearance of fentanyl would have to be reduced by a factor of more than fourfold before clearance moves away from a perfusion-rate limitation to one starting to be controlled by intrinsic clearance. So, although itraconazole at the doses administered probably does inhibit fentanyl metabolism in vivo, the inhibition is not great enough to influence clearance. Evidence supporting this notion is seen by the pronounced reduction in the clearance of fentanyl when coadministered with the protease inhibitor ritonavir, a much more potent inhibitor of CYP3A4 than itraconazole (Fig. 5-22).

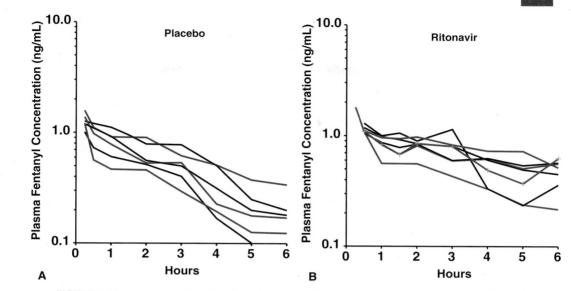

FIGURE 5-22. Mean semilogarithmic plot of plasma fentanyl concentration versus time after an i.v. bolus dose of 5 μg/kg fentanyl alone (**A**), and when coadministered (**B**) with ritonavir (200 mg orally three times daily) to a panel of 11 subjects. Ritonavir is clearly seen to reduce the clearance, and prolong the half-life, of fentanyl. (From: Olkkola KT, Palkama VJ, Neuvonen PJ. Ritonavir's role in reducing fentanyl clearance and prolonging its half-life. Anesthesiology 1999;91:681–685.)

Specifically, in this separate study, clearance of fentanyl was reduced from 0.94 L/hr per kg under control conditions to 0.32 L/hr per kg in the presence of ritonavir. That is, from a high to a low extraction ratio compound ($fu_b \cdot CL_{int} < Q_H$). Furthermore, as ritonavir had no material effect on the volume of distribution of fentanyl (9.4 vs. 7.5 L/kg), the reduction in clearance is reflected in a prolongation in half-life of fentanyl.

Altered Blood Flow. Changes in organ blood flow affect clearance only when extraction ratio is high. This conclusion is based on the concept of a perfusion-rate limitation. It should be borne in mind, however, that effects secondary to an altered blood flow, particularly when decreased, may supersede perfusion considerations alone. For example, a decreased blood flow may produce anoxia, which in turn may affect hepatocellular activity and hence the extraction ratio. The extraction ratio may also be altered by a decreased blood flow, because every blood vessel in the organ may not provide the same exposure of the drug to hepatic parenchymal cells, and the pattern of distribution of blood flow within the eliminating organ may change. This alteration in the degree of shunting or bypassing of the parenchymal cells may occur in certain hepatic diseases and under various conditions.

Good examples of the kinetic consequences of altered blood flow are hard to find. This is not because they are uncommon, but because a number of additional complications always seem to occur concurrently. For example, conditions such as congestive cardiac failure, in which cardiac output is decreased, are often associated with increased third spacing (build-up of fluid in intestinal spaces and body cavities), diminished hepatic and renal functions, and slowed distribution to the tissues. A decrease in hepatic blood flow, brought about by cirrhosis, chronically leads to portal hypertension and extrahepatic shunting of portal blood. Thus, the kinetic consequences of altered blood flow are subsequently examined alone, with the realization that in therapeutic scenarios the effects of changes in more than one physiologic variable need to be considered.

For this theoretical presentation, consider the two drugs given in Table 5-7. Drug L is eliminated in both the liver and the kidneys; its major property is low extraction in both

TABLE 5-7	Pharmacokinetic Parameters of Two Hypothetical Drugs				
				Extraction Ratio	
Drug	Volume of Distribution (L)	Clearance* (L/hr)	Fraction Excreted Unchanged	Hepatic	Renal
L	26	6	0.60	0.03	0.05
H	430	77	0.05	0.95	0.06

*Clearance is based on measurement of drug in blood.

organs. Drug H has a high hepatic extraction ratio and is almost exclusively eliminated by the liver.

Low hepatic extraction ratio. Figure 5-23 shows the effect of a doubling of hepatic blood flow for the poorly cleared drug, drug L. Because drug L has a low hepatic extraction ratio, altered blood flow has little or no effect on the pharmacokinetics of this drug, and with no change in volume of distribution, no change in elimination half-life either.

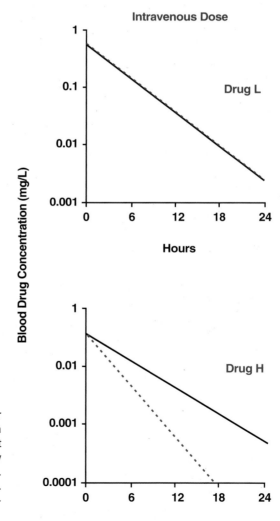

FIGURE 5-23. Increased blood flow to the liver has very little effect on the time course of Drug L, a poorly extracted drug, after an i.v. 15-mg dose but has a pronounced effect on Drug H, a highly cleared drug, following single i.v. (15 mg) dose. Altered condition (----); normal condition (——). See Table 5-7 for other pharmacokinetic properties of these two drugs.

High hepatic extraction ratio. The events following i.v. administration of a drug with a high hepatic extraction ratio, drug H, when hepatic blood flow is increased, are readily apparent. Being perfusion rate-limited, clearance increases, and with no change in distribution, half-life decreases.

An example of a change in kinetics with a change in blood flow is given with lidocaine in Fig. 5-24. Lidocaine is a drug with a high hepatic extraction ratio, and hence, its clearance is perfusion rate-limited. Here, as expected, the concurrent administration of either β-blocker, propranolol or metoprolol, which reduce cardiac output and hepatic blood flow, produces a decrease in the clearance of lidocaine. The change in lidocaine clearance following propranolol administration is larger than that expected for the change in hepatic blood flow, suggesting that one or more other mechanisms may also be operating.

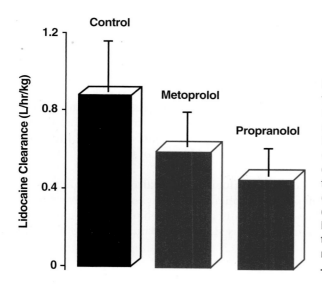

FIGURE 5-24. The clearance of lidocaine following a 4-min i.v. infusion (3 mg/kg) is reduced during metoprolol (50 mg) or propranolol (40 mg) administration (every 6 hr beginning 24 hr before the test dose and continuing for 8 hr thereafter). These drugs decrease cardiac output and hepatic blood flow, the primary mechanism by which the clearance of lidocaine is thought to be reduced. (From: Conrad KA, Byers JM III, Finley PR, Burnham L. Lidocaine elimination: effects of metoprolol and of propranolol. Clin Pharmacol Ther 1983;33:133–138.)

Altered Active Tubular Secretion. Figure 5-25 shows the effect of inhibiting the renal tubular secretion of digoxin by ritonavir, and more. An increase in the *AUC* of digoxin is obvious; it reflects a decrease in clearance, from 409 to 238 mL/min. The inhibition of renal excretion of digoxin by ritonavir, however, only becomes apparent when this pathway is isolated, by also collecting unchanged drug in urine, as was done in the study.

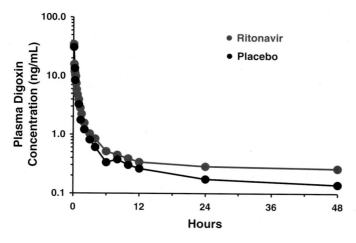

FIGURE 5-25. Semilogarithmic plot of mean plasma digoxin concentration–time profile obtained in 12 subjects after an i.v. dose of digoxin administered alone (●) and on day 3 of an 11-day treatment of 300 mg of ritonavir given orally twice daily (●). (From: Ding R, Tayrouz Y, Riedel KD, et al. Substantial pharmacokinetic interaction between digoxin and ritonavir in healthy volunteers. Clin Pharmacol Ther 2004;76:73–84.)

Renal clearance, given by the ratio of total amount excreted unchanged to AUC ($CL_R = Ae_\infty/AUC$) is reduced by ritonavir, from 194 to 126 mL/min. The substantial renal excretion of digoxin, more than 60% of the i.v. dose, explains why a reduced renal clearance has such a substantive effect on total clearance. To conclude that the reduced renal clearance is caused by inhibition of secretion, several additional pieces of information are needed. First, digoxin is minimally bound to plasma proteins ($fu = 0.8$), and second, ritonavir does not affect glomerular filtration rate. Hence, because filtration clearance is 96 mL/min ($= fu \cdot GFR$), under control conditions there must be some secretion of digoxin ($CL_R > fu \cdot GFR$), which is reduced by ritonavir. An additional important lesson is learned. Ritonavir, like many drugs, interacts at many levels. Previously, we saw that it is a potent inhibitor of CYP3A4 mediated metabolism. Now, we see it is also an inhibitor of renal secretion. Through separate studies, the mechanism of this interaction has been identified. Ritonavir is an inhibitor of the efflux transporter, P-glycoprotein, which resides on the brush border membrane of the proximal cells of the nephron and secretes various compounds, including digoxin, into the lumen.

Altered Plasma Protein Binding. Knowledge of conditions in which the binding to plasma proteins is altered is critical to plasma drug concentration monitoring (Chapter 18, *Initiating and Managing Therapy*). When activities, desired and undesired, relate to the unbound concentration, changes in binding directly affect the interpretation of total concentration data. This problem applies to drugs of both low and high extraction. Whether the altered binding affects the unbound plasma concentration, the concentration at the active site is therapeutically important. These aspects are now addressed in turn.

Low extraction ratio. Shown in Fig. 5-26 is the influence of impaired renal function on the disposition kinetics of the antiepileptic drug, phenytoin (also and formerly referred to as diphenylhydantoin). Normally, one expects disease of an eliminating organ to reduce clearance, but in this case, clearance is increased, by approximately twofold, as can

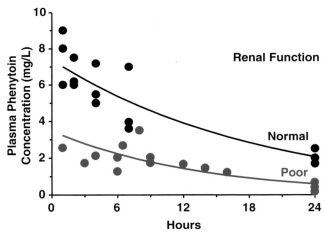

FIGURE 5-26. Semilogarithmic plot of plasma phenytoin concentration–time profile after an i.v. bolus dose of 250 mg of phenytoin to subjects with normal renal function (●) and poor renal function (●). The data are the composite of observations in three nonuremic and five uremic epileptic patients. The lines are the regression of fit of a monoexponential equation to the respective composite data. Notice that both clearance and volume of distribution of phenytoin are higher in the patients with poor renal function. (From: Letteri JM, Mellk H, Louis S, et al. Diphenylhydantoin metabolism in uremia. N Eng J Med 1971;285:648–652.)

be seen by the smaller *AUC* in epileptic patients with poor renal function, classified as uremic owing to the elevated plasma concentration of endogenous urea, which is eliminated almost exclusively by renal excretion. Volume of distribution is also approximately twofold larger in disease, calculated from *Dose/C*(0), increasing from approximately 35 L (250 mg/7 mg/L) to 70 L (250 mg/3.5 mg/L), so that half-life remains almost unchanged. The explanation for these observations lies in a common factor, namely altered plasma binding. One consequence of severe renal impairment, discussed in greater detail in Chapter 15, *Disease*, is diminished binding of some drugs, including phenytoin, to plasma proteins. Specifically, normally 0.1, the fraction unbound of phenytoin is twofold to threefold greater. Phenytoin, a drug primarily eliminated by hepatic metabolism, is a low extraction ratio drug. This is readily seen by dividing dose by *AUC* (500 mg/139 mg-hr/L = 3.6 L/hr). Consequently, total clearance ($fu \cdot CL_{int}$) increases with an increase in *fu*, but because the increase in clearance is in line with the increase in *fu*, intrinsic metabolic clearance remains virtually unchanged, a perhaps not too surprising result given that the kidneys, rather than the liver, are impaired. Furthermore, the twofold increase in volume of distribution is also totally explained by the doubling in *fu*. Given that phenytoin is a drug with a reasonably large volume of distribution ($V \gg 3$ L plasma volume), its value is approximately proportional to *fu*,

$$V \approx V_R \cdot \frac{fu}{fu_R}$$

A twofold increase in *fu* and not in tissue binding (fu_R), explains the observations.

High extraction ratio. Figure 5-27 shows how blood clearance, volume of distribution, and half-life of propranolol vary with the fraction unbound in plasma. Clearance appears

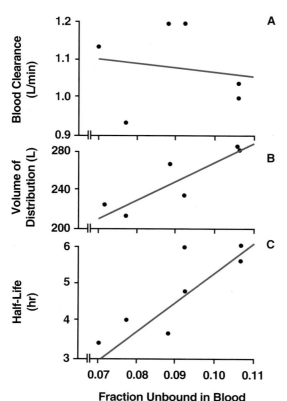

FIGURE 5-27. The clearance of propranolol (**A**), based on its concentration in blood, does not appear to correlate with the fraction unbound in blood of six healthy male volunteers after intravenous administration of 20 mg. On the other hand, the volume of distribution (**B**) and the half-life (**C**) are observed to increase with an increase in the fraction unbound. This kinetic behavior is anticipated for a drug, such as propranolol, that is highly extracted in the liver. Clearance for this drug is perfusion rate-limited. Changes in binding to plasma proteins does not influence blood clearance but does affect the volume of distribution and, therefore, the half-life. The lines are the best fits by linear regression. (From: Evans GH, Shand DG. Disposition of propranolol. VI: Independent variation in steady-state circulating drug concentrations and half-life as a result of plasma drug binding in man. Clin Pharmacol Ther 1973;14:494–500. Reproduced with permission of C.V. Mosby.)

to be independent of protein binding. The volume of distribution (blood) and half-life both increase with an increase in fu. This is the behavior expected for a drug with a large volume of distribution and for which elimination is perfusion rate-limited. The drug is primarily eliminated by hepatic metabolism, and the metabolic (blood) clearance approaches hepatic blood flow (1.35 L/min on average). The increase in volume of distribution with fu is anticipated, as is the increase in half-life.

With the increase in fu and no change in clearance, there must be a corresponding decrease in unbound clearance, since $CL = fu \cdot CLu$. This is reflected in an increase in unbound AUC. An increase in fu therefore raises the unbound concentration and for a given dose the drug's effects. Although there are many drugs with a high hepatic extraction ratio, they are seldom given by the parenteral route under conditions in which binding is altered.

Small volume of distribution. The consequence of altering binding to plasma proteins is illustrated by clofibrate. The half-life of clofibric acid (the active material formed by hydrolysis of the administered ethyl ester, clofibrate) shortens from the usual 16.5 to 8.7 hr in patients with the nephrotic syndrome, a condition involving an extensive loss of plasma proteins in urine (Table 5-8). It is tempting to conclude that metabolism (only 6% of clofibric acid is excreted unchanged) is induced. However, this conclusion is incorrect, as the following shows.

TABLE 5-8	Renal Function Measures, Serum Albumin, Daily Protein Excretion, and Half-Life of the Active Form of Clofibrate, Clofibric Acid, in Patients With and Without the Nephrotic Syndrome

	Creatinine Clearance (mL/min)*	Serum Albumin (g/dL)	Clofibric Acid Half-life (hr)	Protein Excretion (g/day)
Nephrotic group (N = 5)	100 ± 24	2.3 ± 0.5	8.7 ± 3.5	13 ± 12
Control group (N = 8)[†]	98 ± 20	4.4 ± 0.4	16.5 ± 4.7	0

*A measure of glomerular filtration rate.
[†]In healthy subjects, the volume of distribution of clofibric acid is 0.11 L/kg, the fraction unbound in plasma is 0.03 and the fraction excreted unchanged is 0.06. (From: Benet LZ, Williams RL. Appendix II. In: Gilman AG, Rall TW, Nies AS, Taylor P, eds. The Pharmacologic Basis of Therapeutics. 8th ed. New York, Macmillan; 1993.)
From: Goldberg AP, Sherrard DJ, Haas LB, Brunzell JD. Control of clofibrate toxicity in uremic hypertriglyceridemia. Clin Pharmacol Ther 1977;21:317–325.

In the nephrotic syndrome, the loss of plasma proteins results in a twofold drop in serum albumin, the binding protein of clofibric acid. The influence of this drop in serum albumin on fu can be estimated from rearrangement of Eq. 4-19 (Chapter 4, *Membranes and Distribution*), repeated here.

$$fu = \frac{1}{(1 + Ka \cdot fu_p \cdot P_t)}$$

The normal serum albumin concentration reported is 4.3 g/dL and for clofibric acid fu is 0.03. Given that at therapeutic concentrations clofibric acid occupies only a small fraction of the available binding sites, fu_p, the fraction of available binding sites unoccupied, is equal to 1. At a serum albumin concentration of 2.3 g/dL and with a Ka of 7.5 dL/g, the calculated fraction unbound in nephrotic patients is then

$$fu = \frac{1}{(1 + 7.5 \times 2.3)} = 0.055$$

Clofibric acid has a low extraction ratio in that its clearance (calculated from $k \cdot V$) is 0.32 L/hr in healthy subjects, a value much smaller than hepatic blood flow, 81 L/hr. Although one might argue that blood clearance is much larger than plasma clearance (also $C/C_b > 1$), a high hepatic extraction ratio is impossible. Virtually all drug in the body is bound to albumin. Thus, plasma drug concentration can only be greater than blood drug concentration by a factor of 1.7 (1/[1–hematocrit]; see Appendix D, *Plasma-to-Blood Concentration Ratio*).

With clofibric acid being a low-extraction ratio drug, clearance is expected to increase in nephrotic patients. The value of intrinsic clearance, CL/fu, is 10.7 L/hr in healthy subjects. If one assumes the same intrinsic clearance in nephrotic patients, then clearance, $fu \cdot CL_{int}$, in this group is 0.59 L/hr.

The volume of distribution of clofibric acid, given in the footnote to Table 5-8, is 7.7 L/70 kg, indicating that $V = 0.11$ L/kg. This value depends little on changes in plasma protein binding. This is seen from the relationship between V and fu for a drug bound to albumin with a small volume of distribution (Eq. 4-27, Chapter 4, *Membranes and Distribution*), namely,

$$V = 7.5 + Constant \cdot fu$$

With an apparent volume of 7.7 L, the constant is 6.7. If fu is increased to 0.055, then the apparent volume becomes 7.9 L. The volume unbound (V/fu), however, decreases from 257 to 143 L. The calculated half-life (0.693 $\cdot$ V/CL or 0.693 $\cdot$ Vu/CL_{int}) in the nephrotic patients is then about 9.3 hr, a value very close to that observed, 8.7 hr.

The question originally posed is now answered. The half-life is shortened in the nephrotic patients because of decreased binding to albumin; neither metabolism nor intrinsic clearance changed.

The combinations of conditions and scenarios in drug therapy are multitudinous. This chapter has presented approaches and examples toward integrating kinetic principles and physiologic concepts after i.v. bolus administration. To complete this integration, Table 5-9 summarizes the effects expected from increased enzyme activity, inhibition of metabolism, decreased blood flow, and increased fu in blood for a drug eliminated exclusively in the liver. Conditions involving drugs of both low and high extraction ratios are considered. The expectations are similar for a drug eliminated only by the kidneys; however, increased active tubular secretion rather than increased enzyme activity applies.

TABLE 5-9	**Anticipated Effects of Alterations in Selected Physiologic Variables on Various Parameters and Observations for Drugs Eliminated Solely by the Liver Following Intravenous Administration***

	Physiologic Variable Altered			
Parameters or Observations	**Increased Enzyme Activity**[†]	**Inhibition of Metabolism**	**Decreased Blood Flow**	**Increased Fraction Unbound in Blood**
Low hepatic extraction ratio drug				
Half-life	↓[‡]	↑	↔	↔
AUC (blood)	↓	↑	↔	↓
High hepatic extraction ratio drug				
Half-life	↔	↔	↑	↑
AUC (blood)	↔	↔	↑	↔

*$V > 50$ L for all drugs.
[†]Enzyme activity is increased by one of several mechanisms, such as enzyme activation, induction, or increased availability of cofactors, if rate-limiting.
[‡]↑, increased; ↓, decreased; ↔, little or no change.

KEY RELATIONSHIPS

$$CL_{b,R} \quad = \quad Q_R \quad \cdot \quad E_R$$

| Renal blood clearance | Renal blood flow | Renal extraction ratio |

$$CL_{b,H} \quad = \quad Q_H \quad \cdot \quad E_H$$

| Hepatic blood clearance | Hepatic blood flow | Hepatic extraction ratio |

$$Rate\ of\ elimination = CL \cdot C = CL_b \cdot C_b = CLu \cdot Cu$$

$$CL_b = CL \cdot \left(\frac{C}{C_b} \right)$$

$$CLu = \frac{CL}{fu}$$

$$CL = CL_R + CL_H$$

$$CL_{b,H} = Q_H \cdot E_H = Q_H \cdot \left[\frac{fu_b \cdot CL_{int}}{Q_H + fu_b \cdot CL_{int}} \right]$$

$$E_H = \left[\frac{fu_b \cdot CL_{int}}{Q_H + fu_b \cdot CL_{int}} \right]$$

$$Biliary\ clearance = \frac{(Bile\ flow) \cdot (Concentration\ in\ bile)}{Concentration\ in\ plasma}$$

$$CL_R = \frac{Rate\ of\ excretion}{C} = (1 - F_R) \left[\frac{Rate\ of\ Filtration}{C} + \frac{Rate\ of\ Secretion}{C} \right]$$

$$= (1 - F_R) \left[CL_f + CL_S \right]$$

$$CL_R = \frac{Rate\ of\ urinary\ excretion}{Plasma\ concentration}$$

$$Renal\ clearance = fu \cdot Urine\ flow$$

$$k = \frac{Rate\ of\ elimination}{Amount\ in\ body} = \frac{CL}{V}$$

$$t_{\frac{1}{2}} = \frac{0.693}{k} = \frac{0.693 \cdot V}{CL}$$

$$k = \frac{CL}{V} = \frac{CL_b}{V_b} = \frac{CLu}{Vu}$$

$$t_{\frac{1}{2}} = \frac{0.693V}{CL} = \frac{0.693V_b}{CL_b} = \frac{0.693Vu}{CLu}$$

STUDY PROBLEMS

(Answers to Study Problems are in Appendix J.)

1. Define the following terms, which are selected from those listed in the Objectives of this chapter: blood clearance, enterohepatic cycle, filtration clearance, glomerular filtration rate, hepatic acinus, hepatic clearance, intrinsic clearance, perfusion rate-limited elimination, plasma-to-blood concentration ratio, and unbound clearance.

2. The values of selected pharmacokinetic parameters for various drugs are given in Table 5-10. Complete the table by calculating the missing values. Use 80 L/hr as the hepatic blood flow.

TABLE 5-10	Selected Pharmacokinetic Parameters of Drugs A to D						
Drug	Fraction Unbound		Hepatic Clearance (L/hr) Based on Concentration in:			Concentration Ratio (Plasma/Blood)	Hepatic Extraction Ratio
	Blood fu_b	Plasma fu	Blood CL_b	Plasma CL	Plasma water CLu	C/C_b	E_H
A		0.2	1.2	1.6			
B		0.3		90		0.022	
C		0.02				0.37	0.9
D				0.5	5		0.01

3. Comment on the following statements:
   a. A high plasma clearance implies that the drug has a high extraction ratio.
   b. The intrinsic clearance and unbound clearance of a drug by an organ are two terms used to describe the same property.
   c. Clearance by one organ adds to that of another.
   d. Organ clearance is rate-limited either by perfusion or because the drug is a poor substrate for the enzymatic and excretory processes responsible for its elimination.
   e. Enterohepatic cycling effectively reduces the clearance of a drug.

4. a. Complete Table 5-11 (with high, low, ↑, ↓, ↔ in the blank spaces) to indicate the expectation for the drugs listed. Assume that each drug is eliminated exclusively in the liver.

   b. Indicate the expected direction of change in half-life for the conditions given for Drug A and Drug C. Both drugs have a volume of distribution greater than 100 L.

5. The immunosuppressive drug tacrolimus has the following characteristics: plasma clearance = 4.2 L/hr; fraction in plasma unbound = 0.01; plasma-to-blood concentration ratio = 0.03; and essentially the drug is eliminated by CYP3A4-catalyzed hepatic metabolism, with a negligible fraction excreted unchanged in urine.

   a. Comment on whether tacrolimus has a high or low hepatic extraction ratio.
   b. Why is the plasma-to-blood concentration ratio so low?
   c. What are the expected changes in the clearance and half-life of tacrolimus following induction of CYP3A4, which results in an increase in the hepatocellular metabolic activity of the drug?

Drug	Hepatic Extraction Ratio	Hepatic Blood Flow	Unbound Fraction in Blood	Intrinsic Clearance	(Plasma) Clearance
A	High	↑	↔	↔	
B	Low	↔	↓	↔	
C	Low	↔	↔	↑	
D	High	↔	↔	↑	
E	Low	↔		↔	↑
F	High	↔	↓	↔	
G		↓	↔	↔	↔
H		↓	↔	↔	↓

TABLE 5-11   Changes in the Hepatic Handling of Selected Drugs

↑, increase; ↔, little or no change; ↓, decrease.

6. The renal clearances and the fractions unbound in plasma of three drugs in a 70-kg, 20-year-old subject are listed in Table 5-12

   State the likely involvement of filtration, secretion, and tubular reabsorption in the renal handling of each of these drugs, when GFR is 120 mL/min and urine flow is 1.5 mL/min, typical values in a 20-year-old adult man.

TABLE 5-12   Renal Clearance and Fraction Unbound of Phenytoin, Cefonicid, and Digoxin

	Renal Clearance (mL/min)	Fraction Unbound
Phenytoin	0.15	0.10
Cefonicid	20	0.02
Digoxin	100	0.79

7. Table 5-13 lists the renal and total clearance of nicotine (pKa 8.3) in cigarette smokers under normal conditions, sustained low urinary pH (achieved by concurrent and repeated ingestion of ammonium chloride), and high urinary pH (achieved by concurrent and repeated ingestion of sodium bicarbonate) following i.v. administration of nicotine.

   a. Based on the findings, is nicotine an acid or a base?
   b. Is the pKa of nicotine consistent with your expectation of the large pH sensitivity of renal clearance?

TABLE 5-13   Influence of Urinary pH on the Clearance of Nicotine

Treatment	Mean Urine pH	Renal Clearance (mL/min)	Total Clearance (mL/min)
Control	5.8	102	1153
Ammonium chloride	4.5	562	1751
Sodium bicarbonate	6.7	39	1226

From: Benowitz N, Jacobs P. Nicotine renal excretion rate influences nicotine intake during cigarette smoking. J Pharmacol Exp Therap 1985;234:153–155.

c. Under which of the three conditions is renal clearance most likely to be dependent on urine flow rate? The plasma protein binding of nicotine is less than 5%.

d. Under what circumstances would modification of urine pH markedly influence the half-life of nicotine?

8. The following information regarding theophylline is either provided in Problem 10 of Chapter 3, *Kinetics Following an Intravenous Bolus Dose*, or was calculated from the data provided. Clearance is 4 L/hr, volume of distribution is 29 L, half-life 5 hr. It is 40% bound in plasma and freely passes across cell membranes and distributes in all body water spaces. It is also extensively metabolized with only 10% of the dose excreted in the urine unchanged following an i.v. dose.

a. Comment, with justification, on whether theophylline has a low or high hepatic extraction ratio.

b. Comment on whether a definite statement can be made as to whether there is net renal secretion or net renal tubular reabsorption.

c. Knowing the volume of distribution and fraction unbound in plasma, calculate:

   (1) i. The fraction of theophylline in the body unbound at distribution equilibrium.

        ii. The unbound concentration when there is 500 mg of theophylline in the body at distribution equilibrium.

   (2) i. The volume of distribution of theophylline in an individual receiving a 500-mg dose in whom the fraction unbound in plasma is 0.30.

        ii. The unbound concentration in that individual when there is 500 mg of theophylline in the body. Comment on the sensitivity of unbound concentration to changes in fraction unbound in plasma.

9. Meperidine is used as an i.v. analgesic. It is extensively metabolized with only 7% renally excreted. Its blood clearance is 700 mL/min. Using the well-stirred model of hepatic elimination, and a hepatic blood flow of 80 L/min, calculate the expected change in blood clearance and half-life of meperidine had the hepatocellular activity (intrinsic clearance) responsible for its metabolism been:

a. Reduced by a factor of five by metabolic inhibition.

b. Increased by a factor of five by metabolic induction.

Comment on the quantitative changes expected.

10. Table 5-14 summarizes the mean disposition kinetics of propranolol and disopyramide in healthy subjects. The predominant binding protein in plasma for both drugs is α_1-acid glycoprotein. As discussed in Chapter 4, *Membranes and Distribution*, the concentration of this protein is elevated in a number of stress conditions, including surgery, where for example the mean plasma concentration rises from 18 μm before surgery to 34 μm 5 days following surgery.

a. Calculate the anticipated fraction unbound of propranolol and disopyramide 5 days following surgery. Assume that α_1-acid glycoprotein is the only binding protein in plasma and that at therapeutic concentrations the fraction of sites available for binding (fu_p) remains small.

TABLE 5-14	Pharmacokinetic Properties of Propranolol and Disopyramide					
	CL (L/kg)	*V* (L)	*fe*	Plasma-Blood Concentration Ratio	*fu*	Half-life (hr)
Propranolol	60	300	0.02	1.1	0.1	3.5
Disopyramide	3.5	37	0.46	0.9	0.3	7.3

b. Calculate the anticipated half-life of both drugs 5 days following surgery. Assume that the model of distribution represented by Eq. 4-25 (Chapter 4, *Membranes and Distribution*) applies to both drugs.

c. Comment on the statement "The half-life of a drug can be increased by increasing the extent of plasma protein binding."

11. Fexofenadine, a polar compound, clearance 15 L/hr, $fe = 0.3$, $fu = 0.35$, with a plasma-to-blood ratio close to 1, is minimally metabolized. It is a substrate for the hepatic uptake transporter OATP1B1 and the efflux transporter PgP. Comment on the potential of each process to rate limit the hepatic clearance of fexofenadine, and how you might distinguish between these two possibilities.

12. Three drugs are listed in Table 5-15, together with some of their physicochemical properties and disposition characteristics in a 70-kg man.

TABLE 5-15	Selected Physicochemical and Pharmacokinetic Properties of Amoxicillin, Propranolol, and Cyclosporine		
Property or Characteristic	**Amoxicillin**	**Propranolol**	**Cyclosporine**
Polarity of Un-ionized Form and pKa	Polar 2.8 (weak acid)	Nonpolar 9.5 (amine)	Nonpolar (not an acid or a base)
Usual dose (mg)	250	80–120	350
Volume of distribution (L)	29	360	245
Fraction unbound (*fu*)	0.82	0.1	0.06
Half-life (hr)	0.9	4	8
Fraction excreted unchanged (*fe*)	0.56	0.02	<0.01

a. Indicate the drug(s) for which each of the following statements is probably most applicable:

(1) The renal clearance of this drug is the most sensitive to a change in urine pH.

(2) This drug has the highest renal clearance.

(3) This drug is most likely to show the greatest diffusion limitation in crossing the placenta to the fetus.

(4) For 100 mg in the body, the unbound plasma concentration is lowest for this drug after distribution equilibrium is achieved.

(5) This drug has the lowest total clearance.

b. Which one is the most appropriate word, term, or value (of those shown in italics) for the following statements:

(1) The clearance of propranolol will *increase, decrease, show little change* if the drug is significantly displaced from plasma protein binding sites.

(2) For the drug with a renal clearance that is most sensitive to changes in urine pH, *alkalinization, acidification* of the urine should decrease its renal clearance.

(3) Amoxicillin *is, is not* distributed evenly throughout, and accounted for within, the extracellular fluids.

(4) The volume of distribution of cyclosporine *increases, decreases, shows little change* if plasma protein binding is increased.

(5) *Fifty-one percent, 97.6%, and 99.2%* of propranolol in the body is located outside the plasma.

c. Indicate for which drug(s) the following statements is most applicable after a 100-mg i.v. bolus dose.

(1) Twelve percent remains in the body at 12 hr.

(2) This drug has the highest *AUC*.

(3) The plasma concentration of this drug is 0.034 mg/L at 6 hr.

(4) The fraction of the total *AUC* covered by 3 hr is 0.33.

6

Kinetics Following an Extravascular Dose

OBJECTIVES

The reader will be able to:

- Define the following terms: absorption rate constant, absorption half-life, absorption phase, bioavailability, bioequivalence, biopharmaceutics, delayed-release dosage forms, elimination phase, first-order, flip-flop, generic products, extended-release dosage forms, immediate-release dosage forms, lag time, method of residuals, modified-release dosage forms, peak concentration, peak time, relative bioavailability, zero-order absorption.

- Describe the characteristics of, and the differences between, first-order and zero-order absorption processes.

- Determine whether absorption or disposition rate limits drug elimination, given plasma concentration–time data following different dosage forms or routes of administration.

- Anticipate the effect of altering absorption kinetics, extent of absorption, clearance, or volume of distribution on the plasma concentration and amount of drug in the body following extravascular administration.

- Estimate the bioavailability of a drug, given either plasma concentration or urinary excretion data, following both extravascular and intravascular administration.

- Estimate the relative bioavailability of a drug, given either plasma concentration or urinary excretion data following different dosage forms or routes of administration.

- Estimate the renal clearance of a drug from plasma concentration and urinary excretion data following extravascular administration.

ROUTES OF EXTRAVASCULAR ADMINISTRATION

Drugs are more frequently administered extravascularly (common routes listed in Table 2-3 of Chapter 2, *Fundamental Concepts and Terminology*) than intravascularly, and most are intended to act systemically rather than locally. For most drugs then, systemic absorption, the focus of this chapter, is a prerequisite for activity. Delays or losses of drug during systemic input may contribute to variability in drug response and, occasionally, may result in failure of drug therapy. It is primarily in this context, as a source of variability in systemic response and as a means of controlling the plasma concentration–time profile, that systemic absorption is considered here and throughout the remainder of the book. It should be kept in mind, however, that even for those drugs that are used locally (e.g., mydriatics, local anesthetics, nasal decongestants, topical agents, and aerosol bronchodilators), systemic absorption may influence time of onset, intensity, and duration of both local and systemic adverse effects.

This chapter primarily deals with the general principles governing rate and extent of systemic drug absorption, particularly after oral administration. Several oral dosage forms are used. Some are liquids (syrups, elixirs, suspensions, and emulsions), whereas the more common ones are solids (tablets and capsules). Tablets and capsules are generally formulated to release drug immediately after their administration to hasten systemic absorption. These are called **immediate-release products**. Other products are called **modified-release dosage forms**.

Modified-release products fall into two categories. One is **extended-release**, a dosage form that allows a reduction in dosing frequency or diminishes the fluctuation of drug levels, or both, on repeated administration compared with that observed with an immediate-release dosage form. Controlled-release and sustained-release products fall into this category. The second category is that of **delayed-release**. This kind of dosage form releases drug, in part or in total, at a time other than promptly after administration. Enteric-coated dosage forms are the most common delayed-release products; they are designed to prevent drug release in the stomach, where it may decompose in the acidic environment or cause gastric irritation, and then to release the drug for immediate absorption once in the intestine. Modified-release products are also administered by nonoral extravascular routes. For example, repository (depot) dosage forms are given intramuscularly and subcutaneously in the form of emulsions, solutions in oil, suspensions, and tablet implants. While the duration of drug release is limited for orally administered products by the gastrointestinal transit time (typically 12–36 hr), no such limit applies to nonoral routes of administration. Products may be designed to deliver drug over weeks (octreotide acetate for injectable suspension [Sandostatin LAR Depot], used in treating acromegaly, 4 weeks); months (e.g., goserelin acetate implant [Zolodex, 10.8 mg, used in prostate cancer], 3 months); or years (levonorgesterol-releasing intrauterine system [Mirena, contraceptive system], 5 years).

The physiologic and physicochemical factors that influence drug absorption are considered in Chapter 7, *Absorption*. In this chapter, the following aspects are examined: the impact of rate and extent of absorption on the time course of both plasma concentration and amount of drug in the body; the effect of alterations in absorption and disposition on body level-time relationships; and the methods used to assess pharmacokinetic parameters from plasma and urinary data following extravascular administration.

KINETICS OF ABSORPTION

The oral absorption of drugs often approximates first-order kinetics, especially when given in solution. The same holds true for the absorption of drugs from many other extravascular sites, including subcutaneous tissue and muscle. Under these circumstances, absorption is characterized by an **absorption rate constant**, ka, and the corresponding **absorption half-life**, $t_{1/2,a}$. The two are related to each other in the same way that elimination half-life is related to elimination rate constant, that is,

$$t_{1/2,a} = \frac{0.693}{ka}$$

6-1

The half-lives for the absorption of drugs taken orally in solution or in a rapidly disintegrating dosage form usually range from 15 min to 1 hr. Occasionally, they are longer.

When absorption occurs by a **first-order** process,

| *Rate of Absorption* | = | ka | · | Aa | 6-2 |
| | | Absorption
rate constant | | Amount remaining
to be absorbed | |

Restated, the rate is proportional to the **amount remaining to be absorbed**, Aa. First-order absorption is schematically depicted in Fig. 6-1 by the emptying of water from a

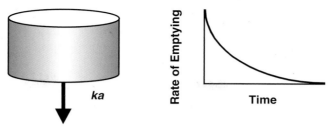

FIGURE 6-1. First-order systemic absorption is analogous to the emptying of water from a hole in the bottom of a cylindrical bucket. The level of water in the bucket decreases with time, as does the rate of emptying. The slowing of the decline of the water level and the rate of emptying are a result of the decrease in water pressure, which depends on the water level (or amount of water) in the bucket. The rate of emptying (g/min), which declines exponentially with time, is proportional to the amount (g) of water in the bucket and the size of the hole. The rate of emptying relative to the amount in the bucket is the fractional rate of emptying, which does not vary with time. In absorption terms, this constant is called the **absorption rate constant**, *ka*.

cylindrical bucket. The rate of emptying depends on the amount of water in the bucket and the size of the hole at the bottom. With time, the level, and hence the head of pressure of water decreases, reducing the rate at which it leaves the bucket. The rate of emptying is directly proportional (*ka*) to the level or amount of water in the bucket.

Sometimes, a drug is absorbed at essentially a constant rate. The absorption kinetics is then said to be **zero order** in nature. Differences between zero-order and first-order kinetics are illustrated in Fig. 6-2. For zero-order absorption, a plot of amount remaining to be absorbed against time yields a straight line, the slope of which is the rate of absorption (Fig. 6-2A). Recall from Chapter 3, *Kinetics Following an Intravenous Bolus Dose*, that the fractional rate of decline is constant for a first-order process; the amount declines linearly with time when plotted semilogarithmically. In contrast, for a zero-order absorption process, the fractional rate increases with time, because the rate is constant but the amount remaining decreases. This is reflected in an ever-increasing gradient with time in a semilogarithmic plot of the amount remaining to be absorbed (Fig. 6-2B).

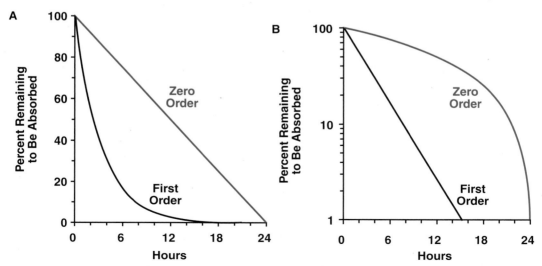

FIGURE 6-2. A comparison of zero-order (*colored lines*) and first-order (*black lines*) absorption processes. Depicted are regular **(A)** and semilogarithmic **(B)** plots of the percent remaining to be absorbed against time. Note the curvatures of the two processes on the two plots.

For the remainder of this chapter, and for much of the book, absorption is assumed to follow first-order kinetics. When absorption is zero order in nature, then the concepts and equations developed in Chapter 10, *Constant-Rate Input*, apply.

EXPOSURE–TIME AND EXPOSURE–DOSE RELATIONSHIPS

The systemic exposure to a drug after a single extravascular dose depends on both absorption and disposition. Consider first how exposure with time after an extravascular dose compares with that seen after an intravenous (i.v.) dose.

COMPARISON WITH INTRAVENOUS ADMINISTRATION

Absorption delays and reduces the *magnitude of the peak* compared with that seen following an equal i.v. bolus dose. These effects are portrayed for aspirin in Fig. 6-3. The rise and fall of the drug concentration in plasma are best understood by remembering (see Eq. 2-2) that at any time,

$$dA/dt = Rate\ of\ absorption - k \cdot A \qquad\qquad 6\text{-}3$$

| Rate of change | Rate of |
| of drug in body | elimination |

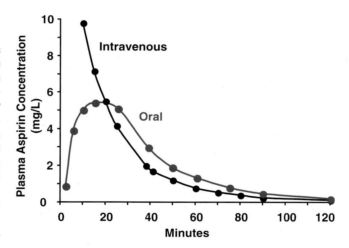

FIGURE 6-3. Aspirin (650 mg) was administered as an i.v. bolus (*black*) and as an oral solution (*colored*) on separate occasions to the same individual. Absorption causes a delay and a lowering of the peak concentration. (From: Rowland M, Riegelman S, Harris PA, Sholkoff SD. Absorption kinetics of aspirin in man following oral administration of an aqueous solution. J Pharm Sci 1972;67:379–385. Adapted with permission of the copyright owner.)

When absorption occurs by a first-order process, the rate of absorption at any time is given by $ka \cdot Aa$.

The scheme in Fig. 6-4 illustrates the expectation. Drug is input into the reservoir by a first-order process and is eliminated in the same manner as that following an i.v. dose (see Fig. 3-3).

Initially, with the entire dose at the absorption site (bucket, see Fig. 6-1) and none in the body (reservoir), rate of absorption is maximal and rate of elimination is zero. Thereafter, as drug is absorbed, its rate of absorption decreases, whereas its rate of elimination, reflecting the amount in the body, increases. Consequently, the difference between the two rates diminishes. As long as the rate of absorption exceeds that of elimination, the plasma concentration continues to rise. Eventually, a time, t_{max}, is reached when the rate of elimination matches the rate of absorption; the concentration (water level) is then at a maximum, C_{max}. Subsequently, the rate of elimination exceeds the rate of absorption and the plasma concentration declines, as shown for aspirin in Fig. 6-3.

The peak plasma concentration is always lower following extravascular administration than the initial value following an equal i.v. bolus dose. In the former case, at the peak time some drug remains at the absorption site and some has been eliminated,

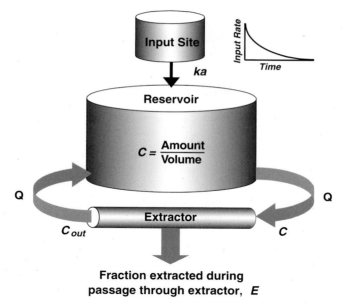

FIGURE 6-4. Scheme for the first-order systemic absorption and elimination of a drug after a single extravascular dose. The systemic absorption is simulated by the emptying of a water bucket (see Fig. 6-1). The rate constant for absorption *ka* is the fractional rate of absorption (i.e., the rate of absorption relative to the amount in the bucket). The elimination of the drug from the body (see Fig. 5-3) depends on the extent of its tissue distribution (volume of reservoir, *V*), and how well the drug is extracted from the fluid going to the eliminating organ (s) (as measured by *CL*). In this integrated model, the amount of water added to the reservoir is negligible as is the amount of drug in the extractor and in the fluid going to the extractor, relative to the amount in the reservoir.

whereas the entire dose is in the body immediately following the i.v. dose. Beyond the peak time, the plasma concentration is expected to exceed that following i.v. administration of the same dose, if the drug is fully bioavailable. This occurs because of continual entry of drug into the body. If bioavailability is low, the plasma concentration may remain lower than that observed after i.v. administration at all times. Frequently, the rising portion of the plasma concentration–time curve is called the **absorption phase** and, the declining portion, the **elimination phase**. As will be seen later, this description may be misleading.

One may observe a delay between drug administration and the beginning of absorption. This is called a **lag time**; it may be particularly important when a rapid onset of effect is desired. The lag time can be anywhere from a few minutes to many hours. Long lag times are frequently observed following ingestion of enteric-coated tablets. Factors contributing to the lag time are the delay in emptying the product from the stomach and the time taken for the protective coating to dissolve or to swell and release the inner contents into the intestinal fluids. However, once absorption begins, it may be as rapid as with uncoated tablets. Because of variability in gastric emptying, enteric-coated products should not be used when a prompt and predictable response is desired.

Absorption influences the time course of drug in the body; but what of the total area under the exposure–time profile, area under the curve (*AUC*)? Recall from Chapter 3, *Kinetics Following an Intravenous Bolus Dose*, that the rate of elimination is:

$$Rate\ of\ elimination = CL \cdot C \qquad 6\text{-}4$$

Integrating over all time,

$$Total\ amount\ eliminated = CL \cdot AUC \qquad 6\text{-}5$$

The total amount eliminated after an oral dose equals the total amount absorbed, $F \cdot Dose$, where the parameter F, **bioavailability**, takes into account that only this fraction of the oral dose reaches the systemic circulation. That is,

$$F \cdot Dose = CL \cdot AUC \qquad\qquad 6\text{-}6$$

| Total amount absorbed | Total amount eliminated |

Absorption kinetics from plasma concentration–time data following an extravascular dose can be calculated when a one-compartment model for drug disposition and first-order kinetics apply (Appendix F, *Absorption Kinetics*). Other less restrictive but generally more complex numeric methods exist to deal with more complicated situations. One of these, the Wagner-Nelson method, is given in Appendix G, *Wagner-Nelson Method*.

CHANGES IN DOSE OR ABSORPTION KINETICS

The concentration–time profile following a change in dose or in the absorption characteristics of a dosage form can be anticipated.

CHANGING DOSE

If all other factors remain constant, as anticipated intuitively, increasing the dose or the fraction of a dose absorbed produces a proportional increase in plasma concentration at all times (Fig. 6-5). The value of t_{max} remains unchanged, but C_{max} increases proportionally with dose.

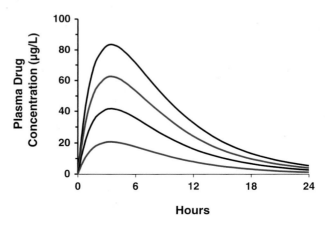

FIGURE 6-5. Effect of change in dose on concentration–time curve. With a decrease in dose (10, 7.5, 5.0, 2.5 mg), note that the peak concentration (C_{max}) and AUC decrease in proportion to the dose, but that the peak time (t_{max}) remains the same.

CHANGING ABSORPTION KINETICS

Alterations in absorption kinetics (e.g., by changing dosage form or sometimes when giving the product with food) produce changes in the time profiles of the plasma concentration. This point is illustrated by the three situations depicted in the semilogarithmic plots of Fig. 6-6, involving only a change in the absorption half-life. All other factors (bioavailability, clearance, volume of distribution, and hence, elimination half-life) remain unchanged.

Disposition is Rate Limiting. In Case A, the most common situation, absorption half-life is much shorter than elimination half-life. In this case, by the time the peak is reached, most of the drug has been absorbed and little has been eliminated. Thereafter, decline of drug in the body is determined primarily by the disposition of the drug, that is, *disposition is the rate-limiting step*. The half-life estimated from the decline phase is, therefore, the elimination half-life.

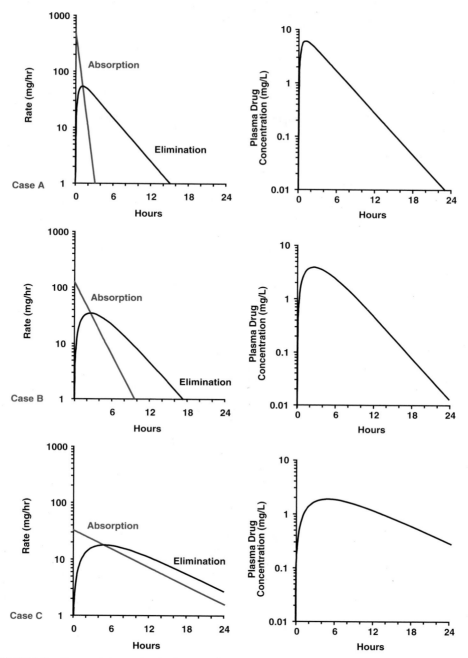

FIGURE 6-6. Rates of absorption (*colored line*) and elimination (*black line*) with time (*graphs on left*) and corresponding plasma concentration–time profiles (*graphs on right*) following a single oral dose of drug under different input conditions. A slowing (from top to bottom) of drug absorption delays the attainment (t_{max}) and decreases the magnitude (C_{max}) of the peak plasma drug concentration. In *Cases A and B* (*top two sets of graphs*), the absorption process is faster than that of elimination. In *Case C* (*bottom set of graphs*), absorption rate limits elimination, so that the decline of drug in plasma reflects absorption rather than elimination; because there is a net elimination of drug during the decline phase, the rate of elimination is slightly greater than the rate of absorption. In all three cases, bioavailability is 1.0 and clearance is unchanged. Consequently, the areas under the plasma concentration–time curves (corresponding linear plots of the top three graphs) are identical. The *AUC*s of the linear plots of the rate data are also equal because the integral of the rate of absorption, amount absorbed, equals the integral of the rate of elimination, amount eliminated.

In Case B, absorption half-life is longer than in Case A but still shorter than elimination half-life. The peak occurs later because it takes longer for the amount in the body to reach the value at which rate of elimination matches rate of absorption; the C_{max} is lower because less drug has been absorbed by that time. Even so, absorption is still essentially complete before most drugs have been eliminated. Consequently, disposition remains the rate-limiting step, and the terminal half-life remains the elimination half-life.

Absorption is Rate Limiting. Occasionally, absorption half-life is much longer than elimination half-life, and Case C prevails (see Fig. 6-6). The peak concentration occurs later and is lower than in the two previous cases, reflecting the slower absorption process. Again, during the rise to the peak, the rate of elimination increases and eventually, at the peak, equals the rate of absorption. However, in contrast to the previous situations, absorption is now so slow that considerable drug remains to be absorbed well beyond the peak time. Furthermore, at all times most of the drug either is at the absorption site or has been eliminated; little is ever in the body. In fact, during the decline phase, the plasma concentration is still falling because the rate of elimination ($k \cdot A$) exceeds the rate of absorption ($ka \cdot Aa$), but now the difference between these rates is small, and therefore, the rate of elimination essentially matches the rate of absorption, that is,

$$k \cdot A \quad\approx\quad ka \cdot Aa \qquad\qquad 6\text{-}7$$

$$\begin{array}{cc} \text{Rate of} & \text{Rate of} \\ \text{elimination} & \text{absorption} \end{array}$$

Elimination of drug during the decline phase is then said to be *absorption rate-limited*. Rearranging Eq. 6-7,

$$A \quad\approx\quad \left(\frac{ka}{k}\right) \cdot Aa \qquad\qquad 6\text{-}8$$

$$\begin{array}{cc} \text{Amount} & \text{Amount} \\ \text{in body} & \text{remaining to} \\ & \text{be absorbed} \end{array}$$

Accordingly, the plasma concentration ($C = A/V$) during the decline phase is directly proportional to the amount remaining to be absorbed. For example, when amount remaining to be absorbed falls by one half, so does amount in body. However, the time for this to occur is the absorption half-life. That is, the half-life of decline of drug in the body now corresponds to the absorption half-life. **Flip-flop** is a common descriptor for this kinetic situation. When it occurs, the terms **absorption phase** and **elimination phase** for the regions where the plasma concentration–time curve rises and falls, respectively, are clearly misleading.

DISTINGUISHING BETWEEN ABSORPTION AND DISPOSITION RATE-LIMITATIONS

Although disposition generally is rate limiting, the preceding discussion suggests that caution may need to be exercised in interpreting the meaning of half-life determined from the decline phase following extravascular administration. Confusion is avoided if the drug is also given intravenously. In practice, however, i.v. dosage forms of many drugs do not exist for clinical use. Absorption and disposition rate-limitations may be distinguished by altering the absorption kinetics of the drug. This is most readily accomplished by giving the drug either in different dosage forms or by different routes. To illustrate this point, consider data for theophylline and penicillin G.

Food and water influence the oral absorption kinetics of theophylline but not the half-life of the decline phase (Fig. 6-7). Here then, disposition rate limits the decline of the theophylline concentration. In contrast, for penicillin, with a very short elimination half-life, intramuscular (i.m.) absorption can become rate limiting by formulation of a sparingly soluble salt (Fig. 6-8).

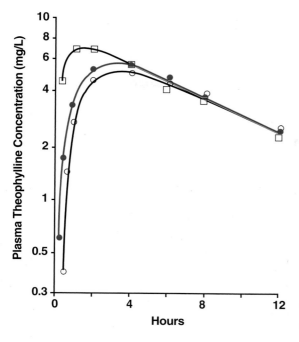

FIGURE 6-7. Two tablets, each containing 130 mg of theophylline, were taken by 6 healthy volunteers under various conditions. Absorption of theophylline was most rapid when the tablets were dissolved in 500 mL of water and taken on an empty stomach (□). Taking the tablets with 20 mL of water on an empty stomach (○) resulted in slower absorption than taking them with the same volume of water immediately following a standardized high carbohydrate meal (●). Despite differences in kinetics of absorption, however, the terminal half-life was the same (6.3 hr), and therefore, it is the elimination half-life of theophylline. (From: Welling PG, Lyons LL, Craig WA, Trochta GA. Influence of diet and fluid on bioavailability of theophylline. Clin Pharmacol Ther 1975;7:475–480.)

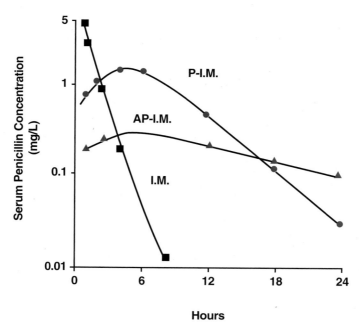

FIGURE 6-8. Penicillin G (3 mg/kg) was administered intramuscularly to the same individual on different occasions as an aqueous solution (*i.m.*), as procaine penicillin in oil (*P-i.m.*) and in oil with aluminum monostearate (*AP-i.m.*). The differing rates of decline of the serum concentration of penicillin G point to an absorption rate-limitation when this antibiotic is given as the procaine salt in oil. Distinction between rate-limited absorption and rate-limited disposition following intramuscular administration of the aqueous solution can only be made by giving penicillin G intravenously. (From: Marsh DF. Outline of Fundamental Pharmacology. Springfield, IL: Charles C. Thomas; 1951.)

CHANGING DISPOSITION KINETICS

What happens to the plasma concentration–time profile of a drug when the absorption kinetics remain constant, but modifications in disposition occur? When clearance is reduced, but bioavailability remains constant, it follows that *AUC* must increase (see Eq. 6-6) and so must both the time and magnitude of the peak concentration. These events are depicted in Fig. 6-9. Recall, a reduction in clearance produces a reduction in elimination rate constant, and hence, prolongation of elimination half-life. With a reduction in the elimination rate constant, a greater amount of drug must be absorbed to reach the time when the rate of elimination equals the rate of absorption. Another view is that, because clearance is decreased, the plasma concentration must be higher, so that the rate of elimination equals the rate of absorption. This occurs at a later time.

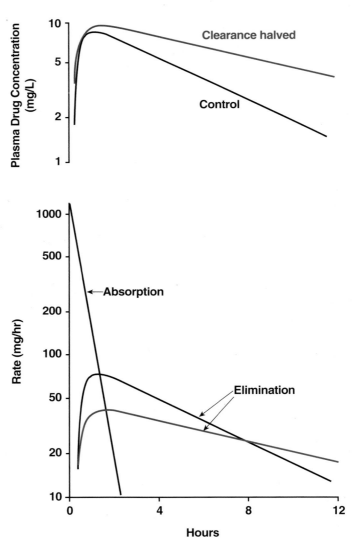

FIGURE 6-9. A twofold reduction in clearance increases the total area under the plasma concentration–time (*colored line*, top graph) twofold compared with that of the control. With no change in absorption kinetics (and hence absorption rate profile with time, bottom graph), the rate of elimination (*colored line*, bottom graph) is observed to be lower at first but to become greater than that of the control (*black line*, bottom graph), as the area under the corresponding linear plots of these rate curves must be equal to the dose (see Fig. 6-6). The decrease in clearance causes the peak concentration to be higher and to occur at a later time (only slightly different here). The peak time occurs when the rate of elimination equals the rate of absorption (bottom graph). The terminal slope reflects the increased elimination half-life.

As shown in Fig. 6-10, the events are different when an increased volume of distribution is responsible for a longer elimination half-life. Under these circumstances, the *AUC* is the same if bioavailability and clearance are unchanged. However, the peak occurs later and is lower. With a larger volume of distribution, more drug must be absorbed before the plasma concentration reaches the value at which the rate of elimination ($CL \cdot C$) equals the rate of absorption. At that time, with less drug remaining at the absorption site, the absorption rate is lower and so is the plasma concentration.

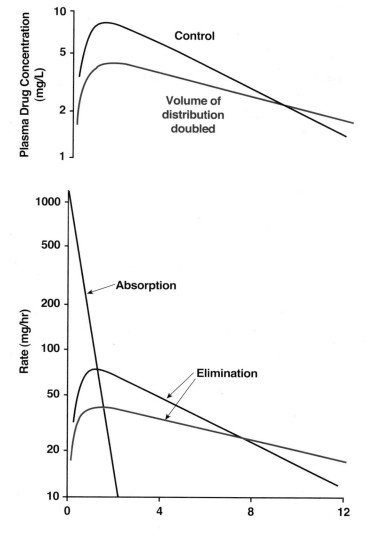

FIGURE 6-10. A twofold increase in the volume of distribution causes a twofold increase in the elimination half-life and delays the time at which the peak plasma concentration occurs (*colored line*, top graph) compared with the control observation (*black line*) after a single extravascular dose. With no change in clearance, *AUC* (under linear concentration–time plot) is unchanged and peak concentration is thereby reduced. Because of a lower concentration, rate of elimination is initially slowed (*colored line*, bottom graph), but because the total amount eliminated is the same (the dose), rate of elimination eventually is greater than that of the control (*black line*, bottom graph).

PREDICTING CHANGES IN PEAK CONCENTRATION AND PEAK TIME

Qualitative changes in C_{max} and t_{max} are not easy to predict when absorption or disposition is altered. To facilitate this prediction, a memory aid has been found to be useful. The basic principle of the method (Fig. 6-11) is simple; absorption increases and elimination decreases the amount of drug in the body. The faster the absorption process (measured by absorption rate constant), the greater is the slope of the absorption line and the converse. The faster the elimination process (elimination rate constant), the steeper is the decline of the elimination line.

When absorption rate constant is increased, the new point of intersection indicates that peak amount is increased and that it occurs at an earlier time. When elimination rate constant is increased, the new point of intersection occurs at an earlier time but at a lower amount.

The graph is designed for predicting changes in t_{max} and peak amount in the body. It applies as well to C_{max} with the exception of when volume of distribution is altered. An increase in volume of distribution causes a decrease in peak concentration, and the converse, as explained in the last section.

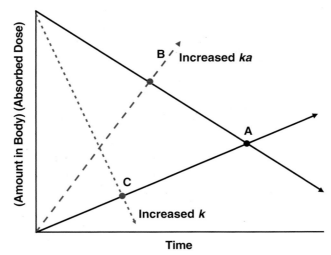

FIGURE 6-11. Memory aid to assess changes in peak time and peak amount in the body after extravascular administration of a single dose when absorption or disposition is altered. The relative peak time and the relative peak amount are indicated by the intersection of the absorption and elimination lines (*colored line* and point A) with slopes representing the absorption and elimination rate constants, respectively. The predictions for an increased absorption rate constant (*colored line* and point B) and an increased elimination rate constant (*colored line* and point C) are shown. (From: Øie S, Tozer TN. A memory aid to assess changes in peak time and peak concentration with alteration in drug absorption or disposition. Am J Pharm Ed 1982;46:154–155.)

The presentation in this chapter uses a one-compartment model. This is often an inadequate approximation of reality, particularly for C_{max}, for which the observed value may be much greater than that predicted by the model. The kinetic consequences of slow distribution to the tissues after a single extravascular dose is discussed in Chapter 19, *Distribution Kinetics*. The therapeutic implication of the slow distribution is discussed in Chapter 8, *Response Following a Single Dose*.

ASSESSMENT OF PRODUCT PERFORMANCE

FORMULATION

Equality of drug content does not guarantee equality of response. The presence of different **excipients** (ingredients in addition to active drug) or different manufacturing processes may result in dosage forms containing the same amount of drug behaving differently in vivo. This is why testing for bioavailability of drug products is essential. Generally, the primary concern is with the extent of absorption. Variations in absorption rate with time may also be therapeutically important. Many factors influence the release of drug from a solid pharmaceutical formulation, and therefore, the rate and extent of systemic absorption. **Biopharmaceutics** is a comprehensive term used to denote the study of pharmaceutical formulation variables on the performance of a drug product in vivo.

The major cause of differences in the rate of systemic absorption of a drug from various solid products is dissolution. There is, therefore, a strong need to control the content and purity of the numerous inactive ingredients used to prepare the drug product; to facilitate manufacture and maintain integrity of the dosage form during handling and storage; and to facilitate, or sometimes control, release of drug following administration of the dosage form. Intended, or otherwise, each ingredient can influence the rate of dissolution of the drug, as can the manufacturing process. The result is a large potential for differences among products in the absorption of drug, especially for those that are relatively insoluble or that poorly permeate membranes.

Assessment of absorption is useful not only to determine the effect of formulation, but also to examine the effects of food, current drug administration, concurrent diseases of the alimentary canal, and other conditions that may alter systemic absorption. One unique kind of bioavailability assessment, which is widely used, is that of **bioequivalence** testing.

BIOEQUIVALENCE TESTING

The purpose of bioequivalence testing is to assess the similarity of products of a given drug. The basic idea is that if the products are pharmaceutically equivalent (same dosage form and dose) and the pharmacokinetics in terms of the exposure–time profile (which reflects rate and extent of absorption) are sufficiently similar, then the therapeutic outcome should be the same, that is, the products would show therapeutic equivalence. Another costly full clinical trial investigating efficacy and safety, often involving hundreds to thousands of patients, is thereby not necessary. In this sense, the bioequivalence trial substitutes for the full clinical trial. In Europe, the term **essentially similar** is used for two pharmaceutically inequivalent dosage forms (e.g., capsules and tablets) that are pharmacokinetically similar. The major concern is the ability of the test product to have the same therapeutic outcome as the product used in the clinical trials. The two products are considered to be bioequivalent or essentially similar if their concentration–time profiles are sufficiently similar, so that they are unlikely to produce clinically relevant differences in both therapeutic and adverse effects. The common measures used to assess differences in exposure are AUC, C_{max}, and t_{max}. In practice, C_{max} and t_{max} are estimated from the highest concentration measured and the time of its occurrence. As the plasma concentration–time curve is quite flat near the peak and because of assay variability and only discrete times of sampling, the value of t_{max} chosen may not be a good representation of the actual value.

Bioequivalence testing usually arises when a patent on an innovator's drug expires. Other manufacturers may then wish to market the drug product. Formulations that are bioequivalent with that of the innovator and bearing the generic name of the drug are called **generic products**. Bioequivalence testing is also performed during the course of development of new drugs when a formulation is changed. For example, because of taste considerations, there may be a desire to market a film-coated tablet instead of a capsule with which the efficacy and safety data have been acquired. A capsule formulation is often chosen for the clinical trial because it is relatively easy to adjust the dose simply by filling different amounts of a given formulation of small drug granules into a larger or a smaller capsule.

A typical bioequivalence trial is usually conducted with about 24 to 36 healthy adult subjects. The number of subjects required is a function of the within subject (intrasubject) variability in the measures used; the larger this variability, the greater the number of subjects needed. Less than 24 subjects may suffice for some drug products, whereas more than 36 may be needed for others. The test and reference products are given in single doses, usually in a crossover design. The AUC and C_{max} are examined statistically. If the 90% confidence interval for the ratio of the measures in the generic or new product (test product) to the innovator's product or product used in full clinical trials (reference product) is within the limits of 0.8 and 1.25 for both AUC and C_{max}, the test product is declared to be bioequivalent. The 90% confidence interval is reduced with an increase in the number of subjects studied; this explains why a greater number of subjects is required when the intrasubject variability is large.

The statistical methods applied in bioequivalence testing are quite different from those applied in bioavailability assessment. In bioavailability studies, questions often asked are of the following type: "Is the oral bioavailability of Drug X in tablet Formulation 1 different from that in tablet Formulation 2?"; "Is the peak exposure following an oral solution greater than that after a capsule dosage form?"; or "What is the oral bioavailability and how

FIGURE 6-12. Declarations possible following the determination of confidence intervals (CI, indicated by *colored arrows*). In bioequivalence testing, the question is: "Are the two products sufficiently similar to call them the same therapeutically?" In bioavailability testing, the question is often "Do the products differ in their systemic delivery of the drug?" Note that the arrow represents 90% CI in bioequivalence studies, whereas it represents the 95% CI in bioavailability studies. From a regulatory perspective, of the products tested only those that are bioequivalent to the innovator's product (reference) are permitted to be marketed. (R, reference; T, test.)

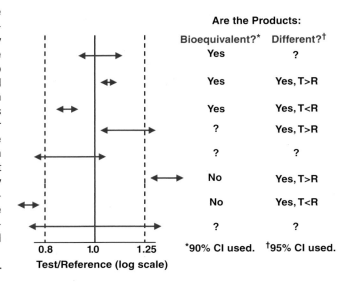

	Are the Products:	
	Bioequivalent?*	Different?†
	Yes	?
	Yes	Yes, T>R
	Yes	Yes, T<R
	?	Yes, T>R
	?	?
	No	Yes, T>R
	No	Yes, T<R
	?	?

0.8   1.0   1.25   *90% CI used.   †95% CI used.
Test/Reference (log scale)

confident are we in its estimate? In bioequivalence testing, the question asked is "are the exposure measures (*AUC* and C_{max}) of the test product no less than 80% or no more than 125% of the reference product?" The question is not whether or not they are different, but rather whether or not they are sufficiently similar. The 80% and 125% values are the criteria used most commonly in regulatory guidances to define how similar the measures must be. The distinction between the two kinds of questions is emphasized in Fig 6-12.

ASSESSMENT OF PHARMACOKINETIC PARAMETERS

How some parameter values are estimated following extravascular administration can be appreciated by considering both the plasma concentration–time curves in Fig. 6-13,

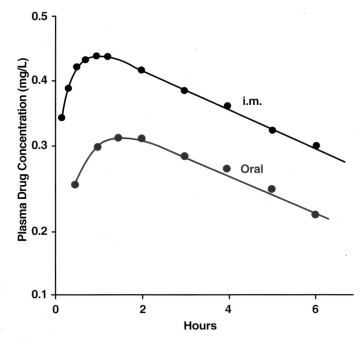

FIGURE 6-13. A 500-mg dose is given intramuscularly (●—●) and orally (●—●) to the same subject on separate occasions. The drug is less bioavailable and is absorbed more slowly from the gastrointestinal tract. A parallel decline, however, implies that disposition rate limit elimination in both instances.

TABLE 6-1	Data Obtained Following Administration of 500 mg of a Drug in Solution by Different Routes		
		Plasma Data	**Urine Data**
Route	**AUC (mg-hr/L)**	**Half-life in Decline Phase (min)**	**Cumulative Amount Excreted Unchanged (mg)**
Intravenous	7.6	190	152
Intramuscular	7.4	185	147
Oral	3.5	193	70

obtained following i.m. and oral administrations of 500 mg of a drug, and the additional information in Table 6-1.

PLASMA DATA ALONE

Bioavailability. Supplemental data from i.v. administration allow calculation of bioavailability, *F*. The total *AUC* following extravascular administration is divided by the area following an i.v. bolus, appropriately correcting for dose. The basis for this calculation, which assumes that *clearance remains constant,* is as follows:

i.v. dose

$$Dose_{i.v.} = CL \cdot AUC_{i.v.} \qquad \text{6-9}$$

Extravascular dose

$$F_{e.v.} \cdot Dose_{e.v.} = CL \cdot AUC_{e.v.} \qquad \text{6-10}$$

Which upon division of Eq. 6-10 by Eq. 6-9 yields

$$F_{e.v.} = \left(\frac{AUC_{e.v.}}{AUC_{i.v.}}\right)\left(\frac{Dose_{i.v.}}{Dose_{e.v.}}\right) \qquad \text{6-11}$$

For example, appropriately substituting the area measurements in Table 6-1 into Eq. 6-11 indicates that the bioavailability of the i.m. dose is 97%. Virtually all drug injected into muscle is absorbed systemically. In contrast, only 46% is bioavailable when drug is given orally in solution.

An alternative method of estimating bioavailability, which gives the same answer, is to substitute the value for clearance directly into Eq. 6-11. Clearance can be estimated from plasma (or blood) data following either an i.v. bolus dose (Chapter 3, *Kinetics Following an Intravenous Bolus Dose*) or a constant-rate i.v. infusion (Chapter 10, *Constant-Rate Input*).

Sometimes, one may wish to determine changes in the bioavailability of a drug under conditions in which the clearance of the drug is altered. Concurrent administration of a drug that inhibits or induces the metabolism of the drug of interest or that inhibits the transport of a drug in the renal tubules are examples of these conditions. Intravenous administration of the drug of interest both in the presence and absence of the coadministered drug is needed to determine the change in bioavailability. The assumption here is that the clearances determined from the i.v. administrations apply when the extravascular dose is administered in the presence and absence of the interacting drug. One approach to assure that this is so is to administer the drug intravenously such as either a radiolabel or a stable isotope in a tracer dose at the same time the extravascular dose is given. The drug concentrations following the i.v. and extravascular administrations can then be followed independently by appropriate techniques that distinguish between the different chemical forms of the drug, in the presence (+) and absence (−) of the interacting drug.

If the i.v. doses are the same, on both occasions, the bioavailability in the presence $F(+)_{e.v.}$ of the interacting drug is then

$$F(+)_{e.v.} = \left(\frac{AUC((-)_{i.v.})}{AUC((+)_{i.v.})}\right) \cdot \left(\frac{AUC(+)_{e.v.}}{AUC(+)_{i.v.}}\right) \cdot \left(\frac{Dose(+)_{i.v.}}{Dose(+)_{e.v.}}\right) \qquad \text{6-12}$$

Relative Bioavailability. Relative bioavailability can be estimated when there are no i.v. data. One may wish to compare the bioavailabilities of different dosage forms, different routes of administration, or different conditions (e.g., effect of food or different diets). As with the calculation of bioavailability, clearance is assumed to be constant.

Thus, taking the general case:

Dosage form A

$$F_A \cdot Dose_A = CL \cdot AUC_A \qquad \text{6-13}$$

$$\begin{array}{cc} \text{Amount} & \text{Total amount} \\ \text{absorbed} & \text{eliminated} \end{array}$$

Dosage form B

$$F_B \cdot Dose_B = CL \cdot AUC_B \qquad \text{6-14}$$

So that,

$$Relative\ bioavailability = \frac{F_B}{F_A} = \left(\frac{AUC_B}{AUC_A}\right) \cdot \left(\frac{Dose_A}{Dose_B}\right) \qquad \text{6-15}$$

The reference dosage form chosen is usually the one with the highest bioavailability, that is, the one having the highest area-to-dose ratio. In the example considered, this is the i.m. dose; the relative bioavailability of the oral dose is then 46%. If only two oral doses had been compared, they may have been equally, albeit poorly, bioavailable. It should be noted that all the preceding relationships hold, irrespective of route of administration, rate of absorption or shape of the curve. Constancy of clearance is the only requirement.

In those conditions in which clearance is altered (drug interactions for example), the relative bioavailability in the presence (+) and absence (−) of the interacting drug can be calculated in a manner analogous to that performed for bioavailability, provided that clearance of drug is the same for both products A and B in each condition. Then,

$$Relative\ bioavailability = \frac{F(+)_B}{F(+)_A} = \left(\frac{AUC(+)_B}{AUC(+)_A}\right) \cdot \left(\frac{Dose(+)_A}{Dose(+)_B}\right) \qquad \text{6-16}$$

and

$$Relative\ bioavailability = \frac{F(-)_B}{F(-)_A} = \left(\frac{AUC(-)_B}{AUC(-)_A}\right) \cdot \left(\frac{Dose(-)_A}{Dose(-)_B}\right) \qquad \text{6-17}$$

A change in the relative bioavailability in the presence compared with the absence of the interacting drug would indicate that the interacting drug causes a change in either the bioavailability of A, B, or both.

Fraction Eliminated. Based on the relationship between area and amount eliminated presented in Chapter 3, *Kinetics Following an Intravenous Bolus Dose*, AUC up to a given time, for example, t_{max}, reflects the amount eliminated up to that time (Fig. 6-14). The area beyond t_{max} reflects the amount remaining to be eliminated. The latter area represents drug in the body if absorption is fast compared with elimination, because absorption is essentially finished. Conversely, the area beyond t_{max} approximates the amount remaining to be absorbed if absorption is rate limiting.

Other Pharmacokinetic Parameters. Given only extravascular data, it is sometimes difficult to estimate pharmacokinetic parameters. No pharmacokinetic parameter can be determined confidently from observations following only a single oral dose. Consider:

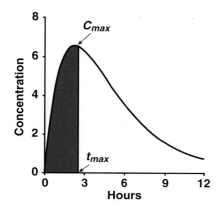

FIGURE 6-14. The *AUC* (*shaded*) up to t_{max}, the time of occurrence of the highest concentration, C_{max}, relative to the total *AUC* represents the fraction of the bioavailable dose that has been eliminated up to t_{max}. The *AUC* (*not shaded*) beyond t_{max}, relative to the total area, equals the fraction of the bioavailable dose that remains to be absorbed and eliminated.

AUC can be calculated without knowing bioavailability, but clearance cannot. Similarly, although a half-life can be ascribed to the decay phase, without knowing whether absorption or disposition is rate limiting, the value cannot be assigned to either absorption or elimination. Without knowing any of the foregoing parameters, the volume of distribution clearly cannot be calculated.

Fortunately, there is a sufficient body of data to determine at least the elimination half-life of most drugs. Failure of food, dosage form, and, in the example in Fig. 6-7, route of administration to affect the terminal half-life indicate that this must be the elimination half-life. Also, small drugs (MW <1000 g/mol) are often fully bioavailable ($F = 1$) from i.m. or subcutaneous sites. Hence, clearance can be calculated knowing area (see Eq. 6-6) and the volume of distribution can be estimated once the elimination half-life is known. Consider, for example, just the i.m. data in Table 6-1. Clearance, obtained by dividing dose (500 mg) by *AUC* (7.4 mg-hr/L), is 67.6 L/hr or 1.1 L/min. Dividing clearance by the elimination rate constant (0.693/185 min) gives the volume of distribution, in this case, 300 L.

URINE DATA ALONE

Cumulative urine data can be used to estimate bioavailability. The method requires that the value of *fe* remains constant. Recall from Chapter 3, *Kinetics Following an Intravenous Bolus Dose*, that *fe* is the ratio of the total amount excreted unchanged (Ae_∞) to the dose given intravenously. More generally, it can be defined as the total amount excreted unchanged relative to the amount systemically absorbed ($Ae_\infty / Dose$). Therefore, for an extravascular dose,

$$fe = \frac{Ae_\infty}{F \cdot Dose} \tag{6-18}$$

Then, using the subscripts A and B to denote two treatments, it follows that

$$F_A \cdot Dose_A = \frac{Ae_{\infty,A}}{fe_A} \tag{6-19}$$

$$F_B \cdot Dose_B = \frac{Ae_{\infty,B}}{fe_B} \tag{6-20}$$

Amount   Amount
Absorbed eliminated

which, upon division of Eq. 6-19 by Eq. 6-20, gives the relative bioavailability:

$$Relative\ bioavailability = \frac{F_A}{F_B} = \left(\frac{Ae_{\infty,A}}{Ae_{\infty,B}}\right) \cdot \left(\frac{Dose_B}{Dose_A}\right) \tag{6-21}$$

The ratio of the dose-normalized cumulative amount excreted unchanged is, therefore, the ratio of the bioavailabilities, the relative bioavailability. When Dose B is given intravenously, the ratio is the bioavailability of the drug. For example, from the cumulative urinary excretion data in Table 6-1, it is apparent that the i.m. dose is almost completely bioavailable; the corresponding value for the oral dose is only 46%. Notice that, as expected, if *fe* is constant, this value is the same as that estimated from plasma data.

Urine data alone can be useful for estimating bioavailability when *fe* approaches 1, that is, when all the absorbed dose is excreted unchanged in the urine. Under this condition, changes in renal clearance (and hence total clearance) affect *AUC*, but do not change the total amount excreted, which is a direct measure of amount absorbed. The major problem here is in ensuring complete urine collection until virtually all the absorbed drug has been excreted, as discussed in Chapter 3, *Kinetics Following an Intravenous Bolus Dose*.

PLASMA AND URINE DATA

The renal clearance of a drug can be estimated when both plasma and urine data exist. The approach is identical to that taken for an i.v. dose (Chapter 3, *Kinetics Following an Intravenous Bolus Dose*). Because no knowledge of bioavailability is required, the estimate of renal clearance from combined plasma and urine data following extravascular administration is as accurate as that obtained following i.v. drug administration.

Now that we have dealt with the kinetics of drugs after administering a single extravascular dose, we might ask what physiologic processes of the body influence the rate and extent of drug absorption and how they do so, the topic of the next chapter (Chapter 7, *Absorption*).

KEY RELATIONSHIPS

$$t_{1/2,a} = \frac{0.693}{ka}$$

$$Rate\ of\ Absorption = \underset{\substack{\text{Absorption} \\ \text{rate constant}}}{ka} \cdot \underset{\substack{\text{Amount remaining} \\ \text{to be absorbed}}}{Aa}$$

$$F \cdot Dose = CL \cdot AUC$$

$$F_{e.v.} = \left(\frac{AUC_{e.v.}}{AUC_{i.v.}}\right)\left(\frac{Dose_{i.v.}}{Dose_{e.v.}}\right)$$

$$Relative\ bioavailability = \frac{F_B}{F_A} = \left(\frac{AUC_B}{AUC_A}\right)\left(\frac{Dose_A}{Dose_B}\right)$$

$$fe = \frac{Ae_\infty}{F \cdot Dose}$$

STUDY PROBLEMS

(Answers to Study Problems are in Appendix J.)

1. List six extravascular routes of administration.

2. Identify each of the statements below that is correct. For the one, or more, that is not correct, state why it is not or supply a qualification.

   a. All other parameters remaining unchanged, the slower the absorption process, the higher the peak plasma concentration after a single oral dose.

b. After a single oral dose, an increase in bioavailability causes the peak time to shorten.

c. For a given drug in a subject, *AUC* is proportional to the amount of drug absorbed.

d. If $ka \ll k$, then the terminal slope of the plasma concentration versus time curve reflects absorption, not elimination.

3. Depicted in Fig. 6-15 are curves of plasma concentration and amount in the body with time following the oral ingestion of a single dose of a drug. First, draw five pairs of curves identical to those in Fig. 6-15. Then, draw another curve on each pair of these curves that shows the effect of each of the following alterations in pharmacokinetic parameters. In each case, the dose administered and all other parameters (among *F, ka, V,* and *CL*) remain unchanged.

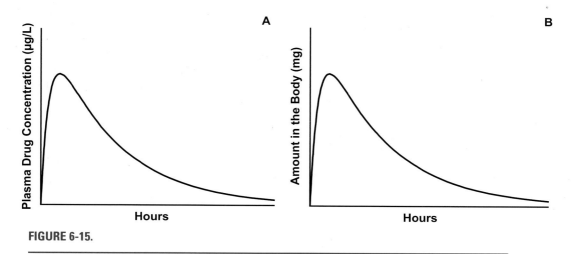

FIGURE 6-15.

a. *F* decreased.

b. *ka* increased.

c. *CL* increased, *k* increased by same factor.

d. *CL* decreased, *k* decreased by same factor.

e. *V* increased, *k* decreased by same factor.

4. Graffner et al. (Graffner C, Johnsson G, Sjögren J. Pharmacokinetics of procainamide intravenously and orally as conventional and slow-release tablets. Clin Pharmacol Ther 1975;17:414–423), in evaluating different dosage forms of procainamide obtained the following *AUC* and cumulative urine excretion data listed in Table 6-2. Plasma and urine were collected for 48 hr following drug administration.

TABLE 6-2	Procainamide Data Following i.v. and Oral Administration		
Route	**Dose (mg)**	***AUC* (mg-hr/L)**	**Amount excreted**
i.v.	500	13.1	332
Oral			
Formulation 1	1000	20.9	586
Formulation 2	1000	19.9	554

a. Estimate both bioavailability and relative bioavailability of Formulation 2 from both plasma and urine data. What are the assumptions made in your calculations?
b. The half-life of procainamide found in this study was 2.7 hr. Was the urine collected over a long enough time interval to obtain a good estimate of the cumulative amount excreted at infinite time?
c. Do the renal clearance values of procainamide vary much among the three treatments?

5. Channer and Roberts studied the effect of delayed esophageal transit on the absorption of acetaminophen. Each of 20 patients awaiting cardiac catheterization swallowed a single tablet containing acetaminophen (500 mg) and barium sulfate, a radio-opaque compound. The first 11 subjects swallowed the tablet while lying down; in 10 of these subjects, transit of the tablet was delayed, as visualized by fluoroscopy. In the other nine subjects who swallowed the tablet while standing, it entered the stomach immediately. In both groups, the tablet was taken with a sufficient volume of water to ease swallowing. Table 6-3 lists the average plasma acetaminophen data obtained over 6 hr after swallowing the tablet.

TABLE 6-3	Plasma Concentration Following Oral Administration of 500 mg of Acetaminophen	
Plasma Acetaminophen Concentration (mg/L)		
Time (min)	Subjects Standing	Subjects Lying Down
0	0	0
10	2.1	0.1
20	5.6	0.3
30	5.8	1.1
40	6.3	1.9
50	4.1	2.8
60	3.5	3.2
90	2.8	3.9
120	2.2	3.1
150	1.7	2.9
180	1.8	1.8
210	1.5	1.7
240	0.75	1.5
360	—	0.7

From: Channer KS, Roberts CJC. Effect of delayed esophageal transit on acetaminophen absorption. Clin Pharmacol Ther 1985;37:72–76.

a. What effect does delayed esophageal transit have on the speed and extent of absorption of acetaminophen?
b. What process, absorption or disposition, rate limits the decline in plasma drug concentration?
c. Acetaminophen is used for the relief of pain. Do the findings of this study affect the recommendation for the use of this drug?

6. Phenylethylmalonide (PEMA) is one of the major metabolites of the antiepileptic drug primidone. As part of a program to assess the potential use of PEMA as an antiepileptic drug itself, its pharmacokinetics were studied following i.v. and oral administration of 500 mg. Table 6-4 lists the resultant plasma concentrations in one subject. Also, 81% of the i.v. dose was recovered in urine unchanged.

TABLE 6-4	Plasma Concentrations following i.v. and Oral Administration of 500 mg of PEMA to a Subject												
Route	**Time (hr):**	0.33	0.5	0.67	1	1.5	2	4	6	10	16	24	32	48
					Plasma PEMA concentration (mg/L)								
i.v.		14.7	12.6	11.0	-	9.0	8.2	7.9	6.6	6.2	4.6	3.2	2.3	1.2
Oral		-	2.4	-	3.8	4.2	4.6	8.1	5.8	5.1	4.1	3.0	2.3	1.3

From: Pisani F, Richens A. Pharmacokinetics of phenylethylmalonamide (PEMA) after oral and intravenous administration. Clin Pharmacokin 1983;8:272–276.

a. From a semilogarithmic plot of the plasma concentration with time, estimate the elimination half-life of PEMA in the subject.
b. Calculate the total AUC following i.v. and oral administration.
c. From the i.v. data, estimate the clearance and volume of distribution of PEMA.
d. Determine the oral bioavailability of the drug.
e. Calculate its renal clearance.

7. Rowland et al. (Rowland M, Epstein W, Riegleman S. Absorption kinetics of griseofulvin in man. J Pharm Sci 1968;57:984–989) gave griseofulvin orally, 0.5 g of a micronized drug formulation, and, on another occasion, intravenously, 100 mg, to volunteers. The plasma concentration–time data obtained in one subject are given in Table 6-5. From appropriate plots and calculations, what can be concluded from these data with respect to:

a. Rate of absorption of griseofulvin with time on an oral administration in this individual?
b. Completeness of absorption?

TABLE 6-5	Plasma Concentration Following i.v. (100 mg) and Oral (500 mg) Administration of Griseofulvin to a Subject													
Route	**Time (hr):**	0	1	2	3	4	5	7	8	12	24	28	32	35	48
						Plasma Griseofulvin concentration (mg/L)								
i.v.		0	1.4	1.1	0.98	0.90	0.80	-	0.68	0.55	0.37	-	0.24	-	0.14
Oral		0	0.4	0.95	1.15	1.15	1.05	1.2	1.2	0.90	1.05	0.90	0.85	0.80	0.50

8. The information in Table 6-6 on cidofovir (Vistide), an antiviral agent, was obtained by Wachsman et al. (Wachsman M, Petty PG, Cundy KC, et al. Pharmacokinetics, safety and bioavailability of HPMPC [Cidofovir] in human immununodeficiency virus-infected subjects. Antiviral Res 1996;29:153–161). Use mean values to answer the following questions.

a. Calculate the bioavailability (extent of systemic absorption) of cidofovir when given by the subcutaneous (s.c.) route using:
(1) The plasma data.
(2) The urine data.

TABLE 6-6   Area, Half-life, and Amount Excreted Unchanged of Cidofovir after Intravenous, Subcutaneous, and Oral Administration

Dose:	1 mg/kg	3 mg/kg		10 mg/kg	
Route of administration:	i.v.	i.v.	s.c.	i.v.	p.o.
AUC(0-∞) (μg-hr/mL)	7.7 ± 2.6	17.9 ± 2.3	17.8 ± 1.5	64.2 ± 8.8	<3.5
Half-life observed (hr)	1.7 ± 0.4	2.5 ± 0.9	2.3 ± 0.7	2.9 ± 0.7	*
Amount excreted un-changed, Ae(∞)(mg/kg)	0.92 ± 0.20	2.38 ± 0.36	2.47 ± 0.25	10.5 ± 1.6	0.24 ± 0.03

p.o., oral.
*Concentration too low to obtain a proper estimate.
From: Wachsman M, Petty PG, Cundy KC, et al. Pharmacokinetics, safety and bioavailability of HPMPC (Cidofovir) in human immununodeficiency virus-infected subjects. Antiviral Res 1996;29:153–161.

b. Calculate the bioavailability of cidofovir when given orally using:
  (1) the plasma data.
  (2) the urine data.
c. Estimate the fraction excreted unchanged after all three i.v. doses.

9. The concentration–time profile following a single 25-mg oral dose of a drug is shown in Fig. 6-16 and is summarized by the equation:

$$C\ (\mu g/L) = 150 \cdot (e^{-0.06t} - e^{-0.5t}); \text{ time in hours.}$$

The elimination half-life (i.v. dose) of the drug is 11.6 hr.

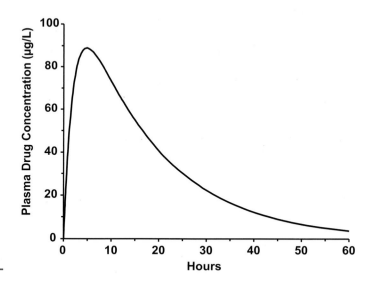

FIGURE 6-16.

a. Is the decline of the concentration rate limited by absorption or elimination?
b. Add lines to Fig. 6-16 (be sure to identify curves as "B1" and "B2") that represent the expected concentration–time profiles (rough approximation) expected when:
  (1) the extent of absorption is halved (Profile B1), but there is no change in absorption kinetics (i.e., ka is constant).
  (2) the absorption process is slowed (ka is 5× smaller), but the extent of absorption (F) is the same (Profile B2). This situation might occur when the dosage form is changed (e.g., from a rapid-release product to a slow-release product).
c. What is the expected peak time (t_{max}) of the concentration in profile B.2?

10. The 90% and 95% confidence intervals of the logarithm of the test/reference ratio of the *AUC* values in Table 6-7 were determined in bioequivalence studies of several immediate-release formulations of a drug during development. Five conclusions are listed below. Identify, in the last column, all the conclusions below that can be applied to each study.

TABLE 6-7	Ninety Percent and 95% Confidence Intervals in Five Separate Studies		
Study	**90% Confidence Interval***	**95% Confidence Interval***	**Conclusions That Apply**
101	0.72–0.94	0.70–0.96	_____
102	0.86–1.20	0.83–1.23	_____
103	1.07–1.23	1.05–1.25	_____
104	1.28–1.46	1.26–1.48	_____
105	0.78–1.11	0.75–1.14	_____

*Confidence interval in the ratio of test/reference values of *AUC* after antilog transformation.

Conclusion:

a. Products are bioequivalent.
b. No declaration of bioequivalence can be made.
c. Products are not bioequivalent.
d. The products differ in their areas.
e. No conclusion of difference in areas can be made.

7

Absorption

OBJECTIVES

The reader will be able to:

- Define the following terms: absorption rate-limited, Biopharmaceutics Classification System (BCS), dissolution, dissolution rate-limited, first-pass loss, gastric emptying, gastrointestinal absorption, intestinal transit, saturable first-pass metabolism.
- Describe the steps involved in the systemic absorption of a drug after extravascular administration generally and specifically after oral administration.
- List five factors influencing dissolution rate of a drug.
- Distinguish between dissolution and permeability-rate limitations in systemic absorption after oral administration.
- State the mean transit times of material in the fasted stomach, small intestine, and large intestine.
- Anticipate for which compounds intestinal permeability is likely to be the reason for incomplete oral bioavailability for a drug absorbed by passive diffusion.
- List possible competing reactions responsible for low oral bioavailability of drugs, together with one example of each possibility.
- Calculate the anticipated maximum oral bioavailability of a drug given either its hepatic extraction ratio or the appropriate information to estimate this value under nonsaturating conditions.
- Anticipate the influence of physicochemical properties of a drug on its absorption from different sites of administration.
- Anticipate the role of gastric emptying and intestinal transit in the systemic absorption of a drug given orally with particular reference to the physicochemical properties of the drug and its dosage form.
- Anticipate the influence of food on the systemic absorption of a drug given orally.
- Describe the rationale underpinning the application of the BCS to the waiver of bioequivalence studies of multisource formulations of the same drug and to deciding which drug transporters are unlikely to affect either their absorption or disposition.
- Describe the influence of decreased permeability and surface area along the intestinal tract on the performance of oral constant-rate release dosage forms.

This chapter deals with the general physiologic and physicochemical principles governing systemic drug absorption, particularly following oral administration. Being a complex structure, many anatomic and physiologic factors affect the overall rate and extent of drug absorption from the gastrointestinal tract, making precise quantitative predictions difficult. Nonetheless, some generalizations can be made on the consequences of many of the events occurring at this and other sites of absorption.

Passage of drug through the membranes dividing the absorption site from the blood is a prerequisite for absorption to occur. To do so, a drug must be in solution. Most drugs are administered as solid preparations (e.g., tablets and capsules). Because solid particles cannot pass through membranes, a drug must dissolve to be absorbed. Many factors influence the dissolution, or release, of drug from a solid pharmaceutical formulation. However, before discussing the factors influencing the release, let us first consider drug absorption from a solution.

ABSORPTION FROM SOLUTION

Systemic absorption is favored after extravascular administration because the body acts as a sink, producing a concentration difference between the diffusible unbound concentrations at the absorption site and in systemic blood. The concentration gradient across the absorptive membranes is maintained by distribution to tissues and elimination of absorbed drug. Physiologic and physicochemical factors that determine movement of drug through membranes in general are presented in Chapter 4, *Membranes and Distribution*. Included among them are the molecular size of the drug, the nature of the membrane involved, presence of transporters, perfusion, and pH. These factors and others are now considered with respect to drug passage through gastrointestinal membranes. In this context, **gastrointestinal absorption** is the term that is subsequently used for this process.

GASTROINTESTINAL ABSORPTION

The first potential site for absorption of orally administered drugs is the stomach. In accordance with the prediction of the pH partition hypothesis, weak acids are absorbed more rapidly from the stomach at pH 1.0 than at pH 8.0, and the converse holds for weak bases. Absorption of acids, however, is much faster from the less acidic small intestine (pH 6.6 to 7.5) than from the stomach. These apparently conflicting observations can be reconciled. Surface area, permeability and, when perfusion rate-limits absorption, blood flow are important determinants of the rapidity of absorption. The intestine, especially the small intestine, is favored on all accounts. The total absorptive area of the small intestine, produced largely by microvilli, has been calculated to be about 200 m^2, and an estimated 1 L of blood passes through the intestinal capillaries each minute. The corresponding estimates for the stomach are only 1 m^2 and 150 mL/min. The permeability of the intestinal membranes to drugs is also greater than that of the stomach. These increases in surface area, permeability, and blood flow more than compensate for the decreased fraction of un-ionized acid in the intestine. Indeed, the absorption of *all* compounds—acids, bases, and neutral compounds—is faster from the small intestine than from the stomach. Because absorption is greater in the small intestine, the rate of gastric emptying can be a controlling step in the speed of drug absorption even when given in solution. In the following discussion, the examples chosen are either drugs administered as solutions or where there is reason to expect, based on solubility considerations for example, that the drug dissolves within the time it spends within the stomach, usually about 30 min or less prior to entering the small intestine. This is especially the case when a drug is taken on an empty stomach with a glass of water.

Gastric Emptying. Food, especially fat, slows gastric emptying, which explains why drugs are frequently recommended to be taken on an empty stomach when a rapid

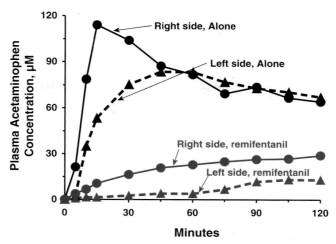

FIGURE 7-1.   Gastric emptying can rate-limit systemic drug absorption. Remifentanil, an ultra short-acting opioid narcotic analgesic, slows gastric emptying as observed by the mean systemic exposure–time profiles of acetaminophen after its oral administration (1.5 g dissolved in 200 mL of water) to 10 healthy volunteers in the presence and absence of the narcotic. The drug was given alone (*black lines*) and 10 min after the start of a constant-rate intravenous infusion of remifentanil of 0.2 μg/kg per minute (*colored lines*). Posture was also shown to minimally influence gastric emptying as observed when acetaminophen was taken while the subjects were lying on their left side with the head lower than the feet by 20 degrees (*dotted lines*) than when the subjects were on their right side with the head higher than the feet by 20 degrees (*solid lines*). (From: Walldén J, Thörn SE, Wattwil M. The delay of gastric emptying induced by remifentanil is not influenced by posture. Anesth Analg 2004;99:429–434.)

onset of action is desired. Drugs that influence gastric emptying also affect the speed of absorption of other drugs, as shown in Fig. 7-1 for acetaminophen, a common analgesic/antipyretic, when remifentanil (Ultiva), a potent ultra short-acting opioid, is concurrently administered. The observed slowing of systemic absorption, which is common to all opioids, is partially a result of slowed gastric emptying, which contributes to the constipation seen with this class of drugs. The figure also shows that gastric emptying may be slightly faster when lying on the right side than when lying on the left side (not statistically significant). Although on first glance it would appear that the extent of absorption (area under the curve [*AUC*]) is affected by remifentanil or the position of the body, one cannot be certain because of the limited time over which blood samples are taken. The total *AUC* (not provided) is needed. Clearly, it is unlikely that one would get a rapid onset of response to a drug when gastric emptying is so slowed.

Retention of acetaminophen in the stomach increases the percentage of a dose absorbed through the gastric mucosa, but this is a minor pathway; the majority of the dose is still absorbed through the intestinal epithelium. In this regard, the stomach may be viewed as a repository organ from which pulses of drug are ejected by peristalsis onto the absorption sites in the small intestine.

Intestinal Absorption and Permeability.   Throughout its length, the intestine varies in its multifaceted properties and luminal composition. The intestine may be broadly divided into the small and large intestines separated by the ileocecal valve. Surface area per unit length decreases from the duodenum to the rectum. Electrical resistance, a measure of the degree of tightness of the junctions between the epithelial cells, is much higher in the colon than in the small intestine. Proteolytic and metabolic enzymes, as well as active and facilitated transport systems are distributed variably along the intestine, often in restrictive regions. The colon abounds with anaerobic microflora. The mean pH, 6.6, in the proximal small intestine rises to 7.5 in the terminal ileum, and then falls sharply to 6.4 at the start of the cecum before finally rising again to 7.0 in the descending colon. Mean transit time of materials is around 3 to 4 hr in the small intestine and from 10 to 36 hr or even longer in the large bowel. Although these and other complexities make precise quantitative prediction of intestinal drug absorption difficult, several general features emerge.

The permeability-surface area ($P \cdot SA$, see Chapter 4, *Membranes and Distribution*) product tends to decrease progressively from duodenum to colon. This applies to all drug molecules traversing the intestine epithelium by non–carrier-mediated processes, whether via the transcellular (through cell) or paracellular (around cell) routes, when drug solutions are placed in different parts of the intestine. How much of this decrease in absorption is a result of a decrease in permeability and how much of the decrease in surface area between small and large intestine is not known for certain. For permeable drugs, absorption is rapid and probably complete within the small intestine. Even if some drugs were to enter the large intestine, the permeability there is still sufficiently high to ensure that all that entered would be absorbed. For these drugs, although absorption across the intestinal epithelia may be perfusion rate–limited, as mentioned previously, the overall rate-limiting step in systemic absorption is likely to be gastric emptying.

Absorption of less permeable, generally more polar, drugs still primarily occurs within the small intestine rather than the large intestine. Evidence supporting this notion is provided with the H_2-antagonist ranitidine (Fig. 7-2). When given intracolonically, the extent of absorption is greatly reduced compared to when placed into the stomach or jejunum, as reflected by the reduced AUC (Fig. 7-2A). Evidently, very little ranitidine is absorbed from the large intestine even though drug can be there for 24 hr or more. Furthermore, absorption from the large intestine appears to become rate limiting in the elimination of drug from the body, as reflected by an increased terminal half-life after colonic administration (Fig. 7-2B).

As discussed in Chapter 4, *Membranes and Distribution*, molecular size is a particularly important determinant of permeability. Small polar substances, such as the antiviral acyclovir (250 g/mol), H_2-antagonist cimetidine (252 g/mol), and atenolol (266 g/mol), primarily move paracellularly across the epithelium. Permeability, in general, and paracellular permeability, in particular, appears to drop off sharply with molecular weights (MWs) above 350 g/mol, a value at which compounds appear to approach the molecular dimensions of the tight junctions between intestinal cells. Drugs with poor permeability characteristics show low oral bioavailability not only for this reason, but also because of the limited time, 2 to 4 hr, they spend in the small intestine where permeability is highest. For example, when given orally, only 60% of ranitidine is absorbed and virtually all within the first 3 to 4 hr after administration; the rest is recovered unchanged in feces. The relationship between fraction absorbed intestinally and jejunal permeability of many drugs is shown in Fig. 7-3 (page 188). Clearly, low permeability drugs are likely to be poorly absorbed. Examples that are particularly poorly absorbed drugs ($F = 0.005$ to 0.14) are listed in Table 7-1. The drugs in the table share the common property of being polar and, with the exception of pyridostigmine, relatively large (MW >400 g/mol). Pyridostigmine is a quaternary ammonium compound with a permanent positive change, which may explain its low oral bioavailability (F about 0.07 to 0.14) despite its relatively small size (181 g/mol).

Most of the compounds in Table 7-1 (page 188) are not reliably active systemically when given orally; they must be given parenterally. Not so much because of their low oral bioavailability, but because of their excessively variable oral absorption and sometimes because there is a need for very large doses to adequately achieve a therapeutic systemic exposure. The bisphosphonates, alendronate, and ibandronate are exceptions. They are given orally in spite of their low oral bioavailabilities (about 0.005 to 0.007). The doses given are not excessively large; only small amounts are apparently needed systemically. The amount of alendronate systemically absorbed when given in a 70-mg weekly regimen

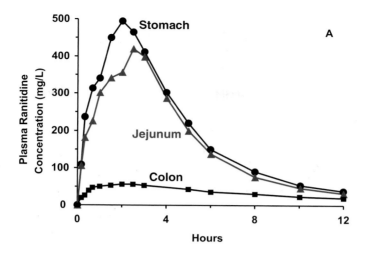

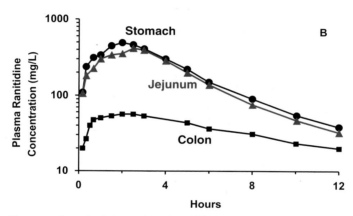

FIGURE 7-2. The gastrointestinal absorption of ranitidine varies with site of application. The variation is shown in linear **(A)** and semilogarithmic **(B)** plots of the mean plasma concentration–time profiles observed after placing an aqueous solution (6 mL) containing 150 mg of ranitidine hydrochloride into the stomach (*black circles*), jejunum (*colored triangles*), and colon (*black squares*) of eight volunteers, via a nasoenteric tube. The much less extensive absorption of this small (MW = 313 g/mol) polar molecule from the colon is consistent with the idea that the $P \cdot SA$ product is much lower in the colon than in the small intestine. Notice that absorption of ranitidine effectively ceases (in terminal decline phase) by 3 hr when placed in the stomach or jejunum, even though the drug is incompletely bioavailable ($F = 0.6$, data not shown), suggesting that the small intestine is the major site of absorption when ranitidine is taken orally. Also, notice in B that the terminal half-life of the decline in the plasma concentration is longer when the drug is administered into the colon. Absorption from the colon thus appears to be slow and rate limiting drug elimination. (From: Williams MF, Dukes GE, Heizer W, et al. Influence of gastrointestinal site of drug delivery on the absorption characteristics of ranitidine. Pharm Res 1992;9:1190–1194.)

is only about 0.42 mg. The amount of ibandronate systemically absorbed from a 150-mg once-monthly dose is only 0.9 mg. Pyridostigmine is also given orally to treat myasthenia gravis, in spite of its low oral bioavailability. Although oral administration is ruled out for many of the antimicrobial agents listed in Table 7-1, occasionally they have utility in treating diseases of the alimentary canal itself. The use of vancomycin in treating pseudomembranous colitis is an example.

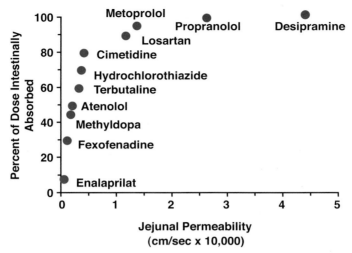

FIGURE 7-3. The fraction of a dose intestinally absorbed after oral administration correlates with human jejunal permeability. Drugs with permeabilities less than 1.0×10^{-4} cm/sec are likely to be incompletely intestinally absorbed. The lower the permeability is below this value, the greater is the likelihood of their being so. (From: Petri N, Lennernäs H. In vivo permeability studies in the gastrointestinal tract. In: van de Waterbeemd H, Lennernäs H, Artusson P, eds. Drug Bioavailability, Estimation of Solubility, Permeability, Absorption and Bioavailability. Berlin, Germany: Wiley-VCH, 2003:345–386.)

TABLE 7-1	Examples of Drugs Showing Low Oral Bioavailability Because of Low Intestinal Permeability*

Alendronate	Gentamicin
Amikacin	Ibandronate
Carbenicillin	Neomycin
Cefamandole	Pyridostigmine
Ceftazidime	Streptomycin
Flumazenil	Vancomycin

*All of the drugs are antimicrobial agents, except the following: alendronate, an agent used in treating rheumatoid arthritis; flumazenil, an agent used to reverse the sedative effects of benzodiazepines; ibandronate, an agent used to treat and prevent osteoporosis; and pyridostigmine, an agent used to treat myasthenia gravis and poisoning by certain nerve gases.

An additional determinant of permeability and hence absorption are transporters, particularly those on the apical side of the epithelial cells (i.e., facing the intestinal lumen). Uptake transporters, such as peptide transporter 1 (PepT1) and organic anion-transporting polypeptide 3 (OATP3), facilitate the absorption of amoxicillin, L-dopa, and antiepileptic/analgesic gabapentin, all of which would otherwise be poorly absorbed. Indeed, as discussed in Chapter 4, *Membranes and Distribution*, it is because the inherent passive permeability of such molecules is low that transporters exert an influence. In contrast, systemic absorption of some drugs is reduced by the presence of efflux transporters (e.g., P-glycoprotein). Drug examples include digoxin, used in treating heart failure and atrial fibrillation; fexofenadine, an antihistamine; paclitaxel, an anticancer drug; and saquinavir, an antiretroviral agent. Low apparent permeability results, not so much from inability to cross intestinal membranes, but from the action of the efflux transporter. Concurrent administration of inhibitors of the transport system (e.g., erythromycin, an

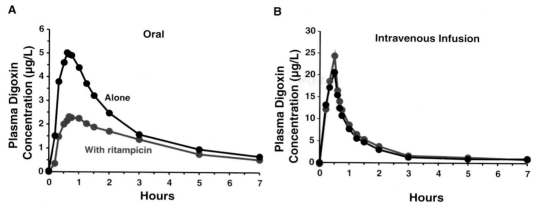

FIGURE 7-4. Rifampicin pretreatment reduces the absorption of digoxin. Shown are plots of mean plasma digoxin concentration–time profiles after oral and i.v. administration (as a 30-min infusion) of 1 mg digoxin alone (●) and after 10 days rifampicin pretreatment (600 mg daily, ●) to seven healthy adults. A clear depression in the oral absorption of digoxin is inferred by the lower concentrations after oral but not i.v. administration after rifampicin pretreatment. This was corroborated by a 30 % decrease in total AUC(0–144hr) (from 54.8 to 38.2 μg-hr/L), corresponding to a fall from 63% to 38% in oral bioavailability. (From: Greiner B, Eichelbaum M, Fritz P, et al. The role of intestinal P-glycoprotein in the interaction of digoxin and rifampin. J Clin Invest 1999;104:147–153.)

antibiotic; ketoconazole, an antifungal agent; quinidine, used in atrial fibrillation; and ritonavir, a protease inhibitor) can increase the oral absorption of these transported substrates, whereas coadministration of inducers of this efflux transporter (e.g., rifampin, an antitubercular drug, and St. John's wort, alleged to be useful for depression and other mental disorders) have the opposite effect. This is clearly illustrated by the effect of rifampicin on digoxin pharmacokinetics (Fig. 7-4). Digoxin, a large (781 g/mol) molecule containing three sugar groups, is absorbed and predominantly renally eliminated unchanged; bioavailability is usually about 70% and most absorption appears to occur within the first 4 hr of administration, in keeping with limited absorption beyond the small intestine. Rifampicin pretreatment has no material effect on the disposition kinetics of digoxin but, rather, reduces its oral bioavailability (based on decreased total AUC). A slowing in the speed of its absorption is also clearly indicated by the decrease in C_{max} and the increase in t_{max}. The mechanism is an increase in the intestinal expression of P-glycoprotein induced by rifampicin. The absorption of digoxin is permeability limited; therefore, a decrease in the effective permeability of digoxin decreases both the speed and extent of its absorption.

An additional consideration is that distribution of transporters along the gastrointestinal tract varies. Certainly, this is true for P-glycoprotein, with activity increasing down along the intestinal tract, being highest in the large intestine. This higher activity may, in part, explain why such drugs as ranitidine have such a much lower permeability in the colon than in the small intestine (see Fig. 7-2).

CAUSES OF LOSS IN ORAL BIOAVAILABILITY

The oral bioavailability (F) of drugs is commonly less than one, even when administered in solution. There are many reasons for the reduced systemic absorption, in addition to low intestinal permeability. Recall from Chapter 2, *Fundamental Concepts and Terminology*, that a drug must pass sequentially from the gastrointestinal lumen, through the gut wall, and through the liver, before entering the general circulation (Fig. 7-5). This sequence is an anatomic requirement because blood perfusing virtually all gastrointestinal tissues drains into the liver via the hepatic portal vein. Drug may also be lost by decomposition in the lumen; the fraction entering the intestinal tissues, F_F, is then the fraction neither lost in the

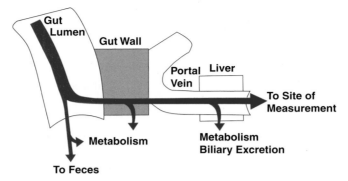

FIGURE 7-5. A drug, given as a solid or a solution, encounters several barriers and sites of loss in its sequential movement from the gastrointestinal tract to the systemic circulation. Dissolution, a prerequisite to movement across the gut wall, is the first step. Incomplete dissolution, slow penetration of the gastrointestinal membranes, or decomposition in the gut lumen are causes of poor bioavailability. Removal of drug as it first passes through gut wall and the liver further reduces the systemic bioavailability.

feces nor decomposed in the lumen. Of this permeating drug, only a fraction may escape destruction within the walls of the gastrointestinal tract, F_G, thereby reducing the fraction of dose reaching the portal vein further to $F_F \cdot F_G$. If drug is also eliminated in the liver, an additional fraction, F_H, of that reaching the liver escapes extraction there, another site of first-pass loss. Accordingly, the measured overall oral systemic bioavailability, F, is then

$$F = F_F \cdot F_G \cdot F_H \qquad \text{7-1}$$

For example, if 50% of the drug is lost at each step, the bioavailability of the drug, measured systematically, would be $0.5 \times 0.5 \times 0.5 = 0.125$, or 12.5%. Note that the drug can be rendered totally unavailable systemically at any one of these steps.

Competing Intestinal Reactions. Any reaction that competes with intestinal uptake reduces the oral bioavailability of a drug. Table 7-2 lists such reactions. They can be either enzymatic or nonenzymatic in nature. Acid hydrolysis in the stomach is a common nonenzymatic one. Enzymatic reactions include those caused by digestive enzymes (from bile and pancreatic fluids), metabolic enzymes within the intestinal epithelium, and microfloral enzymes, predominately resident in the large bowel. Complexation reactions with other drugs also occur; the result may be low drug bioavailability. For example, coadministration of activated charcoal or cholestyramine reduces the absorption of a number of drugs, which include the active metabolite of leflunomide, an agent used to treat rheumatoid arthritis; cephalexin, an antibiotic; and piroxicam, an analgesic agent. When both an adsorbent and an *adsorbable* drug are concurrently used, their administration must be appropriately timed to avoid their concurrent presence in any region of the gastrointestinal tract, particularly the small intestine. Otherwise, the bioavailability of the drug may be greatly reduced.

The complexities that occur in vivo make quantitative prediction of the contribution of a competing reaction to decreased bioavailability difficult. Sometimes, the problem of incomplete absorption can be circumvented by physically protecting the drug from destruction in the stomach or by synthesizing a more stable derivative, which is converted to the active molecule within the gastrointestinal tract or within the body. Similarly, to enhance absorption, more permeable derivatives are made, which are rapidly converted to the active molecule, often during passage through the intestinal wall. For example, absorption of the polar antibiotic ampicillin is incomplete. The systemic delivery of this acidic drug is improved substantially by administering it as a more lipophilic and permeable inactive ester prodrug, pivampicillin, which quickly releases ampicillin. Another example is that of

| TABLE 7-2 | Representative Reactions within the Gastrointestinal Tract that Compete with Drug Absorption from Solution |

Reaction	Drug	Comment
Adsorption	Sumatriptan	Adsorption to charcoal; adsorbed material is not absorbed.
Conjugation		
Sulfoconjugation	Ethinyl estradiol	Concurrent administration of inhibitors of sulfoconjugation (e.g., ascorbic acid and acetaminophen) increase bioavailability of this drug.
Glucuronidation	Morphine	Two glucuronides are formed. The 6-glucuronide has analgesic activity. The 3-glucuronide is inactive.
Decarboxylation	Levodopa	Loss of activity: given with a peripheral dopa decarboxylase inhibitor to reduce gastrointestinal metabolism.
Efflux transport	Fexofenadine	Efflux transporters reduce absorption of this drug.
Hydrolysis		
Acid	Penicillin G	Loss of activity; product is inactive.
	Erythromycin	Loss of activity; product is inactive.
	Digoxin	Products (digitoxides) have variable activity.
Enzymatic	Aspirin	Salicylic acid, an active anti-inflammatory compound is formed.
	Pivampicillin	Active ampicillin formed: pivampicillin (ester) is inactive.
	Insulin	Loss of activity; product is inactive.
Oxidation	Cyclosporine	Loss of activity; products are less active or inactive.
Reduction (microflora)	Olsalazine	Intended for local (colon) anti-inflammatory action; parent drug not systemically absorbed, but is reduced to two molecules of the active metabolite, 5-aminosalicylic acid.

valganciclovir (Valcyte), an antiviral agent. The hydrolysis of this compound by esterases within the gut wall and liver is so rapid that only its active metabolite, ganciclovir, is detected in the systemic circulation. Valganciclovir is therefore, by design, a prodrug as well.

First-Pass Loss. Metabolism during passage across the intestinal wall and through the liver reduces the amount reaching the general circulation. The drug is then said to undergo **first-pass metabolic loss**. A few examples to illustrate first-pass loss follow.

Aspirin (acetylsalicylic acid) is one of the first synthetic prodrugs. It was marketed at the end of the 19th century to help overcome the unpleasant taste and gastrointestinal irritation associated with the anti-inflammatory drug, salicylic acid. Aspirin was originally thought to be inactive, being designed to be rapidly hydrolyzed within the body to salicylic acid. Only subsequently was aspirin itself shown to have some pharmacologic effects of its own, namely an anticlotting effect. Yet the original design worked; upon ingestion, aspirin, a labile ester, is rapidly hydrolyzed, particularly by esterases in the gut wall and liver. Indeed, intestinal and hepatic hydrolysis is so rapid that a sizeable fraction of intestinally absorbed aspirin is converted to salicylic acid in a single passage through these organs, resulting in a substantial loss of oral bioavailability.

Another example of a drug showing first-pass loss is orlistat (Xenical). Apart from having a first-pass loss, one in the gastrointestinal wall (orlistat) and the other primarily in the liver (aspirin), orlistat and aspirin have little in common. They have different chemical structures and possess different pharmacologic activities. Aspirin (MW = 190 g/mol) is a simple acetyl ester of salicylic acid, whereas orlistat is a larger (MW = 496 g/mol), more complex molecule. Aspirin is an anti-inflammatory agent through its active metabolite, salicylic acid, whereas orlistat acts locally as a lipase inhibitor within the gastrointestinal tract to slow fat absorption and help control obesity. The almost complete first-pass metabolism of the small fraction of orlistat that permeates the intestine has, therefore, little impact on its efficacy.

When metabolites formed during the first pass through the intestinal wall and liver are inactive or less potent than the parent drug, the oral dose may need to be larger than the equivalent intravenous or intramuscular dose if the same therapeutic effect is to be achieved. Any drug with a high hepatic extraction ratio (see Table 5-2) has a low and often highly variable oral bioavailability. Being physiologically determined, no amount of pharmaceutical manipulation can improve on this value for an oral dosage formulation. Sometimes, the problem is so severe that either the drug must be given by a parenteral route, or it must be discarded in favor of another drug candidate. Flumazenil, a benzodiazepine receptor antagonist, and naloxone, an opioid antagonist, are examples. These drugs are so highly extracted by the liver that they must be given parenterally to be effective.

Extensive hepatic extraction can be advantageously used in therapy. Talwin (Hospira), a combination product of pentazocine, a potent narcotic analgesic with abuse potential, and naloxone, an analgesic antagonist, is effective as an analgesic when administered orally because naloxone, but not pentazocine, is very extensively metabolized during the first pass through the liver. However, when administered parenterally, the mixture is inactive because of the antagonistic effect of naloxone. The advantage of the combination in the oral product is to prevent its parenteral injection by drug abusers. Another combination product, Suboxone, containing naloxone and the narcotic analgesic buprenorphine, is given sublingually. Naloxone is also found not to be absorbed systemically when given by this route, but presumably a quicker response to buprenorphine is obtained by this dosage form than when given orally. Furthermore, the bioavailability of buprenorphine is greater after sublingual than after oral administration, probably because the vasculature in the mouth drains directly into the superior vena cava, thereby bypassing the liver.

Another example is budesonide, a synthetic corticosteroid used in treating Crohn's disease of the ileum and ascending colon. The drug is given in a modified release dosage form which releases drug in the region where the disease is common. Drug easily permeates the intestinal wall but, owing to extensive first-pass metabolism in gut wall and liver, systemic availability is low, thereby reducing the adverse systemic effects of the corticosteroid. Coadministration of drugs that inhibit metabolism, however, reduces the first-pass loss and increases systemic exposure and therefore adverse events. Coadministration of ketoconazole, a potent inhibitor of metabolism at conventional doses, for example, has been reported to increase by eightfold the AUC of budesonide.

SEPARATING GUT WALL FROM HEPATIC FIRST-PASS LOSS

It is important to distinguish between gut wall and hepatic first-pass loss, as some effects, such as drug interactions to be discussed later in this chapter (see the "grapefruit juice–simvastatin interaction"), occur predominantly in the gut wall, others in the liver, and still others in a combination of both.

Consider an orally administered drug all of which enters the intestinal wall, that is $F_F = 1$, so that $F = F_G \cdot F_H$. An estimate of F_G can be made if F and F_H are known. F is determined experimentally, whereas F_H may be calculated from the hepatic extraction ratio, E_H, since

$$F_H = 1 - E_H$$

Hepatic
extraction ratio

7-2

It is the maximum value of oral bioavailability if the only source of loss is hepatic extraction. Recall, from Chapter 5, *Elimination*, hepatic extraction ratio can be estimated if the hepatic (blood) clearance and hepatic blood flow are known or can be approximated.

To illustrate this, consider the following data obtained after oral and i.v. doses, each 5 mg, of a drug with a plasma-to-blood concentration ratio (C/C_b) of 0.83 and that is eliminated renally and hepatically. After its oral administration, $AUC = 0.21$ mg-min/L. After the i.v. dose, $AUC = 3.53$ mg-min/L, and cumulative amount excreted unchanged ($Ae_\infty = 0.52$ mg). Its clearance (*Dose/AUC*) is then 1.42 L/min; blood clearance ($CL \cdot C/C_b$) is 1.18 L/min; and the fraction excreted unchanged ($Ae_\infty/Dose$) is 0.104. Hence, its renal blood clearance ($fe \cdot CL_b$) is 0.086 L/min. Given that extrarenal elimination occurs only in the liver, by difference, the hepatic blood clearance [$(1 - fe)CL_b$] is 1.09 L/min. Dividing by hepatic blood flow yields the hepatic extraction ratio which, in this example, is 0.81 for a hepatic blood flow of 1.35 L/min. Accordingly,

$$F_H = 1 - \frac{(1 - fe)\, CL_b}{Q_H} = 0.29$$

7-3

The observed oral bioavailability, given by the ratio of *AUC* values, as the same dose was given orally and intravenously, is 0.06. Clearly, this is considerably lower than expected if the loss was only because of hepatic extraction. There must be an additional cause of the low value of *F*. If intestinal absorption is virtually complete, that is, there is no preabsorption loss of drug, then first-pass loss in the gut wall is likely. In this case, the value of F_G is 0.21 (F/F_H), indicating that almost 80% of the oral dose fails to reach the liver. Indeed, gut wall metabolism is then the major contributor to the low oral bioavailability.

The gut contains many of the enzymes found in the liver, in particular cytochrome P450 3A4 (CYP3A4) and several of the glucuronyl transferases (1A8 and 1A10). Table 7-3 lists drugs of moderate-to-low oral bioavailability primarily because of first-pass metabolic loss. All of these drugs are metabolized predominantly by CYP3A4. Despite this commonality, notice that for some, such as tacrolimus and buspirone, there is a substantial gut wall loss, whereas for others, such as triazolam and nifedipine, it is modest. The differences among them are probably because of a combination of intestinal permeability, intrinsic

TABLE 7-3	Bioavailabilities of Various Substrates of CYP3A4 across the Gut Wall and the Liver			
CYP3A4 Substrate	**F**	**F$_F$***	**F$_G$**	**F$_H$**
Tacrolimus	0.14	1	0.14	0.96
Buspirone	-	-	0.21	0.24
Atorvastatin	0.14	1	0.24	0.58
Cyclosporine	0.22–0.36	0.86	0.33–0.48	0.75–0.88
Felodipine	0.14	1	0.45	0.34
Midazolam	0.25–0.41	1	0.40–0.79	0.49–0.74
Triazolam	0.55	0.85	0.75	0.75
Nifedipine	0.41	1	0.78	0.53
Quinidine	0.78	0.95	0.90	0.86
Alprazolam	0.84	0.92	0.94	0.97

*F_F taken as 1 for those drugs for which no other data are available.
From: Galetin A, Hinton LK, Burt H, et al. Maximal inhibition of intestinal first-pass metabolism as a pragmatic indicator of intestinal contribution to the drug–drug interaction of CYP3A4 cleared drugs. Curr Drug Metab 2007;8:685–693.

intestinal metabolic activity, and for some, intestinal transporters, which is discussed below. Notice also, there is relatively little correlation between F_G and F_H. Thus, for nifedipine $F_G > F_H$, for tacrolimus $F_H > F_G$, whereas for midazolam, F_G and F_H contribute almost equally to the low oral bioavailability.

For drugs that undergo extensive first-pass metabolism in the gut wall and the liver, there is often a very large effect of induction or inhibition on their bioavailability. The sequential loss in these organs may partially explain the large effect. For example, consider a drug for which F_G and F_H were both 0.7 and that an inducer is given that increases these values to 0.9. The bioavailability would then be decreased from 0.09 (0.3×0.3) to 0.01 (0.1×0.1), a ninefold reduction. Whereas a threefold reduction would occur if the metabolism only occurred in the liver.

The concurrent administration of grapefruit juice and simvastatin is an example of altered first-pass metabolism primarily within the gut wall (Fig. 7-6). The oral bioavailability of the drug is normally about 0.05 but, when one glass of grapefruit juice is taken once daily for 3 days and concurrently with 40-mg of simvastatin on day 3, its systemic exposure (as reflected by AUC) is increased 3.6-fold. This effect is caused by the presence, within grapefruit juice, of inhibitors of the drug's metabolism.

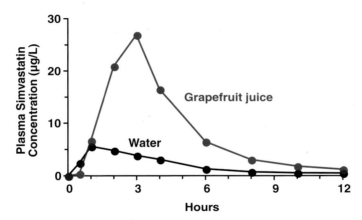

FIGURE 7-6. The mean plasma simvastatin concentration with time after administration of a single 40-mg dose of simvastatin with 200 mL of either water (*black*) or grapefruit juice (*colored*) daily for 3 days. Note the large (3.6-fold) increase in area when grapefruit juice is concurrently given. (From: Lilja JJ, Neuvonen M, Neuvonen PJ. Effects of regular consumption of grapefruit juice on the pharmacokinetics of simvastatin. Br J Clin Pharmacol 2004;58:56–60: Fig. 1.)

The degree of inhibition of simvastatin first-pass intestinal metabolism is a function of how much, as well as when, grapefruit juice is ingested, as illustrated by the data shown in Table 7-4, when "high-dose" grapefruit juice (200 mL of double strength) is given 3 times a day for 3 days. The fall off in the inhibition of the metabolism after discontinuing grapefruit juice is examined by waiting 1, 3, and 7 days before giving the drug. Notice that the high-dose grapefruit ingestion increases the exposure of simvastatin 13.5-fold (compared to 3.6-fold when only one standard glass of grapefruit juice is given daily, see Fig. 7.5). Also note that 24 hr after stopping intake, the increase in AUC is only about 10% of that observed when currently administered, and that the AUC has essentially returned to the control value 1 week later. The therapeutic impact of this interaction is tempered by the fact that several metabolites of simvastatin are also active such that the increase in exposure systemically and within the liver, the site of action, of total active species is less than that observed for simvastatin itself.

| TABLE 7-4 | Mean (±SD) Peak Concentrations (C_{max}) and Total *AUC* after a Single 40-mg Dose of Simvastatin with and without Grapefruit Juice (GFJ)* |

Measure	Control (Water Only)	Concurrent Administration of GFJ	Time After Discontinuing GFJ		
			24 Hr	3 Days	7 Days
Cmax (μg/L)	9.3 ± 4.5 $(100)^{\dagger}$	112 ± 44.8 $(1200)^{\dagger}$	22.0 ± 9.7 $(237)^{\dagger}$	14.2 ± 4.6 $(153)^{\dagger}$	12.4 ± 7.2 $(133)^{\dagger}$
AUC (μg-hr/L)	28.9 ± 14.5 $(100)^{\dagger}$	390 ± 126 $(1350)^{\dagger}$	59.4 ± 27.6 $(206)^{\dagger}$	39.6 ± 11.9 $(137)^{\dagger}$	30.6 ± 15.8 $(106)^{\dagger}$

*The drug was administered with 200 mL water alone (part one of study) or following administration of double strength GFJ 3 times a day, 7:00 a.m., noon, and 8:00 p.m. for 3 days and at 0.5 and 1.5 hr after simvastatin intake (part two of study). In part three, subjects received the GFJ as above, but the dose of simvastatin was withheld for 24 hr, 3 days, or 7 days after discontinuing ingestion of GFJ. (From: Lilja JJ, Kivistö KT, Neuvonen PJ. Duration of effect of grapefruit juice on the pharmacokinetics of the CYP3A4 substrate simvastatin. Clin Pharm Ther 2000;68:384–390.)
†Percent of the control value.

   Some drugs are substrates for both luminal efflux transporters and metabolic enzymes, within the intestinal cells, as shown schematically in Fig. 7-7. Together they reduce the oral bioavailability to a greater extent than if only one of the two processes was involved. Drug examples that appear to include this coupling effect are human immunodeficiency virus 1 (HIV-1) protease inhibitors, indinavir (Crixivan), nelfinavir (Viracept), saquinavir (Invirase), and ritonavir (Norvir); the chemotherapeutic agent, paclitaxel; the cholesterol lowering drug, simvastatin; and the immunosuppressive agent, cyclosporine. The extent to which inhibitors of the enzyme activity and/or the transport system increase systemic availability depends on the contributions of metabolism and transport to first-pass intestinal loss.

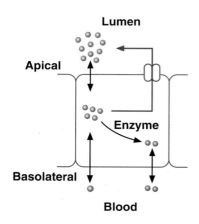

FIGURE 7-7. For some drugs, systemic absorption after oral administration depends on both enzymatic metabolism and efflux transporters (depicted in color) in the intestinal epithelium. The presence of efflux transporters on the apical side in concert with the intracellular metabolism may diminish the movement of drug from the intestinal lumen to blood. Inhibition of either the metabolic activity or the efflux transport leads to an increase in the net movement of unchanged drug into the systemic circulation. Symbols: •, drug; •, metabolite.

   A final note is in order regarding the distribution of drug metabolizing enzymes and transporters along the length of the gastrointestinal tract. Although precise details are currently lacking, it appears that CYP3A has highest activity in the small intestine, and particularly the duodenum, whereas the activity of P-glycoprotein, as previously stated, increases down the intestine, with greatest activity in the large intestine. This could have an impact on the fraction systemically available for some drugs formulated in modified or controlled release products as released drug encounters different absorption environments as it moves down the intestinal tract.

HEPATIC FIRST-PASS PREDICTIONS

As with hepatic clearance itself, we are often interested in predicting the impact of changes in organ blood flow, hepatic intrinsic clearance, or binding within blood on hepatic first-pass extraction of oral drugs. Such predictions can be made using the *well-stirred* model (Chapter 5, *Elimination*) by substituting Eq. 5-15 into the relationship $F_H = 1 - E_H$ (see also Appendix E, *Well-stirred Model of Hepatic Clearance*). That is,

$$F_H = \frac{Q_H}{Q_H + fu_b \cdot CL_{int}}$$ 7-4

It should be re-emphasized that the prediction here, for changes in CL_H, E_H, and F_H with changes in Q_H, CL_{int}, or fu_b, are based on modest alterations. A low extraction ratio drug can become a high extraction ratio drug if CL_{int} or fu_b is increased or if Q_H is decreased by a sufficiently large factor (see Fig. 5-8). The principles here refer to the relative tendencies that modest changes in these factors are likely to produce.

The effect on first-pass extraction can also be visualized by regarding perfusion and protein binding to be in competition with enzymatic activity. An increase in either perfusion ($Q_H \uparrow$) or protein binding ($fu \downarrow$) helps to move drug through the organ, impeding extraction and increasing systemic bioavailability, whereas an increase in enzyme activity ($CL_{int} \uparrow$) more extensively extracts drug from the perfusing blood, decreasing systemic bioavailability.

Consider first the case of a drug with an E_H near zero, that is, Q_H much greater than $fu_b \cdot CL_{int}$. Then F_H is independent of changes in Q_H, CL_{int}, or fu_b. This is not surprising as the extraction is so small that everything presented gets past the liver anyway. Consider next the condition in which $fu_b \cdot CL_{int}$ is much greater than Q_H, so that E_H approaches 1.0. In this case, $F_H = Q_H/(fu_b \cdot CL_{int})$, that is, bioavailability is low and dependent on all three factors. An increase in blood flow increases bioavailability by decreasing the time drug spends in the liver, where elimination occurs. An increase either in enzymatic activity or in fu_b (decreased binding which raises the unbound concentration for a given incoming total concentration) decreases bioavailability by increasing the rate of elimination for a given rate of presentation to the liver.

SATURABLE FIRST-PASS METABOLISM

When absorption is rapid and the first-pass metabolism in the liver is extensive, a common observation is that the extraction ratio, and therefore the bioavailability of the drug, becomes dose dependent; the higher the dose, the greater the bioavailability. Examples of drugs showing this kinetic behavior, called **saturable first-pass metabolism**, are listed in Table 7-5. For several of these drugs, dose dependence in oral bioavailability is observed without an apparent change in elimination half-life. This behavior can be understood by realizing that the concentration of drug reaching the liver during

TABLE 7-5	Examples of Drugs Showing Saturable First-pass Metabolism in the Liver or Gut Wall after Oral Administration of Therapeutic Doses		
Drug	**Indication**	**Drug**	**Indication**
Alprenolol	Hypertension, angina, and cardiac arrhythmia	Niacin	Hyperlipidemia
Atorvastatin	Hyperlipidemia	Nicardipine	Hypertension
Darifenacin	Overactive bladder	Omeprazole	Duodenal ulcers
5-Fluorouracil	Certain cancers	Propafenone	Atrial fibrillation
Fluvastatin	Hyperlipidemia	Propranolol	Hypertension
Hydralazine	Hypertension	Rivastigmine	Alzheimer disease
Isosorbide dinitrate	Angina	Verapamil	Angina and cardiac arrhythmias
Ketoconazole	Select fungal infections	Voriconazole	Select fungal infections

absorption can be much higher than that after absorption is over and especially in the terminal phase of decline where the half-life is measured. Consider, for example, the following conditions: Distribution is instantaneous; all of the administered drug reaches the liver intact; input of drug from the gastrointestinal tract is first-order with a ka of $0.05\ \text{min}^{-1}$ (14-min half-life); oral bioavailability at low doses is 0.1; volume of distribution (blood) is 250 L; total hepatic blood flow, Q_H, is 1.35 mL/min; and absorption is faster than elimination.

The initial rate of input into the portal vein, $ka \cdot Dose$, is also the initial rate of entry of drug into the liver which, on dividing by hepatic blood flow, Q_H, gives the concentration in the arterial blood, $C_{b,initial}$, entering the liver. Consequently, after a 100-mg dose,

$$C_{b,initial} = \frac{ka \cdot Dose}{Q_H} = 3.7\ mg/L \qquad\qquad 7\text{-}5$$

The concentration in the blood entering the liver after absorption is finished, $C_{b,max}$, would have a maximum value of

$$C_{b,max} = \frac{F \cdot Dose}{V_b} = 0.04\ mg/L \qquad\qquad 7\text{-}6$$

The actual $C_{b,max}$ should be less than this value because some of the systemically absorbed drug is eliminated by the time the peak is reached. As can be seen, the concentration entering the liver during the early stages of absorption is much greater than that recycled from the rest of the body, even at the peak. Indeed, the ratio of $C_{b,initial}$ to $C_{b,max}$ in this example is

$$\frac{C_{b,initial}}{C_{b,max}} = \frac{ka \cdot V_b}{F \cdot Q_H} = 92 \qquad\qquad 7\text{-}7$$

The ratio is even larger if one compares the initial concentration entering the liver to the concentration in the decline phase. Thus, the larger the value of ka or V or the smaller the value of F at low (nonsaturating) doses, the greater is the ratio $C_{b,initial}/C_{b,max}$ and more likely there is to be a separation in the degree of saturation of metabolism during absorption and elimination phases. All the drugs listed in Table 7-5 show saturable first-pass metabolism and have pharmacokinetic parameters that favor a high value of $C_{b,initial}/C_{b,max}$. Some, like voriconazole, also show dose-dependent elimination at therapeutic concentrations, a subject further explored in Chapter 16, *Nonlinearities*.

ABSORPTION FROM INTRAMUSCULAR AND SUBCUTANEOUS SITES

In contrast to the gastrointestinal tract, absorption of most drugs in solution from muscle and subcutaneous (s.c.) tissue is perfusion rate–limited. For example, consider the data in Table 7-6 for the local anesthetic lidocaine. Shown are the peak plasma concentrations observed when the same dose of lidocaine is administered parenterally at different sites of the body. Recall from Fig. 6-5 (Chapter 6, *Kinetics Following an Extravascular Dose*), for a given dose, the higher the peak concentration, the faster drug absorption. Large differences in speed of absorption of lidocaine are clearly evident, the speed increasing from s.c. tissue to intercostal muscle, in line with an increasing tissue perfusion rate. The greater the speed of absorption, the more rapidly the exposure at the local site decreases, and consequently, the shorter is the duration of the local anesthetic effect.

The speed of systemic absorption after s.c. administration can be increased by rubbing the area of the injection. Similarly, absorption is faster after i.m. administration during exercise. Increased blood flow to the surrounding tissues is a likely explanation for the increased speed of systemic absorption.

The dependence of rapidity of absorption on local blood flow is taken advantage of when lidocaine is used as a local anesthetic. The addition of epinephrine, a vasoconstrictive

TABLE 7-6	Influence of Site of Injection on the Peak Venous Lidocaine Concentration following Injection of a 100-mg Dose

Injection Site	Peak Plasma Lidocaine Concentration (mg/L)	Perfusion Rate
Intercostal	1.46	↑
Paracervical	1.20	
Caudal	1.18	
Lumbar epidural	0.97	
Brachial plexus	0.53	
Subarachnoid	0.44	
Subcutaneous	0.35	

From: Covino, BG. Pharmacokinetics of local anaesthetic drug. In: Prys-Roberts C and Hug CC, eds. Pharmacokinetics of Anaesthesia. Oxford: Blackwell Scientific Publications, 1984: 270–292.

agent, reduces the blood flow and prolongs the local anesthetic effect. When a drug is administered intramuscularly or subcutaneously and systemic action is desired, reduced local perfusion, and hence drug absorption, may not be an advantage. In extreme cases, such as hemorrhagic shock, perfusion of muscle tissue is drastically reduced. It is therefore appropriate to limit administration of drugs by this route in this condition. Moreover, there is the danger of the absorption of the drug later, perhaps when it is not needed, if the hemorrhagic shock is effectively treated and normal perfusion of muscle tissue is restored.

This dependence of absorption on perfusion may be explained by the nature of the barrier (capillary membrane) between the site of injection (interstitial fluid) and blood. This membrane, generally a much more loosely knit structure than the epithelial lining of the gastrointestinal tract (see Chapter 4, *Membranes and Distribution*), offers little impedance to the movement of drugs into blood, even for polar ionized drugs. For example, vancomycin, a water-soluble, ionized, polar base with an MW of about 1449 g/mol is poorly absorbed when given orally because it has great difficulty penetrating the gastrointestinal mucosa. It also does not pass the blood-brain barrier, nor is it reabsorbed in the renal tubule. However, it is rapidly and completely absorbed systemically from an i.m. site. This low impedance by the capillary membrane in muscle and s.c. tissue applies to all drugs, independent of charge, degree of ionization, and molecular size up to approximately 5000 g/mol. Systemic absorption of macromolecular drugs from i.m. and s.c. sites is examined in Chapter 21, *Protein Drugs.*

ABSORPTION FROM SOLID DOSAGE FORMS

When a drug is taken orally in a solid dosage form (e.g., tablets or capsules), a number of processes must occur before it can be systemically available. The dosage form must disintegrate, deaggregate, and the drug must dissolve, as shown in Fig. 7-8. Dissolution is a key factor, but not the only one. Table 7-7 summarizes factors that determine the release (or dissolution) of a drug from a solid dosage form and the rate and extent of systemic absorption after an oral dose. The factors are classified into four groups, namely release characteristics of the dosage form, physicochemical properties of drug, physiology of gastrointestinal tract, and presence of gastrointestinal tract abnormalities and diseases.

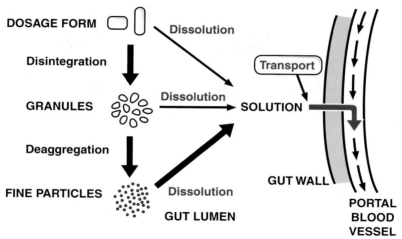

FIGURE 7-8. Following oral administration of a typical immediate-release solid dosage form, tablet or capsule, the product undergoes disintegration to granules. These granules further deaggregate to fine particles. Dissolution of drug occurs at all stages, but usually becomes predominant from the fine particles (see thickness of arrows). The drug, now in solution, must cross the membranes of the gastrointestinal tract to reach the mesenteric blood vessels, which carry the drug via the portal vein and liver to the systemic circulation.

TABLE 7-7	Factors Determining the Release and Absorption Kinetics of a Drug following Oral Administration of a Solid Dosage Form

Release Characteristics of Dosage Form

    Disintegration/Deaggregation

    Dissolution of drug from granules (also dependent on inactive ingredients and formulation variables)

Physicochemical Properties of Drug

    Ionization (acid/base)

    Partition coefficient (octanol/water)

    Solubility in water

Physiology of Gastrointestinal Tract

    Colonic retention

    Gastric emptying

    Intestinal motility

    Perfusion of the gastrointestinal tract

    Permeability of gut wall

Gastrointestinal Tract Abnormalities and Diseases

    Crohn's disease

    Gastric resection (e.g., in obesity)

    Diarrhea

DISSOLUTION

The reason why dissolution is so important may be gained by realizing that absorption following a solid requires drug dissolution.

$$\text{Drug in Product} \xrightarrow{\textit{Dissolution}} \text{Drug in solution} \xrightarrow{\textit{Absorption}} \text{Absorbed drug}$$

Two situations are now considered. The first, less common, depicted in Fig. 7-9A, is one in which dissolution is a much faster process than is absorption. Consequently, most of the drug is dissolved before an appreciable fraction is absorbed. Here, commonly, permeability rather than dissolution rate-limits absorption. An example is the gastrointestinal absorption of sucralfate, an agent used in treating gastric and intestinal ulcers, when given as a tablet. This polar drug dissolves rapidly from the tablet, but has difficulty penetrating the gastrointestinal epithelium. So, little drug is absorbed. The systemic input is **absorption rate–limited** because of poor permeability. Differences in rates of dissolution of sucralfate from different tablet formations have relatively little or no effect on the speed of systemic absorption of this drug.

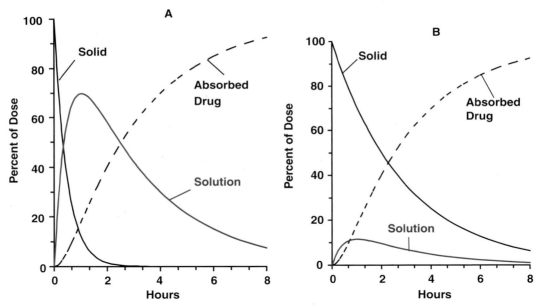

FIGURE 7-9. When absorption is permeability rate–limited **(A)**, most of the drug has dissolved (*colored line*) in the gastrointestinal tract before an appreciable fraction has been absorbed. In contrast, when dissolution rate-limits absorption **(B)**, very little drug is in solution (*colored line*) at the absorption site at any time; drug is absorbed almost as soon as it dissolves. Notice that the majority of drug yet to be absorbed is always found at the rate-limiting step: in solution in *Case A* and as solid in *Case B*.

In the second, and more common, situation shown in Fig. 7-9B, dissolution proceeds relatively slowly, and any dissolved drug readily traverses the gastrointestinal epithelium. Absorption cannot proceed any faster, however, than the rate at which the drug dissolves. That is, absorption is **dissolution rate–limited**. In this case, changes in dissolution profoundly affect the rate, and sometimes the extent, of drug absorption. Evidence supporting dissolution rate–limited absorption comes from the noticeably slower systemic absorption of most drugs from solid dosage forms than from a simple aqueous solution after oral administration. It also comes from modified-release dosage forms in which release, and therefore absorption, is intentionally prolonged.

GASTRIC EMPTYING AND INTESTINAL TRANSIT

Before discussing the role of gastric emptying on absorption of drugs given as solids, consider the information provided in Fig. 7-10. Shown are the mean transit times in the stomach and small intestine of small nondisintegrating pellets (diameters between 0.3 and 1.8 mm) and of large single nondisintegrating units (either capsules, 25 mm by 9 mm, or tablets, 8 to 12 mm in diameter).

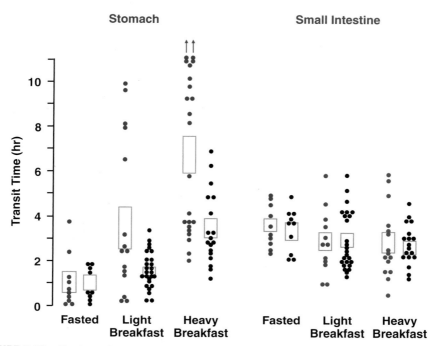

FIGURE 7-10. Food, particularly a heavy meal, increases the gastric transit time of small pellets (*black circles*) and, even more markedly, of large single pellets (*colored circles*). In contrast, neither the food nor the physical size of the solid affects the small intestine transit time. The data (individual points, black or colored circles, and their mean ± S.E., indicated by the rectangles) were obtained in healthy young adults using drug-free nondisintegrating materials. The points with an arrow indicate that the solid was still in the stomach at the time of the last observation, 16 hr. (From: Davis SS, Hardy JG, Fara JW. Transit of pharmaceutical dosage forms through the small intestine. Gut, 1986;27:886–892.)

Gastric Emptying. During fasting, gastric emptying of both small and large solids is seen, on average, to be rapid, with a mean time of around 1 hr, although there is considerable interindividual variability. Gastric emptying of drugs in solution is even faster with a mean time of 10 to 20 min. In the fasting state, the stomach displays a complex temporal pattern of motor activity with alternating periods of quiescence and moderate contraction of varying frequency, the "house-keeping wave," which moves material into the small intestine. The exact ejection time of a solid particle therefore depends on its size, when it is ingested during the motor activity cycle, and where it is located within the stomach. The likelihood of ejection is greatest when the solid particle is in close proximity to the pyloric sphincter when the house-keeping wave occurs. Thus, even for small solid particles, gastric emptying can vary from minutes to several hours in fasting conditions.

The situation is very different after eating. As shown in Fig. 7-10, when taken on a fed stomach, the gastric transit time of solids is increased. This increase is greater after a heavy meal than a light one and is much greater for a large single unit than for small pellets. For example, the mean gastric transit time among subjects for large single unit systems is now almost 7 hr, with some pellets still in the stomach in some subjects 11 hr after ingestion. These observations are explained by the sieving action of a fed stomach. Solids with diameters greater than 7 to 10 mm pass into the small intestine more slowly and less predictably than those of smaller diameter. Some individuals consistently show prolonged gastric emptying of large pellets in the fed state, while for others it is much less apparent. These differences have largely been ascribed to interindividual differences in the size of the pyloric sphincter. This retention of large pellets is generally consistent with the physiologic role of the stomach (i.e., to retain larger food particles until they are reduced in size to facilitate further digestion). With conventional tablets, rapid disintegration and deaggregation into fine particles achieves the same objective. As long as the stomach remains in a fed state, the conditions above prevail. For those persons who eat three hearty meals a day with several snacks in between, gastric emptying of large pellets may be slowed most of the waking hours of the day.

In contrast to events in the stomach, the transit time of solids within the small intestine varies little among subjects, appears to be independent of either the size of a solid or the presence of food in the stomach, and is remarkably short, approximately 3 hr (Fig. 7-10), a time similar to that found for the transit of liquids. Both solids and liquids appear to move down the small intestine as a plug with relatively little mixing. As the mouth-to-anus transit time is typically 1 to 3 days, these data on gastric and small intestinal transit times indicate that, for the majority of this time, unabsorbed materials are either in the large bowel or rectum. Given the previously mentioned physiologic information, the possible role of gastric emptying and intestinal transit on the absorption of drugs given in solid dosage forms can be understood. Consider the following situations.

Rapid Dissolution in Stomach. This is the common situation seen with many permeable and soluble drugs, such as ibuprofen and acetaminophen (see Fig. 7-1), in conventional immediate-release tablets and capsules. Drug dissolves so rapidly in the stomach that most of it is in solution before much of the drug has entered the small intestine. Here, gastric emptying clearly influences the rate of drug absorption, but only to the extent that liquids and deaggregated particles are retained within the stomach. Thus, hastening gastric emptying quickens drug absorption in virtually all circumstances.

Rapid Dissolution in Intestine. Sometimes, drug does not materially dissolve within the stomach, whereas in the intestine it rapidly both dissolves and moves across the intestinal wall. Gastric emptying then also affects the speed of drug absorption. An enteric-coated product is an extreme example of this situation. Proton pump inhibitors, such as omeprazole, lansoprazole, and pantoprazole, and didanosine, an antiviral agent, are examples of drugs that are rapidly hydrolyzed to inactive products in the acidic environment of the stomach. Aspirin, sulfasalazine, used to treat ulcerative colitis, and bisacodyl, a laxative, are gastric irritants. A solution to both types of problems has been to coat these drug products with a material resistant to the acidic environment of the stomach but which breaks down in the intestinal fluids. If such enteric-coated products are large single tablets, the time for an intact tablet to pass from the stomach into the intestine varies unpredictably from 20 min to several hours when taken on an empty stomach, and up to 12 hr, or even more, when taken on a fed stomach (see Fig. 7-10). Accordingly, such enteric-coated products cannot be used when rapid and reliable absorption is required. A product composed of enteric-coated small granules is an improvement because the rate of delivery of the granules to the intestine is more reliable, being less dependent on a single event, a house-keeping wave, and food intake.

Poor Dissolution. Some drugs, such as the oral antifungal broad-spectrum anthelmintic, albendazole, are sparingly soluble or almost insoluble in both gastric and intestinal fluids. When these drugs are administered as a solid, there may already be insufficient time for complete dissolution and absorption. With a fixed short time within the small intestine, slow release from the stomach increases the time for drug to dissolve before entering the intestine, thereby favoring increased bioavailability. As mentioned, food, and fat in particular, delays gastric emptying. This delay may be one of the explanations for the observed fivefold increase in the plasma concentration of albendazole sulfoxide, its primary metabolite, when parent drug is taken with a fatty meal. Subsequently, intestinal fluid and contents move into the large intestine and water is reabsorbed. The resulting compaction of the solid contents may severely limit further dissolution and hence absorption of such drugs.

BIOPHARMACEUTICS CLASSIFICATION SYSTEM

A major advance in anticipating oral bioavailability and bioequivalence problem drug products was made in the last decade by the establishment of the biopharmaceutics classification system (BCS). The system is based on the water solubility of the drug and its ability to pass across membranes, permeability, and applies to immediate-release products (85% dissolved within 15 min in a standardized dissolution test). Those drugs for which the drug content of the dosage form of the highest strength can dissolve in 250 mL of water throughout the pH range of 1 to 7.5 are said to be highly soluble drugs. Those showing complete intestinal absorption (see Fig. 7-3) or rapid movement through epithelial membranes in vitro are said to be highly permeable. With these two criteria, there are four classes of drugs, as listed in Table 7-8. Those drugs in class I, highly soluble and highly permeable, examples listed in Table 7-9, are unlikely to show a bioavailability/bioequivalence problem

TABLE 7-8	Biopharmaceutics Classification System	
	Intestinal Permeability*	
Solubility†	**High**	**Low**
High	Class I	Class II
Low	Class III	Class IV

*Intestinal absorption is complete or compound is shown to be highly permeable in vivo or in vitro.
†Highest available strength is soluble in 250 mL of water throughout pH range 1–7.5.

TABLE 7-9	Examples of Drugs in Class I of the Biopharmaceutics Classification System			
Abacavir	Chlorpheniramine	Ergonovine	Lidocaine	Prednisolone
Acetaminophen	Cyclophosphamide	Ethambutol	Lomefloxacin	Primaquine
Acyclovir	Desipramine	Ethinyl estradiol	Meperidine	Promazine
Amiloride	Diazepam	Fluoxetine	Metoprolol	Propranolol
Amitriptyline	Diltiazem	Imipramine	Metronidazole	Quinidine
Atropine	Diphenhydramine	Ketorolac	Midazolam	Rosiglitazone
Buspirone	Disopyramide	Ketoprofen	Minocycline	Theophylline
Caffeine	Doxepin	Labetalol	Misoprostol	Valproic acid
Captopril	Doxycycline	Levodopa	Nifedipine	Verapamil
Chloroquine	Enalapril	Levofloxacin	Phenobarbital	Zidovudine

From: Wu CY, Benet LZ. Predicting drug disposition via application of BCS: transport/absorption/elimination interplay and development of a biopharmaceutics drug disposition classification system. Pharm Res 2005;22:11–23.

when administered in immediate-release products. Studies in vivo are then felt to be unnecessary as standard dissolution tests can supply adequate information to assure product performance in vivo. For such drug products, biowaivers can be obtained so that full bioavailability/bioequivalence studies in vivo are considered unnecessary. Drugs in Class II, poorly soluble and highly impermeable, and Class III, highly soluble and poorly permeable, may show formulation-dependent differences in their bioavailability/bioequivalence and are therefore not eligible for a biowaiver. Compounds in Class IV (relatively insoluble and impermeable) are particular problems.

Why class I drugs in immediate-release dosage forms are not expected to show bioavailability/bioequivalence problems stems from the belief that drug in these products should rapidly go into solution in the stomach, especially when taken with a glass of water (250 mL). Formulation differences should therefore not impact their intestinal absorption, provided that the products meet appropriate specifications for dissolution in vitro.

An additional benefit of the BCS stems from the observation that small MW drugs in Class I (high solubility, high permeability) tend to be orally absorbed, distributed to the tissues (except, perhaps, in the brain where permeability is very low), and eliminated from the body with little influence by transporters. This does not mean that they are not substrates for transporters, but rather that the rates of facilitated transport by these processes are slower than their passive transport across membranes.

MODIFIED-RELEASE PRODUCTS

The conclusions drawn above for soluble, relatively permeable drugs (BCS Class I) may be particularly pertinent to certain modified-release dosage forms. Some of these products are coated with, or contained within, a nondisintegrating material through which the release rate of drug is independent of both pH and agitation. In such cases, the time of gastric emptying of the dosage form has little effect on the rate of drug absorption. Even though the solid dosage form may be retained in the stomach, the released drug is continuously emptied with the gastric fluid into the duodenum and is available for absorption from the small intestine. Any delay in the gastric emptying of such products, therefore, prolongs the total period for drug release and absorption. For reasons discussed above, this delay is most likely to be seen with large single units taken on a fed stomach. It would be unwise, however, to depend too much on this delay to achieve a prolonged absorption profile given the well-known unpredictability of patients' eating habits and their general lack of compliance in the time of their taking their medications. Furthermore, some concern must exist that compaction in the large intestine may preclude reliable release, and hence input, of drug beyond 12 to 16 hr. This would severely limit the design of controlled-release dosage forms of drugs with short half-lives intended for once-a-day administration. That said, data for some drug-delivery systems indicate that relatively reliable and sustainable absorption for up to 24 hr can be achieved. For drugs in other BCS classes, the properties of the drug can become rate-limiting.

Changing Rate Control. The rate of absorption is controlled by a delivery device as long as release from the device is the rate-limiting step in the absorption process. With the $P \cdot SA$ term for drugs decreasing along the length of the intestinal tract, the rate limitation could change from the device to the intestinal membrane (particularly for BCS class III compounds, i.e., those with high solubility, low permeability) as the device moves down the intestine (Fig. 7-11). In the small intestine, $P \cdot SA$ is at its highest and control may then lie with the delivery device. However, on movement into the colon, $P \cdot SA$ may drop enough so that the rate-limiting step becomes passage across the wall, in which case, control of drug input is lost. This situation is more likely to occur with relatively polar molecules, such as cimetidine and ranitidine, for which permeability may be a problem. Even with rapid-release dosage forms, absorption of these compounds is essentially restricted to the small intestine (e.g., see Fig. 7-2), even if only a portion of the dose is absorbed there.

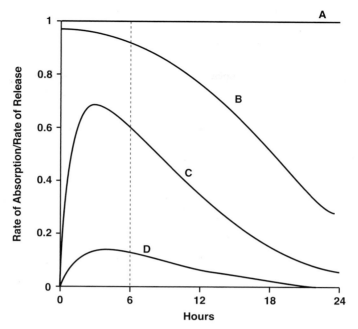

FIGURE 7-11. The rate of absorption relative to the rate of constant release from an oral 24-hr sustained-release delivery device varies with time when movement across the membranes of the gastrointestinal tract, rather than release, becomes rate limiting. The change in rate control from release to membrane occurs for a drug with low membrane permeability. The rate control imposed by permeability is more apparent in the colon (6 hr is shown as the time for the device to leave the stomach and transit the small intestine, *dashed vertical line*), where permeability is much lower than that in the small intestine. The simulations are conducted with the model

$$\frac{dA_R}{dt} \qquad = \qquad R \qquad - \qquad \frac{P \cdot SA}{Va} \cdot e^{-bt} \cdot A_R$$

Net rate of change of $\qquad$ Rate of $\qquad$ Rate of
released drug in lumen $\qquad$ release $\qquad$ absorption

where A_R is amount of released drug residing in the gastrointestinal tract, Va is the volume of luminal fluid into which the released drug is distributed, and b is the rate constant for the decrease in $P \cdot SA/Va$ with time. As the actual changes in P, SA, and Va with time are unknown, an exponential (half-life of 3 hr) decline in the composite is used. The following conditions are simulated: **A.** $P \cdot SA/Va$ is sufficiently high (approaches ∞) to ensure that the rate-controlling step is always in the device with rate of absorption matching rate of release. **B.** $P \cdot SA/Va$ is 10 hr^{-1}, a value for which drug is absorbed virtually as quickly as it is released while in the proximal small intestine but not so further down the gastrointestinal tract where rate control by the device is lost. **C.** $P \cdot SA/Va$ is 1 hr^{-1}. The rate of absorption never matches the rate of release. The product fails to control absorption. **D.** $P \cdot SA/Va = 0.1$ hr^{-1}. Rate control lies almost entirely with the membranes of the gastrointestinal tract at all times. In *Cases B to D*, drug accumulates in the lumen of the intestines. The area under each curve relative to the area under the release curve (curve A) is the fraction of released drug that is absorbed.

Currently, however, it is difficult to make any quantitative prediction of those drugs for which controlled drug delivery can be achieved beyond the small intestine. But clearly, whenever release of drug beyond the stomach continues for 4 hr or more, some of the drug is likely to be released in the large intestine (see Fig. 7-11). More needs to be known about the relationship between the physicochemical properties of a molecule and intestinal permeability. Ultimately, all oral drug delivery systems need to be evaluated in vivo.

Precipitation and Redissolution. Absorption is normally complete within 1 or 2 hr of i.m. or s.c. administration of an aqueous solution of a drug. There are exceptions, as seen with protein drugs (Chapter 21, *Protein Drugs*) and also when injecting a solution of a salt of either a sparingly soluble acid or a base. For example, although, chlordiazepoxide hydrochloride, in solution, is eventually completely absorbed, absorption is slow from the i.m. site. However, large doses sometimes appear to be poorly effective or ineffective. Indeed, absorption is even slower than from the gastrointestinal tract when capsules of chlordiazepoxide hydrochloride are administered (Fig. 7-12). The explanation involves consideration of pH, solubility, perfusion, and stirring.

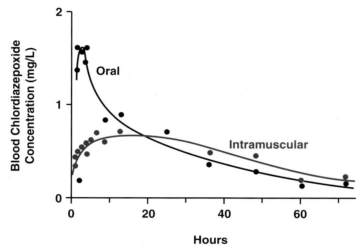

FIGURE 7-12. A delayed and lower peak blood concentration of chlordiazepoxide, when given intramuscularly (●), as compared to when given orally (●), indicates slower absorption from the i.m. than the oral site. On both occasions, 50 mg of chlordiazepoxide hydrochloride were administered. (From: Greenblatt DJ, Shader RI, Koch-Weser J. Slow absorption of intramuscular chlordiazepoxide. N Engl J Med 1974;291:1116–1118.)

In the study referenced in Fig. 7-12, the same dose, 50 mg of chlordiazepoxide hydrochloride, was administered by both routes. The i.m. dose was dissolved in 1 mL of an aqueous vehicle. Chlordiazepoxide is sparingly soluble; its aqueous solubility is approximately 2 mg/mL. To achieve this high concentration of 50 mg of chlordiazepoxide hydrochloride/mL, the vehicle contains 20% propylene glycol and 4% polysorbate 80, both water-miscible materials that permit a greater solubility of the drug. Being the salt of a strong acid and a weak base (pKa 4.5), the final pH is low, approximately 3.0. Upon injection, the buffer capacity of both the tissue and the blood, perfusing it gradually, restores the pH at the injection site to 7.4. This rise in pH and the absorption of the injected water and water-miscible materials cause chlordiazepoxide base to precipitate out of solution. As movement and hence spreading is minimal, a large mass of drug is deposited around the injection site. The rate of absorption now becomes limited by dissolution of the precipitated drug. However, the small surface area, low solubility, limited perfusion, and minimal stirring tend to keep the rate of dissolution down. The result is protracted absorption over many hours or even days. In contrast, absorption following oral administration is relatively rapid. For reasons already discussed, a greater degree of agitation, a larger volume of fluid at the site, and a higher rate of blood flow to the gastrointestinal tract all promote more rapid dissolution and absorption following oral ingestion of chlordiazepoxide hydrochloride. Another example is diazepam, a drug that is sparingly soluble and slowly absorbed when injected intramuscularly. This essentially neutral drug is kept in solution with the aid of propylene glycol. Precipitation at the injection site occurs with dilution and absorption of this water-miscible solvent.

ABSORPTION FROM OTHER SITES

Drugs may be administered at virtually any site on or within the body. In recent years there has been considerable interest in exploiting some of the less conventional sites, such as the lung, nasal cavity, and buccal cavity as a means of delivering drugs both locally and systemically. Polypeptide and protein drugs have received particular attention (see Chapter 21, *Protein Drugs*). Transdermal application has become popular for systemic delivery of small, generally lipophilic, potent molecules that require low input rates to achieve effective therapy.

Inhalation, usually used for treatment of pulmonary diseases, is another route that has received considerable attention. For example, an insulin inhalation product was placed on the market in 2006, but withdrawn in 2007 due to antibody formation. The product had promise as the bioavailability was about 10% of that obtained by rapid-release s.c. injection. It is very difficult to give insulin, or other polypeptide drugs, orally because of its degradation by digestive enzymes in the gastrointestinal tract and because of its being highly impermeable.

The intranasal route is also being used for some protein drugs that cannot readily be administered orally, but that are systemically active (e.g., desmopressin [DDAVP]) used to treat primary nocturnal enuresis. Examples of small MW drugs given by this route are sumatriptan, used to treat migraine attacks, and zanamivir (Relenza), used in treating influenza A and B.

INTEGRATION OF KINETIC AND PHYSIOLOGIC CONCEPTS

Numerous situations exist in which the concentration–time profile after a single extravascular dose may be changed. It may be a result of an alteration in the speed or extent of absorption, or in any pharmacokinetic disposition parameter. The physiologic variables affecting drug disposition are discussed in Chapter 5, *Elimination*. In this exercise, these previously presented concepts are integrated with those affecting drug absorption to predict and evaluate a concentration–time profile after a single extravascular dose. To this end, the dependence of primary pharmacokinetic parameter values on physiologic variables that affect both drug absorption and disposition are summarized in Table 7-10 and six specific conditions are presented and discussed.

TABLE 7-10	**Examples of Physiologic Variables on which Primary Pharmacokinetic Parameters Depend**
Primary Pharmacokinetic Parameter	**Physiologic Variable**
Absorption rate constant	Blood flow at absorption site, rubbing, exercise (i.m. and s.c. administration), gastric emptying, transporters, intestinal motility (oral administration)
Bioavailability	Gastric emptying rate, gastric acid secretion, biliary excretion of hydrolytic enzymes, intestinal motility, extraction in the gut wall and liver, transporters
Hepatic clearance; bioavailability*	Hepatic blood flow, binding in blood, intrinsic hepatocellular activity, enterohepatic cycling
Renal clearance	Renal blood flow, binding in blood, active secretion, active reabsorption, urine pH, urine flow, glomerular filtration rate
Volume of distribution	Binding in blood, transporters, binding in tissues, partitioning into fat, body composition, body size

*Hepatic elimination is assumed to be the only cause of a decrease in oral bioavailability.

CHANGE IN THE SPEED OF ABSORPTION

A change in the speed of absorption can occur when the dosage form is changed, for example, from an immediate-release to a modified-release dosage form. Another situation is when a product is given with food. A change can also be produced by a change in blood flow following s.c. or i.m. administration (e.g., produced by rubbing, by exercise, or by using a different anatomical site for the injection).

Figure 7-13 shows the plasma concentration of growth hormone with time following its s.c. administration at two different sites, abdomen and thigh. Clearly the speed of the hormone's systemic absorption is different from these two sites. Absorption is faster from the abdominal site, as reflected by the higher peak concentration and its earlier occurrence. The slower terminal decline after the injection in the thigh (half-life ~5 hr) indicates that the terminal decline is absorption rate–limited. In actuality, absorption is rate limiting from both sites as the half-life of growth hormone after an i.v. bolus is only 25 min. No data were obtained beyond 12 hr, but if each curve continues to decline with the same half-life, the total areas under the curves would be about the same, indicating that the systemic bioavailability of the drug following administration at both sites is similar.

FIGURE 7-13.   Serum growth hormone concentration–time profile following s.c. administration into the abdomen (*colored*) and thigh (*black*). The speed of the systemic absorption of the hormone is more rapid from the abdominal site (higher and earlier peak), but the amount absorbed (reflected by the total area) may be the same. (From: Beshyah SA, Anyaoku V, Niththyananthan R, et al. The effect of subcutaneous injection site on absorption of human growth hormone: abdomen versus thigh. Clin Endocrinol 1991;35:409–412).

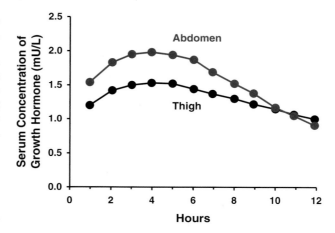

CHANGE IN EXTENT OF ABSORPTION

As previously shown in this chapter, a change in the extent of absorption (F) alone should affect the peak concentration, but not the peak time. In most situations, both F and ka are changed. As an example of the usual situation, consider the data shown in Fig. 7-14 for the oral administration of buspirone taken alone and after grapefruit juice. Notice that C_{max} and AUC are increased during the concurrent administration of grapefruit juice. Buspirone is extensively metabolized in the gut wall and has a low oral bioavailability (0.04). In the presence of grapefruit juice, the gut wall metabolism is inhibited, resulting in a greater fraction of the ingested dose reaching the systemic circulation. There is also an increase in the peak time, which is usually brought about by a slowing of the absorption process. One proposal for this latter observation is a slowing of gastric emptying by the grapefruit juice. Changes in drug disposition are now explored.

CHANGE IN DRUG DISPOSITION

There are many disposition mechanisms responsible for a change in the concentration–time profile. Principles for evaluating and predicting such profiles after an i.v. dose are presented in Chapter 3, *Kinetics Following an Intravenous Bolus Dose*, and Chapter 5, *Elimination*. We will now consider the application of these principles for a single extravascular dose. A key concept for drugs given orally is that elimination and systemic absorp-

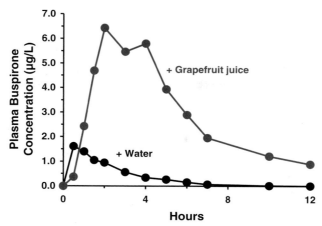

FIGURE 7-14. The ingestion of grapefruit juice alters the systemic exposure to buspirone, a psychotropic drug with anxiolytic properties. Volunteers were given 200 mL of water or 200 mL of double-strength grapefruit juice for 3 days at 7:00 a.m., noon, and 8:00 p.m. and on the day of study at 0, 0.5, and 1.5 hr after oral ingestion of 10 mg of the drug. The *black circles* show the average concentration–time profile when given with water alone; the *colored circles* show the average concentrations when grapefruit juice is given. Components in grapefruit juice inhibit buspirone metabolism; virtually its only route of elimination. (From: Lilja JJ, Kivistö KT, Backman JT, et al. Grapefruit substantially increases plasma concentration of buspirone. Clin Pharmacol Ther 1998;64:655–660.)

tion are linked by first-pass events. A drug that is highly extracted in the gut wall or the liver (high-clearance drug) may then show a change in the extent of systemic absorption when intrinsic clearance, blood flow, or protein binding is altered. To demonstrate the difference in the observations for low and high extraction ratio drugs, let us examine the consequence of coadministration of an inducer of drug metabolism.

Induction, Low Extraction Ratio. Induction of metabolism gives rise to an increase in intrinsic clearance. The manifestation of this condition on the concentration–time profile for a low extraction ratio drug is a decrease in AUC, C_{max}, t_{max}, and half-life and no change in the bioavailability. An example of this is shown by the drug interaction between warfarin and the antitubercular agent, rifampin (Fig. 7-15). Warfarin is predominantly metabolized in the liver; little is excreted in urine unchanged. It is also completely and rapidly absorbed when given orally.

The data in Fig. 7-15 support warfarin having a low hepatic extraction ratio. This conclusion is based on a rough calculation of clearance. Thus, during the control phase clearance, obtained by dividing dose (1.5 mg/kg) by AUC, is 0.0011 L/hr per kg. The plasma/blood concentration ratio is 1.67, so that the corresponding blood clearance is 0.0018 L/hr per kg. This value is low compared to the hepatic blood flow of 81 L/hr per 70 kg or 1.2 L/hr per kg. In the presence of rifampicin, the AUC of warfarin is decreased compared to that of the control value, reflecting a higher clearance. This observation is consistent with induction of hepatic enzymes; the clearance of a drug of low hepatic extraction ratio is expected to be sensitive to changes in hepatocellular enzymatic activity. The data suggest no effect of rifampicin on warfarin distribution. The estimated volumes of distribution, obtained from CL/k, are 0.079 and 0.068 L/kg during the control and rifampicin phases, respectively. These values are probably not significantly different.

The therapeutic consequence of induction can be appreciated from the difference in the response–time curves, shown in the bottom graph of Fig. 7-15. Response here is defined as the elevation in prothrombin time above a baseline value of 14 sec. The overall response, given by the area under the response–time curve after the single oral

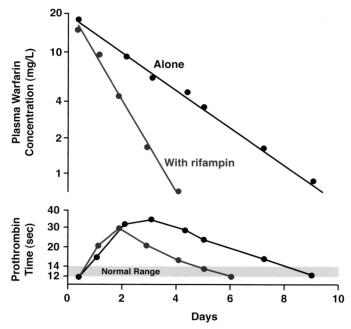

FIGURE 7-15. The half-life of warfarin, a drug with a low extraction ratio, is shortened and clearance is increased when it is given as a single dose (1.5 mg/kg) before (*black*) and while (*color*) the inducer, rifampin, is being administered as a 600-mg dose daily for 3 days prior to warfarin administration. The peak and duration of the elevation in the prothrombin time (response) are decreased when rifampin is coadministered (*lower graph*). (From: O'Reilly RA. Interaction of sodium warfarin and rifampin. Ann Intern Med 1974;81:337–340, with permission.)

dose, is substantially reduced in the presence of rifampin. Consequently, one would expect that the dosage of warfarin must be increased in the presence of rifampin to maintain the same prothrombin time. The reason for the apparently poor correlation between response and plasma warfarin concentration during the first 48 hr after warfarin administration when response is increasing and concentration is falling, lies in its pharmacodynamics, an aspect discussed further in Chapter 8, *Response Following a Single Dose.*

Induction, High Extraction Ratio. Induction always increases intrinsic clearance and hence the extraction ratio and clearance. However, when a drug has a high hepatic extraction ratio, its clearance does not change much (blood flow limited), but the bioavailability $(1 - E_H)$ decreases. Hepatocellular activity and blood flow are competing processes and, with an increase in the former, less drug escapes the liver. This gives rise to a decrease in AUC and C_{max}, but little or no change in the peak time or the half-life, as there is little or no change in either ka or k. The elimination rate constant, k, does not change appreciably because neither CL nor V is changed. Recall from Chapter 6 (Fig. 6-12) that the peak time depends on the values of both k and ka.

The drug interaction observed following the concurrent administration of pentobarbital, an inducer, and alprenolol is an example of this condition (Fig. 7-16). Recall from Chapter 5, *Elimination* (see Fig. 5-19), that the concentration profiles were the same after i.v. administration, but from Fig. 7-16, it is evident that when given orally pentobarbital produces a severalfold decrease in AUC of alprenolol without a change in half-life. Under these circumstances (high hepatic extraction ratio) then, the effect of induction is primarily on F, rather than on CL.

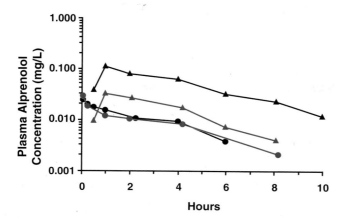

FIGURE 7-16. Induction of alprenolol metabolism by pentobarbital treatment produces marked differences in the plasma concentration when the drug is given orally (200 mg, *solid triangles*), but not when given intravenously (5 mg, *solid circles*). Alprenolol was administered before (*black*) and 10 days into (*colored*) a pentobarbital regimen of 100 mg at bedtime. (From: Alván G, Piafsky K, Lind M, et al. Effect of pentobarbital on the disposition of alprenolol. Clin Pharmacol Ther 1977;22:316–321.)

Impaired Renal Function. For drugs mostly eliminated by renal excretion, a decrease in renal function decreases clearance with a corresponding increase in *AUC*, C_{max}, and half-life, and a consequential lengthening of the peak time. This is shown in Fig. 7-17 with ganciclovir, an antiviral agent that is almost completely dependent on renal excretion for its elimination.

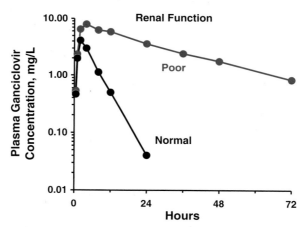

FIGURE 7-17. Mean plasma ganciclovir concentration with time in subjects with normal renal function (*black*) and in those with poor renal function (*colored*). A clear decrease in clearance of ganciclovir is seen (manifested by an increase in *AUC*, peak time, and half-life) in those subjects with reduced renal function. This large dependence of clearance on renal function arises because ganciclovir is totally dependent on renal excretion for its elimination. Each subject received a 900-mg oral dose of valganciclovir, an ester prodrug that is completely hydrolyzed to ganciclovir on passage across the intestinal wall. (From: Czock D, Scholle C, Rasche FM, et al. Pharmacokinetics of valganciclovir and ganciclovir in renal impairment. Clin Pharmacol Ther 2002;72:142–150.)

Increase in Urine pH. When urine pH is increased (for example by a low protein diet, a high intake of an antacid like sodium bicarbonate or when acetazolamide, a carbonic hydrase inhibitor, is given) one expects the renal clearance of a pH sensitive weak base to increase, as the drug is then not as well reabsorbed (less in the diffusible un-ionized form) from the kidney tubule. An example of a drug showing this kinetic behavior is memantine (Fig. 7-18), for which there is a decrease in *AUC*, C_{max}, half-life, and t_{max}.

We have now completed our exploration of the kinetics of a drug following a single dose and the physiologic processes that determine it. In the next chapter (Chapter 8,

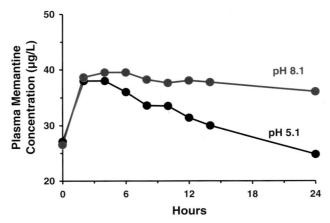

FIGURE 7-18. Plasma concentration–time course for memantine following two treatments: (*black*) acidic urine (mean pH of 5.1); (*colored*) alkaline urine mean pH of 8.1. The low pH was maintained by taking 1 g of ammonium chloride every 3 hr, while the high pH was maintained with 4 g of sodium bicarbonate every 4 h. Memantine is a weak base with a pKa of 10.3. Its un-ionized form is nonpolar and therefore it tends to be reabsorbed in the renal tubule. The higher the urine pH, the greater is the fraction of the drug in the un-ionized form, the greater is reabsorption and the lower is renal clearance, which decreases 10-fold. The fraction excreted unchanged decreases from 0.90 to 0.50. (From: Freudenthaler S, Meineke I, Schreeb KH, et al. Influence of urine pH and urinary flow on the renal excretion of memantine. Br J Clin Pharmacol 1998;46:541–546.)

Response Following a Single Dose), we examine how response varies with time following a single dose. Subsequently, in Section III, we explain how therapeutic regimens are developed to maintain drug exposure and response with time.

KEY RELATIONSHIPS

$$F = F_F \cdot F_G \cdot F_H$$

$$F_H = 1 - (1 - fe)CL_b/Q_H$$

$$F_H = \frac{Q_H}{Q_H + fu_b \cdot CL_{int}}$$

$$\frac{C_{b,initial}}{C_{b,max}} = \frac{ka \cdot V}{F \cdot Q_H}$$

STUDY PROBLEMS

(Answers to Study Problems are in Appendix J.)

1. List at least five reasons why oral bioavailability of drugs is often less than 100%.

2. Indicate the accuracy of the following statements:
   a. When administered orally in solution, gastric emptying rate-limits the absorption of small lipophilic drugs.
   b. For rapidly dissolving products of a drug, differences in rates of dissolution markedly affect the plasma concentration–time profile, when intestinal permeability is the rate-limiting step.

c. Polar drugs are primarily absorbed from the small intestine via the transcellular route.

d. Large nondisintegrating controlled-release dosage forms commonly remain in the stomach for 6 hr when taken just after a heavy meal.

3. Define *saturable first-pass hepatic metabolism,* and describe how this dose-dependent kinetic behavior can be seen after oral administration without observing saturable metabolism after an equivalent i.v. bolus dose.

4. Comment on the statement: Drugs administered in solution are more slowly absorbed from muscle (i.m. administration) than from the small intestine (oral administration).

5. Listed in Table 7-11 are the *AUC* values of ciprofloxacin, a drug with a broad antimicrobial activity, following its delivery (180 mg) in solution to various regions of the gastrointestinal tract. Ciprofloxacin appears to be stable in all parts of the gastrointestinal tract.

a. From which site of the gastrointestinal tract, stomach, small intestine, or large intestine is the majority of ciprofloxacin likely to be absorbed following oral administration of the drug?

b. Based on the difference in *AUC* values following delivery into the stomach and jejunum, suggest a possible primary site of absorption of ciprofloxacin.

c. For drugs that exhibit absorption patterns similar to that of ciprofloxacin, comment on the chances of successfully achieving a constant rate of systemic input for up to 12 hr following administration of an oral drug-delivery system.

TABLE 7-11	Area Under the Plasma Concentration—Time Curve for Ciprofloxacin When Delivered in Solution to Various Regions of the Gastrointestinal Tract				
Region:	Stomach	Jejunum	Ileum	Ascending Colon	Descending Colon
AUC (mg-L/hr)	1.48	0.38	0.24	0.08	0.05

From: Harder S, Fuhr U, Beermann E, et al. Ciprofloxacin absorption in different regions of the human gastrointestinal tract. Investigations with the hf-capsule. Br J Clin Pharmacol 1990;30:35–39.

6. Figure 7-19 (page 214) shows plasma drug concentration–time profiles following oral administration of single doses of two drugs (both are eliminated exclusively by hepatic metabolism and have a *low* hepatic extraction ratio) under the following conditions:

Top Graph. Plasma protein binding is: normal (Case A, shown); halved (Case B, twofold increase in *fu*); and doubled (Case C, twofold decrease in *fu*).

Bottom Graph. Tissue binding is: normal (Case A, shown); halved (Case B, twofold increase in fu_T); and doubled (Case C, twofold decrease in fu_T).

Draw the expected time profiles of the plasma concentration for the two situations for each of the two drugs. Be sure that each graph shows the salient features including relative *AUC*, peak times, and decline of the concentration. The volumes of distribution of both drugs in all conditions are greater than 100 L.

7. Although recognized for many years, the interaction between allopurinol, used in the treatment of gout, and 6-mercaptopurine, an antineoplastic agent, was not well understood until the kinetics of the interaction was elucidated. The *AUC* values of 6-mercaptopurine before and after pretreatment with allopurinol (100 mg orally three times a day for 2 days) following oral and i.v. administrations of 0.8 mmol of 6-mercaptopurine are given in Table 7-13. Both drugs are mostly eliminated by metabolism

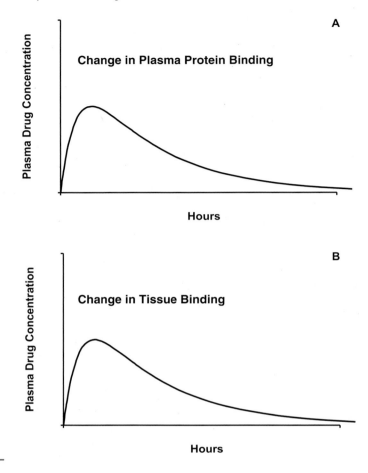

FIGURE 7-19.

in the liver. The half-life of 6-mercaptopurine was not significantly changed by allopurinol treatment. For the purpose of this problem, use a plasma/blood ratio of 1.67.

a. Calculate the clearance and bioavailability of 6-mercaptopurine before and after allopurinol.

b. Provide a logical kinetic explanation for the enhanced efficacy of 6-mercaptopurine in the presence of allopurinol.

TABLE 7-13	Average Areas Under the Plasma 6-Mercaptopurine Concentration–Time Curves (μM-min) Before and After Allopurinol Pretreatment	
	Before	**After**
Oral	142	716
Intravenous	1207	1405

From: Zimm S, Collins JM, O'Neill D, et al. Inhibition of first-pass metabolism in cancer chemotherapy: interaction of 6-mercaptopurine and allopurinol. Clin Pharmacol Ther 1983;34;819–817.

8. The effects of food on the oral bioavailability, systemic clearance, and AUC of propranolol are summarized in Table 7-14. Propranolol is eliminated by hepatic metabolism. The authors suggest that an increase in hepatic blood flow is, in large part, responsible for the observations. Do you agree with the authors or not? Justify your position.

TABLE 7-14	Effect of Food on Bioavailability, Systemic Clearance, and Oral *AUC* of Propanolol	
Parameters	**Fasting**	**High-Protein Meal**
Bioavailability(%)	$27 \pm 2^*$	$46 \pm 4^†$
Clearance‡ (L/min)	1.00 ± 0.06	$1.38 \pm 0.12^†$
Oral $AUC^{††}$ (mg-hr/L)	21.8 ± 2.6	$27.8 \pm 10.0^{‡‡}$

*Mean $\pm$ SEM: N = 6.
†Significantly different; $P < 0.05$.
‡$Dose_{i.v.}/AUC_{i.v.}$ (blood).
††$AUC_{p.o.}$ (blood) of deuterated propranolol given concurrently with the i.v. dose.
‡‡Not significant; $P > 0.05$.
From: Olanoff LS, Walle T, Cowart TD, et al. Food effects on propranolol systemic and oral clearances: support for a blood flow hypothesis. Clin Ther 1986;40:408–414.

9. Comment on the likely influence of a heavy meal, relative to the fasting state, on the rate and extent of oral absorption of a drug in each of the following cases. All of the drugs, except the one in Part C, are chemically stable in the gastrointestinal tract.

   a. A water-soluble highly permeable drug is administered in an immediate-release tablet.
   b. A sparingly soluble lipophilic drug is administered as an intended immediate-release capsule dosage form. Oral bioavailability is typically only 26% because of low solubility.
   c. An acid-labile drug is taken as a single enterically coated (resistant to acidic gastric pH) 0.8-g tablet.

10. Listed in Table 7-15 are some pertinent pharmacokinetic data following administration of a 100-mg dose of a drug orally (tablet) and intravenously to a 68-kg patient. The plasma/blood concentration ratio of the drug is 1.5. Use a hepatic blood flow of 81 L/hr.

TABLE 7-15	*AUC* and Amount Excreted Unchanged (*Ae*∞) of a Drug Following i.v. and Oral Administration	
Route	**AUC (mg-hr/L)**	**$Ae_∞$ (mg)**
Intravenous	1.93	10.5
Oral	0.22	1.22

   a. Calculate the oral bioavailability of the drug.
   b. By appropriate calculation, estimate to what extent the observed bioavailability might be attributed to first-pass hepatic elimination.

Response Following a Single Dose

OBJECTIVES

The reader will be able to:

- Define the following terms: duration of effect, effect compartment, hysteresis, pharmacokinetic–pharmacodynamic modeling, onset of effect, pharmacokinetic rate-limited response, pharmacodynamic rate-limited response, site of action, and time delay.

- Show graphically how one can readily detect when response does not track the plasma drug concentration after a single extravascular dose, and give at least three explanations for the delay.

- Give two examples each of situations in which measured response is rate-limited by pharmacokinetics and pharmacodynamics.

- Explain why a graded response tends to decline linearly with time after a single dose when response lies between 80% and 20% of its maximum.

- Discuss two situations in which response declines more slowly than plasma drug concentration.

- Explain why duration of response is often proportional to the logarithm of dose; and when it is, calculate both the minimum-effective dose and the effective half-life.

In Chapter 2, *Fundamental Concepts and Terminology*, we primarily considered the relationship between systemic exposure and response, that is, the pharmacodynamics of the drug, without much consideration of time. In practice, time always needs to be considered. In this chapter, we integrate pharmacokinetics with response over time following a single dose of drug. Subsequently, in Chapter 10, *Constant-Rate Input*, and Chapter 11, *Multiple-Dose Regimens*, we consider events after continuous and chronic administration. The ensuing discussion is generally restricted to drugs that act reversibly to produce a response. Furthermore, metabolites are considered to be either inactive or not to reach a sufficiently high concentration to contribute to response, although this restriction is lifted in Chapter 20, *Metabolites and Drug Response*.

It is important to realize that the amount of drug involved in producing a response at the site of action is usually only a minute fraction of the total amount in the body. Consequently, drug so involved generally has little to no effect on its own pharmacokinetics, but exceptions do exist as discussed in Chapter 17, *Nonlinearities*, and Chapter 21, *Protein Drugs*.

TIME DELAYS BETWEEN CONCENTRATION AND RESPONSE

Drug response often lags behind plasma concentration. Let us examine how such delays are detected and how they come about.

DETECTING TIME DELAYS

A striking example of a delay in effect is the rise in left ventricular ejection-time index—a measure of effect of digoxin on the heart—while the plasma concentration falls during the first 4 hr after an intravenous (i.v.) bolus dose of digoxin (Fig. 8-1). Certainly, these data do not mean that less drug is needed to produce a greater response. Rather, distribution of digoxin into cardiac tissue with subsequent binding to the target receptor is slow. Therefore, to use plasma concentration as a guide to drug effect, one should wait until distribution equilibrium of drug between plasma and cardiac tissue is reached, which is about 6 hr after a dose of digoxin. When relating response to concentration before 6 hr, an absurd relationship is observed. The response is lowest when the concentration is highest and the converse. We would be foolish to conclude that what is needed for a substantial effect is a low concentration or no drug at all.

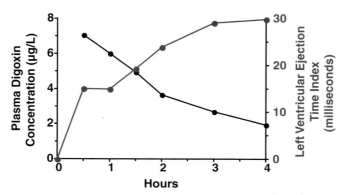

FIGURE 8-1.   The prolongation in the left ventricular ejection-time index (*colored line*), a measure of cardiac effect, increases as the plasma digoxin concentration (*black line*) declines for 4 hr after i.v. administration of a 1-mg dose of digoxin. Average data from six normal subjects. (From: Shapiro W, Narahara K, Taubert K. Relationship of plasma digitoxin and digoxin to cardiac response following intravenous digitalization in man. Circulation 1970;42:1065–1072. Reproduced with permission of the American Heart Association, Inc.)

In contrast to an i.v. bolus dose, plasma drug concentration first rises and then falls following a single oral dose. This may lead to **hysteresis** in the concentration–response relationship—a useful diagnostic of the temporal features of drug response. Hysteresis refers to the condition in which response takes a different path than concentration with time when the concentration rises than when it falls. An example of such behavior is shown in Fig. 8-2 following the oral administration of naproxen, which is an analgesic, antipyretic, and anti-inflammatory agent. Shown in Fig. 8-2A are the plasma concentration and the mean pain relief in a dental-pain model with time after a single 500-mg dose of naproxen. Although there is a suggestion of a delay between plasma concentration and response in this graph, it becomes much more apparent when response is plotted directly against the corresponding plasma concentration (Fig. 8-2B), yielding a characteristic hysteretic loop. Initially, during the absorption phase, response lags behind the rise of naproxen in plasma. Subsequently, while the plasma concentration falls, response continues to rise. Only after 5 hr does response follow the fall in plasma concentration.

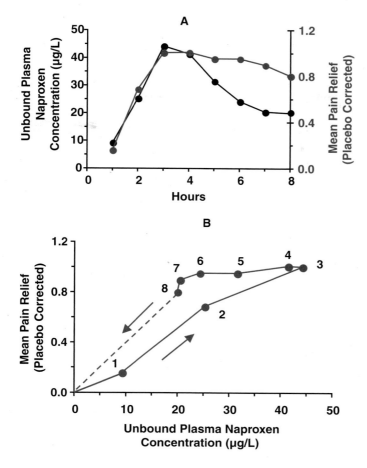

FIGURE 8-2. A. Plot of unbound plasma naproxen concentration (*black line*) and of associated mean pain relief (corrected for placebo response, *colored line*) in a dental pain model with time following an oral 500-mg dose of naproxen. **B.** Pain relief clearly shows hysteresis when plotted directly against the unbound plasma concentration of naproxen, in that different responses are apparent at the same unbound plasma concentration on the rising and falling parts of the concentration–time curve. The time of sampling from 1 to 8 hr is noted next to each point. Notice that the hysteresis is counterclockwise. The extrapolation beyond 8 hr indicates that eventually no benefit is achieved as the plasma-naproxen concentration falls toward zero. (From: Syntex USA Inc., Palo Alto, CA, 1994.)

Notice that the chronologic sequence of the paired concentration–response observations moves in a counterclockwise direction.

CAUSES OF TIME DELAY

There are many reasons, both kinetic and dynamic, for this counterclockwise hysteresis.

Tissue Distribution. In the case of the example of naproxen, as with many drugs, the hysteresis is caused by delayed distribution to the site of action. The therapeutic consequence of such delays depends on the clinical setting. Recall that distribution kinetics depends on tissue perfusion, membrane permeability, and tissue affinity for drug. Many drugs are small lipophilic molecules that equilibrate rapidly across well-perfused tissues (e.g., heart, brain), which are often target organs (i.e., organs containing the site of action). Under these circumstances, because the period of observation in clinical practice is often hours, if not days, a delay in effect in the order of minutes is likely to be minimal, and drug in plasma can be correlated directly with effect, provided that the measured response is rapidly produced by drug at the site of action. This was the case in the study from which the propranolol data in Fig. 2-16 in Chapter 2, *Fundamental Concepts and Terminology*, were obtained. Propranolol was given orally, and measurements were made over several hours, particularly after the peak plasma concentration had been reached. Even if distribution throughout the body has not been achieved, plasma concentration may still track response well; all that is required is that distribution equilibrium of drug between plasma and the active site within the target organ be rapidly achieved.

Emergency admissions and surgical procedures are special settings during which responses are frequently measured in minutes rather than hours. Here, delays in response after drug administration are almost always noticed. Even though plasma concentration monitoring is unlikely to be employed in these circumstances, it is still important to delineate the determinants of the time course of response to improve our general understanding and to optimize treatment procedures and drug use.

Pharmacodynamics. Often, the reason for the hysteresis is pharmacodynamic in origin. Much depends on the underlying dynamics of the affected system and on the closeness of the measured response to the direct action of the drug. Generally, the closer the measured response, the more rapid is that response to changes in drug concentration, which it should be recalled as one of the main reasons why biomarkers are used as early signals of drug action. To expand on these statements, consider the three situations in Fig. 8-3, with drug in Compartment A, the site of action, linked with the rest of the body. The measured response is associated with events in Compartments A, B, and C, respectively. Each downfield compartment reflects upstream changes. In reality, there are often feedback processes whereby a change in a component downstream feeds back on an upstream component to regulate the behavior of the system, sometimes producing oscillations in the level of the component with the time scale varying from minutes, to hours, to days. Also, the components of the body act as a complex three-dimensional interacting network operating in both space and time rather than as a simple linear chain depicted in Fig. 8-3. However, for didactic purposes, such complexities are not considered here.

Consider first the simplest situation, namely where Compartment A is both the site of measurement and the site of the action of a drug, be it a receptor, enzyme, or ion channel. Then, measured response is expected to track drug action instantly, resulting in a fixed relationship between them, independent of time or the shape of the concentration–time

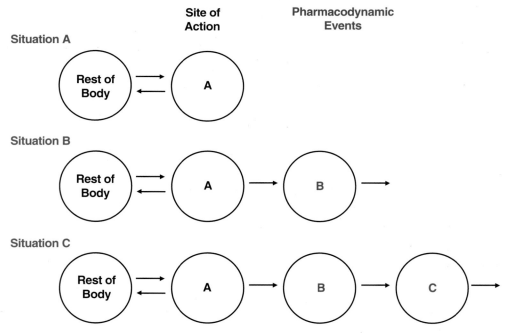

FIGURE 8-3. A drug binds to its active site located in Compartment A, which is linked to drug in the rest of the body. The measured response may relate directly to drug at the active site (Situation A) or to a downstream element in either Compartment B or Compartment C, which changes in response to the initial interaction (Situations B and C).

profile. An example is neuronal conduction; neuromuscular blockage is almost instantaneously reflected by measured paralysis. Another example is seen with acetylcholine esterase inhibitors, which by inhibiting acetylcholine hydrolysis, raise the synaptic concentration of this endogenous neurotransmitter, and thereby, in theory, aid in the treatment of Alzheimer patients. This enzyme resides in many cells, including those in the brain, the site of therapeutic action, and also within red blood cells. In addition, the equilibrium of these drugs with this enzyme is extremely rapid. Hence, drug inhibition can be directly correlated with blood concentration at all times. Occasionally, however, response declines more slowly than concentration bathing the target site in Compartment A. This can occur when a drug binds so tightly to the target site that once bound, it dissociates off very slowly. Given that the magnitude of effect depends on the degree of occupancy of the target, response then declines slowly, rate-limited by the dissociation from the target, as shown in Fig. 8-4. An example, omeprazole, is considered later in this chapter.

Now, consider the situation in which the site of measurement of response is in one of the downstream compartments. The only specific pharmacodynamic characteristic of a

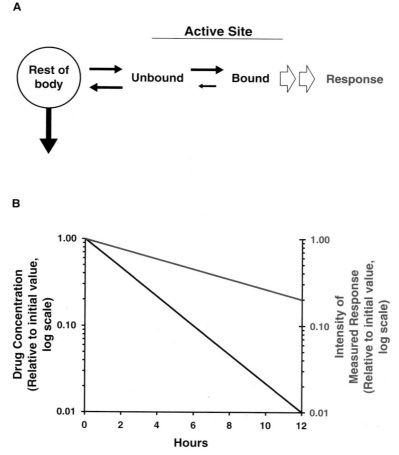

FIGURE 8-4. **A.** A drug reversibly binds to its site of action, and elicits a direct response with intensity dependent on the fraction of the target site occupied. Sometimes, the effect persists much longer than drug in the body. This can occur when drug binds very avidly to the active site, receptor or enzyme, and dissociates from it (*small arrow*) more slowly than elimination of drug from the body. **B.** The drug then continues to elicit its effect (*colored line*) long after drug has been virtually all removed from rest of the body (*black line*), including in the fluid surrounding the target site.

FIGURE 8-5. The site of action of a drug is located in Compartment A of the sequential scheme depicted in Fig. 8-3. Shown is the measured response versus time after than intravenous bolus dose when the measurement relates to drug at the active site (Situation A) or to events produced by the drug downstream (Situations B and C). Notice that the further downstream the measured response is relative to the site of direct action, the more sluggish it is and the later the time of its maximum value.

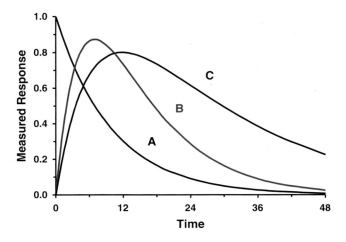

drug is its interaction at its primary site of action, here in Compartment A. All subsequent steps are a property of the affected system within the body and are the same, and independent of drug, for all drugs acting on the target site by the same mechanism. Two aspects now need to be considered: location and dynamics. Recall from Chapter 6, *Kinetics Following an Extravascular Dose*, when considering events in the body following an extravascular dose, plasma concentration reflects the net balance of input and output and always peaks later than that at the absorption site. Extending this concept to the events in Fig. 8-3, response peaks later the more distant the site of measurement is to the initial site of action, as shown in Fig. 8-5. Clearly then, a time delay in response is expected to be seen if plasma concentration corresponds to drug in Compartment A, with the delay being more pronounced as the site of measured response moves down from Compartment B to Compartment C. However, the kinetics of the subsequent events occurring between the initial interaction and the measured response varies greatly, and this will also impact on the ability to see any hysteresis or any clear evidence of a time delay in response. Sometimes, the entire pharmacodynamic system is operating so rapidly, relative to the kinetics of the drug, that measured response changes virtually instantaneously with drug concentration. In such cases, we have a **pharmacokinetic rate-limited response**, and hysteresis may not be seen except, perhaps, at the very earliest moments after drug administration. An example, previously considered, is the β-blockade produced by propranolol. This is essentially the case also with the benzodiazepines, producing central nervous effects, such as sedation, by interacting with the gamma aminobutyric acid (benzodiazepine) receptor. Under these conditions, the time course of response is determined primarily by the pharmacokinetics of these compounds, which differ markedly, varying from triazolam, an ultrashort-acting hypnotic with a half-life of 3 hr, to flurazepam, a long-acting hypnotic with a half-life in the order of 2 or more days. In contrast, many other measured responses are delayed because of the relatively sluggish dynamics of the affected system following direct drug action. That is, the response may be **rate-limited by pharmacodynamics**. Several examples are now considered, and two others, those involving effects of aspirin and omeprazole, are considered later in this chapter.

Systems in Flux. Returning to Fig. 8-3, a delay in measured response occurs when the site of action is say in Compartment A and the site of measurement is in Compartment B. Clearly, the system in Compartment B is in flux, dependent not only on what is happening in Compartment A, but also on events occurring between Compartments B and C. There are many such situations occurring within the body, particularly for those undergoing turnover (Chapter 2, *Fundamental Concepts and Terminology*, and Chapter 10, *Constant-Rate Input*). Two examples are now considered to illustrate this situation.

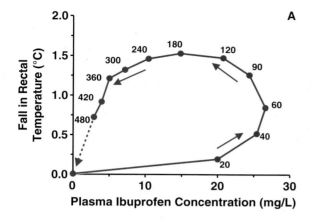

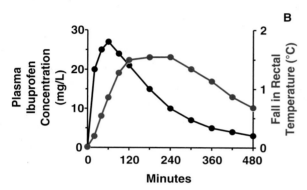

FIGURE 8-6. The fall in rectal temperature (observation minus baseline) in 36 febrile children aged from 6 months through 11 years after a 6-mg/kg oral dose of ibuprofen. **A.** Relationship between the fall in temperature and plasma ibuprofen concentration. Note the large degree of hysteresis present. The time of sampling (min) is indicated next to each point. **B.** Plasma ibuprofen concentration (*black line*) and fall in temperature (*colored line*) as a function of time after dosing. (From: Kelley MT, Walson PD, Edge JH, Cox S, Mortensen ME. Pharmacokinetics and pharmacodynamics of ibuprofen isomers and acetaminophen in febrile children. Clin Pharmacol Ther 1992;52:181–189.)

The first example is ibuprofen, an analgesic and antipyretic agent. Figure 8-6A shows the mean fall in rectal temperature, a measure of body temperature, relative to the plasma concentration when a single dose of drug is administered orally to 36 febrile children. The relationship implies that ibuprofen has little effect at early times when the concentration is high and maximal effect when the concentration has dropped to 15 mg/L. Actually, ibuprofen acts in the brain to affect the heat-control mechanism, causing decreased heat production. With rapid entry into the brain, the effect of ibuprofen there is greatest at early times and has partially worn off by the time the temperature is minimal, reflecting maximal measured response to the drug (Fig. 8-6B). Temperature is a measure of body heat. At any instant, the rate of change in body heat (and body temperature) is the difference between the rates of heat production and heat loss,

$$\begin{matrix} \textit{Rate of Change} \\ \textit{in Body Heat} \end{matrix} = \begin{matrix} \textit{Rate of Heat} \\ \textit{Production} \end{matrix} - \begin{matrix} \textit{Rate of Heat} \\ \textit{Loss} \end{matrix} \qquad \text{8-1}$$

Even if heat production were instantly reduced, time is required for body heat to dissipate and body temperature to fully reflect the reduction. Note that as the concentration of ibuprofen falls, so does its effect, and gradually, the body temperature returns (in this example) toward the preexisting value.

The second example is that of the oral coumarin anticoagulant, warfarin, used in the prevention of deep vein thrombosis. The response to warfarin is monitored clinically by prolongation in the clotting time of blood, which is a function of the prothrombin complex activity in plasma. The components of this complex (clotting factors II, VII, IX, and X) are turning over, being continuously formed and degraded. Figure 8-7 shows a sluggish response–time profile with the maximum occurring 1 to 2 days after the peak warfarin concentration following an oral dose of drug. The sluggishness largely reflects

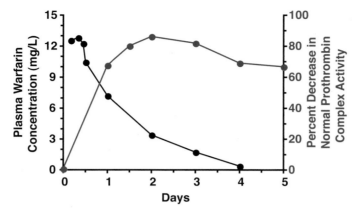

FIGURE 8-7. The sluggish response in the plasma-prothrombin complex activity (*colored line*) to inhibition of its synthesis in the liver by warfarin reflects the indirect nature of the measurement and the slow elimination of this complex. For the first 2 days after giving a single oral 1.5-mg/kg dose of sodium warfarin, response (defined as the percent decrease in the normal complex activity) steadily increases. During the first day, at this dose, the concentration of warfarin is sufficient to almost completely block complex synthesis. As warfarin concentration (*black line*) falls, the synthesis rate of the complex increases and by 48 hr equals the rate of degradation of the complex; the measured response is then at a maximum. Thereafter, as the plasma concentration falls further, with the synthesis rate exceeding the rate of degradation, the response falls. Eventually, when all the warfarin has been eliminated, the plasma-prothrombin complex activity returns—sluggishly—to the normal baseline value. The data points are the averages of five male volunteers. (From: Nagashima R, O'Reilly RA, Levy G. Kinetics of pharmacologic effects in man: the anticoagulant action of warfarin. Clin Pharmacol Ther 1969;10:22–35.)

the slow dynamics of the affected system. The direct effect of warfarin is inhibition of the synthesis in the liver of the prothrombin complex, which actually occurs very rapidly as warfarin, a small lipophilic molecule, readily enters this highly perfused organ. The plasma-prothrombin complex activity then falls, but at a rate determined by its degradation, which is slow with a half-life in the order of 1 to 2 days. Even if synthesis were totally blocked, it would take several days for the prothrombin complex to fall, for example, to 25% of its normal value. As the plasma (and liver) concentrations of warfarin fall, so does the degree of inhibition of synthesis. The prothrombin complex activity then rises and slowly returns to its normal value, determined in substantial part by the half-life of this complex, but not solely. Keep in mind that the return of the measured response to the baseline can be rate-limited by either the pharmacokinetics of the drug or the underlying dynamics of the affected system, whichever is the slowest. This is illustrated in Fig. 8-8, which shows the pharmacokinetics and response with time following the administration of single oral doses of acenocoumarol and phenprocoumon, two other oral coumarin anticoagulants prescribed in several countries. These compounds act by the same mechanism as warfarin but have very different pharmacokinetics. In contrast to warfarin (half-life 1.5 days), acenocoumarol has a half-life of only 15 hr. So that by the time of the maximum response (24 hr), much of acenocoumarol has been eliminated and the subsequent return of clotting factor activity to baseline, by 3 days, is controlled by the turnover of the measured clotting factors. In contrast, the half-life of phenprocoumon is 6 days. Although the time to develop the maximum-observed response is similar to that seen with acenocoumarol, governed primarily by the degradation-rate constant of the clotting factor activity, the return to baseline is very much slower. It takes up to 2 weeks to do so as the return of activity is now rate-limited by the pharmacokinetics of this anticoagulant.

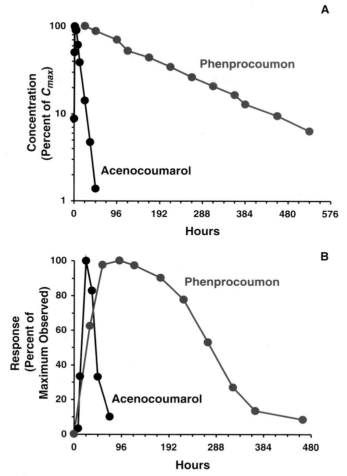

FIGURE 8-8. **A,B.** Either pharmacokinetics or pharmacodynamics can rate limit the decline of response following drug administration. Both acenocoumarol and phenprocoumon are oral anticoagulants that, like warfarin, act by inhibiting the synthesis of the prothrombin complex clotting factors. Notice that although the times for achieving maximum response are similar (1–3 days) for the two compounds, being determined primarily by the degradation-rate constant of the complex, the return of the activity to baseline varies. In the case of acenocoumarol, with a relatively short half-life (15 hr), return to baseline is complete within 3 days being controlled primarily by the kinetics of the complex, a pharmacodynamic rate limitation. In contrast, return to baseline following phenprocoumon administration takes approximately 2 weeks because the return is now rate-limited by the pharmacokinetics of this long half-life compound (5 days). Each drug was given as a single oral dose of the racemate (10-mg acenocoumarol, 0.6 mg/kg [42 mg/70kg] phenprocoumon). To allow comparison, both plasma concentration and response (assessed based on prolongation of the prothrombin time) have been expressed as a percentage of their respective maximum values for each drug. Plasma concentrations are racemic compound for phenprocoumon (kinetics of enantiomers very similar) and the R-enantiomer of acenocoumarol; the S-enantiomer is very rapidly eliminated (half-life 2–4 hr) and contributes negligibly to activity. The data are the mean of 11 subjects for acenocoumarol and 5 subjects for phenprocoumon. (From: Sunkara G, Bigler H, Wang Y, et al. The effect of nateglinide on the pharmacokinetics and pharmacodynamics of acenocoumarol. Curr Med Res Opin 2004;20:41–48; Jähnchen E, Meinertz T, Gilfrich HJ, et al. The enantiomers of phenprocoumon: pharmacodynamic and pharmacokinetic studies. Clin Pharmacol Ther 1976;20:342–349.)

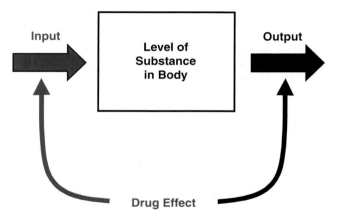

FIGURE 8-9. The level of many systems and endogenous compounds in the body is normally relatively constant, reflecting the balance between the rates of input and output. A drug may act directly to increase or decrease either input or output, thereby perturbing the level. Measurement of the level of the substance in plasma reflects the state of that system at any point in time. The time scale of the change in response can vary from seconds to years; it is often determined by the output-rate constant of the monitored system or endogenous compound.

Generalizing, the level of many substances or measured quantities in the body depends on the difference between rates of input and loss or formation and elimination, as depicted in Fig. 8-9 and expressed in Eq. 8-2.

$$\begin{array}{c} \text{Rate of Change} \\ \text{in Body} \end{array} = \text{Rate of Input} - \text{Rate of Loss} \qquad 8\text{-}2$$

Normally, input and loss are balanced so that the level of the substance or measured quantity remains relatively stable with time, thereby maintaining an internal homeostasis. In addition to body heat and prothrombin complex activity, other examples mentioned in Chapter 2, *Fundamental Concepts and Terminology*, and Chapter 10, *Constant-Rate Input* are body-water content, white and red cell counts, and concentrations of many endogenous proteins, hormones, and serum electrolytes. Drugs act directly by either increasing or decreasing the rates of input or output, thereby changing the level of the quantity being measured. Normally, the direct effect is a graded response, which can be adequately characterized by Eq. 2-4 in Chapter 2, *Fundamental Concepts and Terminology*.

The delay between attainment of a peak plasma concentration and maximal measured response varies widely, being governed by the turnover time of the affected system. The shorter the turnover time, the more rapid the change in the measured response for a change in drug concentration. For example, full response in blood pressure to a change in peripheral resistance or in cardiac output produced by a drug occurs within minutes, whereas the maximal response of the prothrombin complex activity to warfarin, as shown in Fig. 8-7, is not seen for 1 to 2 days after a single oral dose of this anticoagulant. Sometimes, the turnover time of the system is so long and the response so damped that no perceptible response (change from baseline) is seen following a single dose of drug. This is the case with the bisphosphonates, such as alendronate (Fosomax), which increase bone mineral density and ultimately reduce bone fracture rates. Changes in bone mineral density take months to manifest, and in such cases, a drug needs to be given chronically to see a measurable response, as discussed in Chapter 10, *Constant-Rate Iinput*.

REVEALING THE CONCENTRATION–RESPONSE RELATIONSHIP

The approach to revealing the underlying concentration–direct response relationship depends on the reason for the time delay.

Effect Compartment. When a delay in achieving a response is caused by slow distribution to the active site, as reflected by hysteresis in the response–concentration relationship, it can be modeled. To this end, a pharmacodynamic model with the site of action located in an **effect compartment** and linked to the plasma concentration has been used, as depicted in Fig. 8-10. This procedure has been applied to naproxen, which was previously shown to exhibit hysteresis (Fig. 8-2). By adjusting the distribution rate constant leaving the effect compartment, a condition is found in which the hysteresis disappears. The direct relationship between response and concentration in the effect compartment is now exposed, which can often be adequately summarized by the exposure–response model of Eq. 2-4 in Chapter 2, *Fundamental Concepts and Terminology*, as illustrated when applied to naproxen (Fig. 8-11).

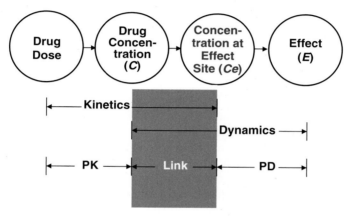

FIGURE 8-10.   The concept of an effect compartment linking plasma concentration with response helps to accommodate the frequently observed delay in time between plasma concentration and response. The delay is caused by the time needed to distribute to the site of action. By accommodating for, and effectively removing, this delay, it is possible to reveal the underlying direct relationship between effect site concentration (*Ce*) and response.

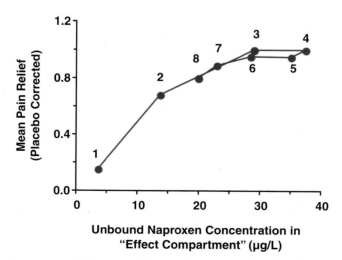

FIGURE 8-11.   Mean pain relief (corrected for placebo response) in a dental-pain model plotted as a function of the unbound plasma concentration of naproxen within the "effect compartment" following an oral 500-mg dose. Notice, when an effect compartment is used, the counterclockwise hysteresis, seen when pain relief is plotted against unbound plasma concentration of naproxen (Fig. 8-2B), is removed. The response can now be related to the effect site concentration at all times. The time of sampling from 1 to 8 hr is noted next to each point. (From: Syntex USA Inc., Palo Alto, CA, 1994).

The distribution half-life accounting for the delay can vary from minutes to hours, as with naproxen.

Systems in Flux. In systems in flux, of the type described by Eq. 8-2, drugs modulate the level of the measured response by increasing or decreasing either the rate of input or output. This creates four possible scenarios, but for illustrative purposes, only one of these is considered here, namely inhibition of input rate, typified by the inhibitory effect of warfarin on the affected clotting factor system. In common with other endogenous substances, the amount of each clotting factor in the body, A, is a result of a difference between its rate of synthesis, R_{syn}, and degradation. Often, as in this case, degradation is a first-order process, with the rate of degradation given $k_t \cdot A$, where k_t is the degradation-rate constant (fractional turnover rate) of the clotting factor. At any moment, whether at steady state or not,

$$\underset{\substack{\text{Rate of change} \\ \text{of clotting factor}}}{\frac{dA}{dt}} = \underset{\substack{\text{Rate of} \\ \text{synthesis}}}{R_{syn}} - \underset{\substack{\text{Rate of} \\ \text{degradation}}}{k_t \cdot A}$$

8-3

Normally, the system is at steady state, $dA/dt = 0$, with synthesis matching degradation. However, in the presence of warfarin, synthesis is inhibited without affecting k_t. The clotting factor concentration (or amount) then falls at a rate that depends on both the degree of inhibition of synthesis and k_t.

To solve this rate equation, without making any assumption about the nature of the warfarin concentration–inhibition relationship, requires an estimate of k_t. One approach in obtaining this value is to give a dose of warfarin that completely blocks synthesis initially ($R_{syn} = 0$). The prothrombin complex activity then falls exponentially, so that a semilogarithmic plot of the prothrombin complex activity against time gives a straight line with a slope of k_t (Fig. 8-12). Subsequently, as the plasma (and liver) concentration of warfarin falls, the degree of inhibition of clotting factor synthesis decreases and the concentration of the prothrombin complex rises (see Fig. 8-7), eventually returning to its

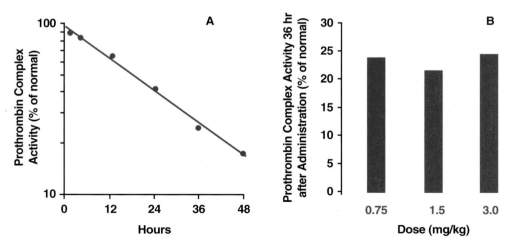

FIGURE 8-12. **A.** A blocking dose of warfarin, 1.5 mg/kg orally as the sodium salt, caused the prothrombin complex activity to decline exponentially over the first 48 hr after administration to a subject. **B.** As expected, higher (oral and i.v.) doses of warfarin produced no further change in the rate of decline of the complex activity, as determined by the activity remaining at 36 hr. (From: Nagashima R, O'Reilly RA, Levy G. Kinetics of pharmacologic effect in man: the anticoagulant action of warfarin. Clin Pharmacol Ther 1969;10:22–35.)

prewarfarin value. The change in synthesis rate, R_{syn}, with time is calculated, from simultaneous measurement of warfarin and prothrombin complex activity on return to the prewarfarin value, as follows:

If A_1 and A_2 are the prothrombin complex activities at the beginning and end of a time interval, Δt, then the rate of change of activity is estimated from $(A_2 - A_1)/\Delta t$ and the average activity within the interval is given by $(A_1 + A_2)/2$. R_{syn} is then calculated from rearrangement of Eq. 8-3

$$R_{syn} = (A_2 - A_1)/\Delta t + k_t \cdot (A_1 + A_2)/2 \qquad 8\text{-}4$$

The percent inhibition of synthesis is then approximated by

$$Percent\ inhibition\ of\ synthesis = 100 \cdot (R_{syn(n)} - R_{syn})/R_{syn(n)} \qquad 8\text{-}5$$

where $R_{syn}(n)$ is the normal prewarfarin synthesis rate. The normal rate is given by $k_t \cdot A(n)$, where $A(n)$ is the normal level of the clotting factor. When the percent inhibition of synthesis is plotted against the logarithm of the warfarin concentration, a classic graded response with no hysteresis is seen, as shown in Fig. 8-13, with the relationship adequately described by Eq. 2-4 in Chapter 2, *Fundamental Concepts and Terminology*. Alternatively, assuming the nature of the concentration–inhibition relationship and having described the warfarin pharmacokinetics by an appropriate equation, Eq. 8-3 may be numerically integrated and fit directly to clotting factor versus time data, to both estimate k_t and the parameters of warfarin concentration–inhibition relationship.

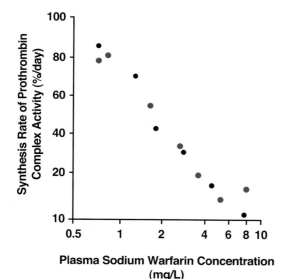

FIGURE 8-13. Pretreatment with heptabarbital (400 mg daily for 15 days, starting 10 days before warfarin) decreased the response to a standard dose of warfarin but failed to alter the linear relationship between synthesis rate of prothrombin complex activity and logarithm of the concentration of warfarin in a 21-year-old normal subject; control experiment (●), with heptabarbital (●) (From: Levy G, O'Reilly RA, Aggeler PM, Keech GM. Pharmacokinetic analysis of the effect of barbiturate on the anticoagulant action of warfarin in man. Clin Pharmacol Ther 1970;11:372–377.)

Responses to standard doses of warfarin change in disease states and following coadministration of other drugs. By ascertaining the relationship between plasma concentration and the direct effect, distinctions can be made between changes in pharmacokinetics of warfarin and changes in responsiveness of the clotting system to this drug. For example, the diminished response to warfarin, when coadministered with heptabarbital (an enzyme inducer), is caused solely by increased clearance of the drug; there is no change in the direct response to the drug (see Fig. 8-13).

DECLINE OF RESPONSE WITH TIME

The response to a drug eventually declines with time after administration of a single dose. For rapidly responsive systems (i.e., the ones involving rapid interaction at the effect site) rapid target distribution, and, if applicable, rapid turnover of an endogenous compound, the rate-limiting and, hence, controlling process is usually the pharmacokinetics of the drug, such that response tracks drug concentration during the decline phase. In other cases, usually because the response system itself is sluggish, the rate-controlling step is pharmacodynamics, and the response then falls more slowly than does plasma concentration; although even for sluggish systems, the rate-limitation may still be pharmacokinetics, if the kinetics of the drug is even slower than that of the pharmacodynamics system. Each of these situations is now considered.

WHEN PHARMACOKINETICS RATE-LIMITS DECLINE

How the intensity of response declines with time depends, as does the duration of effect, on dose and on rate of drug removal from the site of action. It also depends on the region of the concentration–response curve covered during the decline. Here, discussion is limited to the situation in which the response system is so fast that concentration–measured response relationship is essentially maintained at all times.

To appreciate the relationships among dose, intensity of response, and time, consider the events, depicted in Fig. 8-14A, that follow the intravenous administration of a 10-mg bolus dose of a drug with distribution characterized by a one-compartment model, with a half-life of 1 hr. A plot of intensity of response against logarithm of the plasma concentration is shown in Fig. 8-14B. For didactic purposes, it is convenient to divide the plot into three regions. In **Region 1** (up to 20% maximal response), intensity of response is directly proportional to the plasma concentration; in **Region 2** (covering 20%–80% of maximal response), intensity is proportional to the logarithm of concentration; and in **Region 3**, response gradually approaches the maximal value despite large changes in concentration. As the initial concentration lies in Region 3, despite a rapid fall in concentration in the first hour, intensity of response remains almost constant and maximal. Only after 2 hr, when concentration falls below 2 mg/L and response falls below 80% of the maximal value, does response begin to decline more rapidly. Then, for the next 2.5 hr, on passing through Region 2, *response declines almost linearly with time*. The reason for

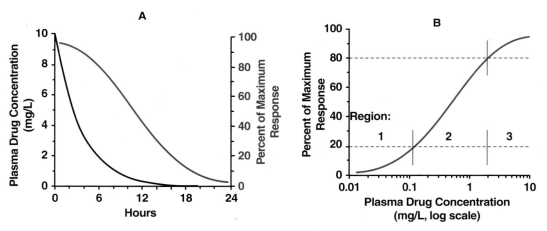

FIGURE 8-14. The decline in the intensity of pharmacologic effect with time (*colored line*, Graph A), following a single large i.v. bolus dose of a drug displaying monoexponential decline (*black line*, Graph A), depends on the region of the concentration–response curve (Graph B). Initially, in Region 3, the response remains almost maximal despite a 75% fall in the concentration. Thereafter, as long as the concentration is within Region 2, intensity of response declines approximately linearly with time. Only when concentration falls into Region 1 does decline in response parallel that of drug in plasma. The concentration–response relationship is defined by $E = E_{max} \cdot C^{\gamma}/(C_{50}{}^{\gamma} + C^{\gamma})$, with $E_{max} = 100\%$, $C_{50} = 0.5$ mg/L, and $\gamma = 1$.

this essentially constant decline in response, while the plasma concentration declines exponentially, is apparent from the inset of Fig. 8-14, because in Region 2

$$Response = m \cdot ln\ C + b \qquad 8\text{-}6$$

where m and b are the slope and intercept of the relationship.

Substituting $ln\ C(0) - k \cdot t$ for $ln\ C$ in Eq. 8-6, where $C(0)$ is the concentration upon entering Region 2 from Region 3, and collecting terms therefore yields:

$$Response = (m \cdot ln\ C(0) + b) - m \cdot k \cdot t \qquad 8\text{-}7$$

Letting $E(0)$ be the intensity of effect $(m \cdot ln\ C(0) + b)$ when the concentration is $C(0)$ gives

$$Response = E(0) - m \cdot k \cdot t \qquad 8\text{-}8$$

Thus, *the intensity of effect falls linearly with time* in Region 2. Note that the rate of decline, $m \cdot k$, depends on both slope of the intensity versus ln concentration relationship and the half-life of the drug. In this instance, for example, $m = 31$ (in Region 2, the intensity of response changes by 31% of the maximal response for a 1-ln change in C), and as $k = 0.7$ hr^{-1}, a constant rate of 22%/hr in the decline of activity is anticipated. Finally, beyond 5 hr, when the concentration falls below 0.1 mg/L and enters Region 1, the fall in response then parallels that of the drug.

The concepts developed above are now illustrated with degree of muscle paralysis produced by the neuromuscular-blocking agent, succinylcholine. Changes in degree of muscle paralysis with time, following a 0.5 mg/kg bolus dose of succinylcholine to a patient, are shown in Fig. 8-15. The 1-min delay before onset of effect is probably accounted for by the time required for blood to circulate from injection site to muscle and, in part, by the time for succinylcholine to diffuse into the neuromuscular junction. However, once at the site and with drug at maximal concentration, as expected with neuronal conduction being so fast, full response ensues very promptly. Total paralysis is then maintained for a full 2 min despite the continual rapid inactivation, by hydrolysis, of this agent (elimination half-life = 3.5 min). Subsequently, the effect subsides. As predicted, between 80% and 20% of maximal response, the effect declines at a constant rate: in this instance, 22%/min. The reason for this very rapid decline in response is a combination of its short half-life of elimination and a steep response–concentration curve. Changes in muscle paralysis can therefore be

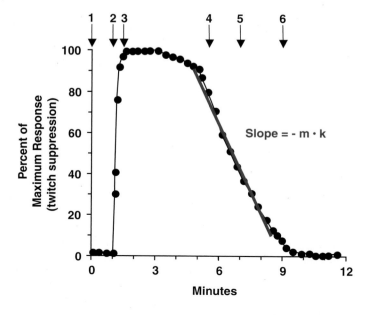

FIGURE 8-15. Changes in the degree of muscle paralysis (assessed as the suppression of a twitch produced in response to ulnar nerve stimulation) with time following an intravenous bolus dose of 0.5 mg/kg succinylcholine to a subject: (1) Time of injection; (2) onset of twitch suppression; (3) complete twitch suppression; (5) recovery of twitch to 50% (T_{50}) of the maximum twitch height. Note that response declines essentially linearly with time between 80% (4) and 20% (6) of maximum effect (*declining colored line*). (From: Walts LF, Dillon JB. Clinical studies on succinylcholine chloride. Anesthesiology 1967;28:372–376.)

produced within a few minutes of changing administration, and once administration is stopped, the patient promptly recovers; both are desirable characteristics. Another example is minoxidil (Rogaine). Although now used topically to promote hair growth, initially, it was investigated as an antihypertensive agent. As seen in Fig. 8-16, the decrease in blood pressure-lowering effect, which almost instantaneously reflects changes in drug concentration, declines essentially linearly with time after an oral dose of this drug.

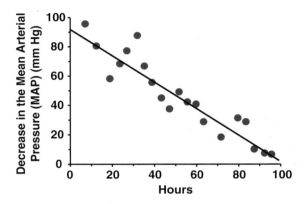

FIGURE 8-16. The degree of lowering of the mean arterial blood pressure (MAP), in a patient with a baseline MAP of 157 mm Hg, falls at a constant rate following a single oral 25-mg dose of minoxidil. (From: Shen D, O'Malley K, Gibaldi M, McNay JL. Pharmacodynamics of minoxidil as a guide to individualizing dosage regimens in hypertension. Clin Pharmacol Ther 1975;17:593–598.)

In the examples of succinylcholine and minoxidil and many other drugs, temporal and quantitative changes in response, which help guide dosage, were obtained without measurement of drug in plasma. The ability to derive such useful information is particularly attractive in situations, such as ocular or pulmonary administration of drugs intended for local action, where there is little to no relationship between events at the site of action and systemic concentration. Nonetheless, whenever possible, it is preferable to also measure drug (and active metabolites) in plasma particularly for systemically acting drugs. This is particularly so when, for example, response varies among individuals or in disease, and one wishes to understand the relative contributions of pharmacokinetics and pharmacodynamics.

WHEN PHARMACODYNAMICS RATE-LIMITS DECLINE

We have seen that response stays essentially constant and maximal and declines more slowly than plasma concentration, as long as the concentration remains in Region 3 of the concentration–response curve. However, there are other situations in which response declines more slowly than plasma concentration for pharmacodynamic reasons. One such situation arises when a drug with a relatively short half-life consumes the target receptor or enzyme, which then has to be resynthesized, which takes time. This explains one action of aspirin. In addition to its long use as an analgesic and anti-inflammatory agent, in more recent years, it has gained widespread use as a prophylactic to reduce the chances of the occurrence of thromboembolic complications, such as reoccurring myocardial infarction, by inhibiting platelet aggregation. Recall from Chapter 6, *Kinetics Following an Extravascular Dose*, that, with a half-life of only 15 min, virtually the entire ingested dose of aspirin has been eliminated within 2 hr of ingestion (see Fig. 6-3). Elimination occurs almost entirely by hydrolysis to form salicylic acid. This metabolite is devoid of antiplatelet activity, yet the antiplatelet activity remains for several days. Aspirin (acetylsalicylic acid) affects platelet aggregation by rapidly and irreversibly inhibiting, by acetylation, prostaglandin cyclooxygenase. This effect lasts for the lifetime of the platelet and prevents the formation of thromboxane B2, which when platelet cells are fractured, promotes platelet adhesion and subsequent clot formation. Once all aspirin has been eliminated, thromboxane B2 and, hence, platelet-adhesion activity return toward the normal baseline with the production of

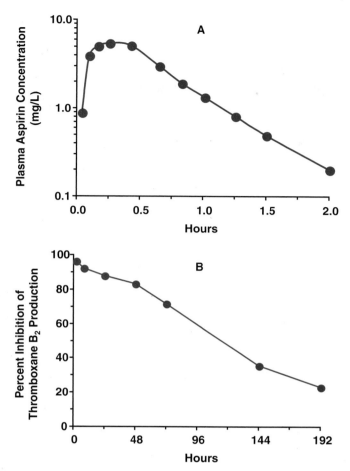

FIGURE 8-17. **A.** Upon oral administration of 650 mg, aspirin is rapidly absorbed and eliminated from the body, caused by rapid hydrolysis, such that little remains after 2 hr. **B.** Despite this, its effect as an inhibitor of platelet thromboxane B2 persists for many days. The slow decline is because of aspirin covalently binding and inactivating prostaglandin, which prevents the formation of thromboxane B2, which in turn has to be resynthesized, a slow process. Note the almost 100-fold difference in the time scales. (From: Ali M, MacDonald JWD, Thiessen JJ, Coates PE. Plasma acetylsalicylate and salicylate and platelet cyclooxygenase activity following plain and enteric coated aspirin. Stroke 1980;11:9–13.)

new platelets, a slow process (Fig. 8-17), because the fractional turnover rate of platelet cells is very low. Once the normal baseline is achieved, the production rate of platelets again matches the rate of their destruction.

A similar situation is seen with omeprazole, but the explanation is somewhat more complicated. Omeprazole, an inhibitor of the proton pump within the acid-secreting parietal cells of the stomach, is used in the treatment of heartburn and gastric and duodenal ulcers. This widely prescribed drug is rapidly absorbed, reaching a peak plasma concentration within 1 hr of oral dosing, and rapidly eliminated largely by conversion to inactive metabolites, with a half-life of just less than 1 hr. Gastric acid production promptly falls but the return to baseline is very slow, taking days (Fig. 8-18). Like aspirin, omeprazole covalently binds and inactivates its receptor, in this case the proton pump, which takes time to be resynthesized. However, this fails to explain completely the observed temporal pattern of gastric acid secretion. It appears that part of the explanation lies in the extremely tight affinity of locally formed omeprazole-derived compounds for the proton pump, from which these dissociate very slowly. In this situation, the plasma concentration rapidly falls below the limit of measurement, giving the impression that response persists when no drug is present in the body, which is not the case.

The last two examples are related to efficacy. Now let us examine an example of an adverse effect, a safety issue. A common and clinically significant toxicity of many anticancer drugs is leukopenia, an abnormal fall in the number of leukocytes in blood. Leukocytes are important in the immunological defense of the body. Most focus clinically is on the

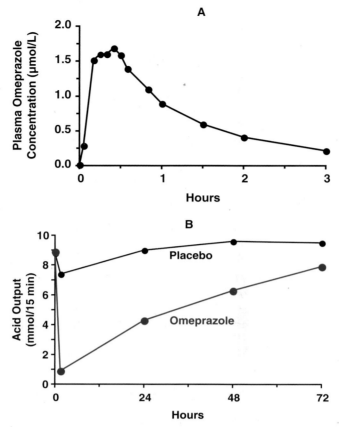

FIGURE 8-18. Despite being very rapidly metabolized within the body, such that little remains in plasma after 3 hr following a 40-mg oral dose of omeprazole **(A)** the inhibition of gastric acid secretion (*colored line*) continues for several days **(B)**. Also shown is the response following a placebo dose (*black line*). The response (expressed as a decrease in acid output over 15 min following a 1-hr infusion of intravenous pentagastrin, which maximally induces gastric acid secretion) was assessed before administration of drug or placebo at 2-hr postadministration, and again at 1, 2, and 3 days. This slow restoration of gastric acid secretion after omeprazole administration is because of a combination of very slow dissociation of tightly bound omeprazole-derived compounds to the proton pump receptor within the parietal cells of the stomach together with the covalent binding and inactivating by omeprazole of this receptor, requiring synthesis of new receptor, which takes time. (From: Lind T, Cederberg C, Ekenved G, Haglund, Oble L. Effect of omeprazole—a gastric proton-pump inhibitor—on the pentagastrin simulated secretion in man. Gut 1983;24:270–276.)

lowest leukocyte count after chemotherapy treatment, but the time course of the fall in count is also important. Shown in Fig. 8-19 is the plasma concentration–time course of one anticancer compound, paclitaxel (A), together with the corresponding time profile of leukocyte count (B) in a patient after single administration of the drug. Notice the large disparity between the relatively rapid elimination of the drug, which is almost completely eliminated within 2 days, and the sluggish changes in the fraction of leukocytes in blood in the patient, only returning to the baseline value 3 weeks after drug administration. Leukocytes in blood reflect the balance between production and destruction. The direct effect of paclitaxel is upstream within the bone marrow reducing the production of mature leukocytes. The exact sequence of events is not fully understood, but it appears that part of the fall in production occurs because certain phases in the development of the mature leukocyte, in particular the mitotic phase, are sensitive to destruction by paclitaxel.

A

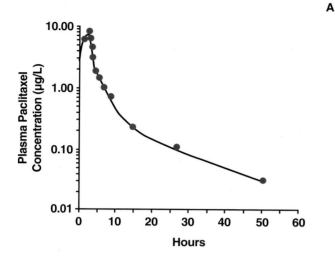

B

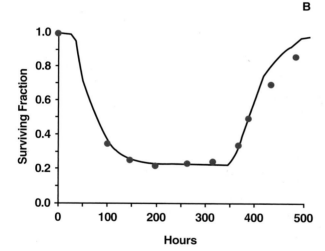

FIGURE 8-19. A. Plasma paclitaxel concentration–time profile; and **B**. the fraction of leukocytes in blood (relative to baseline) with time in a patient receiving an intravenous dose of paclitaxel. The continuous lines are the best-line fits of respective models to the data. (From: Minami H, Sasaki Y, Saijo N, et al. Indirect-response model for the time course of leukopenia with anticancer drugs. Clin Pharmacol Ther 1998;64:511–521.)

Once paclitaxel has been eliminated, a long period of time is needed to produce a sufficient number of mature leukocytes to restore the normal blood pool.

ONSET AND DURATION OF RESPONSE

ONSET OF EFFECT

After a single dose, although an effect may be graded and vary continuously with drug concentration, an effect discernible above baseline can be said to begin when the concentration at the site of action reaches a critical value. The time of onset of effect is governed by many factors, including route of administration, absorption, distribution to target site, and other time delays of pharmacodynamic origin, as discussed previously in this chapter and elsewhere in the book. Additional factors affecting time of onset are dose and the exposure–response relationship.

Increasing the dose shortens the time of onset of effect by shortening the time required to achieve the critical concentration at the site of action.

DURATION OF EFFECT

For a drug with no delays in response, relative to drug at the site of action, and showing a fixed exposure–response relationship (that is one for which response is rate-limited by pharmacokinetics), an effect lasts as long as the minimum effective concentration at the site of action is exceeded. After an intravenous bolus dose, the duration of effect is, therefore, a function of both dose and rate of drug removal from the site of action. Removal can result from either elimination or redistribution from the site to more slowly equilibrating tissues. When a drug distributes rapidly to all tissues, including the site of action, and the response immediately reflects the concentration of drug at the site of action, then the relationship between duration and kinetics is readily conceived following a single bolus dose.

Consider a drug that distributes into a volume (V), and is eliminated by first-order kinetics, characterized by the rate constant (k). After a bolus dose, the plasma concentration falls exponentially, that is

$$C = \frac{Dose}{V} e^{-k \cdot t} \qquad \text{8-9}$$

Eventually, a time is reached (the duration of effect [t_D]) when the plasma concentration falls to a value (C_{min}) below which the response is less than that minimally desired (Fig. 8-20). The relationship between C_{min} and t_D is given by appropriately substituting these quantities into the preceding equation; thus,

$$C_{min} = \frac{Dose}{V} e^{-k \cdot t_D} \qquad \text{8-10}$$

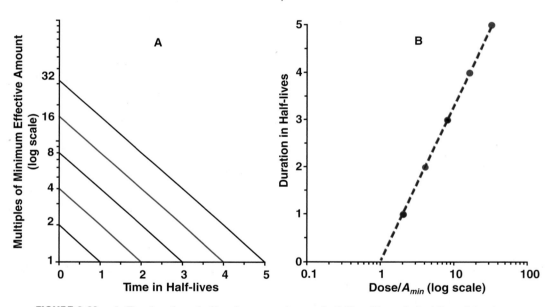

FIGURE 8-20. **A.** The duration of effect increases by one half-life with each doubling of the dose. **B.** Duration is also proportional to the logarithm of the dose. Note in these figures that time is expressed in multiples of half-life and dose is expressed in multiples of the minimum amount of drug needed to produce the desired effect, A_{min}.

Upon rearrangement and taking logarithms, an expression for t_D is obtained,

$$t_D = \frac{1}{k} \ln\left(\frac{Dose}{C_{min} \cdot V}\right) \qquad \text{8-11}$$

where $C_{min} \cdot V$ is the minimum amount needed in the body, A_{min}. According to Eq. 8-11, a plot of duration of effect against the logarithm of dose should yield a straight line with a slope of $1/k$ and an intercept, at zero duration of effect, of $\ln A_{min}$ (Fig. 8-20B). For example, the duration of effect of many local anesthetics is proportional to the logarithm of the injected dose. The muscle relaxant effect of succinylcholine also conforms to this last equation. Figure 8-21 shows the times to 50% (T_{50}) recovery of muscle twitch

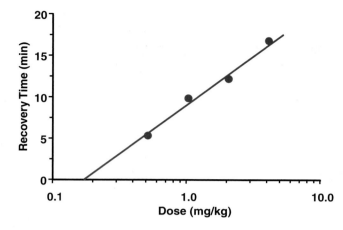

FIGURE 8-21. The time to recover 50% from succinylcholine paralysis (T_{50}) is proportional to the logarithm of the dose injected. (From: Levy G. Kinetics of pharmacologic action of succinylcholine in man. J Pharm Sci 1967;56:1687–1688. The original data are from Walts LF, Dillon JB. Clinical studies of succinylcholine chloride. Anesthesiology 1967;28:372–376.)

(a measure of neuromuscular block after stimulation of a nerve) following i.v. injections of 0.5-, 1-, 2-, and 4-mg/kg bolus doses of succinylcholine. The value of k, estimated from the slope, is 0.2 min^{-1}; the half-life is about 4 min.

To further appreciate the last equation, consider the following statement: "Duration of effect increases by one half-life with each doubling of dose." This must be true. To prove that it is, let a given dose D_O produce a duration of effect, t_D When 2 D_O is given, the amount in the body falls by one half in one half-life, that is, to D_O; the duration of effect beyond one half-life must therefore be t_D. Accordingly, the total duration of effect produced by the larger dose is $t_{1/2} + t_D$. Hence, it follows that the increase in the duration of effect on doubling the dose is one half-life. For example, as 0.5 mg/kg of succinylcholine results in a T_{50} of approximately 6 min, the duration of effect following 1 mg/kg is 10 min (see Fig. 8-21). The increase in the time to recover, 4 min, is the half-life of succinylcholine at the site of action. By inspecting the T_{50} curve in Fig. 8-21, it is apparent that the increase in duration (Δt_D) is the same with each further doubling of the dose.

In the case of succinylcholine, the half-life estimated from the dose–duration-of-action relationship is the elimination half-life of the drug. For some other drugs, such as omeprazole, the situation is more complex. The slow release of drug from the site of action is then a determining factor.

Raising dose to extend duration of effect is not without risks, however, especially for a drug with a short half-life and a narrow window of therapeutic concentrations. For example, to extend the duration of effect by two half-lives, the quadrupled dose required may produce too great an initial response or may substantially increase the chance of toxicity. An alternative and safer approach may well be to prolong the input of drug producing a flatter exposure–time profile. The plasma concentration then remains above the C_{min} for an extended time and the peak concentration is reduced (see Fig. 2-18), both aims of constant-rate infusions (see Chapter 9, *Therapeutic Window*) and some modified-release dosage forms (see Chapter 10, *Constant-Rate Input*), topics of much of the next section, *Therapeutic Regimens.*

KEY RELATIONSHIPS

$$\frac{Rate\ of\ Change}{in\ Body} = Rate\ of\ Input - Rate\ of\ Loss$$

$$Response = E(0) - m \cdot k \cdot t$$

$$t_D = \frac{1}{k}\ ln\left(\frac{Dose}{C_{min} \cdot V}\right)$$

STUDY PROBLEMS

(Answers to Study Problems are in Appendix J.)

1. Define the following terms: effect compartment, direct response, hysteresis, pharmacokinetic rate-limited response, and time delay.

2. Indicate by writing T or F whether the following statements are true or false for the situation in which response is only because of the drug.

    a. Hysteresis in a response versus plasma concentration curve cannot be observed after intravenous bolus administration of the drug.

    b. Between 80% and 20% of maximum effect, a graded response declines exponentially with time after i.v. bolus drug administration.

    c. With quantal responses, response is related to the logarithm of the plasma concentration.

    d. For a drug showing first-order disposition kinetics and producing a graded response, the duration of effect increases linearly with dose.

    e. For responses less than 20% of the maximum, the response is directly proportional to drug concentration only when the steepness factor γ equals one.

    f. One should wait for distribution equilibrium between drug in plasma and that at the site of action to be established before attempting to use plasma monitoring as a guide to therapy.

3. Identify the statements below, if any, that are correct. For those that are not correct or are ambiguous, state why they are so or supply a qualification to make them correct.

    a. Pharmacokinetics, rather than pharmacodynamics, determines the duration of response after an intravenous bolus dose when the response always wears off at the same plasma concentration regardless of the dose given.

    b. For a drug showing one-compartment model characteristic and having a fixed concentration where the effect of the drug drops below some minimum value, halving the dose should always shorten the duration of effect by one half-life.

    c. A common situation in which pharmacodynamics rate limits the change in measured response with time is one in which drug acts directly on either input or output of a sluggish system within the body, and the measured response reflects the state of that system at any point in time.

4. Figure 8-22 shows the relationship between reduction in systolic blood pressure and plasma drug concentration for a drug under steady-state conditions. The line shown is the best fit of the Hill-equation parameters to the data in an individual subject. Estimate the values for E_{max}, C_{50}, and γ.

$$\text{Reduction in Systolic Blood Pressure, mm Hg} = \frac{E_{max} \cdot C^{\gamma}}{C_{50}{}^{\gamma} + C^{\gamma}}$$

5. The following observations displayed in Fig. 8-23A were made for a drug. Clearly, the blood pressure-lowering effect and the plasma concentration do not match in time.

    a. Draw on Fig. 8-23B the relationship you anticipate between measured effect and plasma concentration. Be sure to identify whether the hysteresis is clockwise or counterclockwise.

    b. Give two possible explanations (mechanisms) for the observations in Fig. 8-23B.

6. Give two examples (provided in this chapter) of a situation in which changes in response with time is rate limited by the kinetics of the drug and two that are rate-limited by the dynamics of the affected system.

7. The concentration–response relationship for a drug that produces a graded response is characterized by a C_{50} of 10 mg/L and a γ of 2.5. To be effective, the

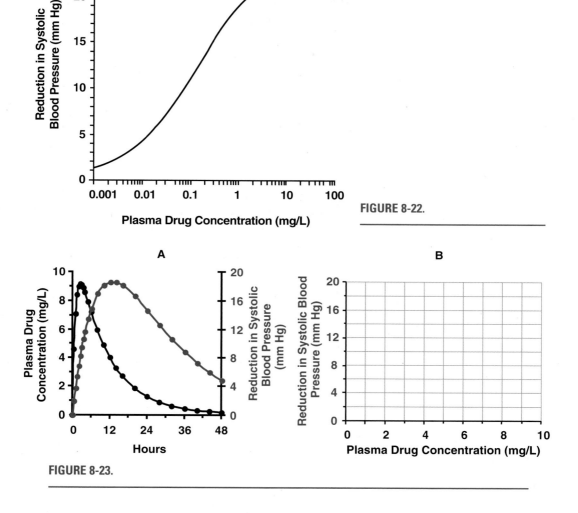

FIGURE 8-22.

FIGURE 8-23.

response to the drug must be kept between 20% and 80% of the maximal value. Calculate the range of concentrations that are needed to achieve this objective. Drug at the site of action equilibrates rapidly with drug in plasma.

8. Propranolol, a β-adrenergic–blocking agent, is used in the treatment of hypertension and angina. One rapid test of its activity is its ability to decrease the heart rate for a given workload, that is reduce exercise tachycardia. McDevitt and Shand (McDevitt DG, Shand DG. Clin Pharmacol Ther 1975;18:708–715) observed a linear relationship between percent reduction in exercise tachycardia and the logarithm of plasma concentration of propranolol. The slope of the line is + 11.5%. Table 8-1 lists the magnitude of effect with time after i.v. bolus administration of 20-mg propranolol.

    a. From the plot of the data in Fig. 8-24, estimate the slope of the response with time and hence the apparent half-life of propranolol in plasma.

    b. Calculate the minimum amount of propranolol needed in the body to achieve a 15% reduction in exercise tachycardia.

TABLE 8-1	Percent Reduction in Exercise Tachycardia with Time Following a 20-mg Intravenous Dose of Propranolol				
Time (hr)	0.25	1	2	4	6
Percent reduction in exercise tachycardia	28	25.5	22	15	8

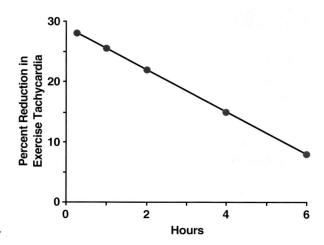

FIGURE 8-24.

c. Calculate how long the reduction in exercise tachycardia is expected to remain above 15% after:
   (1) A 40-mg i.v. bolus dose.
   (2) A 70-mg i.v. bolus dose.

9. A compound is given as an i.v. bolus to a patient requiring a minimum plasma concentration of 4 mg/L for a therapeutic effect. Given that Dose = 100 mg; $k = 0.10$ hr^{-1}; $V = 8$ L, and assuming a one-compartment model,

   a. Calculate how long the clinical effect is expected to last with this dose.
   b. Calculate how long the clinical effect lasts following a 200-mg dose.
   c. Determine the duration of effect following a 100-mg dose, if $k = 0.05$ hr^{-1} and the change in k is a result of
      (1) A twofold decrease in clearance; and
      (2) A doubling of the volume of distribution by increased nonspecific tissue binding.
   d. Does doubling the dose of a drug under the initial conditions ($k = 0.10$ hr^{-1}; $V = 8$ L) yield the same change in duration of clinical effect as doubling the half-life?

10. A drug acts by inhibiting the synthesis of an endogenous substance S (e.g., uric acid, clotting factor); the effect of the drug is measured by monitoring the plasma concentration of S. The scheme of events can be depicted as follows:

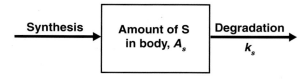

where A_s is the amount of S in the body and k_s is the degradation-rate constant of S. In this scheme, the rate of synthesis of S responds virtually instantaneously to changes in drug concentration.

The times and corresponding plasma concentrations of drug and S when a subject is challenged with a 100-mg i.v. bolus dose of drug are presented in Table 8-2 and data for S are displayed in Fig. 8-25. The pharmacokinetics of the drug are approximated by a one-compartment model in which $k = 0.05 \text{ hr}^{-1}$ and $V = 10$ L. As expected, there is a delay in the maximum lowering of the plasma concentration of S.

TABLE 8-2	Plasma Concentrations of Drug and Endogenous Substance After a Single 100 mg i.v. Bolus of Drug														
Time (hr)	0	2	4	6	8	10	12	16	24	30	36	48	60	72	84
Plasma concentration of drug (mg/L)	10	9.0	8.2	7.4	6.7	6.1	5.5	4.5	3.0	2.2	1.7	0.91	0.5	0.27	0.15
Plasma concentration of endogenous substance, S (% of normal)	100	72	53	40	31	25	21.5	19.1	24.5	32	48	72	88	96	99

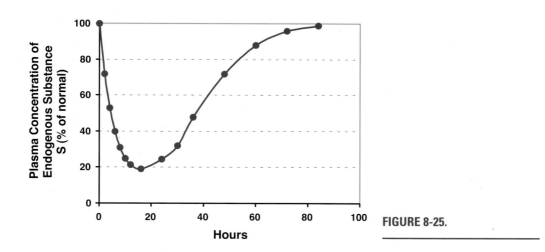

FIGURE 8-25.

Challenging the subject with a 200-mg bolus dose on another occasion did not shorten the time for the concentration of S to initially fall by 50%, it did, of course, cause a deeper and more prolonged depression in the plasma concentration of S.

a. Based on the scheme above and the information given, construct a direct response (inhibition of synthesis) versus plasma drug concentration curve. (Hint: Write the rate equation of S and rearrange it to express the synthesis rate of S as a function of its plasma concentration and its elimination rate constant; you will need to estimate k_s to solve the problem).

b. From the curve produced in part "a," estimate the C_{50} value and comment on the most likely value of γ in the relationship.

$$E = \frac{E_{max} \cdot C^{\gamma}}{C_{50}^{\gamma} + C^{\gamma}}$$

Therapeutic Regimens

9

Therapeutic Window

OBJECTIVES

The reader will be able to:

- Define the terms: dosage regimen, therapeutic effectiveness, therapeutic index, therapeutic utility, therapeutic utility curve, therapeutic window.
- List the factors that determine the dosage regimen of a drug.
- Explain the strategy behind the establishment of a therapeutic window.
- List the range of plasma concentrations associated with therapy within the target patient population for five of the drugs given in Table 9-1.
- Discuss briefly situations in which poor systemic exposure–response relationships may occur.

DOSAGE REGIMENS

The method of drug administration comprising dosage form, dosing rate, size of dose, interval between doses, route of administration, and duration of therapy is called a **dosage regimen**. All substances produce harmful effects if given in high enough amounts, drugs being no exception. Therapeutic dosage regimens are designed to optimize therapy by balancing the risk of ill effects against the benefits achievable with the drug.

In this section, *Therapeutic Regimens*, fundamental aspects of dosage regimens are covered primarily from the point of view of treating a typical patient within the target population with a given disease or condition. It is realized, of course, that individuals vary in their responses to drugs; subsequently, in Section IV, *Individualization*, focus is turned toward optimizing dosage regimens in individual patients.

A dosage regimen is basically derived from the kinds of information shown in Fig. 9-1. This scheme applies essentially to all drugs but particularly to those intended to produce therapeutic effects systemically; for locally acting drugs, local exposure is critical and systemic exposure is more of a safety concern. One consideration is how the body acts on the drug and its dosage form, the essence of pharmacokinetics. Another consideration includes those factors that relate systemic exposure to both efficacy and safety of the drug, pharmacodynamic factors. A third consideration is the clinical state of the patient, which can affect both the pharmacokinetics and the pharmacodynamics of a drug. This includes the disease or condition being treated, other diseases or conditions that the patient may have, as well as associated additional drug therapy—that is, his or her *total* therapeutic regimen. A fourth consideration includes all other factors such as genetics, age and weight, and the extent of adherence by the patient to the dosage regimen. Many of these determinants are interrelated and interdependent. For example, the requirement of

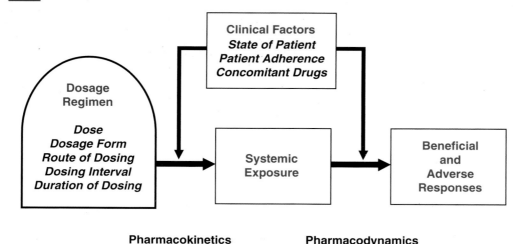

FIGURE 9-1. A dosage regimen of drug comprises dose, dosage form, dosing interval, route of administration, and duration of therapy. These factors are adjusted to achieve an exposure profile that maximizes the benefits compared with adverse effects of the drug. Clinical factors that determine the dosage regimen within a target population include the disease or condition being treated, the presence of other diseases and conditions, and other concomitantly administered drugs. These and other factors affect the regimen by influencing the drug's pharmacokinetics, pharmacodynamics, or both.

frequent dosing can reduce adherence to a regimen and influence clinical outcome, whereas clinical outcome, particularly adverse effects without perceived benefit, can influence adherence even when maintenance of the regimen is critical to the ultimate therapeutic benefit. Also critical to our understanding and to the optimal design and application of dosage regimens are changes in dosage requirements with time. The status of a patient is never static and, in addition to changes that occur soon after drug administration, there are often progressive changes in the disease or condition over the time span of treatment, particularly when the treatment extends over many months, years, or the rest of one's life. Such changes need to be taken into account when assessing the effectiveness and safety of the drug.

Dosage regimens involve using various modalities of drug administration, extending from a single or occasional dose to continuous and constant input. An example of the former is the use of aspirin to treat an occasional headache; the continuous intravenous infusion of heparin to maintain a desired degree of anticoagulation in a patient with deep vein thrombosis is an example of the latter. More commonly, drugs are administered repeatedly in discrete doses. The frequency and duration vary with the condition being treated. For many drugs, maintenance of a relatively constant systemic exposure is needed to maintain a therapeutic effect, which may, for example, be achieved by giving the drug three times daily during the treatment. Other drugs do not require such a strict maintenance of systemic exposure and can be given relatively infrequently, which results in larger fluctuations in the systemic exposure–time profile. Reasons for this latter approach being therapeutically desirable include the development of tolerance to the desired effect of the drug if exposure is maintained; the need to produce high exposure for relatively short periods of time, as occurs in some antibiotic and anticancer chemotherapies; and persistence of drug effect even when the drug has been eliminated, as discussed in Chapter 8, *Response Following a Single Dose*. In all cases, the intent is to achieve effective therapy as safely as possible.

In this chapter, various elements of the dose–response and systemic exposure–response relationships in the context of dosage regimens are explored; these build on principles developed in Chapter 2, *Fundamental Concepts and Terminology* and Chapter 8, *Response*

Following a Single Dose. Principles for achieving a desired exposure–time profile are discussed in the subsequent two chapters of this section, *Constant-Rate Input* (Chapter 10) and *Multiple-Dose Regimens* (Chapter 11).

THERAPEUTIC EXPOSURE

Historically, the range of doses of a drug initially tested in patients has been almost entirely empirical, observing desired and adverse effects and adjusting doses accordingly. Today, the choice of test doses is increasingly based on a combination of prior information on the pharmacokinetics of the drug and concentration–response relationships derived from in vitro and animal studies. However, much uncertainty still remains that can only be addressed through experimentation in the target patient population. During early clinical evaluation, usually involving a few hundred patients at most, detailed systemic exposure–response relationships are developed, which help to define a range of therapeutic useful dosage regimens of a drug. Often, however, much more limited systemic exposure data are gathered during the subsequent large-scale clinical trials, generally involving many thousands of patients. The therapeutic window between ineffective therapy and excessive adverse effects is then defined clinically in terms of the doses of drug administered rather than plasma concentration.

Figure 9-2 displays data that typically might be found for a drug evaluated within the target patient population. Shown are the percent of the patients who did not respond,

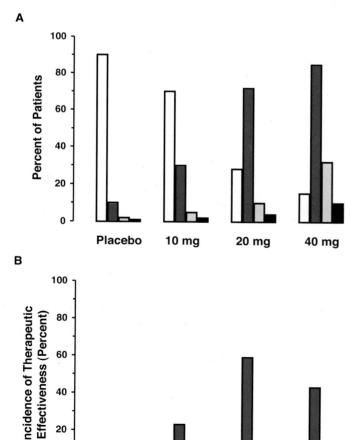

FIGURE 9-2. **A.** Frequencies (percent of patients on each treatment) of ineffective therapy (*white*), effective therapy (*colored*), minor adverse effects (*gray*), and severe toxicity (*black*) observed in a target population in which patients were assigned randomly to receive: a placebo, 10 mg, 20 mg, or 40 mg of a drug once daily. **B.** The incidence of "therapeutic effectiveness" for the four groups of patients displayed in panel A. Therapeutic effectiveness is defined arbitrarily as the difference between the frequency of effective therapy and the frequency of all harmful effects; the therapeutic effectiveness of this drug reaches a maximum at 20 mg.

those who experienced a beneficial effect, those who experienced minor adverse effects, and those who experienced severe adverse responses following daily administration of either a placebo or a 10-, 20-, or 40-mg dose of a drug to different cohorts of patients. As is commonly the case, the drug was considered effective when the desired response reached a given endpoint, such as a lowering of systolic blood pressure by at least 10 mm Hg in hypertensive patients. Adverse effects were considered minor, such as an occasional transient headache, and severe, when the harmful effects necessitated discontinuation of the drug. In practice, there may be finer divisions of adverse effects, such as minor, moderate, serious, and severe.

First, notice that, as is common in clinical practice, a graded response, which is lowering of blood pressure, has been transformed into a quantal response by setting a fixed endpoint as a measure of effectiveness. Along similar lines, an adverse effect, such as increase in heart rate, tachycardia, which is graded, is often divided into degrees of severity, and obviously, a person can only be in one category at a time. Accordingly, it is the sum of all such adverse events that has a maximum probability of 1. Second, it is not uncommon that even on placebo, some patients perceive benefit and some adverse effects even though they have not been exposed to drug. Third, some patients fail to gain clinical benefit even at the highest dose. Next, the incidences of beneficial and harmful responses are all significantly greater in those patients receiving the drug than those receiving the placebo, with the incidence of increasing responses as the daily dose increases. Such information provides an estimate of the likelihood of a patient to experience effective treatment without adverse effects, by subtracting, for example, the sum of the incidences of the adverse responses from that of the beneficial one, a measure of the **therapeutic effectiveness** of the drug (Fig. 9-2B). This difference measure is greater for all doses tested than for placebo, suggesting the drug has merit over the placebo. It also increases up to 20-mg dose and then declines at the 40-mg dose, because the increase in the incidence of harmful effects exceeds that of the beneficial one, suggesting that the optimal dose is 20 mg daily. However, in practice, due regard also needs to be taken of the relative weight to be assigned to measures of benefit and harm when estimating the dose or window of doses, for which therapeutic success is most probable. Obviously, severe adverse effects should be given more weight than minor or moderate ones. For this drug, the incidence may be considered to be so frequent at 40 mg that the upper dose should be limited to 20 mg.

Although helpful in exploring doses, this approach to understanding the therapeutic value of the drug leaves many questions unanswered. Why, for example, did some patients fail to respond beneficially even at the highest dose tested? And, why did others experience benefit with minimal adverse effects even at the highest dose, whereas others experienced severe adverse effects at the 20-mg dose?

These and other questions are often better addressed by exploring response as a function of systemic exposure to the drug, rather than dose administered. Certainly, systemic exposure is better than dose after a single dose of drug, when intensity of a response varies with time, especially for an acute response that correlates directly with drug concentration at all times, because with dose alone, time is not taken into account. It may also be true for long-term drug administration but for a different reason.

The objective of much of drug therapy is to maintain a stable therapeutic response for the duration of treatment, usually by maintaining the same daily dosage of drug. Recalling Fig. 1-7 (Chapter 1, *Therapeutic Relevance*, page 9), it shows the relationship between the plasma concentration and the daily dose/kg body weight of the antiepileptic drug, phenytoin, in a patient population receiving the drug chronically. Notice the large interindividual differences in the plasma concentration at any given daily dose; in the patient cohort studied, the plasma concentration ranged from nearly 0 to 50 mg/L when the daily dose was 6 mg/kg. Had no correction been made for body weight, the deviations at a given dose might have been even greater if body weight captured some of the variability in the pharmacokinetics of the drug. In contrast, plasma concentration correlates reasonably well with effect. Thus, seizures are usually effectively controlled without undue adverse events at plasma phenytoin concentrations between 10 and 20 mg/L. For this drug, plasma concentration is a better correlate than dose during chronic administration because pharmacokinetics is the major source of variability between dose and response. For other drugs, such as atenolol, used to lower blood pressure, pharmacokinetic variability within the patient population is relatively small, and variability in the concentration–response curve is large. In such cases, plasma concentration is no better a correlate with response than dose and indeed may be worse if, for example, metabolites contribute to activity and toxicity (see "Additional Considerations" later). Even then, understanding systemic exposure– response relationships is critically important in anticipating therapeutic outcome when the systemic exposure changes dramatically despite maintaining dose, for example, during some drug interactions and in the presence of diseases, such as hepatic and renal function impairment that may markedly diminish clearance. Moreover, without exploring the systemic exposure–response relationships, one can never know where the source of the major variability lies and how to develop methods for accommodating for it.

Returning to the study reported in Fig. 9-2, consider the same incidence data but now plotted in Fig. 9-3 as a function of the systemic exposure to the drug, rather than daily dose. Note that although concentration is a continuous function, each patient only contributes one value or at most a few values. Advantage is taken here that often, as seen with phenytoin and found in this study, patients have different systemic exposures for the same dose, thereby allowing us to explore concentration–response relationships within the

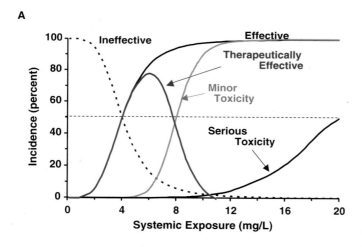

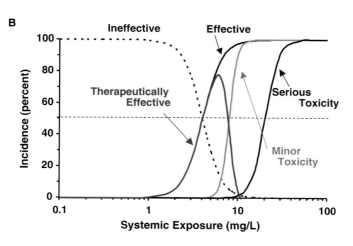

FIGURE 9-3. A,B. Plots of frequency of ineffective therapy, effective therapy, minor adverse effects, serious toxicity, and "therapeutic effectiveness" (effectiveness minus that of the sum of minor and serious toxicity) with systemic exposure of the drug (A: linear scale; B: logarithmic scale) obtained from the same study reported in Fig. 9-2. The therapeutic effectiveness (*colored line*) of this drug, defined as in Fig. 9-2, reaches a peak at about 6 mg/L. To ensure a therapeutic effectiveness of a least 50% of the patient population, the plasma concentration needs to lie between 3 and 11 mg/L.

population over a more continuous and wider range of values than can be achieved with the three doses studied. Clearly, it would have been preferable had each patient been studied on several doses to obtain individual dose–concentration–response relationships, but for various reasons, generally patients are assigned randomly to one of the various treatments in clinical trails, an aspect considered further in Chapter 12, *Variability*. Notice that not all patients were effectively treated even when exposed to the highest concentrations; these are nonresponders. Such nonresponders may unknowingly lack the target receptor, and no amount of exposure to drug will help. Others may have a genetically different target receptor that requires a higher-than-normal exposure to the drug. For them, the solution may be to increase the dose (exposure), provided adverse effects do not become excessive. Here again, the issue may be one of inaccurate diagnosis or misdiagnosis. For example, knowing that a patient suffers from cancer or an inflammatory disease does not guarantee that a particular anticancer or anti-inflammatory drug will be effective. Clearly, improvements in the accuracy of diagnosis should decrease the number of such nonresponders receiving a drug. Alternatively, lack of response may be caused by a very low exposure to the drug even at the highest dose tested (40 mg in this study) because of a very high clearance in these patients, and again for these, a still higher dose may be warranted. Lastly, there are patients who had no or very low systemic exposure because they adhered poorly to the protocol, some even not taking the drug (despite claiming that they did).

It should also be noted in Fig. 9-3 that, as expected, frequency and severity of adverse effects increase with increasing concentration of drug. Thus, serious toxicity begins to appear above 6 mg/L and occurs with increasing frequency at higher concentrations across the patient population. Above 12 mg/L, the major adverse effect may prove fatal in some patients. From these collective data, it can be concluded that for this drug, the range of concentrations associated with effective therapy without undue harm is 3 to 11 mg/L. This range is commonly known as the **therapeutic concentration range** of the drug.

Another important observation made during the study was that not all patients receiving the drug needed plasma concentrations between 3 and 11 mg/L. In a few, the drug was effective at concentrations below 3 mg/L; in others, moderate or severe toxicity occurs before efficacy, and for them, this is certainly not the drug of choice. Accordingly, a therapeutic concentration is most appropriately defined in terms of an individual patient's requirement by varying dose within the patient and observing clinical outcome. Usually, however, this information is unknown, and on initiating therapy, the targeted therapeutic concentration range must be based on that gained from the probability of therapeutic success within the typical patient population.

Also shown in Fig. 9-3 is a curve that represents the frequency of therapeutic effectiveness, that is, the frequency of effective therapy minus the frequency of all adverse effects, showing a maximum around 6 mg/L. At higher concentrations, the increasing risk of harm tends to outweigh increasing benefits of the drug. However, as when considering dose–response data, pay attention to the relative weight to be assigned to measures of benefit and harm.

Let us expand philosophically on this concept of weighting using the information in Fig. 9-3, adding to serious adverse effects hypersensitivity, a potentially life-threatening effect, experienced by the occasional patient as occurs with penicillin and aspirin, and assigning values to the responses according to our best judgment. Figure 9-4 shows the probabilities of the responses, each weighted by a judgmental factor, versus the logarithm of the plasma concentration. The factor is negative for undesirable effects and positive for desirable ones. On algebraically adding the weighted probabilities, a **therapeutic utility curve** is obtained that shows the chance of net therapeutic benefit as a function of the plasma concentration. Note that both low and high concentrations have negative therapeutic utility; that is, at these concentrations, the drug is potentially more harmful than helpful. Again, we see that there is a range of concentrations within which the chances of net benefit are greatest.

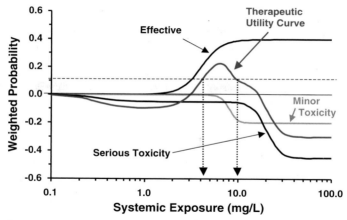

FIGURE 9-4. Schematic diagram of the weighted probabilities of responses versus the plasma concentration of a drug in the target patient population. The probabilities from Fig. 9-3 (plus a hypersensitivity reaction as part of the serious adverse effects) are weighted by the following factors: desired effect, 0.4; minor adverse effect, −0.2; serious toxicity, −1. The line for serious toxicity at low plasma concentrations, which is associated with hypersensitivity, has been exaggerated for illustrative purposes. The algebraic sum of the weighted probabilities versus plasma concentration is the therapeutic utility curve. According to this scheme, which down weights efficacy compared to serious toxicity by a factor of 2.5, the highest weighted probability of therapeutic success occurs at 6 mg/L. The therapeutic window is given by the range of exposures associated with a therapeutic utility being equal or greater than some preset value, in this case, 0.10. For this drug, the therapeutic window is in the region 4 to approximately 10 mg/L, over which range the probability of achieving efficacy rises from approximately 50% and 96% (see Fig. 9-3). Below 4 mg/L and above 10 mg/L, the drug is considered potentially more harmful than beneficial. Obviously, the width of the therapeutic window varies with the assigned relative weightings and the preset value of the therapeutic utility.

The value of the therapeutic utility function mentioned above which therapy is defined as successful depends on the condition or disease being treated. When treating hypertension, the level is set very high because there are many relatively safe and effective antihypertensive drugs already available. Whereas, in the treatment of Alzheimer disease or brain tumors, for which there is a paucity of safe and highly effective drugs, the acceptable level for the therapeutic utility would be much lower. Keep also in mind that ineffective therapy itself has potential adverse consequences. For example, during this period of drug treatment, the underlying disease may continue to progress or, in organ transplantation, rejection may occur. Further, it is important to appreciate that equal values of the therapeutic utility function on either side of the maximum are not clinically equivalent. For a given value, although a greater percent of patients experience therapeutic benefit, more also experience adverse effects at higher than lower systemic exposures to the drug and, one may not wish to go beyond the maximum therapeutic utility. This is not always possible, however. With some cancer chemotherapy, for example, it is not uncommon for patients to receive the maximum tolerated dose because even then not all of them experience the desired benefit.

In the current example, making the assumption that to be of value the therapeutic utility should be above 0.10, we can conclude that there is a range of plasma concentrations (3.5–10 mg/L) associated with successful therapy, the therapeutic plasma concentration window, or simply the **therapeutic window** of the drug. Notice, by reference to Fig. 9-3, over this range of concentration, the probability of achieving efficacy rises from approximately 45% to 96% of the patient population. Also, the window would have been different if we had accepted a different level for the therapeutic utility or restricted it to only the rising part of the curve, although clearly, it would always need to be positive for the drug

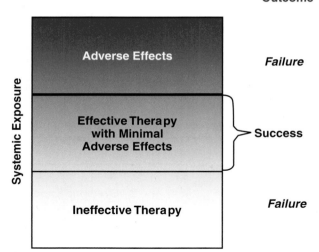

FIGURE 9-5. Schematic diagram depicting the therapeutic window of a drug, which lies between two regions of exposure associated with therapeutic failure. The lower region of failure is principally caused by the absence of adequate efficacy, whereas the upper region is caused by an inability to have adequate efficacy without an unacceptable adverse response.

to have any benefit. Precise limits, of course, are not definable, particularly considering the subjective nature of the utility curve. Each drug produces its own peculiar responses and the weighting assigned to these responses differ, but both the incidence of the drug effects and the relative benefit to risk ratio must be evaluated to determine the therapeutic concentration range. It is always done, but perhaps not so quantitatively. Finally, in practice, considerations are not made in isolation but often involve considering the benefit to risk of one drug against that of another drug operating on the same target, or when the mechanism for the two drugs, for the same indication, are different. This is particularly the case when a reasonable effective treatment is already available. Ethical considerations ultimately require comparison with the standard treatment and not a placebo.

This concept of a therapeutic window based on systemic concentration is depicted in Fig. 9-5. At exposures below the window, therapy is deemed a failure because the probability of efficacy is too low despite the virtual absence of adverse effects. At exposures above the window, therapy is also deemed likely to fail; in this case, although the probability of efficacy is higher, the probability of having adequate efficacy without toxicity is too low. In other words, the risk of harm outweighs the potential benefit from the therapeutic effect. In addition to the weighting of desired and undesired effects, there is also the matter of the intensity of these responses. In general, as discussed in Chapter 8, *Response Following a Single Dose,* intensity tends to increase with increasing exposure to the drug. This is seen, for example, in Fig. 9-6, which shows that the severity or depth of

FIGURE 9-6. The severity of the untoward effects of phenytoin increases (shown as increasing size of solid circle) from nystagmus to mental changes with its concentration in plasma. The values given are the plasma concentrations where the response was first reported. (From: Kutt H, Winters W, Kokenge R, et al. Diphenylhydantoin metabolism, blood levels, and toxicity. Arch Neurol 1964;11:642–648.)

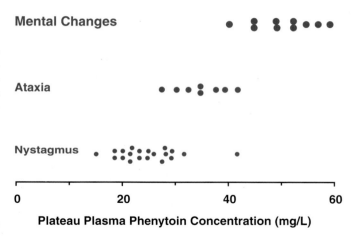

central nervous system depression increases with increasing exposure to phenytoin, which is used in the treatment of epilepsy. The first sign of adverse effects is usually nystagmus (jerky eye movement), which appears above a concentration of approximately 20 mg/L; gait ataxia (unsteadiness) usually appears with a concentration approaching 30 mg/L; and prolonged drowsiness and lethargy may be seen at concentrations greater than 40 mg/L.

There are often problems associated with both the acquisition and interpretation of the incidence, importance, and intensity of the various responses as a function of systemic exposure, especially in clinical practice. For example, in clinical practice, quite frequently patients are titrated with a drug. So a high systemic exposure may result either because the patient failed to respond at a lower dose and the dose was increased without undue toxicity, or because the patient on the usual dosage had diminished clearance due for example to disease, which also predisposed them to toxicity. To avoid this potential bias in interpretation, each patient should be titrated through all the responses. This is, of course, ethically unacceptable. Our information on toxicity must come from the patient who, for one reason or another, exhibits toxicity because the drug concentration is excessive or who has an unusual response at a low concentration.

Therapeutic exposures, expressed in terms of the range of plasma concentrations associated with successful therapy of the patient population with specific conditions, are listed in Table 9-1 for selected drugs. These are drugs that patients are generally taking for relatively long periods of time, measured in months or years, and sometimes a lifetime. The concentrations are generally those obtained just before the next dose (trough concentrations) during such chronic therapy, an aspect discussed in greater detail in Chapter 11, *Multiple-Dose Regimens.* Several points are worth noting. First, for most of

TABLE 9-1	Selected Drugs and Their Plasma Concentrations Usually Associated with Successful Therapy*		
		Therapeutic Window	
Drug	**Disease/Condition**	**(mg/L)**	**(μm)**
Cyclosporine	Organ transplantation	0.15–0.4[†]	0.13–0.34
Digoxin	Cardiac dysfunction	0.0006–0.002	0.0008–0.003
Efavirenz	HIV Infection	1–4	3.2–13
Gentamicin	Gram-negative infection	5–8[‡]	9–14
		1–2[††]	2–3.5
Lithium	Manic and recurrent depression	—	0.6–0.8[‡‡]
Nortriptyline	Endogenous depression	0.05–0.15	0.2–0.6
Phenytoin	Epilepsy	10–20	30–60
	Ventricular arrhythmias	10–20	30–60
Theophylline	Asthma and chronic obstructive		
	Airway diseases	5–15	28–75
	Apnea	5–10	28–55
Warfarin	Thromboembolic diseases	1–4	3–13
Valproic acid	Epilepsy	40–100	280–690

*Generally, a trough concentration during chronic treatment.
[†]Whole blood.
[‡]Thirty min after a 30-min infusion.
[††]Trough concentration.
[‡‡]Trough concentration expressed in milliequivalents/liter.

these drugs, the therapeutic concentration range is narrow; the upper and lower limits differ by a factor of only 2 or 3. Of course, for many other drugs, the range of therapeutic exposures is much wider. Second, some drugs are used to treat several diseases, and the concentration needed may differ with the disease. For example, a lower range of concentrations of theophylline is needed to abolish episodes of recurring apnea in premature infants than is needed to substantially improve pulmonary function in patients with chronic airway diseases. Next, the upper limit of the plasma concentration may be, like the tricyclic antidepressant nortriptyline, a result of diminishing effectiveness at higher concentrations without noticeable signs of increasing toxicity. Or, it may be, like the immunosuppressive agent cyclosporine, used to prevent organ rejection after transplantation, a result of an increased likelihood of renal toxicity. The upper concentration limit may also be caused by the drug being limited in its effectiveness, as with ibuprofen, which is ineffective in relieving pain suffered during severe trauma, when a more potent analgesic is needed. Finally, an adverse effect may be either an extension of the pharmacologic property of the drug, or it may be totally dissociated from its therapeutic effect. The hemorrhagic tendency associated with an excessive plasma concentration of the oral anticoagulant warfarin is an example of the former; the ototoxicity caused by the antibiotic gentamicin is an example of the latter.

It is to be stressed that significant interindividual patient variability occurs in both the efficacy–exposure and adverse response–exposure curves, leading to differences among individuals in the magnitude and location of the therapeutic utility as well as the width of the therapeutic window. This should be kept in mind when considering the data in Table 9-1. The values are derived from patient populations requiring the drugs, and they apply to the typical patient within those populations. Also, the ultimate objective is to treat each patient as efficaciously and safely as possible and not to keep his or her plasma concentrations within the recommended therapeutic window. This window can serve as a useful guide, however, particularly in the absence of additional information about the individual. When combined with pharmacokinetic information, the therapeutic window helps to define the dosage regimen to be used when initiating therapy. Clearly, however, as emphasized previously in this chapter, systemic exposure is particularly informative when pharmacokinetics is the major source of interindividual variability in the dose–response relationships for efficacy and harmful effects, a point considered in greater detail in Chapter 12, *Variability*.

In many therapeutic situations, several drugs are used in combination to treat a given condition or disease. An example is the use of a thiazide diuretic, a β-blocker, and an angiotensin-converting enzyme inhibitor in the treatment of hypertension. Each drug acts on a different part of the cardiovascular system to lower blood pressure. Another is the combination of methotrexate with a nonsteroidal anti-inflammatory agent to relieve pain associated with rheumatoid arthritis. Given that the adverse effects of drugs are often unrelated to their therapeutic effects, the advantage of such combinations is that the dose of each needed to produce a given therapeutic effect may be lower than if given alone, thereby reducing the likelihood of adverse effects. A combination of drugs is also often used in the treatment of infectious diseases, but for a somewhat different reason. For example, in the treatment of human immunodeficiency virus (HIV) infection, patients are likely to receive a combination of one or two nucleoside/nucleotide reverse transcriptase inhibitors (that produce faulty versions of the building block that the virus needs to make more copies of itself thereby stalling its reproduction), together with either a nonnucleoside reverse transcriptase inhibitor or a protease inhibitor (which inhibits the protease enzyme, an essential protein for generating replication competent virus). Each drug acts on a different critical pathway of the viral apparatus such that together they achieve a greater benefit than is possible with any one drug alone, thereby reducing the chances of the emergence of resistant strains. Moreover, the combination allows the use of lower doses of each drug and again reduces the chances of associated adverse effects. Combinations may also allow the use of lower doses of one or more drugs if one of the drugs increases the systemic exposure of the other drugs, as in the case of ritonavir use in combination therapy in HIV treatment (see also Chapter 17, *Drug Interactions*).

THERAPEUTIC INDEX

A concept related to therapeutic window is **therapeutic index**. This index reflects how sensitive *an individual patient* is to the limiting effects of a drug on changing exposure, usually noticed in practice when a dose during chronic therapy is increased. The index is low when the dose giving the desired therapeutic effect is very close to that giving too high a probability of limiting adverse effects. Examples of low therapeutic index drugs are warfarin and digoxin. Minor increases in exposure with these drugs can tip a patient into unacceptable risk. In contrast to these drugs, most other drugs have a moderate-to-high therapeutic index; for them, patients are relatively insensitive to a change in dose, although it is always good practice to use as low a dose as possible commensurate with adequate effectiveness.

ADDITIONAL CONSIDERATIONS

Despite its appeal, measurement of plasma concentration, as an index of systemic exposure, to guide therapy is uncommon in clinical practice (see Chapter 18, *Initiating and Managing Therapy*). One major reason, besides the extra cost and resources required, is that for many drugs, there are direct and simple means of using therapeutic and adverse responses to guide therapy. Furthermore, the concentration may not give a good indication of the response, particularly if there is considerable variability in the concentration–response relationship. Even then, appreciating the relationship among drug administration, systemic exposure, and response over time aids in the rational use of such drugs. Another major reason for not monitoring plasma concentration is the wide margin of safety of many drugs, such as many antibiotics, so that high and effective doses may be given to virtually all patients, the exception being those with a known allergy to the drug, or when a large change in drug disposition (e.g., in a patient with renal or hepatic disease) is anticipated. However, another is that plasma concentration often correlates poorly with measured response. One example, discussed more fully in Chapter 10, *Constant-Rate Input*, is the development of tolerance to the drug whereby response diminishes with time despite maintenance of the plasma concentration. Some other examples of poor correlations with explanations, where known, follow.

MULTIPLE ACTIVE SPECIES

Many drugs are converted to active metabolites in the body. Unless these metabolites are also measured, poor correlations with the drug concentration alone may exist. For example, based on its plasma concentration, alprenolol is more active as a β-blocker when given as a single oral dose than when administered intravenously. This drug is highly cleared on single passage through the liver; so in terms of the parent drug, the oral dose is poorly bioavailable. However, large amounts of metabolites, including an active species, 4-hydroxyalprenolol, are formed during the absorption process, which explains the above apparent discrepancy.

The tricyclic antidepressant amitriptyline offers a second example. Its antidepressant activity correlates poorly with the plasma concentration of parent drug. Only when the contribution of its active desmethyl metabolite, nortriptyline, is also considered can more useful correlations be established. The analgesic activity after administration of codeine is thought to arise from its partial conversion to morphine; clearly, trying to correlate analgesic activity with codeine concentration alone is not likely to be highly successful. Further examples are discussed in Chapter 20, *Metabolites and Drug Response*.

SINGLE-DOSE THERAPY

One dose of aspirin often relieves a headache, which may not return even when the drug has been completely eliminated. Other examples of effective single-dose therapy include albuterol nebulizer to treat an acute asthmatic attack, nitroglycerin to relieve an acute episode of angina, and morphine to relieve acute pain. Although the specific mechanism of action may be poorly understood, the overall effect is known; the drug returns an out-of-balance physiologic system to within normal bounds. Thereafter, feedback control systems within the body maintain homeostasis. The need for drug has now ended. In these instances of single-dose therapy, a correlation between beneficial effect and peak exposure to drug may exist, but beyond the peak, any such correlation is unlikely.

DURATION VERSUS INTENSITY OF EXPOSURE

Another complexity is the relationship between effect, dose, and duration of therapy. Some chemotherapeutic agents, such as methotrexate, exhibit peculiar relationships between response and dose. The response observed relates more closely to the duration of dosing than to the actual dose used or concentrations produced. This behavior for methotrexate can be explained by its activity as an antimetabolite. It inhibits dihydrofolate reductase, an enzyme that plays a critical role in the building of DNA and other body constituents. This enzyme is involved in the synthesis of folic acid, a molecule that shuttles carbon atoms through methylation to enzymes that need them in their reactions. These reactions can be inhibited for short periods of time, such as a few days, without causing irreversible damage, particularly in cells that turnover rapidly, but not longer. Although all attempts are made to minimize the latter risk, occasionally signs of inadvertent methotrexate toxicity are seen in patients. This is particularly true for high-dose methotrexate therapy. Then leucovorin, which is converted to folic acid within the body, is given to prevent any further adverse effect of methotrexate. Another example is seen with corticosteroids. Massive doses can be administered acutely for the treatment of anaphylactic shock without significant adverse effects; yet, when small doses are administered chronically for the treatment of some debilitating inflammatory conditions, some patients develop a cushingoid state, characterized by a moonface and a buffalo hump associated with excessive deposits of fat on the face and back caused by a sustained state of higher-than-normal circulating corticosteroid.

TIME DELAYS

As discussed in Chapter 8, *Response Following a Single Dose* (and again in Chapter 10, *Constant-Rate Input*, and Chapter 11, *Multiple-Dose Regimens*), correlation between systemic exposure and response can be complicated owing to time delays, which are caused by time needed for drug to reach the active site, or because it takes time for the body to respond to the systemic exposure. Both types of complication tend to diminish on chronic medication when exposure and response become relatively stable with time, although this is not always so. It may take decades to develop cancer following the chronic administration of a carcinogenic drug. Furthermore, some effects, such as fetotoxicity, are apparent only in pregnant females and even then only during a specific period of fetal development in utero.

ACHIEVING THERAPEUTIC GOALS

We now look to integrate the concept of therapeutic window with the basic principles for establishing and evaluating dosage regimens for those drugs that show reasonably valid and stable correlations of response with exposure and dose. Chapter 10, *Constant-Rate Input*, examines features of constant-rate input regimens, and Chapter 11, *Multiple-Dose Regimens*, examines the principles underlying the administration of drug in discrete repetitive doses, to attain and maintain successful therapy.

STUDY PROBLEMS

(Answers to Study Problems are in Appendix J.)

1. Define the following terms listed in Objective 1 of this chapter: dosage regimen, therapeutic index, therapeutic utility, therapeutic utility curve, therapeutic window.

2. List and briefly discuss the major factors determining the dosage regimens of drugs.

3. Briefly discuss why response (desired or adverse) is often better correlated with drug exposure than dose.

4. List the plasma concentration ranges commonly associated with successful therapy with cyclosporine, digoxin, gentamicin, lithium, and theophylline. More generally, give three situations that limit the upper bound of the therapeutic window of a drug.

5. State why a combination of drugs may be beneficial in drug therapy to treat a specific disease or condition, and give two examples of such combinations.

6. Give three examples of situations in which a complexity arises in attempting to correlate response to systemic drug exposure.

7. Listed in Table 9-2 are the probabilities of achieving efficacy and experiencing adverse effects as a function of the plasma concentration of a drug in a target patient population.

   a. Complete columns C and D in the table by entering the therapeutic utility (the algebraic sum of the weighted probabilities for efficacy and adverse responses, expressed as a percent) when the weighting for the adverse effect is assigned a value of -1 and the weighting for beneficial response $+1$ (column C) and $+0.6$ (column D), that is down weighted relative to the adverse effect, in essence giving a higher weighting to safety than efficacy.

Column	A	B	C	D
Plasma Drug Concentration (mg/L)	Probability of Efficacy (%)	Probability of Adverse Response (%)	Therapeutic Utility when Weighting Efficacy +1	Therapeutic Utility when Weighting Efficacy +0.6
0	2.5	1.5		
0.5	7.4	1.5		
1.0	20.1	1.9		
1.5	35.7	3.2		
2.0	51.7	5.1		
2.5	65.8	14.9		
3.0	76.3	33.3		
3.5	82.9	53.6		
4.0	86.0	64.6		
4.5	87.5	69.0		
5.0	90.1	70.9		

TABLE 9-2 Plasma Concentration, Probability of Response (Desired, Adverse), and Therapeutic Utility Following Drug Administration

b. Construct a plot of the probability of therapeutic utility versus the plasma drug concentration for the two scenarios (columns C and D), to yield therapeutic utility curves, and calculate the corresponding therapeutic plasma concentration windows when the acceptable therapeutic utility is set at 20%.

c. Discuss your findings with respect to the impact of weighting on the therapeutic window of the drug, and generally, keeping in mind the percent of patients that are likely to be effectively treated when the plasma concentration is kept within the therapeutic window.

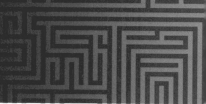

CHAPTER 10

Constant-Rate Input

OBJECTIVES

The reader will be able to:

- Define steady-state (or plateau) plasma concentration and describe the factors controlling it.
- Describe the relationship between half-life of a drug and time required to approach steady state following a constant-rate input with or without a bolus dose.
- Estimate the values of half-life, volume of distribution, and clearance of a drug from plasma concentration data obtained during and following constant-rate intravenous (i.v.) input.
- Determine the bolus dose needed to achieve the same amount in the body, or same plasma concentration, as that achieved at steady state on infusing the drug at a given rate.
- Determine the input rate needed to maintain the bolus amount in the body, or the initial plasma concentration, with time after giving an i.v. bolus dose.
- Use pharmacokinetic parameters to predict the plasma concentration and the amount in the body with time during and following constant-rate input with or without a bolus dose.
- Briefly discuss why short-term infusions are generally used when a single i.v. dose is called for.
- Predict changes in the concentration–time course of a drug during and after a constant-rate infusion when there is an alteration in a physiologic variable that may influence the pharmacokinetics of a drug.
- Briefly discuss how either the pharmacokinetics or pharmacodynamics of a drug can affect the onset of drug effect during a constant-rate i.v. infusion or the continuance of effect after stopping an infusion.

A single dose may rapidly produce a desired therapeutic concentration, but this mode of administration is unsuitable when careful maintenance of plasma or tissue concentrations and effect is desired. To maintain a constant plasma concentration, drug must be administered at a constant rate. This is most often accomplished by infusing drug intravenously. No other mode of administration provides such precise and readily controlled systemic drug input. One major advantage of this method of administration is that drug input can be stopped instantly if adverse effects occur. In contrast to extravascular administration, for which drug input continues, the drug concentration immediately begins to decrease when an i.v. infusion is stopped. A disadvantage of this form of administration is that it is usually restricted to institutional settings. Examples of drugs routinely given by i.v. infusion are listed in Table 10-1. Some, like sedative–hypnotics and analgesics, which

TABLE 10-1	Examples of Drugs Given by Intravenous Infusion	

Drug	Indication	Administration
Bivalirudin	Anticoagulant in patients with unstable angina undergoing percutaneous transluminal coronary angioplasty	Bolus of 1 mg/kg followed by a 4-hr infusion at a rate of 2.5 mg/kg per hour. An additional infusion of 0.2 mg/kg per hr for up to 20 hr may be given if needed.
Cladribine	Hairy cell leukemia	Continuous infusion of 0.09 mg/kg/ per day for 7 days.
Cytarabine	Acute myeloid leukemia	100 mg/m^2 daily by continuous infusion for 7 days.
Eptifibatide	Acute coronary syndrome and for patients undergoing percutaneous coronary intervention	Bolus of 180 μg/kg followed by an infusion of 2.0 μg/kg per min until hospital discharge or initiation of coronary artery bypass graft for up to 96 hr.
Esmolol Hydrochloride	For rapid control of supraventricular and intraoperative and postoperative tachycardia	A loading dose of 0.5 mg/kg infused over 1 min, followed by 0.05 mg/kg per min for 4 min and then increased, as necessary, in steps of at least 4-min duration to a maximum of 0.2 mg/kg per min.
Fentanyl	Treatment of severe chronic pain	Initiate at 5–50 μg/hr and titrate to individual patient's needs.
Heparin	For prevention of venous thrombosis	A loading dose of 5000–10,000 units, followed immediately by a nominal constant-rate infusion of 1000 units/hr, but individualization is required.
Nesiritide	Patients with acutely decompensated congestive heart failure who have dyspnea	Bolus dose of 2 μg/kg followed by continuous infusion of 0.01 μg/kg per min.
Nicardipine Hydrochloride	Short-term treatment of hypertension when oral therapy is not feasible or not desirable	Therapy is initiated with 5 mg/hr. If desired blood pressure reduction is not achieved at this rate, the rate may be increased by 2.5 mg/hr every 5 min up to 15 mg/hr. Once the goal is achieved, the rate is adjusted to maintain the desired response.
Propofol	Sedative-hypnotic for induction and maintenance of anesthesia	Must be individualized. Typically start at 5 μg/kg per min and increase in increments of 5–10 μg/kg per min until desired effect is achieved.
Remifentanil	Pain medicine used before and/or during surgery or other procedure requiring anesthesia	Depends on conditions of use (e.g., for induction of anesthesia through intubation), 0.5–1.0 μg/kg per min and for continuation of anesthesia into immediate postoperative period: 0.1 μg/kg per min.
Tirofiban	Platelet aggregation inhibitor for prevention of early myocardial infarction	0.4 μg/kg per min for 30 min, then 0.1 μg/kg per min.

are used in anesthesia, are given by this route. Others are occasionally administered in this manner in specific situations (e.g., heparin and some barbiturates).

A wider application of constant-rate therapy has become possible with the development and use of constant-rate release devices and systems, which can be ingested or placed at various body sites and which deliver drug for a period extending from hours to years. Some examples of these devices/systems and their applications are given in Table 10-2. Many of the transdermal systems previously presented (Table 10-3) fall into this category as well. When used to produce a systemic effect, absorption is a prerequisite to attain effective

TABLE 10-2   Representative Constant-Rate Devices or Systems and Their Applications

Type of Therapeutic System	Drug	Rate Specifications	Application/Comment
Intramuscular (i.m.) Injection	Haloperidol	Deep i.m. injection (50 and 100 mg/mL in sesame oil). Initial dose of 10–15 times dose of oral immediate-release product. Maintenance with once-monthly injection. Approximately 1/30th of the dose becomes systemically available daily, on average.	Used in treating schizophrenia patients who require prolonged parenteral therapy.
	Leuprolide	Dose depends on age of child (7.5, 11.25, and 15 mg per syringe). Starting dose is 0.3 mg/kg every 4 weeks.	Used in the treatment of children with central precocious puberty.
Oral	Glipizide	2.5, 5, or 10 mg release tablets administered once daily.	Oral blood glucose lowering drug of sulfonylurea class with 24 hr constant-rate release.
	Nifedipine	30, 60, or 90 mg/day administered once daily.	Nondisintegrating system is designed to provide a constant rate of release for 24 hr. Used in treating vasospastic and chronic stable angina and hypertension.
Subcutaneous Implant	Goserelin	Implanted subcutaneously Continuous release of drug for a 12-week period. Product is biodegradable.	Used in treating prostate carcinoma. Potent synthetic decapeptide analogue of luteinizing hormone-releasing hormone.
	Leuprolide acetate	Implant is nonbiodegradable Implanted subcutaneously and removed and replaced once yearly. Contains 72 mg of leuprolide acetate. Delivers 120 μg/day.	Used as palliative treatment of advanced prostatic cancer.

(continued)

TABLE 10-2	Representative Constant-Rate Devices or Systems and Their Applications (*continued*)		
Subcutaneous Injection	Insulin glargine	Exhibits a relatively constant glucose-lowering effect over 24 hr, permitting once-a-day administration.	Treatment of adult and pediatric patients with type I diabetes mellitus or adults with type 2 diabetes mellitus who require long-acting insulin for control of hyperglycemia.
Vaginal Ring	Etonogestrel/ ethinyl estradiol	On average, 0.12 mg of the progestin hormone and 0.05 mg of the estrogen are released per day.	Used to prevent pregnancy. Ring is inserted for 3 weeks. After a 1-week break, another is inserted.

TABLE 10-3	Examples of Transdermal Delivery Systems	
Drug	**Use**	**Delivery**
Clonidine	Treatment of hypertension	Delivery of 0.1, 0.2, or 0.3 mg clonidine per day for 1 week.
Estradiol	Estrogen replacement, menopause	Constant rate of delivery. Applied twice to once weekly. Dosage is individualized.
Fentanyl	Continuous pain relief	Applied every 3 days.
Norelgestromin/ethinyl estradiol	Prevention of pregnancy	Weekly change of patch for 3 weeks. 1 week no patch.
Oxybutynin	Treatment of overactive bladder	Applied every 3–4 days.
Progesterone	Progesterone supplementation, secondary amenorrhea	Vaginally, twice daily for progesterone supplement, every other day for treating amenorrhea.
Scopolamine	Motion sickness	Effect lasts for 3 days (1.0 mg delivered).
Testosterone Patch, Gel Buccal system	Testosterone replacement therapy, male hypogonadism	Once-daily application.

plasma concentrations for all methods that are extravascular in nature. For the purpose of understanding the principles in this chapter, drug delivery from these systems is assumed to be equivalent to a constant-rate i.v. infusion.

This chapter also examines the turnover of the system on which a drug acts. The system affected may be any one of several constituents formed within the body. The subject is included here because the kinetic principles involved in the constant-rate input of drug are the same as those involved in the turnover of body constituents.

EXPOSURE–TIME RELATIONSHIPS

The salient features of the events following a constant-rate infusion are shown in Fig. 10-1 for tissue-type plasminogen activator (t-PA), a substance used to treat myocardial infarctions. The plasma concentration rises toward a constant value and drops off immediately

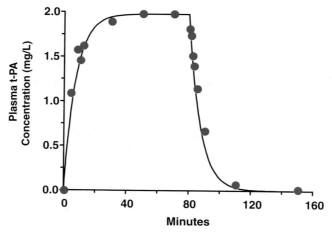

FIGURE 10-1. The plasma concentration of recombinant tissue-type plasminogen activator (t-PA) rapidly approaches a limiting value in a patient who receives 1.4 mg/min by constant-rate infusion for 80 min. At the end of the infusion, the plasma t-PA concentration drops rapidly toward zero with a 5.2-min half-life. The line is the function $C = 1.98 \cdot (1 - e^{-0.133t})$ during the infusion, and $C = 1.98 \cdot e^{-0.133t}$ is the function postinfusion; 0.133 min^{-1} corresponds to a half-life of 5.2 min. (From: Koster RW, Cohen AF, Kluft C, et al. The pharmacokinetics of double-chain t-PA [duteplase]: effects of bolus injection, infusions, and administration by weight in patients with myocardial infarction. Clin Pharmacol Ther 1991;50:267–277.)

after the infusion of 1.4 mg/min is stopped at 80 min. The half-life of the compound in this patient is 5.2 min, so the drug is infused for about 15 half-lives.

A drug is said to be given as a constant (rate) infusion when the intent is to achieve and maintain a stable plasma concentration or amount in the body. In contrast to the input of a bolus dose by a short-term infusion, the duration of a constant-rate infusion is usually much longer than the half-life of the drug. The essential features following a constant infusion can be appreciated by considering the events depicted in Fig. 10-2 in which drug is introduced at a constant rate into the reservoir model previously presented (see Fig. 3-3).

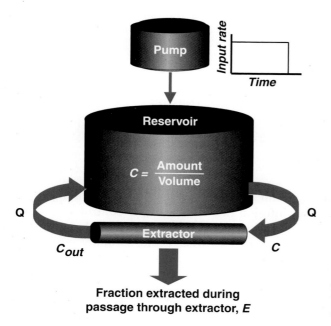

Fraction extracted during passage through extractor, E

FIGURE 10-2. Drug is delivered at a constant rate (pump and rate of input shown) into a well-stirred reservoir (see Fig. 3-3). Fluid from the reservoir perfuses the extractor at flow rate Q. A fraction, E, of that presented to the extractor is removed on passing through it; the remainder is returned to the reservoir. For modeling purposes, the volume of drug solution introduced by the pump and the amount of drug in the extractor are negligible compared with the volume of the reservoir and the amount of drug contained in it, respectively.

THE PLATEAU VALUE

At any time during an infusion, the rate of change in the amount of drug in the body (or reservoir) is the difference between the rates of drug infusion and elimination. Using the model shown in Fig. 10-3,

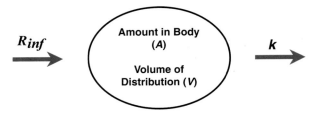

FIGURE 10-3. The time course of the amount of drug in the body during a constant-rate infusion depends on the rate of input and the rate of elimination. The simplest model for examining the time course is shown. The symbols are: R_{inf}, rate of infusion; A, amount in the body; V, volume of distribution; and k, the elimination rate constant. The rate of elimination is equal to $k \cdot A$; the plasma concentration is equal to A/V.

$$\begin{array}{cccc} \textit{Rate of change of} \\ \textit{drug in the body} \end{array} = \begin{array}{c} R_{inf} \\ \text{Constant rate} \\ \text{of infusion} \end{array} - \begin{array}{c} k \cdot A \\ \text{Rate of} \\ \text{elimination} \end{array} \qquad \text{10-1}$$

or expressing the equation in terms of the concentration of drug in plasma,

$$\begin{array}{cccc} \textit{Rate of change of} \\ \textit{drug in the body} \end{array} = \begin{array}{c} R_{inf} \\ \text{Constant rate} \\ \text{of infusion} \end{array} - \begin{array}{c} CL \cdot C \\ \text{Rate of} \\ \text{elimination} \end{array} \qquad \text{10-2}$$

On starting a constant infusion, the amount in the body (reservoir) is zero, and hence, there is no elimination; therefore, amount in the body rises. The rise continues until the rate of elimination matches the rate of infusion. Amount in the body (reservoir) and plasma concentration are then said to have reached a **steady state** or **plateau**, which continues as long as the same infusion rate is maintained. Because the rate of change of amount in the body (reservoir) at plateau is zero, it follows that Eqs. 10-1 and 10-2 simplify to:

$$\begin{array}{ccc} A_{ss} & = & \dfrac{R_{inf}}{k} \\ \\ \text{Amount at} & & \dfrac{\text{Infusion rate}}{\text{Elimination rate constant}} \\ \text{steady state} \end{array} \qquad \text{10-3}$$

$$\begin{array}{ccc} C_{ss} & = & \dfrac{R_{inf}}{CL} \\ \\ \text{Concentration} & & \dfrac{\text{Infusion rate}}{\text{Clearance}} \\ \text{at steady state} \end{array} \qquad \text{10-4}$$

Clearly, the only factors governing amount at plateau are the rate of infusion and the elimination rate constant. Similarly, only infusion rate and clearance control the steady-state plasma concentration. For example, consider the case of eptifibatide (Integrilin), a reversible inhibitor of platelet aggregation, used to treat acute coronary syndrome. Furthermore, suppose, for illustrative purposes, that a steady-state plasma eptifibatide concentration of 1 mg/L is desired in a 70-kg patient. Because the clearance of this drug is 4 L/hr (57 mL/hr per kilogram), the required infusion rate is 4.0 mg/hr. As the elimination rate constant of eptifibatide is 0.28 hr^{-1}, the corresponding amount of drug in the body (reservoir) at steady state is 14.3 mg. Alternatively, the amount can be calculated by multiplying the plateau concentration (1 mg/L) by the volume of distribution of eptifibatide (14.3 L).

To emphasize the factors that control the plateau, consider the following statement: *"All drugs infused at the same rate and having the same clearance reach the same plateau concentration."* This statement is true. The liver and kidneys clear only what is presented to them; the rate of elimination depends only on clearance and plasma concentration. At plateau, rate of elimination is equal to rate of infusion. The plasma concentration must therefore be the same for all drugs with the same clearance if administered at the same rate. However, amount in the body varies with volume of distribution. Only for drugs with the same clearance and volume of distribution are both plasma concentration and amount in the body at plateau the same when infused at the same rate. Now consider the next statement: *"When infused at the same rate, the amount of drug in the body at steady state is the same for all drugs with the same half-life."* This statement is also true, as seen from Eq 10-3. Drugs with the same half-life have the same elimination rate constant. The elimination rate constant is the fractional rate of drug elimination, that is, the rate of elimination divided by the amount of drug in the body. At plateau, rate of elimination equals rate of infusion. Hence, amount in the body at plateau must be the same for all drugs with the same half-life when administered at the same rate. Although the amount in the body is the same, the corresponding plateau concentration varies inversely with the drug's volume of distribution.

During therapy with a drug, it is not uncommon to adjust administration to observed clinical effects. This may require an increase or decrease in dosing rate. Knowledge of the plateau value at one particular infusion rate allows prediction of the infusion rate needed to achieve other plateau values. Thus, provided that clearance is constant, a change in infusion rate produces a proportional change in plateau concentration. Returning to the eptifibatide example, one expects that a rate of 8 mg/hr is needed to produce a plateau concentration of 2 mg/L, because an infusion rate of 4 mg/hr results in a plateau concentration of 1 mg/L.

MEAN RESIDENCE TIME

Conceptually, a useful parameter to describe the sojourn of drug in the body is **mean residence time** (*MRT*). To appreciate its relationship to other pharmacokinetic parameters, consider the infusion situation. For a given constant rate of infusion, the amount of drug in the body at steady state (rate of elimination = rate of infusion) depends on the time an average molecule resides in the body. For example, if 2×10^{20} molecules are eliminated per hour and they reside in the body for 10 hr, then only one tenth of the molecules in the body are removed per hour. Therefore, there must be 20×10^{20} molecules in the body. Thus, *MRT* is related to the infusion rate and the amount in the body by the relationship:

$$MRT = \frac{A_{ss}}{R_{inf}}$$

10-5

From Eq. 10-3, it is evident that

$$MRT = \frac{1}{k}$$

10-6

or, as $k = 0.693/t_{1/2,}$

$$MRT = 1.443 x t_{1/2}$$

10-7

Furthermore, as $k = CL/V$, it follows from Eq. 10-6 that

$$MRT = \frac{V}{CL}$$

10-8

For eptifibatide ($V = 14.3$ L, $CL = 4$ L/hr in the patient example), the *MRT* is 3.58 hr, a value corresponding (Eq. 10-7) to a half-life of 2.5 hr. The *MRT* concept is further discussed in Appendix H, *Mean Residence Time.*

TIME TO REACH PLATEAU

A delay always exists between the start of an infusion and the establishment of plateau. *The sole factor controlling the approach to plateau is the half-life of the drug.* To appreciate this point, consider a situation in which a bolus dose is given at the start of a constant infusion to immediately attain the amount achieved at plateau; clearly, the size of the bolus dose must be A_{ss}. Thereafter, the amount in the body is maintained at the plateau value by constant infusion. Imagine that a way exists to monitor separately drug remaining in the body from the bolus and that accumulating resulting from the infusion. The events are depicted in Fig. 10-4. Drug in the body associated with each mode of administration is eliminated as though the other were not present. The amount associated with the bolus dose declines exponentially and at any time,

$$\text{Amount remaining in the body from bolus dose} = A_{ss} \cdot e^{-kt} \qquad 10\text{-}9$$

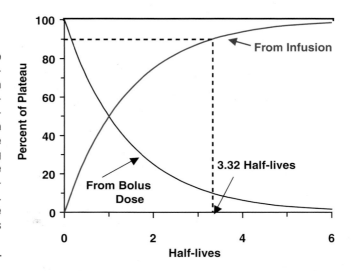

FIGURE 10-4. The approach to plateau is controlled only by the half-life of the drug. Depicted is a situation in which a bolus dose immediately attains and a constant infusion thereafter maintains a constant amount in the body (*solid horizontal line*). As the amount of the bolus dose remaining in the body (*black line*) falls, there must be a complementary rise resulting from the infusion (*colored line*). By 3.32 half-lives, the amount in the body associated with the infusion has reached 90% of the plateau value.

However, as long as the infusion is maintained, this decline is exactly matched by the gain resulting from the infusion. This must be so because the sum always equals the amount at plateau, A_{ss}. Therefore, it follows that the amount in the body associated with a constant infusion (A_{inf}) is always the difference between the amount at plateau (A_{ss}) and the amount remaining from the bolus dose, namely,

$$A_{inf} = A_{ss} - A_{ss} \cdot e^{-kt} = A_{ss}(1 - e^{-kt}) \qquad 10\text{-}10$$

Or, on dividing through by the volume of distribution,

$$C_{inf} = C_{ss}(1 - e^{-kt}) \qquad 10\text{-}11$$

Thus, both the amount in the body and the plasma concentration (C_{inf}) rise asymptotically toward their respective plateau values following constant-rate drug infusion without a bolus dose.

The amount of drug in the body, or plasma concentration, expressed as a percent of the plateau value at different times after initiation of an infusion, is shown in Table 10-4. In one half-life, the value in the body is 50% of the plateau value. In two half-lives, it is 75%

TABLE 10-4	Percent of the Plateau Level at Various Times Following a Constant-Rate Infusion of Drug
Time (in half-lives)	**Percent of Plateau***
0.25	16
0.5	29
1	50
2	75
3	88
3.3	90
4	94
5	97
6	98
7	99

*Values are rounded off to the nearest percentage.

of the plateau value. Theoretically, a plateau is only reached when the drug has been infused for an infinite number of half-lives. *Practically, however, the plateau may be considered to be reached in 3.3 half-lives (90% of the plateau).* Thus, the shorter the half-life, the sooner the plateau is reached. For example, t-PA (half-life of 5 min) reaches a plateau within minutes (3.3 half-lives is 17 min), whereas it takes more than 8 hr of constant eptifibatide administration (half-life of 2.5 hr) before the plateau is reached (3.3 half-lives is 8.25 hr). The important point to remember is that the approach to plateau depends *solely* on the half-life of the drug. This is so whether 8 mg/hr of eptifibatide is infused to attain a plateau concentration of 2 mg/L, or the infusion rate is 4 mg/hr to attain a plateau concentration of 1 mg/L. In the former case, the eptifibatide plasma concentration at 1 half-life is one half the corresponding plateau value of 2 mg/L, or 1 mg/L. So, if one wants to achieve a plateau concentration of 2 mg/L more quickly, one can first infuse at a rate of 16 mg/hr for one half-life (2.5 hr) and then maintain the resulting 2 mg/L by halving the infusion rate to 8 mg/hr.

POSTINFUSION

After stopping an infusion, the amount or concentration in the body falls by one half each half-life. Given only the declining values of a drug, one cannot clearly determine whether a bolus or an infusion had been given. In the example of eptifibatide, 28.6 mg (2 mg/L × 14.3 L) are in the body (reservoir) at plateau following an infusion rate of 8 mg/hr. At 8.25 hr (3.3 half-lives) after stopping the infusion, only one tenth of the plateau value, or 2.86 mg, remains in the body. The same amount of drug would be found in the body 8.25 hr after an i.v. bolus dose of 28.6 mg.

A comment should be made about removing constant-rate devices or systems. After removing some transdermal devices, drug continues to be released from binding sites in skin for appreciable periods of time. In these instances, the plasma drug concentration falls more slowly than after stopping an i.v. infusion because of continued input of drug from the skin.

CHANGING INFUSION RATES

The rate of infusion of a drug is sometimes changed during therapy because of excessive toxicity or an inadequate therapeutic response. If the object of the change is to produce a new plateau, then the time to go from one plateau to another, whether higher or lower, depends *solely* on the half-life of the drug.

Consider, for illustrative purposes, a patient stabilized on a 4-mg/hr infusion rate of eptifibatide, which, with a clearance of 4 L/hr, should produce a plateau concentration of 1.0 mg/L. Suppose that the situation now demands a plateau concentration of 2.0 mg/L. This new plateau value is achieved by doubling the infusion rate to 8 mg/hr. Imagine that, instead of increasing the infusion rate, the additional 4 mg/hr is administered at a different site and that a way exists to monitor drug in the body from the two infusions separately. The events illustrated in Fig. 10-5 show that the eptifibatide concentration associated with the supplementary infusion is expected to rise to 1 mg/L in exactly the same time as in the first infusion; the concentration (1.5 mg/L) halfway toward the new plateau (2.0 mg/L) is achieved in one elimination half-life (2.5 hr) and so on. This expectation can be visualized by adding, at this time, the plasma concentration resulting from the continued initial infusion (1.0 mg/L) to the concentration arising from the supplementary infusion (0.5 mg/L). Clearly, half-life is the sole determinant of the time to go from 1.0 to 2.0 mg/L, or from any initial value to a new steady-state value during constant-rate input.

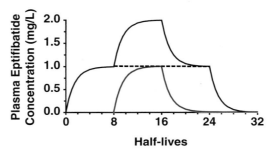

FIGURE 10-5. Situation illustrating that the time to reach a new plateau, whether higher or lower than the previous value, depends only on the half-life of a drug. A plateau concentration of 1 mg/L is reached in approximately 3.3 half-lives after starting a constant infusion of 4 mg/hr of eptifibatide. Doubling the infusion rate is like maintaining 4 mg/hr and starting another constant infusion of 4 mg/hr (*colored line*). In approximately 3.3 half-lives, the eptifibatide concentration rises from 1 to 2 mg/L. Halving an infusion rate of 8 mg/hr is analogous to stopping the supplementary 4-mg/hr infusion. The plasma concentration of eptifibatide returns to the previous plateau concentration of 1 mg/L in approximately 3.3 half-lives. When drug infusion is completely stopped, the concentration falls toward zero at a rate, again, depending on its half-life. The half-life of eptifibatide is about 2.5 hr. The total time span is then about 32 hr.

The decline from a high plateau to a low one is likewise related to the half-life. Consider, for example, the events after stopping the supplementary 4-mg/hr infusion rate discussed above. The eptifibatide concentration associated with this supplementary infusion falls to half of the existing value in one half-life. In 3.3 half-lives, the total concentration has almost returned to the 1.0 mg/L concentration. In addition, it will take another 3.3 half-lives for most of the eptifibatide to be removed from the body once the original 4-mg/hr infusion is also stopped.

An example of the change in plasma concentration on changing from one infusion rate to another is again demonstrated by data on t-PA in Fig. 10-6. The half-life is the determinant of the speed of attaining the new steady state. Clearance determines the steady-state concentration at any given rate of infusion.

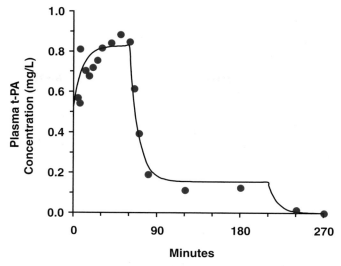

FIGURE 10-6. The plasma concentration of plasminogen activator (t-PA) starts at about 0.6 mg/L and approaches a plateau of 0.8 mg/L following an i.v. bolus of 10 mg and a constant-rate infusion of 1.6 mg/min for 60 min to an individual subject. Subsequently, the plasma concentration drops as the drug infusion is decreased to 0.3 mg/min until 210 min when the infusion is discontinued. The time from the first steady state to the second one (0.16 mg/L) depends on the half-life of the drug, 6.6 min in this subject, as does the decline to zero after drug administration is stopped. (From: Koster RW, Cohen AF, Kluft C, et al. The pharmacokinetics of double-chain t-PA [duteplase]: effects of bolus injection, infusions, and administration by weight in patients with myocardial infarction. Clin Pharmacol Ther 1991;50:267–277.)

BOLUS PLUS INFUSION

It takes 8.25 hr of constant infusion of eptifibatide before 90% of the plateau concentration is reached in the patient with a 2.5-hr half-life. An even longer time is required for drugs with half-lives greater than that of eptifibatide. Situations sometimes demand that the plateau be reached more rapidly, as is the case for eptifibatide. One solution, as previously stated, is to double the infusion rate for the first half-life. Figure 10-2 suggests another solution. That is, at the start of an infusion, give a bolus dose equal to the amount desired in the body at plateau. Usually, the bolus dose is a therapeutic dose, and the infusion rate is adjusted to maintain the therapeutic level. When the bolus dose and infusion rate are exactly matched, as in Fig. 10-2, the amounts of drug in the body associated with the two modes of administration are complementary; the gain from the infusion offsets the loss of drug from the bolus.

Now consider two situations. The first, shown in Fig. 10-7, is one in which different bolus doses are given at the start of a constant-rate infusion. In Case A, drug is infused at a rate of 4 mg/min and the plasma concentration rises, reaching a plateau of 1 mg/L in approximately four half-lives. In Case B, a bolus dose of 15 mg immediately attains, and the infusion rate thereafter maintains the concentration. In Case C, the bolus dose of 30 mg is excessive; because the rate of loss is initially greater than the rate of infusion; consequently, the concentration falls. This fall continues until the same plateau as in Case B is reached. It should be noticed that the time to reach the plateau depends solely on the half-life of the drug. Thus, in Case C at one half-life, the concentration of 1.5 mg/L, composed of 1 mg/L remaining from the bolus and 0.5 mg/L arising from the infusion, lies midway between the values immediately after the bolus dose and the concentration achieved by the infusion. By two half-lives, the concentration of 1.25 mg/L lies 75% of

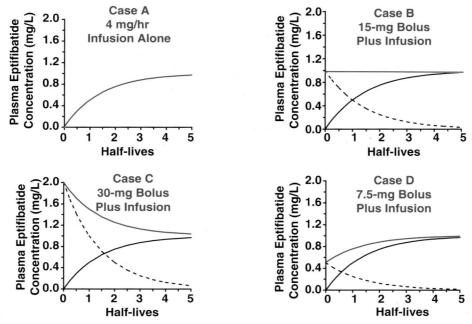

FIGURE 10-7. Situations illustrating that the plateau depends on the infusion rate and not on the initial bolus dose. Whether a bolus dose of eptifibatide is given (*Cases B, C, D*) or not (*Case A*) at the start of the infusion, the plasma concentrations at the plateau are the same when a given infusion rate is used. The plasma concentration associated with the bolus dose declines exponentially (*dashed line*), whereas the concentration associated with the infusion in all cases rises asymptotically toward plateau (*solid line*), as portrayed by *Case A*. In *Cases B, C,* and *D,* the observed concentration (*colored line*) is the sum of the two. When not initially achieved, it takes approximately 3.3 half-lives to reach plateau (*Cases A, C, D*). Note also in *Cases A, C,* and *D* that at one half-life, the plasma concentration lies mid-way between initial and plateau values. The simulation is based on an 83-kg patient given bolus doses of 15 mg (*Case B*), 30 mg (*Case C*), 7.5 mg (*Case D*), and an infusion rate of 4 mg/hr.

the way toward the plateau. By 3.3 half-lives, only 10% of the initial concentration resulting from the bolus remains and the concentration from the infused drug is 0.9 mg/L. We are now (1.1 mg/L) within 10% of the plateau. In Case D, the bolus dose of 7.5 mg is below the plateau amount. Because the rate of infusion now exceeds the rate of drug elimination, the plasma concentration continuously rises until the same plateau, as in the previous cases, is reached. Once again, the time to approach the plateau is controlled solely by the half-life of the drug.

Case D is demonstrated by t-PA in Fig. 10-6. The bolus dose of 10 mg was insufficient to attain the steady state achieved on infusing 1.6 mg/min. This result is expected from the 6.6-min half-life in this patient, because the amount in the body at plateau (R_{inf}/k) is 15 mg.

In the second and more common situation, depicted in Fig. 10-8, the same bolus dose and infusion rate of eptifibatide are administered to three patients, A, B, and C, with different clearance and associated half-life values, but with the same volume of distribution. The half-lives in these patients are 2.5, 5, and 7.5 hr, respectively. All patients start with the same amount of drug in the body and, therefore, plasma concentration. In patient A, the initial concentration is maintained because rate of infusion is exactly matched by rate of elimination. Because elimination is slower, the concentration in patient B rises until rate of elimination equals infusion rate. The time to reach this higher

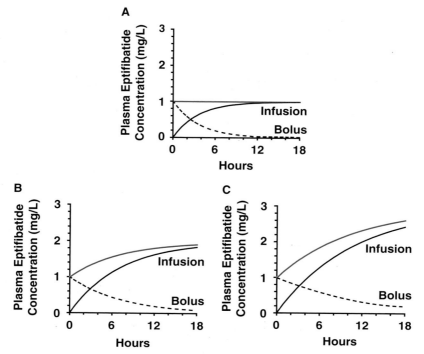

FIGURE 10-8. Situations illustrating that the plateau plasma concentration depends on half-life and clearance. The same bolus dose and constant infusion of eptifibatide are given to patients A, B, and C, with half-lives of 2.5, 5, and 7.5 hr, respectively. The last two patients have decreased renal function, the route of elimination of this dug. Although the initial concentration is the same (1 mg/L) in all three patients, the plateau concentration differs in direct proportion to their respective half-lives, and inversely with clearance. The time course of the plasma concentration associated with the bolus (*dotted line*) depends on the individual's half-life, as does the rise in the plasma concentration associated with the constant infusion (*black solid line*). Only when rate of loss is immediately matched by rate of infusion is the plateau immediately attained and maintained (patient A). Otherwise, the plasma concentration (*colored line*) changes, until after approximately 3.3 half-lives, a plateau is reached (patients B and C). Note for patient C, it would take at least 25 hr (3.3 half-lives) to reach plateau.

plateau value is governed solely by the half-life of the drug in this patient. Thus, by one half-life (5 hr), the plasma concentration in patient B is midway between that from the bolus dose and that at plateau. By the time the plateau is reached, the entire bolus dose has been eliminated. Also, it follows from Eq. 10-4 that for a given infusion rate, concentration at plateau is inversely proportional to the clearance. This is seen in Fig. 10-8C, where the concentration in patient C at plateau is 50% higher than that in patient B. Patient C eliminates the drug even more slowly than does patient B, resulting in a longer time to reach plateau. Clearly, the time to reach plateau is governed solely by the half-life.

SHORT-TERM INFUSIONS

In many therapeutic settings, drugs are said to be given by i.v. infusion when, in fact, they are intended to be given as i.v. bolus doses. Short-term infusions are used because, if the administration were too rapid, the incidence of adverse events increases. Phenytoin, an antiepileptic drug, is one example. This poorly soluble drug, with a pKa of 8.8, is dissolved using a high pH (12) and a high concentration of propylene glycol (40%) in the i.v. dosage form that has been available for many decades. Slow administration is required to avoid precipitation of the drug in the vein, phlebitis, and systemic toxicity. To avoid some of these problems, fosphenytoin, a water-soluble rapidly hydrolyzed phosphate ester prodrug of phenytoin, is now more commonly used.

Another example is propofol, an i.v. anesthetic agent. When given as a true bolus dose, followed immediately by a maintenance infusion, the very high concentration initially reaching the brain, without time to be diluted by fluids of other tissues of the body, produces excessive anesthesia. If the size of the bolus dose is reduced, then the anesthesia is not adequately maintained, because the drug moves quickly from brain out into other tissues. To overcome this problem, the loading dose must be given over at least 40 seconds. Trastuzumab (Herceptin), used to treat metastatic breast cancer in patients whose tumors overexpress the epidermal growth factor receptor 2 protein, is an example of an antibody (molecular weight = 185,000 g/mol) that can produce fever and chills if injected too rapidly. The loading dose of 4 mg/kg is given over a minimum of 90 min and the weekly maintenance dose of 3 mg/kg is given over 30 min, if the loading dose is tolerated in the 90-min period of infusion.

CONSEQUENCE OF SLOW TISSUE DISTRIBUTION

As discussed for an i.v. bolus dose in Chapter 3, *Kinetics Following an Intravenous Bolus Dose*, the body is more complex than the reservoir portrayed in Fig. 10-2. The approach of the plasma concentration toward steady state during a constant-rate infusion, the time course of the decline after discontinuing an infusion, and the time course of the concentration following a combined bolus dose and constant-rate infusion are often not simple functions of the terminal half-life of the drug, because of slow distribution to the tissues.

The i.v. anesthetic agent, propofol, a lipophilic (n-octanol:water partition coefficient of 6760:1) phenol with a pKa of 11, exemplifies what happens when tissue distribution is relatively slow. When infused at a constant rate, the blood concentration rises quickly within the first 20 min, and then continues to rise at a slower rate (Fig. 10-9). A model, in which the drug distributes into three pools (Fig. 10-10), helps to explain the following events: the rapid induction of anesthesia even without a bolus dose, in spite

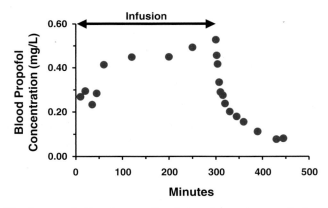

FIGURE 10-9.   Blood concentration–time profile of propofol, an i.v. anesthetic agent, following a constant-rate infusion of 1.0 mg/hr per kilogram for 5 hr (300 min) in a patient after coronary artery bypass surgery. Data for a specific i.v. formulation (Diprivan 10) is shown. (From: Knibbe CAJ, Aarts LPHJ, Kuks PFM, et al. Pharmacokinetics and pharmacodynamics of propofol 6% SA2N versus propofol 1% SAZN and Diprivan-10 for short-term sedation following coronary artery bypass surgery. Eur J Clin Pharmacol 2000;56:89–95.)

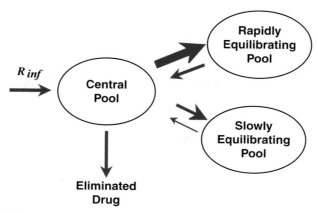

FIGURE 10-10.   Model simulating the effect of distribution to tissues on the approach of the plasma concentration of propofol toward steady state following a constant-rate infusion and its decline when the infusion is stopped. Drug distribution in the body is represented by three body pools. Drug in the central pool, which includes blood, distributes to and from a rapidly equilibrating pool, which includes brain, and a slowly equilibrating pool, which includes fat. The size of the arrows indicate the relative rapidity of the processes.

of a 2-day terminal half-life; the need to decrease the input rate when the drug is infused for long periods of time to avoid oversedation; and the increase in recovery time, after discontinuance, when infused for long periods of time. Each of these events is now considered.

RAPID INDUCTION OF ANESTHESIA

Following an i.v. bolus dose, there is very rapid equilibration of propofol (1–3 min) between the blood and the very highly perfused brain. Even without a bolus dose, anesthesia still develops rapidly because of this rapid equilibration.

DECREASE IN INFUSION RATE ON CHRONIC ADMINISTRATION

The time for equilibration between blood and the rapidly equilibrating pool, including muscle tissue, takes more time than equilibration of propofol between brain and blood and explains the slow rise in the concentration observed in Fig. 10-9. Equilibration of drug in the slowly equilibrating tissue, which includes fat, with that in blood takes much longer and is not shown in Fig. 10-9. As a consequence of the gradual build up in this slowly equilibrating pool when the infusion is maintained, there is a decreased long-term net rate of movement of drug out of blood into the tissues, which in turn results in a slow but continuous rise in the blood concentration. The rise continues as long as the rate of input is greater than the rate of elimination. Accordingly, when the drug is administered for long periods of time, the rate of infusion needs to be reduced at later times. Failure to do so may result in excessive depth of anesthesia as a result of very high blood, and hence brain, concentrations of the drug.

RECOVERY FROM ANESTHESIA

Discontinuation of the infusion rate after the maintenance of anesthesia for approximately 1 hr, or for sedation in an intensive care unit for 1 day, results in a prompt decrease (within a few minutes) in the blood propofol concentration and rapid awakening. Longer infusions (e.g., 10 days of sedation within an intensive care unit) result in accumulation of significant tissue stores of propofol, particularly in fat, so that the reduction in circulating propofol on stopping the infusion is slowed by the return of drug from these slowly equilibrating tissues. Consequently, recovery is slowed.

PHARMACODYNAMIC CONSIDERATIONS

THE DRUG ITSELF

Although an i.v. infusion provides a highly controlled means of delivering drug to the systemic circulation, consideration must also be given to the evolution of the resultant response, which depends on exposure–response relationships. Let us examine a few examples.

Onset of Response. As discussed in Chapter 8, *Response Following a Single Dose*, there are many reasons for a delay in response, including slow specific distribution to the target site (pharmacokinetic in nature) and between the measured response and actual effect of the drug (pharmacodynamic in nature). Under these circumstances, the addition of an i.v. bolus dose to constant-rate therapy to overcome the delay may be of marginal value. An example is that of a leuprolide acetate implant in treating patients with advanced prostatic cancer. The drug inhibits the formation of both follicle-stimulating hormone and luteinizing hormone, which subsequently reduces the levels of testosterone and dihydrotestosterone to below castration values. However, because of the relatively slow kinetics of these systems, it takes 2 to 4 weeks for the pharmacodynamic effect to develop fully. Giving a bolus to start therapy quickly is consequently of little value. Furthermore, treatment often continues for years; there is therefore no urgency for immediately obtaining the response.

Response on Stopping an Infusion. The expected time course of response after stopping an infusion also depends on both pharmacokinetics and pharmacodynamics. Recall that a prolongation of effect occurs, relative to the disappearance of the drug, when the response is delayed (e.g., warfarin, Fig. 8-7); the initial response is in region 3 of the concentration–response relationship (e.g., succinylcholine, Fig. 8-15); or the drug reacts irreversibly with a receptor (e.g., omeprazole, Fig. 8-18).

Response Infusion Versus Single Dose. Concentration–intensity–time relationships after a single i.v. bolus dose are expected to be different from those seen following other modes of administration. A recurring question for drugs of short half-life is whether the cumulative effect for a given amount of drug is greater following a bolus or an infusion. There is no general answer, but it is likely that the outcome may be different. Such a difference is illustrated in Fig. 10-11 with the diuretic furosemide (half-life is about 90 min). The same 40-mg dose is administered as a single i.v. bolus and following an 8-hr constant rate of infusion (4 mg/hr) after a loading bolus of 8 mg. The overall natriuretic effect is clearly greater after the infusion as is the diuretic effect (5.8 vs. 4.6 L of urine in 8 hr) than after the bolus dose. Clearly, concentration–response–time relationships can be more complex following i.v. infusions, multiple-dose regimens, and single extravascular doses than those seen following single i.v. bolus doses.

FIGURE 10-11. Mean cumulative urinary excretion of sodium during an 8-hr period after a single 40-mg bolus dose (*black line*) and after the same amount given as an 8-mg bolus loading dose followed by an 8-hr infusion of 4 mg/hr of furosemide (*colored line*) in eight male volunteers. Although the same amount was given, the rate of delivery of furosemide is clearly a determinant of its cumulative natriuretic effect. (From: van Meyel JJM, Smits P, Russel FGM, et al. Diuretic efficiency of furosemide during continuous administration versus bolus injection in healthy volunteers. Clin Pharmacol Ther 1992;51:440–444.)

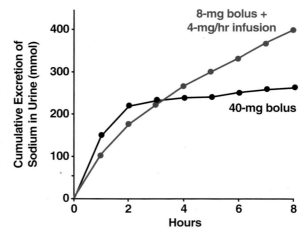

TURNOVER OF AFFECTED SYSTEMS

The response to drugs usually involves the turnover of an endogenous substance or system within the body (Chapter 8, *Response Following a Single Dose*). The concepts involving turnover are important to understand the time course of drug response.

Turnover concepts are similar to those that apply to constant-rate infusion. Consider, for example, the relationship, $k_t = R_t/A_{ss}$ (Eq. 2-5), where R_t is the turnover rate. The analogous equation following constant-rate infusion is $k = R_{inf}/A_{ss}$. Thus, fractional turnover rate, k_t, is synonymous with elimination rate constant for a one-compartment model. Also, pool size (A_{ss}) is synonymous with amount in body at steady state. A major distinction between the two concepts exists with respect to the initial condition. In turnover, the initial condition is one of steady state. With constant-rate infusion, it is not; initially, no drug is in the body. Notwithstanding this and other differences, such as feedback control, many of the concepts of constant-rate input have application in turnover. Selected examples of conditions in which turnover of a system is altered are given in Table 10-5.

TABLE 10-5   Selected Examples of Altered Turnover

Observation	Cause	Turnover Rate	Fractional Turnover Rate	Turnover Time	Example
I. Change in Pool Size					
Increased pool size (or concentration)	Increased synthesis or input	↑	N/C	N/C	Induction of a cytochrome P450 isozyme by phenobarbital
	Decreased ability to eliminate	N/C	↓	↑	Rise in serum creatinine in acute renal function impairment
Decreased pool size (or concentration)	Decreased synthesis or input	↓	N/C	N/C	Decrease in concentration of certain clotting factors after oral anticoagulants
	Increased ability to eliminate	N/C	↑	↓	Decreased renal tubular reabsorption of serum uric acid by a uricosuric agent
II. Little or No Change in Pool Size					
Increased output (or elimination)	Increased input	↑	↑	↓	Increased water consumption in hot weather
Decreased output (or elimination)	Decreased input	↓	↓	↑	Sodium in urine on a low-salt diet

↑, increase; ↓, decrease; N/C, little or no change.

Altered Turnover. The turnover parameters of a system may be obtained if two of the following three are measured: turnover rate, amount in the pool, and fractional turnover rate. None can be obtained from measurement of steady-state plasma concentration alone. The turnover rate can be measured in some circumstances, for example, through the use of tracer amounts of isotopically labeled substances (see Chapter 19, *Distribution Kinetics*), which can be measured independently. Otherwise, fractional turnover rate can only be measured by perturbing steady state.

To appreciate the consequences of altering fractional turnover rate, consider the events in Fig. 10-12A in which elimination is immediately and completely blocked and input is unaltered. The rate at which the substance accumulates depends on its normal turnover. The time required for a doubling of the amount initially present, A_{ss}, is the turnover time (t_t), by definition. Similarly, if concentration is measured, turnover time is that required for the concentration to double the steady-state value. This last statement

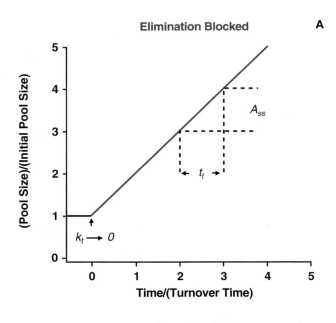

Elimination Blocked **A**

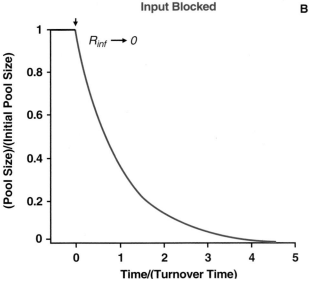

Input Blocked **B**

FIGURE 10-12. A. The pool size increases linearly with time when (*at arrow*) elimination is completely blocked and input rate remains unchanged. The slope is the original turnover rate, A_{ss}/t_t. **B.** The pool size decreases with time when (*at arrow*) input is completely blocked. The decline is exponential when first-order elimination and one-compartment distribution pertain. The rate constant for the decline (slope of semilogarithmic plot) is the fractional turnover rate. In both graphs, pool size is expressed relative to the original value, and time is related to the original turnover time.

assumes that the system acts as a single compartment within the time frame of the measurements. To determine turnover rate, the steady-state amount in the body must be known or the converse.

The consequences of immediately and completely blocking input under conditions in which elimination is first-order, and unaffected, and the body acts as if it were a single compartment are depicted in Fig. 10-12B. The situation is equivalent to stopping a constant-rate i.v. infusion of drug at steady state, namely, that the amount in the body (or plasma concentration) falls exponentially by one half each half-life. The fractional rate of elimination is the elimination rate constant k, and as $t_t = 1/k_t$, it follows that turnover time is related to half-life as follows:

$$t_t = \frac{1}{k_t} = \frac{1}{\frac{0.693}{t_{1/2}}} = 1.44 \cdot t_{1/2} \qquad \text{10-12}$$

or

$$t_{1/2} = 0.693 \cdot t_t \qquad \text{10-13}$$

Warfarin (Chapter 8, *Response Following a Single Dose*) is an example of the consequence of blocking synthesis. Another example is the effect of the xanthine oxidase inhibitor, allopurinol, which decreases the synthesis rate of uric acid, the culprit in gout, and lowers the exposure to the compound throughout the body. Alternatively, degradation or elimination can be increased as is the case with the uricosuric probenecid, which increases renal clearance of uric acid.

Establishment of a New Steady State. Input or elimination is often only partially affected by a drug. Consider now the case when input rate or fractional turnover rate is immediately shifted to a new constant value. It takes time for the pool size to reach a new steady state, and therefore, to reflect the shift in turnover, as illustrated on the next page. Let us examine how quickly the shift occurs in various scenarios.

Turnover rate altered to a new constant value. Changes in pool size with time on increasing or decreasing input (turnover rate) by a factor of 4 are shown, respectively, by the solid lines in Fig. 10-13. The new steady state reflects the change in turnover rate. Notice that, as the elimination half-life is unaltered, the time to reach the new steady state is the same, analogous to the change when altering the infusion rate of a drug. This is seen by the time required to reach one half the way to the new steady state. This statement is true irrespective of the extent of change in turnover rate, as shown in the upper graph of Fig. 10-13. Had the turnover time been 1 hr, then it would have taken 42 min ($0.693 \cdot t_t$) to reach this point; if it had been 1 week, then it would have taken about 5 days. This lack of change in the time to go from one steady state to another distinguishes altered turnover rate from altered fractional turnover rate.

One common example of altered turnover rate is enzyme induction, whereby a compound (the inducer) increases the synthesis rate of a drug-metabolizing enzyme. The result is an increase in the pool size of the enzyme, which in turn is normally reflected by a proportional increase in the Vm, and hence intrinsic clearance, of a substrate. The half-lives of drug-metabolizing enzymes vary from hours to days, so that the full effect of induction may not be seen for some time after an inducing agent is administered.

Fractional turnover rate altered to a new constant value. The consequences of changing elimination rate constant (fractional turnover rate) are quite different from changing input (turnover) rate. The difference is shown in Fig. 10-14 (page 279). It can be seen that a fourfold decrease in the elimination rate constant quadruples pool size, but it takes 4 times as long to reach the same new steady state as it did after quadrupling turnover

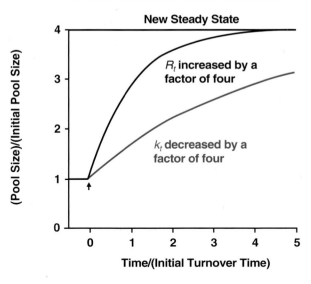

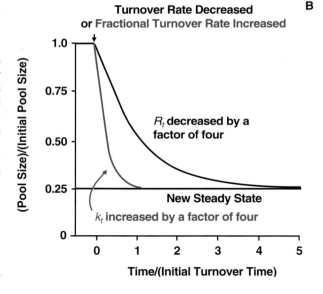

FIGURE 10-13. **A.** Pool size increases to a value four times the original when (*at arrow*) turnover rate (*black line*) increases by four. A fourfold decrease in fractional turnover rate (*colored line*) gives the same end result; however, it takes four times as long to reach the new steady state (*black*). **B.** Pool size decreases to a value one fourth of the original when (*at arrow*) turnover rate decreases (*black line*) by a factor of four. A fourfold increase in fractional turnover rate (*colored line*) again produces the same new steady state; however, the new value is approached four times more rapidly.

rate. On the other hand, a fourfold increase in elimination rate constant reduces pool size by a factor of four, and the new steady state is reached much more quickly than by the former mechanism.

Distinction between decreased turnover rate and increased fractional turnover rate is similar with the analysis above, but here, pool size decreases, as shown in Fig. 10-15 (page 280). The time required to approach the new steady state is the same when production rate is decreased (A), but is shortened when fractional turnover rate is increased (B). The rate of attainment of the new steady state is related to its new value; the lower the value, the more quickly it is achieved, as shown in Fig. 10-15B.

The rate of decline in pool size, on decreasing turnover rate, is limited by the fractional turnover rate itself. The decline in clotting factors, on administering warfarin, serves as a good example, as detailed in Chapter 8, *Response Following a Single Dose*, because it is representative of many other such systems in the body.

Turnover Rate Increased

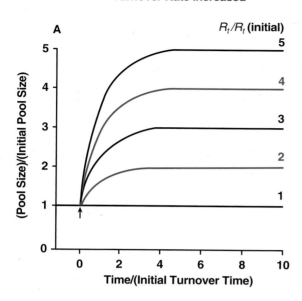

A

R_t/R_t (initial)

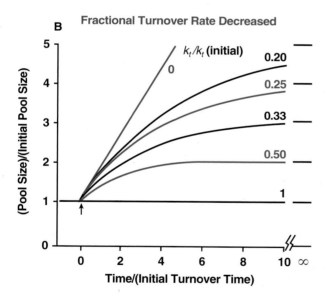

B **Fractional Turnover Rate Decreased**

k_t/k_t (initial)

FIGURE 10-14. A. The pool size is increased from one to five times its original value when (*at arrow*) the turnover increases by the factor R_t/R_t (*initial*). The time (half-life, turnover time) to approach each new steady state is the same. **B.** The approach to the new steady state is prolonged when (*at arrow*) the fractional turnover rate decreases by the factor k_t/k_t (*initial*). When the value of k_t approaches zero (*straight line*), steady state is never achieved. The prolonged approach to the new steady state for the other conditions can be expressed by the time (half-life) required to reach the pool size half-way between the initial and final values.

Interpretation of Non–Steady-State Observations. Frequently, it is necessary to interpret data under nonsteady-state conditions (i.e., when moving from one condition toward a new steady state). This arises following the acute administration of endogenous drugs. Examples are testosterone and L-thyroxine. The number of such drugs is increasing rapidly with developments in biotechnology that enable the expression and production of recombinant human polypeptides and proteins, such as follicle-stimulating hormone, growth hormone, and erythropoietin (see Chapter 21, *Protein Drugs*). With many of these drugs, a basal concentration in plasma exists that must be taken into account when attempting to define the pharmacokinetics of the administered compound. The approach that follows is successful when the basal turnover rate is unaffected by the additional material. Sometimes, this is not so because of feedback control systems that adjust the endogenous turnover rate to maintain homeostasis.

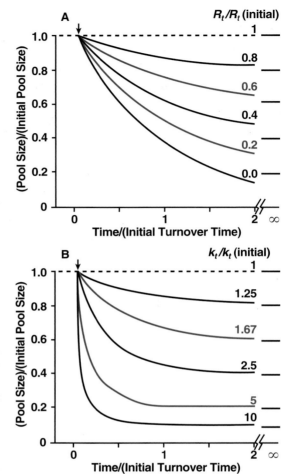

FIGURE 10-15. **A.** Pool size decreases to a new steady state that corresponds to the factor R_t/R_t (*initial*), by which the turnover rate decreases. The new steady state is approached with the same half-life when (*at arrow*) input decreases. **B.** Pool size also decreases when (*at arrow*) fractional turnover rate increases by the factor k_t/k_t (*initial*), but the time (half-life) to achieve the new steady state is shortened.

Cortisol, with feedback control of endogenous levels by the pituitary, is a prime example of this situation.

Figure 10-16A shows the serum concentrations of erythropoietin after i.v. bolus administration of epoetin alfa, a recombinant human erythropoietin, and placebo. Notice the decline of erythropoietin to its basal value. The equation defining the concentration during the decline, $C(t)$, is the sum of two concentrations, the basal concentration and that associated with the bolus dose, C_{bolus}. The difference between $C(t)$ and the basal concentration is seen to be approximated by a monoexponential equation, characterized by C_{bolus} (units/L) $= 1800\ e^{-0.12 \cdot t}$, with time in hours (Fig. 10-16B). The corresponding pharmacokinetic parameters are $V = 4\ \text{L}/70\ \text{kg}$; $CL = 0.5\ \text{L/hr per } 70$ kg and $t_{1/2} = 5.8$ hr.

TOLERANCE

Tolerance can develop, whereby the response is diminished with time for a given concentration. The time course of tolerance can vary from minutes to weeks and probably involves the turnover of one or more endogenous transmitters or receptors to which drug must bind to initiate a response. Tolerance may also be caused by a homeostatic mechanism whereby, through feedback control, the measurement tends to return toward the value before drug administration.

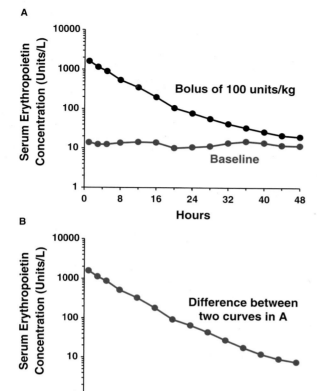

FIGURE 10-16. **A.** Serum erythropoietin concentration with time plotted semilogarithmically after i.v. bolus administration of epoetin alfa (100 units/kg) (●) and placebo (●). **B.** Semilogarithmic plot of the difference between the erythropoietin concentration after the dose of epoetin alfa and the basal value (10 units/L), taken as the average over the period of study following the placebo. Mean data for 21 subjects. (From: Halstenson CE, Macres M, Katz A, et al. Comparative pharmacokinetics and pharmacodynamics of epoetin alfa and epoetin beta. Clin Pharmacol Ther 1991;50:702–712.)

An example of tolerance is that associated with the repeated administration of nicotine (Fig. 10-17). One effect of nicotine is to increase heart rate. When nicotine is re-administered by a 30-min constant-rate infusion within 1 hr, the peak drug concentration, as expected, rises to a higher value, but the peak cardioaccelerating response is less than that following the first short-term infusion. If the administrations are separated by 3.5 hr, the peak concentration after the second infusion is less, but the peak response is now greater than that seen after the first. These results indicate a rapid development of tolerance to the cardioaccelerating effect of nicotine.

When acute tolerance exists, the *rate* at which the concentration changes may be as important as the concentration itself. The effect of nifedipine on hemodynamics illustrates this last statement. Nifedipine, a calcium channel blocking agent, both increases heart rate (tachycardia) and lowers diastolic blood pressure when given to patients as a rapidly disintegrating capsule. Fig. 10-18 (page 282) shows the changes in heart rate and blood pressure, together with the plasma concentrations of nifedipine, following two schedules of i.v. administration to a group of normotensive subjects. When a regimen is employed that promptly attains and then maintains a constant plasma concentration (regimen I), a sustained increase in heart rate but no fall in diastolic blood pressure is observed. In contrast, a fall in diastolic blood pressure but no tachycardia occurs when a constant-rate infusion is employed alone, despite a comparable steady-state concentration of nifedipine. The primary action of nifedipine is arteriolar vasodilation. This causes a reduction in peripheral resistance and blood pressure, followed by an increase in cardiac output and heart rate through activation of the baroreceptor reflex. Apparently, if drug input is slow enough, the adaptive control system has sufficient time to respond and so maintain

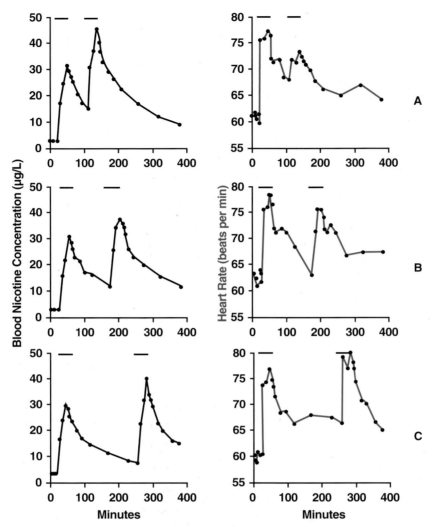

FIGURE 10-17.   Mean blood concentration of nicotine (*in black*) and the corresponding mean heart rate (*in color*) in eight subjects after two 30-min i.v. infusions of 25 μg/min/kg separated by 1 hr **(A)**, 2 hr **(B)**, and 3.5 hr **(C)**. The short bars at the top of each graph indicate the periods during which nicotine was infused. The longer the separation between the doses, the smaller is the increase in the plasma concentration, but the greater the maximum response following the second dose. The effect on heart rate (*colored lines*) is clearly diminished when the doses quickly follow each other, a phenomenon called *tolerance*. (From: Porchet HC, Benowitz NL, Sheiner LB. Pharmacodynamic model of tolerance: application to nicotine. J Pharmacol Exp Ther 1988;244:231–236. The American Society for Pharmacology and Experimental Therapeutics.)

the basal heart rate. Further evidence supporting this hypothesis is the increase in heart rate produced when a small supplementary bolus dose is administered at the end of the constant-rate-alone schedule, which momentarily raises the plasma nifedipine concentration above an already high steady-state concentration. The failure to observe a lowering of blood pressure with the constant-rate-alone regimen is at variance with the consistent lowering achieved in patients. These results underline the need to complement baseline studies in healthy subjects with studies in patients. Nonetheless, the observations described in Fig. 10-18 have a practical application. The primary use of nifedipine is to lower

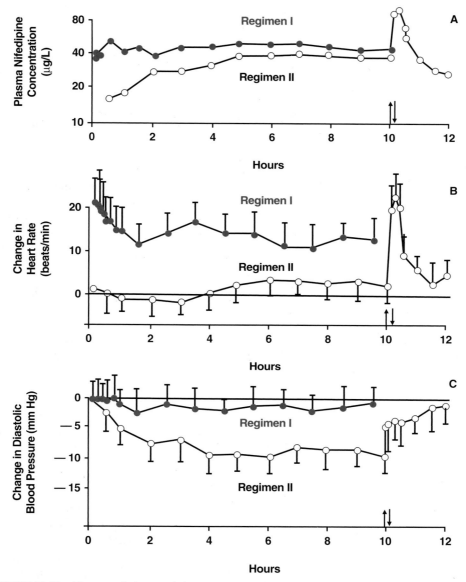

FIGURE 10-18. The rate of change of plasma concentration can be a major determinant of response, as demonstrated here with the hemodynamic effects produced by nifedipine. Each of six subjects received nifedipine in distinct regimens on two different occasions. Regimen I—by means of a computer-controlled infusion pump, the rate was adjusted to immediately attain and then maintain a relatively constant plasma concentration for 9.5 hr. Regimen II—a constant-rate infusion of 1.3 mg/hr for 10 hr at which time the infusion rate was increased 10-fold, to 13 mg/hr for 10 min (the period denoted by ↑↓). **A.** The plasma concentration in one subject associated with regimens I (●) and II (○). **B,C.** The corresponding mean group changes in heart rate and diastolic blood pressure, respectively. The slow approach to plateau associated with regimen II caused a fall in diastolic blood pressure but no tachycardia, whereas with regimen I, the converse was obtained. Further supporting the importance of rate considerations is the sharp rise in concentration and heart rate when the infusion rate was increased sharply and momentarily at the end of regimen I, before which the plasma concentrations produced by the two regimens were comparable. The mechanism for this regimen-dependent difference produced by nifedipine is still not fully understood but may be associated with the time needed for the baroreceptor reflex to respond to a change in arteriolar vasodilation produced by nifedipine. (From: Kleinbloesem CH, van Brummelen D, Danhof M, et al. Rate of increase in the plasma concentration of nifedipine as a major determinant of its hemodynamic effects in humans. Clin Pharmacol Ther 1987;41:20–30. Reproduced with permission of C.V. Mosby.)

blood pressure; tachycardia is an undesirable side effect. The data suggest that the latter effect can be reduced by slowing absorption. Although available in an immediate-release dosage form for specific indications, modified-release dosage forms are used to treat angina and hypertension.

INTEGRATION OF KINETIC AND PHYSIOLOGIC CONCEPTS

As in Chapter 5, *Elimination*, and Chapter 7, *Absorption*, the kinetic principles in this chapter on constant-rate input can be integrated with physiologic concepts previously given to assess how the concentration–time profile during and after a constant rate of input is expected to change when there is an alteration in any physiologic variable that influences the disposition of a drug. Conversely, one can suggest one or more physiologic variables that are likely to explain an observed change in a concentration–time profile in an altered condition. Obviously, changes in response associated with such changes in systemic exposure vary with the affected system and become very case specific. Here, our focus is on kinetic principles.

Clinical examples of the consequences of changing a physiologic variable on events following a constant-rate infusion are uncommon. Because this mode of administration is a good means of controlling systemic input, infusion rates are typically adjusted to achieve the desired response. Studies in conditions such as drug interactions, concurrent disease states, age, and genetic makeup are most frequently performed with either single doses or multiple-dose regimens. Some information on the effect of formulation of certain dosage forms, such as transdermal systems, implants, and modified-release dosage forms, which exhibit something close to zero-order input, as with constant-rate i.v. infusions, might fit into this category, but the primary issue in these studies relates to drug release and systemic absorption rather than changes in disposition. The purpose here is to practice the principles that have much greater usefulness in the subsequent chapters. Therefore, only four simulations are given to help learn the basic concepts.

Consider the expected changes in the pharmacokinetic values of the four drugs in Table 10-6 when there is a threefold change in each of the physiologic variables listed. Figure 10-19 shows the usual concentration–time profile of each of the four drugs on a given infusion regimen and the expected concentration–time profiles under those conditions in which there is a change in the physiologic variable given.

TABLE 10-6   Changes in Kinetic Parameters with Changes in Selected Physiologic Variables

Alteration	Physiologic variable altered*	Change in pharmacokinetic parameter CL	V	Half-life
Drug A: Low hepatic extraction ratio, $fe = 0.05$, $fu = 1.0$, $V = 20L$				
Inhibition of metabolism	$CL_{int} \downarrow$	$\downarrow$	$\leftrightarrow$	$\uparrow$
Drug B: High hepatic extraction ratio, ($E_H = 0.98$), $fe = 0.01$, $fu = 0.02$, $V = 230L$				
Inhibition of metabolism	$CL_{int} \downarrow$	$\leftrightarrow$	$\leftrightarrow$	$\leftrightarrow$
Drug C: Low hepatic extraction ratio, $fe = 0.05$, $fu = 1.0$, $V = 20L$				
Induction of metabolism	$CL_{int} \uparrow$	$\uparrow$	$\leftrightarrow$	$\downarrow$
Drug D: High hepatic extraction ratio, ($E_H = 0.98$), $fe = 0.01$, $fu = 0.02$, $V = 230L$				
Induction of metabolism	$CL_{int} \uparrow$	$\leftrightarrow$	$\leftrightarrow$	$\leftrightarrow$

$\uparrow$, increased; $\leftrightarrow$, little or no change; $\downarrow$, decreased.
*Altered by a factor of three.

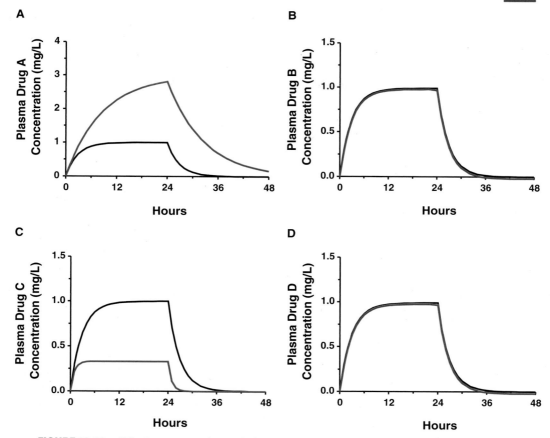

FIGURE 10-19. Whether or not a change in the usual concentration–time profile of Drugs A–D is expected with a change in condition depends on the pharmacokinetic properties of each drug and how it is physiologically handled by the body. Drug A has a low hepatic extraction ratio and is not bound to plasma proteins. Drug B, on the other hand, has a high hepatic extraction ratio and is highly bound to plasma proteins, but like Drug A is almost exclusively eliminated by hepatic metabolism. Drug C is eliminated by hepatic metabolism, but has a low hepatic extraction ratio. Drug D, on the other hand, has a high hepatic extraction ratio. The concentration–time profiles of each of the drugs are shown when given by a 24-hr infusion alone (*black lines*) and when there is a change in a physiologic variable (*colored lines*). Drug A is given concurrently with an inhibitor of drug metabolism as is Drug B. Drugs C and D are given at a time when an enzyme inducer is concurrently administered.

DRUG A. INHIBITION OF HEPATIC METABOLISM, LOW HEPATIC EXTRACTION RATIO

Inhibition of metabolism of Drug A decreases the clearance of this low-extraction ratio drug. The manifestation of this change in the concentration–time profile (Fig. 10-19, Drug A) during and after a constant-rate infusion is that the steady-state concentration is increased (*CL* decreased), the time to achieve it (half-life increased) is lengthened, and the postinfusion decline of the concentration is less steep (half-life increased).

DRUG B. INHIBITION OF HEPATIC METABOLISM, HIGH HEPATIC EXTRACTION RATIO

Inhibition of metabolism has little or no effect on the disposition kinetics of this drug, as long as the inhibition is not too great (Fig. 10-19, Drug B). This is explained by the fact that the hepatic extraction ratio is very high (98%); inhibition may lower the extraction ratio (e.g., to 95%), and consequently there would be some, but very little, change in hepatic clearance ($CL_H = Q_H \cdot E_H$). No adjustment in the i.v. infusion rate would be needed. With little change in CL and V, there is little or no change in half-life. Consequently, the concentration–time curve is essentially unchanged by the interaction. Fentanyl, which is sometimes given by i.v. infusion, is expected to follow this scenario. Recall in Chapter 5, *Elimination*, that the disposition kinetics of fentanyl was not affected by the concurrent administration of itraconazole, a modest inhibitor metabolism of fentanyl metabolism (Fig. 5-19).

DRUG C. INDUCTION OF HEPATIC METABOLISM, LOW HEPATIC EXTRACTION RATIO

Many drugs cause the synthesis of drug-metabolizing enzymes in the liver to increase (see Chapter 17, *Drug Interactions*). When another drug that is metabolized by that same enzyme is concurrently administered, its metabolism is increased. For a drug of low extraction in the liver, this alteration is expected to increase clearance and to shorten the half-life, as shown in Fig. 10-19C. With an increase in clearance, the steady-state plasma concentration is decreased and the time to approach it and to decline after withdrawing the drug is shortened.

DRUG D INDUCTION OF HEPATIC METABOLISM, HIGH HEPATIC EXTRACTION RATIO

An increase in enzyme activity for Drug D results in little or change in clearance because the drug is already almost completely extracted by the liver (Fig. 10-19D). Because clearance and volume are not changed, neither is the half-life. The net result is little or no change in the concentration–time profile.

This chapter has been devoted to constant-rate input of drug and to the turnover of the affected system that results in the measured drug response. We now turn, in the next chapter, to the much more common situation of therapeutic regimens in which drug is repetitively administered in fixed doses at regular intervals.

KEY RELATIONSHIPS

$$\text{Rate of change of drug in the body} = R_{inf} - k \cdot A$$

$$\text{Rate of change of drug in the body} = R_{inf} - CL \cdot C$$

$$A_{ss} = \frac{R_{inf}}{k}$$

$$C_{ss} = \frac{R_{inf}}{CL}$$

$$A_{inf} = A_{ss} - A_{ss} \cdot e^{-kt} = A_{ss}(1 - e^{-kt})$$

$$C_{inf} = C_{ss}(1 - e^{-kt})$$

STUDY PROBLEMS

(Answers to Study Problems are in Appendix J.)

1. Which one or more of the following statements pertaining to constant-rate infusion is correct?

   a. The time for the plasma concentration to reach plateau depends on the rate of infusion.

b. All drugs having the same clearance reach the same plateau concentration when given at the same i.v. infusion rate.

c. Drugs with the same clearance generally reach plateau concentration at the same time.

d. The amount of drug in the body at plateau cannot be the same when drugs with different clearance values are infused at the same rate.

e. All of the above.

f. None of the above.

2. For prolonged surgical procedures, succinylcholine chloride is given by i.v. infusion for sustained muscle relaxation. A typical initial dose is 20 mg followed by continuous infusion of 4 mg/min. The infusion must be individualized because of variation in the kinetics of metabolism of succinylcholine. Estimate the elimination half-lives of succinylcholine in patients requiring 0.4 and 4 mg/min, respectively, to maintain 20 mg in the body.

3. In the graphs in Fig. 10-20 are two multiple infusion-rate scenarios. Sketch the anticipated plasma concentration–time profiles on the graphs on the right using concepts presented in this chapter. The total clearance of the drug is 20 L/hr. Add units to the y-axes of the graphs on the right. Note that the time scales are expressed in half-life units.

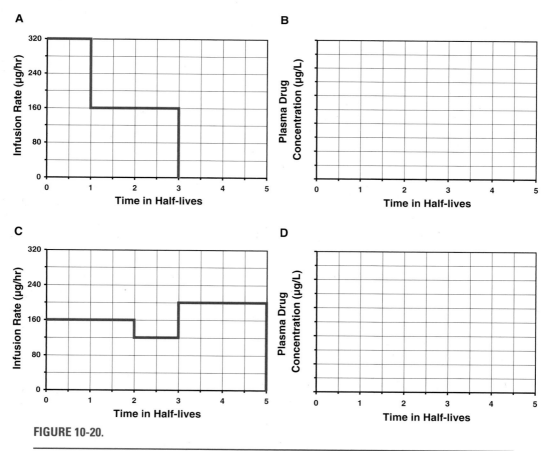

FIGURE 10-20.

4. During an investigational program, the calcium channel-blocking agent nifedipine was infused at a constant rate (1.5 μm/hr) via a rectal osmotic pump device for 24 hr. Table 10-7 lists the plasma nifedipine concentrations during and after the infusion. These data indicate that an average plateau concentration of 21 mg/L was attained.

TABLE 10-7	Nifedipine Kinetics During Rectal Infusion to Steady State with an Osmotic System

Time (hr)	Plasma Nifedipine Concentration (μg/L)
0	0
1	4.2
2	14.5
4	21.0
6	23.0
7.5	19.8
10.5	22.0
14	20.0
18	18.0
24	21.0
25	18.0
26	11.6
27	7.1
28	4.2

Abstracted from Kleinbloessem CH, van Hartenm J, de Leede LGJ, et al. Nifedipine kinetics and dynamics during rectal infusion to steady state with an osmotic system. Clin Pharmacol Ther 1984;36:396–401.

Given that all the infused drugs were systemically absorbed and that nifedipine disposition can be characterized by a one-compartment model:

a. Calculate the clearance, half-life, volume of distribution, and *MRT* of the drug.
b. Is the approach of the concentration to plateau in agreement with the half-life of nifedipine observed on removing the infusion pump?
c. If the infusion rate was 3.0 mg/hr instead of 1.5 mg/hr, what would be the expected concentrations at 1 hr, 2 hr, and at plateau?
d. If the desire is to achieve the plateau concentration associated with the 3.0 mg/hr infusion rate instantly, what is the loading dose required?

5. Droperidol, a butyrophenone derivative, has been used for the prevention and treatment of nausea and vomiting in postoperative patients and in patients undergoing chemotherapy. Droperidol is currently administered intravenously and intramuscularly, both invasive procedures. The oral route creates a problem for patients who are nauseous or vomiting. Gupta et al. (1992) evaluated a continuous-release rectal drug-delivery system as a means of achieving therapy for an extended period. Table 10-8

TABLE 10-8	Mean Plasma Droperidol Concentrations Following an Intravenous Infusion and the Use of Rectal Device in Eight Subjects												
Time (hr):	0	0.5	2	4	6	8	10	14	18	24	26	28	30
	Plasma Droperidol Concentrations (mg/L)												
i.v. infusion	0	0.90	1.80	2.60	2.50	2.50	2.70	2.70	2.90	3.10	1.40	0.61	0.36
Device	0	0	0.49	0.99	1.83	1.84	1.93	1.52	1.43	1.63	0.65	0.29	0.10

From: Gupta SK, Southam M, Hwang S. Pharmacokinetics of droperidol in healthy volunteers following intravenous infusion and rectal administration from an osmotic drug delivery module. Pharm Res 1992;9:694–696.

lists the mean plasma concentrations of droperidol obtained following use of this device, designed to deliver drug at a constant rate for 15 hr. The results are compared with those following a 24-hr constant-rate (0.125 mg/hr) i.v. infusion. The rectal device contained a total of 3-mg droperidol. No drug was found in the recovered device.

a. From the plasma concentration data after stopping the i.v. infusion, estimate the elimination half-life of droperidol.

b. Calculate the expected *MRT* following an i.v. bolus.

c. Estimate the systemic bioavailability of the drug.

d. Calculate clearance.

e. What is the volume of distribution of droperidol?

6. Hadgraft et al. (Hadgraft J, Hill S, Humpel M, et al. Investigators on the percutaneous absorption of the antidepressant rolipram in vitro and in vivo. Pharm Res 1990;7:1307–1312) explored the feasibility of transdermal delivery of a new antidepressant drug, rolipram. Table 10-9 lists the mean plasma rolipram concentrations in the six subjects during and after a 24-hr application of a 25-cm^2 patch made of silicone adhesive, drug, and 5% isopropyl myristate on a polymer backing. The patches (5 × 5 cm), applied to forearm skin areas, were covered for 24 hr. At this time, the patches were removed and the skin area cleaned with alcohol swabs. The average clearance and half-life of rolipram are 8.4 L/hr and 3 hr, respectively.

TABLE 10-9	Mean Rolipram Concentration During and After a Single 24-hr Dermal Application in Six Male Subjects												
Time (hr)	0	1	2	4	6	8	10	12	14	24	25	26	28	30
Plasma concentration (μg/L)	0	0	0.5	0.8	1.1	1.5	1.6	1.5	1.6	1.55	1.45	1.3	0.9	0.55

From: Hadgraft J, Hill S, Humpel M, et al. Investigators on the percutaneous absorption of the antidepressant rolipram in vitro and in vivo. Pharm Res 1990;7:1307–1312.

a. Calculate the average rate that rolipram is being absorbed from the patch between 12 and 24 hr.

b. Determine the total amount of rolipram absorbed during the 24-hr application of the patch. The *AUC* is 39.3 μg-hr/L.

c. Does the approach to steady state follow the expectation of 50% in one half-life, 75% in two half-lives, and so on? If not, briefly discuss how the absorption-time profile differs from that expected following constant-rate input.

7. Figure 10-21 shows the concentration–time profile after constant-rate infusion of a drug from 0 to 6 hr ($R_{inf}[0–6]$) and at another constant rate from 12 to 24 hr ($R_{inf}[12–24]$). In the first infusion, 300 mg was given. Assume a one-compartment model.

a. Determine the clearance, volume of distribution, and half-life of this drug.

b. Calculate the two constant-rates of infusion, (i.e., $R_{inf}[0–6]$ and $R_{inf}[12–24]$).

c. Draw, on the same figure, the concentration–time profile you would expect when a constant rate of infusion of 20 mg/hr is administered from time 0 to 24 hr. Show the full 48-hr profile.

8. Fenoldopam is given by continuous i.v. infusion for in-hospital, short-term (up to 48 hr) management of severe hypertension (diastolic pressure >120 mm Hg) when rapid, but quickly reversible, emergency reduction of blood pressure is clinically indicated. Bolus doses are not recommended because hypotension and too rapid a decrease in blood pressure are to be avoided. The initial infusion rate is

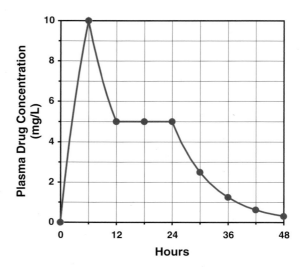

FIGURE 10-21.

titrated upward (or downward), no more frequently than every 15 min to reach the desired therapeutic effect. Constant infusion rates between 0.01 and 1.6 μg/kg per minute are used, with values between 0.025 and 0.3 μg/kg per minute being more common. The half-life of the drug is 5 min and a steady-state plasma concentration of 3.3 ng/mL is obtained on an infusion rate of 0.1 μg/kg per minute. The steady-state fenoldopam concentration is proportional to the infusion rate at all infusion rates.

a. Calculate the clearance of fenoldopam in a 66-kg patient who has a steady-state concentration of 8.25 ng/mL at an infusion rate of 0.25 μg/kg per minute.
b. Estimate the volume of distribution of the drug in this 66-kg patient. Use the typical half-life of the drug.
c. The drug is weakly bound to plasma proteins ($fu = 0.8$). Do you think it is reasonable to conclude that the drug is approximately evenly distributed throughout the extracellular fluids? Briefly discuss.
d. Does the minimum 15-min interval between changes in dosing rate seem reasonable based on the kinetics of the drug? Briefly comment.
e. The fraction excreted unchanged is 0.04. Calculate the renal clearance of the drug and comment on whether you believe it undergoes net secretion or net reabsorption (or neither). Use a glomerular filtration rate of 100 mL/min.

9. The "usual" plasma concentrations of urea and creatinine are 15 mg/100 mL (2.5 mM) and 1 mg/100 mL (0.09 mM), respectively, in young adult patients with normal renal function. The renal clearances of the two compounds are 70 and 120 mL/min, respectively. The volumes of distribution at study state are about the same (42 L). Both compounds are eliminated only by renal excretion.

a. Calculate the usual fractional turnover rates of both compounds.
b. Were the rate of production of these compounds to remain usual, how long would it take for the plasma urea concentration to increase by 30 mg/100 mL (5.0 mM) and the plasma creatinine concentration to increase by 2 mg/100 mL (0.8 mM) in an anephric patient?
c. Urea is an end product of protein metabolism. Its formation can be reduced by decreasing protein in the diet. What is the total amount of urea usually ingested and produced in the body in 24 hr under steady-state conditions?

10. If the turnover time of an enzyme is 4 days and its synthesis rate is instantly increased to a constant value that is three times the normal rate, how long will it take for the enzyme activity (concentration) to double?

11. A drug highly bound to plasma proteins ($fu = 0.01$) has a volume of distribution (based on plasma concentration) of 240 L/70 kg. The liver is the only organ of elimination. The hepatic extraction ratio is 0.95 despite the fact that the fraction in blood unbound, fu_b, is only 0.005. The hepatic blood flow is 81 L/hr.

   a. Estimate the values of the following parameters for this drug (70-kg patient): blood clearance (CL_b), clearance (CL), volumes of distribution based on drug concentrations in plasma water (Vu) and blood (V_b), and half-life.

   b. In uremic patients, the volume of distribution and the ratio Cu/C_b, fu_b, average 143 L and 0.03, respectively. Is there any evidence that the uremic state affects the tissue binding? If so, in what direction and by what factor is tissue binding altered?

   c. When this drug is infused intravenously at the same constant rate to a patient (normal renal function) who is and has been receiving another drug, the value of fu_b is now found to be 0.03. Under steady-state conditions for both drugs, predict the ratio of the unbound concentrations of the drug in the presence and absence of the other drug.

Multiple-Dose Regimens

OBJECTIVES

The reader will be able to:

- Define the meaning of the following words and phrases: drug accumulation, accumulation index, acquired resistance, average level at plateau, loading dose, maintenance dose, multiple-dose regimen, priming dose, relative fluctuation, trough concentration.

- Predict the plasma concentration–time profile following a fixed-dose and fixed–dosing-interval regimen when given the plasma concentration–time profile after a single dose of drug.

- Design a dosage regimen from knowledge of the pharmacokinetics and therapeutic window of a drug.

- Predict the rate and extent of drug accumulation for a given regimen of fixed dose and fixed interval.

- Explain why the time to reach plateau on a multiple-dosing regimen depends only on the half-life of the drug.

- Discuss the rationale behind a loading dose, and calculate the maintenance dose needed to maintain therapeutic levels knowing the half-life and the loading dose of the drug, and vice versa.

- Offer three examples of drugs for which the dosage regimen is conditioned by the half-life of the drug and its therapeutic index.

- Discuss the application of modified-release products to the development of more convenient dosage regimens.

- Explain why the time to reach a plateau of effect following a multiple-dose regimen is sometimes governed more by the pharmacodynamics than the pharmacokinetics of a drug, and give two examples illustrating this situation.

- Discuss how tolerance to the desired or adverse effects of a drug impacts on the optimal design and use of multiple-dose regimens.

- Give an example of a situation that requires intermittent drug administration for optimal therapy.

T he previous chapter dealt with constant-rate regimens. Although these regimens possess many desirable features, they are not the most common ones. The more common approach to the attainment and maintenance of continuous or chronic therapy is to give multiple discrete doses. This chapter covers the pharmacokinetic principles associated with such multiple dosing and, together with pharmacodynamics, the establishment of appropriate multiple-dose regimens. Also covered is the design and application of regimens using modified-release dosage forms.

PRINCIPLES OF DRUG ACCUMULATION

Drugs are most commonly prescribed to be taken on a fixed-dose, fixed–time-interval basis, for example, 50 mg 3 times a day, or 20 mg once a day. Associated with this kind of administration, the plasma concentration and amount in the body fluctuate and, similar to an infusion, rise toward a plateau.

To appreciate what happens when such regimens are taken, consider the plasma concentration–time data over 120 hr (5 days) in Table 11-1, also displayed in Fig. 11-1, following the oral administration of a single 200-mg dose of a drug. This drug is relatively slowly eliminated, is completely absorbed, and because it is very rapidly absorbed, the peak concentration occurs at the first time of measurement, 1 hr after administration. The intention is to give the same dose of this drug once daily. We wish to predict the anticipated concentrations over the first 5 days. To do this, we expect the concentration–time profile associated with each dose to be the same as that following the first dose, except that each profile will be displaced in time by the number of days since the first dose was given, as listed in Table 11-1 and shown as dotted lines in Fig. 11-1. The observed plasma concentration–time profile is then the sum of the concentrations associated with each of the doses. These are listed in the last column of Table 11-1. For example, the concentration at 1 hr after the second dose (25 hr since the first dose) is the

TABLE 11-1	Plasma Concentrations of a Drug following a Regimen of 200 mg Given Once Daily for 5 Days					
	Plasma Concentration Associated with Each Dose (mg/L)					Total Concentration (mg/L)
Time after First Dose (hr)	First Dose	Second Dose	Third Dose	Fourth Dose	Fifth Dose	
0	0					0
1	9.6					9.6
12	6.1					6.1
24	3.7	0				3.7
25	3.5	9.6				13.1
36	2.2	6.1				8.3
48	1.35	3.7	0			5.05
49	1.30	3.5	9.6			14.4
60	0.82	2.2	6.1			9.12
72	0.50	1.35	3.7	0		5.55
73	0.47	1.30	3.5	9.6		14.87
84	0.30	0.82	2.2	6.1		9.42
96	0.18	0.50	1.35	3.7	0	5.73
97	0.17	0.47	1.30	3.5	9.6	15.04
108	0.11	0.30	0.82	2.2	6.1	9.53
120	0.07	0.18	0.50	1.35	3.7	5.80

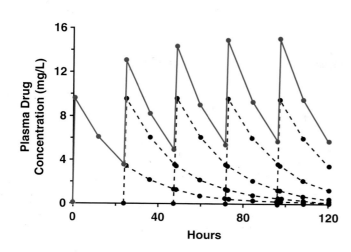

FIGURE 11-1. Accumulation on approach to plateau. When the plasma concentration–time profile is known following a single dose of drug, the anticipated profile following repetitive administration of a fixed dose of drug given at regular intervals can be calculated by replicating the single dose profile after each new dose (*black dashed lines*) and summing at each time the resultant concentrations associated with each dose. The result (*colored lines*) is a typical sawtooth profile rising to a plateau. The data used to generate these profiles are given in Table 11-1.

sum of that remaining from the first dose at 25 hr (3.5 mg/L) plus that associated with the second dose at 1 hr after dosing (9.6 mg/L), or 13.1 mg/L. Similarly, the concentration at 12 hr after the fifth dose, or 108 hr ($4 \times 24 + 12$) after the first dose, is given by

$$\underline{\text{Fifth Dose}} \qquad\qquad\qquad \underline{\text{Single Dose}}$$

$$\text{Total } C_5(12 \text{ hr}) = C_1(12 \text{ hr}) + C_1(36 \text{ hr}) + C_1(60 \text{ hr}) + C_1(84 \text{ hr}) + C_1(108 \text{ hr})$$

$$= 6.1 + 2.2 + 0.82 + 0.30 + 0.11$$

$$= 9.53 \text{ mg/L}$$

where the subscript denotes the dose number, and the value in parenthesis denotes the time since that dose was administered.

Several points are worth noting. First, clear evidence of **accumulation** in the plasma concentration is seen resulting in a characteristic rising sawtooth profile, showing **fluctuation** in concentration within each dosing interval. This accumulation occurs because there is always some drug left in the body from previous doses. Second, accumulation continues until a **plateau** is reached, after which time there is no further increase in the concentration from one dosing interval to the next. Analysis of the data in Table 11-1 shows that this occurs because by that time, about 4 days in the current example, virtually nothing is left in the body from the first dose. This pattern thus repeats itself for each subsequent dosing interval. Lastly, this calculation requires no knowledge of any pharmacokinetic parameter, be it clearance, volume of distribution, or oral bioavailability. All that is needed is the profile after a single dose, irrespective of its shape or complexity. This is the main attraction of this approach. Its limitation is that the calculations are restricted to the same times after each dose as that observed following the single dose. We now consider a direct method of calculating the amount of drug in the body and the plasma concentration *at any time after any number of doses*, starting with repetitive administration of intravenous (i.v.) bolus doses.

MAXIMA AND MINIMA ON ACCUMULATION TO THE PLATEAU

To appreciate further the phenomenon of accumulation, consider what happens when a 100-mg bolus dose is given intravenously (see Chapter 3, *Kinetics After an Intravenous Bolus Dose*) every elimination half-life. To simplify matters, we again start with administration into the well-stirred reservoir model considered in Chapter 5, *Elimination*. The events are depicted in Fig. 11-2. The amounts in the body just after each dose and just before the next dose can readily be calculated; these values correspond to the maximum (A_{max}) and minimum (A_{min}) amounts obtained within each dosing interval. The corresponding values

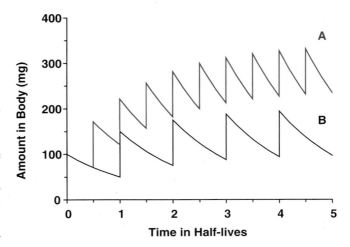

FIGURE 11-2. Dosing frequency controls the degree of drug accumulation. Intravenous bolus dose (100 mg) administered once every half of a half-life (**A**, *colored line*); same bolus dose administered once every half-life (**B**, *black line*). Note that time is expressed in half-life units.

(black line) during the first dosing interval are 100 mg ($A_{max,1}$) and 50 mg ($A_{min,1}$), respectively. The maximum amount of drug in the second dosing interval ($A_{max,2}$), 150 mg, is the dose (100 mg) plus the amount remaining from the previous dose (50 mg). The amount remaining at the end of the second dosing interval ($A_{min,2}$), 75 mg, is that remaining from the first dose, 25 mg (100 mg $\times$ ½ $\times$ ½, because two half-lives have elapsed since its administration) plus that remaining from the second dose, 50 mg. Alternatively, the value, 75 mg, may simply be calculated by recognizing that one-half of the amount just after the second dose, 150 mg, remains at the end of that dosing interval. Upon repeating this procedure, it is readily seen (curve B, Fig. 11-2) that drug accumulation, viewed in terms of either maximum or minimum amount in the body, continues until a limit is reached. At the limit, the amount lost in each interval equals the amount gained, the dose. In this example, the maximum and the minimum amounts in the body at steady state are 200 and 100 mg, respectively. This must be so because the difference between the maximum and minimum amounts is the dose, 100 mg, and because at the end of the interval, one half-life, the amount must be one half that at the beginning.

Recall, following a constant-rate input, that the *plateau* is reached when rate of elimination matches rate of input. Then, the level of drug in the body is constant as long as the input rate is maintained. With discrete dosing, the level is not constant within a dosing interval, but the values at a given time within the interval are the same from one dosing interval to another. The term **plateau** is also applied to this interdosing steady-state condition.

The foregoing considerations can be expanded for the more general situation in which a drug is given at a dosing interval, τ, not equal to the half-life. The general equations are derived in Appendix I, *Amount of Drug in Body on Accumulation to Plateau*, for the maximum and minimum amounts in the body after the Nth dose ($A_{max,N}$; $A_{min,N}$) and at steady state ($A_{max,ss}$; $A_{min,ss}$). These are

$$\text{Maximum amount in body after the Nth dose, } A_{max,N} = Dose \left[\frac{1 - e^{-N \cdot k \cdot \tau}}{1 - e^{-k \cdot \tau}} \right] \qquad \text{11-1}$$

$$= Dose \left[\frac{1 - e^{-N \cdot k \cdot \tau}}{\textit{Fraction lost in interval}} \right]$$

$$\text{Minimum amount in body after the Nth dose, } A_{min,N} = A_{max,N} \cdot e^{-k \cdot \tau} \qquad \text{11-2}$$

$$\frac{\text{Maximum amount in body}}{\text{at steady state, } A_{max,ss}} = \frac{Dose}{(1-e^{-k\cdot\tau})} = \frac{Dose}{\text{Fraction lost in interval}} \qquad \text{11-3}$$

$$\frac{\text{Minimum amount in body}}{\text{at steady state, } A_{min,ss}} = A_{max,ss} \cdot e^{-k\cdot\tau} = A_{max,ss} - Dose \qquad \text{11-4}$$

Recall from Chapter 3, *Kinetics Following an Intravenous Bolus Dose*, that the function $e^{-k\tau}$ is the fraction of the initial amount remaining in the body at time *t*. So that $1 - e^{-k\cdot\tau}$ is the fraction of drug lost during a dosing interval τ. Similarly, the amount in the body at the end of a dosing interval τ of a multiple-dose regimen, $(A_{min,N})$, frequently called the **trough** value, is obtained by multiplying the corresponding maximum amount by $e^{-k\tau}$, that is, $A_{min,N} = A_{max,N} \cdot e^{-k\tau}$ or $A_{min,ss} = A_{max,ss} \cdot e^{-k\tau}$.

The corresponding values for the plasma concentration are obtained by dividing the equations above by the volume of distribution of the drug. Returning to the example in Table 11-1, which approximates an i.v. bolus situation, the half-life of this drug, gained from a semilogarithmic plot of the plasma concentration after the single dose, is 16.7 hr and its volume of distribution is 20 L. Given this information, it is readily seen that the maximum and minimum concentrations anticipated at plateau, $C_{max,ss}$ and $C_{min,ss}$, when the 200-mg dose is given once daily (every 24 hr) are, by substitution

$$C_{max,ss} = \frac{A_{max,ss}}{V} = \frac{200mg}{20\,L \times (1 - e^{-(0.693/16.7hr)\times 24hr})} = 15.82\ mg/L$$

$$C_{min,ss} = \frac{A_{min,ss}}{V} = \frac{200mg \cdot e^{-(0.693/16.7hr)\times 24hr}}{20\,L \times (1 - e^{-(0.693/16.7hr)\times 24hr})} = 5.82\ mg/L$$

Notice that the previously calculated maximum and minimum values after the fifth dose (15.1 and 5.8 mg/L; Table 11-1) are very close to the correspondingly predicted maximum and minimum plateau concentrations, indicating that for all practical purposes (≥90%, as with constant-rate input) a plateau is anticipated to be reached by day 5 of dosing for this drug. Also, it is apparent that Eq. 11-3, upon dividing by *V*, offers a rapid way of calculating the maximum exposure likely to occur with a given dosage regimen, once the pharmacokinetic parameters of a drug following a single dose are known.

Equations 11-1 to 11-4 strictly apply only to intravascular bolus administration. They are reasonable approximations following extravascular administration when, as in the above example, absorption is complete and rapid relative to elimination. The following discussion deals with a less restrictive view of accumulation, which applies to all routes of administration.

AVERAGE LEVEL AT PLATEAU

In many respects, the accumulation of drugs administered in multiple doses is the same as that observed following constant-rate input. The average amount in the body at plateau is readily calculated using the steady-state concept: average *rate in* must equal average *rate out*. The average rate in is $F \cdot Dose/\tau$, where *F* is the bioavailability of the drug. The average rate out is $k \cdot A_{av,ss}$, where $A_{av,ss}$ is the average amount of drug in the body over the dosing interval, τ, at plateau. Therefore,

$$\frac{F \cdot Dose}{\tau} = k \cdot A_{av,ss} \qquad \text{11-5}$$

or

$$\frac{F \cdot Dose}{\tau} = CL \cdot C_{av,ss} \qquad \text{11-6}$$

where $C_{av,ss}$ is the average plasma concentration at plateau. Because $k = 0.693/t_{1/2}$, it also follows that

$$A_{av,ss} = 1.44 \cdot F \cdot Dose \cdot \left(\frac{t_{1/2}}{\tau} \right) \qquad\qquad \text{11-7}$$

while rearranging Eq. 11-6 yields

$$C_{av,ss} = \frac{F \cdot Dose}{CL \cdot \tau} \qquad\qquad \text{11-8}$$

These are fundamental relationships; they show how the average amount in the body at steady state depends on rate of administration ($Dose/\tau$), bioavailability, and half-life, and how the corresponding average concentration depends on the first two factors and clearance. Returning to the first example, with a half-life of 16.7 hr ($= 0.7$ days), $\tau = 1$ day, the average amount in the body at plateau is 200 mg. This amount lies approximately midway between the maximum and minimum amounts of 316 and 116 mg (calculated by multiplying the respective concentrations by the volume of distribution, 20 L). Notice also that, as expected, the difference between the maximum and minimum amounts is the dose, in this case, 200 mg. That $A_{av,ss} = Dose$ in this example is fortuitous. Had, for example, $F = 0.5$ or the dosing interval been changed from 1 day to 12 hr, thereby doubling the frequency of administration, then clearly the equality between $A_{av,ss}$ and $Dose$ would disappear.

Drug accumulation is not a phenomenon that implicitly depends on the property of a drug, nor are there drugs that are cumulative and others that are not. Accumulation, particularly the extent of it, is a result of the frequency of administration relative to half-life ($t_{1/2}/\tau$ or $1/k\tau$) as shown in Fig. 11-2. Here, we see that by halving the dosing interval from one half-life to one half of a half-life (curve A), the extent of accumulation has doubled. Notice, however, that the time to reach the plateau has not changed.

For convenience and to assure adherence to a regimen, drugs are commonly given once or twice a day, with 3 and 4 times daily being less desirable. As a consequence, extensive drug accumulation is more common for those drugs with half-lives greater than 1 day. It is particularly noticeable when the half-life of the drug is much longer than 1 day.

RATE OF ACCUMULATION TO PLATEAU

The amount in the body rises on multiple dosing just as it does following constant-rate input (Chapter 10, *Constant-Rate Input*). That is, *the approach to the plateau depends solely on the drug's half-life*. The simulation for the antiepileptic drug phenobarbital, in Table 11-2, which shows the ratio of the minimum amount during various dosing intervals to the minimum amount at plateau, illustrates this point. This drug has a half-life of 4 days and is given at a dose of 100 mg once daily. Observe that it takes one half-life (4 days), or 4 doses, to be at 50% of the value at plateau, two half-lives (8 days), or 8 doses, to be at 75% of the plateau value, and so on.

TABLE 11-2	Approach to Plateau on Daily Administration of Phenobarbital										
Time (Days)*:	0	1	2	3	4	8	12	16	20	24	∞
Number of Doses (N):	0	1	2	3	4	8	12	16	20	24	∞
$\left[\dfrac{\textit{Minimum Amount}}{\textit{Minimum Amount at Plateau}} \right]^{\dagger}$	0	0.16	0.29	0.40	0.50	0.75	0.875	0.94	0.97	0.98	1.00

*Time after first dose.
$^{\dagger}A_{min,N}/A_{min,ss} = 1 - e^{-0.173N}$

Accumulation of phenobarbital takes a long time because of its long half-life. Although once a day appears to be infrequent, relative to regimens of some drugs, it is frequent relative to phenobarbital's half-life of 4 days. The degree of accumulation is extensive because of relatively frequent administration. The frequent administration also determines the small **relative fluctuation** in the amount of drug in the body at plateau, seen as the difference between the maximum and minimum values relative to the average. At plateau, 100 mg of phenobarbital is lost every dosing interval, the dose, which is small compared with the maximum and minimum amounts (from Eqs. 11-3 and 11-4) in the body at plateau, namely 630 and 530 mg.

The approach to steady state, observed for the minimum amounts of phenobarbital in the body, also holds true for the maximum amounts (proof in Appendix I, *Amount of Drug in Body on Accumulation to Plateau*) that is, on dividing Eq. 11-1 by Eq. 11-3, and Eq. 11-2 by Eq. 11-4:

$$\frac{A_{max,N}}{A_{max,ss}} = \frac{A_{min,N}}{A_{min,ss}} = 1 - e^{-k \cdot N \cdot \tau} \qquad \text{11-9}$$

By recognizing that $N \cdot \tau$ is the total time elapsed since starting administration, expressed in multiples of the dosing interval, the similarity of Eq. 11-9 to the equation describing the rise of drug in the body to plateau following a constant-rate infusion $(1 - e^{-k \cdot t}$; Eq. 10-9) becomes apparent. This point is further illustrated by the events depicted in Fig. 11-3. Here, the average dosing rate is maintained at 100 mg a day, but the drug is given with increasing frequency, which, in the limiting case of the dosing interval becoming infinitesimally small, is a constant-rate input. It is seen that the time course of average amount in the body is the same in all cases, but the less frequent the administration, the greater is the fluctuation.

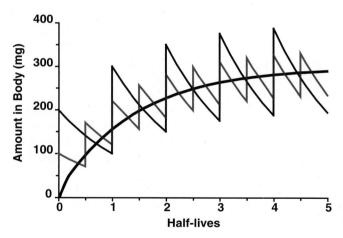

FIGURE 11-3. Plot showing that the time course of approach of amount in the body to the plateau is independent of the dosing interval. Here, the same average dosing rate was administered with increasing frequency, such that ultimately the dosing interval is so short as to approach that of a constant-rate input (*smooth black line*). Although the degree of fluctuation around the average value within a dosing interval varies with the dosing interval, the time to reach the plateau does not.

ACCUMULATION INDEX

When the amounts at steady state are compared with the corresponding values after the first dose, a measure of the extent of accumulation is obtained. This value can be thought of as an **accumulation index** (R_{ac}),

$$\text{Accumulation index } (R_{ac}) = \frac{A_{max,ss}}{A_{max,1}} = \frac{A_{min,ss}}{A_{max,1}} = \frac{1}{(1 - e^{-k \cdot \tau})} \qquad \text{11-10}$$

$$= \frac{1}{\text{Fraction lost in interval}}$$

Thus, the quantity, $1/(1 - e^{-k\tau})$, is the accumulation index. When phenobarbital is given once daily ($k = 0.173$ day^{-1}, $\tau = 1$ day), the accumulation index is 5.8. Thus, the maximum and minimum amounts (and, for that matter, the amount at any time within the dosing interval at plateau) are 5.8 times the values at the corresponding times after a single dose.

CHANGE IN REGIMEN

Sometimes the dose of drug has to be changed, because the response is inadequate or excessive. Suppose, for example, that the decision is made to double the amount of phenobarbital in the body at plateau. The need for a twofold increase in the rate of administration, from 100 to 200 mg/day, follows from Eq. 11-7. However, due consideration has to be given to the time needed to achieve a new plateau on changing the dosing rate. This often guides how long one needs to wait to ensure the achievement of the full response associated with the change, before deciding if any further adjustments in drug therapy are needed. As with i.v. infusion, it takes one half-life to go one-half the way from the original plateau to the new one, two half-lives to go three quarters of the way, and 3.3 half-lives to reach plateau practically. For phenobarbital, it would take about 14 days (3.3 half-lives) to go from the original plateau ($A_{max,ss} = 630$ mg; $A_{min,ss} = 530$ mg) to greater than 90% of the way toward the new one ($A_{max,ss} = 1260$ mg; $A_{min,ss} = 1060$ mg) on doubling the daily dose. Hence, we would not expect to see the full benefits associated with this increase in dose for at least 2 weeks.

RELATIONSHIP BETWEEN INITIAL AND MAINTENANCE DOSES

It is sometimes therapeutically desirable to establish the required amount of drug in the body as soon as possible, rather than wait for this to be achieved by repeatedly giving the same dose at a regular interval. When a larger first or initial dose is given to quickly achieve a therapeutic level, it is referred to as **priming** or **loading dose**. A case in point is sirolimus (Rapamune), an immunosuppressive drug used as part of therapy to prevent rejection following organ transplantation. Sirolimus has a half-life on the order of 2.5 days, and the usual oral maintenance dose is 2 mg once a day. Given in this manner, it would take approximately 1 week to reach the plateau, which is much too long to prevent the increased risk of organ rejection. Instead, patients first receive a loading dose of 6 mg followed by 2 mg daily. Another example is digoxin used in the treatment of chronic atrial fibrillation; it has a half-life on the order of 2 days, and the usual oral maintenance dose is 0.25 mg taken once a day. Taken in this manner, it would take approximately a week to reach the plateau. In some patients, it is important to reach effective levels in the body relatively rapidly. In this case, digoxin is given as a larger initial dose, followed by the regular daily doses. For digoxin, the initial oral dose, up to 1 mg, is often administered in divided doses. Several procedures are followed, but the divided dose is commonly given every 6 hr until the desired therapeutic response is obtained. In this way, each patient is titrated to his or her required initial therapeutic dose.

Instead of determining the loading dose when the maintenance dose is given, it is more common to determine the maintenance dose required to sustain a therapeutic amount in the body. The initial dose rapidly achieves the therapeutic response; subsequent doses maintain the response by replacing drug lost during the dosing interval. The **maintenance dose**, D_M, therefore, is the difference between the loading dose and the amount remaining at the end of the dosing interval, $D_L \cdot e^{-k\tau}$, that is,

$$\frac{Maintenance}{Dose} = \frac{Loading}{Dose} \cdot (1 - e^{-k \cdot \tau}) \qquad \text{11-11}$$

$$= \frac{Loading}{Dose} \cdot [Fraction\ lost\ in\ interval]$$

Likewise, if the maintenance dose is known, the initial dose can be estimated:

$$\frac{Loading}{Dose} = \frac{Maintenance\ Dose}{(1 - e^{-k \cdot \tau})} = \frac{Maintenance\ Dose}{[Fraction\ lost\ in\ interval]} \quad\quad 11\text{-}12$$

$$= R_{ac} \cdot Maintenance\ Dose$$

The relationship between loading dose and accumulation index, R_{ac}, follows from Eq. 11-10. For sirolimus, Eq. 11-12 predicts that a daily maintenance dose of 2 mg requires a loading dose of 8 mg. As noted previously, clinical experience indicates that a slightly lower dose (6 mg) suffices.

The similarity between Eqs. 11-3 and 11-12 should be noted. From the viewpoint of accumulation, Eq. 11-3 relates to the maximum amount at plateau on administering a given dose repetitively. If the maximum amount were put into the body initially, then Eq. 11-11 indicates the dose needed to maintain that amount. The relationships are the same, although they were derived starting from different viewpoints. These equations form the heart of multiple-dose administration.

The ratio of loading to maintenance doses depends on the dosing interval and the half-life and is equal to the accumulation index, R_{ac} (Eq. 11-12). For example, the antibiotic doxycycline has approximately a 1-day half-life, and a dose in the range of 200 mg is considered to provide effective antimicrobial drug concentrations. Therefore, a reasonable schedule is 200 mg (two 100-mg capsules) initially, followed by 100 mg once a day, as shown in Fig. 11-4. (In practice, it is recommended that the initial dose be divided into 100 mg taken 12 hr apart.) A dosage regimen, such as that for doxycycline, consisting of a priming dose equal to twice the maintenance dose and a dosing interval of one half-life, is convenient for drugs with half-lives between 8 and 24 hr. The frequency of administration for such drugs varies from 3 times a day to once daily, respectively. For drugs with half-lives less than 3 hr, or with half-lives greater than 24 hr, this regimen is often impractical.

Although a loading or initial dose greater than the maintenance dose seems appropriate for drugs with half-lives longer than 24 hr, such is often not the case. There are various reasons why this is so, which are discussed at greater length later in this chapter and also in Chapter 18, *Initiating and Maintaining Therapy*. Here, we note a few examples. For piroxicam, an analgesic/antipyretic drug with a half-life of 2 days, the most common adverse effects are gastrointestinal reactions. Such reactions may be increased if a loading dose, which would be 3 to 4 times the maintenance dose (Eq. 11-12, $\tau = 1$ day), is given. Another example is that of protriptyline (an antidepressant with a half-life of 3 days), for which larger doses slow gastric emptying and gastrointestinal activity (anticholinergic effect), resulting in slower and more erratic absorption of this and other drugs.

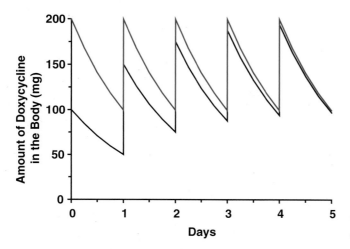

FIGURE 11-4. Sketch of the amount of doxycycline in the body with time in an individual with a 24-hr half-life following i.v. administration of 200 mg initially and 100 mg once daily thereafter (*colored line*). When the initial and maintenance doses are the same, it takes 4 days (four half-lives) before the plateau is practically reached (*black line*). Thereafter, the two curves are essentially the same.

MAINTENANCE OF DRUG IN THE THERAPEUTIC RANGE

Dosage regimens that achieve effective therapy for drugs with both high and medium-to-low therapeutic indices and with various half-lives are listed in Table 11-3.

HALF-LIVES LESS THAN 30 MINUTES

Great difficulty is encountered in trying to maintain therapeutic levels of such drugs. This is particularly true for a drug with a low therapeutic index, for example, heparin and

| TABLE 11-3 | Dosage Regimens for Continuous Maintenance of Levels | | | | |

Therapeutic Index	Half-life	Ratio of Initial Dose to Maintenance Dose	Ratio of Dosing Interval to Half-Life	General Comments	Drug Examples
High	<30 min	—	—	Candidate for constant-rate administration and/or short-term therapy.	Nitroglycerin*
	30 min–3 hr	1	3–6	To be given any less often than every 3 half-lives, drug must have very high therapeutic index.	Cephalosporins Ibuprofen
	3–8 hr	1–2	1–3		Clopidogrel
	8–24 hr	2	1	Very common and desirable regimen.	Doxycycline
	>24 hr	>2	<1	Once daily is practical.	Azithromycin
Medium-to-low	<30 min	—	—	Not a candidate except under very closely controlled infusion.	Esmolol†
	30 min–3 hr	—	—	By infusion or frequent administration; less frequently with modified-release formulation.	Morphine
	3–8 hr	1–2	~1	Requires 3–4 doses per day, but less frequently with modified-release formulation.	Oxycodone
	8–24 hr	2–3	0.5–1	Very common and desirable regimen.	Flecanide‡
	>24 hr	>2**	<1	Daily dosing is the norm.	Sirolimus

*Tolerance to drug prevents continuous administration; see page 319.

†Despite a half-life of 9 min with rapid attainment of steady state, an i.v. bolus loading dose is given because of the use of the drug in emergency settings.

‡As with many other drugs in this category, rather than administering a loading dose, dosage is progressively elevated until the desired response is achieved.

**Loading dose is often not given, or given as smaller divided doses over several days, to avoid acute exposure to high concentrations and excessive adverse effects.

esmolol, which have half-lives of approximately 30 and 10 min, respectively. Such type of drugs must be either infused or discarded unless intermittent systemic exposures are permissible. Drugs with a high therapeutic index may be given less frequently, but the longer the dosing interval, the greater is the maintenance dose required to ensure that drug in the body stays above a minimum effective value, and the greater is the degree of fluctuation. Penicillin is a notable example of a drug for which the dosing interval (4–6 hr) is many times longer than its half-life (~30 min). This is possible because the dose given keeps the plasma concentrations of antibiotic above the minimum inhibitory concentration for most penicillin-sensitive microorganisms for most of a dosing interval. With the dosing interval some 8- to 12-fold longer than the half-life, there is negligible accumulation of drug.

HALF-LIVES BETWEEN 30 MINUTES AND 8 HOURS

For such drugs, the major considerations are therapeutic index and convenience of dosing. A drug with a high therapeutic index need only be administered once every one to three half-lives, or even less frequently. An example is the nonsteroidal anti-inflammatory drug ibuprofen; it has a half-life of around 2 hr, but dosing once every 6 hr, or even 8 hr, is adequate for effective treatment of various inflammatory conditions. A drug with a relatively low therapeutic index must be given approximately every half-life, or more frequently, or be given by infusion. Theophylline, for example, with a half-life of 6 to 8 hr, would need to be given from 3 to 4 times a day; more convenient dosing is achieved by slowing the release of drug from the dosage form (see Modified-Release Dosage Forms discussed on page 311).

HALF-LIVES BETWEEN 8 AND 24 HOURS

Here, the most convenient and desirable regimen is one in which a dose is given every half-life. If immediate achievement of steady state is desired, then, as previously mentioned, the initial dose must be twice the maintenance dose; the minimum and maximum amounts in the body are equivalent to one and two maintenance doses, respectively.

HALF-LIVES GREATER THAN 24 HOURS

For drugs with half-lives greater than 1 day, administration once daily is common, convenient, and promotes patient adherence to the prescribed regimen. For some drugs with very long half-lives, in the order of weeks or more, and which have a moderate to relatively high therapeutic index, once weekly administration is adequate. Examples are mefloquine (half-life of 3 weeks), used as a prophylaxis against malaria, and alendronate, a bisphosphonate (retained and very slowly released from bone, half-life in years) used in the treatment of osteoporosis.

If an immediate therapeutic effect is desired, a therapeutic loading dose needs to be given initially. Otherwise, the initial and maintenance doses are the same, in which case several doses may be necessary before the drug accumulates to therapeutic levels. The decision whether or not to give larger initial doses is often a practical matter. Side effects to large oral doses (gastrointestinal side effects) or to acutely high concentrations of drug in the body may dictate against the use of a loading dose. This is particularly so when, as in many situations, tolerance develops to the adverse effects of a drug (see "Development of Tolerance," later in this chapter, for further discussion).

REINFORCING THE PRINCIPLES

To summarize the foregoing discussion, consider the recommended maintenance dosage regimens given in Table 11-4 for three drugs. The antibiotic amoxicillin, used to treat an infection, the anti-inflammatory agent, naproxen, when used to treat an acute attack of gout, and piroxicam, another anti-inflammatory agent, when used to treat arthritic joint pain. Listed in Table 11-5 are the corresponding fractions of the initial amounts remaining at the end of a dosing interval, the average amounts at steady state,

TABLE 11-4	Dosage Regimens and Half-lives of Three Drugs			
Drug	Loading Dose (mg)	Maintenance Dose (mg)	Dosing Interval (hr)	Half-life (hr)
Amoxicillin	—	250	8	1
Naproxen	750	250	8	14
Piroxicam	20	20	24	50

TABLE 11-5	Amount of Drug in Body (mg) on Regimens Given in Table 11-4			
		Amount in Body		
Drug*	Fraction Remaining at End of Interval[†]	Average at Steady State[‡]	Maximum at Steady State[††]	Minimum at Steady State[‡‡]
Amoxicillin	0.004	45	251	1
Naproxen	0.67	630	765	515
Piroxicam	0.71	60	70.7	50.7

*Bioavailability of all three drugs is 100% ($F = 1$).
[†]Given by $e^{-k\cdot\tau}$
[‡]$1.44 \cdot F \cdot D_M \cdot t_{1/2}/\tau$
[††]$F \cdot D_M/(1 - e^{-k\cdot\tau})$
[‡‡]$A_{ss,max} - F \cdot D_M$

and the maximum and minimum values. Instantaneous and complete absorption is assumed, which are reasonable approximations for these drugs.

The maintenance doses of amoxicillin and naproxen are the same, but the amounts of them in the body with time at steady state are not. Also, despite the difference in dosage regimens, the average amount in the body at plateau is not that different for amoxicillin and piroxicam. The explanation is readily visualized with a sketch.

For naproxen, the amount in the body immediately after the first dose is 250 mg. At the end of the 8-hr dosing interval, with a half-life of 14 hr, the fraction remaining is 0.67, and the amount therefore is 168 mg. The second maintenance dose of 250 mg raises the amount to 418 mg, and so on. Figure 11-5, curve A, is thus readily drawn, from which it is clear that it takes approximately 3 days to reach steady state, when the average amount in the body is 630 mg (Eq. 11-7), and that the accumulation index is 3.06 (Eq. 11-10). Sometimes, a full therapeutic effect needs to be established more quickly, in which case a loading dose of 750 mg is administered. As can readily be seen, following the loading dose, the amount remaining at the end of the first dosing interval is 505 mg (0.67 × 750 mg), and that the amount lost is 245 mg. The maintenance dose of 250 mg then essentially replaces that lost within this first dosing interval, thereby ensuring that steady-state conditions are maintained throughout the regimen (see colored curve of Fig. 11-5).

For amoxicillin, with a half-life of 1 hr and when 250 mg is given every 8 hr, virtually none remains at the end of the dosing interval (eight half-lives), such that a steady state is reached by the time that the second dose is administered. Events in each dosing interval essentially repeat that following the first dose, fluctuation between maximum and minimum amounts is very large, and in contrast to naproxen, for the same dosage regimen, the average amount within a dosing interval at plateau is only 45 mg ($A_{av,ss}/Dose = 2.5$ for naproxen and 0.18 for amoxicillin; Eq. 11-7). Figure 11-6 is a sketch of the amounts of amoxicillin in the body with time.

The results are markedly different for piroxicam than amoxicillin. At the end of each 1-day dosing interval, with a half-life of 50 hr, the fraction remaining for piroxicam is 0.712.

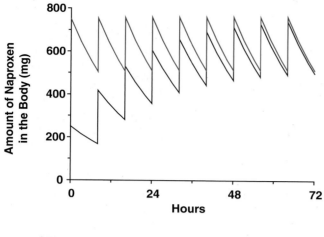

FIGURE 11-5. Sketch of the amount of naproxen in the body with time; simulation of 250 mg given intravenously every 8 hr (*black line*). Because the half-life, 14 hr, is somewhat longer than the dosing interval, the degree of accumulation is extensive, but the fluctuation is modest. Notice that a loading dose of 750 mg immediately achieves the conditions at steady state (*colored line*).

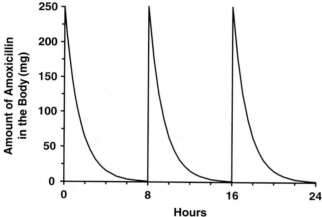

FIGURE 11-6. Sketch of the amount of amoxicillin in the body with time when 250 mg is given intravenously every 8 hr. Because the half-life, 1 hr, is very short relative to the dosing interval, the degree of accumulation is negligible and the fluctuation is extremely large.

Accumulation then occurs until the 29% lost in each interval is equal to the dose, and the maximum amount in the body at steady state is therefore about 3.53 times the 20-mg maintenance dose, for example, 71 mg. The minimum amount at steady state is 51 mg. From the calculated value of the maximum amount at plateau and the half-life, it is apparent that a sketch must be scaled to at least 71 mg and to about 7 days (Fig. 11-7). The amount in the body at its half-life, 50 hr, is one-half of the steady-state amount, at 100 hr

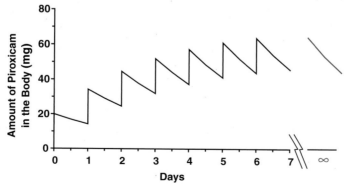

FIGURE 11-7. Sketch of the amount of piroxicam in the body with time; simulation of 20 mg given intravenously once daily. Because the half-life, 50 hr, is long relative to the dosing interval, the degree of accumulation is large, and the fluctuation at plateau is low, a result similar to that seen with naproxen in Fig. 11-5. The maximum and minimum values during a dosing interval at steady state, 71 and 51 mg, are shown by the colored line.

the level it is 75% of the plateau amount, and so on. Practically, fluctuations are relatively minor, and the average amount at plateau of 60 mg is now comparable to that obtained with amoxicillin, despite the 12-fold difference in the maintenance dose.

ADDITIONAL CONSIDERATIONS

So far, consideration has been given primarily to the amount of drug in the body following multiple i.v. bolus injections, or their equivalent, at equally spaced intervals. In practice, chronic administration is usually by the oral route. Furthermore, only drug concentration in plasma or in blood can be measured and not the amount of drug in the body. These aspects are now considered. Issues related to unequal doses and dosing intervals and to missed doses, as arises when adherence to the dosage regimen is poor, are covered in Chapter 18, *Initiating and Managing Therapy*.

EXTRAVASCULAR ADMINISTRATION

The oral (also intramuscular, buccal, subcutaneous, and rectal) administration of drugs requires an added step, absorption. Equations 11-1 to 11-4 apply to extravascular administration, provided that absorption has essentially ended within a small fraction of a dosing interval, a condition similar to i.v. bolus administration. Even so, a correction must be made if bioavailability is less than 1. For example, the maximum amount of drug in the body at plateau, $A_{max,ss}$ is then

$$A_{max,ss} = \frac{F \cdot Dose}{(1 - e^{-k \cdot \tau})} \qquad 11\text{-}13$$

Equations 11-9, 11-10, 11-11, and 11-12 also still apply even if bioavailability is less than 100% provided that absorption is much faster than elimination, so that the bolus approximation assumption holds.

When absorption becomes slower, within each dosing interval the peak becomes lower and the trough (minimum) concentration higher, tending thereby to decrease the degree of fluctuation seen around the average value. This decrease in fluctuation is apparent when extravascular administration is contrasted with i.v. bolus dose administration, as demonstrated in Fig. 11-8. Notice, that the impact of absorption kinetics is greater on the peak than the trough. This occurs because the peak reflects the condition when rate of input matches the rate of output, and hence is very sensitive to changes in input rate. In contrast, the trough better reflects the amount of drug in the body once absorption is over, and as such is relatively insensitive to changes in absorption kinetics.

The therapeutic impact of differences in absorption kinetics, but not in bioavailability, of extravascularly administered drug products given continuously also depends on

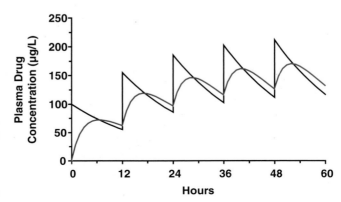

FIGURE 11-8. Compared with an i.v. bolus regimen (*black line*), when given orally the impact of absorption kinetics lowers the peak and raises the trough (*colored line*). In this example the bioavailability of the drug is 100%, so the average concentration at steady state is the same.

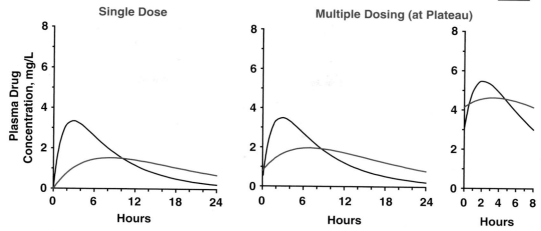

FIGURE 11-9. Differences in the absorption kinetics between two dosage forms following a single extravascular dose *(left panel)* may have a major therapeutic impact at plateau during multiple dosing, depending on the relative frequency of administration. The impact is greater when the products are given infrequently *(middle panel)* than when given frequently *(right panel)*. The colored line represents the dosage form showing the slower absorption.

the frequency of their administration. As illustrated in Fig. 11-9, major differences in absorption kinetics seen following a single dose only persist, and are of potential therapeutic concern, at plateau when the drug products are given infrequently relative to the half-life of the drug. The differences between them almost disappear at plateau when the products are given frequently. In the latter case, as stated previously, with extensive accumulation of drug, the concentration at plateau is relatively insensitive to variations in the absorption rate with time.

When absorption continues throughout a dosing interval or longer, then Eqs. 11-1 to 11-4 do not strictly apply, but the relationships of Eqs. 11-7 and 11-8 still hold. These relationships allow estimation of the average plateau amount in the body and the average plateau concentration, respectively. The slowness of drug absorption affects the degree of fluctuation around, but not the value of, the average level. The exception is when absorption becomes so slow that there is insufficient time for complete absorption, for example, when limited by the transit time within the gastrointestinal tract, in which case bioavailability becomes dependent on absorption kinetics.

PLASMA CONCENTRATION VERSUS AMOUNT IN BODY

During multiple dosing, the plasma concentration can be calculated at any time by dividing the corresponding equations defining amount by volume of distribution. However, distribution equilibrium between drug in the tissues and that in plasma takes time, as further discussed in Chapter 19, *Distribution Kinetics*. Thus, observed maximum concentrations may be appreciably greater than those calculated by dividing Eqs. 11-1 and 11-3 by V, which assume that distribution equilibrium is complete.

The average plateau concentration may be calculated using Eq. 11-8. This equation is applicable to any route, method of administration, or dosage form, as long as bioavailability and clearance remain constant with both time and dose.

DESIGN OF DOSAGE REGIMENS USING PLASMA CONCENTRATION

Dosage regimens can be designed to maintain concentrations within a therapeutic window. The window is defined by a lower limit (C_{lower}) and an upper limit (C_{upper}). The maximum dosing interval, τ_{max}, and maximum maintenance dose, $D_{M,max}$, can be readily computed from these limits as follows:

$$C_{lower} = C_{upper} \cdot e^{-k \cdot \tau_{max}} \qquad \text{11-14}$$

where τ_{max} is the maximum time interval over which these upper and lower concentrations can occur. By rearrangement of Eq. 11-14, the value of τ_{max} is

$$\tau_{max} = \frac{ln\left(\dfrac{C_{upper}}{C_{lower}}\right)}{k} \qquad \text{11-15}$$

and, from the relationship, $k = 0.693/t_{1/2}$,

$$\tau_{max} = 1.44 \cdot t_{1/2} \cdot ln\left(\frac{C_{upper}}{C_{lower}}\right) \qquad \text{11-16}$$

The corresponding maximum maintenance dose, $D_{M,max}$, that can be given every τ_{max} is

$$D_{M,max} = \frac{V}{F} \cdot (C_{upper} - C_{lower}) \qquad \text{11-17}$$

When $D_{M,max}$ is administered every τ_{max}, there is an average concentration produced within the dosing interval, defined by

$$\frac{D_{M,max}}{\tau_{max}} = \frac{CL}{F} \cdot C_{ss,av} \qquad \text{11-18}$$

By dividing Eq. 11-17 by Eq. 11-15 and comparing this ratio to Eq. 11-18, it is apparent that the value of $C_{ss,av}$ is given by

$$C_{ss,av} = \frac{(C_{upper} - C_{lower})}{ln\left(\dfrac{C_{upper}}{C_{lower}}\right)} \qquad \text{11-19}$$

A dosage regimen may be designed by setting the dosing rate to achieve the average concentration, $C_{ss,av}$. Choosing the average concentration within the dosing interval at plateau to be $C_{ss,av}$ allows the greatest possible dosing interval. This dosing interval (Eq. 11-15) and the corresponding maintenance dose (Eq. 11-17) may not be practical, however. Both values may need to be adjusted to make the frequency of administration convenient for patient compliance and to accommodate the dose strengths of the drug products available. The guiding principle is to maintain the same rate of administration and therefore the same chosen average steady-state concentration.

Having chosen a convenient dosing interval, τ smaller than τ_{max}, the maintenance dose is

$$D_M = \frac{D_{M,max}}{\tau_{max}} \cdot \tau \qquad \text{11-20}$$

and the loading dose, appropriate to attain the peak steady-state concentration, initially, is

$$D_L = \frac{D_M}{(1 - e^{-k \cdot t})} \qquad \text{11-21}$$

If more (or less) vigorous therapy is desired, resulting in the setting of the average targeted concentration to be higher (or lower) than $C_{ss,av}$, the dosing rate can be increased (or decreased) proportionately. However, one may wish to adjust the dosing interval to ensure that concentrations remain within the therapeutic window.

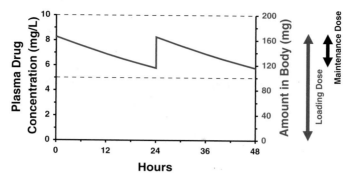

FIGURE 11-10. The dosage regimen design of a drug is designed to maintain the same average concentration as that obtained when the concentration fluctuates between the upper (10 mg/L) and lower (5 mg/L) limits. The regimen shown is for a 24-hr dosing interval. A loading dose is required to achieve the steady-state concentration immediately. The loading and maintenance doses are indicated on the right side of the graph.

For example, consider a drug with a therapeutic window of 5 to 10 mg/L, a volume of distribution of 20 L and a 46-hr half-life ($k = 0.015$ hr^{-1}). The maximum dosing interval is then 46 hr (ln (10/5)/0.015 hr^{-1}), the maximum dose is 100 mg (20 L × (10 − 5 mg/L), and the dosing rate needed to stay within these bounds is 2.17 mg/hr (100 mg/46 hr). If an interval of 24 hr is chosen, then the maintenance dose needed is about 50 mg (*2.17 mg/hr* × *24 hr*). The loading dose (*50 mg/*(1 − $e^{-k\tau}$)) is 165 mg. Figure 11-10 illustrates the expected concentration–time profile when a loading dose of 165 mg and a maintenance dose of 50 mg is given every 24 hr.

Following extravascular administration, fluctuations in the plasma concentration of drug are less than those after intravascular administration. Depending on the slowness of the absorption process, it may be possible to administer the drug less frequently than indicated in the regimens designed above.

WHEN BIOAVAILABILITY AND VOLUME ARE UNKNOWN

Oral dosage regimens can also be designed without determining bioavailability. This is accomplished using the area under the plasma concentration–time curve (*AUC*), following a single dose. From the relationship $F \cdot Dose = CL \cdot AUC$ after a single dose (Eq. 6-6) and the relationship $F \cdot Dose/\tau = CL \cdot C_{av,ss}$ during steady state after multiple doses (Eq. 11-6), it follows that

$$C_{av,ss} = \frac{AUC\ (single\ dose)}{\tau} \qquad \text{11-22}$$

Consequently, either the dosing interval necessary to achieve a desired average steady-state concentration or the average concentration resulting from administering the dose every dosing interval can be calculated.

By definition of $C_{av,ss}$, the value of $\tau \cdot C_{av,ss}$ is the *AUC* within a dosing interval at steady state. Thus, this area is equal to that following a single dose. This principle is shown in Fig. 11-11, and a practical illustration is shown in Fig. 11-12. Given the plasma concentrations with time after a single oral dose, the concentration at any time during repeated administration of the same dose can be readily calculated by adding the concentrations remaining from each of the previous doses. For example, if doses are given at 0, 12, and 24 hr, then the concentration at 30 hr is equal to the sum of the values at 30, 18, and 6 hr after a single dose.

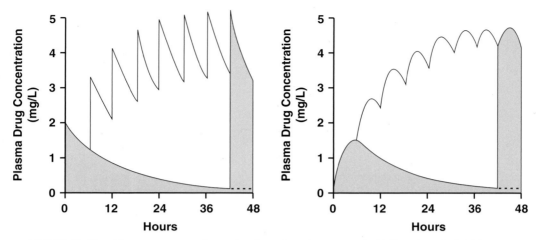

FIGURE 11-11. Plasma concentrations of a drug given intravenously (*left*) and orally (*right*) on a fixed dose of 50 mg and fixed dosing interval of 6 hr. The half-life is 12 hr. Note that the *AUC* during a dosing interval at steady state (42–48 hr, *colored*) is equal to the total *AUC* following a single dose (0–∞, *colored*). The fluctuation of the concentration is diminished when given orally (absorption half-life is 1.4 hr), but the average steady-state concentration is the same as that after i.v. administration, when, as in this example, $F = 1$.

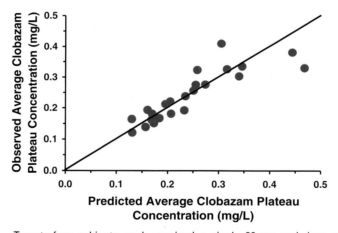

FIGURE 11-12. Twenty-four subjects each received a single 20-mg oral dose of the benzodiazepine, clobazam, followed 1 month later by an oral regimen of 10 mg of clobazam daily for 22 consecutive days. The observed average plateau clobazam concentration was well predicted by the value calculated from the single-dose data, obtained by dividing the *AUC* by the dosing interval and correcting for dose. The solid line is the perfect prediction. (From: Greenblatt DJ, Divoll M, Puri SK, et al. Reduced single-dose clearance of clobazam in elderly men predicts increased multiple-dose accumulation. Clin Pharmacokinet 1983;8:83–94. Reproduced with permission of ADIS Press Australasia Pty Limited.)

TABLE 11-6 **Relationships for Evaluating Dosage Regimens[†]**

			Extravascular		
		i.v. Bolus	Rapid Absorption $(ka \gg k)$	Slow Absorption $(ka > k)$	$(k > ka)$
Maintenance dose	$D_M = D_L \cdot (1 - e^{-k \cdot \tau})$	***	***	**	N
Accumulation index	$R_{AC} = \dfrac{1}{(1 - e^{-k \cdot \tau})}$	***	***	**	N
Average amount at plateau	$A_{av,ss} = 1.44 \cdot F \cdot Dose \dfrac{t_{1/2}}{\tau}$	****	****	****	****
Average concentration	$C_{av,ss} = \dfrac{F \cdot D_M}{CL \cdot \tau}$	****	****	****	****
	$C_{av,ss} = \dfrac{AUC \,(\text{single dose})}{\tau}$	***	***	***	***
Maximum concentration	$C_{ss,max} = \dfrac{F \cdot D_M \cdot e^{-k \cdot \tau}}{V \cdot (1 - e^{-k \cdot \tau})}$	*‡	**‡	**	**
Minimum concentration	$C_{min,ss} = \dfrac{F \cdot D_M \cdot e^{-k \cdot \tau}}{V \cdot (1 - e^{-k \cdot \tau})}$	**	***	**	N

****, very reliable; ***, generally useful; **, a reasonable approximation; *, limited usefulness; N, not valid.
[†]For regimens of equal doses and dosing intervals.
[‡]Should not be encouraged because distribution is not instantaneous.

Useful relationships have been derived for designing and evaluating a dosage regimen in which the dose and the dosing interval are fixed. Table 11-6 summarizes some of the more important relationships and their limitations.

MODIFIED-RELEASE PRODUCTS

One way of maintaining a relatively constant response is by constant-rate administration. Although some constant-rate release systems have been developed (Chapter 10, *Constant-Rate Input*), other dosage forms exist from which drug release is not constant but is much slower than from conventional immediate release dosage forms. Such **modified-release products** do not completely obliterate but do reduce considerably the relative fluctuation in the plasma concentration at plateau, when compared with conventional therapy for a given dosing interval. They are particularly useful when maintenance of a therapeutic level requires frequent dosing of the immediate release dosage form, such as 3 or 4 times a day. The dosing interval may then be increased (same daily dose) to give a more convenient once- or twice-daily regimen. This is illustrated in Fig. 11-13, which shows events at plateau for morphine, with a half-life of approximately 2 hr. With an immediate release dosage form, absorption is rapid and, to maintain effective concentrations, the drug would need to be given very frequently, perhaps every 4 hr, for the relief of chronic severe pain. Whereas, effective concentrations can be maintained throughout the day and night with a modified release dosage form given as infrequently as once daily. This would appear to be made possible in the particular case of morphine, because this drug slows gastrointestinal motility thereby retaining the product in the gastrointestinal tract for longer than normal from which release with subsequent absorption continues.

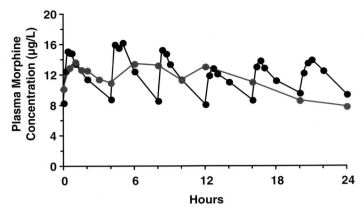

FIGURE 11-13. A modified release dosage form allows for once daily dosing of morphine, despite its short half-life of approximately 2 hr. Mean steady-state plasma concentrations following once-daily dosing of a modified release product (Avinza, *colored*) compared with 6-times daily administration of morphine solution (*black*). (From: Physicians' Desk Reference, 2004).

To maintain the same exposure at plateau for the 24-hr interval, because it is given less frequently, the maintenance dose contained in a modified-release product must be proportionally larger than that in the conventional immediate release product. Obviously, modified-release products must therefore perform reliably, and in particular should not be sensitive to food which, through increased gastric retention and agitation, severely tests such products. If the entire dose were released immediately, unacceptability high plasma concentrations would result. Other examples of useful modified-release dosage forms are theophylline, oxycodone, and lithium.

For oral administration, once or twice daily is desirable. Accordingly, for drugs with half-lives greater than 12 hr, oral modified-release products may be of little value, not only because the usual regimen is already convenient but because protracted release may put drug into the large intestine or perhaps out of the body before release is complete. Decreased bioavailability then becomes a major concern, especially in patients with diseases in which gastrointestinal transit is shortened, such as in an acute flare up in patients with Crohn's disease or ulcerative colitis.

For a drug that is usually given intramuscularly, or subcutaneously, multiple injections are inconvenient and a modified-release injectable dosage form may be advantageous. Depending on the total dose required and on the local effects of the injection mixture, it may only be necessary to administer the injection weekly, monthly, or perhaps even as a single dose. For example, leuprolide (a synthetic nonopeptide analog of naturally occurring gonadotropin-releasing hormone) has a half-life of approximately 3 hr, yet it is effective as once-a-month intramuscular depot therapy, comprising a slowly releasing dosage form, for the management of endometriosis and as a treatment for advanced-stage prostate cancer. Indeed, even a once-a-year implant is available.

EVALUATION OF A MULTIPLE-DOSE REGIMEN

With respect to its pharmacokinetic features, the development of dosage regimens proceeds in two stages. The first involves establishing whether the events on multiple dosing are predicted from single-dose data. Often there is good accord between observation and prediction, indicating that the pharmacokinetic parameters have not changed upon multiple dosing. Sometimes, prediction is poor, signifying a change in one or more pharmacokinetic parameters. This is evidence of and defined as a dose or time dependency (see Chapter 16, *Nonlinearities*). If prediction is good, the second stage is relatively straightforward. It involves varying the regimen to achieve particular plasma concentration–time profiles, which can be evaluated against therapeutic response and toxicity. The task is much more difficult when dose and time dependencies prevail.

The second stage, the subject of this section deals with how to both evaluate a multiple-dose regimen, with or without single-dose data, and estimate pharmacokinetic parameters. It builds on what has been covered in the preceding parts of the chapter.

CLEARANCE/BIOAVAILABILITY

Stability in this ratio (CL/F) on multiple dosing is present when $AUC_{ss} = AUC$ *(single)*, where AUC_{ss} is the AUC within a dosing interval at plateau. A plateau is taken to be reached when several consecutive trough concentrations, determined from blood samples taken just before the next dose, show no consistent trend up or down with time. The accuracy of the estimates of AUC_{ss} and AUC (single) are heavily dependent on the number and timing of blood samples. If needed, the estimate of AUC_{ss} can be improved using several dosing intervals, which in turn improves the estimate of CL/F at plateau. As shown in Fig. 11-12 for clobazam, CL/F does not change on multiple dosing.

HALF-LIFE

This parameter may be difficult to estimate during multiple dosing. Certainly, half-life cannot be estimated within a dosing interval with any confidence when the dosing interval is shorter than the half-life, as the decline in plasma concentration is too small over this time interval. The problem is made impossible if absorption continues throughout the dosing interval as often occurs with modified-release products. Theoretically, half-life could be estimated from trough values taken on the approach to plateau, in much the same way as done with plasma data obtained on the rise to plateau following a constant-rate input regimen (Fig. 10-4). In practice, however, this method is generally not very precise, especially when the dosing interval approaches the half-life, resulting in only a few trough values before plateau is reached.

The best way to estimate half-life is after stopping drug administration. At plateau, plasma concentrations are often much higher than those achieved after a single dose and so can be measured over much longer periods of time after stopping dosing, thereby facilitating an accurate estimate of half-life.

DEGREE OF ACCUMULATION

Accumulation always occurs. The major question is whether the degree of accumulation differs from that anticipated. One predictor of the degree of accumulation, given in Eq. 11-10, is the quantity $1/(1 - e^{-k\tau})$, the accumulation index (R_{ac}). This quantity predicts the ratio of the amount in the body at some time within the dosing interval at plateau to that at the same time after the first dose. However, plasma concentrations and not amounts are measured, and the ratio of amount to concentrations is only constant when the body acts as a single compartment. In practice, because distribution equilibrium between drug in tissues and that in plasma takes time, discrepancies arise between observed concentration and calculated values, assuming complete distribution. The discrepancy is greatest at early times. For this reason and because the value is difficult to estimate in practice, C_{max} is a poor choice to estimate the degree of accumulation. A trough value is a better choice, as distribution equilibrium is more likely to have been achieved at the end of the dosing interval. The observed degree of accumulation is $C_{ss,min}/C_{1,min}$, where $C_{1,min}$ is the trough concentration at the end of the first dosing interval. However, this last method relies on values obtained at only one time. This limitation is avoided using a commonly employed method based on AUC considerations, namely observed accumulation index $= AUC_{ss}/AUC_{1,\tau}$, where $AUC_{1,\tau}$ is the area under

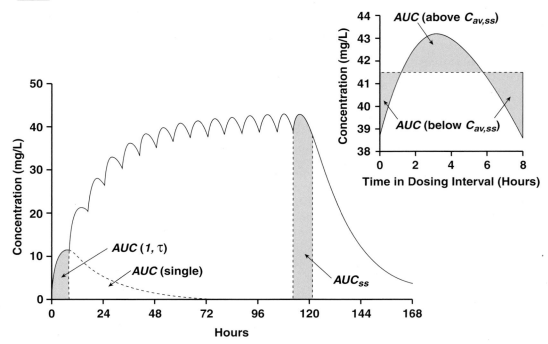

FIGURE 11-14. Evaluation of a multiple-dose regimen. The stability of the CL/F ratio with dosing can be assessed by comparing the area during a dosing interval at plateau (AUC_{ss}) with that of the total area after a single dose (AUC [single]). The degree of accumulation is taken as the ratio of AUC_{ss} to the area during the first dosing interval to time τ (AUC [1, τ]). The half-life is best determined after stopping drug administration. The inset shows the method for estimating the degree of fluctuation based on AUC (Eq. 11-23) above and below the average concentration, $C_{av,ss}$, within the dosing interval at plateau. Alternatively, it can be calculated from the observed maximum and minimum concentrations at plateau, $C_{max,ss}$, $C_{min,ss}$; degree of fluctuation = $(C_{max,ss} - C_{min,ss})/C_{min,ss}$.

the plasma concentration–time profile during the first dosing interval to time τ. The procedure, analogous to the use of $A_{av,ss}$ values (Eq. 11-7), is illustrated in Fig. 11-14. Obviously, a prediction based on the ratio AUC (single)$/AUC_{1,\tau}$ will match the observed ratio if $AUC_{ss} = AUC$ (*single dose*). The last term is the total AUC after a single dose. The value is approximately equal to $1/(1 - e^{-k\tau})$ if absorption is virtually complete at time τ after a single dose.

DEGREE OF FLUCTUATION AT PLATEAU

Fluctuation is an important consideration of any dosing regimen. It is usually evaluated at plateau. One common measure of the degree of fluctuation is the ratio ($C_{ss,max}$ − $C_{min,ss})/C_{min,ss}$. An advantage of this measure is that it deals with direct observations, $C_{max,ss}$, $C_{min,ss}$, which are thought to have relevance with respect to correlates of safety and minimum efficacy. A disadvantage of this measure, however, is that it relies on only two observations, one of which ($C_{max,ss}$) is often difficult to estimate accurately, unless many blood samples are taken within the dosing interval, a relatively uncommon clinical practice. Another more stable measure of fluctuation, which is less dependent on single observations, is given by

$$Fluctuation = \frac{AUC\,(above\ C_{av,ss}) - AUC\,(below\ C_{av,ss})}{AUC_{ss}} \qquad 11\text{-}23$$

where AUC (*above* $C_{av,ss}$) and AUC (*below* $C_{av,ss}$) are the areas above and below the average concentration at plateau (AUC_{ss}/τ), respectively. Estimation of these values is shown in the inset to Fig. 11-14.

OTHER PARAMETERS

As the amount entering the systemic circulation $(F \cdot Dose)$ equals the amount eliminated $AUC(0 - \tau)$ in each dosing interval, the relative bioavailability of a drug administered extravascularly in two different dosage forms or by two different routes (identified by A and B) can be readily determined under conditions of constant clearance from the relationship

$$F_{rel} = \frac{AUC(0 - \tau)_A}{AUC(0 - \tau)_B} \cdot \frac{(Dose)_A}{(Dose)_B} \qquad \text{11-24}$$

Renal clearance can be estimated from the amount of drug excreted unchanged in a dosing interval at steady state, $Ae_{ss,\tau}$ and the value of $AUC(0 - \tau)$,

$$CL_R = \frac{Ae_{ss,\tau}}{AUC_{ss}} \qquad \text{11-25}$$

PHARMACODYNAMIC CONSIDERATIONS

In the examples listed in Table 11-3, the main driving force for defining appropriate multiple-dosing regimens, and particularly the dosing interval and time to achieve full therapeutic effect, is pharmacokinetics. This is because, as is often the case, response tracks plasma concentration with relatively little time delay. However, even then, the dosing interval is also determined by what part of the exposure–response relationship is needed for therapeutic efficacy, commensurate with being within the therapeutic window, as illustrated in Fig. 11-15 during maintenance therapy at steady state, for a drug with a half-life of 8 hr. Based on pharmacokinetic considerations alone, a reasonable dosing interval might be 8-hourly, which would maintain the level within a twofold range. This may well be appropriate if the required response lies at or below 50% of the maximum response, E_{max} as then for the most part response is in the range where it varies in direct proportion to the logarithm of the level (Fig. 11-15A). However, if the peak response is closer to E_{max}, then as large changes in level produce minimal changes in response, the 8-hr dosing interval will maintain essentially the same response throughout the interval (Fig. 11-15B). Alternatively, it may well be possible to extend the dosing interval to 24 hr, permitting once-daily administration, and still maintain response within an acceptable range (Fig. 11-15C). For example, although the elimination half-life of atenolol is approximately 6 hr, a dose of 50 or 100 mg can be administered once daily because both the degree of beta-blockage and antihypertensive effect associated with the maximum plasma concentration are each close to the maximum response produced by this drug (higher doses producing no further increase), such that these therapeutic effects persist throughout the 24-hr interval.

Sometimes, response declines more slowly than the plasma concentration, which also allows for a longer dosing interval than based on pharmacokinetics. For example, as discussed in Chapter 8, *Response Following a Single Dose*, although both omeprazole and aspirin have very short half-lives, of 1 hr or less, the decline in response is very sluggish and for these drugs, once-daily administration, for the sustained reduction in secretion of gastric acidity and in platelet adhesion, respectively, is adequate. In addition, there are aspects of the pharmacokinetic–pharmacodynamic relationship of drugs and drug classes that influence the ultimate therapeutic regimen. These may argue for the need of a fluctuating or even an intermittent exposure profile rather than constant exposure, and for the need to wait for many days or even weeks or months before the full therapeutic effect of the drug, despite a relatively short half-life of a drug. We now consider some examples.

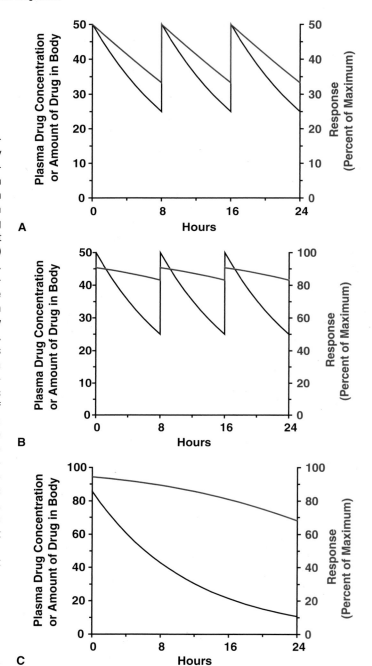

FIGURE 11-15. The dosing interval on maintenance therapy depends not only on the pharmacokinetics of a drug, but also on its pharmacodynamics, even when response tracks the plasma concentration or amount of drug in the body, shown here at plateau (using an arbitrary scale) for a drug with a half-life of 8 hr. *Case A*, when the therapeutic response corresponding to the maximum plasma concentration of a given drug lies at or below 50% of the maximum response, response (*colored line*) declines similarly to that of the plasma concentration (*black line*), although less so, as response is proportional to the logarithm of plasma concentration. Here, a dosing interval of 8 hr may well be reasonable. *Case B*, when the therapeutic response corresponding to the maximum plasma concentration of a drug now lies close to the maximum response, then because response changes little with plasma concentration, it remains relatively constant within the 8-hr dosing interval, and it may well be possible to increase the dose and lengthen the dosing interval to 24 hr, allowing once-daily administration, and still maintain adequate response within the entire interval (*Case C*).

TIME TO ACHIEVE THERAPEUTIC EFFECT

Statins are widely used to reduce the risk of coronary heart disease and cardiovascular events by lowering the concentration of cholesterol by inhibiting its synthesis in the liver. One such statin is atorvastatin, which has a relatively short half-life, in the order of 12 hr, yet the drug is given once daily. One needs to wait for at least 3 to 4 weeks before considering any dose adjustment, rather than the 2 days that might be expected based solely on its pharmacokinetics. The reason lies in the sluggish response of cholesterol to a decrease in its rate of synthesis, as seen in Fig. 11-16, because of the slow turnover of cholesterol within the body creating a pharmacodynamic rate limitation, as discussed in Chapter 8, *Response*

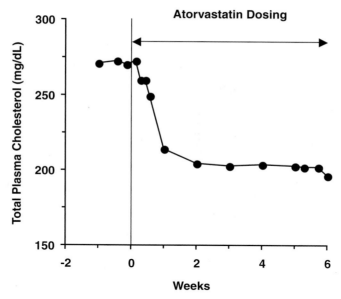

FIGURE 11-16.   Plot of total plasma cholesterol against time following oral administration of 5 mg ator-vastatin once daily for 6 weeks. Atorvastatin is a selective, competitive inhibitor of HMG-CoA reductase, the rate-limiting enzyme that converts 3-hydroxy-3-methylglutaryl-coenzyme A to mevalonate, a precur-sor of sterols, including cholesterol. Note, despite the relatively short half-life of atorvastatin (14 hr), it takes almost 2 weeks to see the full effect of inhibition of cholesterol synthesis. (From: Stern RH, Yang BB, Hounslow NJ, et al. Pharmacodynamics and pharmacokinetic-pharmacodynamic relationships of ator-vastatin, an HMG-CoA reductase inhibitor. J Clin Pharmacol 2000;40:616–623.)

Following a Single Dose. The rate at which cholesterol is normally eliminated is small relative to the total pool in the body, that is, its turnover is slow (Chapter 2, *Fundamental Concepts and Terminology*). This situation is analogous to the slow approach to the new lower steady state when the constant rate of input of a drug with a long half-life is decreased during chronic administration (Chapter 10, *Constant-Rate Input*).

In the case of statins, the response is not well related to the plasma concentration at any given time, especially just after starting therapy. The same applies to the bisphos-phonates, agents used to treat osteoporosis. Long-term effects to both classes of drugs are, however, closely related with the average steady-state concentration $(AUC[0 - \tau]/\tau)$ or total drug intake, so the daily dose is important. In these kinds of situations, it is some-times said that there is no relationship between the plasma concentration and the re-sponse. There is one; it is just a long-term one.

The second example is erythropoietin, an antianemic agent given to patients with end-stage renal disease, who have developed anemia because the kidney is the source of syn-thesis of endogenous erythropoietin, which stimulates red cell production. Erythropoietin has a short half-life of only 9 hr and reaches steady state on chronic administration within 2 days. Yet, it is commonly given 2 to 3 times weekly, but even then, as the data in Fig. 11-17 show, following chronic administration of the drug the hematocrit rises for about 70 days, and sometimes longer, before it levels off. Accordingly, adjustment in dosage is gen-erally no more frequent than once a month, and sometimes longer. One might be tempted to conclude that the effect of the drug takes time to develop. In fact, the drug in-creases the rate of production of red blood cells throughout the entire course of its ad-ministration. What is observed is the accumulation of newly formed cells until they have reached their lifetime potential, around 70 days, and begin to die. The rates of production and death of the cells subsequently come into balance; the hematocrit now fully reflects the increased production of red blood cells induced by the drug.

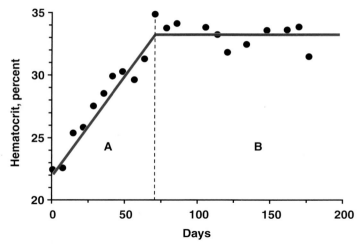

FIGURE 11-17.   The hematocrit in a uremic patient undergoing dialysis and receiving erythropoietin after dialysis 3 times a week increases for 70 days and then levels off. **A.** The drug increases erythrocyte production rate; hematocrit increases because the newly produced erythrocytes do not die at this early stage. **B.** Erythropoietin continues to stimulate production of erythrocytes. However, after reaching one life span, 70 days, erythrocytes die at the current production rate, and a new steady state is reached. (From: Uehlinger DE, Gotch FA, Sheiner LB. A pharmacodynamic model of erythropoietin therapy for uremic anemia. Clin Pharmacol Ther 1992;51:76–89.)

INTERMITTENT ADMINISTRATION

Intermittent administration is relatively common in cancer chemotherapy, with the gap between administrations often being two to three weeks, essentially independent of the pharmacokinetics of the drug, whose half-lives are often in the order of hours. Many of these agents kill proliferating cells, especially cancerous ones, which are the most rapidly proliferating. However, there is also unavoidable death of rapidly proliferating healthy cells, including those of the erythropoietic system, such as leukocytes, neutrophils, and platelets. The gap between administrations is to allow the number of these healthy cells to recover. The recovery is sluggish, in the order of weeks rather than days, as seen with red cells and leukocytes following administration of erythropoietin and paclitaxel (Fig. 8-19, Chapter 8, *Response Following a Single Dose*), respectively.

ONSET, DURATION, AND INTENSITY

In situations in which response is closely related to the plasma concentration, extending the duration of effect by increasing the dose rapidly results in a condition of diminishing returns, especially for a drug with a short half-life and a narrow therapeutic index. For example, when duration of effect is extended by two half-lives, the quadrupled dose required may produce too great an initial response or may substantially increase the chance of toxicity. Multiple smaller doses are then called for.

Instead of fixing the dose and dosing interval, a safer approach is to give the same dose each time the effect reaches a predetermined value, for example, just when the effect wears off (Fig. 11-18). The amount in the body at this time is A_{min}. This approach can be used when there is a good biomarker to determine the response to the drug. It is common for drugs used in anesthesia, but is not practical for most situations. With this approach, an increase in duration and, if the response is graded, an increase in intensity is expected with the second dose. The reason is readily apparent for i.v. doses. Immediately after giving the second dose, the amount in the body is not the dose, but *Dose* + A_{min}. How much intensity or duration of effect increases, therefore, depends on the relative

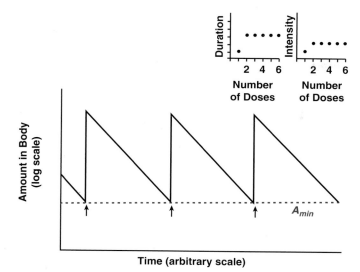

FIGURE 11-18. Both the duration and the intensity of a graded response increase with the second, but not with subsequent doses when each dose is given, indicated by an arrow, at the time the effect reaches a predetermined level (occurs at A_{min}, dashed colored line).

magnitude of dose and A_{min}. If A_{min} is small relative to dose, very little remains from the first dose when the second one is given, and little increase in response, or duration of effect, is expected. In contrast, large increases in both response and duration are expected when the response from the first dose wears off before much drug is lost.

No further increase in intensity or duration of effect is anticipated with third or subsequent doses, because the amount in the body always returns to the same value, A_{min}, before the next dose is given. Stated differently, from the second dose onward, during each dosing interval, the amount lost equals the dose given.

DEVELOPMENT OF TOLERANCE

The effectiveness of a drug can diminish with continual use. Acquired resistance denotes the diminished sensitivity of a population of cells (microorganisms, viruses, neoplasms) to a chemotherapeutic agent; tolerance denotes a diminished pharmacologic responsiveness to a drug. The degree of acquired resistance through mutation varies; it may be complete, thereby rendering the agent, for example, an antibiotic or antiviral agent, ineffective against a microorganism or virus. The degree of tolerance also varies but is never complete. For example, within days or weeks of its repeated use, subjects can develop a profound tolerance but not total unresponsiveness to the pharmacologic effects (euphoria, sedation, respiratory depression) of morphine. Tolerance can develop slowly; for example, tolerance to the central nervous system effects of ethanol takes weeks. Tolerance can also occur acutely; it is then called **tachyphylaxis**. For example, tolerance, expressed by a diminished cardiovascular responsiveness, seen as a decrease in the degree of tachycardia, develops within minutes following repetitive intake (through smoking) of nicotine (see Fig. 10-12). At any moment, a correlation might be found between the intensity of response and the plasma concentration of the drug, but the relationship varies with time.

The therapeutic implication of tolerance depends on whether it involves the beneficial or harmful effects of the drug. The development of tolerance to desired responses may require adjustment in the manner of delivery of a drug. For example, nitroglycerin, a drug used in treating or preventing angina, has an elimination half-life of just minutes and is very quickly absorbed when given sublingually, producing an effective pulse in its systemic response. When placed in a transdermal constant-rate release patch, a normally therapeutic systemic concentration can be maintained for 24 hr or more. Such products, however, are no longer used. They were shown to be ineffective chronically because of the development of tolerance to the prophylactic effects of the drug. The current recommendation is to remove the patch overnight (when occurence of an anginal attack is less probable) to allow the concentration of nitroglycerin to fall, and thereby reduce the development of tolerance.

Tolerance to the harmful effects of drugs, such as a headache or a sense of nausea, can be an advantage. As mentioned previously, while a loading dose may seem appropriate for a drug with a long half-life, acutely high concentrations can produce excessive adverse effects, which may limit the tolerability of an otherwise useful drug. Such adverse effects are less frequently encountered when drug is allowed to slowly accumulate in the body with a regimen that comprises only the maintenance dose. This is certainly the case with the antidepressant protriptyline. Recall that this drug has a long half-life (3 days), yet no loading dose is given. The reasons for this are severalfold. In addition to the previously mentioned adverse gastrointestinal effects experienced with large doses, many of the adverse central nervous system effects are mitigated against owing to tolerance to these effects as drug in the body builds up slowly on maintenance therapy. Also, in common with many other antidepressants, independent of the pharmacokinetics of the drug, the development of the full benefit of the therapeutic effect is delayed, usually for 2 to 4 or even more weeks, for pharmacodynamic reasons related to the kinetics of the underlying affected system within the brain.

MODALITY OF ADMINISTRATION

Figure 11-19 illustrates another situation, this time with antimicrobial agents, for which modality of administration can influence therapeutic outcome. Shown are major differences in the effect of dosing frequency on the daily dose of ceftazidime and gentamicin required to produce 50% of maximal efficacy in pneumonia that is caused by *Klebsiella pneumoniae* in neutropenic mice. Whereas decreasing the frequency of administration, and hence increasing the degree of fluctuation in plasma concentration, drastically diminished the effectiveness of ceftazidime, it had minimal effect on gentamicin. The explanation lies in the different pharmacodynamic profiles of these two drugs.

Ceftazidime, like other β-lactam antibiotics, exhibits only minimal concentration-dependent bactericidal activity, so that bacterial killing is more dependent on time above

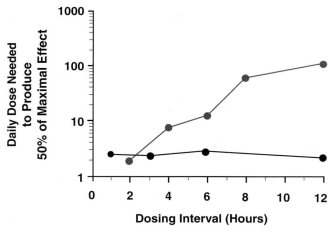

FIGURE 11-19. The influence of lengthening the dosing interval on the daily dose needed to produce 50% of maximal efficacy in treating pneumonia because of *Klebsiella pneumoniae* in neutropenic mice varies with the antimicrobial agent. Whereas, no change in daily dose is needed with gentamicin (*black line*), much larger daily doses of ceftazidime (*colored line*) are needed when administered less frequently. (From: Leggett JE, Fantin B, Ebert S, et al. Comparative antibiotic dose-effect relations at several dosing intervals in murine pneumonitis and thigh-infection models. J Infect Dis 1989;159:281–292.)

the minimal inhibitory concentration (MIC) than on the magnitude of the drug concentration. Greater benefit is therefore achieved with more frequent administration that minimizes the possibility of the plasma concentration falling too low. An additional reason for frequent administration is that the duration of the postantibiotic effect—whereby bacterial growth is suppressed for some time after intermittent exposure of bacteria to the antimicrobial agent—is very short with the β-lactam antibiotics.

In contrast to ceftazidime, gentamicin and other aminoglycosides produce a prolonged postantibiotic effect. They also exhibit marked concentration-dependent killing over a wide range of concentrations with higher values having a more pronounced effect on the rate and extent of bactericidal activity. Accordingly, for the same daily dose, large infrequent doses of gentamicin are as effective as smaller more frequent ones.

Although data in patients with infections, of necessity, are more variable than those obtained in the experimental mouse model, they do tend to bear out the findings in Fig. 11-19. First, for the antibiotics exhibiting minimal concentration dependence, a long half-life has proved to be a distinct advantage in allowing longer dosing intervals while maintaining efficacy. Second, studies indicate that for the same daily dose, once-daily regimens of aminoglycosides are as effective as more frequent ones, despite the short (in the order of 2–4 hr) half-lives of these compounds. This explains the increasing move from a previous thrice-daily administration, which was based almost solely on half-life considerations, to once-daily administration of gentamicin. However, irrespective of the mode of action of the antibiotic, if treatment is to be effective in eradicating the infection and increasing the probability of the microorganism remaining susceptible to the antibiotic, because of lack of emergence of resistant strains, evidence, such as that shown in Fig. 11-20, indicates that the ratio of 24-hr unbound *AUC* of antibiotic to the *AUC* below the unbound MIC of the microorganism (commonly referred to as the area under the unbound inhibitor curve, *AUIC*) needs to be in excess of 100 throughout treatment, in the case of patients who are seriously ill with enteric Gram-negative infections. The *AUIC* ratio varies with the type of infection. For example, a ratio of 35 appears adequate for the successful treatment with fluoroquinolone antibiotics of respiratory infections with *Pseudomonas pneumoniae*.

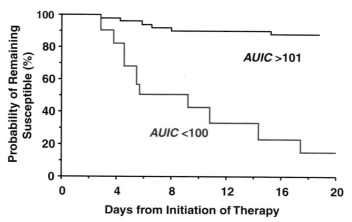

FIGURE 11-20. Area under the microbiological inhibitory curve (*AUIC*) and organism resistance. At *AUIC* values above 101 (*black line*), only 9% of patients developed resistant organisms. Whereas, at *AUIC* below 100 (*colored line*), only 50% of the organisms remained susceptible after 5 days of antibiotic therapy. Inadequate concentrations, particularly if these fall below the organism's MIC, increases the likelihood of resistant strains emerging. (From: Thomas JK, Forrest A, Bhavnani SM, et al. Pharmacodynamic evaluation of factors associated with the development of bacterial resistance in acutely ill patients during therapy. Antimicrob Agents Chemother 1998;42:521–527.)

WHEN ABSORPTION OR DISPOSITION IS ALTERED

We have now covered the principles of drug accumulation following repeated administration of single doses of a drug at fixed intervals, for example, multiple-dose regimens. Let us now consider how systemic exposure to a drug after multiple dosing would change when absorption or disposition is altered. This, of course, requires integration of physiologic concepts with the kinetic principles of this chapter. The anticipated change in the exposure profile depends on whether we are dealing with drugs of high or low hepatic extraction and whether the drugs are administered intravenously or orally. We previously examined what happens to a single i.v. dose (Chapter 5, *Elimination*) and to a single extravascular dose (Chapter 7, *Absorption*). Pertinent to this chapter is what happens when a multiple-dose regimen is administered.

SKETCH OF CONCENTRATION–TIME PROFILES

It is helpful to construct exposure–time profiles to show the consequences of altered absorption or disposition. To adequately show the salient kinetic features of drug accumulation in these situations, the y-axis of an exposure–time profile needs to be scaled to the maximum concentration (or amount in body) that is achieved. The time axis needs to be scaled to show the accumulation of drug to steady state, generally this means to four to five half-lives (of the longer half-life, control or altered condition).

Model of Multiple Intravenous Doses. In situations in which accumulation is extensive, common to long half-life drugs, absorption is rapid compared with elimination and a model of multiple i.v. doses is reasonable, as long as the extent of absorption is taken into account. The peak amount in the body after the first dose is then $F \cdot Dose$. The fraction remaining at the end of the interval of duration τ is $e^{-k\tau}$. Let us prepare a quick sketch of the amount of digoxin in the body with time for an individual on a regimen of 0.25 mg (250 µg) once daily. The key parameters for the drug in this patient are $F = 0.8$, $k = 0.345$ days^{-1}, $V = 400$ L. The amount absorbed from each is $F \cdot Dose$ (0.8 × 250 µg = 200 µg); the fraction remaining at the end of a dosing interval is 0.708 ($e^{-0.345 / \text{day} \times 1 \text{ day}}$). The amount remaining at the end of the first dosing interval is 142 µg. Following the second dose, the peak amount is 342 µg. This accumulation continues until steady state (peak = 685 µg, trough = 485 µg) is achieved. The results of these calculations are shown in Fig. 11-21. If plasma concentration rather than

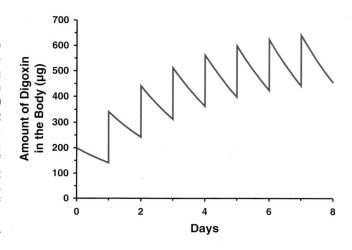

FIGURE 11-21. Sketch of the amount of digoxin in the body following the oral administration of 0.25 mg once daily in an individual in whom $F = 0.8$, $k = 0.345$ day^{-1}, and $V = 400$ L. An i.v. bolus model, with adjustment for bioavailability, is used in sketching the amount–time profile. The y-axis is scaled to the maximum amount of digoxin achieved in the body at steady state. The x-axis is scaled to 4 half-lives to show the approach of amount to steady state.

amount in body is desired, the calculated values above should be divided by the volume of distribution, 400 L in this case.

Extravascular Administration. Recall (from Fig. 11-1), that the expectation after multiple oral doses can be predicted from single-dose data. The expectation in the second dosing interval is simply the sum of the observations in the first and second intervals following a single dose. The expectation in the third interval is the sum of the observations in the first, second, and third intervals after a single dose, and so on. This applies to either multiple i.v. or extravascular doses. The maximum value on the y-axis would then accommodate the steady-state maximum value. The x-axis would need to be scaled to the time after a single dose when the area under the curve is at least 90% of the total area.

Two conditions are subsequently used to illustrate how this might be done for an oral dose. First, we consider a drug that is coadministered during a period of time when another drug, which is an inhibitor of its hepatic metabolism, is given (Condition A). The exposure to the other drug is at steady state when the drug of interest, which has a low hepatic extraction ratio, is repetitively administered orally. In the second scenario (Condition B), a drug with a high hepatic extraction ratio is given orally during a period of time when an inducer of drug metabolism is administered. Again, assume that the inducer, and its effect, are at steady state.

INHIBITION OF HEPATIC METABOLISM (CONDITION A)

For a low hepatic extraction ratio drug, a decrease in the hepatic metabolic activity causes a decrease in clearance, which, in turn, increases the half-life and the average concentration at steady state (Fig. 11-22). Thus, it takes longer to reach steady state as is evident from the profile following a single dose. The difference between peak and trough at steady state is not changed substantially as the volume of distribution is unchanged, and the differences in amounts of drug in the body at peak and trough are nearly the same in the absence and presence of the inhibitor, $F \cdot Dose$. This is especially true when absorption is rapid.

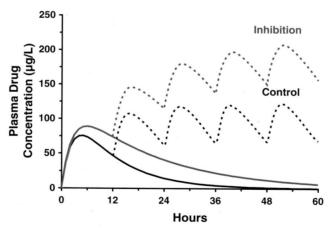

FIGURE 11-22. Concentration–time profile of a drug following single (*solid lines*) and multiple (*dashed lines*) oral doses when given alone (*black line*) and during a period of time when another drug that inhibits its metabolism is concurrently administered (*colored line*). The drug is exclusively eliminated by hepatic metabolism and has a low hepatic extraction ratio; therefore, its bioavailability is unaffected by the presence of the inhibitor. Clearance, on the other hand, is reduced and half-life increased by the inhibitor. Simulated is a drug with the following properties: *Dose* = 12 mg, $F = 1$, $ka = 0.4$ hr^{-1}, $k = 0.1$ hr^{-1}, $V = 100$ L. In the presence of the inhibitor, k is reduced to 0.05 hr^{-1}.

INDUCTION OF METABOLISM (CONDITION B)

Induction of hepatic metabolism after oral administration causes a decrease in the steady-state concentration for a high extraction ratio drug (Fig. 11-23). Recall that, as a result of increased intrinsic clearance, the bioavailability is decreased, but the clearance shows little or no change for a high extraction drug. The half-life is unchanged, because neither clearance nor volume of distribution is affected. The difference between peak and trough is reduced because of the decrease in bioavailability.

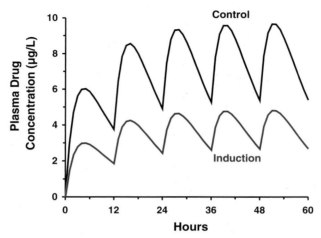

FIGURE 11-23. Concentration–time profile of a drug following multiple oral doses when given alone (*black line*) and during a period of time when another drug that induces its metabolism is concurrently administered (*colored line*). The drug is exclusively eliminated by hepatic metabolism and has a high hepatic extraction ratio; therefore, the bioavailability is appreciably reduced by the presence of the inducer. On the other hand, clearance and half-life are not materially affected by the inducer. Simulated is a drug with the following properties when given alone: *Dose* = 45 mg, F = 0.04, ka = 0.4 hr^{-1}, k = 0.1 hr^{-1}, V = 778 L.

OTHER SITUATIONS

There are many other causes of changes in the concentration–time profile after a single dose, as discussed in Chapter 5, *Elimination*, and Chapter 7, *Absorption*. A change in formulation or route of administration, renal disease, and hepatic disease are among them. These, and other conditions, are extensively discussed in subsequent chapters. Such situations can readily be analyzed or predicted from the observation after a single dose.

Multiple dosing has been presented using a one-compartment description of distribution characteristics. However, when the therapeutic or adverse effects develop or wear off during distribution, attention needs to be given to the kinetics of the distribution process. This aspect is discussed more fully in Chapter 19, *Distribution Kinetics* .

This section of the book deals with the principles surrounding the design and application of dosage regimens intended for the treatment or amelioration of a condition or disease in a typical patient. However, patients vary in their response to drugs. Consequently, the next section of the book covers the issue of individualization of drug therapy. It starts with a chapter that puts variability into perspective, then proceeds through the various sources of variability, and finishes with a chapter on how one accommodates for variability to optimize the initiation and management of drug therapy.

STUDY PROBLEMS

(Answers to Study Problems are in Appendix J.)

1. Define the meaning of the following words and phrases, which are selected from those listed in the first objective at the beginning of this chapter: drug accumulation, accumulation index, average level at plateau, loading dose, maintenance dose, plateau relative fluctuation, and trough concentration.

2. Comment on the accuracy of the following statements with regard to drugs given as an oral multiple-dose regimen of fixed dose and fixed dosing interval.

   a. Accumulation always occurs.

   b. The extent of accumulation increases when drug is given less frequently.

   c. The time to reach plateau following multiple-dose regimen depends on the frequency of drug administration.

   d. At plateau, the amount of drug lost within a dosing interval equals the oral maintenance dose.

   e. The average plateau concentration depends on the volume of distribution of the drug.

   f. The average plateau concentration depends on the absorption kinetics (changes in ka) of the drug.

3. The population pharmacokinetics of the oral diuretic agent, chlorthalidone, for a 70-kg person are:

$$F = 0.64 \qquad V = 280 \text{ L} \qquad CL = 4.5 \text{ L/hr}$$

   a. Given that absorption is instantaneous relative to elimination, calculate the following when a 50-mg dose of chlorthalidone is taken daily at breakfast.

   (1) The maximum and minimum amounts of drug in the body at plateau.

   (2) The accumulation ratio, based on trough concentration.

   (3) The minimum plasma concentration at plateau.

   (4) The time required to achieve 50% of plateau.

   b. Complete the table below (Table 11-7) for the dosage regimen of chlorthalidone given in (a).

TABLE 11-7	Maximum and Minimum Amounts of Chlorthalidone in the Body when 50 mg is Taken Daily							
	Amount of Chlorthalidone in Body (mg)							
Dose Number	1	2	3	4	5	6	7	∞
$A_{max,N}$								
$A_{min,N}$								

   c. Prepare a sketch on regular graph paper of the amount of chlorthalidone in the body with time. Show the salient features of accumulation of this drug during therapy.

   d. If required, what is the loading dose of chlorthalidone that would be needed to immediately attain the condition at plateau?

4. Mr. J.M., a nonsmoking, 60-kg patient with chronic obstructive pulmonary disease, is to be started on an oral regimen of aminophylline (85% of which is theophylline).

The pharmacokinetics parameter values for a typical nonsmoking patient with this disease are:

$$F = 1.0 \text{ (for theophylline)} \quad V = 0.5 \text{ L/kg} \quad CL = 40 \text{ mL/hr/kg}$$

Design an oral dosage regimen of *aminophylline* (available as 100- and 200-mg tablets) for this patient to *attain and maintain* a plasma theophylline concentration within the therapeutic window, 10 to 20 mg/L. The oral absorption of theophylline is complete and rapid.

5. Table 11-8 lists a typical plasma concentration–time profile obtained following an oral 500-mg dose of a drug. The *AUC* is 80.6 mg-hr/L, and the terminal half-life is 5 hr.

TABLE 11-8	Plasma Concentration-Time Profile of a Drug After a Single 500-mg Oral Dose								
Time (hr)	0	1	2	4	8	12	24	36	48
Plasma drug concentration (mg/L)	0	2.3	4.7	5.2	4.0	2.8	0.6	0.14	0.03

a. What oral dosing rate of drug is needed to maintain an average plateau concentration of 10 mg/L?
b. The decision has been made to give the drug once every 12 hr. What is:
(1) The unit dose strength of product needed?
(2) The plateau trough concentration expected.

6. The therapeutic dose of a rapidly (compared with elimination) and completely absorbed drug is 50 mg. A controlled-release dosage form to be given every 8 hr is designed to release its contents *evenly* and *completely* (no loading dose) over this dosing interval. Given that the half-life of the drug is 4 hr,

a. How much drug should the controlled-release dosage form contain?
b. To achieve a prompt effect, a rapidly absorbed dosage form is administered initially. When should the first controlled-release dosage form be given?
c. Following the dosage regimen in (b), what is the total dose on Day 1 and on Day 2?
d. In tabular form or on the same graph, provide the amounts of drug in the body versus time curves expected when the controlled-release preparation only is given (i) every 4 hr (ii) every 8 hr, or (iii) every 12 hr.

7. Adinazolam is a drug under investigation for the treatment of depression and panic disorders. Table 11-9 summarizes some of the salient pharmacokinetic information following single and multiple doses of immediate-release and modified-release products.

a. What rate-limits the decline of plasma adinazolam concentration following the administration of the modified-release product?
b. On multiple dosing, have the immediate-release and modified-release products been given long enough to ensure that a plateau should have been reached? In your answer, indicate whether any difference is expected in the time to reach plateau between the two products.
c. For both products, are the plasma concentration data observed on multiple dosing (see Table 11-9) those predicted from single-dose data?
d. What is the relative bioavailability of adinazolam of the modified-release product compared with the immediate-release product?

| TABLE 11-9 | Mean Adinazolam Pharmacokinetic Information following Single and Multiple Doses of Immediate-Release and Modified-Release Preparation to a Group of 16 Subjects |

	Immediate Release		Modified Release	
	Single Dose 40 mg	Multiple Doses 40 mg every 8 hr	Single Dose 60 mg	Multiple Doses 60 mg every 12 hr
AUC(mg-hr/L)	0.57*	1.72†	0.88*	1.57†
C_{max} (mg/L)	0.15	0.20	0.07	0.11
t_{max} (hr)	1.00	-	2.50	-
Terminal $t_{1/2}$ (hr)	2.20	-	5.50	-

*AUC(0–∞).
†AUC(0–24) after 7 days of dosing.
From: Fleishalker JC, Wright CE. Pharmacokinetic and pharmacodynamic comparison of immediate-release and sustained-release adinazolam mesylate tablets after single- and multiple-dose administration. Pharm Res 1992;9:457–463.

e. Are the pharmacokinetics of adinazolam after administration of the immediate-release and modified-release products such that the terminal half-life can be determined within the respective dosing intervals at plateau?

f. What are the degrees of accumulation associated with the immediate-release and modified-release regimens, given that the AUC (0–8 hr) and AUC (0–12 hr) following the single 40-mg immediate-release product and the 60-mg modified-release products are 0.45 and 0.44 mg-hr/L, respectively? Base your calculations on AUC considerations.

8. Table 11-10 lists typical pharmacokinetic parameter values and dosage regimens frequently used for acetaminophen, ibuprofen, and naproxen, three nonprescription analgesic/antipyretic agents.

| TABLE 11-10 | Pharmacokinetic Parameters and Common Regimens of Acetaminophen, Ibuprofen, and Naproxen |

Drug	F	V(L)	CL(L/hr)	Common Oral Dosage Regimen
Acetaminophen	0.9	67	21	1000 mg/6 hr
Ibuprofen	0.7	10	3.5	400 mg/6 hr
Naproxen	0.95	11	0.55	500 mg/12 hr

a. Calculate the average plateau plasma concentrations of these three drugs when subjects are on the regimens given in Table 11-10.

b. For which of the three drugs is the plateau reached the fastest?

c. For which of the three drugs is the degree of accumulation the greatest on the common regimens given in Table 11-10?

d. Assuming instantaneous absorption and distribution, calculate the maximum plateau plasma concentration of ibuprofen and naproxen on the regimens given in Table 11-10.

e. Assuming instantaneous absorption, calculate the minimum plateau plasma concentration for ibuprofen and naproxen on the regimens given in Table 11-10.

f. Assuming instantaneous absorption, calculate the relative fluctuations of ibuprofen and naproxen on the regimens given in Table 11-10. How do you rationalize the difference between these two drugs?

9. It has been said that maintenance of an effect requires the maintenance of a constant systemic exposure (plasma concentration) to a drug. Do you support this view? Discuss briefly.

10. Table 11-11 lists key pharmacokinetic parameters and measures of mefloquine (MQ), an antimalarial agent effective against many strains of multidrug-resistant plasmodium vivax and plasmodium falciparum. The drug is administered as a race-mate. The values given in the table are for the racemate and each of the enantiomers after oral administration of the racemate.

TABLE 11-11	**Mean (± SD) Pharmacokinetic Measures and Parameters Obtained for Racemate (rac) and (±) and (−) Isomers of Mefloquine (MQ)**		
	Rac-MQ	**(+)-MQ**	**(−)MQ**
After a Single 250-mg dose of the Racemate:			
C_{max} (mg/L)	0.52 (± 0.18)	0.12 (± 0.02)	0.36 (± 0.09)
t_{max} (hr)	27 (± 24)	18 (± 16)	30 (± 31)
AUC (0-∞) (mg-hr/L)	223 (± 118)	20 (± 5)	190 (± 63)
Half-life (hr)	400 (± 275)	128 (± 50)	409 (± 166)
AUC (0–7 days) (mg-hr/L)	56 (± 14)	12 (± 2)	45 (± 12)
At Steady State (13 weeks) after Weekly 250-mg Doses of the Racemate:			
$C_{max,ss}$ (mg/L)	1.68 (± 0.24)	0.26 (± 0.05)	1.42 (± 0.19)
$C_{min,ss}$ (mg/L)	1.12 (± 0.29	0.11 (± 0.04)	1.01 (± 0.26)
$C_{av,ss}$ (mg/L)	1.35 (± 0.27)	0.18 (± 0.05)	1.17 (± 0.22)
t_{max} (hr)	12 (± 8)	15 (± 11)	12 (± 0.26)
AUC (0–7days) after last dose (mg-hr/L)	227 (± 45)	30 (± 9)	197 (± 37)
Half-life (hr)	421 (± 157)	173 (± 57)	430 (± 255)

From: Gimenez F, Pennie RA, Koren G, et al. Stereoselective pharmacokinetics of mefloquine in healthy Caucasians after multiple doses. J Pharm Sci 1994;83:824–827.

Answer the following questions, given that the drug follows first-order kinetics and a one-compartment disposition model. Use the mean values only, except for Part d.

a. Is the drug rapidly absorbed? Justify your answer.
b. Does a difference in clearance or volume of distribution, or both, explain the observed kinetic differences between the enantiomers?
c. Using the single-dose data, estimate the peak concentration ($C_{max,ss}$) you would expect from (−)-MQ on a once-weekly regimen. Assume i.v. bolus doses for this problem. Show your calculations. How does your estimate compare with the observed $C_{max,ss}$?
d. The drug (racemate) was given for 13 weeks. Is this time long enough to assure achievement of steady state for both enantiomers in *all* subjects? Briefly discuss.
e. Based on the single-dose data, calculate an accumulation index for (−)-MQ on administering the racemate once weekly.
f. Determine the relative fluctuations of the plasma concentrations for (+)-MQ, and (−)-MQ at steady state. How do you explain the difference in the values for the two enantiomers?
g. When given to treat patients with malaria, the dosage regimen is five 250-mg tablets (1250 mg) in a single dose. For prevention of malaria, it is recommended that a traveler take 250 mg once weekly for 2 to 3 weeks before going to the endemic area and

to continue weekly doses while traveling and after returning home. Do these regimens seem reasonable to you? Briefly discuss from a pharmacokinetic point of view.

11. Ampicillin has the following average pharmacokinetic parameter values in a 70-kg subject.

$$F(\text{oral}) = 0.6 \quad V = 20 \text{ L} \quad CL = 160 \text{ mL/min} \quad fe = 0.8$$

Determine the minimum oral maintenance dose of ampicillin, to be given every 6 hr, to keep the urinary drug concentration (in ureters) above 50 mg/L. This value is the minimum inhibitory concentration against an antibiotic-resistant organism believed to be producing the patient's urinary tract infection. Use an average urine flow of 1 mL/min. Instantaneous absorption and distribution of ampicillin and steady-state conditions apply.

12. Discuss three situations in which pharmacodynamics, rather than pharmacokinetics, drives the choice of the dosage regimen, particularly the dosing interval.

Individualization

Variability

OBJECTIVES

The reader will be able to:

- Define the terms: adherence to prescribed dosage regimen, bimodal frequency distribution, coefficient of variation, chronopharmacology, intraindividual variability, interindividual variability, persistence, population pharmacokinetics, population pharmacodynamics, unimodal frequency distribution.
- List six major sources of variability in drug response.
- Evaluate whether variability in drug response is caused primarily by variability in pharmacokinetics, pharmacodynamics, or both, given response and pharmacokinetic data.
- State why variability around the mean and shape of the frequency distribution histogram of a parameter are as important as the mean itself.
- Explain how variability in hepatic enzyme activity manifests itself in variability in both pharmacokinetic parameters and plateau plasma drug concentrations for drugs of high and low hepatic extraction ratios.
- Describe an approach to the design of the number of dose strengths of a drug needed to cover the target patient population when response is primarily determined by the pharmacokinetics of the drug, and response is directly correlated to the average exposure to drug at steady state.

T hus far, in the context of drug dosage, all patients have been assumed to be alike. Yet, we know that people differ in their responsiveness to drugs. Accordingly, there is often a need to tailor drug administration to the individual patient. A failure to do so can lead to ineffective therapy in some patients and undue harm in others.

This section of the book is devoted to treating the individual patient. A broad overview of the subject is presented in this chapter. In particular, evidence for and causes of variation in drug response are examined. Before proceeding, a distinction needs to be made between an individual and the population. Substantial differences in response to drugs commonly exist among patients. Such between or **interindividual variability** is often reflected by various marketed dose strengths of a drug. For example, diazepam, used in the management of some anxiety disorders, is marketed as 2-, 5-, and 10-mg tablets. Because variability in response within a subject from one occasion to another (**intraindividual variability**) is generally smaller than *inter*individual variability, there is usually little need to subsequently adjust an individual's dosage regimen, once well-established, unless the condition or treatment of the patient changes. Clearly, if intraindividual variability were large and unpredictable, finding and maintaining dosage for an individual would be an extremely difficult task, particularly for a drug with a low therapeutic index.

Many patients stabilized on one medicine receive another for the treatment of the same or concurrent condition or disease. Sometimes, the second drug affects the response to the first. The change in response may be clinically insignificant for most of the patient population, with the recommendation that no adjustment in dosage be made. However, a few individuals may exhibit an exaggerated response, which could prove fatal unless the dosage of the first drug given to them is reduced. The lesson is clear: Average data are useful as a guide; but ultimately, information pertaining to the individual patient is all-important.

EXPRESSIONS OF INDIVIDUAL DIFFERENCES

Evidence for interindividual differences in drug response comes from several sources. Variability in the dosage required to produce a given response is illustrated in Fig. 12-1, which shows the wide range in the daily dose of warfarin needed to produce a similar degree of anticoagulant control, a consequence of variability in both pharmacokinetics

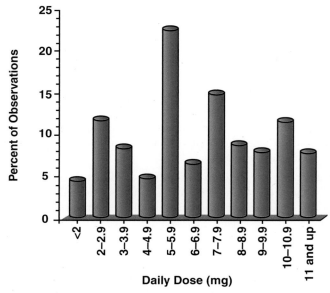

FIGURE 12-1. The daily dose of warfarin required to produce a similar degree of anticoagulation in 200 adult patients varies widely. (From: Koch-Weser J. The serum level approach to individualization of drug dosage. Eur J Clin Pharmacol 1975;9:1–8.)

and pharmacodynamics. Figure 12-2, which shows frequency distribution histograms of the plateau plasma concentration of the antidepressant drug nortriptyline to a defined daily dose, demonstrates interpatient variability in the input–exposure (pharmacokinetic) relationship. Variability in pharmacokinetics is also illustrated by the wide scatter in the plateau plasma concentration of phenytoin seen following any fixed daily dose of this drug (see Fig. 1-7, page 9). Because the pharmacokinetics of a drug reflects the body's ability to handle drugs, it is not surprising that clearance values within the population associated with the oxidation of certain drugs strongly cosegregate. For example, a patient who is a poor metabolizer of midazolam is also a poor metabolizer of alfentanil; both drugs are eliminated predominantly by the same enzyme, in this case CYP3A4 (Fig. 12-3). Similarly, a rapid metabolizer of one of these drugs is a rapid metabolizer of

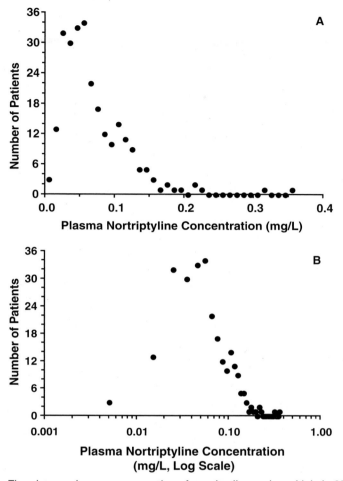

FIGURE 12-2. The plateau plasma concentration of nortriptyline varies widely in 263 patients receiving a regimen of 25 mg nortriptyline orally 3 times daily. **A.** Plot of the frequency against the plasma concentration shows a skewed distribution. **B.** The same data plotted against the logarithm of the concentration showing an essentially symmetrical distribution, indicating that the distribution is log-normal. (From: Sjoqvist F, Borga O, Orme MLE. Fundamentals of clinical pharmacology. In: Avery GS, ed. Drug Treatment. Edinburgh: Churchill Livingstone; 1976:1–42.)

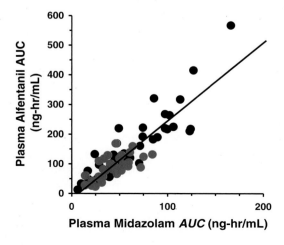

FIGURE 12-3. A high degree of cosegregation exists between midazolam and alfentanil exposure after intravenous (●) and oral (●) administration of these drugs to 12 subjects. Both drugs are primarily eliminated by CYP3A4 catalyzed metabolism, and reflect variation in the functional activity of this enzyme within this group of subjects. (From: Kharasch ED, Walker A, Hoffer C, et al. Sensitivity of intravenous and oral alfentanil and papillary miosis as minimally invasive and noninvasive probes for hepatic and first-pass CYP3A4 activity. J Clin Pharmacol 2005;45:1187–1197.)

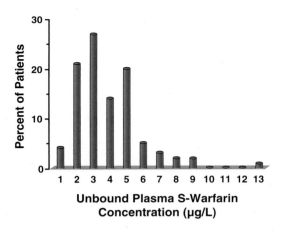

FIGURE 12-4. There is considerable interindividual pharmacodynamic variability in response to the oral anticoagulant warfarin as demonstrated by the substantial spread in the unbound concentration of the active S-isomer associated with a similar degree of anticoagulation in a group of 97 patients on maintenance therapy. (From: Scordo MG, Pengo V, Spina E, et al. Influence of CYP2C9 and CYP2C19 genetic polymorphisms of warfarin maintenance dose and metabolic clearance. Clin Pharmacol Ther 2002;72:702–710.)

the other. The data in Fig. 12-4, showing the plateau unbound plasma concentration of the more active S-warfarin enantiomer required to produce a similar degree of anticoagulant control following maintenance therapy with (racemic) warfarin, demonstrate substantial interpatient variability in exposure–response (pharmacodynamics) for this drug. Many drugs produce their effects by competing with endogenous agonists or antagonists, and in such cases part of the observed interindividual variability in pharmacodynamics, which can be substantial, is likely to arise from differences among patients in the concentrations of these endogenous compounds at the target site(s).

Clearly, variability exists in both pharmacokinetics and pharmacodynamics, and measurement of drug in plasma is a prerequisite for separating the two. The characterization of pharmacokinetic and pharmacodynamic variabilities within the population is called **population pharmacokinetics** and **population pharmacodynamics**, respectively.

Some patients fail to respond to treatment even when systemic exposure to the drug is within the range associated with therapeutic response. The causes of such nonresponders are manifold, but all center around either misdiagnosis of the disease or because the individual lacks the therapeutic target or expresses one that fails to produce an adequate response (see Chapter 13, *Genetics*).

The examples of variability in drug response so far have been of the therapeutic effect of the drug, but the situation equally applies to adverse effects. For some relatively minor adverse effects, variability may be as great as, or even greater than, that for the therapeutic effect, particularly when they are associated with the inherent pharmacologic property of the drug (side effects), such as dryness of mouth experienced with some sympathomimetic nasal decongestants. Frequent side effects are also invariably experienced by patients undergoing chemotherapy during cancer treatment. However, in many other therapeutic settings, moderate to severe side effects are much less frequently experienced. Occasionally, the frequency of an adverse effect is so low that it is only detected with any significance when tens of thousands, if not millions, of patients have been treated with the drug. Even so, there is still some relationship between the likelihood and severity of an adverse effect and the exposure to the drug, although establishing it with any confidence may be difficult.

QUANTIFYING VARIABILITY

The magnitude and relative contribution of pharmacokinetics and pharmacodynamics to variability in response within a patient population vary with the drug. In clinical practice, an attempt to assign the relative contribution to pharmacokinetics and pharmacodynamics is often based on direct observations of plasma concentration and response. Such an assignment could be strongly influenced, however, by the timing of the observations and the magnitude of the response, as illustrated in Fig. 12-5 following a single dose. Here, a drug that displays little interpatient variability in C_{max}, t_{max}, and in maximum effect, E_{max}, but

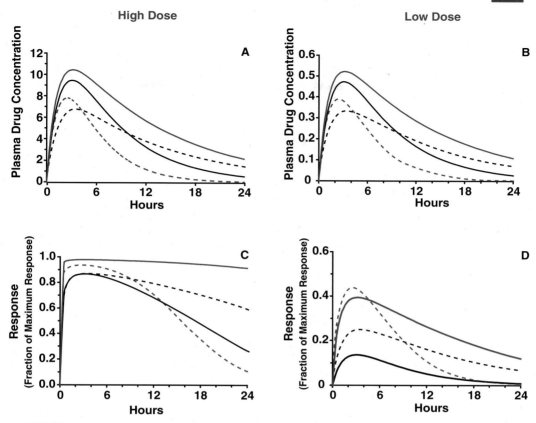

FIGURE 12-5. The interindividual variability in concentration and response varies with dose and time of observation. Shown are plasma concentrations (**A** and **B**) and responses (**C** and **D**) following large (*left*) and small (*right*) doses of a drug that displays little interpatient variability in C_{max}, t_{max}, and maximum response, E_{max}. but large interpatient variability in half-life and concentration needed to produce 50% maximum response. High dose (*top*): at t_{max}, the maximum response in all patients is produced with little variability in either C_{max} or response. Greater variability in concentration and response is seen at later times. Low dose (*bottom*): at t_{max}, variability in C_{max} is still low, but that in response is now considerable. Each line corresponds to a different patient.

large variability in half-life and concentration needed to produce 50% maximum response (C_{50}), is given orally at two dose levels. The higher dose achieves close to maximal response in all patients, whereas the lower dose does not. At the higher dose, observations made at t_{max} would suggest little variability in either concentration or pharmacodynamics, with perhaps a greater assignment of variability to the former, as variation in plasma concentration produces relatively little change in response. At later times after this higher dose, substantial variability is observed in both concentration and response. In contrast, for the lower dose, at t_{max} there is still little interpatient variability in C_{max}, but now there is considerable variability in response. This dependence on dose and time in the assignment of variability is minimized by expressing variability not in terms of observations but rather in terms of the parameter values defining pharmacokinetics and pharmacodynamics, that is, in F, ka, CL, and V for pharmacokinetics, and in E_{max}, C_{50}, and the factor defining the steepness of the concentration–response relationship (γ) for pharmacodynamics (Chapter 2, *Fundamental Concepts and Terminology*). Once variability in these parameters is defined, the expected variability in concentration and response within the patient population at any time associated with a given dosage regimen can be calculated.

DESCRIBING VARIABILITY

Knowing how a particular parameter varies within the patient population is important in therapy. To illustrate this statement, consider the frequency distributions in, for example, clearance of the four hypothetical drugs shown in Fig. 12-6. The mean, or central tendency, for all four drugs is the same, but variability about the mean is very different. For Drugs A, B, and C, the distribution is **unimodal** and log normal; here, the mean represents the typical value of clearance expected in the population. As variability about the mean is much greater for Drugs B and C than for Drug A, one has much less confidence that the mean of Drug C, in particular, applies to an individual patient. For Drug D, distribution in clearance is **bimodal**, signifying that there are two major groups within the population: those with high and low clearances. Obviously, in this case, the mean is one of the most unlikely values to be found in this population.

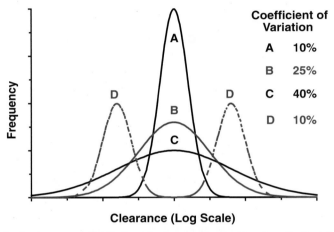

FIGURE 12-6. As the frequency distributions for the clearance of four hypothetical drugs (*A, B, C, D*) show, it is as important to define variability around the mean and the shape of the frequency distribution curve as it is to define the mean itself. Drugs A, B, and C exhibit unimodal log-normal distributions with coefficients of variation of 10%, 25%, and 40%, respectively. The distribution for Drug D is bimodal, with a low frequency of individuals in whom clearance is the mean value for the entire population.

A comment on the quantitation of variability is needed here. One measure of variability is variance; it is defined as the sum of the squares of the deviations of observations from their means. Although useful to convey variability within a particular set of observations, variance does not allow ready comparison of variability across sets of observations of different magnitude, or of different dimensions, such as those of clearance and volume of distribution. To illustrate this point, suppose the clearance of a drug within a population has a mean of 100 mL/min and a variance of 2500 (mL/min)^2. If instead clearance had been quoted in L/min, numerically the mean value would be a 1000-fold smaller (i.e., 0.1 L/min), and variance would be a millionfold smaller (i.e., 0.0025 L^2/min^2). **Coefficient of variation**, the square root of variance (the standard deviation) normalized to the mean, overcomes this problem. In the example above, the coefficient of variation is 0.25 or 25%, independent of the units of clearance. Subsequently, the terms *high* and *low variability* refer to distributions that have high and low coefficients of variation, respectively. Typically, a coefficient of variation of a pharmacokinetic parameter of 10% or less is considered low, 25% is moderate, and above 40% is high. Although these values do not appear too dissimilar, examination of the three unimodal distributions in Fig. 12-5 with these respective coefficients of variations illustrates, however, just how variable a distribution with a coefficient of variation of 40% (Drug C) truly is.

A practical illustration of interindividual variability in a parameter among drugs is seen in Fig. 12-7, which shows that the coefficient of variation in oral bioavailability among subjects increases as bioavailability of a drug decreases, from about 10% when bioavailability is close to 100% to 50% as bioavailability tends toward zero. That is, there is an increasing tendency to be less confident in the application of the population mean bioavailability to an individual as bioavailability decreases. The low variability when bioavailability is 100% is as expected, because this is the upper limit of this parameter, but what is equally informative is how the magnitude of variability changes with decreasing bioavailability.

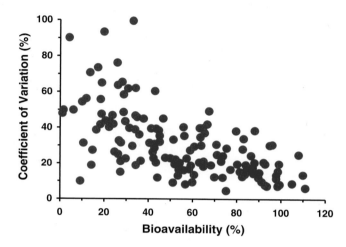

FIGURE 12-7. There is a trend for intersubject variability (expressed as percent CV) in oral bioavailability to increase as the bioavailability of a drug decreases. Data obtained from a total of 149 studies covering 100 drugs. There was no discernible difference between healthy volunteers and patients. (From: Hellriegel ET, Bjornsson TD, Hauck WW. Interpatient variability in bioavailability is related to the extent of absorption: Implications for bioavailability and bioequivalence studies. Clin Pharmacol Ther 1996;60: 601–607.)

A cautionary related note to variability is the danger of misinterpreting the results of averaging of data. Figure 12-8 contains three extreme scenarios aimed at illustrating this point. Shown are individual profiles together with the average profile obtained by taking the arithmetic mean of the individual observations (y-axis) for given values of the horizontal axis, concentration in Fig. 12-8A and time in Fig. 12-8B,C. As is clearly apparent, the mean line in each case gives a distorted view as what might be expected in an individual. In Fig. 12-8A, the value of the steepness factor, γ, of the concentration–response relationship is much smaller than observed in any individual. In Fig. 12-8B, although the decline in concentration with time is monoexponential in each subject, the mean line is polyexponential giving the illusion that distribution kinetics prevails, whereas in Fig. 12-8C, the mean profile gives the illusion that the plasma concentration is constant for up to 10 hr, whereas in any individual it is seen to be relatively constant for only about 2 hr. Clearly, to avoid such problems, whenever possible, it is better to obtain individual profiles and appropriately average the parameters while maintaining the same model for all individuals.

WHY PEOPLE DIFFER

The reasons why people differ in their responsiveness to a given dose of a drug are manifold and include genetics, disease, age, gender, body weight, drugs given concomitantly, and various behavioral and environmental factors. Age, body weight, disease, and concomitantly administered drugs are important because they are measurable sources of variability that can be taken into account. Gender-linked differences in hormonal balance, body composition, and activity of certain enzymes manifest themselves in differences in both pharmacokinetics and responsiveness, but overall, the effect of gender is small. Although inheritance accounts for a substantial part of the differences in response among individuals for many drugs, much of this variability is

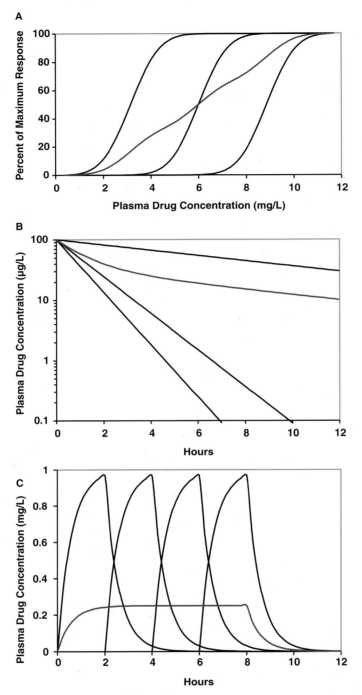

FIGURE 12-8. A simple averaging of data can result in a mean profile (*in color*) which is not representative of events in the individual (*black line*). **A.** The average line for the concentration–response relationship is much shallower than seen in the individual. **B.** The mean line is polyexponential while concentration declines monoexponentially in the individuals. **C.** Here, while in each subject the 2-hr constant-rate input is not long enough to result in a plateau, the staggering of the inputs among subjects (as might occur with ingestion of a constant-rate device that only starts releasing drug once it enters the intestine) creates a mean profile that gives the illusion that the plasma concentration remains constant for at least 6 hr. Notice also that the mean maximum concentration is much lower than seen in any individual.

still largely unpredictable, particularly in regard to pharmacodynamics, although as discussed in Chapter 13, *Genetics*, our understanding of this source of variability is improving rapidly.

Disease can be an added source of variation in drug response. Usual dosage regimens of many drugs may need to be modified substantially in patients with renal function impairment and hepatic disorders, whereas adjustment in others may be needed in patients suffering from congestive cardiac failure, thyroid disorders, gastrointestinal disorders, and other diseases. The modification may apply to the drug being used to treat the specific disease and may apply equally well to other drugs the patient is receiving. For example, to prevent excessive accumulation and so reduce the risk of toxicity, the dosage of the antibiotic gentamicin used to treat a pleural infection of a patient must be reduced if the patient also has compromised renal function, the major route of elimination of this antibiotic. Similarly, patients with hyperthyroidism require higher than usual doses of digoxin, a drug used to decrease the likelihood of atrial fibrillation. Moreover, a modification in dosage may arise not only from the direct impairment of a diseased organ but also from secondary events that accompany the disease. Drug metabolism, for example, may be modified in patients with renal disease; plasma and tissue binding of drugs may be altered in patients with uremia and hepatic disorders.

Table 12-1 lists examples of additional factors known to contribute to variability in drug response. The most important of these is lack of **adherence** to the prescribed regimen. This includes the taking of drug at the wrong time, the omission or supplementation of the prescribed dose, and the premature stopping of therapy, a problem of **persistence** in adhering to the full course of treatment, which may last for a lifetime. The pattern of nonadherence appears to be unrelated to the disease. For example, as shown

TABLE 12-1	**Additional Factors Known to Contribute to Variability in Drug Response**
Factors	**Observations and Remarks**
Lack of adherence to, and persistence in taking, a dosage regimen	A major problem in clinical practice; solution lies largely in patient motivation.
Route of administration	Patient response can vary on changing the route of administration. Particularly noticed when speed of absorption and bioavailability is route dependent.
Food and diet	Rate and occasionally extent of absorption can be affected by eating. Effects depend on composition of food, in particular the presence of a high fat meal, which markedly slows gastric emptying. Severe protein restriction may reduce the rate of drug metabolism, and increase urine pH, which will affect the renal clearance of pH-sensitive drugs. Constituents in grapefruit juice are inhibitors of intestinal CYP3A4.
Herbs	Herbs contain many constituents some of which can enhance or antagonize the effect of drugs, or act as inhibitors or inducers of drug-metabolizing enzymes.
Pollutants	Drug effects are sometimes less in smokers and workers occupationally exposed to pesticides, the result of enhanced metabolism particularly those metabolized by CYP1A2.
Time of day and season	Circadian variations are seen in pharmacokinetics and response of some drugs. These effects have been sufficiently important to lead to the development of a specialty, chronopharmacology.

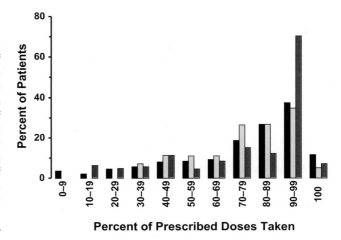

FIGURE 12-9. The pattern of nonadherence is relatively independent of disease. Shown are the similar frequency histograms of the percentage of prescribed doses taken by patients receiving drug therapy for treatment of glaucoma (*black*), epilepsy (*gray*), and ankylosing spondylitis (*colored*). (From: Urquhart J, De Kerk E. Contending paradigms for the interpretation of data on patient compliance with therapeutic regimens. Statist Med 1998;17: 251–267.)

in Fig. 12-9, similar patterns were seen in patients with: glaucoma treated twice daily with timolol eyedrops; epilepsy with occasional seizures treated with oral phenytoin and/or carbamazepine once/twice daily, and painful ankylosing spondylitis treated with either of two once-daily analgesic nonsteroidal anti-inflammatory agents (piroxicam or tenoxicam). This would suggest that the problem has a strong behavioral component, with some patients by nature adhering closely to the prescribed regimen, and others less so, to varying extents. There is also the matter of patients' satisfaction with the medicine itself, which has a strong influence on the persistence of drug therapy, that is, the time between the first-taken dose and the last-taken dose, however well or poorly the patient executes the regimen in between. If patients suffer adverse effects, particularly if they perceive that they are deriving no benefit, or if they perceive that the cause of the original problem has resolved, they tend to stop medication before the end of the prescribed treatment, even if continuing to take the medication is important. Whatever the reason, if adherence to the full course of treatment is important, the solution, in large part, lies in the area of patient counseling to improve motivation. This may involve explaining to the patient, perhaps with visual aids, the consequence of not persisting with the treatment.

Pharmaceutical formulation and the process used to manufacture a product can be important because both can affect the rate and extent of release, and hence entry, into the body (Chapter 7, *Absorption*). A well-designed formulation diminishes the degree of variability in the release characteristics of a drug in vivo. Good manufacturing practice, with careful control of the process variables, ensures the manufacture of a reliable product. Drugs are given by numerous routes including oral, topical, parenteral, and by inhalation (Table 2-3, page 24). Route of administration can affect the concentration locally and systemically. All these factors can profoundly affect the response to a given dose or regimen.

Food, particularly fat, slows gastric emptying and so decreases the rate of systemic drug absorption after oral administration. The extent of absorption is not usually affected by food, but there are many exceptions to this statement. Food is a complex mixture of chemicals, each potentially capable of interacting with drugs. For example, alendronate, a bisphosphonate used to reduce the risk of bone fracture in the elderly, needs to be taken on a fasted stomach because food significantly reduces its oral bioavailability. In contrast, nelfinavir (Viracept), used in the treatment of acquired immune deficiency syndrome, needs to be taken with food because food substantially improves its bioavailability. Recall also that grapefruit juice contains compounds that inhibit intestinal CYP3A4 and so increases the hepatic and systemic exposure of compounds, such as simvastatin (an agent used to reduce cholesterol) and felodipine (a calcium channel blocking agent used in the treatment of hypertension) that normally exhibit a low oral bioavailability caused by extensive CYP3A4-catalyzed metabolism during absorption across the intestinal wall and passage through the liver (Fig. 7-6, page 194). Diet may also affect drug metabolism. Enzyme synthesis is ultimately dependent on protein intake. When protein intake is severely reduced for prolonged periods, particularly because of an imbalanced diet, drug metabolism may be impaired. Conversely, a high protein intake may cause enzyme induction.

To many, herbal preparations and other plant extracts are believed to be both efficacious in ameliorating or curing diseases and devoid of adverse effects, because they are "natural products." However, it is well to remember that these preparations contain many constituents about which little to nothing is known, and that many potent, and potentially toxic, compounds, including morphine, atropine, and digoxin are derived from plants, namely opium poppy, deadly nightshade, and foxglove, respectively. Many plant constituents also have the potential to interact with prescribed drugs. Figure 12-10 illustrates the magnitude of such an interaction with St. John's wort (*Hypericum perforatum*), a popular herbal preparation used to treat depression. The substantial decrease in systemic exposure of midazolam arises because this herb contains compounds that are powerful inducers of CYP3A4. The result is a tendency for a decrease in the effectiveness of CYP3A4 substrate drugs that can have severe consequences. For example, taking St. John's wort has been reported to precipitate organ rejection in patients stabilized on cyclosporine, an immunosuppressive agent used to minimize the risk of organ rejection. Cyclosporine has a narrow therapeutic window and is eliminated almost entirely via CYP3A4-mediated metabolism; its metabolites are either less active than cyclosporine itself or inactive. St. John's wort also induces P-glycoprotein, particularly in the intestinal wall, and in doing so decreases the oral bioavailability of compounds such as fexofenadine, a relatively polar nonmetabolized drug, whose absorption is limited because of efflux by this transporter (Fig.12-9B).

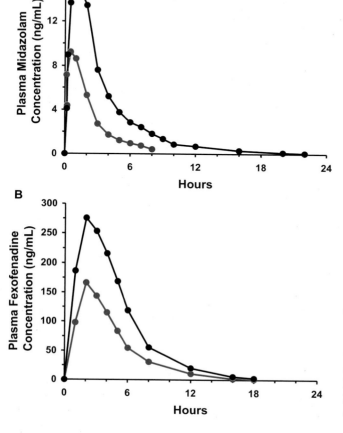

FIGURE 12-10. **A.** Mean plasma concentrations with time of midazolam and **(B)** fexofenadine following a single oral dose of 4-mg midazolam and 180-mg fexofenadine, respectively, alone (control, *black*) and after 11-day treatment with 300-mg St. John's wort 3 times daily (*colored*). Notice the reduction in the *AUC* of both midazolam (2.7-fold) and fexofenadine (1.9-fold) caused by St. John's wort, inducing CYP3A4 and P-glycoprotein, respectively. (From: Dresser GK, Schwarz UI, Wilkinson GR, et al. Coordinate induction of both P4503A and MDR1 by St. John's wort in healthy subjects. Clin Pharmacol Ther 2003;73:41–50.)

Heavy cigarette smoking tends to reduce clinical and toxic effects of some drugs, including theophylline, caffeine, and olanzapine. The drugs affected are extensively metabolized by hepatic oxidation catalyzed by CYP1A2; induction of this enzyme is the likely cause. Many environmental pollutants exist in higher concentrations in the city than in the country; they can also stimulate synthesis of hepatic metabolic enzymes.

Although on average the body maintains homeostasis, many biological functions (e.g., cardiovascular function) and many endogenous substances (e.g., hormones) undergo temporal rhythms. The period of the cycle is often circadian, approximately 24 hr, although there may be both shorter and longer cycles upon which the daily one is superimposed. The menstrual cycle and seasonal variations in the concentrations of some endogenous substances are examples of cycles with a long period. Drug responses and pharmacokinetics may therefore change with time of the day, day of the month, or season of the year. **Chronopharmacology** is the study of the influence of time of day (or month) on drug response. Epidemiologic studies have demonstrated the heightened morning-time risk of angina, myocardial infarction, and stroke, and there is a case for a varying, rather than constant, input rate or dosing pattern of some drugs during the day to ensure adequate systemic exposure at the time of greatest need. Particular note of this phenomenon of circadian rhythms is taken in cancer chemotherapy. Many chemotherapeutic agents have very narrow margins of safety and are given in combination. Appropriate phasing in the timing of administration of each drug during the day can improve the margin of safety considerably. For example, administering a schedule of 5-fluorouracil (with leucovorin) from 10 p.m. to 10 a.m. and oxaliplatin from 10 a.m. to 10 p.m. to patients with metastatic colorectal cancer produced a better therapeutic response and lower incidence of various adverse effects, with lower withdrawal rates caused by excessive toxicity, compared with a combined continuous constant-rate regimen (Fig. 12-11). The higher tolerability to 5-fluorouracil during the night is a result of

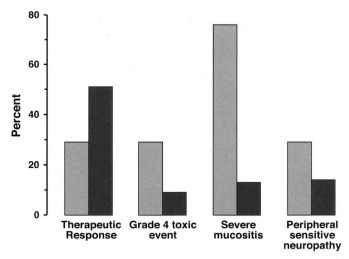

FIGURE 12-11. Chronotherapy (■) produced a higher incidence of therapeutic response (defined as disappearance of symptoms and signs of disease for a minimum of 4 weeks) and lower incidence of severely limiting adverse effects (grade 4 toxicity, severe mucositis, peripheral sensitive neuropathy) compared to constant-rate administration (■) in patients receiving chemotherapy (5-fluorouracil, leucovorin, oxaliplatin) for the treatment of metastatic colorectal cancer. Chronotherapy comprised a schedule of 5-fluorouracil (with leucovorin) from 10 p.m. to 10 a.m., and oxaliplatin from 10 a.m. to 10 p.m., and the constant-rate regimen comprised a continuous infusion of the three drugs, each treatment given as 5-day courses with 16-day intervals. (From: Lévi F, Zidani R, Misset JL. Randomised multicentre trial of chronotherapy with oxaliplatin, fluorouracil, and folinic acid in metastatic colorectal cancer. Lancet 1997;350:681–686.)

a combination of higher cellular activity of dihydropyrimidine dehydrogenase, the enzyme responsible for intracellular deactivation of this drug, and fewer of the rapidly turning over normal cells (e.g., bone marrow, oral mucosa, intestine) being in the susceptible S-phase of growth. With tumor cells tending to show little chronosensitivity to chemotherapeutic agents, the advantage of giving oxaliplatin during the afternoon appears associated with higher levels of reduced glutathione in blood and bone marrow, which protects against oxaliplatin toxicity.

DEFINING THE DOSE–RESPONSE RELATIONSHIP

Variability has an important bearing on the estimation of dose–response relationships in clinical trials. A common procedure is to randomly divide patients into several groups, each group receiving a different dose of drug such as 5, 10, or 20 mg. An attempt to establish a dose–response relationship is then made on the mean data for each group, using variability within groups to test for levels of statistical significance. A problem arises when much of the variability between dose and response resides in pharmacokinetics such that there is considerable overlap in the plasma concentrations among the groups despite receiving different doses. Thus, in a given clinical trial, individuals from the high-dose and low-dose groups can have the same plasma concentration (and response); those in the low-dose group have a low clearance and those in the high-dose group a high clearance of the drug. The greater the variability within each group, the weaker is the ability to detect a dose–response relationship although a clear concentration–response may be clearly evident, as seen in Fig. 12-12.

One solution to this problem of demonstrating a dose–response relationship is to increase the number of subjects in each group to increase the certainty of estimating the true mean response at each dose level. This, however, increases the expenses involved. Another solution is to expose each patient to several dose levels of the drug. This approach has the distinct advantage of not only increasing the chances of establishing a dose–response relationship, but also of providing an estimate of interpatient variability in the relationship. Unfortunately, in practice, this design is not always practical to implement, especially for drugs for which the full effect only occurs after several months or longer into drug administration. A third solution is the concentration-controlled clinical trial. In this approach, the pharmacokinetics of the drug is first evaluated in the patient cohort and then, based on this information, doses are adjusted so that the plasma concentration in each patient lies within one of several tightly defined bands. This more elaborate, and sometimes more expensive, design enables much clearer statements to be made about the concentration–response relationship and about interpatient variability in pharmacokinetics and pharmacodynamics. However, it may have limited utility for dose recommendations when a poor correlation is found between plasma drug concentration and response. Many other designs, varying in complexity, each with advantages and disadvantages, can be envisaged. In all cases, variability is a central issue.

THERAPEUTIC EXPOSURE

Variability also impacts on the estimation and interpretation of a therapeutic window, previously discussed in Chapter 9, *Therapeutic Window*. Recall that the therapeutic window of a drug for a patient population was determined by evaluating the frequency of both beneficial and adverse effects for predefined endpoints, as a function of the plasma concentration of the drug, each patient providing at least one measurement of each effect. Recall also the statement made that such a therapeutic window has limited value when most of the interpatient variability in the dose–response relationship lies in pharmacodynamics. To appreciate this last statement and how variability impacts on the

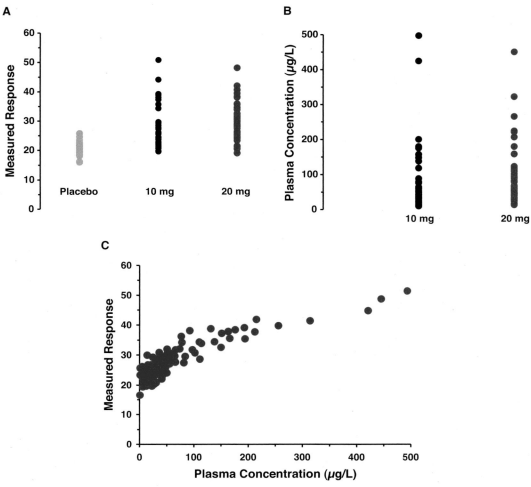

FIGURE 12-12. A clinical trial is undertaken in which patients are randomly assigned to once-daily dosing for 4 weeks of either placebo, 10 or 20 mg of a drug, with assessment made at the end of the trial by which time response is relatively stable. **A.** An attempt to establish a dose–response relationship, for this drug for which pharmacokinetics is the major source of variability, is difficult because some patients, with a low clearance, have a systemic exposure with the low dose that overlaps with that in some patients with high clearance receiving the higher dose, as seen in **(B)**. **C.** A clear concentration–response relationship is seen however when response in each patient is plotted directly against the patient's corresponding plasma concentration of the drug.

steepness of the frequency–concentration relationship, as well as on the degree of overlap between the beneficial and adverse effects curves, consider the situations simulated in Fig. 12-13. Displayed are expected intensity of response versus steady-state exposure relationships within a patient population for four drugs for which response (E/E_{max}, expressed in percentage) is graded, characterized by a C_{50} and a steepness factor, γ. To simplify matters, for each drug toxicity is an extension of its pharmacologic property, in the same way that internal hemorrhage with warfarin is a result of overanticoagulation (although the conclusions drawn would be the same if effectiveness and toxicity were manifestations of different properties of the drugs). Arbitrarily, each drug is taken to be clinically effective when E/E_{max} equals 50% and toxic when the value exceeds 90%. For Drugs A and B, interpatient variability in pharmacodynamics (C_{50}) is small, whereas for Drugs C and D, it is large. The only other difference between them is in γ, which is

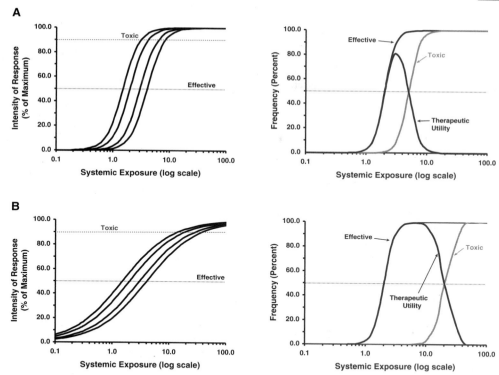

FIGURE 12-13. Impact of interpatient variability in pharmacodynamics on the utility of systemic exposure as a guide to therapeutic outcome in the patient population. *Left-hand panels*: Intensity of response–exposure relationships within a patient population for four drugs (A, B, C, D) for which response (E/E_{max}, expressed in percentage) is graded, characterized by a C_{50} and a steepness factor, γ. For each drug, toxicity is an extension of its pharmacologic property; it is clinically effective when E/E_{max} equals 50% and toxic when the value exceeds 90%. For Drugs A and B, interpatient variability in pharmacodynamics (C_{50}) is small, whereas for Drugs C and D (on page 348), it is large. The only other difference between them is in γ, which is much greater for Drugs A and C than for Drugs B and D. *Right-hand panels*: Frequency of effectiveness and toxicity, together with therapeutic utility, versus logarithm of plasma concentration. Notice that despite the difference in the response intensity steepness factor γ between Drugs A and B, the frequency–exposure relationships for both effectiveness and toxicity are both very steep, because there is little difference in the parameters defining the pharmacodynamics (C_{50}) among patients. However, while the maximum value of therapeutic utility (the difference in incidence between effectiveness and toxicity) is high in both cases, the therapeutic window is wider for Drug B than Drug A because there is a wider separation of concentrations between those associated with effectiveness and toxicity. In contrast, for Drugs C and D the frequency–exposure relationships for both effectiveness and toxicity are now shallow because interpatient variability in pharmacodynamics is large, irrespective of the difference in the value of γ. Moreover, for both drugs the maximum therapeutic utility is low and the therapeutic window narrow, although again it is wider for Drug D because of the wider separation of concentrations for each patient between effectiveness and toxicity. Clearly, systemic exposure has little value as a guide to therapy within the population when interpatient variability in pharmacodynamics is large. *(continued)*

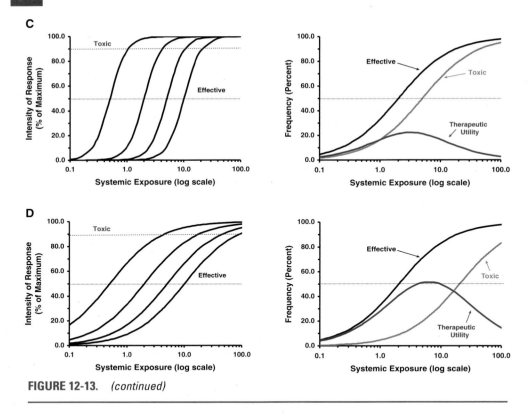

FIGURE 12-13. *(continued)*

much greater for Drugs A and C than for Drugs B and D. Notice, in the panels on the right, that despite the difference in the steepness factor between Drugs A and B, the frequency–exposure relationships for effectiveness and toxicity are both very steep because there is little difference in the parameters defining the pharmacodynamics among patients. However, while the maximum value of therapeutic utility (the difference in incidence between effectiveness and toxicity) is high in both cases, the therapeutic window is wider for Drug B than for Drug A because there is a wider separation of concentrations between those associated with effectiveness and toxicity. Now consider Drugs C and D. For these drugs, the frequency–exposure relationships, panels on the right, for both effectiveness and toxicity are now shallow because interpatient variability in pharmacodynamics (C_{50}) is large, irrespective of the difference in the value of γ. Moreover, for both drugs, the maximum therapeutic utility is low and the therapeutic window narrow, although again it is wider for Drug D because of the wider separation of concentrations for each patient between effectiveness and toxicity. This does not mean that patients cannot be adequately and safely treated with Drugs C and D, but rather that systemic exposure is a poor guide to therapeutic outcome in the population when interpatient variability in pharmacodynamics is large. It may still be a useful guide in the individual patient, particularly for addressing questions related to the drug's bioavailability or disposition. In general, the key to unraveling the optimal dosage regimen for the individual lies in determining whether variability is greater in pharmacokinetics or pharmacodynamics in that patient, aspects of which are discussed further in Chapter 18, *Initiating and Managing Therapy.*

KINETIC MANIFESTATIONS

Considerable variability in enzymatic activity and, to a lesser extent, in plasma and tissue binding exists even among healthy individuals. How such variability manifests itself, in

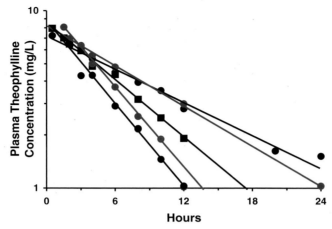

FIGURE 12-14. Five healthy subjects each received 350-mg theophylline orally, in solution as an elixir. Large differences in *AUC* are seen, but in contrast to propranolol (Fig. 12-13), the peak concentrations are almost identical. These observations are as expected for theophylline, a drug of low hepatic extraction that is extensively metabolized in the liver. Variability in hepatic enzyme activity is manifested primarily in variability in clearance, and hence half-life; the weight-corrected volume of distribution of theophylline is relatively constant. Oral bioavailability is close to 100% in all subjects, and because absorption occurred much faster than elimination, peak concentrations are similar. Each symbol refers to a different subject. (From: S. Toon, personal observations.)

pharmacokinetic parameters and in such measurements as plateau plasma concentration, depends on the hepatic extraction ratio and route of administration of the drug, particularly for drugs that are eliminated predominantly by hepatic metabolism. For example, the large interindividual variability in half-life of theophylline (Fig. 12-14) can be explained primarily by variations in hepatic enzyme activity, probably associated with variations in the amounts of the enzymes, particularly CYP1A2, responsible for metabolism of this compound. This conclusion is based on theophylline being predominantly metabolized in the liver, having a low extraction ratio, and being only moderately bound to plasma and tissue components. In contrast, such a high degree of variability in enzymatic activity is expected to be masked in the clearance of a drug having a high hepatic extraction ratio, because clearance tends to be perfusion rate–limited and hepatic blood flow is relatively constant among healthy individuals. Moreover, unless plasma and tissue binding are highly variable, volume of distribution and disposition kinetics of such a drug is much the same for all healthy individuals. This is so for propranolol (Fig. 12-15), a drug of high hepatic clearance.

As described in Chapter 7, *Absorption*, when considering induction and inhibition, changes in hepatic enzyme activity result in variations in oral bioavailability for a drug with a high hepatic extraction ratio. Accordingly, with subsequent disposition being controlled by hepatic perfusion, a series of similarly shaped plasma drug concentration–time profiles, but reaching different peak concentrations, should be seen among individuals with varying enzyme activity receiving the same oral dose of drug. This is indeed seen with propranolol (see Fig. 12-15). In contrast, for a drug with a low hepatic extraction ratio, such as theophylline, variation in enzymatic activity is reflected by variation in clearance (and half-life) rather than in oral bioavailability (and maximum plasma concentration), which is always high (see Fig. 12-14).

The impact of variability in oral bioavailability, because of a high first-pass hepatic effect, depends on the intended use of a drug. It may result in patients' needing

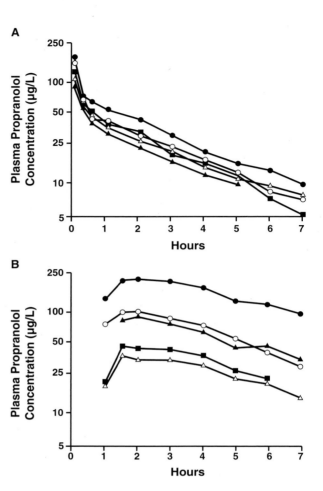

FIGURE 12-15. Five healthy subjects each received propranolol intravenously (10 mg over 10 min) and orally (80 mg) on separate occasions. The plasma concentration–time profiles were very similar following i.v. administration **(A)**, but showed large differences, particularly in peak concentration and *AUC*, following oral administration **(B)**. Such differences in variability with the two routes of administration are expected for propranolol, a drug of high hepatic extraction. Variability in hepatic enzyme activity among the group is manifested primarily in variability in oral bioavailability (16%–60%), rather than in differences in clearance (1 L/min), which is perfusion rate–limited, or hence in half-life. (From: Shand DG, Nuckolls EM, Oates JA. Plasma propranolol levels in adults, with observations in four children. Clin Pharmacol Ther 1970;11:112–120. Reproduced with permission of C.V. Mosby.)

different single oral doses to produce the same effect, as might be the case if the drug is to be used as a sedative hypnotic or to relieve a headache. However, if the drug is intended for chronic use, the degree of variability in average plateau concentration should not be inherently different from that which exists for a drug of low hepatic clearance and having the same degree of variability in enzymatic activity (Fig. 12-16). This statement is based on the following reasoning. At plateau, the average concentration ($C_{av,ss}$) is given by

$$C_{av,ss} = \frac{F \cdot Dose}{CL \cdot \tau}$$

12-1

where τ is the dosing interval. For a drug of high hepatic clearance, variability in $C_{av,ss}$ reflects variability in enzyme activity through F_H; whereas, for a drug of low hepatic clearance, variability in $C_{av,ss}$ reflects variability in enzyme activity through CL (with $F_H \simeq 1$). In both cases, the oral dosing rate (Dose/τ) would need to be adjusted by the same degree to maintain a common $C_{av,ss}$ within subjects. This is achieved by adjusting the dose for the high-clearance drug (as half-life is relatively constant) and perhaps by a mixture of adjusting dose and dosing interval (given that half-life varies) for the low-clearance drug. Of major importance is the underlying variation in enzyme activity, which differs from one enzyme system to another. Obviously, if pharmacokinetics was

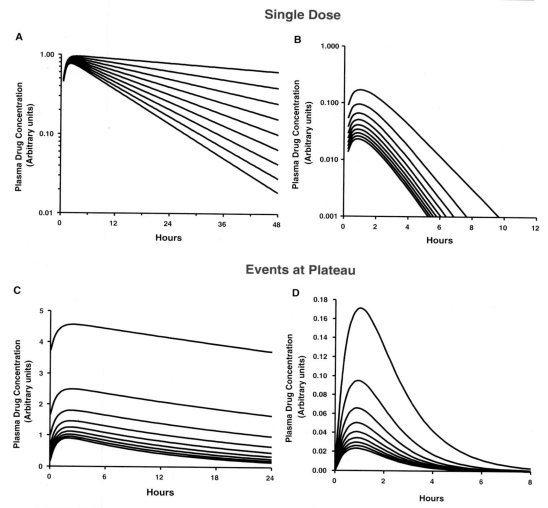

FIGURE 12-16. The impact of variation in hepatic intrinsic clearance within the population on the systemic exposure–time profile after oral administration depends on the extraction ratio of the drug and whether it is given as a single dose or chronically to achieve steady-state conditions. **A,B.** Semilogarithmic plots of plasma concentration–time profile following a single dose of a low **(A)** and a high **(B)** extraction ratio drugs. **C,D.** Regular plot of plasma concentration–time profile within a dosing interval at plateau after multiple dosing of the same two drugs. As expected (and seen with theophylline in Fig. 12-13) variation in intrinsic clearance manifests itself in variations in *AUC* and half-life for a drug of low extraction ratio, and in C_{max} and *AUC*, but not half-life, for a drug of high extraction ratio (as seen with propranolol, Fig. 12-14). However, within a dosing interval at plateau both drugs show an equal degree of variation in the *AUC*, and hence average concentration, reflecting equally the inherent variability in intrinsic clearance. In this simulation both drugs are substrates for the same enzyme, the concentration (and intrinsic clearance) of which varies ninefold. Prediction is based on the well-stirred model of hepatic elimination, when the liver is the only organ of elimination and both drugs are exclusively eliminated by the enzyme.

the major source of variability in drug response and a choice of drugs within a therapeutic class existed, to minimize variation in pharmacokinetics and response, molecules would need to be selected which, if metabolized, are substrates of enzyme systems that show the least variability among subjects. Unfortunately, current information is insufficient to make this selection.

It follows from the foregoing that there is no inherent reason to believe that a set variation in hepatic enzyme activity (caused by a variation in concentration of enzymes, inhibitors, or inducers) should cause a greater interindividual variation in $C_{av,ss}$, for a drug of high hepatic extraction than for one of low hepatic extraction, as long as the drug is eliminated by the same enzyme. Clearly, the situation is more complicated when there is also substantial loss of oral bioavailability caused by gut wall metabolism, as the more extensive this component is, the greater will be the added variability to systemic exposure above that because of hepatic metabolism.

DOSE STRENGTHS

Products are frequently marketed as unit doses of defined strength, such as 50 or 100 mg. If the therapeutic index is high, all patients can receive the same dose strength almost irrespective of any differences in pharmacokinetics among the patient population. However, a narrow therapeutic index necessitates the manufacture of several dose strengths. Although the final number of strengths chosen depends on many practical issues, a rough estimate of the number can be calculated in the following manner for drugs intended for chronic maintenance therapy, and for which pharmacokinetics is the major source of variability in drug response.

Suppose that the upper and lower clearance values encompassing 95% of the patient population, designated CL_{upper} and CL_{lower}, respectively, differ by a factor of six. That is, $CL_{upper} = 6 \cdot CL_{lower}$. It would then follow from Eq. 12-1 that the range of dosing rates needed would be sixfold if the object was to obtain the same $C_{av,ss}$ in all patients. In practice, the therapeutic index is sufficiently wide to allow some tolerance. Let average plateau concentrations within 33% (0.67–1.33) of the optimal value be acceptable. Accordingly, the highest dosing rate that could be given to a patient with a clearance value of CL_{lower} is one that produces a $C_{av,ss}$ that is 1.33 times the optimal value; the lowest dosing rate that could be given to a patient with a clearance of CL_{upper} is one that produces a $C_{av,ss}$ that is 0.67 times the optimal value. The range of associated dosing rates (and hence doses, if the dosing interval is kept constant) is threefold ($6 \times 0.67/1.33$). Now, usually, adjacent dose strengths differ by a factor of 2. Therefore, in the current example, if the smallest dose strength is 50 mg, it would be reasonable to market three dose strengths, 50-, 100-, and 200-mg products, which would suffice for more than 95% of the population. Of the outstanding patients, those with a particularly high clearance may be accommodated with a larger-than-usual maintenance dose, comprising a combination of the marketed unit dose strengths, or they may receive a marketed dose strength more frequently. Those with a particularly low-clearance value may be accommodated by taking the lowest available dose strength less frequently than usual, because the half-life in this group is likely to be the longest in the population.

Variability is a major issue in drug therapy. This chapter has provided evidence for, and identified causes of, variability in drug response. Subsequent chapters deal in much greater detail with *Genetics* (Chapter 13), *Age, Weight, and Gender* (Chapter 14), *Disease* (Chapter 15), *Nonlinearities* (Chapter 16), and *Drug Interactions* within the body (Chapter 17). However, it is important to keep in mind that the separation is for didactic purposes only. In reality, these and other factors each not only affect to varying degrees the underlying processes controlling the pharmacokinetics (and some also the pharmacodynamics) of a drug, as indicated in Fig. 12-17, but many are themselves significantly correlated, such as advancing age and cardiovascular disease, resulting in a complex interplay that determines both interpatient and intrapatient variability. How this information is used in practice is the focus of Chapter 18, *Initiating and Managing Therapy*.

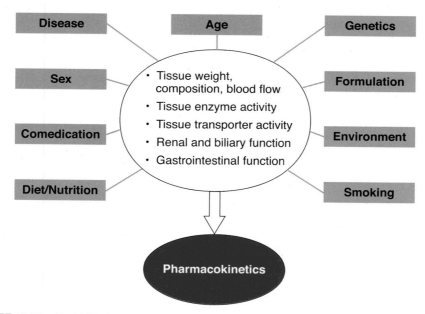

FIGURE 12-17. Variability in observed pharmacokinetics (and pharmacodynamics) of a drug within and between patients is influenced to varying degrees by many factors that not only impact on the underlying controlling processes but also are often themselves highly correlated (such as predisposition of chronic diseases in the elderly).

STUDY PROBLEMS

(Answers to Study Problems are in Appendix J.)

1. Define the following terms, which are selected from the list in Objective 1 at the beginning of the chapter: adherence, coefficient of variation, intrapatient variability, persistence, and population pharmacokinetics.

2. Describe six major sources of variability in drug response.

3. Why is variability in response so important in drug therapy, and why does distinction need to be made between intraindividual and interindividual variability?

4. Do all drugs with a low therapeutic index show low intersubject and intrasubject variability? Briefly discuss.

5. The data in the Table 12-2 were obtained in a study to provide a preliminary assessment of the pharmacokinetic variability of a drug that is predominantly excreted

TABLE 12-2	Observations of a Drug in 5 Subjects Following Intravenous Infusion (20 mg/hr for 48 hr)				
Subject	1	2	3	4	5
Steady-state plasma concentration (mg/L)	2.5	1.6	3.0	1.5	2.3
Postinfusion half-life (hr)	1.4	1.9	1.7	3.0	2.8
Fraction unbound	0.1	0.15	0.09	0.16	0.12

unchanged, $fe = 0.99$. The drug was infused intravenously in five subjects at a constant rate of 20 mg/hr for 48 hr. The fraction unbound was independent of drug concentration but did vary among the subjects.

a. From the values above, calculate the values of Cu_{ss}, CL, CLu, V, and Vu in each of the patients by completing Table 12-3.

TABLE 12-3	Unbound Steady-State Concentration, Clearance, and Volume of Distribution in 5 Subjects				
Subject	1	2	3	4	5
Cu_{ss} (mg/L)	0.25	0.24			0.28
CL (L/hr)		12.5	6.7	13.3	
V (L)		34.2		57.6	35.2

b. The coefficients of variation (standard deviation/mean) for the measured and derived values in the two previous tables are summarized in Table 12-4 below.

TABLE 12-4	Coefficient of Variation of Selected Measures and Pharmacokinetic Parameters					
Measure or Parameter	C_{ss}	$t_{1/2}$	fu	Cu_{ss}	CL	V
Coefficient of Variation	0.29	0.32	0.25	0.07	0.44	0.53

(1) Which of the measures or parameters is the most variable and which is the least variable?

(2) What do these data imply with respect to the source of the most variable pharmacokinetic parameter in this subject population? (Hint: Which physiologic variable most likely explains the variability seen?)

c. Discuss briefly the therapeutic implications of these data with regard to the rate of attainment and maintenance of a "therapeutic" concentration in the various subjects during a constant-rate intravenous infusion?

6. In a group of healthy subjects, the average pharmacokinetic parameters of the β-adrenergic blocking agent alprenolol, which is eliminated almost exclusively by hepatic metabolism, were found to be: volume of distribution, 230 L; clearance, 1.06 L/min; and half-life, 2.5 hr. After i.v. administration, values of these parameters differed little within this group; yet, when the drug was ingested orally, both peak plasma concentration and AUC varied over a fivefold range. Suggest why variability in the observed plasma concentration–time curve is much greater after oral than after i.v. administration.

7. The 95% confidence interval of clearance of a drug within a patient population is 1.5 to 7.5 L/hr, a difference of fivefold. Other pharmacokinetic parameters, F and V, vary much less. Therapeutic activity resides exclusively with the drug, and not the metabolites.

a. Discuss the potential impact of this variability in clearance on the attempt to define a dose–response relationship within a patient population, using a design in which patients are randomly assigned to one of three groups receiving a multiple-dose regimen of either 50, 100, or 200 mg daily of the drug.

b. Suggest and justify a more efficient design to establish the dose–response relationship and the intersubject variability in the parameters.

8. Propofol is used as intensive care unit sedation infusions. Figure 12-18 shows the relationship between the propofol plasma concentration and absence of response to verbal command, somatic response (pain originating from skeletal muscle or ligaments) to gastroscopy, and gag response to gastroscopy, in a group of 70- to 89-year-old outpatients who were undergoing elective upper gastrointestinal endoscopy. In terms of graded or quantal responses, how do you explain both the difference in the C_{50} value and the steepness of the plots for the three measured responses?

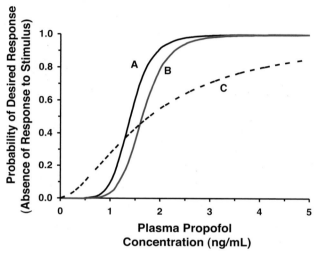

FIGURE 12-18. Relationship between the plasma propofol concentration and response to: verbal command (—) **(A)**, somatic response to gastroscopy (—) **(B)**, and gag response to gastroscopy (---) **(C)** in a group of 70- to 89-year-old outpatients who were undergoing elective upper gastrointestinal endoscopy following i.v. propofol administration. The horizontal line corresponds to 0.5 probability of no response. (From: Kazama T, Takeuchi K, Ikeda K, et al. Optimal propofol plasma concentration during upper gastrointestinal endoscopy in young, middle-aged, and elderly patients. Anesthesiology 2000;93:662–669.)

13

Genetics

OBJECTIVES

The reader will be able to:

- Define the terms: allele, dominant allele, genotype, genetic polymorphism, haplotype, homozygous, heterozygous, drug idiosyncrasy, monogenic, pharmacogenetics, pharmacogenomics, phenotype, polymodal frequency distribution, polygenic, poor metabolizers, recessive allele, unimodal frequency distribution.

- Give three examples of inherited variability in pharmacokinetics and three in pharmacodynamics.

- Demonstrate how population studies and studies in twins can be used to indicate the existence of genetic polymorphism.

- State under what circumstances phenotype status is of therapeutic value.

- Describe at least two ways, other than twin studies, in which genetic polymorphism can be demonstrated and list two examples of each.

nheritance accounts for a large part of both the striking and the subtle differences among individuals, including much of the variation in response to an administered drug. Unlike other sources of variability, inherited traits remain an individual's characteristic for a lifetime. Our knowledge of this area is expanding very rapidly with the characterization of the human genome. **Pharmacogenetics** is the study of inherited variations in drug response. **Pharmacogenomics** is the application of genomic information to the identification of putative drug targets and to the causes of variability in drug response. Before proceeding to consider specific examples, some definitions are important to an understanding of the subject.

The basic biological unit of heredity is the gene. **Genotype** is the fundamental assortment of genes of an individual, the blueprint, whereas **phenotype** is the outward characteristic expression of an individual, such as the color of one's eyes. The mode of inheritance is either monogenic or polygenic, depending on whether it is transmitted by a gene at a single locus or by genes at multiple loci on the chromosomes. Monogenically controlled conditions are often detected as a dramatic and abnormal drug response, that is, a **drug idiosyncrasy**. They may also be detected in population studies by a **polymodal frequency distribution** of the characteristic or some measure of it, as depicted for the clearance of Drug D in Fig. 12-6 (Chapter 12, *Variability*). Polygenically controlled variations tend to have the appearance of a **unimodal frequency distribution**.

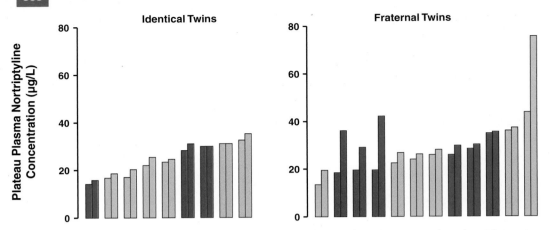

FIGURE 13-1. The much smaller intrapair variability in plateau plasma concentration of nortripty-line between nine identical twins than between 12 fraternal twins indicates that genetics plays a major role in nortriptyline pharmacokinetics. Female (*dark color*); male (*light color*). (From: Alexanderson B, Evans DA, Sjöqvist F. Steady-state plasma levels of nortriptyline in twins: influence of genetic factors and drug therapy. Br Med J 1969;4:764–768.)

Historically, the role of genetics in drug response has been demonstrated by showing that interindividual variation in phenotypic behavior in identical twins is much smaller than that between nonidentical, gender-matched twins, or in any two randomly selected age-, gender-, and weight-matched subjects (Fig. 13-1). Although this approach in identifying the relative importance of genetics is helpful, today, more definitive data concerning mechanisms are obtained by genomic profiling using molecular biology techniques.

The human genome comprises over 1.5 million single-nucleotide polymorphisms (SNPs), locations along DNA where a difference exists among individuals in the nucleotide. The alternate forms, each occupying corresponding positions on paired chromosomes, one inherited from the male and the other from the female, are called **alleles**. Different alleles produce variation in inherited characteristics such as hair color, blood type, or drug metabolizing ability. An allele is **dominant** if it expresses itself phenotypically and **recessive** if it does not. An individual possessing a pair of identical alleles is said to be **homozygous** for the gene and **heterozygous** when the individual has different alleles for the gene. Both homozygous and heterozygous individuals containing the dominant allele may show the same phenotype, and homozygous individuals with recessive alleles may show another. Alleles are often characterized using the * notation. For example, a gene denoted by *1/*1 is homogenous, and one by *1/*3 is heterogeneous, for allele 1, where allele 1 is often the wild-type, or the most common allele, for the gene found in the population studied. The numbering generally follows the chronologic order in which an allele was identified. Sometimes, it is a set of nearby SNPs on the same chromosome that is inherited as a block, a **haplotype**, rather than a single SNP, which determines phenotypic behavior.

Because the approximately 30,000 genes contain multiple SNPs, identifying the most relevant ones affecting disease susceptibility, drug metabolism and transport, and drug response holds the promise of predicting these for individual patients. Although there are a myriad of possible polymorphisms, historically, a **genetic polymorphism** has been defined clinically as the condition in which the frequency of the variant occurs in greater than 1% of the population. Tables 13-1 and 13-2 (page 360) list genetic polymorphisms that affect the pharmacokinetics and pharmacodynamics of some drugs. Although focus is on factors determining therapeutic efficacy and adverse effects, the inability of approximately 30% of Caucasians to taste certain drugs such as

TABLE 13-1	Frequency of Genetic Polymorphisms Producing Slow Metabolism in Some Drug-Metabolizing Enzymes and Representative Substrates*

Enzyme	Frequency of Poor Metabolizer Status	Drug Substrates[†]
Phase I Reactions		
CYP2D6	5%–10% Caucasians 3.8% African Americans 0.9% Asians 1% Arabs	Bufurolol, codeine, dextromethorphan, encainide, flecainide, metoprolol, nortriptyline, timolol
CYP2C9	1%–3% Caucasians	Celecoxib, fluvastatin, glyburide, S-ibuprofen, tolbutamide, phenytoin, S-warfarin
CYP2C19	3%–5% Caucasians 16% Asians	Diazepam, lansoprazole, omeprazole, pantoprazole.
Butylcholinesterase	Several abnormal genes; most common disorder 1 in 2500	Succinylcholine
Phase II Reactions		
Thiopurine S-methyltransferase	0.3% Caucasians 0.04% Asians	Azathioprine, mercaptopurine
N-Acetyltransferase (NAT2)	60% Caucasians, African Americans 10%–20% Asians	Amrinone, hydralazine, isoniazid, phenelzine, aminosalicylic acid
Uridine diphosphate glucuronyl transferase	11% Caucasians 1%–3% Asians	Irinotecan

*Generally results in enhanced or prolonged effect following standard dose of drug.
[†]A major pathway for the elimination of compound.

propylthiouracil, which contains a thiocyanate group, illustrates how genetics also contributes to variability in the senses.

Before considering specific examples, a final general comment is warranted. Commonly, individuals are classified demographically by their ethnicity, such as Caucasians, African American, or Asian. Although, as we shall see, such classification does sometimes help in characterizing differences in response within the population to drugs, it is well to remember that this classification relates essentially to external features, and within each ethnic group, there is often almost as much interindividual variability as between the groups. Clearly, the most important genetic characteristics are those of the individual receiving the drug.

INHERITED VARIATION IN PHARMACOKINETICS

Examples of inherited variability in pharmacokinetics have been almost exclusively restricted to drug metabolism. Comparatively, there is little clinically significant genetic polymorphism currently identified in drug absorption, distribution, and renal or biliary excretion. Nonetheless, genetic polymorphisms have been identified in drug transporters, such as the hepatic uptake transporter, organic anion-transporting polypeptide 1B1 (OATP1B1), and it is likely that clinically important changes in pharmacokinetics will be found especially for those substrates, such as pravastatin, for which hepatic uptake rate limits clearance. When polymorphism in a transporter affects the distribution into a target

TABLE 13-2	Some Genetic Polymorphisms in Pharmacodynamics	

Target	Drug(s)	Drug Effect Linked with Polymorphism
Therapeutic Effects		
ACE*	ACE inhibitors (e.g., enalapril)	Lowering of blood pressure, renoprotective effects
VKORC1†	Warfarin	Variation in sensitivity to anticoagulation; pronounced resistance very occasionally seen
β_2-Adrenergic receptor	β_2-Agonists (e.g., albuterol)	Bronchodilatation, cardiovascular effects
Dopamine receptors (D1, D2, D3)	Antipsychotics (e.g., clozapine)	Antipsychotic response
Estrogen receptor	Conjugated estrogens	Increase in bone mineral density
Adverse Effects		
Glucose-6-phosphate dehydrogenase (G6PD)	Variety of drugs (e.g., primaquine, nitrofurantoin)	Favism or drug-induced hemolytic anemia in those with G6PD deficiency; affects approximately 100 million worldwide; high frequency in African Americans.
HLA-B*1502	Carbamazepine	Dangerous or even fatal skin reactions; exclusively in broad areas of Asia, including South Asian Indians
Bradykinin B2 receptor	ACE* inhibitors	ACE-inhibitor induced cough
Dihydropyridine receptor Ca^{+2} channels	Volatile anesthetics	Malignant hyperthermia, a rare potentially fatal reaction

*Angiotensin-converting enzyme.
†Vitamin K epoxide reductase.

organ, such as liver or brain, or a site of potential toxicity, modifying the ratio of local unbound drug or metabolite to that in plasma, the effect would be defined as an inherited variation in pharmacodynamics, in efficacy or safety, even though the cause is a pharmacokinetic one. Clearly, in the absence of knowing the unbound concentration at the active site, which is rarely determined clinically, the mechanism for such variability in response cannot be ascribed with confidence.

Several genetic polymorphisms of drug metabolism have now been identified, primarily involving oxidation, but also S-methylation, acetylation, and hydrolysis (see Table 13-1). Most were initially detected by adverse reactions occurring in a distinct group within the population termed, **poor metabolizers**, following normal doses of the archetypic drugs. Some examples follow.

OXIDATION

Debrisoquine, an antihypertensive agent no longer in use, was the first drug shown to exhibit genetic polymorphism in oxidation. There is a deficiency in the metabolism of this drug in 5% to 10% of Caucasians, poor metabolizers, with wide differences in frequency in other ethnic groups (see Table 13-1). It is a recessive trait, caused by a specific variant of cytochrome P450 2D6 (CYP2D6). Of the remainder of the population, often referred to as **extensive metabolizers**, some are ultrafast metabolizers, because they possess up to 13 copies of the normal gene within the population, commonly referred to as the wildtype, which is clearly expressed phenotypically in a strong inverse correlation between the number of copies and the area under the curve (*AUC*) for nortriptyline,

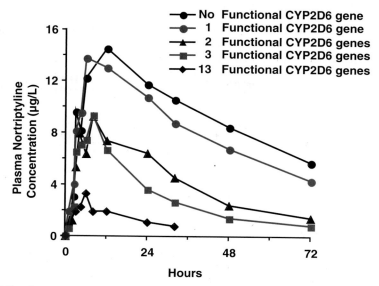

FIGURE 13-2. Strong genetic influence in the pharmacokinetics of nortriptyline is clearly demonstrated by the high correlation between the plasma concentration–time profile and the number of functional CYP2D6 genes possessed by an individual; the larger the number of functional genes, the higher is the clearance and the lower is the exposure profile following a single 25-mg dose of nortriptyline. (From: Dalén P, Dahl ML, Bernal Ruiz ML, et al. 10-Hydroxylation of nortriptyline in white persons with 0, 1, 2, 3, and 13 functional CYP2D6 genes. Clin Pharmacol Ther 1998;63:444–452.)

which predominantly cleared via CYP2D6 oxidation (Fig. 13-2). This variation in the metabolizing enzyme(s) is the predominant reason for the widespread steady-state plasma nortriptyline concentrations among patients receiving the same dosage regimen of nortriptyline (Fig. 13-2). It is also expressed in the large difference in metoprolol profiles between poor and extensive metabolizers (Fig. 13-3). Recall from Chapter 5, *Elimination*, although comprising only approximately 2% of the total cytochrome P450 (CYP450)

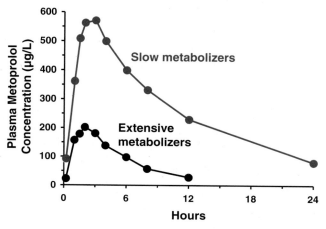

FIGURE 13-3. Plasma metoprolol concentrations after a single oral dose of 200-mg metoprolol tartrate were much higher in poor (*colored line*) than in extensive (*black line*) CYP2D6 metabolizers. Because metoprolol is a drug of high hepatic clearance, the difference between poor and extensive metabolizers is expressed in the large difference in oral bioavailability, because of differences in first-pass hepatic loss. (From: Lennard MS, Silas JH, Freestone S, et al. Oxidative phenotype—a major determinant of metoprolol metabolism and response. Reprinted by permission of New Eng J Med 1982;307:1558–1560.)

content in the liver, CYP2D6 is responsible for the metabolism of approximately 25% of prescribed drugs, particularly basic compounds, including the β-blocker bufurolol, and the antidepressants, doxepin and paroxetine. With all these drugs, CYP2D6-catalyzed metabolism is the major pathway for elimination.

Genetic polymorphism is not restricted to CYP2D6. Although the wide variation in the daily maintenance dose of warfarin has been known for many years, only recently has it become clear that a significant contribution to this variability is mutation of the cytochrome P450 2C9 (CYP2C9) gene, primarily responsible for the metabolism of the more potent S-isomer of this racemic drug (Fig. 13-4). Other drugs that are predominantly metabolized by CYP2C9, and for which clearance is reduced between 3- to 10-fold of the wild type in poor metabolizers, include tolbutamide, glyburide, and phenytoin.

Many drugs are oxidized with widely differing efficiencies by the different forms of CYP450 in addition to CYP2D6 and CYP2C9, such as cytochrome P450 2C19 (CYP2C19) (see Table 13-1). There is also considerable overlap in the structural specificity of some of these enzymes, such that a drug may be a substrate for more than one of them. The majority of oxidatively metabolized drugs are substrates for cytochrome P450 3A4 (CYP3A4), the most abundant drug metabolizing cytochrome. Commonly, there is marked variability in clearance of such substrates within the population, with a

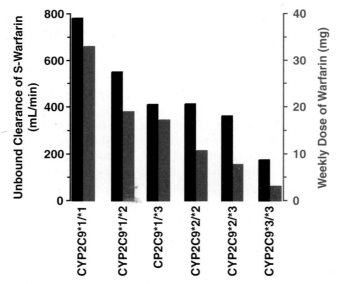

FIGURE 13-4. Genetics plays a significant role in the maintenance dose requirement of warfarin used in the treatment of various cardiovascular diseases. Shown are the unbound clearance of S-warfarin (*black*) in groups of patients with different CYP2C9 genotypes, all titrated and stabilized to a narrow target INR (International Normalization Ratio) range, a measure of anticoagulation, of between 2 and 3, and the mean weekly maintenance dose (obtained by summing the daily dose over 1 week, *in color*). Warfarin is administered as the racemate, with most of the therapeutic effect associated with the more active S-isomer, which is primarily eliminated by CYP2C9-catalyzed metabolism. Homozygous patients with two wild-type alleles (denoted by CYP2C9*1/*1) have the highest S-warfarin clearance and require the highest maintenance dose, and those with two of the most deficient alleles (CYP2C9*3/*3) have the lowest clearance and need the smallest maintenance dose. Heterozygous patients have intermediate clearance. However, as noted in Fig. 12-4 (Chapter 12, *Variability*), in addition to pharmacokinetic variability, there is also considerable interindividual variability in pharmacodynamics of this compound. (From: Scordo MG, Pengo V, Spina E, et al. Influence of CYP2C9 and CYP2C19 genetic polymorphisms of warfarin maintenance dose and metabolic clearance. Clin Pharmacol Ther 2002;72:702–710.)

coefficient of variation in the order of 30% to 40%, because of variation in enzymatic activity. One might expect to demonstrate a genetic influence in the clearance of substrates of this enzyme, but no such relationship to explain much of this variability has been clearly demonstrated to date. Unlike CYP2D6 and CYP2C9, CYP3A4 (and P-glycoprotein [PgP]) is inducible by various environmental factors, weakening any ability to detect genetic factors. However, even when there is a genetic influence involved in the formation of a metabolite, whether one is likely to detect it based on measurement of drug alone, depends on the importance of the affected pathway to the overall elimination of the compound and the frequency of its occurrence within the population. Very low frequency events are by definition difficult to detect in a randomly selected population. Also, examining only half-life or total clearance of the unchanged drug may fail to detect a genetically controlled source of variability of a minor pathway of metabolism. Yet, if the affected metabolite is very potent or toxic, identifying this source of variation may be therapeutically important. This appears to be the case with codeine. Although a minor pathway of codeine metabolism, formation of morphine via CYP2D6 catalyzed oxidation, contributes substantially to the analgesic effect following codeine administration. Accordingly, poor metabolizers of this enzyme receive relatively little analgesic benefit taking codeine. In contrast, ultrafast metabolizers of CYP2D6 form larger than normal amounts of morphine from codeine. One particularly vulnerable group to such high amounts of morphine are suckling neonates and infants, with the risk of respiratory depression, such that taking of codeine by breastfeeding women who are ultrafast metabolizers is contraindicated. Although quite rare in Caucasians (1%), this characteristic is relatively common (28%) among some North African communities.

S-METHYLATION

Thiopurine methyltransferase (TPMT) is the predominant enzyme within hematopoietic cells that inactivates thiopurines by catalyzing their S-methylation. Thiopurine drugs include azathioprine, mercaptopurine, and thioguanine, which are used in the treatment of several conditions, such as leukemia and inflammatory bowel disease. TPMT exhibits genetic polymorphism. Approximately 90% of patients inherit high activity; they are homozygous with two high-activity TPMT alleles. Another 10% have intermediate activity; they are heterozygous with one high-activity and one essentially nonfunctional TPMT allele. And, 0.3% has minimal to no detectable activity, associated with the inheritance of two nonfunctional TPMT alleles. The last group is at particular risk when given standard doses of the above drugs, resulting in an excessively high intracellular concentration of the corresponding active thioguanine nucleoside. The high concentration results from the failure to remove the nucleoside by S-methylation, with attendant severe hematopoietic toxicity, even sometimes when giving just one dose of the thiopurine. Fortunately, subjects receiving these drugs can be readily genotyped prior to treatment, and the dose reduced in the deficient patients, sufficient to achieve adequate therapy without the toxicity, as depicted in Fig. 13-5.

CONJUGATION

Irinotecan (Camptosar), used in the treatment of metastatic colorectal cancer, is a prodrug hydrolyzed to an active species (SN-38). Some patients manifest severe neutropenia and diarrhea, which can be life threatening, on standard doses of irinotecan, whereas others do not, a difference which appears to be a result of genetic polymorphism in uridine diphosphate-glucuronosyltransferase 1A1 (UGT1A1), the enzyme that catalyzes the conjugation of SN-38 to its inactive glucuronide, its primary route of elimination. The specific mutation (UGT1A1*28) has been identified; it has a lower catalytic activity than that of the wild type, resulting in lower clearance of SN-38 and higher exposure in patients who are homozygous for this mutation.

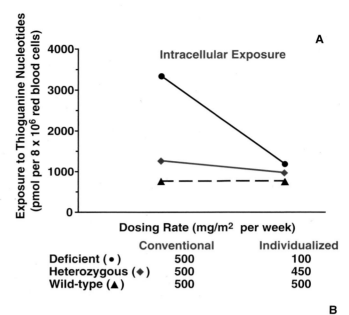

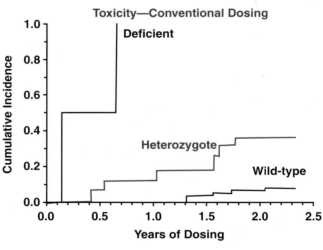

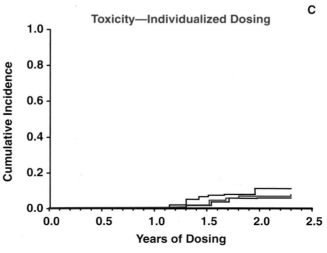

FIGURE 13-5. Genetic polymorphism of TPMT plays a major role in determining the dose of thiopurine drugs (azathiopurine, mercaptopurine, and thioguanine) required for optimal therapy. When all patients receive the same conventional dose of these drugs, the systemic exposure of the active thioguanine nucleotides in blood cells is 10-fold higher in the homozygous TPMT-deficient patients **(A)**, with an associated much higher toxicity experienced by such patients. Heterozygous patients have an intermediate systemic exposure and toxicity **(B)**. In contrast, when the dosage is individualized based on genotypic status prior to therapy, systemic exposure is similar across all patients **(C)**, and severe acute toxicity is avoided. (From: Evans WE. Thiopurine S-methyltransferase: a genetic polymorphism that affects a small number of drugs in a big way. Pharmacogenetics 2002;12:421–423.)

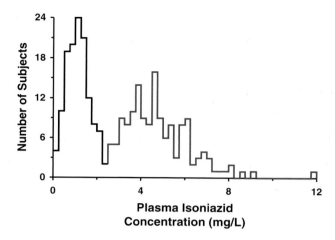

FIGURE 13-6. The bimodal distribution of the 6-hr plasma isoniazid concentration in 483 subjects after 9.8 mg/kg isoniazid orally results from acetylation polymorphism. (From: Evans DA Manley KA, McKusick VA. Genetic control of isoniazid metabolism in man. Br Med J 1960;2:485–491.)

ACETYLATION

Individuals vary widely in their elimination kinetics of the antitubercular drug isoniazid. The bimodality of the frequency distribution histogram of the 6-hr plasma isoniazid concentration following a single oral dose (Fig. 13-6) was the first observation of genetic control of drug metabolism. Although subsequent evidence confirmed that polymorphic isoniazid elimination exists and is under monogenic control, the use of a single time–point measurement could have been misleading. One does not know, a priori, whether a low concentration reflects poor bioavailability, slow absorption with perhaps the concentration still rising, or rapid elimination with the concentration falling. Moreover, if the measurements had been taken at 2 hr, when the concentration primarily reflects absorption rather than elimination, one might have obtained a unimodal frequency distribution and therefore not have identified monogenic control of elimination.

Isoniazid is primarily acetylated in the liver to N-acetylisoniazid, a precursor of a hepatotoxic compound; differences in the elimination kinetics of isoniazid reflect polymorphism of a particular N-acetyltransferase, NAT2, a cytosolic enzyme, of which there are many variants. As shown in Table 13-3, large genetically controlled ethnic differences exist in the distribution of acetylator status. Both Caucasians and African Americans have approximately equal numbers of slow and fast acetylators, while in Asian and Eskimo populations the percentage of slow acetylators is much smaller. Slow acetylators are genetically homozygous with a recessive allele pair, and because acetylator status is under

		Slow Acetylators	Fast Acetylators (%)	
Population	**Number**	**(%)**	**Heterozygotes**	**Homozygotes**
South Indians (Madras)	1477	59	35.6	5.4
Caucasians	1958	58.6 (52–68)	35.9	5.5
African Americans	531	54.6 (49–65)	38.6	6.8
Eskimos	485	10.5 (5–21)	43.8	45.7
Japanese	2141	12.0 (12–15)	45.3	42.7
Chinese	685	22	49.8	28.2

TABLE 13-3   Distribution of Acetylators of Isoniazid in Different Populations

From: Kalow W. Ethnic differences in drug metabolism. Clin Pharmacokinet 1982;7:373–400. Reproduced with permission of ADIS Press Australasia Pty Limited.

monogenic control, it is possible to calculate the frequency of heterozygous and homozygous fast acetylators from gene frequencies. The results displayed in Table 13-3 for each ethnic group are calculated in the following manner: if p and q are the frequencies of two alleles, so that $p + q = 1$, then the frequencies of the three genotypes (consisting of a combination of the alleles) are $p^2 + 2pq$, and q^2. The sum of these frequencies is 1.0. For example, in the data in Table 13-3 for Caucasians, p^2 (for the homozygous slow acetylators) is 0.586, so that $p = 0.766$, that is, 76.6% of Caucasians have one slow acetylator allele. Hence, the frequency for the fast acetylator allele is 0.234, which leads to distributions for heterozygous and homozygous fast acetylators of 0.359 ($2pq$) or 35.9% and 0.055 (q^2) or 5.5%, respectively.

Isoniazid is an exception. Generally, the frequency of occurrence of an allele is linked with other factors, such as gender. Also, several subgroups within the general population are often of a given ethnicity. These effects make it difficult to calculate the genotype frequency. However, notwithstanding the difficulties in making precise calculations, knowledge of the existence of large ethnic differences in pharmacokinetics, such as seen with isoniazid and some other drugs including desipramine (see later), is clearly important for the optimal use of drugs. This is particularly true for drugs prescribed worldwide or used in a multiracial society.

Interest in acetylation polymorphism is not just academic. Peripheral neuropathy, associated with elevated concentrations of isoniazid, occurs more prevalently in slow acetylators, unless an adjustment is made in the dosage of isoniazid or vitamin B_6, to offset this effect, is concomitantly administered. Awareness of the prevalence of homozygous and heterozygous rapid acetylators may also be clinically relevant, because they appear to differ in their susceptibility to adverse reactions, such as isoniazid-induced hepatic damage. Acetylation polymorphism also occurs and is important for several other drugs, such as hydralazine and amrinone (see Table 13-2). For both drugs, the N-acetyl derivative is the major metabolite. A systemic lupus erythematosus-like syndrome, a generalized inflammatory response, can limit the use of hydralazine; it develops more rapidly in slow rather than rapid acetylators. The mechanism remains obscure, but does appear to be associated with elevated plasma concentrations of parent compound. In contrast, rapid acetylators require higher doses of hydralazine to control hypertension.

HYDROLYSIS

A rare phenotype is seen with succinylcholine. Typically, muscle paralysis wears off within minutes of discontinuing an infusion of this neuromuscular blocking agent, because it is rapidly hydrolyzed to inactive products, choline and monosuccinylcholine, by plasma and hepatic butylcholinesterases. In an occasional patient, however, neuromuscular blockade may last several hours after stopping the infusion, because hydrolysis is much slower than usual. The reason is the existence of an atypical enzyme rather than a lower concentration of the typical butylcholinesterase; the atypical esterase has only 1/100th of the usual affinity for succinylcholine, and it behaves differently from the typical cholinesterase to various enzyme inhibitors. Many aberrant forms of this enzyme are now known to exist.

ADDITIONAL CLINICAL CONSIDERATIONS

Several additional points need to be made. First, the clinical implications of genetic polymorphism in drug metabolism (Table 13-4) depend on whether activity lies with the affected substrate or the metabolite, as well as the importance of the pathway to overall elimination. For drugs such as nortriptyline, activity resides predominantly with the drug, and elimination occurs almost completely via the affected pathway. In such cases, unless the dose is reduced, more pronounced and sustained effects may occur together with potentially more frequent adverse reactions in poor metabolizers. Recall, the contrasting and interesting situation seen with codeine. Part of its analgesic activity is because of

TABLE 13-4 | **Potential Consequences of Genetic Polymorphism Involving Drug and Metabolite for Poor Metabolizers***

Case[†]	Drug Is Active	Metabolite Is Active
D →(b) M →	Exaggerated response, potential toxicity. Example[‡]: Metoprolol	Diminished response, unless this is only route of drug elimination. Example: Proguanil**
D → M →	No change in response.	Exaggerated response, potential toxicity. Example: Imipramine[††]
D → M →	Little change in response. Example: Dapsone	Diminished response. Example: Codeine
D → M →	No change in response. Example: Caffeine[‡‡]	Small increased response in toxicity. Example: Clobazam***

*Affected pathway shown in color.
[†]Major pathway in rapid metabolizer (large arrow); minor pathway (small arrow).
[‡]Where known, examples are given and either discussed further in the text or presented in Table 13-1.
**Proguanil, a prodrug, is metabolized to the active drug, cycloguanil.
[††]Imipramine is N-demethylated to desipramine, both compounds are 2-hydroxylated by CYP2D6. As both are active, the dose of imipramine may need to be reduced in poor metabolizers.
[‡‡]Caffeine is converted to a minor metabolite, which then undergoes acetylation polymorphism.
***There is a greater systemic exposure and occurrence of adverse effects seen during clobazam treatment in poor metabolizers of CYP2C19.

morphine formed from codeine by CYP2D6-catalyzed metabolism. Accordingly, subjects born with the deficient gene may derive less analgesic benefit from codeine. Another example is that of tamoxifen, used in the treatment of metastatic breast cancer. Tamoxifen is effectively a prodrug and needs to be converted to the highly active metabolite, endoxifen, to be effective. This conversion occurs via CYP2D6, so women who are poor metabolizers have a compromised clinical benefit. Many other scenarios can be envisaged depending on the relative importance of the affected pathway to elimination and whether drug, metabolite, or both, contribute to activity and toxicity.

Second, genetic polymorphism in drug metabolism has implications in clinical trials during drug development. Relatively few subjects are studied in the early phases of clinical evaluation of a potentially new therapeutic agent. Accordingly, if the frequency of an important drug-metabolizing enzyme deficiency is very low, an important source of interpatient variability in pharmacokinetics, and response, may be missed until the drug becomes widely prescribed, with potentially serious consequences. Fortunately, with the increasing availability of pure human drug-metabolizing enzymes, produced using biotechnology, preclinical in vitro screens are increasingly used to characterize the enzymes primarily responsible for metabolism of a drug. If the enzyme involved is one known to display genetic polymorphism, the drug can be evaluated in a preselected group of subjects with the enzyme deficiency to examine whether serious problems might arise during its subsequent use in patients of this type. The same consideration applies to situations of known polymorphism in pharmacodynamics, examples of which are now discussed.

INHERITED VARIABILITY IN PHARMACODYNAMICS

It is not uncommon for a significant fraction of a patient population to fail to respond to drug treatment. Reasons for this are many, but one of them is lack, or much lower affinity, of the target receptor in nonresponders. For example, trastuzumab (Herceptin) is a humanized monoclonal antibody used in the treatment of primary breast cancer. It has a high affinity for, and effectively inhibits, the proto-oncogene human epidermal growth factor receptor 2 (HER2), a promoter of cancer. However, HER2 protein overexpression is only observed in 24% to 30% of primary breast cancers. Because trastuzumab is not without adverse effects and is expensive, it is inappropriate to administer this drug to the 65% to 70% of patients who would derive no benefit from the drug. The solution has been to screen all patients with a diagnostic genomic test, and only give the drug to patients in whom tumor cells overly express the receptor. Another is gefitinib (Iressa) used in the treatment of patients with non–small-cell lung cancer. This drug inhibits epidermal growth factor receptor tyrosine kinase (EGFR-TK), an important mediator of growth factor signaling pathways that regulate key cellular functions. Patients with tumors that have certain somatic mutations of EGFR-TK show a much more marked beneficial response to gefitinib. These susceptible mutations occur with higher frequency in Japanese than in Caucasians.

Another example of genetically determined variation in pharmacodynamics is illustrated in Fig. 13-7, which shows differences in the forced expiratory volume in 1 sec (FEV$_1$), a measure of respiratory function, in patients following a single oral dose of the β-adrenergic agonist albuterol. Yet another example is seen with warfarin. As previously noted, patients vary in the dosage requirements of warfarin needed to produce adequate anticoagulant control of which only a part is explained by differences in pharmacokinetics; some is because of differences in pharmacodynamics (Fig. 12-4). Warfarin acts by lowering the concentration of reduced vitamin K within the liver by decreasing its regeneration from the inactive vitamin K epoxide pool in the vitamin K cycle, through inhibition of vitamin K epoxide reductase (VKOR). Vitamin K is an essential cofactor for the synthesis of the vitamin K-dependent clotting factors (Factors II, VII, IX, and X) as well as the anticoagulant proteins C and S. Certain polymorphisms in the vitamin K epoxide reductase complex subunit 1 (VKORC1) gene have now been associated with lower dose requirements for warfarin. Although, understandably, attention has been focused on patients needing low doses to minimize the risk of overanticoagulation, some patients are resistant to warfarin and require massive doses (up to 180 mg weekly, compared with the normal range of 7–50 mg) to achieve a therapeutic response; failure to do so brings the risk of a thromboembolism. A normal pharmacokinetic

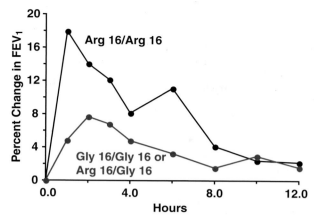

FIGURE 13-7. Functional pharmacodynamic consequences of genetic polymorphisms in the β_2-adrenoreceptor are seen by differences in FEV_1, a measure of respiratory function, in patients in response to a single 8-mg oral dose of the β-agonist albuterol. Note, that the response is greater in those homozygous with arginine (*black*), than with glycine, or heterozygous with arginine and glycine (*colored*), on position 16 of the gene encoding for the receptor. (From: Lima JJ, Thomason DB, Mohamed MH, et al. Impact of genetic polymorphisms of the β_2-adrenoreceptor on albuterol bronchodilator pharmacodynamics. Clin Pharmacol Ther 1999;65:519–525.)

profile of warfarin in the resistant patients points to a pharmacodynamically based resistance. The high resistance is conferred by a particular abnormal variant of the VKORC1 haplotype, which while rare among most populations is relatively common (15%) in specific ethnic groups (of Jewish or Ethiopian ancestry). However, while helpful in identifying the ultrasensitive and resistant patients, VKORCl and CYP2C9 genotypes, even when taken together with other significant covariates, particularly age and body weight, still explains only about 60% of the variability in the warfarin maintenance dose within the population (Fig. 13-8). Consequently, while genotyping helps to identify the extremes, ultrasensitive and resistant patients, adjustment of dosage continues to be based on measures of the individual's degree of anticoagulation.

Genetic control is not restricted to therapeutically beneficial effects, but increasingly is being identified as a major source of variability in adverse effects. One clear example is

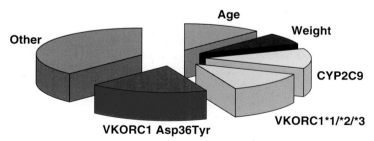

FIGURE 13-8. Pie chart showing the percentage of the total variance in dose of warfarin needed to maintain the INR between 2 and 3 in a population of Jewish Israelis. Note that together genotyping (for CYP2C9, VKORC1, and VKCORC1 Asp36Tyr, the variant haplotype that confers resistance) captures 43% of the total variance, with age and body weight capturing an additional 19%, leaving 38% unexplained. These percentages will vary depending on the composition of the patient population receiving warfarin. Note also that in terms of dose range categories the CYP2C9*2,*3 and VKORC1 *2,*3 polymorphisms mark the low dose range (<25th percentile: <20 mg/wk), whereas the Asp36Tyr polymorphism marks the high dose range (>75th percentile: >70 mg/wk). (From: Loebstein R, Dvoskin I, Halkin H, et al. A coding VKORC1 Asp36Tyr polymorphism predisposes to warfarin resistance. Blood 2007;109:2477–2480.)

seen with abacavir (Ziagen), a guanosine reverse-transcriptase inhibitor used as part of anti-HIV treatment. In Caucasians, 5% to 8% experience severe, and potentially fatal, immunologically determined adverse reactions, including fever, rash, and severe gastrointestinal and respiratory distress when treated with abacavir. These patients carry the HLA (human leukocyte antigen)-B*5701 allelic variant, which is highly predictive of these severe reactions. HLA-B*5701 has been proposed as a screening biomarker to limit the use of abacavir to HLA-B*5701-negative patients, in whom it is relatively safe.

Other examples of genetically determined variation in pharmacodynamics are given in Table 13-2. Although the number of examples is currently small, the importance of such sources of variability in response, when coupled with an appropriate diagnostic test, is likely to play a more dominant role in future drug therapy.

METABOLIC PHENOTYPING

Phenotyping patients for a particular metabolic pathway, such as acetylation or oxidation, prior to drug administration has been proposed based on the ratio of drug and metabolite concentrations in urine following a single dose of a marker. For example, sulfamethazine has been used to phenotype for slow acetylation; and sparteine, for CYP2D6 slow oxidation. This approach aims to better anticipate the dosage regimen of a drug required in an individual. Its appeal is greatest in those situations in which: the therapeutic index of the drug is low; the analyses of drug and its metabolites in plasma are difficult; the marker is relatively safe, easy to measure, and its phenotypic characteristic is highly correlated with that of the drug.

Despite its appeal, metabolic phenotyping is not widely employed in clinical practice for many reasons. One is the inconvenience associated with taking of the marker and collecting urine; another is assay costs; and yet others are the possibility of false positives that arise because of other currently administered drugs, such as quinidine, inhibiting the enzyme and the complication introduced by poor renal function, which can affect the renal clearance of both drug and metabolite. Genotyping, based on DNA analysis of a small sample of blood or any other tissue, holds promise of providing a more direct approach toward predicting metabolic phenotype in situations where the correlation with the clearance of the drug is very high. Currently, DNA tests have correctly predicted the phenotypes for both N-acetylation and CYP2D6 in 95% to 97.5% of healthy volunteers, which clearly indicates the importance of genetics as the major source of variability here. To facilitate application of such type of information to individualization of drug therapy, a commercial genomic kit is now available to classify an individual's genetic status of an array of drug-metabolizing enzymes and transporters, including CYP2D6, CYP2C19, and PgP. The application of phenotyping to predict dosage depends on the relative contribution of other factors, such as disease and concurrent drugs, to the overall variability in drug metabolism and variability in response in the patient population.

STUDY PROBLEMS

(Answers to Study Problems are in Appendix J.)

1. Define the following terms: allele, genotype, genetic polymorphism, haplotype, heterozygous, pharmacogenomics, and phenotype.

2. Discuss how pharmacodynamic sources of variability can be distinguished from pharmacokinetic sources, and give three examples of inherited variability in pharmacokinetics and three in pharmacodynamics.

3. Discuss briefly how an inherited source of variation in pharmacokinetics can be identified within the patient population.

4. A drug developed for worldwide use is extensively metabolized by N-acetyltransferase (NAT1). What are the potential implications of this finding?

5. Subjects genotyped for CYP2D6 status (poor or extensive metabolizers) ingested one of the following four β-adrenergic blocking drugs; atenolol, metoprolol, propranolol, and timolol. Table 13-5 lists the mean values of various pharmacokinetic parameters for each drug and whether the correlation with CYP2D6 status was weak or strong. Discuss briefly possible reasons for the observed correlations.

TABLE 13-5	Pharmacokinetic Parameters and Correlations with CYP2D6 Status of Several β-adrenergic Blocking Drugs			
	Pharmacokinetic Parameters (Mean Value)			**Correlation with CYP2D6 Metabolic Status**
Drug	CL (L/hr)	V (L)	CL_R (L/hr)	
Atenolol	5.0	38	4.3	Weak
Metoprolol	63.0	290	6.0	Strong
Propranolol	50.0	280	<0.3	Weak
Timolol	31.0	150	4.7	Strong

6. a. Give two examples, in addition to metoprolol and timolol, of drugs that are oxidized and that exhibit genetic polymorphism in their clearance.

   b. Briefly discuss each of the following statements:
   (1) Flecainide, an antiarrythmic agent ($fe = 0.43$), is a substrate for CYP2D6, yet only in patients with severe renal dysfunction is genetic polymorphism in clearance readily apparent.
   (2) Dapsone and codeine are two examples of drugs that form minor metabolites via pathways that exhibit genetic polymorphism, but only for codeine is there a potential therapeutic implication.
   (3) Quinidine converts extensive metabolizers of substrates of CYP2D6 to poor metabolizers.
   (4) Genetics poorly explains interindividual variability in clearance of substrates extensively metabolized by CYPA4.

7. The frequency within the population of an allele associated with slow oxidation of a drug is 0.15. If slow oxidizers are homozygous with a recessive allele pair, what are the expected frequencies of slow and fast oxidizers in the population? Assume that oxidation status is under monogenic control and that all the variability in oxidation within the population is of genetic origin.

14

Age, Weight, and Gender

OBJECTIVES

The reader will be able to:

- Define what is meant by a typical patient and a usual adult dosage regimen of a given drug.
- Define adolescent, adult, body mass index, body surface area, creatinine clearance, elder, ideal body weight, infant, lean body mass, and neonate.
- Determine those drugs for which loading dose, normalized for body weight, is likely to be independent of age, given the volume of distribution and fraction unbound.
- Describe the likely changes in the pharmacokinetics of a drug predominantly excreted unchanged, from neonate to elderly patients.
- Explain the general trend of metabolic clearance of drugs with age, from neonate to elderly patients.
- Discuss the general gender differences observed in pharmacokinetics and pharmacodynamics.
- Given the usual adult dosage regimen of a drug in a typical patient, estimate the dosage to be given to patients from 1 to 100 years of age (without considering other sources of variability).

Aging, characterized by periods of growth, development, and senescence, is an additional source of variability in drug response and, as a result, the usual adult dosage regimen may need to be modified, particularly in the young and the old, if optimal therapy is to be achieved. Furthermore, it is the very young and the aged, in particular, who often are in most critical need of drugs. It is against this background in which an attempt is made in this chapter to develop a framework for making dosage adjustments for age. Body weight and gender are also examined.

The life of a human is commonly divided into various stages. In this book, the various stages are defined as follows: **neonate**, up to 1 month post utero; **infant**, between the ages of 1 month and 2 years; **child**, between 2 and 12 years of age; **adolescent**, between the ages of 13 and 19 years; **adult**, between 20 and 75 years; and **elder**, older than 75 years of age. It is recognized, however, that this stratification of human life is arbitrary. Life is a continuous process with the distinction between one period and the next often ill defined. Furthermore, society's view of who is "elderly" is changing as the general health of the population improves with new therapies and as the baby boom generation ages. It is also recognized that chronologic age does not necessarily define functional age, and accordingly, statements made in this chapter pertain to the average person within the age bracket rather than to the individual.

Expediency and practicality dictate against the wide use of longitudinal studies in individuals to examine the influence of age on pharmacokinetics or pharmacodynamics. Rather, single observations are made in individuals of differing ages. The information obtained therefore pertains to the population sampled at the time of the observations and does not necessarily reflect how an individual may change with age.

THE TYPICAL PATIENT AND USUAL DOSAGE REGIMEN

WHO IS "THE TYPICAL PATIENT"?

The typical patient is the individual who usually receives a drug of interest for a given indication. The age of the typical patient may therefore vary with the drug and the indication of its use. Figures 14-1 to 14-3 show different age trends for selected diseases in the United Kingdom. Some diseases (e.g., congestive cardiac failure, hypertension, diabetes, arthritis or rheumatism [Fig. 14-1], and cancer) tend to be much more common in the elderly. The incidence of others, such as asthma, back problems, epilepsy, and migraine (see Fig. 14-2), tend to be spread across the entire lifespan. Still others primarily occur in childhood or early adulthood, like hay fever (see Fig. 14-3), Duchenne muscular dystrophy, and cystic fibrosis. For a few diseases, there is a decided gender difference, as seen with migraine in Fig. 14-2D. Some, of course, are decidedly gender specific, such as benign prostatic hyperplasia, breast cancer, prostate cancer, and testicular cancer.

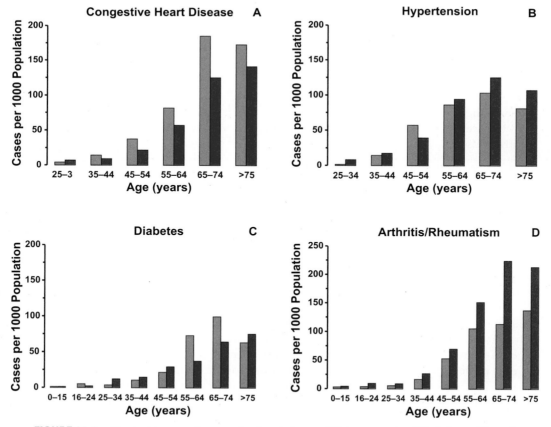

FIGURE 14-1. The incidences of congestive heart disease **(A)**, hypertension **(B)**, diabetes **(C)**, and arthritis/rheumatism **(D)** in 2003 are much greater in the elderly population (up to 200 cases per 1000 people) than in children or young adults in the United Kingdom. Males, (*gray bars*); Females, (*colored bars*). (From: General Household Survey & Key Health Statistics from General Practice, U.K. Office for National Statistics.)

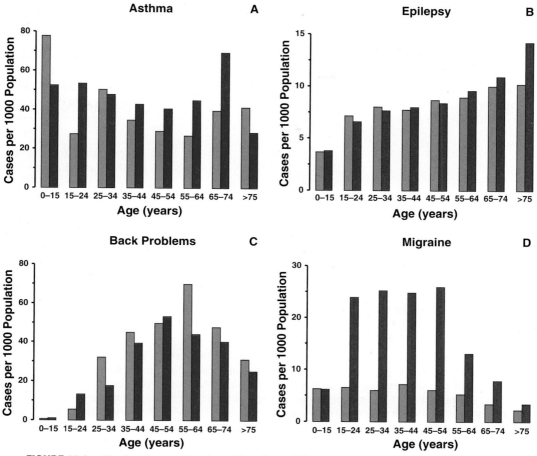

FIGURE 14-2. The incidences of asthma (**A**), epilepsy (**B**), back problems (**C**), and migraine (**D**) are relatively evenly spread across the population in the United Kingdom in 2003, except for epilepsy for which the data are for 1998. Note the incidences are all lower than in those listed in Fig. 14-1, and that the incidence of migraine is higher in females than males. Males, *gray bars*; Females, *colored bars*. (From: General Household Survey & Key Health Statistics from General Practice, U.K. Office for National Statistics.)

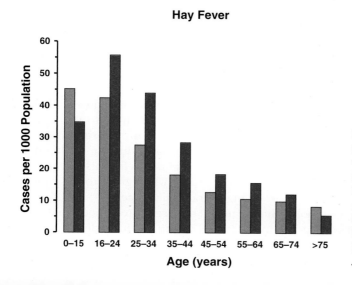

FIGURE 14-3. The incidence of hay fever is much greater in children and young adults than in the elderly population in the United Kingdom in 2003. Males, *gray bars*; Females, *colored bars*. (From: General Household Survey & Key Health Statistics from General Practice, U.K. Office for National Statistics.)

Most drugs tend to be, on average, given to either older adults or the elderly. This is evidenced by the number of prescriptions written for various age groups as shown in Fig. 14-4, which summarizes data from the Third National Health and Nutrition Examination Survey (1988–1994). Overall, a majority of 62% of the U.S. population took no prescription drugs, but it is evident that the percentage drops off with advancing years (Fig. 14-4A). Also apparent is the increase in the number of prescribed drugs concurrently taken by the elderly (Fig. 14-4B), giving rise to a much greater use of drugs in this age group.

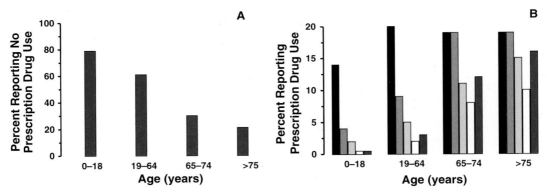

FIGURE 14-4. Patterns of prescription drug use in the United States, 1988 to 1994. **A.** Sixty two percent of the general population took no prescribed drug, but when broken down into four age groups, the percent receiving no drug greatly decreased with advancing years. **B.** Also apparent is a large increase in the number of drugs concurrently taken in those 65 years of age and older. Key: On one drug (*black*); on two drugs (*dark gray*); on three drugs (*gray*); on four drugs (*white*); on five or more drugs (*colored*). (From: National Health and Nutrition Examination Survey, Department of Health and Human Services, Center for Disease Control and Prevention, National Center for Health Statistics. Retrieved from http://www.cdc.gov/nchs/data/nhanes/databriefs/preuse.pdf. Accessed September 3, 2009.)

There are exceptions (Figs. 14-2 and 14-3) to greater drug use in the elderly, particularly for those drugs given to treat diseases more common to children or young adults. However, because drug utilization is, in general, more frequent in the older adult, a typical patient will subsequently be considered to be 60 years of age and to weigh 70 kg. For many frequently prescribed drugs, this may be an underestimate of the average age of the "typical" patient, particularly for the drugs used in diseases such as benign prostatic hyperplasia, heart disease, incontinence, Parkinson's disease, and prostate cancer. These patients may, on average, be even older (e.g., 70–80 years).

WHAT IS "THE USUAL DOSAGE REGIMEN"?

Throughout this chapter, reference is made to the **usual adult dosage regimen**. Before proceeding, this phrase needs to be defined. The word *adult* refers here to the typical adult patient with the disease or condition requiring the drug. For drugs primarily used in children, such as hay fever, or for a condition common to young adults (e.g., rheumatoid arthritis), the typical patient is younger, and the usual regimen is for this age group. The "*usual*" *adult dosage regimen* is defined as the regimen that when given to the typical patient, on average, has the best chance of achieving therapeutic success.

The data in Table 14-1 illustrate a point about age and disease. Listed are estimates of the population pharmacokinetics of digoxin in a group of young, healthy adults and in a

TABLE 14-1	Population Pharmacokinetic Parameters of Digoxin in Young, Healthy Subjects and Inpatients With Severe Congestive Cardiac Failure					
	Age (Years)	Weight (kg)	Oral Bioavailability	Volume of Distribution (L)	Renal Clearance (L/hr)	Extrarenal Clearance (L/hr)
Young, healthy subjects	28	71	40–70	760	8.5	3.5
Inpatients, severe congestive cardiac failure	54	68	60	476	3.5	1.4

From: Koup JR, Greenblatt DJ, Jusko WJ, et al. Pharmacokinetics of digoxin in normal subjects after intravenous bolus and infusion dose. J Pharmacokinet Biopharm 1975;3:181–192; and Sheiner LB, Rosenberg B, Marthe VV. Estimation of population characteristics of pharmacokinetic parameters from routine clinical data. J Pharmacokinet Biopharm 1977;5:445–479.

group of inpatients receiving digoxin for treatment of severe congestive cardiac failure. Notice the differences in the values of the estimates, particularly for renal clearance, between the two groups. Evidently, estimates obtained in the young, healthy group have limited application to therapy in patients.

Part of the difference in renal clearance of digoxin between the two groups is accounted for by the disease. Part, however, is accounted for by age. One objective of this chapter is to suggest means of correcting values of pharmacokinetic parameters for age. The intent, thereby, is to permit a better estimate to be made of the initial dosage required to treat a disease in an individual patient or in a patient population whose age differs substantially from the mean age of the patient population in which the usual adult dosage regimen was established. For didactic purposes, the influence of all other factors—such as disease being treated, concurrent diseases, and other drugs—on pharmacokinetics or pharmacodynamics are assumed to be accounted for independently. In practice, these factors are often highly correlated.

PHARMACODYNAMICS

Throughout this chapter, the range of unbound plasma drug concentrations associated with successful therapy is assumed to be independent of age. This is the case for anti-infective agents. For antiepileptic drugs and digoxin, effective plasma drug concentrations also appear to be the same in both children and adults, although children appear to tolerate higher unbound concentrations of these drugs before any toxic manifestations become apparent. Differences in response with age are likely to exist for certain drugs. For example, the observed increased sensitivity of elderly patients to the central nervous effects of benzodiazepines cannot be explained on the basis of differences in pharmacokinetics of this group of drugs. Also, the elderly show reduced response to β-adrenergic drugs, such as propranolol, and are more sensitive to the adverse effects of neuroleptic drugs and anesthetic agents, as shown in Fig. 14-5 for the general inhalation anesthetic, desflurane (Suprane). The systemic exposure of desflurane required to give the same depth of anesthesia needs to be reduced in the elderly. The minimum alveolar concentration is used to measure systemic exposure to the drug in much the same way that a breath test is used to assess blood–alcohol levels.

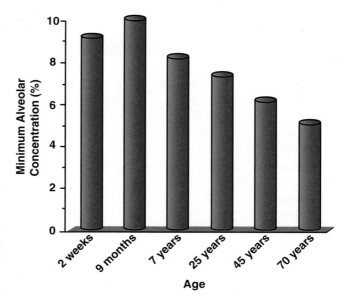

FIGURE 14-5. The minimum alveolar concentration (%) of desflurane required for general anesthesia varies with age. Elderly patients are clearly more sensitive to the anesthetic effect of the drug. (From: Physician's Desk Reference, 2003;867.)

PHARMACOKINETICS

ABSORPTION

Drug absorption does not appear to change dramatically with age. Nonetheless, all the factors discussed in Chapter 7, *Absorption*, that affect drug absorption, including gastric pH, gastric emptying, intestinal motility, and blood flow, do change with age. Thus, in the neonate, a condition of relative achlorhydria persists for the first week of life, and only after 3 years of age does gastric acid secretion approach the adult value. Gastric emptying is also prolonged, and peristalsis is irregular during the early months of life. The diet of the neonate (restricted to milk) is also unique. Skeletal–muscle mass is much reduced, and muscle contractions, which tend to promote both blood flow and spreading of an intramuscularly administered drug, are relatively feeble.

A delay in gastric emptying and both diminished intestinal motility and blood flow are seen in the elderly. Although generally still acidic, a more elevated gastric pH and a slower return to acidic gastric conditions on ingestion of meals, because of a decrease of acid-secreting parietal cells, are observed in the elderly. Differences in oral drug absorption among adults, the very young, and the elderly are therefore expected. Generally, changes in rate rather than in extent of absorption are observed. Children often appear to absorb drugs completely and, if anything, more rapidly than adults. Accordingly, in subsequent calculations of dosage, extent of absorption is assumed not to change with age.

DISPOSITION

Body Weight and Composition. One aspect of aging is body weight. Weight, 3.5 kg at birth, increases rapidly in childhood and adolescence and then declines slowly in the elderly (Fig. 14-6). Because body-water spaces, muscle mass, organ blood flow, and organ function are related to body weight, so too should volume of distribution, clearance, and hence, dosage regimens of drugs. Owing to large variability, however, a weight adjustment is generally considered only if the weight of an individual differs by more than 30% from that of the typical patient (70 kg). In practice, then, adjustments for weight are made only for neonates, infants, and children and for adults who are petite, emaciated, or have a very large frame. For individuals who are obese, adjustment in dosage for body weight may be inappropriate as renal and hepatic functions do not increase with the extra fat-related weight.

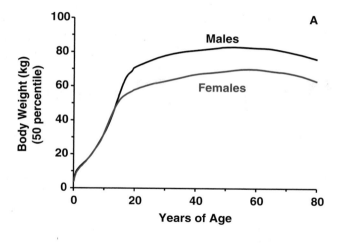

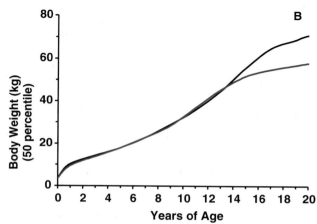

FIGURE 14-6. A. Variation in average weight with age in males (*black*) and females (*colored*), from the neonate to the elder. Weight increases rapidly in the young, particularly during the first year of life, and during puberty. It declines slowly after 50 years of age. **B.** Same data as in A for the age range 0 to 20 years. (From: National Center for Health Statistics in collaboration with the National Center for Chronic Disease Prevention and Health Promotion. Retrieved from http://www.cdc.gov/growthcharts. Accessed September 3, 2009.)

Loading Dose. Clinically, correcting the adult loading dose proportionally with body weight appears reasonable. The volume of distribution based on unbound drug, *Vu*, is frequently both directly proportional to body weight and independent of age, but not always so. Much depends on the physicochemical properties of the drug and on the reason for the difference in weight.

Shown in Table 14-2 are values for degree of plasma protein binding, volume of distribution (*V*), unbound volume of distribution (*Vu*), and percent of drug in the body unbound, for three drugs in neonates and adults. The last two parameters were calculated from fraction of drug from plasma unbound (*fu*) and *V* (see Chapter 4, *Membranes and Distribution*). As commonly found, plasma binding is lower in neonates than adults. Yet, for phenobarbital, *Vu*, corrected for body weight, is the same because most of the drug is unbound in the body. Clearly, for this drug, a weight-normalized initial dose is expected to produce a similar unbound peak drug concentration in both neonates and adults or in any other age group. Digoxin is extensively distributed to the tissues and is only weakly bound to plasma proteins, yet there appears to be little or no change in the unbound volume of distribution, implying no change in tissue binding with age. For phenytoin, there is a decrease in binding to plasma proteins (*fu* doubles) in the neonate, but most of the drug is located in the tissues as well, so that again no change in the weight-normalized dose is needed. For all three drugs then, a given amount in the body per kilogram gives the same unbound concentration in both groups. Consequently, the same weight-corrected loading dose, if required, should suffice.

TABLE 14-2	Plasma Protein Binding and Distribution Data for Some Drugs in Neonates and Adults

Drug	Fraction Unbound in Plasma (*fu*)		Volume of Distribution (*V*, L/kg)		Unbound Volume of Distribution (*Vu*, L/kg)*		Percent of Drug in Body Unbound[†]	
	Neonate	Adult	Neonate	Adult	Neonate	Adult	Neonate	Adult
Phenobarbital	**0.68**	0.53	**1.0**	0.55	**1.5**	1.0	**67**	60
Digoxin	**0.80**	0.70	**5–10**	7.0	**6–12**	10	**6–12**	6
Phenytoin	**0.20**	0.10	**1.3**	0.63	**6.5**	6.3	**12**	10

*Calculated from *V/fu*.
[†]Calculated from $100 \times V_{TBW}/Vu$, where V_{TBW} is the total body water (0.6 L/kg in adults and 0.8 L/kg in neonates), assuming unbound drug distributes through body water and is in equal concentration in all body water spaces.
From: Morselli PL. Clinical pharmacokinetics in neonates. Clin Pharmacokinet 1976;1:81–98.

A loading dose correction should also be considered for emaciated and obese adult patients. The difference in loading dose may not be as great as anticipated from body weight alone. However, as with age-related changes in distribution, much depends on the physicochemical properties of the drug. Digoxin and polar drugs, for example, do not partition well into fat. Accordingly, for these drugs, *Vu* correlates better with **lean body mass** (body weight minus fat content), which is similar in obese and average persons of the same height and frame, than with total body weight.

Maintenance Dosing Rate. Because renal and hepatic functions (and body weight) change dramatically with age, especially in early childhood, some adjustment in dosing rate is clearly needed. The primary question is how much the usual adult dosage regimen should be adjusted. To maintain the same systemic exposure, the rate of administration must be adjusted to match the change anticipated in elimination, the subject of the next section.

CHANGE IN PHYSIOLOGIC FUNCTIONS AND DRUG DISPOSITION WITH AGE

CREATININE CLEARANCE AND RENAL FUNCTION

Figure 14-7 shows changes with age in half-life and clearance of creatinine expressed per kilogram of body weight. Creatinine distributes into total body water spaces, is negligibly bound to tissue or plasma constituents, is eliminated almost entirely by renal excretion, and has a clearance essentially equal to the glomerular filtration rate (*GFR*). The example of creatinine is chosen because changes in total body water and glomerular filtration rate with age are well understood. To the extent that creatinine clearance mimics that of other drugs, the data displayed in Fig. 14-7 further our understanding of age-related changes in pharmacokinetics and suggest a means of individualizing dosage regimens for age. Let us consider the various parts of Fig. 14-7 in some detail.

Neonates and Infants. Clearance, if normalized for body weight, is depressed in the neonate, but increases rapidly to reach a maximum value at 6 months, when it is more than twice that in the typical 60-year-old adult patient. The change is particularly rapid in the first week after birth, as shown in Fig. 14-8 and is often referred to as postnatal maturation of renal function. Thus, creatinine clearance in this age range can be thought of as the product of an adjustment based on body size and a maturation component. After

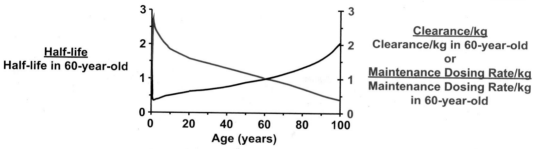

FIGURE 14-7. How half-life (left scale, *black line*) and both clearance and maintenance dosing rate (right scale, *colored line*) of a drug might vary with age. The values were calculated from data on creatinine. The drug, like creatinine, distributes into total body water, is not bound in plasma or tissues, and is eliminated entirely by renal excretion with a clearance equal to the glomerular filtration rate. Half-life is expressed as a fraction of the average value for a typical 60-year-old adult patient; the dosage regimen is calculated assuming that the desired average plateau unbound concentration remains constant throughout life. Notice that because of poor renal function, elimination is slow in the neonate, but improves rapidly such that, by 1 year, half-life is about one half the adult value. During childhood and adolescence, the half-life becomes longer because clearance, a function of surface area, increases more slowly with growth than does volume of distribution, a function of body weight. Although body weight, and therefore, volume of distribution change only slightly beyond 30 years, half-life is longer in the elderly, because renal function, and therefore, clearance progressively diminish. By 90 years, half-life is 1.6 times the typical adult value. These changes in clearance and weight with age explain why the maintenance dose per kilogram of body weight is higher in the child and lower in both the neonate and the aged than in the typical adult patient.

The data used in the calculations were obtained as follows: half-life—calculated from volume of distribution and clearance. Half-life in an average adult (60 years) is 5.9 hr. Volume of distribution: taken as 78% of body weight at birth, 67% of body weight at 6 months, and 60% of body weight thereafter (Friis-Hansen B. Changes in body water compartments during growth. Acta Paediatr 1956;110:1–68). Clearance: at birth, taken as inulin clearance, 3 mL/min (Weill WB. The evaluation of renal function in infancy and childhood. Am J Med Sci 1955;229:678–694); between 6 months and 20 years, calculated by multiplying creatinine clearance, 120 mL/min/per 1.8 m^2 in an average, healthy, young adult of 21 to 29 years, by body surface area; between 30 and 99 years, taken from the data of Siersbaek-Nielsen (From: Siersbaek-Nielsen K, Hansen JM, Kampmann J, Kristensen M. Rapid evaluation of creatinine clearance. Lancet 1971;1:1133–1134). Surface area—calculated from body weight (kg) using the relationship: surface area (m^2) = 1.73 · (Weight/70)$^{0.75}$.

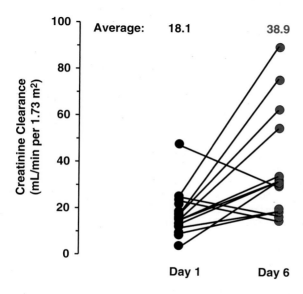

FIGURE 14-8. Creatinine clearances of neonates on Day 1 and Day 6 after birth. Although three of the neonates showed a decrease in creatinine clearance, the average was essentially doubled in this short postnatal period. (From: Sertel H, Scopes J. Rates of creatinine clearance in babies less than 1 week of age. Arch Dis Child 1973;48:717–720.)

about 6 months of age, weight-normalized clearance begins to fall but still remains, throughout childhood, considerably above the adult value.

Because total body water as a percent of body weight, and hence distribution, changes relatively little during life (78% in neonates to 60% in adults), the change in creatinine half-life inversely reflects the change in clearance. That is, the half-life is shortest around 1 year of age; it is longer in both newborn and elderly patients. Similar age-related trends in renal clearance of drugs are observed.

In the *premature* newborn, creatinine clearance is even more depressed per kilogram of body weight than in full-term neonates. Creatinine clearance appears to increase exponentially by a factor of 8 between weeks 28 and 40, as shown in Fig. 14-9. The data indicate that creatinine clearance during the first few weeks after birth is predicted by conceptional age (time since conception). Dosing requirements for a drug that is primarily excreted unchanged during this period may be approximated from knowledge of the conceptional age; however, the requirements, as reflected by creatinine clearance, are rapidly changing and must be continually updated.

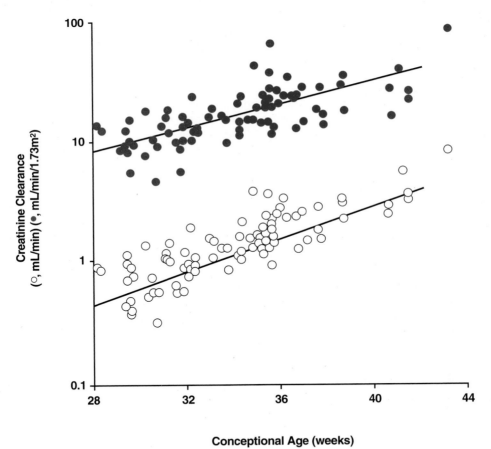

FIGURE 14-9. Creatinine clearance, corrected (*colored circles*) and uncorrected (*open circles*) for body surface area, plotted versus conceptional age. The normal full term is 40 weeks. The lines represent the best fit of an exponential equation to the data. For the upper and lower curves, the equations are CL_{cr} (mL/min/1.73 m^2) = 0.373 $e^{0.111 \cdot Age}$ and CL_{cr} (mL/min) = 0.00462 $e^{0.161 \cdot Age}$, respectively, with age expressed in weeks. Even after correcting for surface area, clearance is greatly depressed in neonates, especially those of earlier conceptional age. Recall that creatinine clearance from 6 months to 20 years is about 120 mL/min/1.73 m^2. (From: Al–Dahhan J, Haycock GB, Chantler C, Stimmler L. Sodium homeostasis in term and preterm neonates. Arch Dis Child 1983;58:335–342.)

Children. As previously stated, creatinine clearance per kilogram of body weight tends to be greater in children than in adults. It has been found that creatinine clearance correlates better with **body surface area** (*BSA*) than with weight in this age group. For this reason, creatinine clearance in children is often expressed relative to body surface area. Traditionally, 1.73 m² has been the nominal surface area of a typical young adult, and therefore, creatinine clearance is given in units of milliliter per minute per 1.73 m² (mL/min/1.73 m²). A major advantage of doing so is that the nominal values of 120 mL/min/1.73 m² for men and 108 mL/min/1.73 m² for women are the same from about 1 to 20 years of age. Reduced renal function can then be readily deduced after normalization of an observed value to body surface area.

Body surface area can be estimated from the weight and height of a child using one of several relationships, including the following:

$$BSA \ (m^2) \ = \ 0.0243 \times Weight \ (kg)^{0.538} \times Height \ (cm)^{0.396} \qquad \text{14-1}$$

Another approximation takes body weight only into account, provided that body weight is close to that expected for body height,

$$BSA \ (m^2) \ = \ 1.73 \left(\frac{Weight \ (kg)}{70} \right)^{0.75} \qquad \text{14-2}$$

Adults and the Elderly. An often forgotten point is that throughout adulthood many functions decrease with age (Fig. 14-10). This is certainly so for creatinine clearance (glomerular filtration rate), which, by rule of thumb, diminishes in adults at a rate of about 1% per year.

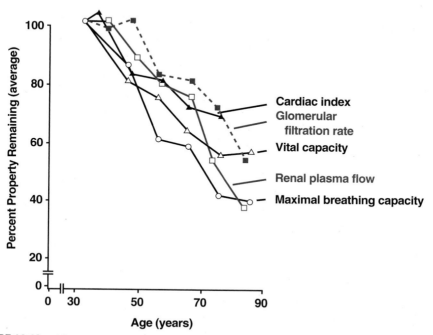

FIGURE 14-10. Many physiologic functions diminish by approximately 1% per year with increasing age during adulthood. (From: Shock NW. Age changes in physiological functions in the total animal: the role of tissue loss. In: Strehler BL, ed. The Biology of Aging. Washington, DC: American Institute of Biological Sciences, 1960;250–264.)

Taking into account the differences observed in male and female adults, the change in creatinine clearance beyond 20 years of age for individuals of near-normal weight for height can be approximated by:

$$\textbf{Men: } \textit{Creatinine Clearance (mL/min)} = (140 - Age) \cdot \left(\frac{Weight}{70}\right)^{0.75} \qquad \text{14-3}$$

$$\textbf{Women: } \textit{Creatinine Clearance (mL/min)} = 0.85 \cdot (140 - Age) \cdot \left(\frac{Weight}{70}\right)^{0.75} \qquad \text{14-4}$$

where age is expressed in years and weight in kilograms. Thus, in an average 90-year-old, 70-kg adult, clearances (50 mL/min for men and 43 mL/min for women) are 0.63 times those of a typical 60-year-old patient (80 mL/min for men and 68 mL/min for women), whereas the values in a 20-year-old, 70-kg adult (120 mL/min for men and 102 mL/min for women) are 1.5 times these values. More global relationships that incorporate serum creatinine, a reflector of both creatinine production and renal excretion, as well as age, weight, and gender, are given in Chapter 15, *Disease*. In general, gender differences are not taken into account, and a value of 70 mL/min may be used as the creatinine clearance of a typical 60-year-old patient. How the value of 70 mL/min is obtained is explained in Chapter 15.

An additional comment is pertinent here with regard to the elderly patient. The elderly tend to show greater variability (coefficient of variation) in renal function than young or middle-aged adults. This increase in variability is a result of several factors,

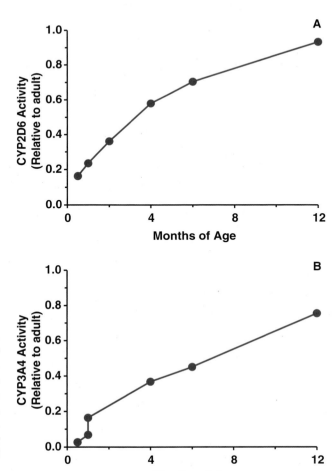

FIGURE 14-11. Mean changes in CYP2D6 (**A**) and CYP3A4 (**B**) activity (relative to adult values during the first year after birth, with both in vitro enzyme activity and liver weight taken into account). (From: Johnson TN, Tucker GT, Rostami-Hodjegan A. Development of CYP2D6 and CYP3A4 in the first year of life. Clin Pharmacol Ther 2008;83: 670–671.)

including the concurrent presence of multiple diseases and a host of changes related to the aging process. This is particularly true for the frail elderly patient.

METABOLISM

Neonates and Infants. As with renal function, the ability of neonates to metabolize drugs matures within the first 6 to 12 months of life. Shown in Fig. 14-11 are, for example, the activities of CYP2D6 and CYP3A4, expressed per gram of liver and relative to adult values, of children from birth to 12 months of age. Liver size also increases rapidly in this age group. The rapid change in metabolism during this age range makes it difficult to predict the appropriate dosage for the individual patient, especially for neonates.

The metabolic activity of CYP3A4 within the gut wall has also been shown to mature rapidly during the first few months after birth (Fig. 14-12). Those drugs showing extensive first-pass metabolism in the gut wall and liver in adults, therefore, show a much smaller first-pass loss in the neonate.

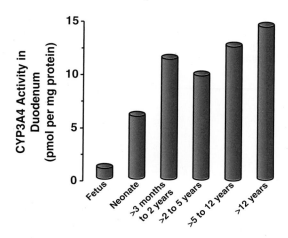

FIGURE 14-12. Changes in the activity of CYP3A4 per milligram of protein in the duodenum of pediatric patients as a function of their age. (From: Johnson, TN, Tanner MS, Taylor CJ, Tucker GT. Enterocytic CYP3A4 in a paediatric population: developmental changes and the effect of celiac disease and cystic fibrosis. Br J Clin Pharmacol 2001;51:451–460.)

Children. From about 6 months to 20 years of age, metabolism follows the same general trend as does the renal function. Clearance relative to body surface area remains relatively constant. Clearance per kilogram of body weight is considerably higher in children, especially at the lower end of this age group.

Adults and the Elderly. Metabolic clearance, in general, decreases with age in adults. Taking substrates of CYP3A as an example, Fig. 14-13 shows the results of 19 studies (on 10 drugs) in which data were separated by sex and in 24 studies (on 15 drugs) in which it was not. It is clear from these studies that, on average, the clearance in the elderly is decreased to about 60% to 70% of that in the young adult group for substrates of CYP3A. The average age of the elderly groups was typically 65 to 75 years of age, whereas that of the young was about 25 to 35. The rule of 1% loss per year for creatinine clearance is pertinent here, on average, as the difference in the ages of the two groups was about 30 to 40 years.

Entire Lifespan. To examine the trends for metabolism with age, consider the data on diazepam, a drug metabolized primarily by CYP2C19 and that reflects drug metabolism in general. As seen in Fig. 14-14, diazepam's half-life is longest in the premature neonate and in adults older than 55 years of age. Infants, 1 to 10 months of age, eliminate the drug most rapidly. With creatinine, the long half-life in the neonate is caused by depressed renal function, which takes several months to mature. With diazepam, the long half-life in the neonate reflects a lack of maturation in drug-metabolizing activity.

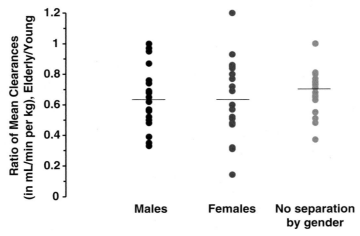

FIGURE 14-13. Changes in CYP3A metabolism with age. Whether separated by gender (19 studies of 10 different drugs) or not (24 studies of 15 different drugs), it is apparent that the clearances (mean [—] and individual values [•]) of these drugs, primarily eliminated by CYP3A metabolism, in the elderly groups is only approximately 60% that of young adults. (From: Cotreau MM, von Moltke LL, Greenblatt DJ. The influence of age and sex on the clearance of cytochrome P4503A substrates. Clin Pharmacokinet 2005;44:33–60.)

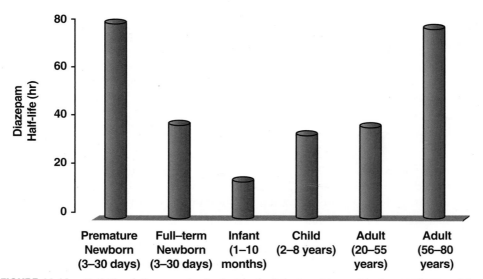

FIGURE 14-14. Half-life of diazepam is shortest in the infant and longest in the newborn and the aged. (From: Morselli PL. Drug Disposition During Development. New York: Spectrum Publications, 1977;311–360,456; Klotz U, Avant GR, Hoyumpa A, et al. The effect of age and liver disease on the disposition and elimination of diazepam in adult man. J Clin Invest 1975;55:347–359.)

Figure 14-15 shows how the CYP2C19 activity per gram of liver develops over the first few months after birth. That the premature neonate has the longest half-life of diazepam is not surprising and stresses a point made earlier: chronologic and functional age must be distinguished, especially in neonates.

The shorter half-life of diazepam in the infant than in the 20- to 55-year-old adult reflects differences in clearance per kilogram, because volume of distribution of this drug is approximately the same (1.2 L/kg) in both groups. The further prolongation in half-life in the most elderly group, clearly shown to be age related (Fig. 14-16), requires some

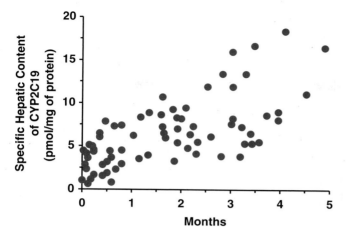

FIGURE 14-15. Developmental expression pattern of CYP2C19 activity during neonatal period and early infancy. Enzymatic activity is expressed per milligram of protein. (From: Koukouritski SB, Manro JR, Marsh SA, et al. Developmental expression of human hepatic CYP2C9 and CYP2C19. J Pharmacol Exp Therap 2003;308:965–974.)

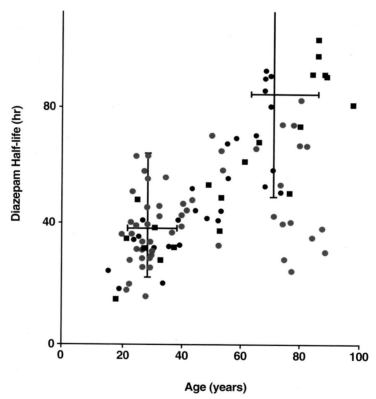

FIGURE 14-16. The half-life of diazepam increases with age, from 20 to 80 years. (From: [●]: Klotz U, Avant GR, Hoyumpa A, et al. The effects of age and liver disease on the disposition and elimination of diazepam in adult man. J Clin Invest 1975;55:347–359; [*bars*, mean and range]: Greenblatt DJ, Allen MD, Harmatz JS, Shader RI. Diazepam disposition determinants. Clin Pharmacol Ther 1979;23:301–312; [●]: Macleod SM, Giles HG, Bengert B, et al. Age- and gender-related differences in diazepam pharmacokinetics. J Clin Pharmacol 1979;19:15–19; [■]: Macklow AF, Barton M, James O, Rawlins MD. The effect of age on the pharmacokinetics of diazepam. Clin Sci 1980;59:479–483.)

discussion. Clearance remains essentially constant, and volume of distribution is increased with age from 20 to 80 years, but only because of the tendency for lower plasma binding of drug with advancing age. Diazepam is a drug of low hepatic extraction and moderately large volume of distribution, and both its clearance and volume of distribution are dependent on protein binding. The unbound volume of distribution changes relatively little with age. However, the all-important unbound clearance is reduced (Fig. 14-17), probably reflecting diminished capacity for hepatic metabolism.

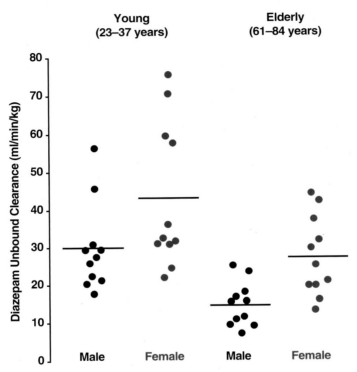

FIGURE 14-17. The unbound clearance of diazepam tends to be reduced in elderly patients compared with young adults. Differences also exist between males and females. The reduced unbound clearance ([–] mean values; [•, •] individual values) is the primary reason for a prolonged half-life of diazepam in the elderly patient. (From: Greenblatt DJ, Allen MD, Harmatz JS, et al. Diazepam disposition determinants. Clin Pharmacol Ther 1980;27:301–312. Reproduced with permission of Nature.)

For some metabolized drugs, no change in clearance or half-life has been observed in the elderly. These drugs have generally been shown to have decreased binding to plasma proteins in the elderly. Thus, although total clearance shows little change, unbound clearance is decreased. In the absence of information on a specific drug, the best current prediction is that metabolism (unbound clearance) is decreased in the elderly. To be on the conservative side and as a rough approximation, the unbound metabolic clearance should be considered to decline with age like that for creatinine clearance, 1% per annum, regardless of the metabolic pathway. As with other factors, specific information on the change with age for a given drug is preferred.

Studies have shown that the daily dosage requirements of warfarin decrease with age regardless of one's genetic makeup (Fig. 14-18) . The individuals in this study are classified by their genetic variant of CYP2C9, the enzyme primarily responsible for metabolism of the active S-warfarin. Clearly, for all genetic groups and for both men and women, the dosage requirements to achieve the same anticlotting activity decrease with

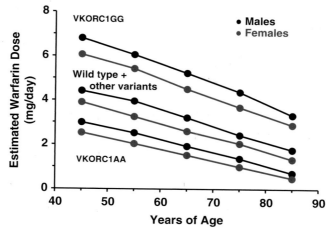

FIGURE 14-18. Estimated daily maintenance doses (milligram per day) of warfarin for males and females using a web-based online estimator that incorporates age, sex, weight, height, and CYP2C9 and VKORC1 genotype data for estimations. Estimates were based on a target INR of 2.2 using mean weight and height data for the U.S. population. Note how the daily dose of warfarin decreases with age for all genotypes and is lower in females than in males. (From: Schwarts JB. The current state of knowledge on age, sex, and their interactions on clinical pharmacology. Clin Pharmacol Ther 2007;82:87–96.)

age, presumably primarily due to a gradual decline in metabolism toward the end of the human lifespan.

GENDER DIFFERENCES

PHARMACOKINETICS

Gender-specific differences in creatinine clearance and renal function occur, as noted in Eqs. 14-3 and 14-4 above. Creatinine clearance, and presumably renal clearance of drugs, in women tends to be about 85% of that in men for individuals of the same age and body weight. It has been suggested that much of this difference can be accounted for by the greater proportion of fat in women. With the usual 25% to 30% variability in drug disposition, this small difference has minimal clinical relevance. Therefore, the recommended usual adult dosage of renally excreted drugs is essentially the same for both men and women.

But what about metabolism? Figure 14-19 shows the results of 23 studies performed on 11 different drugs for which CYP3A is the major metabolic enzyme. The clearances of

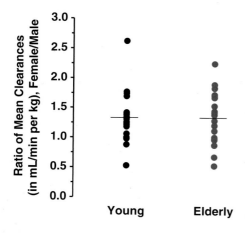

FIGURE 14-19. Effect of gender on CYP3A metabolism. When separated by gender (19 studies of 10 different drugs), it is apparent that, on average, the clearances per kilogram of these drugs, primarily eliminated by CYP3A metabolism, are approximately 30% greater in women than in men, in both young adults and the elderly. However, taking weight into account (see Table 14-3), there is very little difference in clearance between the sexes ([–] mean ratio across studies; [•, •] mean ratio for individual studies). (From: Cotreau MM, von Moltke LL, Greenblatt DJ. The influence of age and sex on the clearance of cytochrome P4503A substrates. Clin Pharmacokinet 2005;44:33–60.)

TABLE 14-3	Median Weights (Kilogram) of Caucasian Men and Women in the United States of America					
Age Group	20–29	30–39	40–49	50–59	60–69	70–80
Men	76.0	80.0	82.6	83.0	82.0	78
Women	60.0	65.0	67.7	70.0	68.9	66
Ratio	1.27	1.24	1.22	1.17	1.21	1.18

*Values at 50% percentile.
From: NHANES III Survey, conducted in the United States from 1988 to 1994. Retrieved from http//www.halls.md/chart/height-weight.htm. Accessed September 3, 2009.

the drugs in milliliter per minute per kilogram in women are compared (ratio of values) with those of men. Note that the ratio of clearances in both young and elderly is higher (1.31 and 1.31, women/men) per kilogram of body weight. However, when differences in body weight (about 1.27 in the 20- to 29-year-old and 1.21 in the 60- to 69-year-old groups) are taken into account (Table 14-3), there is very little difference in the actual clearance values between the sexes in both age groups. On average then, one would not expect to adjust the dosage of drugs metabolized by CYP3A based on gender per se. There are individual drugs, such as nimodipine, however, for which the metabolism is much faster in women and for which an adjustment in dosage may be prudent. Some of the variability observed in general for the CYP3A substrates in Fig. 14-19 may be because of differences in its isoforms, as not all CYP3A enzymes are alike with respect to substrate specificity.

A gender-specific change in the binding of drugs to albumin occurs in pregnant women. By the time of parturition, the serum albumin drops to about 50% to 60% of the value before pregnancy. This results in less binding for those drugs that bind to this protein. Lower total exposures are therefore seen during pregnancy, but the unbound drug concentration does not generally seem to be affected. There is, therefore, no need to adjust dosage because of the reduction in plasma albumin.

PHARMACODYNAMICS

For a few drugs, such as female and male contraceptives, and agents used to treat benign prostatic hyperplasia, breast cancer, and prostate cancer, there are decided gender-specific differences in their pharmacodynamics. Gender differences also exist in the sensitivity to adverse effects of some drugs. On the whole, however, there are few drugs that show large quantitative or qualitative gender-specific differences in their pharmacodynamics. Gender is, therefore, generally not a major consideration in drug therapy.

ADJUSTMENT OF DOSAGE FOR AGE

Figure 14-20 summarizes the dosage changes with age beyond 1 year required to maintain the same average unbound plateau concentration for a drug that is primarily eliminated by renal excretion. The maintenance dosing rate increases almost linearly between 1 and 12 years of age. These predictions are based on changes in body surface area with age, which are estimated from average weights, and the general correlation observed between clearance and body surface area in children. Because clearance increases up to 20 years of age and then declines thereafter, there are pairs of age values for which the same rate of administration is required. For example, on average, a 4-year-old child (16 kg) requires the same rate of drug administration as a 90-year-old person (60 kg). Similarly, a 12-year-old child (39 kg) requires the same daily dose as the reference 70-kg patient, namely, the usual maintenance dose.

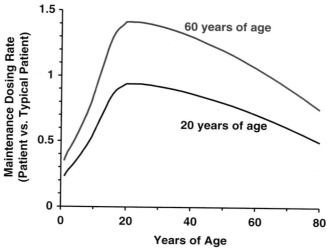

FIGURE 14-20. Variation in the maintenance dosing rate expressed as a fraction of the maintenance dosing rate of a typical adult as a function of age, from 1 to 90 years. The colored line represents the values when the typical patient is 60 years of age; the black line represents the values when the typical patient is 20 years of age. Note the increase in maintenance dosing rate with age from 1 to 20 years, associated primarily with an increase in body size, and the decline between 30 and 80 years, associated primarily with diminished organ function with advancing years. Also note that the dosing rate in the 20-year-old is only about fourfold greater than that for the 1-year-old, even though their weights differ 6.5-fold (65 kg vs. 10 kg). Values for children (1–20 years of age) are calculated using the average of the weights given for males and females in Fig. 14-6 and Eq. 14-6 (when the typical patient is 60 years old) and letting the factor 1.5 in the equations be 1.0 when the typical patient is 20 years old. Values for adults (20–80 years of age) are calculated from Eqs. 14-10 and 14-11 using age and the average of the weights given for male and female adults in Fig. 14-6. Again, typical patients of 60 and 20 years of age are considered.

The rules for those drugs that are primarily renally excreted unchanged also appear to apply, in general, to drugs that are primarily eliminated by metabolism. There is much less certainty in applying the general rules here, however. Drug-specific information on age-related changes in metabolism should be sought whenever possible, which in turn demands knowledge of the quantitative contribution of the enzymes and transporters involved in the elimination of the drug. Let us now examine dosage adjustments, whether excretion or metabolism is involved, in various age groups in further detail.

Neonates and Infants. The lack of maturation of renal and hepatic function necessitates that the rate of administration of drugs to both neonates and young infants be reduced, even on a body-weight basis, if toxicity is to be avoided. Unfortunately, changes occur so rapidly in these early stages of life that it is impossible to predict clearance with confidence and, hence, the dosage regimen required in an individual. Caution must clearly be exercised in administering drugs to this patient population. Besides carefully noting response, monitoring of the plasma concentration of drugs with a narrow therapeutic index may be helpful. Information in this area is increasingly becoming available for newly developed drugs, as regulatory agencies are requiring studies in this age group.

In passing, noteworthy is the incidental exposure of fetus and suckling infant to drugs. For those drugs that can pass the placenta, the unbound plateau concentration in the fetus is likely to equal that in the pregnant mother receiving chronic therapy. With eliminating capacity generally poorly developed, the fetus acts for the most part as an additional "tissue" of distribution, with half-life in the fetus being virtually the same as that in the mother. A drastic change occurs, however, on delivery. Deprived of access to the fully developed eliminating organs of the mother, elimination of drug from the newborn child, especially the premature, can be very slow.

The suckling infant is exposed to those drugs taken by its mother. As suckling occurs regularly, of concern are events over an extended period of time. The risks are greatest for drugs that are poorly cleared by the infant, and that have a narrow therapeutic index.

The primary factors determining the concentration in maternal milk, relative to that in plasma, are the lipophilicity, degree of ionization, and plasma protein binding. Lipophilicity is important for two reasons: ease of passing across membranes and partitioning into the fat in milk. Ionization may play a role because the pH of milk (about 7.2) is lower than that in plasma (7.4). Furthermore, the concentration in milk is often delayed relative to that in plasma, particularly for short half-life drugs, because the measured concentration in milk is a function of the time required to obtain a milk sample and the past history of the plasma concentration. Such a delay is shown for the antidepressant bupropion in Fig. 14-21. A more meaningful ratio of milk-to-plasma concentrations may be obtained from the ratio of the areas under the respective concentration–time curves.

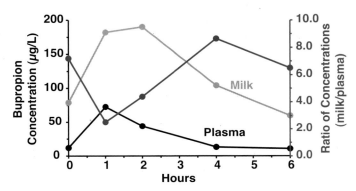

FIGURE 14-21. Plasma (*black*) and breast milk (*gray*) concentrations of bupropion after 100-mg oral doses every 6 hr. Also shown is the milk-to-plasma concentration ratio with time (*colored*). The ratio varies with time for at least two reasons: the time required to obtain a milk sample may be considerably longer than that to obtain a plasma sample; and distribution of the drug from plasma to milk may be delayed. (From: Begg EJ, Duffull SB, Hackett LP, et al. Studying drugs in human milk: time to unify the approach. J Hum Lact 2002;18:323–332.)

Children. The evidence in Figs. 14-7 and 14-22 suggests that a maintenance regimen, calculated by correcting the adult dosage for body weight, would prove inadequate for children, especially for the very young. Dosage requirements, cardiac output, hepatic and renal blood flow, and glomerular filtration rate in children and in young adults of widely differing sizes have been found to correlate better with body surface area than body weight. Because clearance relates dosing rate to plateau plasma concentration and because, for most drugs, renal clearance is proportional to glomerular filtration rate (see Chapter 15, *Disease*), the choice of surface area over weight as the method of calculating maintenance therapy has some justification. Taking a 60-year-old man (or woman) as the typical patient receiving the drug, the clearance expected for a 70-kg, 20-year-old man (or woman) is 1.5 times that for the reference patient (Eqs. 14-3 and 14-4). According to this concept, a child's maintenance dosage is calculated from the formula:

$$\begin{matrix} \text{Child's} \\ \text{maintenance dose} \end{matrix} = 1.5 \times \left[\frac{\begin{matrix} \text{Surface area} \\ \text{of child } (m^2) \end{matrix}}{1.73 \ m^2} \right] \cdot \begin{matrix} \text{Typical adult} \\ \text{maintenance dosage} \end{matrix} \qquad \text{14-5}$$

where 1.73 m^2 is the surface area of an average 70-kg adult. The surface area of a child can be determined from its body weight using the observation that surface area is proportional to body weight to the 0.75 power (weight$^{0.75}$). Using this observation, Eq. 14-5 may be rewritten as

$$\begin{array}{c} \text{Child's} \\ \text{maintenance dose} \end{array} = 1.5 \times \left[\dfrac{\begin{array}{c}\text{Weight of}\\\text{child (kg)}\end{array}}{70} \right]^{0.75} \cdot \begin{array}{c}\text{Typical adult}\\\text{maintenance dosage}\end{array} \qquad 14\text{-}6$$

Tha ratio of (*weight*/70)$^{0.75}$ (Eq. 14-2) is an estimate of the ratio of body surface areas. The factor of 1.5 accounts for a 20-year-old having a creatine clearance about 50% greater than that of a typical 60-year-old patient. To illustrate the use of the relationship expressed in Eq. 14-6, consider the example of the use of digoxin in a child; the usual adult maintenance dose is 0.25 mg daily. The typical patient is at least 60 years old. Using this age as the reference point, let us examine what we might expect to be the maintenance dosage requirements in a 15-kg, 3.5-year-old male child with a congenital heart problem, but with normal renal function for his age. The daily dose can be estimated using Eq. 14-6, from the factor by which the elimination of the drug by a young adult is greater than that of the typical patient and the ratio of surface areas (estimated from body weight).

$$\text{Child's dosage of digoxin} = 1.5 \times \left(\dfrac{15}{70}\right)^{0.75} \times 0.25 \text{ mg} = 0.12 \text{ mg}$$

Notice that the weight-normalized daily dose of digoxin in the child, 0.008 mg/kg (0.12 mg/15 kg), is much higher than that in the typical 60-year-old adult, 0.0036 (0.25 mg/70 kg).

In general, the need for a higher maintenance dose per kilogram body weight, the smaller and, hence, usually the younger the child, is seen in Fig. 14-22 for children between 6 months and 12 years. Note the complementary decrease in the half-life with decreasing size and age. Thus, not only may a 1-year-old child require a larger maintenance dosing rate per kilogram body weight than an adult, but because of a shorter half-life, the drug may also need to be given more frequently. This is especially so if the drug has a low therapeutic index and large fluctuations around the average plateau concentration are to be avoided.

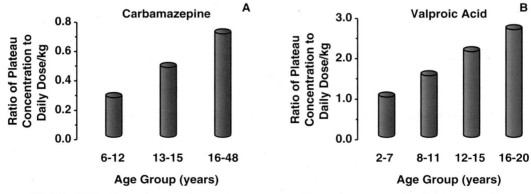

FIGURE 14-22. The plateau plasma drug concentrations of two antiepileptic drugs, carbamazepine **(A)** and valproic acid **(B)**, are measured after chronic oral medication in children. An increase in clearance per kilogram of body weight explains the lower ratio of concentration to daily dose per kilogram in the youngest children. (From: Morselli PL. Antiepileptic drugs. In: Morselli PL, ed. Drug Disposition During Development. New York: Spectrum Publications, 1977;11:311–360.)

Next, consider the intramuscular administration of tobramycin, an antibiotic, to a 15-kg, 3.5-year-old male child with an infection for which a typical patient is 20 to 30 years of age. The recommendation would then require adjustment of the usual regimen of 3 mg/kg (210 mg/70 kg) per day in divided doses based only on surface area.

$$\begin{matrix} Child's \\ maintenance\ dose \end{matrix} = \left[\cfrac{\begin{matrix} Weight\ of \\ child\ (kg) \end{matrix}}{70} \right]^{0.75} \cdot \begin{matrix} Typical\ adult \\ maintenance\ dosage \end{matrix} \qquad 14\text{-}7$$

Therefore,

$$Child's\ dosage\ of\ tobramycin = \left(\frac{15}{70}\right)^{0.75} \times 70\ kg \times 3\ mg/kg = 66\ mg$$

Note in this case that the child's daily dose per kilogram (66 mg/15 kg = 4.4 mg/kg) is not that much larger than that in the typical patient (3 mg/kg), compared to that seen previously for digoxin. A better approach yet to individualize dosage requires taking renal function into account, the subject of Chapter 15, *Disease*.

Adults. For most adult patients, there is generally no need to adjust dosage for age, as most of the patients are expected to be near that of the typical patient. A need may exist when the difference between the individual and the typical patient exceeds 20 years, for example, in young adults less than 40 years of age and in those individuals beyond 80 years of age, when the typical patient is 60 years old. An approximation of dosage requirements in adults outside the usual age range and who do not differ greatly in weight from 70 kg is:

$$\begin{matrix} Individual's \\ maintenance\ dose \end{matrix} = \frac{(140 - Age)}{(140 - Age\ of\ typical\ patient)} \cdot \begin{matrix} Typical\ adult \\ maintenance\ dosage \end{matrix} \qquad 14\text{-}8$$

Generally, dosage is not changed based on gender. The "usual" adult dose is derived from clinical studies in a mixed population. Consideration of adjusting for gender becomes more important at the extremes (i.e., for elderly women and young men). As shown in Table 14-4, creatinine clearances of 60-year-old male and female patients are expected to be fairly close, but a 90-year-old woman and a 20-year-old man differ by threefold in their creatinine clearances. A 20-year-old woman, however, differs only twofold from that of a 90-year-old man. Weight is also a factor here, as the average 20-year-old man may be close to 70 kg in weight, whereas the average 90-year-old woman is probably frail and only weighs 60 kg or less (see Table 14-3). The difference may then be even greater than that noted in Table 14-4. Thus, added attention might be given to reducing maintenance dosage in elderly women and increasing dosage in young men for drugs for which the typical patient is 60 years old.

Dosage adjustment in obese, highly muscular, and emaciated patients should be considered when maintenance of the same average systemic exposure (unbound plasma

TABLE 14-4	Expected Creatinine Clearances for 70-kg Adult Men and Women at Three Selected Ages*	
	Creatinine Clearance (mL/min)	
Age	**Men**	**Women**
20	120	102
60	80	68
90	50	43

*Calculation based on Eqs. 14-3 and 14-4.

concentration) is desired. Usually, drug elimination (e.g., renal clearance) is not increased because of either added adipose or muscle tissue. People with larger body frames (height and build) probably have higher clearances, and the converse. A quick method of assessing whether an adult has an appropriate weight for height, except for those who are highly muscular, is obtained from the **body mass index** (*BMI*). It is calculated from the ratio of an individual's weight (in kilogram) to the square of the individual's height (in meters).

$$BMI = \frac{Body\ weight\ (in\ kg)}{(Height\ (in\ meters))^2} \qquad 14\text{-}9$$

Thus, for an 85-kg man with a height of 192 cm, the *BMI* is 23 kg/m², a value in the range (20–25) for a healthy weight for height. *BMI* values below 20 kg/m² indicate that the person is underweight. Values between 25 and 30 kg/m² indicate that the individual may be overweight, whereas values above 30 kg/m² indicate obesity. Much also depends on body composition. For example, an individual with a *BMI* of 32 kg/m² would be considered to be obese, but not a muscle builder who may actually have a very low fat content.

In overweight and obese patients, creatinine clearance can be estimated, to a first approximation, from **lean body weight**. Lean body weight (body weight minus fat content) in kilograms can be estimated from the following relationships, incorporating body weight and height.

$$Lean\ body\ weight\ (male) = 1.10 \times Weight\ (kg) - \frac{128 \times (Weight\ (kg))^2}{(100 \times Height\ (m))^2} \qquad 14\text{-}10$$

$$Lean\ body\ weight\ (female) = 1.07 \times Weight\ (kg) - \frac{148 \times (Weight\ (kg))^2}{(100 \times Height\ (m))^2} \qquad 14\text{-}11$$

The expected clearance of creatinine can then be calculated from Eqs. 14-3 and 14-4 for adults. Again, these relationships do not apply to highly muscular individuals.

The Elderly. The elderly constitute an increasingly greater proportion of the total population. They also consume more prescription drugs per capita than do people at any other age (see Fig. 14-4). As a broad generalization, dosage should be reduced in elderly patients, reflecting the general decline in body functions with age (see Fig. 14-10). A reduction in dosage is needed particularly in weak and frail elderly patients.

Certainly, the marked and progressive decrease in renal function implies that the dosage regimens of drugs that are predominantly excreted unchanged should be reduced in the elderly population. For example, an 80-year-old patient requires, on average, only 70% of the usual adult dosage expressed relative to 70 kg of body weight. The dose required may be even less when the elderly patient is frail. In addition to a lower weight, a depressed clearance without dose adjustment and the use of multiple drugs probably explains a good part of the increased frequency and degree of adverse drug effects often noted in elderly patients.

DOSAGES EXPRESSED PER KILOGRAM BODY WEIGHT OR PER 1.73 m²

In some therapeutic areas, such as cancer, dosages are often expressed in milligram per kilogram (mg/kg) or milligram per 1.73 m² (mg/1.73 m²) for all age groups with the belief that the same dosage can then be used across a range of patients. Such a means of expressing dosage has the advantage of the clinician being able to prescribe a single dose of a medication and then to adjust to body size. In children, expressing the dose per 1.73 m² is helpful because renal function (specifically creatinine clearance) varies with body surface area. Expressing dosage in mg/kg or mg/1.73 m² is reasonable if the limits (age, body composition, renal function) of its application are specified. However, the broader use of such rules is suspect. Does a grossly obese patient really need more of a drug because of his or her extra body fat? Does a bodybuilder need more drug because of his or her muscle mass? In these cases, there is a danger that too high a dose is calculated adopting this procedure. A more reasonable approach is one that takes the pharmacokinetics (i.e., renal function, phenotyping, genotyping, if needed) and pharmacodynamics into account. Phenotyping and genotyping were discussed in the last chapter. In Chapter 15, *Disease*, the use of renal function is examined.

A final note is in order with regard to changes in physiologic parameters with age and their implications for drug administration. Physiologic parameters such as cardiac output, hepatic blood blow, renal blood flow, and glomerular filtration rate decrease with age (see Fig. 14-10). The values most widely quoted (e.g., glomerular filtration rate = 100–120 mL/min) and hepatic blood flow = 1.35 L/min, are typical for young healthy adults, not for the typical patient who may be 60 to 70, or more, years of age. Whenever comparisons are made in typical patients, they should be made carefully. For example, a hepatic blood clearance of 0.7 L/min for a given drug may indicate high hepatic extraction in an 80-year-old patient population in whom the hepatic blood flow may be 0.8 L/min instead of 1.35 L/min. Similarly, a value of 50 mL/min for renal clearance may be equal to the GFR of an elderly patient population. One must be careful, however, in these interpretations, as there is variability in all of these renal and hepatic functions, not only with age and weight, but across a given patient population of the same age and weight.

KEY RELATIONSHIPS

$$\text{Men: } Creatinine\ Clearance\ (mL/min)\ =\ (140 - Age) \cdot \left(\frac{Weight}{70}\right)^{0.75}$$

$$\text{Women: } Creatinine\ Clearance\ (mL/min)\ =\ 0.85\ (140 - Age) \cdot \left(\frac{Weight}{70}\right)^{0.75}$$

$$BSA\ (m^2)\ =\ 0.0243 \times Weight\ (kg)^{0.538} \times Height\ (cm)^{0.396}$$

$$BSA\ (m^2)\ =\ 1.73 \left(\frac{Weight\ (kg)}{70}\right)^{0.75}$$

Typical patient is 60 years of age

$$\frac{Child's}{maintenance\ dose}\ =\ 1.5 \times \left[\frac{Weight\ of\ child\ (kg)}{70}\right]^{0.75} \times \frac{Typical\ adult}{maintenance\ dosage}$$

Typical patient is 20 years of age

$$\frac{Child's}{maintenance\ dose}\ =\ \left[\frac{Weight\ of\ child\ (kg)}{70}\right]^{0.75} \times \frac{Typical\ adult}{maintenance\ dosage}$$

$$\frac{Individual's}{maintenance\ dose}\ =\ \frac{(140 - Age)}{(140 - Age\ of\ typical\ patient)} \cdot \frac{Typical\ adult}{maintenance\ dose}$$

$$BMI = \frac{Body\ weight\ (kg)}{(Height\ (m))^2}$$

$$Lean\ body\ weight\ (male) = 1.10 \times Weight\ (kg) - \frac{128 \times (Weight\ (kg))^2}{(100 \times Height\ (m))^2}$$

$$Lean\ body\ weight\ (female) = 1.07 \times Weight\ (kg) - \frac{148 \times (Weight\ (kg))^2}{(100 \times Height\ (m))^2}$$

STUDY PROBLEMS

(Answers to Study Problems are in Appendix J.)

1. Comment on whether each of the following statements is true or false. Qualify your answer when you think it appropriate.

   a. Oral bioavailability increases with increasing body weight.
   b. Volume of distribution varies in direct proportion to body weight.
   c. In children, clearance per kilogram of body weight decreases with increasing age beyond 1 year of age.
   d. Beyond 20 years of age, renal function decreases by approximately 0.3% per year.
   e. For humans between 1 and 90 years of age, the half-life of a drug tends to be the shortest in young adults.

2. a. Discuss the pharmacokinetic and pharmacodynamic issues involved in dosing a drug to a 1-month-old infant.

   b. From the data in Fig. 14-18:
   (1) Discuss the role of age, genetic makeup, and gender in determining the daily dosage of warfarin needed to maintain an International Normalized Ratio (INR) of 2.2.
   (2) Do the data exclude the possibility that an increased sensitivity to warfarin (change in pharmacodynamics) with age could explain the decreased dosage needed to have the same effect? Briefly discuss. What further information would you like to have to confirm your conclusion?

3. Simons et al. studied the pharmacokinetics of the antihistamine diphenhydramine in children and in both young and elderly adults after intravenous (i.v.) administration. Their findings are listed in Table 14-5.

   a. Are the differences in volume of distribution across the age groups those expected?
   b. Are the differences in clearance across the age groups those expected?

TABLE 14-5	Average Demographic and Pharmacokinetic Data for Diphenhydramine		
	Children	**Young Adults**	**Elderly Adults**
Age (year)	8.9	32	69
Weight (kg)	32	70	71
Clearance (L/hr)	93	98	50
Volume of distribution (L)	690	1223	966

From: Simons KJ, Watson TA, Martin TJ, et al. Diphenhydramine: pharmacokinetics and pharmacodynamics in elderly adults, young adults and children. J Clin Pharmacol 1990;30:665–671.

4. The usual adult dosage regimen of a drug is 20 mg once a day. What daily dose would you recommend for a typical 3-year-old, 15-kg child?

5. An adult dose of gentamicin often recommended to treat a severe infection in a typical 60-year-old, 70-kg patient is 5 mg/kg daily administered intramuscularly. This antibiotic is almost completely renally excreted unchanged (let *fe* = 1). Calculate a maintenance dosage regimen of gentamicin to treat a severe infection caused by *Pseudomonas aeruginosa* with the objective of maintaining the same average plateau plasma concentration in:

    a. A child, 4 years of age, weighing 15 kg, with normal renal function for its age.

    b. An elderly female patient, 87 years of age, weighing 63 kg, with normal renal function for her age.

    c. A premature infant with conceptional age of 36 weeks.

6. Figure 14-23 shows the variation in clearance per square meter (m^2) of body surface area of the cephalosporin antibiotic ceftriaxone in individuals from 1 day to 92 years of age. Renal and biliary excretions are about equally involved in the elimination of this drug in normal adults.

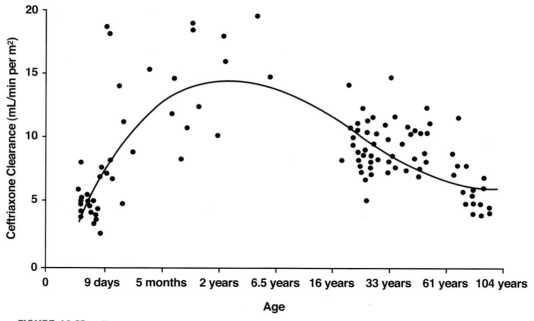

FIGURE 14-23. Clearance of ceftriaxone in subjects from 1 day to 92 years of age. Each symbol represents a value in an individual. Note the scale for age, which is age raised to the power of 0.25 (age$^{0.25}$). (From: Hayton WL, Stoeckel K. Age-associated changes in ceftriaxone pharmacokinetics. Clin Pharmacokinet 1986;11:76–86. Reproduced with permission of ADIS Press Australasia Pty Limited.)

    a. Discuss briefly the changes observed.

    b. Given that no change in volume of distribution (L/kg) with age is observed, state the expected trend of half-life with age.

    c. What are the general implications of the finding for the administration of ceftriaxone?

7. Blychert et al. studied the pharmacokinetics of the calcium antagonist felodipine, used in the management of hypertension, in a group of 140 subjects. All subjects received either 5 or 10 mg orally twice daily for 6 to 30 days. Forty two of them also received the drug intravenously (either 0.04 or 1.5 mg). The subjects were divided

TABLE 14-6	Mean Demographic Data and Felodipine Pharmacokinetic Parameters and Measures

Age Group (Years)	Number	Age (Years)	Weight (kg)	Number Receiving i.v. Dose	CL (L/min)	Half-life (hr)	Oral Dosing AUC_{ss} (0–12 hr)* (mg · hr/L)	F (%)
20–39	70	26	76	17	0.82	18	0.028	14
40–59	30	52	88	12	0.64	24	0.041	14
60–80	40	68	77	13	0.45	29	0.052	16

*AUC data normalized to a 10-mg twice daily oral dose.
From: Blychert E, Edgar B, Elmfeldt D, et al. A population study of the pharmacokinetics of felodipine. Br J Clin Pharmacol 1991;31:15–24.

into three age groups: 20 to 39 years, 40 to 59 years, and 60 to 80 years. Table 14-6 summarizes the demographic data and pharmacokinetic findings. Clear age dependencies in AUC_{ss} (0–12 hr), clearance, and half-life are seen.

In answering the questions below, the clearance values estimated from the i.v. data in the three subgroups apply to all those in each of the respective age groups.

a. With activity residing only in the parent drug, comment on the need to adjust the dose of felodipine for age.
b. Comment on whether the distribution of felodipine varies with age.
c. Estimate the corresponding oral bioavailability for each group.
d. Given that little felodipine is found in urine after i.v. administration and that the drug undergoes extensive hepatic metabolism, comment on the likely reason for the oral bioavailability values.
e. Which parameter, F or CL, most likely explains the increase in AUC_{ss} (0–12 hr) with increasing age?
f. What mechanism might explain your answer to part e?

8. When administering drugs to obese patients, a concern exists whether dose should be weight corrected. Table 14-7 lists information on the volume of distribution of three drugs in control and obese patients; an individual was classified as obese if his or her weight for height was in excess of 150% of lean body weight. Neither theophylline nor digoxin, relatively polar drugs, showed a difference in the volume of distribution between normal and obese individuals; the weight-corrected values were lower in the obese individuals. In contrast, the volume of

TABLE 14-7	Volume of Distribution of Three Drugs in Control and Obese Adult Patients

Drug	Volume of Distribution (L)		Weight Corrected Volume of Distribution (L/kg)		Average Ratio of Weight to Lean Body Weight (%)	
	Obese	Control	Obese	Control	Obese	Control
Theophylline	29	27	0.32	0.47	165	91
Digoxin	981	937	10.7	14.3	162	98
Diazepam	292	91	2.81	1.53	164	95

From: Abernethy DR, Greenblatt D. Drug disposition in obese humans, an update. Clin Pharmacokinet 1986;11:199–213.

distribution of diazepam, a nonpolar drug, was much greater in the obese group, even after correcting for differences in body weight. No significant difference in plasma binding of these three drugs has been found between obese and normal-weight subjects.

    a. What explains the difference in the effect of obesity on the volume of distribution for each of the drugs?

    b. What impact do such findings have on the dosage regimens of these drugs?

9. Montelukast sodium (Singulair) is a leukotriene receptor antagonist, used to treat asthma and seasonal allergic rhinitis. The package insert recommends once-daily administration of the drug as shown in Table 14-8.

TABLE 14-8   **Daily Dose of Montelukast Sodium Recommended for Various Age Groups**

Patient	Typical Weight (kg)	Typical Surface Area (m^2)	Daily Dose*
Adolescent and adult ≥15 years	70 (25 years)	1.73	10-mg tablet
Child			
6–14 years of age	33 (10 years)	1.13	5-mg chewable tablet
2–5 years of age	16 (3.5 years)	0.66	4-mg chewable tablet or 4-mg oral granules
12–33 months of age	12 (18 months)	0.52	4-mg oral granules

*From package insert, 2008.

    a. Compare the package-insert recommendations for the dosage in children with those you would predict based on the adult dose. Make your comparison by completing the following table. Show calculations.

	Recommended Daily Dose (mg)	Predicted Daily Dosage (mg)
Adult (≥15 years of age)	10 mg	10 mg
Child (6–14 years)	5 mg	
Child (2–5 years)	4 mg	
Child (12–24 months)	4 mg	

    b. In the case of many diseases, the typical age of an adult patient is close to 60 years old. Do you think a typical patient on montelukast is 60 years old? Briefly comment.

    c. To obtain the same average systemic exposure to a drug, the daily dose for a 3-year-old child (15 kg, on average) should be about 0.21 times that of a young adult (70 kg, 20 years old). Is this correct?

10. The usual adult oral dose of levofloxacin, a fluoroquinolone antibacterial agent, usually recommended for a typical 60-year-old, 70-kg patient with community-acquired pneumonia is 500 mg once daily. The drug is available in 250-mg, 500-mg, and 750-mg tablets. This antimicrobial agent is almost completely eliminated by renal excretion. Calculate an oral *maintenance dosage regimen* of levofloxacin to treat the following individuals, with the objective of maintaining the same average plasma concentration at plateau as in the typical 60-year-old patient. The renal and hepatic functions of all the individuals are normal for their age and weight.

    a. A 4-year-old, 15-kg girl.

    b. A 20-year-old, 82-kg man.

c. A 92-year-old, 63-kg woman.

d. Considering the practical side of drug administration, for which of the patients above would you consider *not* giving the typical dosage regimen? Briefly discuss.

11. Figure 14-24 shows the minimum alveolar concentration (MAC) at one atmospheric pressure that produces immobility to an obnoxious stimulus in 50% of subjects of four different inhaled anesthetic agents.

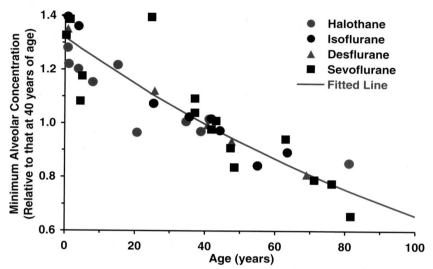

FIGURE 14-24.   The minimum alveolar concentration (MAC) at one atmosphere of pressure that produces immobility to an obnoxious stimulus in 50% of subjects of four different inhaled anesthetic agents. The data were obtained from several studies. Each value of MAC was divided by the value at 40 years of age. The line was obtained by least-squares regression of the log of the MAC values with age. (From: Eger EI. Age, minimum alveolar anesthetic concentration, and minimum alveolar anesthetic concentration-awake. Anesth Analg 2000;93:947–953.)

a. The equation of the colored line (least-squares fit of all the data) is:

$$\text{MAC (Fraction of the value at age 40)} = 1.32 \times 10^{-0.00303 \cdot \text{Age}}$$

(Age in years)

Calculate the percent decrease in MAC with each decade of life.

b. Does it appear that young children (1–4 years of age) are more susceptible to the anesthetic effects of these agents than young adults (20 years of age)? Briefly comment.

c. Halothane undergoes metabolism in the body. Briefly discuss how much you would expect the rate of metabolism to change in a 70-kg, 80-year-old patient compared to that in a 70-kg, 20-year-old patient when they both show the same anesthetic effect. Use the fitted line to answer this question.

15

Disease

OBJECTIVES

The reader will be able to:

- List at least four diseases in which the pharmacokinetics of drugs is known to be altered.
- List and briefly discuss the pharmacokinetic parameters that are often altered in patients with hepatic and renal diseases.
- Judge, using pharmacokinetic principles, on when alteration of drug administration should be considered for patients with hepatic or renal diseases.
- Estimate how much the clearance of a drug of known fraction excreted unchanged is decreased in a patient with known renal function.
- Estimate the creatinine clearance of a patient from the patient's age, weight, gender, and serum creatinine.
- List the assumptions that underlie the application of renal function tests in dosage regimen adjustment for patients with renal disease.
- Establish, from pharmacokinetic principles, a dosage regimen for a drug with no active metabolites in a patient of a given age, weight, gender, and serum creatinine, when the fraction excreted unchanged is known.
- Sketch the amount of drug in the body with time following the dosage regimen recommended for the patient in the previous objective.
- Discuss the pertinence of issues, such as diminished metabolism and transport in multiple organs, and metabolism in the kidneys, on the adjustment of drug administration in renal disease.
- Define clinical dialyzability, continuous ambulatory peritoneal dialysis, dialysis, dialysis clearance, dialyzer, dialyzer efficiency, extracorporeal dialysis, and hemodialysis.
- Calculate the changes in clearance and half-life of a drug and predict the kinetic events brought about by hemodialysis or continuous ambulatory peritoneal dialysis, given the clearance by the procedure, together with the total (body) clearance and the half-life in the absence of the dialysis treatment.
- Given dialysis clearance and the pharmacokinetic parameters of a drug in the absence of the dialysis procedure, anticipate if a supplementary dose is desirable immediately after dialysis. Also, determine what the supplementary dose should be.

D isease is a major source of variability in drug response. For many diseases, this variability is primarily a result of differences in pharmacokinetics, the area of principal focus in this chapter. Needless to say, drug therapy in each disease state may need to be tailored to the severity of the disease and the specific needs of the individual being treated. One must also be cognizant of the presence of diseases other than the one for which a given drug is taken. Concurrent diseases such as hepatic cirrhosis, congestive cardiac failure, and renal function impairment can alter dosage requirements as well. It is in this context that the effect of disease on drug therapy is examined in this chapter. Hepatic, cardiovascular, and renal disease are of primary importance, especially renal disease for which adjustment in dosage is the most quantitative.

Hemodialysis and related procedures have become established treatments for patients with end-stage renal disease. These procedures are designed to remove toxic waste products that accumulate in patients with this disease. However, they also remove drugs. Thus, such procedures may require adjustment of drug administration, in addition to that required by the loss of renal function. This chapter provides information needed to decide when and how to make such an adjustment. Continuous ambulatory peritoneal dialysis is also discussed, because it is regarded as the treatment of choice for some patients. The chapter ends with a discussion of hemodialysis of overdosed patients to help remove drugs or other substances from the body.

HEPATIC DISEASES

Because the liver is the major site for drug metabolism, an impression prevails that special care should be taken when administering drugs to patients with disease states in which hepatic function is modified. Objective data, although generally supporting this impression, are occasionally in conflict.

One reason for the conflict arises from an attempt to classify hepatic disorders as a single entity. However, disorders of the liver, local or diffuse, are caused by many diseases; each disease affects various levels of hepatic organization to a different extent. With few exceptions, the hepatic clearance of drugs is, on average, decreased in cirrhosis. In contrast, in acute viral hepatitis, there appears to be a fairly even division between those drugs for which metabolic clearance is decreased, or half-life prolonged, and those for which no significant change is detected. Existing data suggest that drug elimination is diminished in obstructive jaundice. The effect is expected to be more extensive for those drugs eliminated predominantly by biliary excretion.

Another potential pitfall is to equate prolongation of half-life with diminution of hepatic drug-metabolizing activity. Half-life is controlled by both total clearance and volume of distribution, two independent parameters (Chapter 5, *Elimination*). To assess clearance and volume of distribution, the drug should be given intravenously to ensure complete bioavailability. When so studied, the volumes of distribution of some drugs remain unaltered in hepatic disease, but those of others are increased. An increase in volume of distribution is found particularly with drugs bound to albumin in patients with cirrhosis. The explanation lies in the depressed synthesis of albumin in these patients. The resultant fall in albumin concentration is responsible for a decreased plasma binding, an associated increase in volume of distribution, and an associated increase in clearance for a drug of low extraction. A fall in hepatic enzymes is responsible, in large part, for a diminished hepatic unbound clearance of many drugs. Oxidized drugs appear to be more affected than those eliminated by conjugation.

The influence of hepatic disease on drug absorption is incompletely understood. The problem is complicated by the need to separate disposition from absorption when analyzing plasma concentration–time data. However, it is likely that the oral bioavailability of drugs that are usually highly extracted by the liver is increased in cirrhosis (Fig. 15-1). There are two reasons for this increase. One is a diminished first-pass hepatic loss resulting from depressed hepatocellular activity. The other is that many cirrhotic patients develop portal bypass, a condition in which a significant fraction of the portal blood bypasses the functional liver cells and enters the superior vena cava via esophageal varices. These porta-caval shunts, formed as a consequence of the portal hypertension brought about by the diseased liver, and the changes in the liver itself, can greatly increase oral bioavailability.

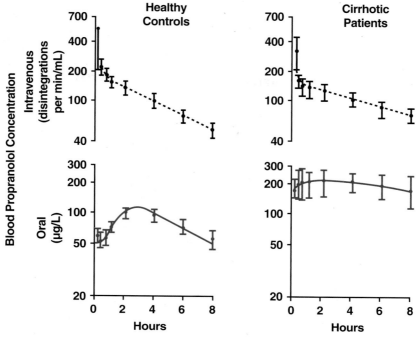

FIGURE 15-1. In cirrhosis, the oral bioavailability of propranolol is greatly increased, as evidenced by comparison of the blood concentration of unlabeled drug after oral administration (*colored line*) with that of tritiated drug after intravenous administration (*dashed black line*), following simultaneous determination of the kinetics of propranolol during the seventh dosing interval of an oral 8-hr dosing regimen in 9 normal subjects and 7 patients with cirrhosis (mean ± SE). (From: Wood AJJ, Kornhauser DM, Wilkinson GR, et al. The influence of cirrhosis on steady-state blood concentrations of unbound propranolol after oral administration. Clin Pharmacokinet 1978;3:478–487. Reproduced by permission of ADIS Press Australasia Pty Limited.)

From the foregoing discussion, it is apparent that drug dosage may need to be reduced in patients with hepatic function impairment as a result of both decreased clearance and increased oral bioavailability. An adjustment in dosage is particularly warranted when the usual regimen results in the unbound drug concentration at plateau approaching or exceeding the upper limit of the therapeutic concentration window. This condition arises when the clearance based on unbound drug is substantially depressed, because it is this clearance that controls the average unbound drug concentration at plateau, as $\frac{F \cdot Dose}{\tau} = CLu \cdot Cu_{av,ss}$.

To illustrate these points, consider the data in Table 15-1. The observations on three different drugs studied in healthy subjects and in cirrhotic patients are shown. For cefetamet, a cephalosporin antibiotic, there is virtually no significant change in any of the pharmacokinetic parameters measured. This lack of an effect can be explained by this drug being primarily eliminated via renal excretion ($fe = 0.85$) and by its being only weakly bound to plasma proteins ($fu = 0.85$ in control subjects). Thus, changes in elimination and protein binding are not expected. On the other hand, meptazinol, an opioid analgesic, shows a dramatic increase in its bioavailability (400+ %) and about a 50% increase in half-life. This change resulting from hepatic cirrhosis, too, may be anticipated. One might expect meptazinol to have a high hepatic extraction ratio, for two reasons—the low oral bioavailability and the high plasma clearance. The increase in

TABLE 15-1 **Comparison of the Pharmacokinetics of Selected Drugs in Healthy Subjects with that in Patients with Hepatic Cirrhosis**

Drug	F	CL (L/hr)	V (L/kg)	fu	$t_{1/2}$ (hr)
Pharmacokinetic Parameter					
Cefetamet*					
Healthy controls	$0.45\pm0.09^{\dagger}$	7.7 ± 0.6	0.33 ± 0.03	0.82 ± 0.11	2.4 ± 0.21
Hepatic cirrhosis	0.50 ± 0.13	7.5 ± 0.7	0.32 ± 0.07	0.85 ± 0.12	2.4 ± 0.41
Meptazinol‡					
Healthy controls	0.07 ± 0.01	83 ± 10	4.3 ± 0.5	ND**	2.7 ± 0.2
Hepatic cirrhosis	$0.28\pm0.005^{\dagger\dagger\dagger}$	72 ± 8	5.7 ± 0.5	ND**	$4.2\pm0.6^{\dagger\dagger\dagger}$
Verapamil††					
Healthy controls	0.22 ± 0.08	76 ± 12	6.8 ± 2.0	$0.10\pm0.02^{\ddagger\ddagger}$	$3.7***$
Hepatic cirrhosis	$0.52\pm0.13^{\dagger\dagger\dagger}$	$37\pm17^{\dagger\dagger\dagger}$	$12.1\pm4.5^{\dagger\dagger\dagger}$	$0.16\pm0.16^{\dagger\dagger\dagger}$	$14.2^{\dagger\dagger\dagger}$

*From: Hayton WL, Kneer J, Blouin RA, Stoeckel K. Pharmacokinetics of intravenous cefetamet and oral cefetamet pivoxil in patients with hepatic cirrhosis. Antimicrob Agents Chemother 1990;34:1318–1322.
†Bioavailability of cefetamet following the oral administration of the prodrug, cefetamet pivoxil.
‡From: Birnie GG, Thompson GG, Murray T, et al. Enhanced oral bioavailability of meptazinol in cirrhosis. Gut 1987;28:248–254.
**ND, not determined in this study.
††From: Somogyi A, Albrecht M, Kliems G, et al. Pharmacokinetics, bioavailability and ECG response of verapamil in patients with liver disease. Br J Clin Pharmac 1981;12:51–60.
‡‡From: Giacomini KM, Massoud N, Wong FM, Giacomini JC. Decreased binding of verapamil to plasma proteins in patients with liver disease. J Cardiovasc Pharmacol 1984;6:924–928.
***Harmonic mean.
†††Statistically significantly different.

half-life is a result of a small, although not significant, change in both clearance and volume. With a high extraction ratio, the bioavailability reflects a decrease in hepatocellular activity and increased portacaval shunting of blood, common to hepatic cirrhosis. For verapamil, an antihypertensive and antiarrhythmic agent, significant changes occur in all of the pharmacokinetic parameters listed in the table. The drug has a high extraction ratio in controls, which decreases to an intermediate value in cirrhosis, as evidenced by the increase in F and the decrease in CL (determined from intravenous data). The volume of distribution based on the unbound drug (V/fu) is basically unchanged. The increase in half-life is then a consequence of a large decrease in unbound clearance (CL/fu).

Hepatic dysfunction is a graded phenomenon, and theoretically, a correlation should exist between changes in the pharmacokinetic parameters of drugs, especially hepatic clearance, and an appropriate measure of hepatic function. Attempts to establish such relationships, although encouraging, have not been highly successful. One example of an approach that has been partially successful is to relate clearance to the status of the hepatic function in hepatic cirrhosis.

In cirrhosis, a correlation between the severity of the condition (Child-Pugh Classification, Table 15-2) and the likelihood of depressed metabolism by oxidation, as shown for amprenavir (Agenerase, now also commercially available as a prodrug, fosamprenavir [Lexiva or Telzir]) in Fig. 15-2, and some conjugation reactions have been reported. Drug metabolism is often decreased in severe cirrhosis, signified by the combination of a low albumin (<28 g/L), an elevated clotting time (INR >2.2), refractory ascites, and the presence of Grade III or IV hepatic encephalopathies. The decreased metabolism frequently requires reducing the dose and monitoring the patient for adverse reactions.

TABLE 15-2	Child-Pugh Score for Assessing the Prognosis of Chronic Liver Disease (Mainly Cirrhosis)

Scoring

Measure	1 Point	2 Points	3 Points	Units
Bilirubin*	<2 (<34)	2–3 (34–50)	>3 (>50)	mg/dL (μmol/L)
Serum albumin	>35	28–35	<28	g/L
INR	<1.7	1.71–2.20	>2.20	None
Ascites	None	Suppressed with medication	Refractory	None
Hepatic encephalopathy	None	Grade I–II (or suppressed with medication)	Grade III–IV (or refractory)	None

Interpretation

Total Points	Class	1-year survival	2-year survival
5–6	A	100%	85%
7–9	B	81%	57%
10–15	C	45%	35%

*Total bilirubin in parantheses.
From: Child CG, Turcotte JG. Surgery and portal hypertension. In: Child CG, ed. The Liver and Portal Hypertension. Philadelphia: Saunders; 1964:50–64; and Pugh RN, Murray-Lyon IM, Dawson H, et al. Transection of the oesophagus for bleeding oesophageal varices. Br J Surgery 1973;60:646–649.

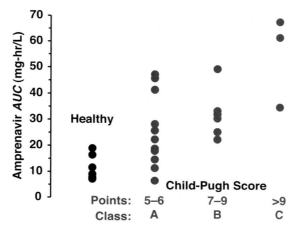

FIGURE 15-2. Relationship between amprenavir *AUC* and the Child-Pugh score. No subject with a Child-Pugh score greater than 12 was enrolled in the study. Amprenavir is eliminated primarily by CYP3A4 metabolism. Although there is considerable variability in patients with hepatic disease, there appears to be a trend toward an increased *AUC*, and therefore reduced clearance, in those with more severe hepatic disease. (From: Veronese L, Rautaureau J, Sadler BM, et al. Single-dose pharmacokinetics of amprenavir, a human immunodeficiency virus type 1 protease inhibitor, in subjects with normal or impaired hepatic function. Antimicrob Agents Chemother 2000;44:821–826.)

One needs to consider if an extensively metabolized drug is truly needed or if an alternative (renally excreted) drug is available.

One reason why the correlation with the Child-Pugh score often fails is because, unlike renal excretion, there are numerous pathways of drug metabolism, each with a different set of cofactor requirements and each affected to a different degree in hepatic disorders.

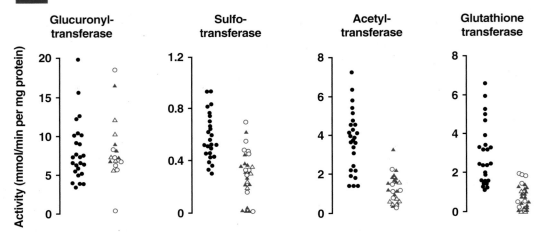

FIGURE 15-3.   Activities of the conjugating enzymes, glucuronyltransferase, sulfotransferase, acetyl-transferase, and glutathione transferase, in normal (*black*) and abnormal (*colored*) human livers vary widely. Open circles, filled triangles, and open triangles refer to biopsied samples from patients with chronic persistent hepatitis, chronic active hepatitis, and cirrhosis, respectively. The substrates were 2-naphthol for glucuronyl transferase and sulfotransferase, p-aminobenzoic acid for acetyltrans-ferase, and benzo(a)pyrene-4,5-oxide for glutathione transferase. In contrast to the other enzymes, glucuronyl transferase does not appear to be affected by any of the hepatic conditions. Also appar-ent is a virtual lack of activity of the last three enzymes in some patients. The implications for drugs pri-marily eliminated by the conjugation pathways are great. (From: Pacifici GM, Viani A, Franchi M, et al. Conjugation pathways in liver disease. Br J Clin Pharmacol 1990;30:427–435.)

Variability in metabolism is apparent from the activities of four hepatic enzymes responsi-ble for conjugation reactions (Fig. 15-3). The enzyme activities were measured in liver samples obtained by biopsy. Glucuronyl transferase appears to be unaffected by hepatic disease. Supporting this observation, the pharmacokinetics of the benzodiazepine ox-azepam, which is eliminated almost entirely by glucuronidation, appears to be affected only in severe hepatic disease. It is also apparent that although the activities of the other three enzymes are on average decreased, there are some individuals within the normal range of activity and others in whom very little or no activity remains. Altered metabolism in chronic persistent hepatitis, chronic active hepatitis, and cirrhosis is also dependent on transporters, if involved.

CARDIOVASCULAR DISEASES

Circulatory disorders, which include shock, malignant hypertension, and congestive car-diac failure, are generally characterized by diminished vascular perfusion to one or more parts of the body. Because blood flow may influence drug absorption, distribution, and elimination, it is not surprising that the pharmacokinetics of drugs may be altered in cir-culatory disorders.

A diminished perfusion of absorption sites (e.g., gastrointestinal tract and muscle) with associated protracted and erratic drug absorption, tends to be seen in patients with depressed cardiovascular states; it may be necessary to give the drug intravenously if a prompt response is desired. However, in these conditions, the kinetics of distribution is also affected, with perfusion to many organs diminished. Exceptions are the brain and the myocardium, which consequently receive an increased fraction of an intravenous (i.v.) bolus dose, particularly in the earlier moments. For centrally acting and cardioactive agents, the rate of administration of a bolus dose to patients with circulatory depression

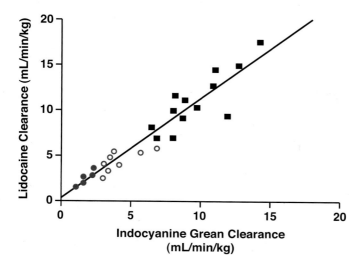

FIGURE 15-4. A strong positive correlation exists between the clearances of lidocaine and indocyanine green in patients without (■) and with both mild (○) and severe (●) congestive cardiac failure. (From: Zito RA, Reid PR. Lidocaine kinetics predicted by indocyanine green clearance. Reprinted, by permission of New Engl J Med 1978;298:1160–1163.)

must be tempered if the risk of toxicity is to be reduced. In these depressed circulatory states, cardiac output and therefore hepatic blood flow and, to a much lesser extent, renal blood flow are also reduced. Thus, a decrease in clearance of highly extracted drugs is expected. Evidence supporting this concept is illustrated in Fig. 15-4 by a strong positive correlation between the clearances of lidocaine, a drug eliminated hepatically by metabolism, and indocyanine green, a diagnostic agent rapidly picked up by active transporters within the liver, and excreted into bile, in patients with varying degrees of congestive cardiac failure. Both indocyanine green and lidocaine are high hepatic extraction ratio drugs whose clearances should therefore reflect a diminished hepatic blood flow. Notice in Fig. 15-4 the almost 16-fold variation in clearance of both lidocaine and indocyanine green. This range is almost certainly greater than the range of hepatic blood flows in these patients. The hepatic flow, usually about 18 mL/min per kilogram, is unlikely to fall to a value as low as 2 mL/min per kilogram, because severe anoxia is expected to result at even higher flow rates. Hepatocellular metabolism and transport are most probably also depressed when perfusion is severely diminished; this would further depress the clearances of both lidocaine and indocyanine green. Exposure to lidocaine is increased in patients with congestive cardiac failure, and the risk of toxicity is therefore increased.

RENAL DISEASES

There are many diseases of the kidneys. Some affect the glomerulus; others primarily affect the tubules. To a first approximation, the renal clearance of virtually all small molecules is reduced to the same degree regardless of the location of the disease. This general observation supports the "unit nephron hypothesis," that is, there appears to be a corresponding decrease in filtration, secretion, and reabsorption. Stated differently, the decrease in renal clearance of a drug that is filtered and neither reabsorbed nor secreted is reduced in approximately the same proportion to one that is either highly secreted or extensively reabsorbed.

THE PHARMACOTHERAPEUTIC PROBLEM

In patients with compromised renal function, renal clearance of drugs is diminished. The degree of reduction depends on the reduction in renal function, as shown in Fig. 15-5 for cefepime, a fourth-generation cephalosporin antibiotic. The lower the renal function, the longer also is the half-life of the drug.

When a usual intramuscular (i.m.) regimen of amikacin (7.5 mg/kg) is administered to a 67-kg patient with renal function that is only 17% of a typical patient (colored line of

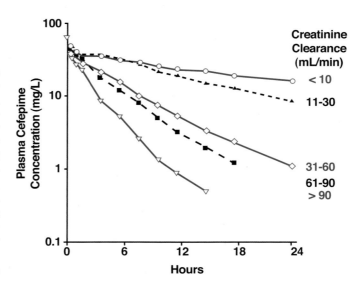

FIGURE 15-5. The mean plasma concentration–time profiles of cefepime, a cephalosporin antibiotic, are different in patients with varying degrees of renal function after i.v. infusion of a 1000-mg dose over 30 min. The subjects were grouped according to their measured creatinine clearance values (in mL/min). (From: Barbhaiya RH, Knupp CA, Fargue ST, et al. Pharmacokinetics of cefepime in subjects with renal insufficiency. Clin Pharmacol Ther 1990;48:268–276.)

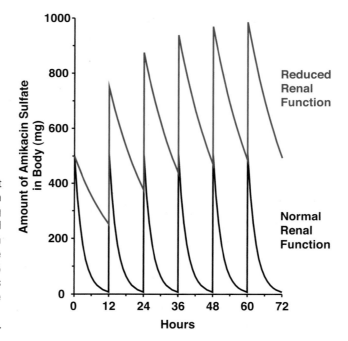

FIGURE 15-6. Sketch of the amount of amikacin sulfate in the body with time following a regimen of 500 mg every 12 hr in a patient whose renal function is normal (*black line*) and in a patient whose age and weight are the same but whose renal function is 17% of normal (*colored line*). Intravenous bolus administration is simulated. The normal half-life is assumed to be 2 hr.

Fig. 15-6), the drug accumulates extensively, relative to that in a typical patient (black line). Note also that the average amount in the body at steady state increases sixfold, whereas the peak amount only doubles. The trough value increases many fold. The figure reminds us that the extent of accumulation depends on both frequency of administration and half-life, and that the time required to approach plateau is a function of half-life only (Chapter 11, *Multiple-Dose Regimens*). Having a much longer half-life than usual, the time to reach steady state is much longer in this patient than in a individual with renal function of the typical patient. Obviously, to avoid excessive exposure, dosage must be reduced in the patient with renal dysfunction. The therapeutic questions to be asked here are whether the effects of the drug relate to the peak or average exposures to the drug. The former would suggest only a twofold reduction in dosage; the latter would require a sixfold decrease in dosage.

The clinician needs information on which drugs result in excessive exposures in renal dysfunction and, more importantly, how to adjust drug administration to achieve an optimal therapeutic response. The basic principles that permit this calculation follow. These are developed with the view that drug effect, and therefore unbound drug concentration, needs to be maintained and that metabolites, if any, are inactive. The issue of active metabolites is further considered in Chapter 20, *Metabolites and Drug Response*.

DECREASE IN UNBOUND CLEARANCE

The elements of the problem of renal dysfunction are shown in Fig. 15-7. Ceftazidime clearance, unbound clearance here because the drug is not bound to plasma proteins, is low when renal function, measured by creatinine clearance, is low and increases linearly with renal function. Note that some unbound clearance remains (y-intercept) even when there is no renal function, as measured by creatinine clearance. This represents elimination by nonrenal pathways. The magnitude of change in unbound clearance depends on the renal function remaining and the fraction excreted unchanged.

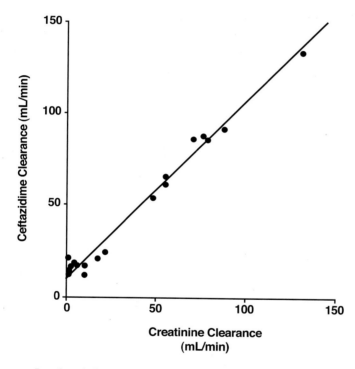

FIGURE 15-7. The total clearance of the cephalosporin, ceftazidime, varies linearly with creatinine clearance in a group of 19 patients with varying degrees of renal function. Note that some clearance remains (y-intercept) when there is no renal function. (From: van Dalen R, Vree TB, Baars AM, et al. Dosage adjustment for ceftazidime in patients with impaired renal function. Eur J Clin Pharmacol 1986;30:597–605.)

In what follows, emphasis is placed on unbound rather than total clearance. This is not only because the all-important unbound concentration is related to unbound clearance but also because, for many drugs, fu varies in renal disease, making interpretation based on total plasma concentration more problematic. Our goal is to devise a relationship that allows estimation of the maintenance regimen in a patient with renal impairment. The first step is to relate unbound renal clearance in the patient with renal disease (d), $CLu_R(d)$, to unbound renal clearance in the typical (t) 60-year-old, 70-kg patient, $CLu_R(t)$.

$$CLu_R(d) = RF \cdot CLu_R(t) \tag{15-1}$$

The ratio of the two is the renal function (RF) in the patient relative to that in the typical patient. This relative value is subsequently simply called *renal function*.

In the typical patient, $CLu_R(t)$ is a fraction, $fe(t)$, of unbound (renal + nonrenal) clearance, $CLu(t)$.

$$CLu_R(t) = fe(t) \cdot CLu(t) \tag{15-2}$$

By combining Eqs. 15-1 and 15-2, the unbound renal clearance in the patient can be related to $CLu(t)$, the unbound clearance (by all routes) in the typical patient, by

$$CLu_R(d) = RF \cdot fe(t) \cdot CLu(t) \qquad \text{15-3}$$

The next step is to consider the unbound clearance by nonrenal routes, CLu_{NR}. In the typical patient, it is

$$CLu_{NR} = [1 - fe(t)] \cdot CLu(t) \qquad \text{15-4}$$

CLu_{NR} is usually not materially changed because of renal disease. This is not always the case as will be subsequently discussed. Its value is, however, expected to change with age and weight. On the assumption that it does so like renal function, then $CLu_{NR}(d)/CLu_{NR}(t)$ is just the ratio of expected renal clearances with age and body weight. From Eq. 14-3 (Chapter 14, *Age, Weight, and Gender*) this ratio, the factor by which renal clearance deviates from that in the typical patient, is $\dfrac{(140 - Age) \cdot Wt(d)^{0.75}}{1936}$, where the denominator is the value of the numerator when age is 60 years and weight is 70 kg. Based on these considerations, the factor by which *nonrenal* clearance ($CLu_{NR}[d]$) deviates from that in the typical patient ($CLu_{NR}[t]$) then becomes

$$CLu_{NR}(d) = [1 - fe(t)] \cdot CLu(t) \cdot \frac{(140 - Age(d)) \cdot Wt(d)^{0.75}}{1936} \qquad \text{15-5}$$

where age and weight are in years and kilograms, respectively. Now, under any condition,

$$CLu(d) = CLu_R(d) + CLu_{NR}(d) \qquad \text{15-6}$$

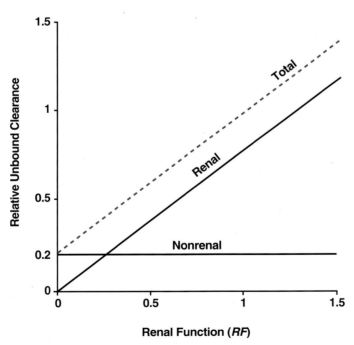

FIGURE 15-8. Renal, nonrenal, and total unbound clearances, expressed relative to the total unbound clearance of a typical patient, versus renal function (*RF*) for a drug with an *fe*(*t*) value of 0.8. Unbound nonrenal clearance remains constant and independent of renal function. In contrast, unbound renal clearance increases in direct proportion to renal function. The resulting (total) unbound clearance (*colored dashed line*) increases in parallel with renal clearance from a value of 0.2, represented by non-renal clearance, to a value of 1.0, when the renal function is that of the typical patient. In this illustration, renal function varies in a group of 60-year-old, 70-kg patients. Nonrenal clearance is, of course, expected to change with age and weight (Chapter 14, *Age, Weight, and Gender*). Note that *RF* values greater than 1.0 are shown to include those individuals with creatinine clearances greater than the average.

For a given age and weight, $CLu_{NR}(d)$ is expected to be constant, independent of renal function; whereas $CLu_R(d)$ is expected (Eq. 15-4) to change in direct proportion to renal function (RF). Thus, the unbound clearance in the patient, $CLu(d)$, increases linearly with RF. The extent of the increase depends on $fe(t)$, the contribution of the renal route to all routes of elimination in the typical patient. This relationship is shown in Fig. 15-8 for a drug with an $fe(t)$ of 0.8.

On substituting Eqs. 15-1 to 15-5 into Eq. 15-6, the following useful relationship is derived for R_d, the unbound clearance ratio, $CLu(d)/CLu(t)$.

$$R_d = \frac{CLu(d)}{CLu(t)} = RF \cdot fe(t) + [1 - fe(t)] \cdot \frac{(140 - Age) \cdot Wt(d)^{0.75}}{1936} \qquad 15\text{-}7$$

The first term, $RF \cdot fe(t)$, does not incorporate age and weight directly, because RF is estimated from creatinine clearance (next section) in the renally impaired patient relative to that of the typical patient. For a patient whose age and weight do not deviate far from that of a typical patient,

$$Rd = RF \cdot fe(t) + 1 - fe(t) \qquad 15\text{-}8$$

Figure 15-9A illustrates how R_d, ratio of unbound clearances, depends on both the renal function remaining in a patient and the value of $fe(t)$ in a typical 60-year-old, 70-kg

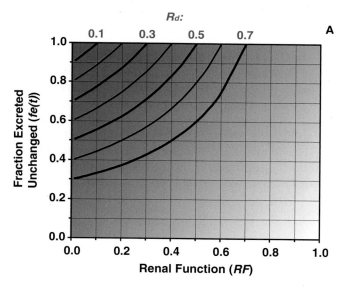

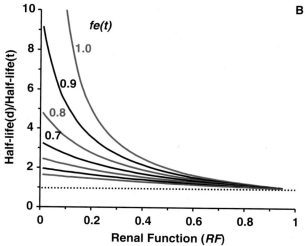

FIGURE 15-9. **A.** In patients with renal disease, the extent of decrease in R_d, the ratio of unbound clearances, depends on both the fraction excreted unchanged, $fe(t)$ in typical patients and on the renal function (RF) remaining in an individual patient. The value of R_d is lowest (shown by deepest shading) when $fe(t)$ approaches 1.0 and RF approaches zero. The lines show the combinations of $fe(t)$ and RF that give the same R_d. **B.** The half-life of a drug, relative to the typical value, is expected to be the highest when RF approaches zero and $fe(t)$ approaches 1.0. The lines indicate the ratio of half-lives for various values of $fe(t)$ as a function of RF. Both panels are simulations based on Eq. 15-7 for a 70-kg, 60-year-old patient.

patient. It is apparent that R_d changes the most with renal function when $fe(t) = 1$ and is unchanged when $fe(t) = 0$. The value of $fe(t)$ is, by definition,

$$fe(t) = \frac{CLu_R(t)}{CLu(t)} = \frac{CL_R(t)}{CL(t)} \qquad \text{15-9}$$

where $CLu_R(t)$ and $CLu(t)$ are the unbound renal and total clearances, and $CL_R(t)$ and $CL(t)$ are the corresponding values based on the total plasma concentration of the drug in the typical patient for whom the usual regimen is intended. Experimentally, $fe(t)$ is the fraction of an i.v. dose recovered unchanged in urine in a typical patient.

Recall that $t_{1/2} = \dfrac{0.693 \cdot Vu}{CLu}$. The half-life in a patient with renal function impairment, $t_{1/2}(d)$, compared with that in a typical patient with fully functioning kidneys, $t_{1/2}(t)$, is then

$$\frac{t_{1/2}(d)}{t_{1/2}(t)} = \frac{Vu(d)}{Vu(t)} \cdot \frac{1}{R_d} \qquad \text{15-10}$$

where $Vu(d)$ and $Vu(t)$ are the unbound volumes of distribution in the patient with renal disease and in the typical patient, respectively. Also, recall that Vu tends to vary in direct proportion to body weight. If renal function does not affect Vu, then

$$\frac{t_{1/2}(d)}{t_{1/2}(t)} = \frac{Wt(d)}{Wt(t)} \cdot \frac{1}{R_d} \qquad \text{15-11}$$

Figure 15-9B illustrates the dependence of half-life on both renal function and fraction excreted unchanged. Notice that half-life changes the most when renal function approaches zero and $fe(t)$ approaches 1.0.

Before leaving this section, an additional point needs to be made with respect to data in Fig. 15-7 in which each point represents an observation from a different patient. The x-axis, creatinine clearance, is a function of age, weight, gender, and renal disease. One might expect that nonrenal clearance may also be related to age and weight. Higher values of nonrenal clearance occur in younger and larger patients, who have higher creatinine clearances, and smaller values are expected in older and smaller patients. This positive correlation of nonrenal clearance with creatinine clearance may distort the regression, so that the y-intercept is lower and the slope is greater than expected. Ideally, renal clearance should be correlated with creatinine clearance, and the nonrenal clearance should be examined separately for its dependence on age, weight, and perhaps renal disease.

DECREASE IN BINDING TO PLASMA PROTEINS

Renal disease is often associated with a decrease in binding to plasma proteins, especially those drugs that bind to albumin. The decreased binding is because of several factors, the most important of which is a decrease in albumin concentration. The accumulation of endogenous substances that may displace drug from the binding sites and the carbamylation of albumin (because of high levels of urea), that decrease its affinity for drugs, may also contribute. As a result of the decreased binding, clearance of metabolized drugs with a low hepatic extraction ratio tends to increase. Although the clearance of those drugs that are primarily excreted unchanged and bound to albumin also tends to increase, it is not as extensive as the decrease resulting from the decrease in renal function. Clearance of such drugs therefore decreases in renal disease, but it is only the unbound clearance that reflects unbound concentration, the correlate of drug response. This is the reason why the equations above (Eqs. 15-1 to 15-11) were derived using unbound drug.

ESTIMATION OF RENAL FUNCTION

Many methods have been developed over the years, since the physiology of the kidneys was originally worked out, to assess renal function. Two particularly useful methods that use serum creatinine are currently in common use.

Estimation of Glomerular Filtration Rate. An estimate of glomerular filtration rate (*GFR*) is useful to assess the ability of the kidneys to handle drugs and other substances. Table 15-3 lists the *GFR* values used to define the stages of loss of renal function with age (see also Chapter 14, *Age, Weight, and Gender*) and concurrent diseases, such as diabetes and hypertension.

TABLE 15-3	Staging System and Action Plan for Chronic Kidney Disease		
Stage	Description	GFR (mL/min per 1.73 m²)	Action*
—	At increased risk for CKD	≥90 with risk factors[†]	Screening, CKD risk reduction
1	Kidney damage[‡] with normal or increased *GFR*	≥90	Diagnosis and treatment Slow progression of CKD Treat comorbidities Cardiovascular disease risk reduction
2	Mild decrease in *GFR*	60–89	Estimate progression
3	Moderate decrease in *GFR*	30–59	Evaluate and treat complications
4	Severe decrease in *GFR*	15–29	Prepare for renal replacement therapy
5	Kidney failure	<15 or dialysis	Replacement if uremic

CKD, chronic kidney disease.
*Includes actions from previous stages.
[†]Risk factors: hypertension, dyslipidemia, diabetes mellitus, anemia, systemic lupus erythematosis, chronic analgesic ingestion.
[‡]Kidney damage as manifested by abnormalities noted on renal pathology, blood, urine, or imaging tests.
From: National Kidney Foundation (NKF) Kidney Disease Outcome Quality Initiative (K/DOQI) Advisory Board. K/DOQI clinical practice guidelines for chronic kidney disease: evaluation, classification, and stratification. Kidney Disease Outcome Quality Initiative. Am J Kidney Dis 2002;39S:565. With permission from Elsevier Science.

A method was recently developed using serum creatinine to determine *GFR*. *GFR* was directly assessed from the renal clearance of ^{125}I-iothalamate. The procedure is known as the *modification of diet in renal disease* (MDRD) method. There are now two relationships used. The original procedure contains six variables; an adaptation, and now the more common one, contains four, as shown in Table 15-4. The calculated value is an estimate of the patient's *GFR* and is normalized to 1.73 m². Body weight is therefore not one of the variables. Although a valuable procedure for assessing renal function, it has not yet been

TABLE 15-4	"Modification of Diet in Renal Disease" Relationships for Estimating the Glomerular Filtration Rate

The 6-Variable Relationship*

$$GFR = \frac{161.5 \times Albumin^{0.318} \times (1.18 \ if \ black; \ 0.762 \ if \ female)}{Serum \ Creatinine^{0.999} \times Age^{0.176} \times SUN^{0.17}}$$

The 4-Variable Relationship

$$GFR = \frac{175 \times (1.212 \ if \ black; \ 0.742 \ if \ female)}{Serum \ Creatinine^{1.154} \times Age^{0.203}}$$

*Abbreviations and units: albumin (g/dL); serum creatinine (mg/dL); age (years); serum urea nitrogen (SUN, mg/dL)
From: Levey AS, Coresh J, Greene T, et al. Using standardized serum creatinine values in the modification of diet in renal disease study equation for estimating glomerular filtration rate. Ann Intern Med 2006;145:247–254.

extensively applied pharmacokinetically to adjust dosage in renal disease. Furthermore, for this purpose, *GFR* needs to be expressed in milliliters per minute, not milliliters per minute per 1.73 m². Most of the literature to date on dosage adjustment uses creatinine clearance, a value which is typically about 15% to 20% greater than *GFR*.

Estimation of Creatinine Clearance. The usefulness of creatinine clearance lies in the observation that renal clearance of many drugs varies linearly with creatinine clearance (e.g., see Fig. 15-7), regardless of whether the drug is filtered only, secreted extensively, or reabsorbed in the renal tubule. Creatinine is virtually only eliminated from the body by renal filtration.

Under Chronic, Relatively Stable Conditions. In clinical practice, creatinine renal clearance is usually estimated from serum creatinine alone rather than from creatinine measurements in both plasma and urine. Apart from the extra analysis and inconvenience involved, incomplete urine collection is a major problem in the clinical setting often resulting in an underestimate of creatinine clearance. Serum creatinine alone is a reasonable indicator of renal function, because the daily production of creatinine is matched by its elimination under normal circumstances. Consequently, serum creatinine is related to creatinine clearance by

$$Serum\ creatinine = \frac{Rate\ of\ creatinine\ production}{Creatinine\ clearance} \qquad 15\text{-}12$$

Table 15-5 summarizes relationships commonly used to approximate creatinine clearance from serum creatinine in adults and children. The first two relationships for

TABLE 15-5   Cockcroft-Gault Method for Estimation of Creatinine Clearance in Adults* and the Schwartz Method for Estimation of the Value in Children[†]

	Creatinine Clearance (mL/min)	
Population	**Serum Creatinine in mg/dL**	**Serum Creatinine in μM**
Adults (20–100 years of age)[‡]		
Men	$\dfrac{(140 - Age) \times Weight}{72 \times Serum\ Creatinine}$	$\dfrac{1.23\,(140 - Age) \times Weight}{Serum\ Creatinine}$
Women	$0.85 \times \dfrac{(140 - Age) \times Weight}{72 \times Serum\ Creatinine}$	$\dfrac{1.04\,(140 - Age) \times Weight}{Serum\ Creatinine}$
Children (0–20 years of age)**		
CL_{cr} (/1.73 m²)	$\dfrac{Factor^{\dagger\dagger} \times Height}{Serum\ Creatinine}$	$\dfrac{88.3 \times Factor \times Height}{Serum\ Creatinine}$
CL_{cr} (mL/min)	$\dfrac{Factor \times Height}{Serum\ Creatinine} \times \left(\dfrac{Weight}{70}\right)^{0.75}$	$\dfrac{88.3 \times Factor \times Height}{Serum\ Creatinine} \times \left(\dfrac{Weight}{70}\right)^{0.75}$

*Adults 20 years of age and older. Poor estimates are obtained for obese and emaciated patients. (From: Lott RS, Hayton WL. Estimation of creatinine clearance from serum creatinine concentration. Drug Intell Clin Pharm 1978;12:140–150.)

[†]Children 0–20 years of age. (From: Schwartz GJ, Haycock GB, Edelman CM Jr, Spitzer A. A simple estimate of glomerular filtration rate in children derived from body length and plasma creatinine. Pediatrics 1976;58:259–263.) The last term is added to express creatinine clearance in mL/min instead of mL/min per 1.73 m².

[‡]Age in years; body weight in kilograms.

**Height in centimeters; body weight in kilograms. The equation given by the authors, giving the creatinine clearance per 1.73 m², has been modified, using weight, to give the actual creatinin clearance in mL/min. A child of or near normal weight for height is assumed.

[††]Factor: premature to 1 year: 0.33; full term to 1 year: 0.43; children and adolescent girls: 0.55; adolescent boys: 0.70.

adults include corrections of creatinine production for age, weight, and gender. It should be emphasized that they are most accurate for adults with an average muscle mass (source of creatinine) for their age, weight, and height. For emaciated, highly muscular, or obese adult patients, poor estimates are obtained. The same is true for the estimation of *GFR* by the *MDRD* method. For such patients, an actual creatinine clearance measurement may be more appropriate than an estimate of its value from serum creatinine alone. Finally, on passing, it should be noted that both rate of production and clearance of creatinine decline with age. Consequently, serum creatinine only changes with age to a minor degree (Fig. 15-10). As noted, there are gender differences with adult women and men having serum creatinines of about 1.0 mg/dL and 1.2 mg/dL, respectively.

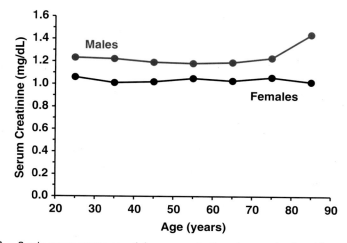

FIGURE 15-10. Crude mean serum creatinine concentrations for men (*colored line and circles*) and women (*black line and circles*) per decade of life (values shown at middle of decade). To avoid the inclusion of data for individuals with severe renal function impairment, all values greater than the 95th percentile have not been included for each gender. Note the consistency of the values with age in both men and women with the exception of the 80 to 90 decade for men. (From: Cullerton BF, Larson MG, Evans JC, et al. Prevalence and correlates of elevated serum creatinine levels. Arch Intern Med 1999;159:1785–1790, Fig. 1.)

A measure of renal function in the individual patient that can be used to adjust dosage remains to be determined. Renal function was previously defined (Eq. 15-1) as the ratio of the unbound renal clearance of a drug in the individual patient ($CLu_R[d]$) relative to that of a 60-year-old typical patient ($CLu_R[t]$). This ratio is also given by

$$RF = \frac{CL_{cr}(d)}{CL_{cr}(t)} = \frac{CLu_R(d)}{CLu_R(t)} \qquad 15\text{-}13$$

where $CL_{cr}(d)$ and $CL_{cr}(t)$ are the corresponding creatinine clearances, respectively. As stated in Chapter 14, *Age, Weight, and Gender*, the value of $CL_{cr}(t)$ for a typical 60-year-old is approximately 70 mL/min, 74 mL/min in men and 66 mL/min in women. These values are determined from the Cockcroft-Gault relationships. Typical 60-year-old men are 80 kg in weight (Fig. 14-6) and have a serum creatinine of 1.2 mg/dL (see Fig. 15-10), whereas women are 70 kg in weight and have a serum creatinine of 1.0 mg/dL. In general, gender differences are not taken into account and the average value of 70 mL/min may be used as the creatinine clearance of a typical 60-year-old patient.

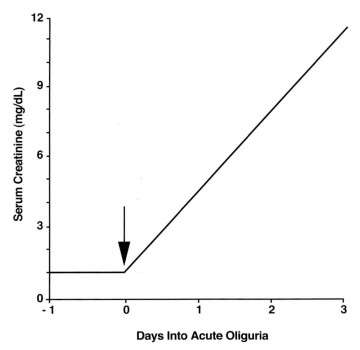

FIGURE 15-11. Acute renal failure (at time shown by arrow) causes the serum concentration of creatinine to rise at a constant rate of 3.5 mg/dL per day.

When Renal Function Changes Acutely. Creatinine is almost totally excreted unchanged. Accordingly, as shown in Fig. 15-11, serum creatinine is expected to rise linearly, not exponentially, with time in a patient with acute renal shutdown, as might be seen following a violent accident, a severe infection, or the accidental ingestion of a nephrotoxic substance. Notice that the actual rate of rise (dC/dt) is about 3 mg/dL per day (0.31 mM/day) in a typical 60-year-old patient, from which the turnover of creatinine can be calculated as follows:

Equation 15-14 expresses the interrelationships between turnover time (t_t, amount in the body relative to the rate of input) and rate of rise of plasma creatinine on completely blocking its elimination.

$$t_t = \frac{A_{ss}}{R_t} = \frac{V \cdot C_{ss}}{V \cdot dC/dt} = \frac{C_{ss}}{dC/dt} \qquad 15\text{-}14$$

where A_{ss} and C_{ss} represent the amount in the body and plasma concentration of creatinine under normal steady-state conditions, and R_t is its turnover rate (rate of production). Clearly, to define the normal turnover of creatinine, both its volume of distribution (V) and normal plasma concentration (C_{ss}) are needed. Although neither value is known for a patient, the usual values, which do not vary widely among normal healthy individuals, are likely to apply. The volume of distribution of creatinine is 42 L/70 kg, because it distributes into total body water and is unbound within the body. A typical plasma concentration is 1.1 mg/dL (11 mg/L or 0.1 mM). Hence, the turnover rate of creatinine, R_t, is 1260 mg/day (3 mg/dL per day × 42 L), and the turnover time is 9.6 hr. But what happens to the serum creatinine when renal function abruptly decreases?

If renal function drops immediately to a value that is 50%, 33%, 25%, or 20% of normal, the plasma creatinine concentration rises to a new steady state that is 2, 3, 4, or 5 times the normal value, respectively, as shown in Fig. 15-12 (also see Fig. 10-14, page 279).

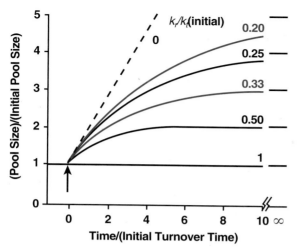

FIGURE 15-12. The approach to the new steady state is prolonged when (*at arrow*) the fractional turnover rate decreased by the factor k_t/k_t(*initial*). When the value of k_t approaches zero (*dashed line*), steady state is never achieved. The prolonged approach to the new steady state for the other conditions can be expressed by the time (half-life) required to reach the pool size half-way between the initial and final values.

The new steady-state concentration is directly proportional to the turnover time. The turnover time and the half-life of creatinine elimination at various degrees of renal function are shown in Table 15-6.

The time required for a plasma creatinine concentration to reflect a change in renal function can be greatly prolonged with severe renal function impairment. Interpretation of a plasma creatinine value in a clinical situation is therefore dependent on the acuteness of the change in renal function and on the degree to which renal function is impaired. Furthermore, muscle mass is typically decreased in bedridden or only partially ambulatory patients with severe renal dysfunction, leading to a reduced production rate of creatinine and a rise of only about 1 to 2 mg/dL (0.09–0.18 mM) per day in plasma creatinine between hemodialysis treatments, instead of a 3 mg/dL per day rise when renal function is acutely and totally impaired.

TABLE 15-6	Calculated Turnover Time and Half-Life of Creatinine when Renal Function is Decreased	
Renal function (percent of "normal")*	**Turnover time (hr)**	**Half-life (hr)**
100	6	4
50	12	8
33	18	12
25	24	17
20	30	21
10	60	42

*Based on an expected creatinine clearance of 7 L/hr for a 20-year-old, 70-kg man and a creatinine volume of distribution of 0.6 L/kg.

ADJUSTMENT OF DOSAGE REGIMENS

The alternatives for adjustment of maintenance and loading doses in patients with renal function impairment apply, in principle, to all disease conditions in which drug elimination is altered. For no other condition, however, is the required adjustment as readily predicted and assessed.

Maintenance Rate. On the assumption that the pharmacodynamics is unchanged (no change in response at a given Cu), the simplest way of conceiving the adjustment of a maintenance regimen for a patient with renal insufficiency is to maintain the same average unbound concentration at steady state, $Cu_{av,ss}$:

$$F \cdot \frac{D_M}{\tau} = CLu \cdot Cu_{av,ss} \qquad \text{15-15}$$

Rate of administration in renal insufficiency, $\left(\dfrac{D_M}{\tau}\right)_d$, compared with the usual rate of administration to the typical patient, $\left(\dfrac{D_M}{\tau}\right)_t$ is then

$$\frac{\left(\dfrac{D_M}{\tau}\right)_d}{\left(\dfrac{D_M}{\tau}\right)_t} = \frac{CLu(d)}{CLu(t)} \cdot \frac{F(t)}{F(d)} \qquad \text{15-16}$$

where $F(d)$ and $F(t)$ are the bioavailabilities of drug in the patient with renal insufficiency and in the typical patient, respectively. When bioavailability does not change, which appears to be commonly the case, the required rate of administration in a patient with renal dysfunction is

$$\left(\frac{D_M}{\tau}\right)_d = R_d \cdot \left(\frac{D_M}{\tau}\right)_t \qquad \text{15-17}$$

The reduction in dosing rate is therefore seen to depend only on the ratio of unbound clearances, R_d. Associated with the reduction in renal function is a prolongation in half-life, which means that the time to achieve the desired plateau is longer the more severe the impairment of renal function (Eq. 15-10). This last feature is illustrated in Fig. 15-13 for constant-rate administration. In practice, administration is by discrete doses and adjustment of a maintenance regimen may be made by decreasing the frequency of administration, decreasing the maintenance dose, or a combination of both. The outcomes of these approaches are different. To appreciate the differences, consider the adjustment of a usual regimen of amikacin sulfate 7.5 mg/kg injected intramuscularly every 12 hr, to a 23-year-old, 68-kg patient with an estimated creatinine clearance of 12 mL/min.

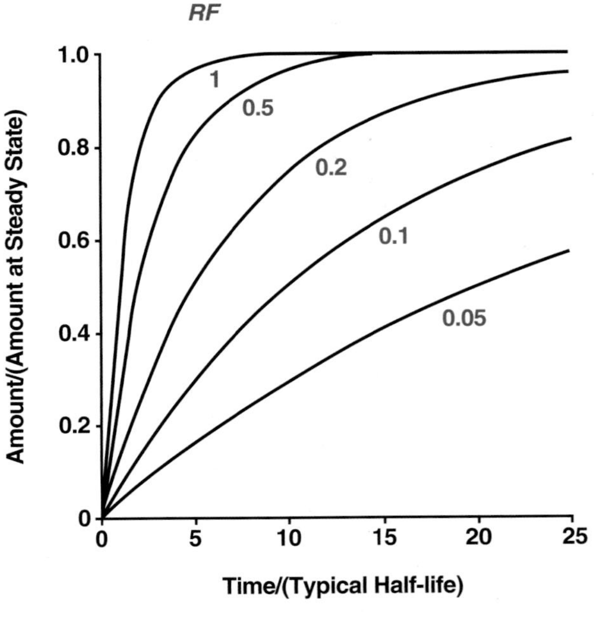

FIGURE 15-13. It takes longer to reach plateau following constant-rate administration of a drug as renal function (*RF*) falls because half-life is correspondingly increased. The effect of renal insufficiency is particularly marked if *fe*(t) = 1, as is the case in this figure. No effect is expected if *fe*(t) = 0. Note that time is expressed in units of half-life for a typical patient.

As the expected creatinine clearance in a typical 60-year-old patient is 70 mL/min, the value of *RF* in the 23-year-old patient is 0.17. Using Eqs. 15-8 and 15-17, it is apparent that the maintenance dosing rate of amikacin sulfate should be decreased by a factor of about six. Thus, the maintenance regimen might be one of the following: (a) dosing interval increased sixfold, regimen: 500 mg (7.5 mg/kg × 68 kg) every 72 hr; (b) the maintenance dose may be reduced by a factor of six, regimen: 83 mg every 12 hr; or (c) both dosing interval and maintenance dose may be adjusted to reduce the average dosing rate sixfold, regimen: 167 mg every 24 hr.

The typical half-life of amikacin is 2 hr, so for the patient under consideration, the half-life is prolonged sixfold to 12 hr (Eq. 15-10). Figure 15-14A is a sketch of the amount in the body with time for the three maintenance regimens considered, given that absorption from the i.m. site is complete and instantaneous. Although both time to reach plateau and average amount in body at plateau are the same for all three regimens, the picture is very different for each one. Clearly, changing the interval to 3 days (dashed line) results in the greatest fluctuation, with many hours at both high and low levels. Changing the maintenance dose (colored line) reduces fluctuation but suffers from the inconvenience of frequent i.m. injections. Finally, changing both maintenance dose and dosing interval (dotted line) reduces both fluctuation and inconvenience to the patient and as such may be preferred for this drug and for many others.

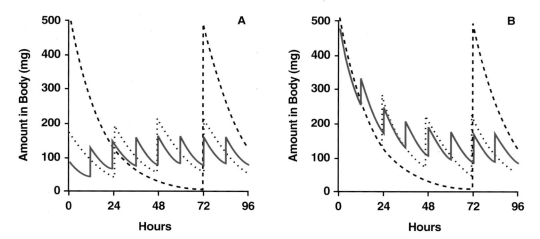

FIGURE 15-14. Sketch of the amount of amikacin sulfate equivalents in the body with time in a patient whose renal function is 17% of the typical value. Shown are regimens without **(A)** and with **(B)** a 500-mg loading dose. The maintenance regimens are: (*dashed heavy black line*)—500 mg every 72 hr; (*colored line*)—83 mg every 12 hr; (*dashed light black line*)—167 mg every 24 hr. Note: i.v. bolus administration is simulated.

In this example with amikacin, administration of the usual dosage regimen to the patient with renal dysfunction at plateau results in a twofold increase in the maximum amount in the body and a sixfold increase in the average amount at plateau (see Fig. 15-6). It is important, however, to consider whether the maximum amount (or concentration) or the average amount is more closely related to efficacy and toxicity of the drug. Only a twofold reduction in the maintenance dose would be required (see also Fig 15-6) if the former were true.

Loading Dose. Particularly large differences in the amount of amikacin in the body exist following the first dose of the three regimens just considered (Fig. 15-14A). With the regimen of 500 mg given every 72 hr to a patient with renal dysfunction, as with the regimen of 500 mg given every 12 hr to a typical patient, there is little accumulation because the dosing interval is much longer than the half-life. Accordingly, effective levels are reached after the first dose. In contrast, appreciable accumulation occurs with the relatively frequent regimens of once every 12 or 24 hr in patients with renal dysfunction. The initial dose is now much less than the average amount in the body at plateau. Under these circumstances, a case may be made for a loading dose. Giving a usual dose of 500 mg can lead to high levels in the body for an extended period after initiating therapy (Fig. 15-14B), which may increase the chance of an adverse effect. A smaller loading dose might be prudent. In the particular case of amikacin, based on experience, a large loading dose, perhaps the usual dose, is often helpful to initiate a therapeutic response at the outset.

GENERAL GUIDELINES AND ADDITIONAL CONSIDERATIONS

Except for drugs with very low therapeutic indices, a reduction of less than 30% in the dosing rate, based on a change in renal function alone, is probably unwarranted for individuals in the usual patient population. Variability in absorption, distribution, and extrarenal elimination is usually at least of this magnitude, and the therapeutic range is often sufficiently large to make adjustment here unnecessary. Consequently, as long as the fraction excreted unchanged in typical patients, $fe(t)$, is 0.30 or less and the metabolites are inactive, no change in a regimen is called for, based on renal function, regardless of the function. Similarly, regardless of the contribution of the renal route, if renal function is 0.70 or more of the typical value, no change is needed (see Eq. 15-7). These concepts are summarized in Fig. 15-9A.

As renal function approaches zero, the importance of nonrenal clearance increases. However, nonrenal clearance usually varies widely within the population, making prediction of the optimal dosage difficult for an individual with marginal renal function. When $fe(t)$ approaches one and RF approaches zero, total clearance is small, and the dosing rate must be drastically reduced. Three particularly difficult problems are encountered here. One is a relatively large change in the chronic maintenance requirements of a drug with only a small change in renal function, (e.g., a change from 0.20–0.05 in renal function reduces the required rate of administration fourfold). The second problem is associated with accuracy of measurement of the contribution of the renal route to drug elimination. A difference in the estimated fe of only 5%, from 1.0 to 0.95, in the scenario above (RF decreased from 0.2 to 0.05) reduces the required dosing rate by 2.5-fold, rather than fourfold. The third relates to the stability of renal function with time. The function may be improving during convalescence or deteriorating with a worsening disease condition. All three problems create uncertainty in predicting dosage requirements under these circumstances.

A further complication in patients with severe renal disease is the concurrent and regular use of a dialysis technique to remove unwanted endogenous toxic substances, which would otherwise accumulate and cause problems. Dialysis sometimes hastens elimination of drugs, complicating drug therapy in these patients, a topic covered subsequently in this chapter.

The foregoing recommended adjustments are based on several assumptions. The method falters when bioavailability changes in renal dysfunction, which is relatively uncommon; when compromised renal function alters the ability to metabolize drug, which obviously occurs when the kidney is an organ of metabolism as well as excretion; or when metabolism or renal excretion exhibits concentration-dependent kinetics, as the relationship between total clearance and renal function then becomes extremely complex. A problem also exists if renal function varies with time, or renal clearance is not directly proportional to the measure of renal function.

Amplifying on the last qualification, regardless of whether the drug is excreted by glomerular filtration or active secretion, renal clearance is assumed to decrease in direct proportion to creatinine clearance. This assumption appears to be valid as a first approximation in chronic renal disease. Para-aminohippuric acid, cephalosporins, and penicillins are examples of actively secreted compounds with renal clearances directly proportional to endogenous creatinine clearance. Finally, interpatient differences in absorption, distribution, metabolism, the response to a given unbound plasma concentration (pharmacodynamics), and concurrent disease states have not been considered. Renal function is only one of several sources of variability. Adjustment of drug administration based on renal function alone must be put into perspective.

Renal disease often affects more than just renal clearance. Furthermore, concurrent diseases may alter dosage requirements. Digoxin distributes much less extensively to tissues in uremia, resulting in a smaller volume of distribution and a shorter half-life than that predicted from loss of renal function. This decreased tissue distribution reduces the loading dose required but has little or no effect on the maintenance dose. However, the presence of severe congestive cardiac failure, a condition for which the drug is used, is associated with decreased hepatic clearance and with a daily maintenance dosage requirement reduced beyond that expected based on renal function impairment alone. The changes in digoxin clearance and volume of distribution with renal function and congestive cardiac failure, obtained from population pharmacokinetic studies, are summarized in Table 15-7.

TABLE 15-7	Estimation of Clearance and Volume of Distribution of Digoxin in Patients with Mild and Severe Congestive Cardiac Failure	
Congestive Cardiac Failure	**Clearance (L/hr per kg)**	**Volume of Distribution (l/kg)**
Mild	CL_{cr}* $+ 0.048^{\dagger}$	$3.8 + 52 \cdot CL_{cr}$
Severe	$0.9 \cdot CL_{cr} + 0.02$	$3.8 + 52 \cdot CL_{cr}$

*CL_{cr}, Creatinine clearance in L/hr/kg.
†Approximation of nonrenal (metabolic) clearance.
From: Sheiner LB, Rosenberg B, Marathe VV. Estimation of population characteristics of pharmacokinetic parameters from routine clinical data. J Pharmacokinet Biopharm 1977;*5*:445–479.

Phenytoin (see Fig. 5-25 in Chapter 5, *Elimination*) and many other acidic drugs are two to three times less well-bound to plasma proteins in uremic than in normal subjects. Part of this change is a result of a decreased concentration of plasma albumin. The mechanism accounting for the rest of the change is uncertain, although displacement by an endogenous compound(s) that accumulates in renal impairment has been suggested. Even so, the unbound values of both clearance and volume of distribution of these principally metabolized drugs remain essentially unchanged, and no change in dosage regimen is anticipated in renal function impairment. The total plasma clearance, however, increases twofold to threefold, giving rise to a corresponding drop in the steady-state plasma concentration on chronic dosing. This change must be carefully considered when interpreting plasma concentrations of these drugs in patients with renal disease.

Another less common, but potential, complication to adjusting drug administration in renal disease is metabolism in the kidney. An example is that of imipenem, an antibiotic that undergoes hydrolysis during excretion by a renal brush border dehydropeptidase. Patients with renal disease have a decreased ability to renally metabolize as well as excrete the drug. The changes in both total and renal clearances are shown in Fig. 15-15 for adult patients with varying degrees of renal function. The expectation, as noted in Fig. 15-8, is that total plasma clearance and renal clearance increase in parallel when nonrenal clearance remains constant. Instead, it is apparent that the difference between them becomes smaller in patients with lower renal function. Here, a component of the

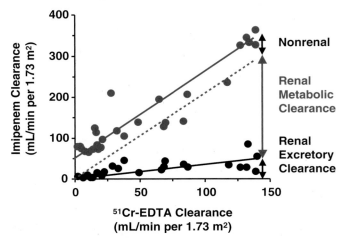

FIGURE 15-15. Total plasma (*colored*) and renal (*black*) clearances of the antibiotic imipenem increase with the renal clearance of ^{51}Cr-ethylenediaminetetraacetic acid (EDTA) (normalized to 1.73 m^2 of body surface area), a marker of glomerular filtration rate. Surprisingly, the two clearances do not increase in parallel as expected (see Fig. 15-7), indicating that the *nonrenal* clearance of the drug must be decreasing with decreased renal function. The explanation is that the drug is metabolized by renal brush border dehydropeptidase and that this activity (renal metabolic clearance) decreases with decreasing renal function. The intercept indicates that some nonrenal elimination must be occurring. (From: Verpooten GA, Verbist L, Buntinx AP, et al. The pharmacokinetics of imipenem (thienamycin-formamidine) and the renal dehydropeptidase inhibitor cilastatin sodium in normal subjects and patients with renal failure. Br J Clin Pharmacol 1984;18:183–193.)

so-called nonrenal clearance occurs in the kidney even though it involves metabolism. Furthermore, the positive intercept value, presumably where no kidney function is present, shows that nonrenal metabolism must occur as well. Many protein drugs with a molecular size less than 30,000 g/mol also fall into this category. They are filtered at the glomerulus and then metabolized within the tubules. This area is expanded upon in Chapter 21, *Protein Drugs*.

The approach to adjusting dosage in renal disease patients has been based on the assumption that metabolism and drug transport in the gut wall, liver, and other organs is unchanged in this disease. In recent years, this assumption has been shown to not hold up well for several drugs. Examples are listed in Table 15-8. The drugs listed were chosen to represent those that are both partially and totally metabolized. This area is relatively new, and there are many questions that remain to be answered, such as, "Are all metabolic pathways similarly affected?"; Is the change predictable?"; "Does renal metabolism account for some of the differences seen?"; and "Are the changes essentially restricted to those patients with severe renal function impairment?" Although generally not greater than a factor of two, the observations to date strongly suggest that even those drugs that are not excreted unchanged should be studied in patients with renal disease.

Perhaps, the *most* common invalid assumption is that metabolites are pharmacologically and toxicologically inactive. For example, the metabolite of morphine, morphine-6-glucuronide, is also active. Prediction of the total activity of the drug and of dosage adjustment needed in end-stage renal disease can be much more complex. Nonetheless, there are ways of treating such situations, as discussed in Chapter 20, *Metabolites and Drug Response*.

In this chapter, so far, approaches have been presented for predicting changes in the clearance of drugs in various disease states and rules for estimating renal clearance of a drug from creatinine clearance or serum creatinine have been given. This kind of

TABLE 15-8	Total, Renal, and Nonrenal Clearances and Half-lives of Selected Drugs in Patients with Normal and Severe Chronic Renal Disease (SCRD)

Drug	fe	Renal Function	CL (L/hr)	CL_R (L/hr)	CL_{NR} (L/hr)	Half-life (hr)
Cervastatin*	0	Normal	22.2	NR[†]	NR	2.3
		SCRD[‡]	13.3	NR	NR	3.4
Bupropion**	0.005	Normal	414	NR	NR	8.1
		SCRD	155	NR	NR	19.4
Telithromycin[††]	0.11	Normal	4.75	0.55	4.20	12.6
		SCRD	3.0	0.16	2.84	14.6
Cyclophosphamide[‡‡]	0.19	Normal	4.74	0.89	3.84	4.8
		SCRD	2.82	0.14	2.68	7.3
Felbamate***	0.30	Normal	2.1	0.63	1.47	19.2
		SCRD	1.05	0.08	0.97	33.9

*From: Vormfelde SV, Muck W, Freudenthaler SM, et al. Pharmacokinetics of cervistatin in renal impairment are predicted by low serum albumin concentration rather than by low creatinine clearance. J Clin Pharmacol 1999;39:147–154.
†Not reported.
‡Severe chronic renal disease (creatinine clearance <30 mL/min).
**From: Terpeinen M, Koivuviita N, Tolonen A, et al. Effect of renal impairment on the pharmacokinetics of bupropion and its metabolites. Br J Clin Pharmacol 2007;64:165–173.
††From: Shi J, Montay G, Chapel S, et al. Pharmacokinetics and safety of the ketolide telithromycin in patients with renal impairment. J Clin Pharmacol 2004;44:234–244.
‡‡From: Haubitz M, Bohnenstrengel F, Brunkhorst R, et al. Cyclophosphamide pharmacokinetics and dose requirements in patients with renal insufficiency. Kidney Int 2002;61:1495–1501.
***From: Glue P, Sulowicz W, Colucci R, et al. Single-dose pharmacokinetics of felbamate in patients with renal dysfunction. Br J Clin Pharmacol 1997;44:91–93.
From: Nolin TD, NaudJ, Leblond FA, Pichette V. Emerging evidence of the impact of kidney disease on drug metabolism and transport. Trans Med 2008;83:898–903.

information is useful for initiating drug therapy in an individual patient, but the variability remaining is often sufficiently large that monitoring of plasma concentration may be prudent, especially for a drug with a narrow therapeutic window and when renal function is very low.

Let us now turn our attention to those patients who have end-stage renal disease (CL_{cr} generally <15 mL/min per 1.73 m^2) and who require dialysis to remove waste products that accumulate in this condition. The most common method of doing so is hemodialysis.

HEMODIALYSIS

Basically, **dialysis** is a process that involves separating diffusible from less diffusible substances by the use of a semipermeable membrane with little or no net movement of fluid across the membrane. When the semipermeable membrane is that of the peritoneal cavity, the dialysis is termed **peritoneal dialysis**. The common dialysis technique, **hemodialysis**, involves passage of blood through a system containing an artificial semipermeable membrane. Because of the large area of membrane required, such a system is, by necessity, outside the body. Accordingly, this method is termed **extracorporeal dialysis**. The dialysis system itself is called a **hemodialyzer** or an **artificial kidney**. One prevalent kind of system used today is the hollow-fiber dialyzer. It contains hundreds of hollow fibers bundled within a compact cylinder. Blood flows through the semipermeable hollow fibers, whereas dialysate fluid flows outside the fibers in a generally countercurrent direction.

These systems are small, efficient, relatively easy to use, and are sometimes reusable. In the following discussion on quantitative procedures, **dialysis** and **dialyzer** are terms used to describe the general method and the apparatus of hemodialysis, respectively.

A typical period of dialysis is 2 to 4 hr. Even shorter times (1–2 hr) are used for the most efficient systems. The actual time required is a compromise between the time needed to adequately remove fluids and metabolic waste products and the comfort and convenience to patients in general. The efficiency of the dialyzer is a major determinant of both.

Various hemodialysis systems are used. The ability of a dialysis system to remove drugs from the body depends on many factors. These include drug characteristics (MW, protein binding, volume of distribution); mechanical properties of the dialysis system (surface area and thickness of membrane, porosity, geometry of the system [e.g., whether blood and dialysate flows are countercurrent or concurrent]); and dialysis conditions (e.g., blood and dialysate flow rates). Because of the various systems and conditions used in literature studies, quantitative extrapolation of data from one study to another may be difficult. Nonetheless, a body of principles applies to all systems and to the removal of both endogenous substances and drugs from the body by them. These principles and considerations of possible adjustment in drug administration in patients undergoing these procedures follow.

DIALYSIS CLEARANCE

As with many other applications of pharmacokinetics, the most useful concept when dealing with dialysis of drugs is clearance. **Dialysis clearance** is a measure of how effectively a dialyzer can remove a drug from blood. It is the rate of removal relative to the concentration in the blood entering the dialyzer. The use of the concentration in blood, rather than in plasma, has an advantage in relating blood clearance to blood flow and in relating rate of removal to rate of presentation to the dialyzer, principles previously developed for hepatic and renal extraction (Chapter 5, *Elimination*).

To appreciate how dialysis clearance is measured, consider the schematic representation of a dialyzer shown in Fig. 15-16. At steady state (i.e., when there is no net change in the amount of drug in the dialyzer), the rate of its removal from blood can be determined in several ways.

Extraction from Blood. One method is by taking the difference between the rates at which the substance enters ($Q_{b,in} \cdot C_{b,in}$) and leaves ($Q_{b,out} \cdot C_{b,out}$) the dialyzer, where $Q_{b,in}$ and $Q_{b,out}$ are the blood flows, and $C_{b,in}$ and $C_{b,out}$ are the concentrations in the arterial blood entering and venous blood leaving the dialyzer.

Dialysis blood clearance, CL_{bD}, is then given by

$$CL_{bD} = \frac{Q_{b,in} \cdot C_{b,in} - Q_{b,out} \cdot C_{b,out}}{C_{b,in}} \qquad 15\text{-}18$$

Dialysis clearance, CL_D, based on drug concentration in plasma entering the dialyzer, C_{in}, can be determined from $CL_D = \dfrac{Q_{bD} \cdot C_{b,in}}{C_{in}}$.

The values of $Q_{b,in}$ and $Q_{b,out}$ are not exactly equal, because there is often a 2- to 3-L loss of fluid during a typical 3- to 4-hr dialysis period. However, this loss is small relative to the volume of blood (~50–100 L) that has passed through the dialyzer. The value of $Q_{b,in}$ is determined accurately with flow sensors. The value of $Q_{b,out}$ is calculated by multiplying $Q_{b,in}$ by the ratio of hematocrit values across the dialyzer.

Rate of Recovery in Dialysate. A second method uses the net rate at which the substance leaves in the dialysate fluid, $Q_{D,out} \cdot C_{D,out} - Q_{D,in} \cdot C_{D,in}$, where $Q_{D,out}$ and $Q_{D,in}$ are

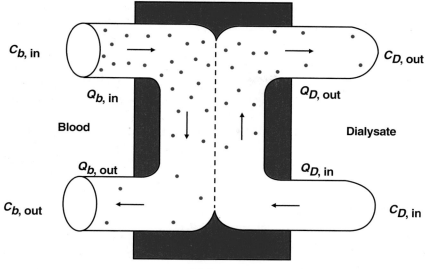

Dialyzer

FIGURE 15-16. Schematic representation of a hemodialysis system in which drug is passively transferred across a semipermeable membrane (---) from blood to dialysate. Drug is delivered to the system at rate $Q_{b,in} \cdot C_{b,in}$ and is returned to the body at rate $Q_{b,out} \cdot C_{b,out}$. The difference between these rates is the net rate of loss into the dialyzing fluid. This rate of removal is the same as the difference between the rates leaving, $Q_{D,out} \cdot C_{D,out}$, and entering, $Q_{D,in} \cdot C_{D,in}$, the dialyzer in the dialysate. Within the dialyzing system, blood and dialysate flows may be essentially concurrent, countercurrent, or crosscurrent, depending on the system design. Flows in the most common dialyzer, hollow fiber, are countercurrent, as shown. $C_{b,in}$; $C_{b,out}$ = drug concentrations in blood entering and leaving dialyzer, respectively. $C_{D,in}$; $C_{D,out}$ = drug concentrations in dialysate entering and leaving dialyzer, respectively. $Q_{b,in}$; $Q_{b,out}$ = blood flows (usually 200–400 mL/min) entering and leaving the dialyzer. $Q_{D,in}$; $Q_{D,out}$ = dialysate flows (usually 300–600 mL/min) entering and leaving the dialyzer.

the dialysate flows leaving and entering the dialyzer, and $C_{D,out}$ and $C_{D,in}$ are the respective concentrations.

$$CL_{bD} = \frac{Q_{D,out} \cdot C_{D,out} - Q_{D,in} \cdot C_{D,in}}{C_{b,in}} \qquad \text{15-19}$$

Loss of water to the dialysate is accounted for here. With the common nonrecirculating (single-pass) dialysis systems, $C_{D,in} = 0$. Equation 15-19 then reduces to

$$CL_{bD} = \frac{Q_{D,out} \cdot C_{D,out}}{C_{b,in}} \qquad \text{15-20}$$

Amount Recovered in Dialysate. A third, and generally the most accurate, method of determining dialysis clearance is to calculate the ratio of amount recovered in the dialysate ($V_D \cdot C_D$) to the area under the arterial blood concentration–time curve, $AUC_{b,in}(0 - \tau)$ within the collection period, τ. That is,

$$CL_{bD} = \frac{V_D \cdot C_D}{AUC_{b,in}(0 - \tau)} \qquad \text{15-21}$$

where V_D is the volume of dialysate collected during the collection interval, and C_D is the drug concentration in the dialysate after mixing. The plasma dialysis clearance is obtained by relating the amount recovered in the dialysate to the area under the plasma concentration–time curve, that is,

$$CL_D = \frac{V_D \cdot C_D}{AUC(0 - \tau)}$$

15-22

Dialysis clearance depends on the dialysis system, the fraction unbound in blood, and the molecular size of the substance. An approximation can be predicted from

$$\frac{Blood\ dialysis}{clearance} = \frac{Dialysis\ clearance}{of\ creatinine} \cdot \sqrt{\frac{113}{MW}} \cdot fu_b$$

     or   15-23

$$\frac{Plasma\ dialysis}{clearance} = \frac{Dialysis\ clearance}{of\ creatinine} \cdot \sqrt{\frac{113}{MW}} \cdot fu$$

where fu_b is the ratio of concentrations in plasma water and whole blood (fu is the fraction unbound in plasma), and MW is the molecular weight of the substance (a measure of molecular size), and 113 is the MW of creatinine.

Because protein binding is often altered in dialysis patients, a more useful parameter than blood or plasma dialysis clearance is

$$\frac{Unbound\ dialysis}{clearance} = \frac{Dialysis\ clearance}{of\ creatinine} \cdot \sqrt{\frac{113}{MW}}$$

15-24

The dialysis clearance of creatinine, a readily dialyzable endogenous compound not bound to plasma proteins, is a means of assessing the capability of a given dialysis system to remove drug from the body. With current dialyzers, dialysis clearance values for creatinine are usually between 80 and 200 mL/min. The unbound dialysis clearance for drugs and most other substances is usually lower than this because their MWs are greater than that of creatinine and, in the case of (total) dialysis clearance, because they are often bound to plasma proteins or blood cells. Adjustment based on the square root of MW recognizes that aqueous diffusion tends to be proportional to the square root of the size of the molecule.

The predictions of dialysis clearance based on concentrations in whole blood, plasma, or plasma water (Eqs. 15-23 and 15-24) tend to be underestimates of the respective clearances of drugs in systems with high flux membranes. This underestimation occurs because the dialysis clearance of creatinine, a low-MW endogenous substance, is limited by and approaches blood flow. The greater the efficiency of the dialyzer, the more this last statement applies. In addition, for drugs with higher MW, the tendency for clearance to be blood-flow limited is less.

There is usually little, if any, correlation of dialysis clearance with either ionization or lipophilicity, because the membranes used are porous rather than lipoidal barriers.

A large range of dialysis clearance values have been observed (Fig. 15-17). Part of this variability is caused by differences in binding of drug to plasma proteins, as shown for CLu_D versus CL_D in Fig. 15-17. MW differences, even though relatively small in the range observed for most drugs, also contribute to this variability, as shown when CLu_D is further adjusted for its molecular size. When both of these sources are accounted for, there is still considerable variability in dialysis clearance, owing, in large part, to the wide range of dialyzers and dialysis conditions used to acquire the information shown. Relating dialysis clearance to that of creatinine for each dialyzer should adjust for more of this remaining variability. In the absence of such information, Eqs. 15-23 and 15-24 can be used but should be treated as rough approximations.

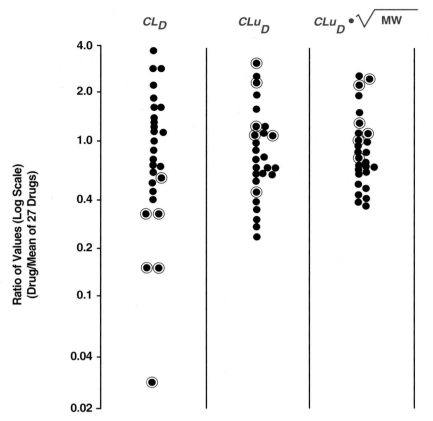

FIGURE 15-17. Plasma dialysis clearance and unbound dialysis clearance with an adjustment for molecular size for 27 different drugs show considerable variability. Variability is greatest for (total) dialysis clearance CL_D. On correcting for protein binding to give unbound dialysis clearance, CLu_D, variability is decreased, and those drugs that are highly bound (◉) are brought into the range of unbound dialysis clearance values of the other drugs. Correction of unbound dialysis clearance with the square root of the molecular weight (MW) appears to diminish variability further, but prediction using both molecular weight and fraction unbound is still not too accurate. Presumably, further adjustment for dialyzer and dialysis conditions by relating dialysis clearance of the drug to that of creatinine should be helpful. The data in this figure were obtained before the advent of systems with greater efficiencies and the use of high-flux membranes. Because the results are expressed relative to the mean of the values obtained, the observations on more recent systems would probably remain similar to those shown here. However, the dispersion of the values because of the different systems may not be as great. For comparative purposes, in each column the value for a drug has been expressed relative to the average value for all 27 drugs on a logarithmic scale. (From: Lee CC, Marbury TC. Drug therapy in patients undergoing haemodialysis: clinical pharmacokinetic considerations. Clin Pharmacokinet 1984;9:42–66.)

EXTRACTION COEFFICIENT

Under steady-state conditions, rate of removal relative to the rate of presentation is a measure of the **efficiency** of a dialysis system. By this definition, efficiency is the dialyzer extraction ratio, or more commonly called the **extraction coefficient**. Its value can be calculated from dialysis blood clearance and blood flow. That is,

$$Extraction\ Coefficient = \frac{CL_{bD}}{Q_{b,in}}$$

15-25

where CL_{bD} is estimated from Eqs. 15-18, 15-19, or 15-21. Dialysis clearance and efficiency are measures of the ability of the dialyzer to remove drug from blood, but they do not indicate how readily it is removed from the body. A measure of the latter is the fraction of drug initially in the body removed by dialysis during a period of treatment. This value is a measure of the **clinical dialyzability** of the drug.

Pharmacokinetic evaluation of hemodialysis and related procedures requires information on the parameters CL_b, CL_{bD}, and V_b (or the corresponding sets of values based on unbound drug or on drug in plasma) and the duration of the procedure. In the following derivation and throughout the remainder of this chapter, the set of parameter values based on measurement of unbound drug is emphasized.

DRUG ELIMINATION

During dialysis, drug is removed by the dialyzer and by the body's own elimination mechanisms, therefore,

$$\textit{Rate of elimination from body during dialysis} = (CLu + CLu_D) \cdot Cu \qquad \text{15-26}$$

If the clearance values are constant with time then, on integration, the unbound concentration at any time t after starting dialysis is

$$Cu = Cu(0) \cdot e^{-k_D \cdot t} \qquad \text{15-27}$$

where $Cu(0)$ is the unbound drug concentration in plasma at the start of dialysis and k_D is the elimination rate constant $[(CLu + CLu_D)/Vu]$ during dialysis. Thus, $e^{-k_D \cdot \tau}$ is the fraction of drug remaining at the end of a dialysis period τ, and so

$$\textit{Fraction lost from body during a dialysis period} = 1 - e^{-k_D \cdot \tau} \qquad \text{15-28}$$

The contribution of dialysis to total drug elimination remains to be determined. Of the total drug eliminated during a dialysis period, the fraction removed by dialysis, f_D, is

$$f_D \quad = \quad \frac{CLu_D}{(CLu + CLu_D)} \qquad \text{15-29}$$

Fraction of total elimination
occurring by dialysis

The fraction of drug in the body at the start of dialysis that is eliminated by the dialysis procedure depends on the fraction of total elimination that dialysis represents, Eq. 15-29, and the fraction of drug lost by all routes of elimination, Eq. 15-28. Therefore,

$$\begin{array}{l} \textit{Fraction of drug initially in} \\ \textit{the body eliminated by dialysis} \end{array} = f_D \cdot (1 - e^{-k_D \cdot \tau}) \qquad \text{15-30}$$

The important parameters, which control f_D and k_D, are CLu, CLu_D, and Vu.

EFFECTIVENESS OF PROCEDURE

Figure 15-18 demonstrates the effectiveness of hemodialysis as a function of unbound (nondialysis) clearance (CLu) and unbound volume of distribution (Vu) for a typical 3-hr dialysis period. An unbound dialysis clearance of 150 mL/min, a common value for drugs with high-flux dialyzers, is used. It is apparent from this figure that hemodialysis is ineffective (<20% of drug initially in body is removed by dialysis treatment) if the unbound volume of distribution is large (>120 L). Also, if CLu is much greater than CLu_D, dialysis becomes less effective in eliminating the drug. When CLu is 400 mL/min or greater, the amount removed by the treatment must be less than 20% (regardless of the value of Vu.

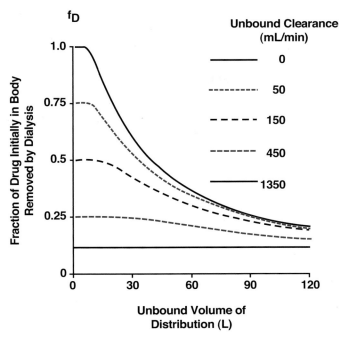

FIGURE 15-18. Displayed is the fraction of drug in the body at the start of dialysis that is eliminated by 3 hr of dialysis treatment as a function of unbound clearance (nondialysis elimination) and unbound volume of distribution. The unbound dialysis clearance is set at 150 mL/min, a common value for drugs in high-flux systems. The y-axis is f_D, the fraction of total elimination occurring by dialysis. Each line represents the expected fraction eliminated at a given unbound clearance as a function of the unbound volume of distribution. Clearly, either a small f_D ($CLu > CLu_D$) or an unbound volume of distribution greater than about 120 L would produce a recovery in the dialysate during a 3-hr dialysis treatment with the high-flux system of less than 20% of the original amount in the body. The unbound volume of distribution has a lower limit, that of the extracellular volume (about 16 L). Only those conditions in which Vu is greater than 16 L therefore apply.

The effectiveness of dialysis may also be evaluated by comparing the half-lives during $(t_{1/2,during})$ and between $(t_{1/2})$ dialysis treatments. During dialysis,

$$t_{1/2}(during) = \frac{0.693 \cdot Vu}{(CLu + CL_D)} \qquad \text{15-31}$$

and between dialysis treatments,

$$t_{1/2} = \frac{0.693 \cdot Vu}{CLu} \qquad \text{15-32}$$

The change in the half-life during dialysis is a function of how much dialysis clearance contributes to the body's own clearance of a drug, that is,

$$\frac{t_{1/2}(during)}{t_{1/2}} = \frac{CLu}{(CLu + CLu_D)} = 1 - f_D \qquad \text{15-33}$$

However, a dramatic reduction in half-life during dialysis does not guarantee that the procedure effectively removes drug during a single-dialysis treatment. Take, for example, phenobarbital in a 70-kg end-stage renal disease patient whose pharmacokinetic parameters are $Vu = 77$ L, $CLu = 0.4$ L/hr, $k = 0.005$ hr^{-1}, and $t_{1/2} = 137$ hr. Using a value of 150 mL/min (9 L/hr) for unbound dialysis clearance, the half-life of phenobarbital is reduced to 5.7 hr during dialysis. Thus, dialysis accounts for 96% of drug elimination (Eq. 15-29); but only

29% (Eq. 15-30) of the drug present in the body at the start of dialysis is removed during a 3-hr dialysis period. Even though the half-life of phenobarbital is decreased 24-fold, the fraction removed in the 3-hr dialysis period is small, because the half-life during dialysis is still considerably longer than the dialysis period.

DRUG ADMINISTRATION TO DIALYSIS PATIENTS

One approach to dosage adjustment is to replace the amount lost in the dialysate during the treatment period. This amount can be calculated from Eq. 15-30, knowing the amount in the body at the start of dialysis, $V \cdot C(0)$. A more appealing approach is to restore the amount in the body at the end of dialysis to the value that would have occurred had the patient not been dialyzed; this procedure permits the patient's existing regimen to be maintained (Fig. 15-19). The amount to be replaced is calculated as follows. The amount remaining in the body at time τ had no dialysis been employed is $V \cdot C(0) \cdot e^{-k \cdot \tau}$; the corresponding amount when dialysis is employed is $V \cdot C(0) \cdot e^{-k \cdot \tau}$. The difference between these two terms provides an estimate of the supplemental dose needed to achieve the objective.

$$Supplemental\ dose = V \cdot C(0) \cdot (e^{-k \cdot \tau} - e^{-k_d \cdot \tau}) \qquad 15\text{-}34$$

This kinetic approach toward dosage adjustment is subsequently illustrated for drugs with properties such as those of gentamicin and phenobarbital.

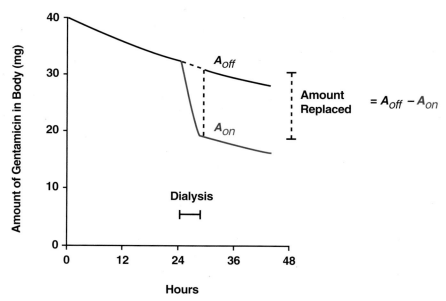

FIGURE 15-19. The dose of gentamicin needed to return the amount in the body at the end of dialysis to the value that would have been present at that time, had the patient not been dialyzed, is the difference between the amounts in the body at the end of the interval in the absence (A_{off}) and presence (A_{on}) of dialysis. The replacement dose (12 mg) in this example of an anephric patient is close to the amount in the dialysate because little has been lost by the body's own mechanisms during the dialysis interval.

The pharmacokinetic parameters of gentamicin in the typical 60-year-old, 75-kg patient are: $CL = 4.2$ L/hr, $V = 16$ L, $t_{1/2} = 2.6$ hr, and $fe > 0.95$. As fe is greater than 0.95 and probably close to 1.0, the kinetics of this drug are drastically altered in a patient without renal function. From the relationship $\dfrac{t_{1/2}(d)}{t_{1/2}(t)} = \dfrac{Vu(d)}{Vu(t)} \cdot \dfrac{1}{R_d}$ (Eq. 15-10), and given that $Vu(d) = Vu(t)$, the half-life of this drug in anephric patients is greater than 40 hr.

Needless to say, administration of this drug to an anephric patient requires extreme caution. For purposes of the example below, assume a half-life of 72 hr in an anephric patient on gentamicin alone. This half-life corresponds to a clearance of 2.4 mL/min; the rate of administration to maintain the same average steady-state concentration should therefore be 30 times less than usual. A common regimen of gentamicin for a patient with normal renal function is 350 mg (5 mg/kg), intramuscularly or intravenously, once daily; the initial dose and the maintenance doses are the same. But a strong argument exists for a larger initial dose than maintenance dose for an anephric patient. Accordingly, a recommendation for an anephric patient might be a 175- to 350-mg loading dose followed by 12 mg every other day. The loading dose alone may suffice.

The expected amount in the body with time following this recommended regimen, in the absence of dialysis, is shown as Curve A in Fig. 15-20. The anephric patient is dialyzed for 4 hr on days 2, 4, and 6 between doses on days 1, 3, and 5. Consideration of a supplementary dose requires an estimate of the fraction lost in the dialysate during each treatment period. The dialysis clearance of gentamicin, a drug not bound in plasma, in a common dialyzer is 30 mL/min. The combined clearance in this patient is therefore 32.4 mL/min. The corresponding elimination rate constant, k_D, is 0.13 hr^{-1} ($t_{1/2} = 5.3$ hr). Using Eq. 15-29, the fraction lost during a 4-hr dialysis period is 0.4.

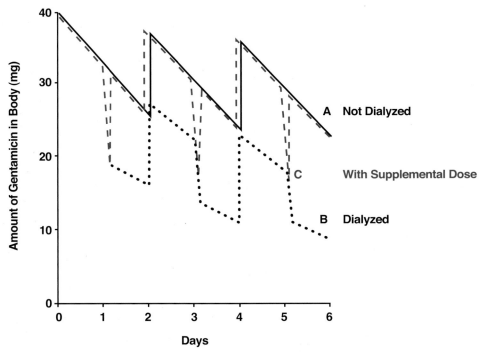

FIGURE 15-20. Sketch of amount of gentamicin in the body with time in an anephric patient on an i.m. dosage regimen of 40 mg initially and 12 mg every other day. Curve A (——)—patient not dialyzed. Curve B (·····)—patient undergoing dialysis (for 4 hr) on Days 2, 4, and 6. Curve C (-----)—patient undergoing dialysis is given a supplementary dose of 12 mg just after each dialysis period. A one-compartment model with instantaneous absorption is used.

Thus, hemodialysis every 2 or 3 days would result (1 week later) in very little gentamicin being in the anephric patient (Curve B, Fig. 15-20) if the suggested regimen above were not adjusted. Clearly, a supplementary dose at the end of each dialysis period is warranted.

The supplementary dose should be sufficient to return the amount in the body to the value that would have occurred had the patient not been dialyzed, the condition simulated in Curve C of Fig. 15-20. The amount continues to decline with dialysis every other day after a loading dose of 40 mg. The amount in the body at the time of the first dialysis on Day 2 $(40 \times e^{-0.693 \times 24/72})$ is 32 mg. The supplementary dose is then 12 mg (Eq. 15-34).

For a drug that is readily dialyzed and is required by the patient at all times, consideration might be given to administering it during dialysis treatment. Another approach is to use a therapeutic (unbound) concentration of the drug in the dialysate. Although theoretically more logical, the latter approach may be very expensive. The total volume used is 144 L when a typical dialysate flow rate of 600 mL/min is continued for 4 hr. For gentamicin, a therapeutic concentration of 2 mg/L in the dialysate would therefore require the addition of almost 300 mg. If the drug is an antibiotic, one might argue that doing this would help to prevent infection.

Although only about 29% of phenobarbital initially present was previously calculated to be removed in a single 3-hr session with a high-flux dialysis system, the steady-state phenobarbital concentration may be considerably reduced during repeated sessions. The amount of phenobarbital in a patient who has a half-life of 5.5 days and a volume of distribution of 38 L is decreased by 12% $(1 - e^{-\frac{CL \cdot \tau}{V}})$ during the dosing interval (1 day). The additional loss of 29% every other day (on dialysis) would more than double the average percent lost (12% per day between dialysis treatments and about 40% on dialysis day). In this patient, the dosage would have to be doubled to keep the same average amount in the body at steady state. Clearly, the effect of dialysis should also be examined at steady state, the therapeutically relevant situation for phenobarbital.

PERITONEAL DIALYSIS

Peritoneal dialysis is accomplished by introducing dialyzing fluid into the peritoneal cavity via a catheter. After a period, the **dwell time**, the fluid is drained and discarded. Although several chronic peritoneal dialysis procedures have been used clinically, the one that has become the most common is **continuous ambulatory peritoneal dialysis** (CAPD). The subsequent discussion is restricted to this dialysis modality.

DIALYSIS CLEARANCE

In CAPD, dialysis clearance, CL_{PD}, is most frequently expressed as the amount of a drug or substance recovered in the drained dialysate relative to the plasma AUC during the dwell time, τ, after administration by any route, $AUC(0 - \tau)$. Analogous to Eq. 15-22 and with the subscript PC meaning peritoneal cavity,

$$CL_{PD} = \frac{C_{PC} \cdot V_{PC}}{AUC(0 - \tau)}$$

15-35

where V_{PC} is the dialysate volume in the peritoneal cavity. The plasma and dialysate concentrations of the cephalosporin, cefsulodin, during a commonly employed 5-hr dwell time, after i.v. and intraperitoneal (i.p.) administrations are shown in Fig. 15-21. At the end of the dwell time, the peritoneal concentration approaches that of plasma after i.v. administration, and the plasma concentration approaches that of dialysate after i.p. administration. Clearance, obtained by Eq. 15-35, then reflects the net movement of the drug during the dwell time. This clearance term is not strictly a measure of the ability of a drug to pass from blood into the peritoneal cavity as its value decreases with dwell time. This situation is in contrast to the clearance term for nonrecirculating hemodialysis for which sink conditions are maintained. A unidirectional measure can be obtained for peritoneal dialysis if the dialysate is exchanged at sufficient frequency to ensure that sink conditions are approximated.

The unbound (peritoneal) dialysis clearance value for most drugs lies between 2 and 7 mL/min. The reason for this low value can be explained as follows. There is negligible protein in the dialysate fluid (1–2 g/2 L, relative to that in plasma, 86 g/2L) at the end of the

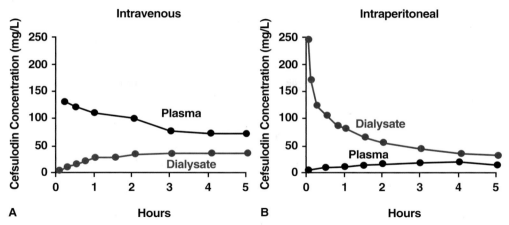

FIGURE 15-21. The plasma (●) and dialysate (●) concentrations of cefsulodin, a cephalosporin antibiotic that is virtually unbound in plasma, after i.v. administration **(A)** and i.p. administration **(B)** to a patient with end-stage renal disease tend to approach an equilibrium within a 5-hr dialysate dwell time. The concentration in plasma after i.v. administration does not decline much because of the patient's renal disease and because the amount distributing into the 2-L dialysate volume from the 16-L extracellular fluid volume of distribution is small. In contrast, the concentration in the dialysate drops dramatically as it distributes from the 2-L volume into the 16-L volume. (From: Brouard R, Tozer TN, Merdjan H, et al. Transperitoneal movement and pharmacokinetics of cefotiam and cefsulodin in patients on continuous ambulatory peritoneal dialysis. Clin Nephrol 1988;30:197–206.)

dwell time. Consequently, when equilibrium is achieved ($C_{PC} = Cu$), the amount in the dialysate is $Cu \cdot V_{PC}$, where Cu is the unbound concentration in plasma and C_{PC} is the unbound concentration in dialysate. If the plasma concentration is constant with time, then the unbound AUC is $Cu \cdot \tau$. Thus, the unbound dialysis clearance value is $Cu \cdot V_{PC}/Cu \cdot \tau$ or V_{PC}/τ. With a usual dialysate volume of 2000 mL and a τ of 300 min, the net clearance value is 6.7 mL/min. This low clearance means that drug elimination by peritoneal dialysis is not a major consideration for patients on CAPD. When CAPD is the only route of elimination and drug is distributed in extracellular fluids (0.25 L/kg or 17,500 mL/70 kg, the smallest volume possible for unbound drug), the half-life is then 1810 min ($t_{1/2} = 0.693 \times$ 17,500 mL/6.7 mL/min) or 1.26 days. Other routes of elimination or therapeutic maneuvers to remove drug are generally of greater importance than CAPD.

Dialysis clearance values for other dialysis methods (e.g., intermittent peritoneal dialysis and continuous cycling peritoneal dialysis) can be 10 to 40 mL/min, values much greater than those for CAPD, because sink conditions tend to be maintained when using short dwell times. For this reason, removal of a significant fraction of drug in the body can occur during a treatment period just as with hemodialysis, but dialysis is then not continuous. The methods of analysis and prediction of drug removal are the same, except that the intermittent nature of the modality must be incorporated.

ROUTE OF ADMINISTRATION

Although little drug is lost into the peritoneal cavity during CAPD after parenteral administration, most (>60%) of a dose administered into the peritoneal cavity is absorbed into the body during a typical 3- to 6-hr dwell time. Because of the continuous nature of CAPD, this route of administration has a potential application for systemic purposes, especially for drugs that cannot be absorbed when taken orally because of poor intestinal permeability, as is the case for many antibiotics. Dwell time becomes particularly important here as a determinant of systemic bioavailability. Not all the drug instilled into the cavity reaches the systemic circulation. This is shown in Fig. 15-22 for teicoplanin, a

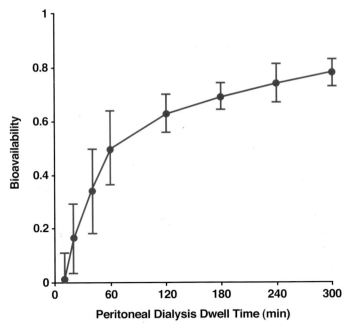

FIGURE 15-22. Relationship between systemic bioavailability (mean ± SD of five patients) and dwell time when teicoplanin is administered intraperitoneally. Two liters of peritoneal dialysis solution were instilled into the peritoneal cavity for 5 hr in patients undergoing continuous ambulatory peritoneal dialysis. Bioavailability was calculated by comparison of *AUC* values following single intraperitoneal and intravenous doses as well as from the amount of drug remaining within the peritoneal cavity with time. At 5 hr (300 min), the bioavailability was about 0.78 by both methods. The coefficient of variation (SD/mean) was much greater at early than at late times. Longer dwell times therefore give more complete and less variable bioavailability. (From: Brouard RJ, Kapusnik JE, Gambertoglio JG, et al. Teicoplanin pharmacokinetics and bioavailability during peritoneal dialysis. Clin Pharmacol Ther 1989;45:674–681, with permission.)

glycopeptide antibiotic. Bioavailability increases with dwell time and is about 78% at 5 hr. The data also indicate a much greater coefficient of variation in bioavailability at earlier times. Thus, to ensure consistent absorption, a short dwell time is not recommended.

Peritonitis has been a major issue in CAPD. A major question here is whether direct administration of an antibiotic into the peritoneal cavity to treat peritonitis might be more effective than systemic administration. Although i.p. administration would appear to be superior, drug may be delivered to the site of infection more readily via the capillaries than through the peritoneum. In some situations, a combination of both i.p. and other routes of administration may be advantageous.

DIALYSIS IN DRUG OVERDOSE

Assessment of the contribution of hemodialysis or hemoperfusion (where blood is passed by an absorbent, often charcoal) to the reduction of the morbidity and mortality of drug intoxication is facilitated by quantitative information on drug removal. Measurement of the amount of drug in the dialysate or on the absorbent alone is inadequate. For example, a recovery of 2 g may be unimportant if more than 20 g were in the body at the start of the procedure. Information on the fraction of the amount initially in the body that is eliminated by the procedure is needed.

Several factors associated with the overdosed patient may affect the pharmacokinetics of a drug (e.g., anoxia, metabolic acidosis, carbon dioxide retention, hypotension, depressed renal function, and hypothermia). Furthermore, complications may arise because of slow tissue distribution of a drug (Chapter 19, *Distribution Kinetics*) and because of the concentrations of drug and active metabolites attained (Chapter 20, *Metabolites and Drug Response*). Brief comments on a few of these complications are in order here.

TOXIC METABOLITES

Little correlation may exist between the drug concentration and the patient's clinical status for drugs for which a metabolite is primarily responsible for toxicity. Clinical response is then expected to be more closely related to the concentration of the metabolite. The removal of active metabolite, as well as unchanged drug, should be considered. Often, there is a paucity of information of this nature.

OTHER CONSIDERATIONS

Determination of the overall benefit-to-risk ratio of hemodialysis or hemoperfusion requires weighing of many factors. The severity of the poisoning, the value of other procedures such as forced diuresis (Chapter 5, *Elimination*), control of urine pH, and the risks of the procedure to the patient, in addition to other clinical variables must all be considered.

KEY RELATIONSHIPS

$$R_d = \frac{CL_u(d)}{CL_u(t)} = RF \cdot fe(t) + [1 - fe(t)] \cdot \frac{(140 - Age) \cdot Wt(d)^{0.75}}{1936}$$

$$R_d = RF \cdot fe(t) + 1 - fe(t)$$

$$\frac{t_{1/2}(d)}{t_{1/2}(t)} = \frac{Vu(d)}{Vu(t)} \cdot \frac{1}{R_d}$$

$$Serum\ Creatinine = \frac{Rate\ of\ creatinine\ production}{Creatinine\ clearance}$$

$$RF = \frac{CL_{cr}(d)}{CL_{cr}(t)} = \frac{CLu_R(d)}{CLu_R(t)}$$

$$\left(\frac{D_M}{\tau}\right)_d = R_d \cdot \left(\frac{D_M}{\tau}\right)_t$$

$$CL_{bD} = \frac{Q_{b,in} \cdot C_{b,in} - Q_{b,out} \cdot C_{b,out}}{C_{b,in}}$$

$$CL_{bD} = \frac{Q_{D,out} \cdot C_{D,out} - Q_{D,in} \cdot C_{D,in}}{C_{b,in}}$$

$$CL_D = \frac{V_D \cdot C_D}{AUC(0 - \tau)}$$

Fraction lost from body during a dialysis period $= 1 - e^{-k_D \cdot \tau}$

$$f_D = \frac{CLu_D}{(CLu + CLu_D)}$$

Fraction of total elimination occurring by dialysis

$$\frac{\text{Blood dialysis}}{\text{clearance}} = \frac{\text{Dialysis clearance}}{\text{of creatinine}} \cdot \sqrt{\frac{113}{MW}} \cdot fu_b$$

or

$$\frac{\text{Plasma dialysis}}{\text{clearance}} = \frac{\text{Dialysis clearance}}{\text{of creatinine}} \cdot \sqrt{\frac{113}{MW}} \cdot fu$$

$$\frac{\text{Unbound dialysis}}{\text{clearance}} = \frac{\text{Dialysis clearance}}{\text{of creatinine}} \cdot \sqrt{\frac{113}{MW}}$$

$$\text{Extraction Coefficient} = \frac{CL_{bD}}{Q_{b,in}}$$

$$\frac{\text{Fraction of drug initially in}}{\text{the body eliminated be dialysis}} = f_D \cdot (1 - e^{-k_D \cdot \tau})$$

$$\frac{t_{1/2}(during)}{t_{1/2}} = \frac{CLu}{(CLu + CLu_D)} = 1 - f_D$$

$$\text{Supplemental dose} = V \cdot C(0) \cdot (e^{-k \cdot \tau} - e^{-k_D \cdot \tau})$$

STUDY PROBLEMS

(Answers to Study Problems are in Appendix J.)

1. a. Briefly discuss the administration of drugs, in general, to patients with diseases of either the liver or the cardiovascular system.

   b. Define dialysis, extracorporeal dialysis, hemodialysis, continuous ambulatory peritoneal dialysis, dialysis clearance, dialyzer, dialyzer efficiency, and clinical dialyzability of a drug.

2. a. Rank the situations in Table 15-9, from most important to least important, for considering a change in a dosage regimen of the cephalosporins listed in adult patients with varying degrees of renal function. Given that all these drugs have comparable therapeutic indices, use anticipated change in clearance as the basis of your ranking.

   b. Name the situations in Table 15-9 for which you would recommend that consideration be given to a change in the usual dosage regimen.

TABLE 15-9	Percent Excreted Unchanged and Renal Function for Selected Drugs and Patients		
Situation	**Drug**	**Percent of Dose Normally Excreted Unchanged ($fe(f)$)**	**Renal Function (percent of typical patient)**
A	Ceftizoxime	28	10
B	Cefonicid	98	5
C	Cefamandole	96	40
D	Ceforanide	80	20
E	Ceftazidime	84	60

3. Table 15-10 summarizes pharmacokinetic observations of two different opioid analgesics in patients with and without hepatic cirrhosis.

   a. Knowing that pentazocine and meperidine are eliminated primarily by hepatic metabolism, suggest a mechanism to explain the altered kinetics in hepatic cirrhosis.

   b. Explain why the oral bioavailability of pentazocine is affected much more than that of meperidine.

TABLE 15-10	Oral Bioavailability and Blood Clearance of Pentazocine and Meperidine in Control Groups and Cirrhotic Patients			
	Pentazocine		Meperidine	
	Control	Cirrhotic	Control	Cirrhotic
Oral bioavailability*	0.18	0.68	0.48	0.87
Blood clearance† (L/min)	1.25	0.68	0.90	0.57

*From ratio of *AUC* values after oral and i.v. administrations on separate occasions.
†From dose/AUC_b after an i.v. dose.
From: Neal EA, Meffin PJ, Gregory PB, Blaschke TF. Enhanced bioavailability and decreased clearance of analgesics in patients with cirrhosis. Gastroenterology 1979;77:96–102. Mean values are listed.

4. In Table 15-11, various data on four patients with varying degrees of renal function are listed. None of them is undergoing a dialysis procedure.

   a. Estimate the creatinine clearance in each of these individuals.

   b. Calculate the renal function in each of these patients. Express renal function as a ratio of creatinine clearance in the patient to the value expected in a typical 60-year-old, 70-kg patient.

TABLE 15-11	Demographic Data of 4 Patients			
Patient	SW*	BJ	DA	BT
Gender	M	F	F	M
Age (years)	25	82	3	15
Weight (kg)	84	60	15	68
Height (cm)	182	160	96	169
Serum creatinine (mg/dL)	1.0	2.5	1.6	3.0

*Identification of specific patient.

5. a. For each of the 4 patients listed below, estimate his/her creatinine clearance from the information given. For three of the patients, the calculated value is likely to be different from the true value (purposefully so). For them, state whether you think the calculated value is likely to be an overestimate or underestimate of the true value and why you think so.

   b. Determine the body mass index of each of the 3 adult patients.

   Patient I. Mr. DT is a 29-year-old, 85-kg, 175-cm tall construction worker who is admitted to the hospital with a high fever and a severe headache that developed after an afternoon workout in the gym to which he regularly goes. His serum creatinine is found to be 3.1 mg/dL.

Patient II. Mrs. PF is an 84-year-old, 52-kg, 168-cm tall patient who has been bedridden (in the hospital or in an assisted living facility) for several months because of several fractures of her arm, leg, and hip bones. Her serum creatinine is 1.2 mg/dL.

Patient III. LB is a 3-year-old, 95-cm tall, 17-kg boy who is being examined during a routine yearly checkup. His serum creatinine is 0.40 mg/dL. Also compare your value with the value you would estimate for a typical 3-year-old using the surface area rule (CL_{cr}[child] $= CL_{cr}$ [20-year-old] $\times$ [Wt./70]$^{0.75}$).

Patient IV. Mrs. TS is a 49-year-old, 105-kg, 165-cm tall woman with diabetes. Her serum creatinine was found to be 1.8 mg/dL.

6. Vancomycin is chosen for the therapy of a 17-kg, 4-year-old, 108-cm tall boy with staphylococcal pneumonia, which is refractory to other antibiotics. The child has impaired renal function as indicated by a serum creatinine of 2.7 mg/dL. Approximately 95% of a dose of vancomycin is normally excreted unchanged. Its half-life and volume of distribution are 6 hr and 0.4 L/kg, respectively, in a typical 60-year-old patient.

    a. Estimate the maximum and minimum steady-state concentrations associated with therapy in a typical 60-year-old 70-kg patient who receives a 1000-mg i.v. bolus dose every 12 hr.

    b. Determine a dosage regimen for the 4-year-old patient to attain and maintain the amount (or concentration) within the limits you derived in "a" above to minimize the likelihood of the child developing ototoxicity and a further decrease in renal function, both toxic manifestations of excessively high concentrations of vancomycin.

    c. Prepare sketches of the anticipated amount of vancomycin in the body with time had the usual maintenance dose been adjusted for:
    (1) The child's age and weight only (no adjustment for renal disease).
    (2) The child's age, weight, and renal function.
    No loading dose is given in either situation.

7. The kinetics of pentoxifylline, a hemorrheologic agent prescribed for the treatment of peripheral arterial disease and intermittent claudication, is affected by cirrhosis. Table 15-12 shows the changes in half-life and *AUC* following i.v. and oral (modified-release tablet) administrations. Less than 1% is excreted unchanged in the urine. For the purpose of this problem, use only mean values.

    a. Determine differences in pentoxifylline kinetic parameter values between healthy subjects and cirrhotic patients with respect to the following:
    (1) Absorption
    (2) Distribution
    (3) Elimination

    b. Briefly discuss how hepatic cirrhosis is likely to produce the changes calculated for the absorption, distribution, and elimination parameters of this drug.

TABLE 15-12   Half-Life and *AUC* of Pentoxifylline in Healthy Subjects and Cirrhotic Patients

	Healthy Subjects		Cirrhotic Patients	
	Half-life (hr)	*AUC* (mg-hr/L)	Half-Life (hr)	*AUC* (mg-hr/L)
i.v. dose (100 mg)	0.8 ± 0.3	0.41 ± 0.08	2.1 ± 1.2	1.14 ± 0.15
Oral dose (400 mg) (modified-release tablet)	—	0.52 ± 0.17	—	3.36 ± 1.76

From: Rames A, Poirier JM, LeCoz F, et al. Pharmacokinetics of intravenous and oral pentoxifylline in healthy volunteers and in cirrhotic patients. Clin Pharmacol Ther 1990;47:354–358.

8. The pharmacokinetics of lorazepam, a benzodiazepine with demonstrated efficacy as an anxiolytic, anticonvulsant, antiemetic, and sedative hypnotic, was studied in patients with spinal cord injury. The drug (2-mg dose) was given as a single short-term (1–2 min) i.v. infusion. The results of the study in tetraplegics, paraplegics, and controls are summarized in Table 15-13. The drug is bound to albumin ($fu = 0.09$).

TABLE 15-13	Lorazepam Pharmacokinetic Parameters in Patients with Spinal Cord Injury and in Controls		
Subjects	CL (mL/min/m²)	V (L/kg)	$t_{1/2}$ (hr)
Tetraplegic (n = 9)	26 ± 6	1.6 ± 0.4	31 ± 13
Paraplegic (n = 6)	37 ± 11	1.6 ± 0.5	25 ± 9
Controls (n = 9)	42 ± 19	1.5 ± 0.5	20 ± 12

From: Segal JL, Brunnemann SR, Eltorai IM, et al. Decreased systemic clearance of lorazepam in humans with spinal cord injury. J Clin Pharmacol 1991;31:651–656.

a. When given orally, the bioavailability of lorazepam is 90%. Using the kinetic data in Table 15-13 and assuming instantaneous absorption, calculate the mean peak and trough concentrations expected on orally administering 2 mg twice daily (every 12 hr), a typical regimen for treatment of anxiety, in the tetraplegic and able-bodied (no spinal injury) patients. Use an average weight of 70 kg and $F = 0.9$ for all subjects.

b. Lorazepam is primarily eliminated by hepatic glucuronidation; the conjugate is extensively secreted into the bile. Discuss each of the following mechanisms as a possible explanation for the decreased clearance of lorazepam in patients with spinal cord injury.
   (1) Decreased hepatic blood flow.
   (2) Decreased hepatocellular metabolic activity.
   (3) Enterohepatic cycling of drug through its glucuronide with less loss of drug or metabolite in feces.
   (4) Increased binding to plasma proteins.

9. Phenytoin, an antiepileptic drug, is extensively bound to serum albumin ($fu = 0.1$ in the typical patient) and is eliminated by hepatic metabolism. The therapeutic window typically observed for the drug is about 10 to 20 mg/L. In a patient with renal disease, protein binding in plasma is greatly reduced (fu about 0.25). On the assumption that responses (beneficial and harmful) are related to the unbound concentration, what is the therapeutic window of plasma concentrations for the drug in this patient?

10. In a study of the removal of phenytoin by hemodialysis (Adapted from Martin E, Gambertoglio JG, Adler DS, et al. Removal of phenytoin by hemodialysis in uremic patients. JAMA 1977;238:1750–1753), the following data were obtained in one of the subjects. Sodium phenytoin (350 mg of acid form of drug) was administered intravenously over 30 min, 2 hr before hemodialysis treatment. The average blood and dialysate flows through the dialyzer were 305 and 267 mL/min, respectively. The plasma phenytoin concentration dropped from 3.9 to 3.5 mg/L during the 6-hr dialysis treatment. The fraction unbound was 0.21, and the amount of phenytoin collected in the 6-hr dialysate was 14 mg. The dialysis clearance of creatinine was 83 mL/min. The concentrations in blood and plasma were virtually identical.

a. Calculate the dialysis clearance of phenytoin.
b. What is the efficiency (extraction coefficient) of the dialyzer used?
c. The blood concentrations into and out of the dialyzer could have been used to determine dialysis clearance. If they had been used, what would the ratio (out/in)

have been to give the clearance observed in "a"? Assume no net loss of fluid from the body into the dialysate. Do you think clearance could have been determined accurately from the blood concentrations into and out of the dialyzer?

    d. Calculate the fraction of drug initially in the body that is eliminated by dialysis.

    e. Is the observed dialysis clearance of phenytoin (MW = 252 g/mol) close to the value predicted by Eq. 15-24 in the text?

11. a. Complete Table 15-14 by estimating unbound and total dialysis clearance values, the ratio of half-lives between and during dialysis treatments, and the half-life between dialysis treatments for each of the three drugs listed. Use a creatinine dialysis clearance of 150 mL/min and a one-compartment model.

TABLE 15-14	Pharmacokinetic Information and Estimated Unbound Dialysis Clearances and Half-Life Ratios (During/Between Dialysis Treatments) During Hemodialysis of Specific Patients With End-Stage Renal Disease

	V (L)	fu	CL (L/hr)	Unbound Dialysis Clearance (L/hr)	Dialysis Clearance (L/hr)	$\left(\dfrac{t_{1/2}}{t_{1/2,during}}\right)$	$t_{1/2}$ (hr)
S-Naproxen (MW = 230 g/mol)	11	0.003	0.55				
Tobramycin (MW = 468 g/mol)	23	0.95	0.3				
Verapamil (MW = 455 g/mol)	350	0.10	105				

    b. Using Eq. 15-30, assess the *clinical dialyzability* of the three compounds listed in Table 15-14 using a 4-hr dialysis treatment. For any drug of questionable dialyzability, briefly discuss the one kinetic property that is most likely responsible for its being a poor candidate for removal by dialysis.

12. The data in Table 15-15 on vancomycin were acquired in patients receiving CAPD treatment. Vancomycin was given intravenously and intraperitoneally in doses of 10 mg/kg on separate occasions. The first dwell time after vancomycin administration was 4 hr. Two additional 4-hr exchanges and an overnight 12-hr dwell time were used.

    a. The authors claim that the value of vancomycin peritoneal dialysis clearance, calculated after i.p. instillation, differs from that after i.v. administration. Do you agree? Defend your answer.

TABLE 15-15	Vancomycin Clearance and Peritoneal Clearance Values After i.v. and i.p. Administration	
Route of Administration	**Clearance* (mL/min)**	**Peritoneal Dialysis Clearance (mL/min)**
Intravenous	9	1.5[†]
Intraperitoneal instillation	15	2.5[‡]

*Includes peritoneal dialysis clearance. Calculated from *Dose/AUC*.
[†]Amount in dialysate between 0 and 72 hr divided by *AUC* within the same interval.
[‡]Amount in dialysate between 4 and 72 hr divided by *AUC* within the same interval.
From: Bunke CM, Aronoff GR, Brier ME, et al. Vancomycin kinetics during continuous ambulatory peritoneal dialysis. Clin Pharmacol Ther 1983;34:631–637.

    b. Can you explain the differences observed in the estimates of clearance from the two routes of administration?

13. With the introduction of membranes with high MW cut-off values, high dialysis clearances of relatively large molecules became possible. Vancomycin (MW = 1448 g/mol) is an example of a drug that had been shown to be essentially nondialyzable with previous conventional membranes. Böhler et al. examined the dialyzability of vancomycin with high-flux, high MW cutoff membranes. Table 15-16 lists the plasma concentrations of vancomycin with time in one patient following i.v. infusion of 1 g over 1 hr. Blood samples were taken at the times (after end of infusion) indicated.

    a. Prepare a semilogarithmic plot of the data.

    b. What is the half-life of vancomycin during dialysis?

    c. Vancomycin is usually given only once a week to hemodialysis patients. Maintenance of a plasma concentration above 5 mg/L is desired. Does dialysis 3 times a week with the dialyzer used appear to suggest the need for additional doses of vancomycin?

    d. This patient was dialyzed using a blood flow of about 125 mL/min. Would you expect the removal of vancomycin to be increased if the blood flow to the dialyzer were increased to 220 mL/min, a value used for other patients in the study? Focus your answer on the apparent distribution of the drug.

TABLE 15-16	Plasma Vancomycin Concentration at Various Times Over 1 Week in a Patient Who Received an Intravenous Infusion of 1 g over 1 hr and Who Was Hemodialyzed on Days 3, 5, and 7
Time (hr)	**Vancomycin Concentration (mg/L)**
0.17	43.0
1.0	31.3
4.0	22.0
6.0	18.7
24	12.5
66*	10.0
66.5	8.65
67.5	8.02
70	6.40
71	8.01
73	8.50
76	8.74
110*	7.33
114	5.22
120	6.72
158*	5.64
162	3.74
167	4.75

*Periods of hemodialysis: 66–70 hr, 110–114 hr, and 158–162 hr.

From: Böhler J, Reetze-Bonorden P, Keller E, et al. Rebound of plasma vancomycin levels after hemodialysis with highly permeable membranes. Br J Clin Pharmacol 1992;42:635–640.

14. Cefprozil, a broad-spectrum oral cephalosporin antibiotic, is composed of cis and trans geometric isomers in an approximate ratio of 9:1. Both isomers are primarily excreted unchanged in urine in patients with normal renal function. Table 15-17 lists selected pharmacokinetic parameters of the cis isomer after a 1000-mg single oral dose of the mixture in subjects with varying degrees of renal function, including a group (Group V) undergoing intermittent hemodialysis. The kinetic behavior of the trans isomer was virtually identical to that of the cis. Hemodialysis was performed with (what appears to be) a high-flux dialyzer for 3 hr approximately 18 hr after administration of the drug. The half-life during dialysis was 2.05 hr. The average amount of the mixture recovered in the 3-hr dialysate was 30 mg, during which time the AUC was 5.75 mg-hr/L.

| **TABLE 15-17** | **Mean Pharmacokinetic Parameters and Observations of the Cis Isomer of Cefprozil After a Single 1000-mg Oral Dose in Patients With Varying Degrees of Renal Function** | | | | |

	Group				
	I	**II**	**III**	**IV**	**V**
Creatinine clearance (mL/min)	>90	61–90	31–60	<31	Hemodialysis*
Parameter/observation	13.3[†]	16.1	22.6	30.4	36.7
	(1.61)	(3.1)	(2.4)	(9.5)	(6.2)
t_{max} (hr)	2.1	1.8	2.7	3.7	4.0
	(0.7)	(0.3)	(0.8)	(1.0)	(1.3)
$t_{1/2}$ (hr)	1.7	2.1	3.4	5.2	5.9
	(0.6)	(0.6)	(1.1)	(1.1)	(1.1)
AUC_{0-8} (mg-hr/L)	46	72	117	260	373
	(7)	(17)	(14)	(96)	(51)

*Patients with low renal function who regularly received intermittent hemodialysis.
[†]Mean (SD).
From: Shya WC, Pittman KA, Wilber RB, et al. Pharmacokinetics of cefprozil in healthy subjects and patients with renal impairment. J Clin Pharmacol 1991;31:362–371.

a. Explain why C_{max} and t_{max} tend to increase on going from Group I to Group V.
b. Calculate the hemodialysis clearance of cis cefprozil.
c. What fraction of drug (*cis* isomer) in the body at the beginning of dialysis is removed during a 3-hr procedure?
d. Predict the dialysis clearance (based on plasma concentration) expected from knowledge of the drug's MW (407 g/mol), its protein binding ($fu = 0.7$) and the dialysis clearance of creatinine (158 mL/min).
e. How well does the hemodialysis clearance of cefprozil (part "b") agree with your prediction (part "d")? If they are not in agreement, suggest a reason for the discrepancy.

16

Nonlinearities

OBJECTIVES

The reader will be able to:

- Define the following terms: autoinduction, capacity-limited metabolism, dose dependence, dose-dependent kinetics, inhibition by a metabolite, linear pharmacokinetics, maximum rate of metabolism, maximum rate of transport, mechanism-based autoinhibition, Michaelis-Menten constant, Michaelis-Menten kinetics, nonlinear pharmacokinetics, principle of superposition, saturability, saturable plasma protein binding, saturable facilitated transport, saturable first-pass metabolism, saturable metabolism, saturable tubular reabsorption, saturable tubular secretion, target-mediated drug disposition, time-dependent kinetics.

- List at least 10 physiologic processes of drug absorption, distribution, and elimination in which dose or time dependence is known to occur.

- Recognize dose- or time-dependent kinetics from either plasma or urine data showing such behavior.

- Given data showing nonlinear renal clearance, determine if saturable tubular secretion or saturable active tubular reabsorption is responsible for the kinetic behavior.

- Graphically depict the tendencies in the kinetic behavior of a drug when the situation and the cause of a dose or time dependence are given.

- On analyzing data in which a dose or time dependence occurs, identify which pharmacokinetic parameters are affected, and assign probable causes to the observation.

- Demonstrate the kinetic consequences at steady state of a change in rate of input, Vm, or Km, of a low extraction ratio drug showing saturable Michaelis-Menten metabolism.

- Describe how saturable first-pass metabolism and saturable transport can occur, and discuss their kinetic consequences.

A n epileptic patient who has not responded to phenytoin after 2 weeks on 300 mg/day is observed to have a plasma concentration of 4 mg/L. Twenty days after the daily dose is subsequently increased to 500 mg, the patient develops signs of toxicity, nystagmus, and ataxia; the plasma concentration of phenytoin is now 36 mg/L. Why should only a 67% increase in daily dose give rise to a ninefold increase in plasma concentration? The answer lies in the **dose-dependent** metabolic behavior of this drug (provided adherence is not an issue).

Similarly, at a daily intake of 75 mg of ascorbic acid (vitamin C), the steady-state plasma concentration is 9 mg/L, whereas at a daily dose of 10,000 mg, the steady-state concentration is only approximately doubled to 19 mg/L in a study subject. The renal clearance of ascorbic acid is less than 0.5 mL/min at the plasma concentration of 9 mg/L, whereas the renal clearance is 21 mL/min at 19 mg/L, a greater than 42-fold increase for only a 171% increase in plasma concentration. Why is the increase in the steady-state concentration of ascorbic acid so small for a 133-fold increase in daily dose? Why is renal clearance increased at all? The answer to these questions again lies with the **nonlinear** behavior of this vitamin. Let us now address what nonlinearities are and how they come about.

DEFINITION OF NONLINEAR KINETIC BEHAVIOR

Normally, observations, such as plasma (or blood) concentration, unbound concentration, and amount of drug and its metabolites excreted in urine, all increase in direct proportion to dose, when drug is administered as a single dose or in multiple doses. Therefore, on correcting such observations for the dose administered, the values are expected to superimpose at all times. This is referred to as the **principle of superposition**. When superposition occurs, the pharmacokinetics of a drug is said to be **dose-independent**, or **linear**. When it does not, the pharmacokinetics is **dose-dependent** or **nonlinear**. In addition to a lack of superpositioning of dose-normalized observations, **nonlinearity** or **dose-dependence** can be defined as a change in one or more pharmacokinetic parameters with size of dose administered or dosing rate. The term *nonlinear* derives its name from the properties of the differential equation(s) needed to model the observed kinetic behavior. Dose-dependence refers to the condition in which parameter values depend on the dose administered.

There are many reasons why the principle of superposition may not hold. Among them are the administration of a drug by different routes (intramuscular versus oral), in different dosage forms (tablets versus capsules), or by different methods (intravenous [i.v.] bolus versus infusion). These are examples of dependencies on route, dosage form, and method of administration. They are not the subject of this chapter.

When there is a lack of superposition on administering a drug (by the same route, dosage form, and method) on separate occasions or a lack of predictability following repeated or continuous dosing, based on single-dose data, the drug is said to show **time-dependent kinetics**. One or more of the pharmacokinetic parameters must then be changing with time. Both dose-dependent and time-dependent behaviors are sources of variability in drug response—the reason for the placement of this chapter in Section IV, *Individualization*. Although relatively uncommon, such kinetic behavior occurs frequently enough in drug therapy to warrant particular consideration.

CAUSES OF NONLINEARITY

Nonlinear kinetics occurs when one or more processes of absorption, distribution, metabolism, or excretion are **saturable**. Saturability refers to situations in which the rate or extent of a process fails to increase in direct proportion to dose or concentration and approaches an upper limit. Figure 16-1 shows four different processes that exhibit **saturability**. For example, the concentration in an aqueous solution increases in proportion to the amount of drug added to a given volume until the solution becomes saturated. This concentration is called the solubility of the drug. Drug metabolism, facilitated transport, and plasma protein binding also can show a tendency to approach an upper limit (i.e., to show saturability). Let us now examine each of these saturable processes in greater detail.

SATURABLE PROCESSES

SATURABLE METABOLISM

Most of our present knowledge of enzymatically mediated metabolism is derived from studies in vitro in which substrate, enzyme, and cofactor concentrations are controlled. The Michaelis-Menten model, developed from in vitro data, can apply in vivo as well.

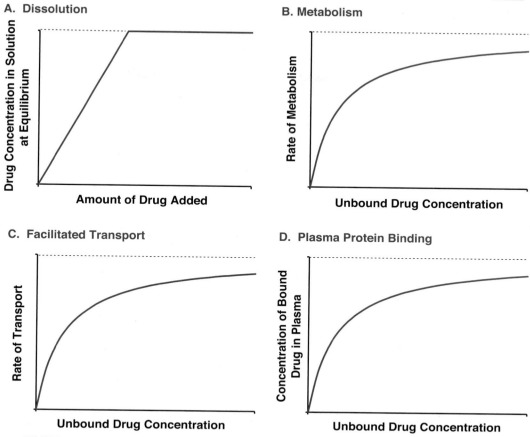

FIGURE 16-1. Processes that show saturation characteristics include: **A. Dissolution**. The concentration in the solution has an upper limit, the solubility. No matter how much more is added to a given volume, the concentration remains the same. **B. Metabolism**. The rate of enzymatic metabolism approaches an upper limit as the substrate concentration is increased. **C. Facilitated transport**. The rate of transport by a facilitative transporter has an upper limit. **D. Plasma protein binding**. The concentration of bound drug is limited by the concentration of sites available for binding.

The curve in Fig. 16-2B is characteristic of hepatic metabolism of a drug by a given enzyme. The behavior displayed is typical of **Michaelis-Menten kinetics**, where the rate of formation of a metabolite approaches a maximum, *Vm*, by the relationship:

$$\frac{Rate\ of\ metabolite}{formation} = \frac{Vm \cdot Cu_H}{Km + Cu_H} \qquad\qquad 16\text{-}1$$

in which *Km* is a constant, the **Michaelis-Menten constant** and Cu_H is the unbound intracellular concentration of drug at the enzymatic site. The value of *Vm* is directly proportional to the total concentration of enzyme, and *Km*, with units of concentration, is an inverse measure of the affinity of the drug for the enzyme. The lower the value of *Km*, the greater the affinity. Note in Eq. 16-1 that a value of Cu_H equal to *Km* gives a rate that is one half the maximum; this is a convenient way of defining the constant *Km*. It is also, according to the Michaelis-Menten model, the drug concentration that results in the occupation of half of the enzyme sites. Drugs typically have *Km* values in the micromolar range. At unbound plasma concentrations well below *Km*, rate and concentration vary in direct proportion, a condition in which the kinetics is linear. At concentrations above *Km*, the rate approaches the value of *Vm* and the kinetics become nonlinear and show saturability.

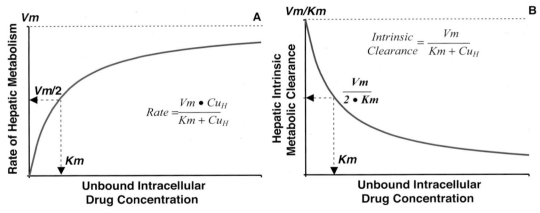

FIGURE 16-2. **A.** When hepatic metabolism follows Michaelis-Menten kinetics, the rate of metabolism increases toward a maximum value, *Vm*, as the unbound intracellular drug concentration, Cu_H, is increased. The concentration at which the rate is one half the maximum is the *Km* value. **B.** The intrinsic metabolite clearance falls with increasing intracellular concentration. The concentration at which intrinsic metabolic clearance is one half the maximum is also the *Km* value. The equations for the relationships are shown.

Because intrinsic metabolic clearance in the well-stirred model of the liver (see Chapter 5, *Elimination*) is defined as the rate of metabolism relative to the unbound hepatic intracellular concentration, it follows that

$$CL_{int,m} = \frac{Vm}{Km + Cu_H} \qquad \text{16-2}$$

Intrinsic metabolic
clearance

At low concentrations, $Km \gg Cu_H$, the intrinsic clearance associated with the formation of the metabolite is nearly constant, maximal, and equal to *Vm/Km*, which is often the case in drug therapy. The kinetics of metabolite formation is then said to be linear in that intrinsic clearance is virtually independent of drug concentration. However, its value decreases at drug concentrations that approach or exceed the value of *Km*, producing nonlinear kinetics. This is shown in Fig. 16-2B.

SATURABLE TRANSPORT

A behavior similar to that of metabolism is also seen with facilitated transport of drugs. Transport occurs with the maximum rate, the **transport maximum**, *Tm*, and with a corresponding concentration at which the transport rate is one half the maximum, K_T.

$$Rate\ of\ Transport = \frac{Tm \cdot Cu}{K_T + Cu} \qquad \text{16-3}$$

SATURABLE BINDING TO PLASMA PROTEINS

A similar model is used to model the nonlinear binding to plasma proteins, namely:

$$Bound\ Concentration = \frac{n \cdot P_t \cdot Cu}{K_d + Cu} \qquad \text{16-4}$$

where $n \cdot P_t$ is the total concentration of sites available for binding, P_t is the concentration of the protein, and K_d (an inverse function of the affinity constant, *Ka*, presented in the protein binding discussion in Chapter 4, *Membranes and Distribution*) is the concentration producing half saturation of the total binding sites. The bound concentration then depends on the capacity, $n \cdot P_t$, and affinity ($Ka = 1/K_d$) for binding.

TABLE 16-1 Processes and Mechanisms Showing "Saturability" at Therapeutic Doses and the Pharmacokinetic Parameter Affected

Process	Mechanism	Pharmacokinetic Parameter Typically Affected (and Direction) as Dose is Increased	Selected Examples
Dissolution	Limited solubility	$F\downarrow$	Griseofulvin
Transport			
Intestinal	Active absorption	$F\downarrow$	Amoxicillin
	Efflux transport	$F\uparrow$	Protease inhibitors, fexofenadine
	P-glycoprotein induction*	$F\downarrow$	Tipranavir
Renal	Tubular secretion	$CL_R\downarrow$	Penicillin G
	Active tubular reabsorption	$CL_R\uparrow$	Ascorbic acid
Hepatic	Biliary secretion	$CL_H\downarrow$	Sulfates, glucuronides
Metabolism	Capacity-limited metabolism	$CL\downarrow$	Phenytoin, paroxetine, voriconazole
	Saturable first-pass metabolism	$F\uparrow$	Nicardipine, mesalamine, niacin
	Autoinduction*	$CL\uparrow$	Carbamazepine
	Mechanism-based autoinhibition*	$CL\downarrow$	Clarithromycin, ticlopidine, clopidogrel
Binding	Saturable plasma protein binding	$V\uparrow$, CL ($\uparrow$ or $\leftrightarrow$, depends on E)	
	Nonspecific	Binding to albumin or α_1-acid glycoprotein	Salicylate, disopyramide, naproxen
	Receptor	Binding to specific protein (site of action)	Angiotensin-converting enzyme inhibitors
	Saturable tissue binding	$V\downarrow$	
	Nonspecific	Binding to nonactive site in tissues	—
	Target-mediated drug disposition*	Much of drug in body is bound to active site	Bosentan, imirestat, draflazine

*Time-dependent as well.

There are many physiologic processes that have a potential to exhibit saturability. Table 16-1 lists examples of representative processes together with the pharmacokinetic parameters affected. Let us now consider the processes by which drugs show nonlinear behavior in their absorption or disposition. For many of these processes, therapeutic implications and means of accommodating or circumventing the problems are discussed.

PHARMACODYNAMICS

Another saturable process is that of the relationship between response and systemic exposure. Indeed, pharmacodynamics is inherently nonlinear in nature as shown by the equations defining the models typically used to quantify drug response (Chapter 2, *Fundamental Concepts and Terminology*), namely,

$$E = \frac{E_{max} \cdot C^{\gamma}}{C_{50}{}^{\gamma} + C^{\gamma}}$$

This relationship is structurally analogous to the saturable kinetic processes previously discussed.

The reason pharmacodynamic relationships generally exhibit nonlinearity, while pharmacokinetic relationships do not, can be explained by the typical values of C_{50} relative to the values commonly encountered for Km (metabolism), K_T (transport), and K_d (protein binding), as shown for Km in Fig. 16-3. Midazolam is an example. It is almost exclusively eliminated by CYP3A with a Km of about 3.3 μM, whereas its C_{50} (unbound) for sedation in humans is closer to 0.05 μM. This difference for drugs in general may partially be explained by the search for ever more potent agents, which, by definition, have lower values of C_{50}. It also appears that to achieve a therapeutic response, the concentration of most drugs must be at or above the C_{50}, where nonlinearity in response is expected. Occasionally, unbound therapeutic concentrations are at or above the values for Km, K_T, or K_d (e.g., phenytoin and alcohol), because they are not very potent. For phenytoin, the Km and C_{50} values are comparable; alcohol is a rare example of a drug with a Km (about 100 mg/L) below its C_{50} value for depression of the central nervous system. Drugs (e.g., bosentan, draflazine, and imirestat) that exhibit target-mediated drug disposition are additional exceptions with comparable Km and C_{50} values. They are discussed later in the chapter.

FIGURE 16-3. Nonlinearity is common to drug response but less common to drug metabolism. This is a result of C_{50} values being below those of Km, based on the unbound drug concentration. As a result, the pharmacokinetics of drugs is generally linear because therapeutic concentrations are below those producing nonlinear metabolism.

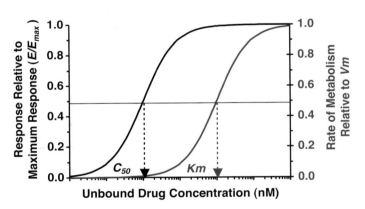

NONLINEAR ABSORPTION

Dose or time dependencies in systemic drug absorption may be reflected by a change in either bioavailability or rate–time profile of absorption. These dependencies most often arise from three sources following oral administration. First are solubility and dissolution limitations in the release of drug from a dosage form in the gastrointestinal tract. Second and third are saturabilities in a transport mechanism or metabolism on passage across the gastrointestinal membranes and through the liver.

SOLUBILITY

Dissolution can be the cause of dose dependency in bioavailability for drugs with low aqueous solubility, when given orally in relatively large doses. With a fixed transit time through the gastrointestinal tract, the amount of drug dissolved and hence absorbed is unlikely to increase in proportion to the dose administered. An example is griseofulvin (Fig. 16-4). For this sparingly soluble drug (solubility is about 10 mg/L), bioavailability decreases as the dose is increased from 250 to 500 mg.

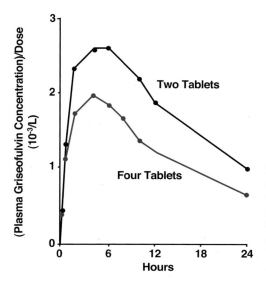

FIGURE 16-4. Plasma concentration, normalized to dose, as a function of time following the oral administration of two tablets (●) and four tablets (●) of ultramicronized griseofulvin (125 mg/tablet). (From: Barrett WE, Bianchine JR. The bioavailability of ultramicronized griseofulvin (GRIS-PEG) tablets in man. Curr Ther Res 1975;18:501–509.)

SATURABLE ACTIVE TRANSPORT

For a few drugs, absorption from the gastrointestinal tract occurs by a capacity-limited transport mechanism. An example is that of amoxicillin, a polar β-lactam antibiotic. This drug is absorbed by a peptide transport mechanism in the small intestine. This conclusion is supported by the observation that bioavailability decreases with increased oral dose, but the peak time changes little (Fig. 16-5). The decrease in bioavailability, reflected

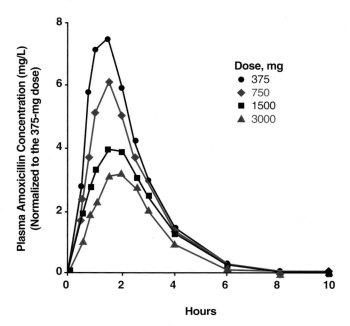

FIGURE 16-5. Mean amoxicillin plasma concentrations after single oral doses of 375 (●), 750 (◆), 1500 (■), and 3000 (▲) mg. The concentrations are normalized to those expected for a 375-mg dose ($C = C$ [observed] $\times$ 375/Dose [mg]). Note the decrease in the C_{max} and AUC values, and the similarity in t_{max}, on increasing the dose. The observations are explained by oral bioavailability decreasing with dose with little or no change in peak time. (From: Sjövall J, Alván G, Westerlund D. Dose-dependent absorption of amoxycillin and bacampicillin. Clin Pharmacol Ther 1985;38:241–250. Interpretation from: Reigner BG, Couet WR, Guedes JP, Fourtillan JB, Tozer TN. Saturable rate of cefatrizine absorption after oral administration to humans. J Pharmacokinet Biopharm 1990;18:17–34.)

by the decreased area under the curve (AUC) relative to dose, is explained by the capacity-limited nature of the transport process. The lack of a major change in the peak time is a consequence of the limited region in the small intestine from which absorption can occur. The dose size does not influence the time between ingestion and movement past the site of absorption.

SATURABLE FIRST-PASS METABOLISM

Nicardipine, a dihydropyridine calcium-channel blocker, exhibits dose dependence in its oral bioavailability (Table 16-2) because of saturability in its metabolism on first pass through the liver. The data in the table were acquired during an 8-hr dosing interval at steady state (3 days into regimen). An i.v. radiolabeled tracer dose (0.885 mg) was given concurrently with the 30-mg dose to determine oral bioavailability.

TABLE 16-2	Saturable First-Pass Metabolism of Nicardipine Observed at Steady State Following Oral Doses of 10 to 40 mg Every 8 Hr	
Dose (mg)		**Bioavailability (%)**
10		19(4)*
20		22(5)
30		28(5)
40		36(6)

*Mean and standard error (SE) of data from six subjects.
From: Wagner JG, Ling TL, Mroszczak EJ, et al. Single intravenous dose and steady-state oral dose pharmacokinetics of nicardipine in healthy subjects. Biopharm Drug Dispos 1987;8:133–148.

Saturable first-pass metabolism occurs for a number of orally administered drugs that are highly extracted by the liver or intestinal tissues. Additional examples were given in Table 7-5, Chapter 7, *Absorption*. For several of these drugs, dose dependence in oral bioavailability is observed without an apparent change in elimination half-life, as explained in the text of the chapter.

An interesting example of a drug that undergoes saturable first pass is that of methylphenidate. The drug is available in the racemic form, a mixture of the two enantiomers. Figure 16-6A shows the concentration of (+)-methylphenidate and (−)-methylphenidate after the oral administration of 30 mg of the racemate. The systemic exposure to the (+)-isomer is much greater than that to the (−)-isomer. Both enantiomers are extensively extracted during the first pass through the gut wall and the liver, but the fraction reaching the systemic circulation is much greater for the (+)-isomer (about 20%) than for the (−)-isomer (about 4%). Although the bioavailability of the (+) and (−) isomers are very different, the amounts of the corresponding ritalinic acid metabolites formed during the first pass and during elimination of absorbed drug are the same (top two curves of Fig. 16-6A), a topic further discussed in Chapter 20, *Metabolites and Drug Response*. Furthermore, it is evident in Fig. 16-6B that the first-pass metabolism of the (+)-isomer depends on dose administered, as the AUC increases disproportionally with an increase in dose, a consequence of saturable first-pass metabolism.

CAPACITY-LIMITED METABOLISM

Perhaps the most dramatic dose-dependent elimination mechanism is that of **capacity-limited metabolism** commonly well characterized by Michaelis-Menten–type kinetics.

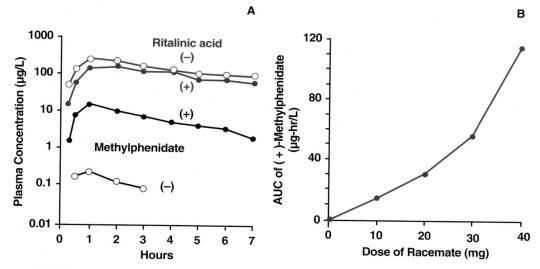

FIGURE 16-6. **A.** The plasma concentrations of (+)-methylphenidate (●), (−)-methylphenidate (○) and their respective metabolites, (+)-ritalinic acid (●), and (−)-ritalinic acid (○) after the oral administration of 30 mg of racemic methylphenidate hydrochloride to a volunteer. **B.** The relationship between the *AUC* of (+)-methylphenidate and dose following oral administration of 10, 20, 30, and 40 mg of the racemate to the same volunteer. No appreciable difference is seen for the metabolites. (From: Aoyama T, Kotaki H, Sasaki T. Nonlinear kinetics of threo-methylphenidate enantiomers in a patient with narcolepsy and in healthy volunteers. Eur J Clin Pharmacol 1993;44:79–84.)

The therapeutic consequences of Michaelis-Menten kinetics are now explored with two examples, alcohol and phenytoin. Both compounds rapidly permeate the hepatocyte and achieve distribution equilibrium, with unbound drug in the circulating plasma virtually equal to that in the hepatocyte. From Eq. 16-1 and letting $Cu = Cu_H$,

$$Rate\ of\ metabolism = \frac{Vm \cdot Cu}{Km + Cu}$$

for a drug showing saturable Michaelis-Menten kinetics. Also, recall from Eq. 16-2 that in this case

$$CL_{int,m} = \frac{Vm}{Km + Cu}$$

ALCOHOL

At usual doses, the metabolism of alcohol becomes capacity limited and can be approximated by a Michaelis-Menten model with a single enzyme, alcohol dehydrogenase, responsible for its elimination. This simplified kinetic model is subsequently presented.

The maximum rate of metabolism, *Vm*, and the Michaelis constant, *Km*, are approximately 10 g/hr and 100 mg/L, respectively. The pharmacologic effects of alcohol, which does not bind to plasma proteins, become apparent when the plasma concentration is about 200 mg/L, concentrations above 5000 mg/L are potentially lethal. Thus, the concentration range in which alcohol exerts its pharmacologic effects is well above its *Km*. For comparison, the legal concentration above which one is said to be "driving under the influence" of alcohol in most countries is 800 mg/L (0.08 g/dL) or close to this value.

Table 16-3 shows the calculated rate of metabolism and clearance of alcohol as a function of the concentration at the metabolic site. Note that rate of metabolism of alcohol is essentially constant, zero-order, and close to *Vm* throughout the range of concentrations

TABLE 16-3	Calculated Rate of Metabolism and Clearance of Alcohol as a Function of the Concentration at the Metabolic Site

Concentration at Metabolic Site (mg/L)	Rate of Metabolism (g/hr)*	Clearance (L/hr)†
7000	9.9	1.4
5000	9.8	2.0
3000	9.7	3.2
1000	9.1	9.1
500	8.3	17
200	6.7	33
100	5.0	50
50	3.3	67
10	0.91	91

*Rate of metabolism $= Vm \cdot Cu/(Km + Cu)$, $Vm = 10$ g/hr, $Km = 100$ mg/L.
†Clearance $= Vm/(Km + Cu)$.

associated with activity. Accordingly, clearance decreases at high concentrations. At low concentrations, the intrinsic clearance (Vm/Km) approaches 100 L/hr or 1.6 L/min, a value in excess of hepatic blood flow. Thus, at very low concentrations, the extraction ratio is sufficiently high so that the rate of metabolism is partially limited by hepatic perfusion. Under these latter conditions oral bioavailability is expected to be reduced.

The consequences of zero-order elimination can be dramatic. The usual-size drink, 45 mL, of 40% v/v whiskey contains about 18 mL, or 14 g, of alcohol. Drinking this quantity of alcohol each hour exceeds the capacity for its elimination from the body. Consequently, alcohol accumulates until ultimately either coma or death intervenes. The production of coma, by preventing further drinking, keeps the latter from being commonplace.

Alcohol distributes evenly throughout total body water without appreciable binding to either plasma proteins or tissue components; its volume of distribution is therefore about 42 L/70 kg. Accordingly, approximately 200 g of alcohol are needed in the body to achieve a concentration, about 5000 mg/L, that can produce death. But, since the rate of ingestion, 14 g/hr, exceeds the rate of metabolism, 10 g/hr, by only 4 g/hr, this rate of drinking must be maintained for at least 2 days (a total of 48 drinks) to accumulate 200 g of alcohol. This degree of accrual can occur within 5 hr (20 drinks) when four drinks are consumed every hour, because this rate of ingestion, 56 g/hr, exceeds the maximum metabolic capacity by 46 g/hr. The times given above are for the average person. People do vary in size and metabolic capabilities and therefore more conservative rules should be used to predict systemic exposures from alcohol ingestion.

If the rate of ingestion in the average person is reduced to one-half drink (or 7 g/hr), then, with respect to the effect of alcohol, the person can drink with virtual impunity as now shown. By definition, at steady state, rate of elimination matches rate of administration (or input), R_o.

$$R_o = \frac{Vm \cdot Cu_{ss}}{Km + Cu_{ss}}$$

16-5

or on rearrangement

$$Cu_{ss} = \frac{Km \cdot R_o}{Vm - R_o}$$

16-6

Using the previously given values for *Km* and *Vm* and an R_o value of 7 g/hr, the plateau concentration of alcohol is 230 mg/L, which produces only a marginal effect.

Reflect on the preceding calculations. Chronically imbibing one half a drink of whiskey per hour produces little or no effect, but consuming one drink hourly would eventually become lethal. There can be no standard dosage regimen to maintain the effects of alcohol. Maintenance of effect requires titration of dosage with time to the effect itself.

The consequence of capacity-limited metabolism on the time-course of a drug in the body when input rate is changed is also demonstrated with alcohol. When alcohol is administered 10 min after ingesting water, light cream, or a glucose solution (80 g/240 mL), the plasma concentration–time profiles differ profoundly (Fig. 16-7). Compared to water, administration of light cream and 33% glucose, foods that delay gastric emptying, lower both *AUC* and peak concentration and increase time to reach the peak. These observations can be explained by the nearly zero-order metabolism at this dose of alcohol.

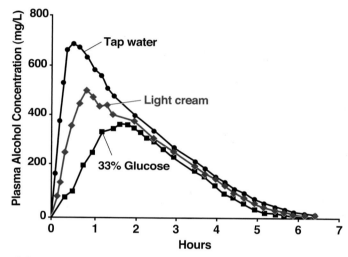

FIGURE 16-7. A decrease in the absorption rate of alcohol, produced by slowing gastric emptying, causes peak concentrations and *AUC* to decrease and time to reach the peak to increase. The effect differs from that expected of first-order elimination kinetics by the observed decrease in *AUC*. This observation is explained by a constant rate of elimination at almost all concentrations, as illustrated schematically in Fig. 16-8. Alcohol, 45 mL of 95% ethanol in 105 mL of orange juice, was administered 10 min after 240 mL of tap water (●); 240 mL of light cream (◆); or 240 mL of a 33% glucose solution (■). (From: Sedman AJ, Wilkinson PK, Sakmar E, et al. Food effects on absorption and metabolism of alcohol. J Stud Alcohol 1976;37:1197–1214. Reprinted with permission of Journal of Studies on Alcohol, Inc., Rutgers Center of Alcohol Studies, New Brunswick, NJ.)

To emphasize the point, assume that both elimination and input are strictly zero-order, as shown in Fig. 16-8. Decreasing the input rate, for a given total dose administered, lowers *AUC* and peak concentration as well as increases the peak time. Clearly, oral bioavailability in the presence of zero-order elimination and variable input rates cannot be assessed by conventional area ratio methods.

PHENYTOIN

Therapeutic problems encountered with capacity-limited metabolism are classically exemplified by phenytoin. Typical *Vm* and *Km* values of this drug are 500 mg/day and 0.4 mg/L, although the values vary widely. The value of *Km* is usually expressed in terms of total, rather than unbound, concentration. Since *fu* is typically 0.1, the apparent *Km* for total concentration, *Km'*, is equal to 4 mg/L.

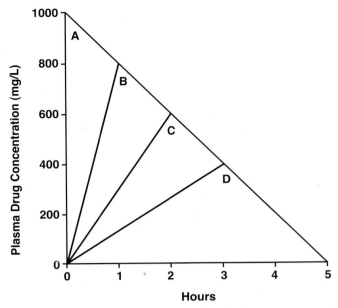

FIGURE 16-8. As a consequence of zero-order elimination, the plasma concentrations at the end of a 1000-mg dose of a drug by bolus injection (**A**) and constant-rate infusions of 1-hr (**B**), 2-hr (**C**), and 3-hr (**D**) durations are quite different from those expected with first-order kinetics. The amount in the body at the end of each infusion is the difference between dose and amount lost during the infusion period. Consequently, the concentration at the end of each of the infusions is the same as that expected at that time following the i.v. bolus dose. Note that the slower the input rate, the smaller is *AUC* and the lower is peak concentration. The time to peak is, of course, increased. Furthermore, if the dose had been infused over a 5-hr period (i.e., at 200 mg/hr) output would have matched input and there would have been no *AUC* in this hypothetical example.

Plateau. Perhaps the most striking consequence of the kinetics of this drug is the relationship observed between steady-state plasma concentration and rate of administration, as shown in Fig. 16-9. A greatly disproportionate increase in concentration is observed in, and above, the therapeutic concentration range, 10 to 20 mg/L. As a result, the difference between the daily dose giving ineffective therapeutic concentrations, less than 10 mg/L, and that producing potentially toxic concentrations, above 20 mg/L, is narrow.

The observed increase in concentration can be explained by rearrangement of Eq. 16-6.

$$\frac{Cu_{ss}}{R_o} = \frac{K_m}{Vm - R_o} \qquad 16\text{-}7$$

The consequences of Michaelis-Menten metabolism result when either the desired steady-state unbound concentration is above Km (Km' for total concentration) or the rate of administration required to achieve these concentrations approaches Vm.

Because of its kinetics, only small changes in phenytoin input caused, for example, by a change in salt form (acid and sodium salt are used) or in bioavailability can produce relatively large changes in the steady-state concentration. To illustrate this point, consider a male patient with Km' and Vm values of 3 mg/L and 425 mg/day, respectively, and who has an average steady-state concentration of 12 mg/L when taking 200 mg orally every 12 hr. On switching from his current dosage form (bioavailability = 0.85) to one with a bioavailability of 0.95, it is seen, by setting $R_o = F \cdot D/\tau$ in Eq. 16-7, that the average steady-state concentration is expected to increase to 25 mg/L. Thus, a 12% change in bioavailability (0.85 to 0.95) causes a doubling (200%, 12 to 25 mg/L) in the steady-state concentration when the dosing rate approaches the Vm value.

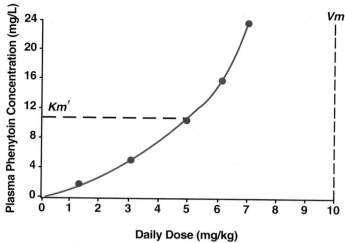

FIGURE 16-9. The steady-state plasma concentration increases disproportionately with rate of administration (given twice daily) of phenytoin, a drug that is virtually eliminated by a single metabolic pathway that exhibits typical Michaelis-Menten enzyme kinetics. The estimated *Vm*, the maximum rate of metabolism, and *Km'*, the total plasma concentration at which the rate is half of the maximum (*dashed line*), are shown. All the data were obtained in the same individual whose *Km'* and *Vm* values are considerably higher than the typical ones of 4 mg/L and 7 mg/kg per day. (From: Martin E, Tozer TN, Sheiner LB, Riegelman S. The clinical pharmacokinetics of phenytoin. J Pharmacokinet Biopharm 1977;5:579–596. Reproduced with permission of Springer.)

Time to Plateau. Because of capacity-limited metabolism, the time to reach steady state varies with the rate of administration. To show this point, consider the model for the situation of having a constant rate of input of phenytoin, R_o. The rate of change of drug in the body, $\dfrac{V \cdot dC}{dt}$, is then

$$\frac{V \cdot dC}{dt} = R_o - \frac{Vm \cdot C}{Km' + C} \qquad \text{16-8}$$

On integrating,

$$\frac{Km' \cdot Vm}{(Vm - R_o)} \cdot \ln\left[\frac{R_o \cdot Km'}{R_o \cdot Km' - (Vm - R_o) \cdot C}\right] - C = \frac{(Vm - R_o)}{V} \cdot t \qquad \text{16-9}$$

Defining the time to reach steady state as the time to reach 90% of the steady-state value, that is,

$$C = 0.9 \frac{Km' \cdot R_o}{(Vm - R_o)}$$

The time to steady state becomes

$$t_{90} = \frac{Km' \cdot V(2.303 \cdot Vm - 0.9\,R_o)}{(Vm - R_o)^2} \qquad \text{16-10}$$

Figure 16-10 shows the approach to plateau during each of four dosing rates, which increase by small increments from 300 to 425 mg/day, in a patient with typical *Vm* and *Km'* values. Note that the calculated time (arrows) to reach 90% of plateau increases progressively with the rate of administration. These disproportionate changes in the steady-state concentration and the time required to reach them are major problems in optimally

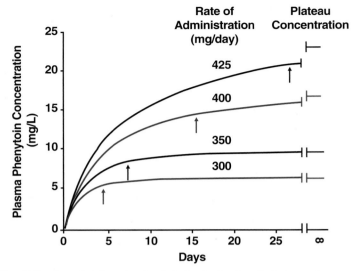

FIGURE 16-10.   Following administration (i.v. infusion is simulated) of phenytoin at constant rates of 300, 350, 400, and 425 mg/day, the plasma concentration approaches steady-state values (on right) of 6, 9.3, 16, and 22.7 mg/L, respectively. Not only are the steady-state concentrations disproportionately increased, but so also is the time required to approach the plateau. The arrows indicate the time required to reach 90% of the plateau value. The following parameter values were used: Km', 4 mg/L; Vm, 500 mg/day; V, 50 L. (Reproduced by permission of publisher. From: Winter ME, Tozer TN. Phenytoin. In: Burton ME, Shaw LM, Schentag JJ, Evans WE, eds. Applied Pharmacokinetics and Pharmacodynamics: Principles of Therapeutic Drug Monitoring. 4th ed. Philadelphia: Lippincott Williams and Wilkins, 2006.)

dosing phenytoin and interpreting its concentrations. Even though the approach to plateau is usually somewhat quicker on reducing doses than on increasing them, it can still take a long time, as shown in Fig. 16-11.

Because clearance, and hence half-life, are functions of the plasma concentration, the meanings of these parameters are lost when capacity-limited metabolism occurs. For this reason, these parameters should not be used for predicting or summarizing the kinetics of drugs showing this kind of behavior. The parameters of choice are those of the appropriate nonlinear model (Km and Vm for Michaelis-Menten kinetics and V).

Alterations in Metabolism.   Another therapeutically important facet of the kinetics of phenytoin is altered metabolism brought about by other drugs and disease states. Either Km' or Vm can be altered, but the effect on plasma concentration is different. From Eq. 16-7 it can be seen that the phenytoin concentration at steady state is directly proportional to Km'. Thus, an increase in the Km' value, for example by competitive inhibition (discussed in Chapter 17, *Drug Interactions*), produces a corresponding change in the steady-state phenytoin concentration. For example, when cimetidine inhibits phenytoin metabolism, thereby increasing Km' from 4 to 6 mg/L, the steady-state unbound and total phenytoin concentrations are expected to increase by 50% as well.

In contrast, either an increase in Vm, brought about by enzyme induction, or a decrease in Vm, caused by the presence of hepatic cirrhosis, is expected to produce a disproportionate change in the steady-state phenytoin concentration. This is seen by taking the ratio of the two different concentrations, $Cu_{ss,1}$ and $Cu_{ss,2}$ (Eq. 16-7), that result from the unaltered, Vm_1, and altered, Vm_2, values, respectively.

$$\frac{Cu_{ss,2}}{Cu_{ss,1}} = \frac{Vm_1 - R_o}{Vm_2 - R_o}$$

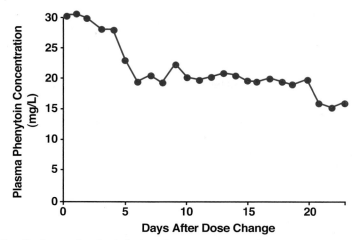

FIGURE 16-11. On decreasing the daily dose from 250 to 200 mg/day, the plasma phenytoin concentration (obtained daily just before the morning dose) declines slowly toward a new steady state in a patient. Note that a 20% reduction in the daily dose leads to a 50% decrease in the concentration at steady state (the concentration stabilized after day 23). (From: Theodore WH, Qu ZP, Tsay JY, et al. Phenytoin: the pseudosteady-state phenomenon. Clin Pharmacol Ther 1984;35:822–825. Reproduced with permission of C.V. Mosby.)

For example, when R_o = 300 mg/day, Vm_1 = 500 mg/day, and Vm_2 = 400 mg/day, the unbound concentration at steady state is doubled, $Cu_{ss,2}/Cu_{ss,1}$ = 2. If Vm_2 is 600 mg/day, the ratio is 0.67. Thus, a 20% decrease in Vm doubles the steady-state concentration; whereas a 20% increase in Vm reduces the steady-state concentration by 33%. Note that a Vm of 300 mg/day results in a concentration approaching infinity, and that with a Vm below 300 mg/day, steady state can never be achieved. The input rate would then always exceed Vm, and Eqs. 16-5 to 16-7 would not be applicable.

Alcohol and phenytoin represent extreme cases in that almost all the elimination of each drug occurs by a single saturable pathway. More commonly, a drug is metabolized by several pathways, and only one or two of them approaches saturation. Then, saturation has less effect on total clearance. The extent of the effect depends on fm, the fraction of drug eliminated by the saturable pathway at low drug concentrations. Only if fm is 0.5, or greater, under nonsaturating conditions is total clearance materially affected by saturation of the pathway. Examples of drugs in this category include propranolol, many protease inhibitors, and salicylic acid. In this situation, the clearance of a drug can be thought of as having linear, CL_{lin}, and nonlinear components. With one pathway in each category,

$$CL = CL_{lin} + \frac{Vm \cdot C}{Km + C}$$

16-11

And, as half-life = $0.693 \cdot V/CL$,

$$Half\text{-}life = \frac{0.693 \cdot V}{CL_{lin} + \dfrac{Vm}{Km + C}}$$

16-12

Clearance then has two limiting values, CL_{lin} when the concentration is well above the Km of the saturable pathway and $CL_{lin} + Vm/Km$ when the concentration is well below Km. Similarly, half-life has two limiting values, $0.693 \cdot V/CL_{lin}$ and $0.693 \cdot V/(CL_{lin} + Vm/Km)$. Salicylic acid is a good example. At low concentration, for example those after a 300-mg dose, the half-life is about 2 to 3 hr, whereas in overdose conditions (>10 g in the body), the half-life appears to be linear with a value of about 24 hr, a result of a substantial part of salicylate metabolism showing saturability.

CONCENTRATION-DEPENDENT RENAL EXCRETION

Renal clearance can vary with plasma concentration. Filtration is a passive process, and when reabsorption is passive, the rates of both processes are directly related to plasma concentration. In contrast, active secretion and active reabsorption are saturable processes with maximum capacities. This is shown in Fig. 16-12, for active secretion.

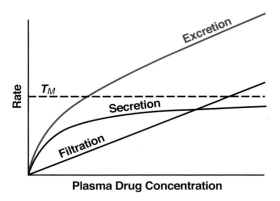

FIGURE 16-12. The rate of renal secretion has a limiting value, the maximum transport rate (T_M), whereas the rate of filtration increases in direct proportion to the plasma concentration of a drug. Consequently, the rate of excretion of a drug that is both filtered and secreted, but not reabsorbed, increases with its plasma concentration. The increase, however, is not in direct proportion. Drug is either not bound in plasma or fu remains constant throughout the range of plasma concentrations.

The rate of tubular secretion increases in direct proportion to the plasma concentration until the transport approaches an upper limit, the T_M value. Consequently, clearance by secretion decreases as plasma concentration increases. This is observed for the antimicrobial agent dicloxacillin (Fig. 16-13). On increasing the dose from 1 to 2 g, the renal clearance, assessed by Ae_∞/AUC, is reduced. Extrarenal clearance is unaffected.

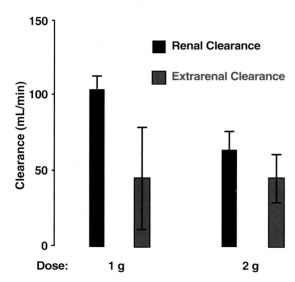

FIGURE 16-13. Renal clearance of dicloxacillin, as measured by Ae_∞/AUC, is decreased following a 2-g i.v. dose relative to that observed after a 1-g i.v. dose. The extrarenal clearance is not affected by dose. Saturable secretion of drug into the renal tubule explains the decrease in renal clearance. Mean ± SD (*bars*). (From: Nauta, EH, Mattie H. Dicloxacillin and cloxacillin: pharmacokinetics in healthy and hemodialysis subjects. Clin Pharmacol Ther 1976;20:98–108.)

With an fu of 0.04, renal clearance, 104 mL/min following the 1-g dose, greatly exceeds the expected value of filtration clearance, $fu \cdot GFR$, indicating that this drug is extensively secreted into the tubular lumen (see Chapter 5, *Elimination*). At these doses, secretion shows concentration dependence and, as a consequence, the *AUC* increases more than proportionately with dose. The body's exposure to the drug and the half-life are disproportionately increased, considerations in the therapeutic use of large doses.

Secretion never occurs alone; filtration is always a component, and passive reabsorption may or may not be. Figure 16-12 also demonstrates how the rate of excretion of a drug that undergoes filtration and secretion, such as penicillin, always increases with plasma concentration. Even though the rate of secretion approaches an upper limit, the rate of filtration continues to increase directly with unbound plasma concentration.

Renal clearance is the rate of drug excretion (left panel) divided by its plasma concentration. A drug that is only filtered and not bound in plasma (curve A), has the same renal clearance at all concentrations, as shown schematically in curve A of Fig. 16-14 (right panel). Curve B depicts the events that occur for a drug that is actively secreted. In the region of plasma concentrations well below those required to approach saturation, renal clearance is highest and is relatively insensitive to changes in drug concentration. The therapeutic concentrations of most actively secreted drugs lie within this region. At higher plasma concentrations, renal clearance decreases; the lower limiting value is that contributed by both filtration and passive reabsorption.

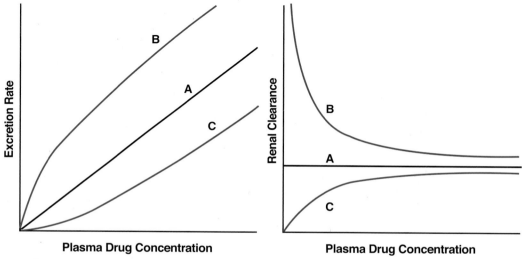

FIGURE 16-14. Relationships between either rate of excretion (*on left*) or renal clearance (*on right*) and plasma concentration depend on whether the drug undergoes filtration only (curve A), filtration and secretion (curve B), or filtration and active reabsorption (curve C). The drug is either not bound to plasma proteins, or *fu* remains constant throughout the range of plasma concentrations.

The renal clearances of ascorbic acid and disopyramide exhibit the properties of curve C in Fig. 16-14. They both increase with increasing concentrations, but for different reasons. Ascorbic acid (vitamin C) is normally conserved in the body by active reabsorption from the renal tubule. When the plasma concentration is excessive, the capacity of the reabsorption mechanism is exceeded, and the vitamin appears in large amounts in the urine (Fig. 16-15). The consequence of nonlinear excretion following oral administration of ascorbic acid is illustrated by the data in Table 16-4. Although statistically significant, note that the plasma concentration does not increase much even when megadoses are given. Another nonlinear mechanism also contributes to this observation. The bioavailability of the vitamin decreases with increasing dose (not shown) because it is absorbed in the intestine by a saturable process. The combined effect of saturable gastrointestinal absorption and saturable renal tubular reabsorption is that only a relatively small change in the steady-state plasma concentration occurs, even when the daily oral dose is increased greatly, thereby maintaining the level of the vitamin in the body within relatively narrow bounds.

Rather than saturable reabsorption, nonlinear binding to α_1-acid glycoprotein causes renal clearance (based on total concentration) of disopyramide to be greater at

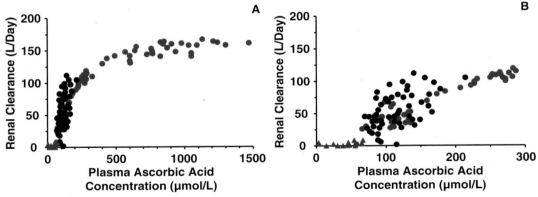

FIGURE 16-15. **A.** The renal clearance of ascorbic acid increases with its plasma concentration. The increase occurs because the rate of filtration exceeds the capacity of a facilitated transport mechanism to reabsorb the vitamin from the tubular lumen. At high concentrations, the renal clearance of ascorbic acid approaches *GFR*. **B.** The renal clearance data in the limited concentration range of 0 to 300 μmol/L. (From: Blanchard J, Tozer TN, Rowland M. Pharmacokinetic perspectives on megadoses of ascorbic acid, Am J Clin Nutr 1997;66:1165–1171. The original data were obtained from three sources: [●], Ralli EP, Friedman GJ, Rubin SH. The mechanism of the excretion of vitamin C by the human kidney. J Clin Invest 1940;17:765–770; [●], Melethil S, Mason WD, Chang CJ. Dose-dependent absorption and excretion of vitamin C in humans. Int J Pharmaceut 1986;31:83–89; and [▲], Kallner AB, Hartmann D, Hornig D. Steady-state turnover and body pool of ascorbic acid in man. Am J Clin Nutr 1979;32:530–539.)

TABLE 16-4	Steady-State Trough Plasma Ascorbic Acid Concentrations in Healthy Adults Taking Various Doses of the Vitamin Twice Daily for 3 to 4 Weeks

Group	Plasma Ascorbic Acid Concentration* (mg/L)
1. No supplementary dose, 6 subjects. Daily dietary intake of 50–70 mg expected.	$9 \pm 0.6^{\dagger}$
2. 1 to 3 g/day, 11 subjects	$15.4 \pm 1.6^{\ddagger}$
3. 8 to 12 g/day, 6 subjects	$19.5 \pm 2.0^{\ddagger}$

*Blood sampled in the morning before the next dose.
†Mean ± SE of the mean.
‡Significantly different from group 1.
From: Yew, MLS. Megadose vitamin C supplementation and ascorbic acid and dehydroascorbic acid levels in plasma and lymphocytes. Nutr Rep Intem 1984;30:597–601.

---

earlier times after a 1.5-mg/kg i.v. dose (Fig. 16-16A). Unbound renal clearance, on the other hand, shows no evidence of nonlinearity (Fig. 16-16B). The greater total clearance coincides with a higher total concentration and a lower plasma binding ($fu \uparrow$) at earlier times.

Renal clearance may also show concentration dependence when a drug (a) produces changes in pH and its tubular reabsorption is pH-dependent (e.g., salicylate); (b) is a diuretic and renal passive clearance is flow-dependent (e.g., theophylline); or (c) causes nephrotoxicity (e.g., an aminoglycoside). The mechanisms of the last two drugs are also time-dependent. Theophylline produces diuresis soon after its administration, but this effect, and consequently its renal clearance, decrease with time. The nephrotoxic effect of aminoglycosides, on the other hand, develops with dose and duration of exposure to the drug.

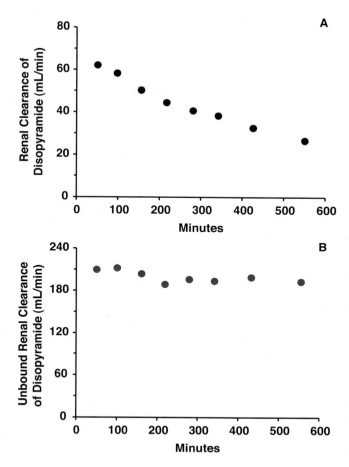

FIGURE 16-16. A. The renal clearance of disopyramide in an individual subject shows changes with time after a single 1.5-mg/kg i.v. dose. **B.** Unbound renal clearance, on the other hand, does not appear to change over the corresponding time period. The initial plasma concentrations were in the range of 2 to 4 mg/L. These total concentrations are expected to produce nonlinear binding to α_1-acid glycoprotein, the protein to which this drug primarily binds in plasma. (From: Giacomini KM, Swezey SE, Turner-Tamiyasu K, Blaschke TF. The effect of saturable binding to plasma proteins on the pharmacokinetic properties of disopyramide. J Pharmacokinet Biopharm 1982;10:1–14.)

SATURABLE TRANSPORT

Transport systems to facilitate movement across cell membranes or to concentrate substances within or without cells are common throughout the body. These processes are potentially saturable. For example, the absorption of amoxicillin shows saturability after oral administration (see Fig. 16-5), as does the systemic absorption of vitamin B_{12} (Table 16-5). For vitamin B_{12}, absorption is primarily limited by the production of an "intrinsic factor" formed within the stomach. The transporter, however, is located in the terminal ileum.

TABLE 16-5	Gastrointestinal Absorption of Vitamin B_{12}	
Dose (μg)	**Amount Absorbed (μg)**	**Percent of Dose Absorbed**
0.5	0.4	80
2.0	0.9	45
5.0	1.3	26
10	1.5	15
50	2.0	4
200	3.3	1.6
500	6	1.1

From: Diem K. Documenta Geigy Scientific Tables. 7th ed. Hoboken, NJ: John Wiley & Sons; 1970:484.

The renal clearance of ascorbic acid (vitamin C) is a prime example of saturable transport producing nonlinear elimination. For vitamin C (see Table 16-4 and Fig. 16-15), the nonlinearity occurs in the reabsorption of the compound from the renal tubule, leading to a dramatic increase in renal clearance with plasma concentration. Saturable transport also occurs for tubular secretion as shown in Fig. 16-13 for dicloxacillin. Here, as the plasma concentration (or *AUC* following a single dose) is increased, the renal clearance is decreased.

SATURABILITY OF PLASMA PROTEIN AND TISSUE BINDING

BINDING TO PLASMA PROTEINS

A limited number of binding sites exist on each plasma protein to which drugs bind. Recall from Tables 4-5 and 4-6 (Chapter 4, *Membranes and Distribution*) that the average plasma concentration of albumin is about 43 g/L or 600 μM (molecular weight [MW] = 67,000 g/mol). At one binding site per albumin molecule, there is then a limiting concentration of 600 μM for the bound drug. For α_1-acid glycoprotein, the limitation occurs at about 15 μM, a much lower concentration. The sites to which drugs bind in the tissues may be similarly limited. Consequently, the volume of distribution depends on drug concentration, a **concentration-dependent** behavior. Changes in binding tend to become appreciable when more than 20% of the available sites are occupied. This number, corresponding to 120 μM for one binding site on albumin, is arbitrary but useful for predicting the likelihood of concentration-dependent binding. For a drug with a MW of 250, 120 μM corresponds to a concentration of 30 mg/L. For basic drugs of comparable size and bound to α_1-acid glycoprotein, nonlinearity in binding is expected to begin at about 0.75 mg/L (20% $\times$15 μM $\times$ 250 μg/μmol).

For drugs that show saturable binding to plasma proteins, the volume of distribution is expected to increase significantly with *fu*, except when the volume of distribution is small (less than 0.2 L/kg, see Chapter 4, *Membranes and Distribution*). Conversely, for drugs that show saturability in binding to tissues, the volume of distribution decreases as plasma concentration is increased. Because of the potential dependence on the fraction unbound in plasma and the dependence of half-life on both clearance and volume of distribution, dose dependence in distribution may be difficult to identify and quantify, unless plasma protein binding is measured. Consider the example of naproxen.

The *AUC* of naproxen following single doses fails to increase linearly with dose when doses above those maximally recommended (500 mg) are given (Fig. 16-17). Without any other information, this nonlinear observation might be explained by either a decrease in bioavailability or an increase in clearance, in that

$$AUC = \frac{F \cdot Dose}{CL}$$

The increase in clearance may be due to induction of metabolism or saturable binding to plasma proteins. As naproxen is a drug of low clearance (*Dose/AUC* calculated from data in Fig. 16-15A varies from 0.3 to 1.3 L/hr), the peak concentrations observed at doses approaching 4 g (Fig. 16-15B) provide information to distinguish between these possibilities. If one approximates a concentration of 110 mg/L when most of a 1000-mg dose is in the body, a value of *V/F* of approximately 9 L can be estimated. This small volume suggests that most naproxen in the body is strongly bound to plasma proteins. The maximum concentrations obtained are in the region where nonlinear binding is expected for naproxen, a weak acid that binds to albumin. With a MW of 230 g/mol, 100 and 200 mg/L correspond to concentrations of 430 and 870 μM, values approximating that (600 μM) of serum albumin. This is the condition in which *fu* is expected to increase with higher doses. Thus, with minimal information, a probable source of nonlinearity, saturable binding to plasma albumin, can be deduced.

The therapeutic consequence of decreased binding to plasma proteins at higher daily doses of a drug of low extraction ratio differs dramatically from that of drug-induced

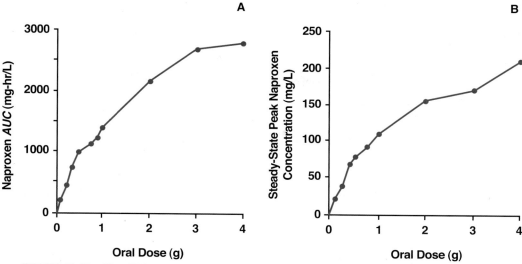

FIGURE 16-17. The *AUC* of naproxen increases with the size of a single oral dose but not in direct proportion; the *AUC* appears to approach a limiting value (**A**). Nonlinearity is also observed in the peak concentration at steady state following multiple doses (**B**). These observations are consistent with either a decrease in *F* or an increase in *CL* with decreasing dose. As explained in the text, saturable binding to plasma albumin is most probably responsible. (From: Runkel R, Chaplin MD, Sevelius H, et al. Pharmacokinetics of naproxen overdoses. Clin Pharmacol Ther 1976;20:269–277.)

increased enzyme activity (**autoinduction**). When binding decreases (*fu* increases), the steady-state total plasma concentration is not increased much on doubling the rate of administration. The steady-state unbound concentration, however, doubles as a consequence of no change in unbound clearance. The intensities of toxic and therapeutic responses are expected to increase accordingly. In contrast, an increase in enzyme activity would affect both unbound and total concentrations proportionally. Thus, if autoinduction occurs, only a minor increase in response would be expected at higher rates of administration.

The expected change in the time-course of a drug in plasma when plasma protein binding exhibits saturable behavior is complex. Changes can occur in both volume of distribution and clearance. The magnitude of the changes depends on both the volume of distribution and the extraction ratio of the drug at concentrations below saturation. Furthermore, because with saturation volume of distribution changes with amount in body, the decline of the plasma concentration does not reflect, in direct proportion, the disappearance of drug from the body. The slope of the semilogarithmic decline in the concentration–time curve is then not a good measure of the fractional rate of elimination. The qualitative effect of saturable binding to plasma proteins for a drug with a small volume of distribution is demonstrated by the decreasing slope of the unbound cefonicid concentration with time on a semilogarithmic plot (Fig. 16-18) after a single 30-mg/kg i.v. dose. The difference between the decline of the total and unbound concentrations (Fig. 16-18A) is explained by the decrease in the fraction unbound with time (Fig. 16-18B). The apparent one-compartmental nature of the total concentration decline is explained by virtually all drug in the body being bound to albumin.

Saturable binding to plasma proteins (see Fig. 16-18) has been given as one explanation for the observation of an oral bioavailability of greater than 1.0, based on *AUC* comparisons and hence, assumption of constancy of clearance. For a low extraction ratio drug, saturation associated with the high initial concentrations leads to a higher clearance and hence, lower overall *AUC* then occurs with an equal fully available oral dose, especially when absorption is relatively slow resulting in plasma concentrations, even at C_{max}, below that causing saturation.

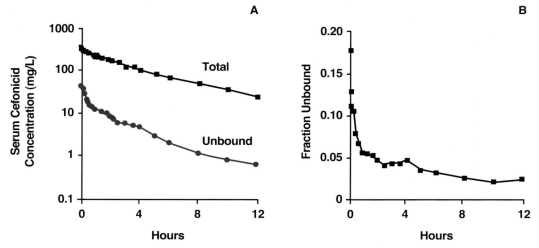

FIGURE 16-18. **A.** Mean total (■) and unbound (■) plasma cefonicid concentrations with time in six volunteers after a single i.v. dose of 30 mg/kg given over 5 min. Note the much more rapid decline of the unbound concentration during the first 2 hr. **B.** The difference between the declines of the two curves in **A** is explained by a rapid decrease in the fraction unbound with time. As a consequence of the limited capacity of serum albumin to bind cefonicid, the high total concentrations at early times tend to approach the capacity for binding. (From: Dudley MN, Shyu WC, Nightingale CH, Quintiliani R. Effect of saturable serum protein binding on the pharmacokinetics of unbound cefonicid in humans. Antimicrob Agents Chemother 1986;30:565–569, with permission.)

The ACE (angiotensin-converting enzyme) inhibitor trandolaprilat, formed following oral administration of trandolapril (the ethyl ester prodrug), shows nonlinear plasma and tissue protein binding, as do other agents in this pharmacologic class. Evidence of nonlinearity in trandolaprilat kinetics is provided in Fig. 16-19. Both AUC (Fig. 16-19A) and plasma concentration (Fig. 16-19B), particularly during the terminal phase, fail to increase in direct proportion to the oral dose of trandolapril, over the eightfold range (0.5–4.0 mg) studied. Also, contrary to the expectation of linear kinetics, dosing daily, which is relatively frequent compared to the long terminal half-life, does not lead to extensive accumulation (Fig. 16-19C). Thus, when a 2-mg dose of trandolapril is administered orally for 10 days, the accumulation ratio of trandolaprilat ($AUC_{ss}/AUC_{1,\tau}$), see "Degree of Accumulation," Chapter 11, *Multiple-Dose Regimens*) is only 1.49. Direct evidence of concentration-dependent plasma protein binding of trandolaprilat is shown in Fig. 16-19D. It should be noted that the range of concentrations, 0.5 to 5.0 μg/L, over which the fraction unbound changes fourfold, covers most of the plasma trandolaprilat concentrations obtained following the oral doses of trandolapril (Fig. 16-19B,C).

The observations above can be rationalized as follows. The extremely low plasma concentration at which saturable binding occurs suggests a binding protein of much lower concentration, and hence capacity, than albumin or α_1-acid glycoprotein (see Table 4-6, Chapter 4, *Membranes and Distribution*). The body of evidence points to *ACE* itself as responsible. This high-affinity, low-capacity enzyme resides in both plasma and the endothelial linings of the vasculature, the latter site being interpreted as tissue binding when viewed from plasma data. Trandolaprilat, a relatively polar molecule, is restricted in its distribution mainly to extracellular spaces and is cleared systemically, mostly by renal excretion. Renal excretion is primarily via glomerular filtration, so that renal clearance shows concentration dependence associated with saturable protein binding. At high concentrations of trandolaprilat, which saturate ACE, renal clearance is high and elimination is rapid. As the plasma concentration falls, the fraction bound to plasma and tissue ACE increases, thereby diminishing the unbound pool and lowering renal clear-

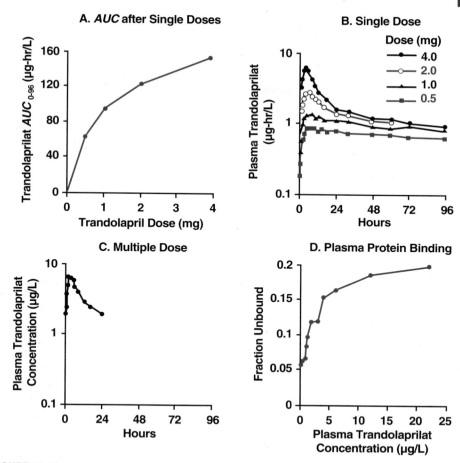

FIGURE 16-19. Trandolaprilat, the active metabolite of trandolapril, exhibits nonlinear kinetic behavior. **A.** The *AUC* (0 to 96 hr) of the metabolite does not increase in direct proportion to the dose of trandolapril over the dose range of 0.5 to 4.0 mg. **B.** A semilogarithmic plot of mean plasma trandolaprilat concentrations after oral trandolapril doses of 0.5, 1.0, 2.0, and 4.0 mg shows nonlinearity in that the curves are not equally spaced by a factor of 2 in the vertical direction for each of the successive doses. The lack of proportionality with dose is particularly evident at later times. **C.** Administration of 2 mg of trandolapril daily for 10 days fails to produce the degree of accumulation of trandolaprilat, as viewed from the concentration–time profile within a dosing interval at steady state (24 hr), that is predicted based on the long terminal decline in plasma concentration observed following a single 2-mg dose (see **B**). **D.** Binding of trandolaprilat to plasma proteins shows nonlinearity in that the fraction unbound increased with increasing concentration. (**A** and **B** from: Lenfant B, Mouren M, Bryce T, et al. Trandolapril: pharmacokinetics of single oral doses in male healthy volunteers. J Cardiovasc Pharmacol 1994;23[Suppl 4]:S38–S43; **C** from: Arner P, Wade A, Engfelt P, et al. Pharmacokinetics and pharmacodynamics of trandolapril after repeated administration of 2 mg to young and elderly patients with mild-to-moderate hypertension. J Cardiovasc Pharmacol 1994;23[Suppl 4]:S50–S59; **D** from: Lenfant B. Personal communication.)

ance. The net effect is a much slower elimination of material from the body. Thus, the biphasic decline of plasma trandolaprilat, seen in the semilogarithmic plots (Fig. 16-19B) is caused by concentration-dependent protein binding in plasma and not tissue distribution kinetics. Notice, that had only 1 dose of drug been administered, one could not have readily distinguished between concentration-dependent binding and distribution kinetics as the cause of the apparent biexponential decline of the plasma data. Finally, the lack of appreciable accumulation on multiple dosing arises because after each dose, most of the systematically available trandolaprilat is eliminated before reaching the terminal phase. Thus, nonlinear binding to the active site, ACE, within plasma appears to explain virtually all of trandolaprilat's odd kinetic behavior.

TISSUE BINDING

The nonlinear kinetics of bosentan, used in the treatment of pulmonary hypertension, is explained by saturable binding to tissues as shown in Fig. 16-20. Again, as with the ACE inhibitors, the nonlinear binding of bosentan occurs at the active site, endothelin receptors in the tissues. The drug is a competitive inhibitor. At low concentrations, much of the drug in the body is on these receptors.

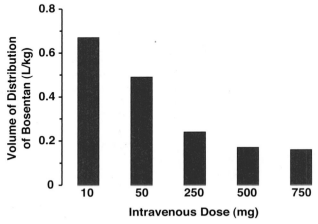

FIGURE 16-20. The steady-state volume of distribution of bosentan, calculated using model-independent methods (see Chapter 19, *Distribution Kinetics*), decreases with the size of an intravenous dose, a result of saturable tissue binding. Binding to plasma proteins is concentration independent. Tissue binding occurs primarily at the site of action, the endothelin receptor. (From: Weber C, Schmitt R, Birnboeck H, et al. Pharmacokinetics and pharmacodynamics of the endothelin-receptor antagonist bosentan in healthy human subjects. Clin Pharmacol Ther 1996;60:124–137.)

Another example, Fig. 16-21, of saturable tissue binding is imirestat, an aldose reductase inhibitor. The time course of the drug depends on the dose administered because the volume of distribution is decreased at higher plasma concentrations. Again, the decreased tissue binding is associated with binding at the active site.

A third example of saturable tissue binding is of that of draflazine, a compound with cardioprotective properties. The blood and plasma concentration–time courses are quite different for this drug (Fig. 16-22) as a consequence of saturable binding to nucleoside transporters located on erythrocytes. On measuring drug concentration in plasma, binding to erythrocytes would be viewed as tissue binding. The relationship between blood and plasma concentrations of this drug is shown in Fig. 16-23. Trandoloprilat, imirestat, bosentan, and draflazine all demonstrate what has been called **target-mediated drug disposition**, because their nonlinear pharmacodynamic and pharmacokinetic behaviors are a result of a common mechanism, saturable binding to the target site.

TIME-DEPENDENT DISPOSITION

The study of changes in response to drug administration or kinetics with time of day, month, or year is an area called chronopharmacology (see Chapter 12, *Variability*). The pharmacokinetic component is **time-dependent kinetics** or **chronopharmacokinetics**. Although enzyme induction is perhaps the most common cause of time-dependent

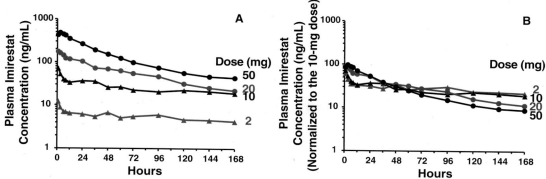

FIGURE 16-21. **A.** Mean plasma imirestat concentration–time profiles following 2-mg, 10-mg, 20-mg, and 50-mg single oral doses. **B.** The concentration–time profiles in graph A normalized to the dose administered. Note that the order of the normalized values between 6 and 36 hr in Fig.16-20B reverses after about 96 hr, a result of an increase in the volume of distribution with time as the plasma concentration drops. The total area under the dose-normalized concentration–time curve in this graph tends to remain much the same. One cannot be sure of this conclusion, however, because the sampling only continued to 168 hr; a large percentage of the normalized area remains under the curve after this time, especially at low concentrations. (From: Brazzell RK, Mayer PR, Dobbs R, et al. Dose-dependent pharmacokinetics of the aldose reductase inhibitor imirestat in man. Pharm Res 1991;8:112–118.)

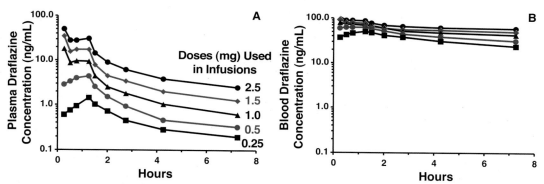

FIGURE 16-22. **A.** Mean plasma concentrations of draflazine as a function of time after a 15-min intravenous infusion of 0.25- (■), 0.5- (●), 1.0- (▲), 1.5- (◆), and 2.5- (●) mg draflazine followed by a 1-hr infusion of the same dose in eight healthy male subjects. **B.** Mean whole blood concentrations of draflazine in the same studies. (From: Snoeck E, Plotrovskij V, Jacqmin P, et al. Population analysis of the nonlinear red blood cell partitioning and the concentration–effect relationship of draflazine following various infusion rates. Br J Clin Pharmacol 1997;43:603–612.)

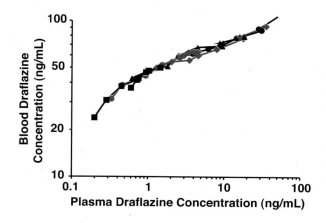

FIGURE 16-23. Relationship (full logarithmic plot) between draflazine concentrations in whole blood and plasma in the studies summarized in Fig. 16-22. Note the relatively small change in whole blood concentration of draflazine compared to that in plasma. The symbols are the same as those in Fig. 16-22 for the 5 doses administered.

kinetics, there are many other reasons for this behavior. For example, circadian variations in renal function, urine pH, α_1-acid glycoprotein concentration, gastrointestinal physiology (food and drink), and cardiac output all occur.

An example of circadian changes in drug absorption and disposition is shown in Fig. 16-24. Median data are shown (because of skewed distribution of values) for eight subjects who received an oral 80-mg dose of verapamil at various times during the day. Note that administration in the evening produces a lower peak drug concentration and, as such, may produce less effect than does administration in the morning.

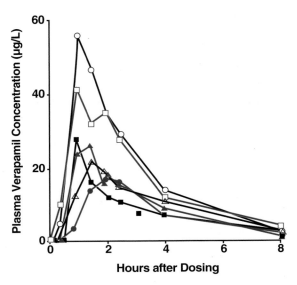

FIGURE 16-24. Median plasma verapamil concentration–time profiles for eight subjects, each given a single 80-mg tablet of drug at the following times: 4:00 A.M. (▲); 8:00 A.M. (○); noon (□); 4:00 P.M. (△); 8:00 P.M. (●); and midnight (■). Food was withheld 2 hr before to 2 hr after drug administration, as food is known to affect verapamil absorption. To minimize a delay in esophageal transit, subjects took the tablets while standing and remained so for 15 min. The kinetics of the drug appears to change with the time of administration during the day. Factors other than food and posture may be responsible (e.g., changes in hepatic blood flow [verapamil has a high hepatic extraction ratio], enzyme activity, or protein binding). (From: Hla KK, Latham AN, Henry JA. Influence of time of administration on verapamil pharmacokinetics. Clin Pharmacol Ther 1922;51:366–370.)

Chronic effects of a drug on its own renal and hepatic elimination have also been seen, as previously mentioned. For example, aminoglycosides can produce renal toxicity with chronic administration. Because these antibiotics are primarily eliminated by renal excretion, a diminishing renal function with time may cause greater drug accumulation and therefore more toxicity. There is clearly a need to monitor therapy and to limit the duration of therapy, especially in patients who already have compromised renal function.

Food is a major cause of circadian variations, with patients tending to eat much more at the evening meal than at breakfast. Gastric emptying is slowed or delayed by food, often resulting in a decrease in the peak concentration and an increase in the time of its occurrence following a single dose, as seen with verapamil (Fig. 16-24). When absorption is slowed by food, the rate of input into the liver and the concentration of verapamil entering the liver are lower and prolonged. Because metabolism is more complete at lower concentrations, bioavailability is therefore reduced by the

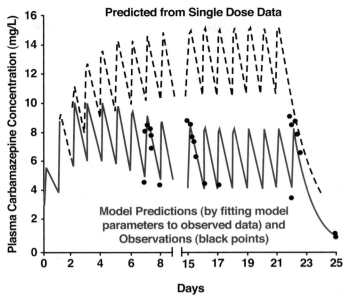

FIGURE 16-25. Carbamazepine undergoes autoinduction as evidenced by the declining plasma concentration (•), assessed on days 7, 8, 15, 16, 22, and 23 of an oral multiple-dose regimen of 6 mg/kg taken by a subject once daily in the morning for 22 consecutive days. Predictions based on single-dose pharmacokinetic data, obtained previously in the subject and based on the assumption that no induction occurs, are shown by the *stippled line*. Predictions assuming an autoinduction model for carbamazepine, in which the turnover time of the affected enzyme is approximately 5 days, are indicated by the *solid colored line*. Notice the break between days 8 and 15. (Copyright 1976 by the American Pharmaceutical Association, Clinical Pharmacokinetics: Concepts and Applications, 2nd ed. Reprinted with permission of the American Pharmaceutical Association.)

concurrent intake of food and, as expected, the effect is greater after the heavy evening meal than after breakfast.

Carbamazepine shows time dependence in its disposition (see Fig. 16-25). The decrease in its peak concentration on repetitive oral administration indicates that either oral bioavailability decreases or clearance increases with time. The latter has been shown to explain the observation caused by carbamazepine inducing its own metabolism. This autoinduction is also dose- and concentration-dependent, a property common to many time-dependent processes.

Autoinduction has a number of therapeutic consequences. It reduces the time to achieve steady state and limits one's ability to use information from a single dose to predict kinetics after repeated doses or continuous administration. Furthermore, it may be associated with the induction of metabolism (same enzymatic pathway) of coadministered drugs, producing a drug interaction.

Another time-dependent mechanism is mechanism-based autoinhibition. The mechanism is discussed more fully in Chapter 17, *Drug Interactions*. Suffice it to say here that the drug destroys its own metabolizing enzyme. Such compounds have been called "suicide substrates." The net result is that the larger the dose and the longer the time of exposure, the greater the apparent inhibition. Clarithromycin (Fig. 16-26) shows this nonlinear behavior. Note that on increasing a single dose from 250 to 500 mg, there is a disproportionate increase in *AUC* (see Fig. 16-25A) and an increase in half-life (see Fig. 16-25B). The same occurs on multiple dosing. By the seventh dose, the half-life is considerably longer than that seen after a single dose at both the 250- and 500-mg dose levels.

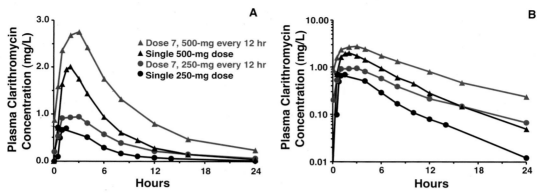

FIGURE 16-26. Mean plasma clarithromycin concentrations with time after a single 250-mg dose (●—●), after dose 7 of a regimen of 250 mg every 12 hr (●—●), after a single 500-mg dose (▲—▲), after dose 7 of a regimen of 500 mg every 12 hr (▲—▲). Both linear (**A**) and semilogarithmic (**B**) plots are shown. (From: Chu S, Wilson DS, Deaton RL, et al. Single- and multiple-dose pharmacokinetics of clarithromycin, a new macrolide antimicrobial. J Clin Pharmacol 1993;33:719–725.)

RECOGNITION OF NONLINEARITIES

Nonlinearities are often apparent in graphic and tabular presentations of data. The interpretation of such kinetic behavior often requires a methodical analysis of the information. This analysis may be accomplished using the following steps:

1. Compare the observation to that expected for linear kinetics. This is most easily accomplished by normalizing the observations with time or the pharmacokinetic parameters to the dose given. With linear kinetics, the observations with time should superimpose and the parameter values should not change with dose.
2. Identify the kinetic parameter(s) that appear(s) to be altered and the direction of the change.
3. Determine the primary pharmacokinetic parameter(s) CL_H, CL_R, V, ka, and F that appear(s) to be affected. Also evaluate if fu is altered.
4. Consider if the mechanism(s) is (are) consistent with the changes observed.

URINARY RECOVERY

Nonlinearities are often first identified from recovery of drug and metabolites in urine. This is the case for salicylic acid, as shown in Table 16-6.

TABLE 16-6	Urinary Recovery of Salicylic Acid and Its Metabolites as a Percentage of a Single Oral Dose*		
Dose (mg)	Salicylic Acid	Salicyluric Acid	Salicyl Phenolic and AcylGlucuronides
192	3	83	17
767	5	70	24
1533	17	59	24
3000	14	50	30

*Dose and recovery expressed in equivalents of salicylic acid. (From: Levy G. Pharmacokinetics of salicylate elimination in man. J Pharm Sci 1965;54:959–967.)

Analysis. Step 1. Dose dependence in salicylic acid is apparent from changes in the fraction of a single oral dose recovered in urine as unchanged drug and as the metabolites, salicyluric acid and glucuronide conjugates. With linear kinetics, the fraction of each compound recovered remains the same regardless of dose.

Steps 2 to 4. The increased percent recovered as unchanged drug on increasing dose could be explained by an increased bioavailability, an increased renal clearance, or a capacity limitation in its metabolism. This is seen from the relationships $Ae_\infty/Dose = fe \cdot F$ and $fe = CL_R/(CL_R + CL_{NR})$. Without further information, these possibilities cannot be distinguished. The decreased recovery of the major metabolite, salicyluric acid, and the nearly complete total recovery (as drug and metabolites) at all of the doses suggest that increased bioavailability may not be the explanation (see Chapter 5, *Elimination*). Increased bioavailability would increase metabolite recovery as well, which was not the case.

CONCENTRATION–TIME PROFILE

Figure 16-27 is a semilogarithmic plot of plasma salicylic acid concentration with time after a single 3-g oral dose. It is generally preferred to have observations following more than 1 dose, but let us examine the single-dose data.

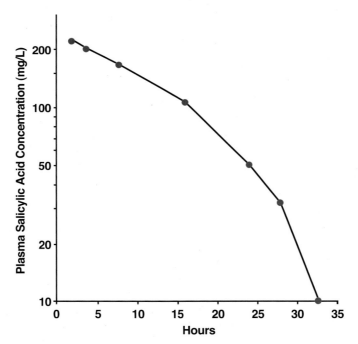

FIGURE 16-27. Semilogarithmic plot of the plasma concentration of salicylic acid in a subject following a single oral dose of 3 g of sodium salicylate. The steadily increasing decline with time is caused by the concentration falling from the region that saturates metabolic pathways to one below saturation. (From: Salassa RM, Bollman JL, Dry TJ. The effect of para-aminobenzoic acid on the metabolism and excretion of salicylate. J Lab Clin Med 1948;33:1393–1401.)

Analysis. Step 1. The slope of the decline is greater at low than at high concentrations. When linear kinetics operates, there is either no change in slope or a greater slope at early times while distribution is occurring (Chapter 19, *Distribution Kinetics*).

Step 2. The half-life shortens as time passes or as concentration declines.

Step 3. It appears that either *CL* increases or *V* decreases with time or with falling concentration.

Step 4. From the dose and maximum concentration (around 200 mg/L) and the conclusion based on urinary data (and independent i.v. data) that salicylic acid is totally absorbed after oral administration, the volume of distribution is estimated to be about 15 L. Being so small, *V* is unlikely to decrease much with either time or decreasing concentration. An increase in *CL* with time or at lower concentrations would occur if elimination of salicylic acid is capacity-limited. The data in Table 16-6 indicate that salicylic acid is extensively converted to several metabolites. However, the pronounced increase in frac-

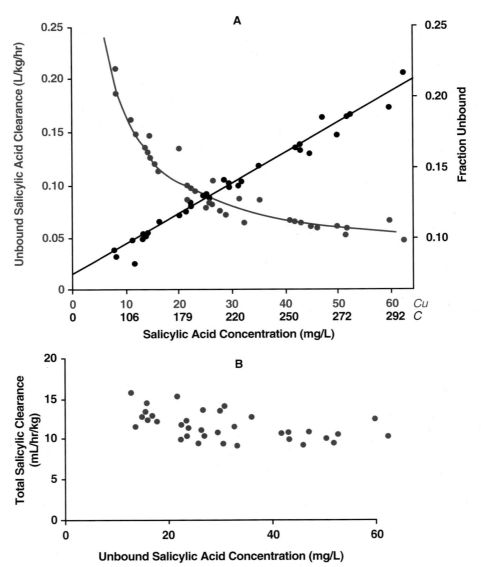

FIGURE 16-28. **A.** The clearance of unbound drug (●, *colored line*), determined under steady-state conditions, and the fraction unbound in plasma (●) vary inversely with each other as the salicylic acid concentration is increased. The corresponding total plasma concentrations are superimposed on the linear scale of the unbound drug concentration. (From: Furst DE, Tozer TN, Melmon KL. Salicylate clearance: the result of protein binding and metabolism. Clin Pharmacol Ther 1979;26:380–389. Reproduced with permission of Nature Pub. Group.) **B.** The total clearance of salicylic acid, determined under steady-state conditions, remains relatively constant within the range of therapeutic concentrations; a fortuitous consequence of the essentially equivalent and opposing effects of saturable plasma protein binding and saturable metabolism.

tion excreted as unchanged salicylic acid with increasing dose (see Table 16-6) implies that saturability of a major metabolic pathway is likely at the 3-g dose level.

PROTEIN-BINDING DATA

The incorporation of binding data further clarifies the nature of nonlinearities present, as shown in Fig. 16-28.

Analysis. Step 1. As observed in Fig. 16-28A, *fu* increases with increasing concentration, indicating nonlinearity of salicylic acid binding to plasma proteins. Nonlinearity in CLu (and hence CL_{int}, as $Dose/AUC$ calculations shows it to be a low extraction ratio drug) is also uncovered. As shown in Fig. 16-28B, salicylic acid has a low clearance even at low concentrations. As such, CL_{int}, should remain constant if elimination processes are unaffected by the concentration (dose) of salicylic acid.

Steps 2 to 3. The parameters affected are identified in this case, *fu* and CL_{int}.

Step 4. The mechanisms involved appear to be saturable binding to plasma proteins and some form of capacity-limited elimination. From the additional information in Table 16-6 and Fig. 16-28, the capacity limitation must lie with metabolism.

Interestingly, total clearance is relatively constant throughout the therapeutic range of salicylic acid (*Cu* between 10 and 60 mg/L). This is a consequence of the opposing tendencies of the two forms of nonlinearity. Clearance decreases with concentration because of capacity-limited metabolism. Saturable binding, on the other hand, tends to increase clearance at higher concentrations, $CL = fu \cdot CL_{int}$. The decrease in unbound clearance, the consequence of saturability in two major metabolic pathways of salicylic acid (formation of salicyluric acid and salicyl phenolic glucuronide) leads to a disproportionate increase in unbound concentration with increasing dosing rate (Fig. 16-29). Further information on the specific nonlinear metabolic pathways requires isolating the metabolic pathways. This has been accomplished by comparing the rates of urinary

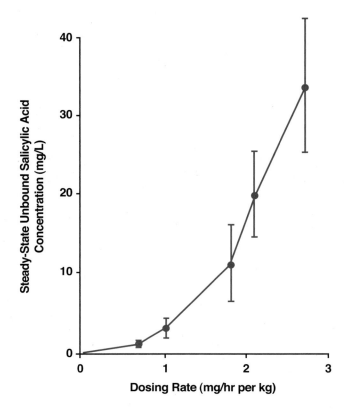

FIGURE 16-29. The steady-state unbound concentration of salicylic acid in plasma (mean ± standard deviation [SD]) increases disproportionately with the dosing rate of aspirin. Aspirin is completely hydrolyzed to the measured metabolite, salicylic acid. The disproportionate increase reflects the saturability of two of salicylic acid's major pathways of elimination, formation of salicyl phenolic glucuronide and salicyluric acid. (From: Tozer TN, Tang-Liu DD-S, Riegelman S. Linear vs. Nonlinear kinetics. In Breimer D, Speiser P, eds. Topics in Pharmaceutical Sciences. New York: Elsevier, 1981:3–17.)

excretion of each metabolite to the amount of salicylic acid in the body, a procedure analogous to the determination of renal clearance. The method is applicable if the rate of excretion of metabolite equals its rate of formation, as is the case for salicylic acid after a single dose and for all drugs under steady-state conditions.

KINETICS IN DRUG OVERDOSE

Nonlinear kinetics is perhaps more the rule than the exception in drug overdose. Either the volume of distribution or the total clearance, or both, are often changed in the overdose situation. Ethchlorvynol, a generally superseded sedative–hypnotic used only when intolerance or allergic responses to other agents exists, shows such concentration-dependent kinetic behavior (Fig. 16-30) in cases of drug overdose. At normal therapeutic doses, the half-life is 25 hr; in overdose cases, it is increased to more than 100 hr, probably because of a decreased metabolic clearance at the higher concentrations. Similar to lithium (Chapter 19, *Distribution Kinetics*) and many other drugs, ethchlorvynol also shows plasma rebound after dialysis as the concentration at the beginning of the first two dialysis treatments is higher than that at the end of the previous dialysis sessions. The redistribution here is a consequence of the high affinity of ethchlorvynol for fat, a poorly perfused tissue.

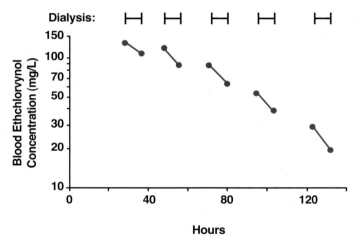

FIGURE 16-30. The overall decline of ethchlorvynol concentration in blood on this semilogarithmic plot shows concentration dependence in an intoxicated patient. During each 8-hr dialysis period (*indicated by the bars*), the concentration (●—●) was reduced but tended to rise again when dialysis was discontinued, indicative of redistribution. (From: Tozer TN, Witt LD, Gee L, et al. Evaluation of hemodialysis for ethchlorvynol (Placidyl) overdose. Am J Hosp Pharm 1974;31:986–989. Original data from: Gibson PF, Wright N. Ethchlorvynol in biological fluids: specificity of assay methods. J Pharm Sci 1972;61:169–174.)

THERAPEUTIC CONSEQUENCES OF NONLINEARITIES

The therapeutic consequences of dose-dependent kinetics are perhaps best considered under steady-state conditions. Here, dose dependence in rate–time profile of absorption is of little or no consequence unless bioavailability (extent) is also altered. Alterations in bioavailability are important in that unbound concentration and amount in the body at steady state may change disproportionately on changing dose. Conditions that cause dose dependence in bioavailability may also produce increased variability in this parameter at the same dose. For example, consider two drugs, a dissolution rate-limited one, such as griseofulvin, and one that is highly extracted on passing across the gastrointestinal membranes or through the liver, such as alprenolol. Changes in gastric emptying and in other physiologic factors can produce large variations in the bioavailability of these drugs. The effect of rapid gastric emptying may be a decrease in bioavailability of griseofulvin because of less time for mixing and dissolution but an increase in bioavailability of alprenolol because of saturability in intestinal and hepatic metabolism.

Clinically, the most dramatic source of dose dependence is capacity-limited metabolism. Only small changes in bioavailability may produce large changes in the steady-state concentration. Under these conditions, careful titration of an individual patient's dosage requirement is needed, especially if the drug has a narrow therapeutic index. Moreover, this source of dose-dependence also produces large interpatient variability in steady-state concentration, as observed for phenytoin in Fig. 1-7 (page 9).

Time-dependent kinetics is perhaps best typified by both autoinduction and mechanism-based inhibition. Another cause is decreased renal function on continued administration of a nephrotoxic drug. If the drug is primarily renally eliminated, the therapeutic consequence of the latter cause is clear and opposite to that of autoinduction.

In general, if two drugs are equivalent in all respects except for one showing either a dose- or time-dependent kinetic behavior, then the one showing linear kinetics is the drug of choice. On the other hand, just because a drug in development shows nonlinear kinetic behavior does not mean it should be discarded. There are many useful agents that show nonlinearity in their absorption or disposition.

KEY RELATIONSHIPS

$$Rate\ of\ metabolism = \frac{Vm \cdot Cu}{Km + Cu_H}$$

$$CL_{int,m} = \frac{Vm}{Km + Cu_H}$$

Intrinsic metabolic
clearance

$$Rate\ of\ transport = \frac{Tm \cdot Cu}{K_T + Cu}$$

$$Bound\ Concentration = \frac{n \cdot P_t \cdot Cu}{K_d + Cu}$$

$$Cu_{ss} = \frac{Km \cdot R_0}{Vm - R_0}$$

$$\frac{Cu_{ss}}{R_0} = \frac{Km}{Vm - R_0}$$

STUDY PROBLEMS

(Answers to Study Problems are in Appendix J.)

1. Circle the number(s) of the one or more *correct* answers to each of the following multiple-choice questions. Briefly discuss those answers that may be ambiguous (situations in which the statement may be true or false).

   a. Capacity-limited metabolism of a drug is associated with:

   (1) A less than proportional increase in the steady-state plasma concentration on increasing the total daily dose.

(2) An apparent half-life that is longer at low than at high concentrations.

(3) A decrease in the rate of metabolism as the amount of drug in the body is increased.

(4) All of the above.

(5) None of the above.

b. A mean steady-state plasma concentration obtained after 30 doses that is much higher than that predicted from the value of clearance obtained after a single dose suggests that:

(1) Induction has occurred.

(2) The volume of distribution has decreased.

(3) A metabolite may be acting as an inhibitor of parent drug elimination.

(4) None of the above.

c. The following steady-state plasma drug concentrations have been observed in a subject following various constant daily oral dosages:

Dosing Rate (mg/day)	Steady-State Plasma concentration (mg/L)
500	45
1000	56
1500	62

These data are consistent, on increasing the dosing rate, with and may be explained by:

(1) Decreased bioavailability.

(2) Increased clearance.

(3) Decreased plasma protein binding.

(4) Increased volume of distribution.

d. The total cumulative amounts of drug collected in the urine within 48 hr (essentially Ae_∞) following various single oral doses of a drug, administered on separate occasions, are shown below.

Dose (mg)	Amount Excreted Unchanged in 48 hr (mg)
50	1.1
100	2.8
200	9.0

These data are consistent with and may be explained by:

(1) Saturable active transport in the wall of the gastrointestinal tract.

(2) Saturable first-pass metabolism.

(3) Saturable active renal tubular secretion.

(4) Saturable active renal tubular reabsorption.

2. a. Define *mechanism-based autoinhibition.*

b. Ticlopidine has a half-life of 2 hr after a single 250-mg dose and a half-life of 4 to 5 days after a few weeks of daily dosing. Is this observation consistent with mechanism-based autoinhibition of metabolism? Briefly discuss.

3. For *each* of the following tables, indicate *all* of the possibilities in the following list that might explain the dose-dependent kinetics observed for each drug.

List of Explanations

I. Saturable hepatic metabolism.

II. Saturable renal tubular reabsorption.

III. Saturable renal active secretion.

IV. Saturable plasma protein binding with extraction ratio approaching one in organs of elimination.

V. Saturable plasma protein binding with extraction ratio approaching zero in organs of elimination.

VI. Saturable metabolism during first pass of drug through the intestines or the liver.

VII. Saturable gastrointestinal transport.

A.

TABLE 16-7   *AUC* with Increasing Dose of Drug

Single oral dose (mg)	300	600	900
Area under blood concentration–time curve (mg-hr/L)	3	10	19

B.

TABLE 16-8   Steady-State Plasma Concentration with Increasing Rate of Infusion of Drug

Rate of i.v. infusion (mg/hr)	5	10	15
Steady-state plasma concentration (mg/L)	2	6.5	14

C.

TABLE 16-9   Events in Plasma Seen with a Drug Exhibiting One-Compartment Disposition Following i.v. Bolus Dose Administration*

Single i.v. dose (mg)	50	100	200	400
Initial blood concentration (mg/L)	1.1	2.0	4.3	8.7
Area under blood concentration–time curve (mg-hr/L)	20	55	160	410

*One-compartment drug.

4. The relationship between glucose urinary excretion rate and its plasma concentration in a healthy individual is displayed in Table 16-10. Prepare a graph of glucose renal clearance in milliliters per minute as a function of its plasma concentration, and briefly explain the observation.

TABLE 16-10   Glucose Excretion Rate at Various Plasma Glucose Concentrations

Excretion rate (mg/min)	5	66	151	256	400	520	631
Plasma glucose concentration (g/L)	2.00	3.01	3.98	5.03	6.05	7.08	7.99

5. The data in Table 16-11 were observed for disopyramide (M.W. = 339.5 g/mol) in two different subjects, each receiving various rates of i.v. infusion. Approximately 55% of disopyramide, a basic drug that binds to α_1-acid glycoprotein, is normally excreted unchanged in urine. The remainder is metabolized. Based from the information above, give two possible explanations for the dose-dependence of disopyramide clearance.

TABLE 16-11	Steady-State Concentrations of Disopyramide Following Various Intravenous Rates in Each of Two Subjects	
Subject	**Infusion Rate (mg/min)**	**Steady-State Concentration (mg/L)**
J.J.	0.039	0.70
	0.077	1.15
	0.154	2.01
	0.309	2.48
B.H.	0.08	0.82
	0.16	1.30
	0.32	2.30
	0.64	2.90
	1.05	4.09
	1.94	5.56

6. Four mechanisms that produce dose-dependent kinetics together with supplemental information obtained under linear conditions are listed below. Graphically show, on the plots requested, the kinetic consequences of each of these mechanisms. Draw a *solid line* for the observation expected when the kinetics is linear and a *dashed line* for the situation in which dose-dependent behavior occurs. General tendencies, rather than specific functionalities, are sought.

    a. Saturable first-pass metabolism (oral administration of a single dose)

    Plot: *Dose/AUC* versus *Dose*

    b. Saturable reabsorption in the renal tubule ($F = 0.9$; $fe = 0.5$; drug given as single oral dose)

    Plot: *Ae$_\infty$/AUC* versus *Dose*

    c. Capacity-limited metabolism ($fe = 0.01$, drug infused intravenously at a constant rate)

    Plot: C_{ss} versus Infusion rate

    d. Saturable binding to plasma proteins (single oral dose)

    Plot: *Cu* versus *C*

7. Table 16-12 is intended to summarize the direction of change expected in the disposition parameters and in total and unbound steady-state blood concentrations of a drug, relative to the rate of i.v. administration, when there is a dose dependency in absorption, distribution, or elimination. Complete the table by indicating ↑ for increase, ↓ for decrease, or ↔ for little or no change.

TABLE 16-12	**Disposition Kinetics and Total and Unbound Steady-State Blood Drug Concentrations as a Function of Dose-Dependency in Each of Several Sources following Oral and Intravenous Administration**

Source of Dose Dependency	Direction of Change with Increased Total Daily Dose*	$V^\dagger$	CL	$t_{1/2}$	$\left[\dfrac{\text{CONCENTRATION}}{\text{RATE OF ADMINISTRATION}} \right]^\ddagger$ Total	Unbound
Oral Administration						
Bioavailability	↓	↔				
Absorption rate constant	↓	↔				
Intravenous Administration						
Fraction unbound in blood						
Low extraction ratio drug	↑	↑				
High extraction ratio drug	↑	↑				
Fraction unbound in tissue	↑		↔			
Metabolic clearance	↑		↑			
Renal clearance	↓		↓			

*Only one example of each direction of change is shown.
†The volume of distribution is at least 10 times the blood volume.
‡The average steady-state total and unbound blood drug concentration relative to the rate of administration.

8. The data in Fig. 16-11 for dicloxacillin were presented without associated plasma protein binding information (not provided in the article). The renal clearance of the drug, as assessed from Ae_∞/AUC, decreased on increasing the dose from 1 to 2 g. Dicloxacillin, a weak acid with a MW of 470 g/mol, is extensively bound to albumin ($fu = 0.04$ at 10 mg/L) and produces a peak concentration of about 60 mg/L after oral administration of 2 g. Could saturable binding to a plasma protein explain the decrease in Ae_∞/AUC with the larger dose?

9. Table 16-13 lists plasma heparin activity determined by the amount of hexadimethrine bromide required to neutralize heparin activity using thrombin-induced coagulation as an endpoint.

   a. Plot both sets of activity–time data on the same semilogarithmic graph.
   b. Do the data suggest dose-dependent kinetic behavior? If so, which pharmacokinetic parameters appear to be affected?
   c. Could the kinetic behavior be explained by capacity-limited elimination of the Michaelis-Menten type? Briefly discuss.

		Heparin Activity*	
Time (min)	Dose (Units/kg)	25	75
0		0.313	-
15		-	0.872
20		0.238	-
30		0.175	-
40		0.106	-
45		-	0.592
60		0.06[†]	0.420
90		-	0.249
120		-	0.228
150		-	0.161
180		-	0.083

TABLE 16-13 Heparin Activity in Plasma after Single Intravenous Injections of 25 and 75 U/kg of Heparin on Separate Occasions in a Healthy Subject

*Activity in units per milliliter.
[†]Point added for didactic purposes.
From: Bjornsson TD, Wolfram KM, Kitchell BB. Heparin kinetics determined by three assay methods. Clin Pharmacal Ther 1982;31:104–113.

d. Heparin is a natural heterogeneous mucopolysaccharide consisting of polymeric units of different chain length and chemical composition with MW ranging from 3000 to 40,000 g/mol. Could the nonlinear kinetic behavior be explained by the simultaneous assay of multiple components? Briefly discuss.

10. Comment on the accuracy of the following statements:

a. Capacity-limited metabolism of a drug is associated with a less than proportional increase in the steady-state concentration on increasing the daily dose.

b. Saturable reabsorption in the renal tubule of drugs with an fe close to 1.0 leads to longer half-lives at higher drug concentrations.

c. A drug that undergoes "target-mediated drug disposition" shows an increase in clearance as the dose is increased.

17

Drug Interactions

OBJECTIVES

The reader will be able to:

- Define the following terms: additivity, antagonism, displacer, combination products, competitive inhibition, drug interaction, inhibition constant, isobologram, mechanism-based inhibition, noncompetitive inhibition, synergism, therapeutic drug interaction.

- Discuss the graded nature of drug interactions, and provide two examples involving reversible inhibition, two involving mechanism-based inhibition, and one involving induction.

- Explain mechanistically and kinetically the difference between reversible and mechanism-based inhibition.

- Ascertain whether pharmacokinetics or pharmacodynamics of a drug, or both, is altered by another drug, given response and unbound plasma drug concentration–time data following chronic administration.

- Anticipate the likely changes in plasma and unbound concentrations with time when the pharmacokinetics of a drug is altered by concurrent drug administration.

- Explain why displacement of plasma protein binding is unlikely to produce a clinically significant drug interaction.

- Explain why the degree of interaction tends to be greater when the affected drug is administered orally than when administered parenterally, for drugs that are normally subjected to a high oral first-pass metabolic loss.

- Explain why the risk of a severe interaction resulting from inhibition is greater in poor than extensive metabolizers, when the fraction of drug metabolized polymorphically in extensive metabolizers is high, and the inhibitor inhibits elimination via the other pathway(s).

- Anticipate the likely changes in plasma and unbound concentrations with time when the pharmacokinetics of a drug is altered by concurrent drug administration.

- Show graphically the consequence of a pharmacokinetic drug interaction when the mechanism and the circumstances of its occurrence are given.

- Explain why the combination of two agonists or two antagonists of the same receptor may not produce a greater response than that achieved with any one of them.

Patients commonly receive two or more drugs concurrently; indeed, inpatients on average receive five drugs during a hospitalization, and many, particularly elderly, patients may be taking concurrently eight or more drugs, as discussed in Chapter 14, *Age, Weight, and Gender*, Fig. 14-4. In addition, with an increasingly aged population, the issue of polypharmacy is of ever greater concern. The reasons for multiple-drug therapy are many. One reason, as discussed in Chapter 9, *Therapeutic Window,* is that drug combinations have been found to be beneficial in the treatment of some conditions, including various cardiovascular diseases, infections, and cancer. Another reason is that patients frequently suffer from several concurrent diseases or conditions, and each may require the use of one or more drugs, in which case the number of drug combinations is huge. Furthermore, drugs may be prescribed by clinicians in different medical specialties each of whom may be not fully aware of the therapeutic maneuvers of the others. Finally, patients may also self-medicate with over-the-counter medicines or herbal preparations. All of these reasons lead to a high probability of a **drug interaction** during drug therapy, especially in the elderly.

A drug interaction occurs when either the pharmacokinetics or pharmacodynamics of one drug is altered by another. In addition, constituents of some foods and herbal preparations may alter the pharmacokinetics or pharmacodynamics of drugs. Examples are inhibition by grapefruit juice of gut wall CYP3A and induction of this enzyme by St. John's wort, discussed in Chapter 7, *Absorption,* and Chapter 12, *Variability.* As the principles are the same as for drugs, such food and herbal drug interactions are not considered further, although they can be therapeutically important.

The potential for interactions among drugs within the body are almost limitless and are a source of variability in drug response. Many regard drug interactions as all-or-none, viewing them either as occurring or not, whereas in reality, most drug interactions, whether pharmacokinetic or pharmacodynamic in nature, are graded, depending on the concentration of the interacting drugs, and hence on the dosage regimens and pharmacokinetics of the drugs. Few of these interactions are of a type or of a sufficient magnitude to be clinically important. However, a number are and the risk of them occurring increases with the number of drugs that the patient is taking. A **therapeutic drug interaction** has then occurred. It is prudent to provide a cautionary note for those situations in which the two (or more) drugs need to be coprescribed. Some examples are listed in Table 17-1; in most cases, the interaction results in an exaggerated response of the affected drug, but not always so. Reduced activity can arise because the perpetrating drug either is an antagonist, reduces bioavailability, or increases clearance. Occasionally, the magnitude of the interaction is so great as to contraindicate the simultaneous use of the drugs. Very occasionally, the interaction has been so much more severe than anticipated and the likelihood of the combination being inadvertently given so great to cause either the affected or offending drug to be removed from the market. Examples are the antihistamines terfenadine and astemizole, the antihypertensive mebifredril, the statin cerivastatin, and cisapride, used to treat heartburn. However, the drugs were not removed from the market until some major clinical adverse events, sometimes fatal, occurred. Inadvertent, and potentially avoidable, adverse drug interactions also comprise a significant source of hospital admissions.

Not all patients receiving several interacting drugs elicit a therapeutically significant interaction. Often, it is just a few. The reasons for these differences in response among patients are manifold. Included are individual differences in the dosage regimen and duration of administration of each drug, in the sequence of drug administration, and in patient adherence. Pharmacodynamic and pharmacokinetic differences in genetics, concurrent disease states, and many other factors also contribute. Thus, the circumstances associated with a clinically significant interaction in an individual should always be carefully documented.

A pharmacodynamic interaction can arise for various reasons. These include the interacting drug complementing the action of the other, such as the use of a thiazide diuretic and a β-blocker, each acting by a different mechanism to lower blood pressure. Alternatively, the interacting drug may act as an antagonist or agonist at the same receptor site as the other drug, and, if an agonist, it may act additively or synergistically. The effect is

TABLE 17-1	**Classification and Examples of Drug Interactions to Be Avoided**

Pharmacodynamic Interactions

Response		Example	Comment
	↑*	Diphenhydramine ↔ Alcohol[†]	Mutual sedative effects.
	↓	Naloxone → Fentanyl[‡]	Naloxone antagonizes the analgesic effect of the opioid fentanyl and can precipitate withdrawal symptoms.

Pharmacokinetic Interactions

Parameter			
Oral Bioavailability	↑	Saquinavir → Midazolam	Saquinavir inhibits intestinal CYP3A4-mediated metabolism of midazolam.
	↓	Antacids → Chloroquine	An interval of at least 4 hr is needed to avoid reduced absorption of chloroquine.
Volume of Distribution	↓	Quinidine → Digoxin	Quinidine reduces the tissue distribution of digoxin, causing need to reduce loading dose.
Metabolic Clearance	↑	Rifampin → Warfarin	Rifampin strongly induces hepatic microsomal enzymes.
	↓	Erythromycin → Sildenafil	Erythromycin strongly inhibits CYP3A4; major enzyme responsible for sildenafil metabolism.
Renal Clearance	↓	Diuretics → Lithium	By causing sodium loss, diuretics can reduce the renal clearance of lithium, and increase lithium retention, with potential toxicity.

*↑ Denotes increase, ↓ decrease in pharmacodynamic response or pharmacokinetic parameter value.
[†]↔ Denotes a mutual interaction, each affecting the other.
[‡]→ Denotes a unidirectional interaction; the arrow points to affected drug.

additive if the combined effect is that expected based on the concentration–response curves for each drug given independently. **Synergism** occurs when the effect produced with the two drugs is even greater than expected had the effect been additive.

In the case of pharmacodynamic interactions, for which the mechanism of action of each compound is known, the interaction is generally predictable and, if undesirable, is avoidable. The same is increasingly true of pharmacokinetic interactions, and when the interaction is desirable, the interacting drugs are often prescribed as combinations of fixed doses, although in such cases, there is commonly only one active principle; the second compound interacts to overcome an existing limitation in one or more aspects of the pharmacokinetics of the affected drug to increase its exposure–time profile at the target site for a given dose. Examples of pharmacokinetically driven beneficial combination products are listed in Table 17-2. Detailed aspects of some of these are discussed later in this chapter. Furthermore, most attention clinically in the area of drug interactions has been directed to changes in systemic exposure of drugs, and this forms the major emphasis of the current chapter.

Before considering drug interactions in greater detail, two final general comments need to be made. The first concerns the sequence of drug administration. A drug interaction is most likely to be detected in clinical practice when the interacting drug is initiated or withdrawn. For example, given the usual variability in patients' responses to

TABLE 17-2	Pharmacokinetically Driven Combination Products	

Drug combination	Indication	Rationale for combination
Lopinavir/Ritonavir	AIDS	Ritonavir increases the systemic exposure, and decreases interpatient variability, of lopinavir by increasing its oral bioavailability and decreasing its clearance by inhibiting its CYP 3A4-catalyzed metabolism. It also allows for a reduced daily dose of lopinavir and a decrease in the frequency of dosing, every 12 hr versus 8 hr.
L-Dopa/Carbidopa	Parkinson's disease	Carbidopa increases the systemic exposure, and decreases interpatient variability, of L-dopa by inhibiting the decarboxylase enzyme responsible for L-dopa metabolism in intestinal, hepatic, and renal tissues. It allows for a reduced dosage of L-dopa and a more prolonged systemic exposure.
Imipenem/Cilastatin	Urinary tract infection	By inhibiting renal dehydropeptidase, responsible for metabolism of imipenen in the kidney, cilastatin increases the urinary tract concentrations of this antibiotic.
Amoxicillin/Cavulanate	Systemic infection	Some microorganisms are resistant to amoxicillin; they produce β-lactamases that destroy this antibiotic locally. Cavulanate overcomes this resistance by inhibiting β-lactamases, thereby increasing the local antibiotic exposure.

drugs, it is unlikely that a drug interaction would be detected if the affected drug is titrated to response in a patient already stabilized on the drug causing the interaction. Certainly, the dosage regimen of the affected drug would be different in *that* patient than would otherwise be the case, but the resulting regimen may still be within the normal range. In this case, only if the offending drug is withdrawn first, when the patient is stabilized on the drug combination, would the interaction be seen. The interaction would also have been detected if the interacting drug had been administered to the patient already stabilized on the original drug. However, sometimes the delay in full expression of the interaction may take so long that the clinician may not associate a change in patient response to the addition or withdrawal of the offending drug.

The second final comment concerns interactions involving drug transporters. Recall from Chapter 7, *Absorption*, that drugs that belong to class 1 of the Biopharmaceutics Classification System are highly soluble and permeable (e.g., Table 7-9); their absorption, and most of their disposition, is unaffected by transporters. The reason is that passive permeability tends to predominate. For analogous reasons drug interactions involving inhibition or induction of transporters, certainly in relation to intestinal absorption and probably hepatic processes, are not anticipated to affect the pharmacokinetics of such drugs. A clear potential exception exists at the blood-brain barrier, because there, owing to a low passive permeability, even for class 1 compounds, distribution may be permeability rate-limited. Inhibition of transporters there could result in altered brain permeability, and hence changes in both rate and extent of brain distribution, even of class 1 compounds. However, examples to date are rare. Class 1 drugs can nonetheless be inhibitors or inducers of transporters, and so potentially may affect the pharmacokinetics of drugs in classes 2 to 4 of the Biopharmaceutics Classification System.

CLASSIFICATION

One system of classifying drug interactions is to note whether drug response is increased or decreased. While perhaps clinically useful, this classification does not help to define the mechanism of the interaction. In this book, interactions are classified based on whether pharmacokinetics or pharmacodynamics is altered; occasionally, both are changed. Distinction between the two is made by relating response to the unbound plasma concentration of the pharmacologically active species. No change in the unbound concentration–response curve implies a pharmacokinetic drug interaction, which can arise either through a chemical interaction, such as inhibition of metabolism, or through a physiologic process, such as altered blood flow at an absorption site. The result is a change in one, or more, of the primary pharmacokinetic parameters, ka, F, V, CL_R, CL_H, that in turn alters the secondary pharmacokinetic parameters, such as half-life and fe.

Before proceeding, a discussion of what is meant by the word *interaction* is worthwhile. Strictly speaking, this word implies a *mutual effect*. The interaction between two drugs, A and B, might thus be denoted by A $\leftrightarrow$ B. An example is the competition between two drugs for a common binding site on albumin, one drug displaces but is also displaced by the other. Generally, however, the term **interaction** is interpreted more broadly to indicate any situation in which one drug affects another. For example, phenobarbital appears to reduce the absorption of the diuretic, furosemide, but the renal clearance of phenobarbital is increased by the diuresis produced by furosemide. This might be regarded as a **bidirectional interaction** and may be denoted by A $\rightleftharpoons$ B. Clearly, in the case of mutual and bidirectional interactions, the measured response of one drug cannot be considered without also defining the level of the other.

When given in sufficient quantities, two drugs almost always affect each other; this may not be the case, however, at concentrations achieved in therapy. For example, the antibiotic enoxacin inhibits the metabolism of theophylline, but theophylline, at doses normally given, does not affect the response or the pharmacokinetics of enoxacin. This interaction is *unidirectional* and may be denoted by A $\rightarrow$ B. In a unidirectional interaction, the unaffected Drug A (e.g., enoxacin) can be considered independently, but the change in response of the affected Drug B (e.g., theophylline) cannot be adequately defined without also considering the concentration–response curve of the effect of Drug A on Drug B. Examples of different types of drug interactions are listed in Table 17-1.

Finally, various terminologies have been used to describe the drugs involved in an interaction. The one producing the interaction has been called the offending drug, the precipitant, the perpetrator, or the villain (when the outcome is adverse). The one affected has been called the affected drug, the object, or the victim. In this chapter, these terms are used interchangeably.

Emphasis in this chapter is on pharmacokinetic drug interactions, although some aspects of pharmacodynamic interactions are considered toward the end. The physiologic concepts developed in Chapter 4, *Membranes and Distribution*, Chapter 5, *Elimination*, and Chapter 7, *Absorption*, together with the kinetic principles developed in Chapter 9, *Therapeutic Window*, Chapter 10, *Constant-Rate Input*, and Chapter 11, *Multiple-Dose Regimens*, form the basis for discussing many aspects of pharmacokinetic drug interactions. For convenience, in this chapter, the effect of one drug on another is examined under the separate headings of altered absorption, altered distribution, and altered clearance. However, it should be borne in mind that several pharmacokinetic parameters can be, and sometimes are, altered simultaneously, examples of which are subsequently discussed.

ALTERED ABSORPTION

It was stated in Chapter 6, *Kinetics Following an Extravascular Dose*, and Chapter 11, *Multiple-Dose Regimens*, that the more rapid the absorption process, the higher and earlier is the peak plasma concentration and that neither total area under the curve (*AUC*) after a single dose nor *AUC* within a dosing interval at plateau after chronic dosing changes unless the bioavailability of the drug is altered. Therapeutic consequences of a change in either rate or extent of drug absorption were discussed in Chapter 11, *Multiple-Dose Regimens.*

Considered now are situations in which bioavailability is altered, with emphasis on changes in average plasma concentration with time during chronic dosing; an altered speed of absorption *(ka)* changes only the degree of fluctuation around the average value. The events with respect to a constant rate of drug input are illustrated in Fig. 17-1.

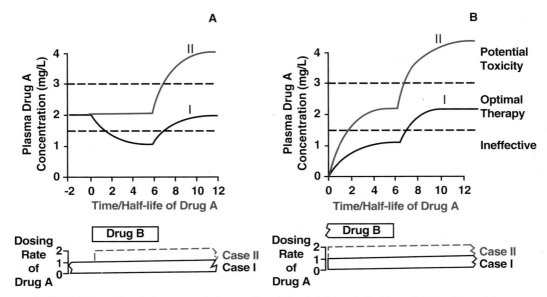

FIGURE 17-1. Altered absorption. As long as Drug B is administered, the bioavailability of Drug A is reduced by one half. For simplicity, Drug A is assumed to be given at a constant rate. The therapeutic concentration range of Drug A lies between 1.5 and 3 mg/L. **A.** Patient stabilized on Drug A. The plasma concentration of Drug A falls by one half (*Case I*), unless the dosing rate is doubled (*Case II, color*), when Drug B is concurrently administered. A problem potentially arises if administration of Drug A is not reduced to its preexisting rate when Drug B is removed (*Case II, color*). **B.** Patient stabilized on Drug B. An adequate concentration of Drug A is not achieved (*Case I*), unless the usual dosing rate of this drug is doubled (*Case II, color*). When Drug B is withdrawn, there is a potential problem similar to that considered in *A*. In both **A** and **B**, the time course of events for Drug A is determined by its half-life.

Figure 17-1A depicts the situation in which a patient stabilized on Drug A, now receives Drug B, which reduces the bioavailability of Drug A. It is apparent that if no steps are taken to change the dosing rate of Drug A, its concentration falls to a lower plateau, *the time being determined by the elimination half-life of this drug.* Suppose that it is then noticed that the patient is no longer being treated effectively with Drug A, and that, having recognized the problem, the offending drug is withdrawn. The concentration of Drug A would then return to the previous plateau value in 3.3 elimination half-lives. Therapeutic control would again be restored. Alternatively, on another occasion, in anticipation of the problem but desiring to give the two drugs together, the dosing rate of Drug A is increased appropriately at the time that Drug B is introduced. As long as Drug B continues to be administered, therapeutic control is satisfactory. A problem arises, however, if Drug B is subsequently withdrawn, but the dosing rate of Drug A is not correspondingly reduced. Then, in 3.3 elimination half-lives, the concentration of Drug A reaches a higher plateau where toxicity is likely.

Another possible situation is one in which Drug A is added to the regimen of a patient stabilized on Drug B (Fig. 17-1B). Here, as before, optimal therapy with Drug A in the presence of Drug B is achieved only if the usual dosing rate of Drug A is appropriately increased. However, the danger of the concentration of Drug A rising too high, if the dosing rate of Drug A is not readjusted when Drug B is withdrawn, must always be kept in mind.

The situations just considered emphasize the dependence of time course of events on the half-life of the affected drug. Thus, for affected drugs with very long half-lives, such as phenobarbital (4-day half-life), changes in response are insidious, occurring over several weeks, and the clinician may not associate the interaction with the causative drug, which was either initiated or stopped quite some time previously.

ALTERED DISTRIBUTION

One drug can affect the kinetics of tissue distribution of another, for example, by changing tissue perfusion, a hemodynamic interaction. This occurs during general anesthesia when perfusion to many tissues is reduced. However, primary consideration here is directed to changes in the extent of distribution, reflected in changes in volume of distribution, V. Recall the relationship for drugs of $V \geq 50$ L (≥ 0.7 L/kg)

$$V = V_P + V_T \frac{fu}{fu_T} \qquad 17\text{-}1$$

from which it is seen that V can be altered by changes in either fu or fu_T, the fraction unbound in that tissue space. Although theoretically possible, changes in V_P, the volume of plasma, and V_T, the volume of aqueous space of tissues into which drug distributes, are extremely unlikely to occur. Recall also when $V < 50$ L, and particularly for very low volume of distribution drugs ($V < 15$ L or < 0.20 L/kg), we need to take into account that changes in fu give rise to corresponding changes in binding to the same plasma protein residing in the interstitial spaces. Another cause of an altered distribution, considered later, is one in which a drug inhibits the uptake or efflux by a transporter of another drug whose distribution is permeability rate-limited.

The most common explanation for altered distribution in a drug interaction is displacement. Displacement is the reduction in the binding of a drug to a macromolecule, usually a protein, caused by competition of another drug, the **displacer**, for common binding site(s). The result is a rise in fu or fu_T, or in both. Sometimes, binding is diminished through an allosteric effect. The second drug, binding at another site, induces a conformational change in the protein, thereby reducing the affinity of the first drug for the protein. Occasionally, an allosteric effect causes an enhanced affinity between drug and protein; drug binding is then increased.

CONDITIONS FAVORING DISPLACEMENT

Two conditions must be met before substantial displacement occurs. First, in the absence of a displacer, the drug must be bound mostly to a protein, that is, its fu or fu_T must be low. Obviously, if a drug is not bound, it cannot be displaced. Second, the displacer must occupy most of the binding sites, thereby substantially lowering the number of sites available to bind drug.

Table 17-3 lists two groups of acidic drugs that bind to albumin. As can be seen, not all drugs bind to, and hence compete for, the same primary binding site on albumin. Albumin and some other proteins have several binding sites, each exhibiting some degree of specificity. Hence possessing an acidic function is not in itself a sufficient criterion for predicting the ability of one acidic drug to displace another. Moreover, even though almost all those drugs that compete for the same site have a high affinity for albumin, only a few are generally listed clinically as displacers, such as salicylic acid, valproic acid, and ibuprofen. This list is limited because the bound plasma concentration achieved during therapy must approach or exceed 0.6 mM (140 g/3 L), the molar concentration of plasma albumin. For a substance with a molecular weight of 250, this concentration corresponds

TABLE 17-3	Binding of Selected Drugs to Albumin

Drugs That Bind to and Compete for One of Two Sites, Designation I and II, on Albumin

Site 1*	Site 2†
Chlorothiazide	Benzodiazepines
Furosemide	Cloxacillin
Indomethacin‡	Dicloxacillin
Naproxen‡	Glibenclamide
Phenytoin	Ibuprofen
Sulfadimethoxine	Indomethacin‡
Salicylic acid	Naproxen‡
Tolbutamide‡	Oxacillin
Valproic acid	Probenecid
Warfarin	Tolbutamide‡

*Archetype: warfarin.
†Archetype: diazepam.
‡These drugs bind to both sites.

to 150 mg/L, but even a concentration 20% of this value, 30 mg/L, may increase *fu* significantly. These concentrations are approached during salicylate and valproic acid therapy and during high-dose ibuprofen therapy, because these drugs are given in doses approaching 1 g, they are of low molecular weight (138, 144, and 204 g/mol, respectively) and they possess relatively small volumes of distribution, 10 to 15 L/70 kg. High molar concentrations could also be achieved with lower daily doses if the compound has a long half-life relative to dosing interval, thereby resulting in extensive accumulation. For example, approximately 40% of a 25-mg daily dose of leuflonamide is converted to a very highly albumin-bound active metabolite (molecular weight = 270 g/mol), which, because of its very low clearance (0.01 L/hr) and long half-life (~10 days), yields plateau plasma metabolite concentrations in the order of 50 mg/L.

Displacers share an expected common property (i.e., their *fu* values change with plasma concentration). With most sites occupied by the displacer, the fraction unoccupied is sensitive to a change in the concentration of displacer. Therefore, displacers must show concentration-dependent disposition kinetics (Chapter 16, *Nonlinearities*).

So far, distinction has been made between displacer and displaced drug, but it should be apparent that this classification is arbitrary. Valproic acid is said to displace warfarin from albumin, but only because the therapeutic plasma concentration of valproic acid (70 mg/L; 0.48 mM) approaches the molar concentration of albumin (0.6 mM), whereas that of warfarin (1–4 mg/L; 0.003–0.01 mM) does not. Both drugs have high affinity for the same site on albumin, and if the concentrations were reversed, warfarin would be called the displacer.

The conclusions drawn from the interactions between acidic drugs and albumin are generally applicable to all drug–protein interactions, bearing in mind the widely differing molar concentrations of the various binding proteins in plasma (Chapter 4, *Membranes and Distribution*). For example, the molar concentration of α_1-acid glycoprotein, which avidly binds many basic drugs, is low (0.009–0.023 mM), and therefore displacement interactions can occur at plasma concentrations much lower than those required for displacement of acidic drugs from albumin (600-mM concentration). Substantial displacement of bases from tissue binding, observed as a decrease in *V*, is less likely, however, because unlike in plasma, where α_1-acid glycoprotein is the primary binding protein, there are relatively high concentrations of the major binding proteins, the acidic phospholipids, in tissues. Or, stated differently, the unbound tissue concentrations of many bases are well below the K_d of the binding constituents.

THERAPEUTIC IMPLICATIONS

Displacement interactions in plasma have been studied primarily in vitro. The potential displacer is added at therapeutic concentrations to a sample of plasma containing the drug, and changes in its binding are measured. Substantial displacement is frequently demonstrated, yet this may be of little therapeutic consequence. Much depends on whether the events are acute or occur at plateau during chronic therapy.

Acute Events. Two situations can be envisaged. One involves the administration of a loading dose of drug to a patient already stabilized on a displacer. The other involves the administration of a dose of displacer to a patient already stabilized on a drug. In both situations, the question of altering the usual dose of drug arises only if the unbound drug concentration increases above the therapeutic range, in the presence of the displacer. The extreme situation is one in which the displacer is administered as an intravenous (i.v.) bolus, which initially is restricted essentially to plasma, causing a transient rise in the unbound displaced drug there, before falling back as both displacer and unbound displaced drug moves down their respective concentration gradients into tissues. Accordingly, if response tracks unbound plasma concentration more rapidly than the kinetics of redistribution, a transient increase in response might be anticipated. In practice, this last situation is unlikely to arise, because to minimize the risk of adverse reactions, most intravenously administered drugs are given as a short-term infusion rather than as a bolus.

Less transient events are expected if, after redistribution, the unbound volume of distribution (Vu) of displaced drug decreased significantly, because this will produce a sustained increase in unbound drug for a given amount in the body. Such a decrease in Vu occurs only if, in the absence of the displacer, the drug is substantially bound in the body and the displacer causes significant displacement of drug from the major binding sites. For example, the unbound concentration rises if displacement occurs from sites on a plasma protein for a drug with a small volume of distribution, around 10 L/70 kg, or if displacement occurs from tissue-binding sites for a drug with a large volume of distribution. An example of the former situation is the displacement of warfarin from albumin-binding sites by naproxen. Displacement from tissue-binding sites would be expected to occur with high doses of bosentan and imirestat coadministered with drugs that bind to the same sites, given that these sites are saturated at such high doses (Chapter 16, *Nonlinearities*). However, these situations are relatively uncommon. More common is displacement from plasma-binding sites of a drug with a large volume of distribution. Then, because so little drug resides in plasma, relative to that in the body as a whole, only a minimal change in the unbound drug concentration, and hence response, occurs even when all the drug on the proteins are displaced, as discussed in Chapter 4, *Membranes and Distribution*. For example, if the volume of distribution is 100 L and 99% of the drug in plasma is bound ($fu = 0.01$), then only 3% ($100 \times [1 - fu]$) $\cdot$ ([plasma volume]/V) of that in the body resides bound in plasma. Even if completely displaced, the small amount affected would redistribute throughout the rest of the body and so would only marginally increase the unbound body pool.

Returning to the example of warfarin, because the clinical response (prothrombin time) is so delayed and insensitive to acute changes in warfarin concentration (Fig. 8-7, Chapter 8, *Response Following a Single Dose*), no adjustment in dosage of this oral anticoagulant would be contemplated in the event of acute displacement, even though Vu is reduced. A more important consideration for most other drugs is the effect of displacement on events at plateau, because most drugs, including displacers, are given chronically.

Events at Plateau. The influence of displacement on the unbound concentration at steady state (Cu_{ss}) depends on extraction ratio and route of administration of the affected drug.

Consider a drug with a *low extraction ratio*. Recall that clearance depends on fu, but unbound clearance (CLu) does not. Also recall the equalities (Eq. 5-2, Chapter 5, *Elimination*)

$$CLu \cdot Cu = CL \cdot C \qquad 17\text{-}2$$

and that for this class of drug, CLu approximates CL_{int}. When drug is infused at a constant rate, R_{inf}, and steady state is achieved,

$$R_{inf} = CL_{int} \cdot Cu_{ss} = CL \cdot C_{ss} \qquad 17\text{-}3$$

However, because intrinsic clearance is unaffected by displacement, the same is true of the value of Cu_{ss}. Thus, although displacement by increasing fu increases clearance (and hence causes the total plasma concentration to fall), no change in response and therefore in dosing rate is anticipated at steady state. Neither is any change anticipated in $Cu_{av,ss}$ upon chronic multiple dosing.

Now consider a drug with a *high extraction ratio*. Because blood clearance is unaffected by displacement, the steady-state blood concentration is also unaffected following a constant-rate i.v. infusion. However, as binding is diminished, ($fu_T \uparrow$), Cu_{ss} and therefore response to the drug must be increased as $Cu_{ss} = fu_b \cdot C_{b,ss}$. The maintenance dosing rate of the drug may need to be reduced. Although an extremely uncommon situation, conceivably the opioid fentanyl, which has a high extraction ratio, is reasonably highly bound ($fu = 0.15\text{--}0.2$) and administered both intravenously and transdermally, fulfills the condition, but no clinically significant displacement interaction has been reported.

Prediction of the outcome when a drug with a high extraction ratio is given orally and when elimination occurs predominantly in the liver is difficult. In the presence of the displacer, both unbound drug clearance and oral bioavailability decrease (see Chapter 7, *Absorption*); the effect of displacement on the unbound drug concentration at plateau is therefore likely to be relatively small. Irrespective of any effect of displacement, however, the unbound concentration at plateau is lower than that achieved following an equivalent i.v. infusion.

The events predicted at plateau before and after displacement for drugs of low and high extraction are shown in Fig. 17-2. Shown in Fig. 17-3 are the total and unbound plateau plasma concentrations of the antiepileptic drug phenytoin in patients before and after receiving valproic acid, another antiepileptic drug, which displaces phenytoin from albumin binding sites. As predicted for a drug of low extraction, the unbound concentration is unaltered, whereas the total plasma concentration is decreased. Accordingly, based on these observations, there is no need to alter the dosing rate of phenytoin in patients receiving valproic acid.

Kinetic Features. Both acute events and events at plateau have been discussed. Remaining to be discussed are the kinetic consequences of displacement on approach to plateau under the usual condition in which both drug and displacer are given chronically. To do so, first consider the expected changes in disposition kinetics of a drug upon displacement.

Disposition Kinetics. The subsequent points summarize those made in Chapter 5, *Elimination*. Because clearance of a drug with a high extraction ratio is unaffected by displacement, the half-life changes with volume of distribution. In contrast, for a drug of low extraction, because unbound clearance, CLu (CL_{int}) does not change, half-life either remains constant (when Vu does not change) or shortens (if Vu decreases) with displacement from plasma proteins.

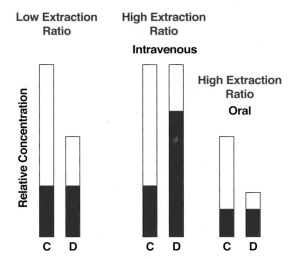

FIGURE 17-2.   Changes, at plateau, in the total (□ and ■) and unbound (■) concentrations (D = displaced; C = control) depend on the extraction ratio of the drug and route of drug administration. For a drug of low extraction ratio, diminished binding ($fu \uparrow$) reduces the total, but not the unbound, concentration regardless of the route of administration. For a drug of high hepatic extraction ratio, clearance, and so total concentration, is unaffected by diminished binding when the drug is given intravenously. The unbound concentration, however, is elevated. Because diminished binding decreases oral bioavailability of the highly cleared drug, the likely outcome of displacement after oral administration is a decrease in the total concentration and little or no change in the unbound concentration. The actual change depends on whether the effect on oral bioavailability or clearance predominates.

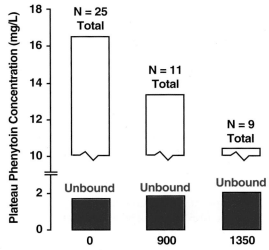

FIGURE 17-3.   The valproic acid–phenytoin interaction involves displacement only. Although plasma protein binding of phenytoin is decreased when sodium valproate is administered chronically to a group of patients stabilized on phenytoin, with a resultant fall in the steady-state plasma phenytoin concentration, there was no substantial change in the unbound phenytoin concentration (*colored*). These observations are consistent with a displacement interaction of phenytoin by valproic acid. Note that the degree of phenytoin displacement depends on the dose of sodium valproate. Of the 25 patients stabilized on phenytoin, 11 received 900-mg sodium valproate per day; 9 received a 1350-mg daily dose; and some received both regimens. (From: Mattson RH, Cramer JA, Williamson PD, Novelly, RA. Valproic acid in epilepsy: clinical and pharmacological effects. Ann Neurol 1978;3:20–25.)

Plasma Concentration–Time Profile. Although there are many possible combinations of events, only one common situation is considered. In this case (Fig. 17-4), the displacer, which has a longer half-life than that of the drug, is added to the regimen of a patient stabilized on a low extraction ratio drug. To simplify matters, both drug and displacer are administered by constant-rate infusion and both are assumed to always be at distribution equilibrium. Although these conditions are somewhat restrictive, the situation chosen does illustrate the importance of both kinetics and the manner of drug administration on the likely therapeutic outcome on approach to plateau.

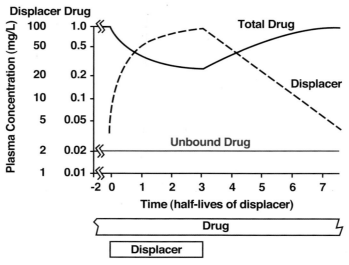

FIGURE 17-4. When constantly infused, the unbound concentration (*color*) of a drug with a low extraction ratio remains virtually unchanged if a displacer with a long half-life, relative to the drug, is either infused or withdrawn. The change in total plasma drug concentration reflects the displacement.

Notice in Fig. 17-4 that slow accumulation and correspondingly slow elimination of the displacer results in insignificant changes in the unbound drug concentration and therefore response. This is a consequence of the kinetics of the displacer being slower than that of the drug. The concentration of the displacer is changing so slowly relative to that of the drug that at all times the drug is at a virtual steady state, with rate of elimination ($CL_{int} \cdot Cu_{ss}$) matching the rate of input. That is, although there is a tendency for the unbound drug concentration to rise above the concentration at steady state during accumulation of the displacer, there is an opposing tendency for the unbound concentration to fall because the rate of elimination ($CL_{int} \cdot Cu$) would then exceed the rate of administration ($CL_{int} \cdot Cu_{ss}$). The reverse tendencies occur on stopping the displacer, but once again, they balance each other out. Accordingly, although the unbound concentration remains essentially unaltered, the total plasma drug concentration changes inversely with that of the displacer, reflecting the changing degree of displacement. A transient change in unbound concentration might occur if the kinetics of the drug, rather than that of the displacer, had been the slower.

In the case just discussed, no change in effect, and hence in the dosage regimen of the drug, is anticipated even though displacement has occurred. If only response were monitored, displacement would not have been suspected.

ALTERED CLEARANCE

A reduction in unbound clearance is potentially the most dangerous type of drug interaction. The unbound drug concentration can then rise to a toxic level, unless a reduction in dosage is made. Consequently, it is extremely important to be able to identify, characterize, and, where possible, avoid this type of adverse interaction. Interactions involving an increase in unbound clearance, because of induction, also occur causing the unbound drug concentration to fall, potentially resulting in a diminished response. Although generally of less concern, a diminished response can sometimes lead to failure of therapy with its attendant risks. Both inhibition and induction often have a high degree of specificity involving a specific enzyme. Examples of inhibitors and inducers of the major drug-related CYP enzymes are illustrated in Fig. 17-5. Inhibition and induction of transporters also occurs, but currently far less is known about specific transporters than enzymes.

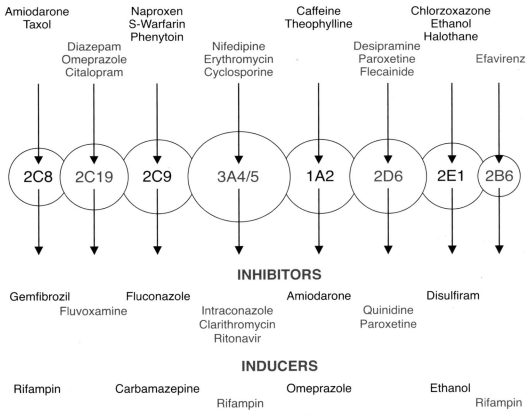

FIGURE 17-5. Graphic representation of the different forms of cytochrome-P450 (*circles*) in humans with different but some overlapping substrate specificities. The arrows indicate single metabolic pathways. Representative substrates are listed above for each enzyme. Also listed are relatively selective inhibitors and inducers of the enzymes.

INHIBITION

Inhibition of drug metabolism is the major cause of reduced unbound clearance. A reduction can also occur on inhibition of biliary and renal secretion and on inhibition of an uptake transporter, when uptake permeability rate-limits, or becomes the rate-limiting step in, organ clearance. Inhibition is of two general types, **competitive** and **noncompetitive**. Competitive inhibition occurs when inhibition can be overcome by raising sufficiently high the concentration of the substrate. It is the most common type of inhibition. The net effect is an increase in the apparent Km of the substrate but no change in its Vm. The term is normally applied to enzyme metabolism, but, more broadly, can be applied also to transport processes, with an associated increase in observed K_T but no change in Tm. Noncompetitive inhibition, which although less common is no less important, involves independent inhibition of an enzyme and, unlike competitive inhibition, cannot be overcome by raising the concentration of the substrate; it is characterized by a decrease in Vm but no change in Km of the substrate. One common type of noncompetitive inhibition is **mechanism-based inhibition** involving the formation of a reactive metabolite that effectively covalently binds to, and permanently inactivates, the enzyme. We first focus on competitive inhibition and then mechanism-based inhibition.

Competitive Inhibition

A Case Study. Some patients receiving theophylline develop nausea when enoxacin, an anti-infective quinoline, is added to the theophylline regimen. The nausea is associated with an elevated concentration of theophylline caused by enoxacin inhibiting the metabolism of theophylline.

The dramatic rise in the trough plasma concentration of theophylline when enoxacin is added to the regimen, and the return to the pre-enoxacin value when enoxacin is withdrawn, are illustrated in Fig. 17-6. Notice that it takes approximately 4 days of enoxacin

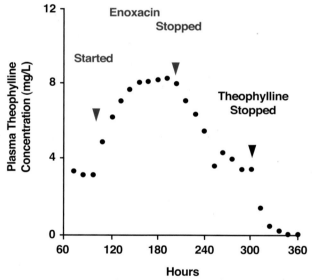

FIGURE 17-6. Enoxacin inhibits theophylline elimination. Subjects received 150-mg theophylline (in a controlled-release dosage form) orally every 12 hr for 12 days (288 hr). By 72 hr, as expected, the trough has reached a plateau with an average concentration within a dosing interval of 4.8 mg/L (*not shown*). Enoxacin was given, 400 mg orally every 12 hr for 4 days, starting 96 hr into the theophylline regimen. On addition of enoxacin, the mean trough theophylline concentration rose to a new and higher plateau (average interdose concentration of 9 mg/L, *not shown*). The time course of the rise was determined by the half-life of theophylline in the presence of enoxacin (22 hr). Although, on withdrawal of enoxacin, the plasma theophylline concentration fell toward the pre-enoxacin value (average interdose concentration of 4 mg/L, *not shown*), the concentration of enoxacin must have been sufficient to maintain appreciable inhibition for some time. Otherwise, the return of theophylline to the pre-enoxacin concentration would have been much quicker, being determined by the normal half-life of theophylline, 8.8 hr. (From: Rogge MC, Solomon WR, Sedman AJ, et al. The theophylline-enoxacin interaction: II. Changes in the disposition of theophylline and its metabolites during intermittent administration of enoxacin. Clin Pharmacol Ther 1989;46:420–428.)

administration for theophylline concentration to rise to the new plateau and a similar time for it to return to the pre-enoxacin value after enoxacin is withdrawn.

A more quantitative picture of the events may be gained from two equations. One, previously examined (Eq. 11-8, Chapter 11, *Multiple-Dose Regimens*), defines the average concentration of drug at plateau

$$C_{ss,av} = \frac{F \cdot Dose}{CL \cdot \tau}$$

17-4

The other equation defines the new (and longer) half-life of theophylline ($t_{1/2,inhibited}$) in relation to the normal half-life ($t_{1/2,normal}$).

$$t_{1/2,inhibited} = t_{1/2,normal} \cdot \frac{CL_{normal}}{CL_{inhibited}}$$

17-5

where CL_{normal} and $CL_{inhibited}$ are the clearances of theophylline in the absence and presence of the inhibitor, respectively. Equation 17-5 follows from the equation $k = CL/V$ and from the knowledge that enoxacin does not affect the volume of distribution of theophylline, a drug only weakly bound in plasma and tissue.

The half-life of theophylline in the absence of enoxacin is 8.8 hr, estimated from the declining concentration when theophylline administration is stopped (day 13). As expected, with such a short half-life, the plateau concentration ($C_{av,ss}$), approximately 4 mg/L, is reached within 2 days of starting the theophylline regimen.

Enoxacin is rapidly absorbed and immediately inhibits theophylline metabolism when administered on the fifth day into the theophylline regimen. With continual administration of the same dosage regimen of theophylline, its plasma concentration rises to a new plateau, approximately 9 mg/L, determined by the new, and lower, clearance value ($CL_{inhibited}$). Accordingly, by reference to Eq. 17-4,

$$\frac{CL_{inhibited}}{CL_{normal}} = \frac{C_{ss,av,normal}}{C_{ss,av,inhibited}}$$

17-6

and on substituting 4 mg/L and 9 mg/L for $C_{av,ss,normal}$ and $C_{av,ss,inhibited}$, one obtains $CL_{inhibited} = 0.44 \times CL_{normal}$. That is, enoxacin reduces the clearance of theophylline by 56%. This calculation is based on the assumption that the bioavailability of theophylline, which is usually well absorbed, is unaffected by enoxacin.

The new half-life of theophylline in the presence of the inhibitor can now be calculated by appropriately substituting into Eq. 17-5; it is 22 hr (8.8 L × 1/0.44). This longer half-life explains why it takes 4 days, rather than the usual 2 days, to reach the new plateau. It is also consistent with the observation that the plasma concentration of theophylline (6.5 mg/L) midway between the previous and new plateaus occurs 1 day after administering enoxacin.

The slow return of the plasma theophylline concentration to the pre-enoxacin value on withdrawal of enoxacin remains to be explained. Although withdrawn, the concentration of enoxacin in plasma ($t_{1/2}$ = 4–5 hr) persists at a sufficiently high value to continue to inhibit the metabolism of theophylline for a considerable period of time. As such, the half-life of theophylline, which controls the return of theophylline to its pre-enoxacin concentration, remains elevated for some time. Had inhibition ceased immediately upon withdrawing enoxacin, the half-life of theophylline would have reverted to its control value, 8.8 hr, and the return of theophylline concentration to the pre-enoxacin value would have been much quicker.

A Graded Effect. The last statement needs some amplification. The inhibition of theophylline by enoxacin is not an all-or-none effect, but rather, as with all interactions, a graded one. The degree of inhibition varies with the plasma concentration, and hence dose, of enoxacin, as illustrated in Fig. 17-7. Shown are both the plasma

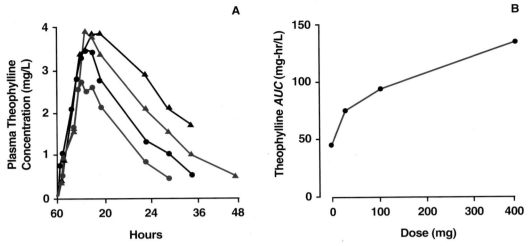

FIGURE 17-7. The inhibition of theophylline elimination by enoxacin is graded, as evidenced by the prolongation in half-life of decline of plasma theophylline concentration (**A**) and increase in *AUC* (**B**) when a 200-mg dose of theophylline is administered alone (●) and during 7-day regimens of 25-mg (●), 100-mg (▲), and 400-mg (▲) enoxacin given every 12 hr. Data are the means of four subjects. (From: Rogge MC, Solomon WR, Sedman AJ, et al. The theophylline-enoxacin interaction: I. Effect of enoxacin dose size on theophylline disposition. Clin Pharmacol Ther 1988;44:579–587.)

concentration–time profiles and *AUC* of theophylline following a single dose of theophylline taken alone and at steady state during regimens of 25, 100, and 400 mg of enoxacin given every 12 hr. As expected for a drug of low clearance, both *AUC* and half-life of theophylline increase with inhibition. Notice that inhibition is evident even with the 25-mg enoxacin regimen and then increases, tending to approach an upper limit with the 400-mg regimen. Restated, even though the plasma enoxacin concentration falls after a 400-mg dose, inhibition persists, to varying degrees, for some time thereafter. Clearly, the longer the half-life of an inhibitor, the more persistent is inhibition on withdrawing it.

To appreciate more fully the graded nature of inhibition of metabolism, consider the following. Recall (Chapter 16, *Nonlinearities*) that for each metabolic pathway operating–according to Michaelis-Menten–type kinetics

$$Rate\ of\ metabolite\ formation = \frac{V_m}{K_m} \cdot Cu_{cell} \qquad 17\text{-}7$$

when the unbound drug concentration at the (intracellular) enzyme site, Cu_{cell}, is well below the Michaelis-Menten constant, K_m. Or, expressed in terms of intrinsic clearance associated with metabolite formation, $CL_{int,f}$.

$$CL_{int,f} \cdot Cu_{cell} = fm \cdot CL_{int} \cdot Cu_{cell} \qquad 17\text{-}8$$

where *fm* is the fraction of the drug that is converted to the metabolite. Inhibition decreases $CL_{int,f}$ of a metabolite. A common model to describe metabolism in the presence of the inhibitor is

$$Rate\ of\ metabolism = \frac{CL_{int,f} \cdot Cu_{cell}}{1 + Cu_I/K_I} = \frac{fm \cdot CL_{int} \cdot Cu_{cell}}{1 + Cu_I/K_I} \qquad 17\text{-}9$$

where Cu_I is the unbound concentration of the inhibitor and K_I is the **inhibition constant**, given by the unbound inhibitor concentration that decreases $CL_{int,f}$ of the affected pathway by twofold. Clearly, the lower the K_I, the more potent is the inhibitor.

Two main conclusions may be drawn from Eq. 17-9. First, the degree of inhibition of a particular pathway depends on the unbound inhibitor concentration relative to its K_I. Many a compound has been shown to inhibit drug metabolism in vitro but fails to do so in vivo, because the unbound concentrations associated with therapeutic regimens of the inhibitor are well below its K_I value. Also, given that the concentration of the inhibitor generally varies with time after its administration, so does the degree of inhibition. Clinically, it is useful to classify an inhibitor as strong, moderate, or weak (Table 17-4), because this helps to decide whether the combination with a susceptible drug is either contraindicated or requires a reduction or no change in dosage. Clearly, this classification depends as much on the therapeutic concentration range of the inhibitor as on its K_I. If another clinical indication for the inhibitor requires a much lower or higher concentration, then its classification as an inhibitor when used for this indication may be different.

Second, the impact of inhibition on drug elimination depends on f_m and whether response lies with drug or metabolite formed. Inhibition has the most profound effect when the affected pathway is either obligatory for the elimination of the drug, that is

TABLE 17-4	**Classification of Inhibitors by the Magnitude of Their Effect at Therapeutic Doses***	
Strong (≥fivefold increase in *AUC*)	**Moderate (≥two- but <fivefold increase in *AUC*)**	**Weak (≥1.25- but <twofold increase in *AUC*)**
CYP3A		
Clarithromycin[†]	Amprenavir	Cimetidine
Itraconazole	Aprepitant	
Ketoconazole	Diltiazem[†]	
Ritonavir[†]	Erythromycin[†]	
Telithromycin[†]	Fluconazole	
	Grapefruit juice[†]	
	Verapamil	
CYP1A2		
Fluvoxamine	Ciprofloxacin	Norfloxacin
	Propafenone	Verapamil
CYP2C9		
	Amiodarone	Sulfinpyrazone
	Fluconazole	
CYP2D6		
Fluoxetine	Terbinafine	Amiodarone
Paroxetine		Sertraline
Quinidine		

*Strong, moderate, and weak inhibitors are those that, in clinical evaluations, cause a ≥fivefold, a two- to fivefold, and 1.25- to twofold increase in the *AUC*, or more than an 80%, 50% to 80%, 20% to 50% decrease in clearance, of substrates in which $f_m \simeq 1$, respectively.
[†]Mechanism-based inhibitor.
From: FDA Draft Guidance. Drug Interaction Studies—Study Design, Data Analysis, and Implications for Dosing and Labeling. September, 2006.

when $fm \approx 1$, and the drug is active, or when the metabolite formed by a minor pathway is active. In the former case, higher drug exposures result in increased response; in the latter case, lower active metabolite exposures and reduced response are expected. Often there are multiple pathways, of which only one may be inhibited, in which case the effect of inhibition will be less profound. Expanding on this thought, and recognizing that $fm \cdot CL_{int} \cdot Cu_{cell} = fm \cdot CL \cdot C$ and that clearance is additive, it follows from Eq. 17-9 that

$$CL_{inhibited} = CL_{normal} \left[\frac{fm}{1 + \dfrac{Cu_I}{K_I}} + (1 - fm) \right] \qquad 17\text{-}10$$

For example, even at the highest dose, enoxacin is only able to reduce the (total) clearance of theophylline by approximately threefold, with a corresponding tripling of theophylline half-life. Theophylline is eliminated by demethylation, ring oxidation, and renal excretion. Evidently, enoxacin inhibits only approximately 67% of the total pathways (i.e., $fm = 0.67$). The antidepressant desipramine, metabolized by the CYP2D6 to form 2-hydroxydesipramine, is another example. Quinidine, a potent inhibitor of CYP2D6 ($Cu_I/K_I \gg 1$) that essentially blocks this enzyme, effectively converts (genetically defined) extensive metabolizers of desipramine, in whom this pathway is a major one ($fm \approx 0.75$), to poor metabolizers, with a pronounced fourfold reduction in clearance ($(1 - fm)CL_{normal}$) and a corresponding fourfold prolongation in half-life. In such cases, the clinical consequences of an interaction depend on the relative contributions of drug and metabolite to efficacy and toxicity. With desipramine, the dose in extensive metabolizers should be reduced to avoid toxicity, if quinidine, or any other strong inhibitor of CYP2D6, is coadministered. As might be expected, quinidine has little effect on the pharmacokinetics of desipramine in the already poor CYP2D6 metabolizer phenotype, because the affected pathway is a minor one in such an individual.

It is important to be able to estimate the potential increase in exposure associated with a drug interaction involving inhibition, especially for drugs with a narrow therapeutic index. This estimate can be obtained for a given dose of drug by appropriately substituting Eq. 17-10 into Eq. 17-4, rearranging, and realizing that $AUC = C_{av,ss} \cdot \tau$, to yield

$$\frac{AUC_{inhibited}}{AUC_{normal}} = \frac{F_{inhibited}}{F_{normal}} \left[\frac{1}{\dfrac{fm}{1 + \dfrac{Cu_I}{K_I}} + (1 - fm)} \right] \qquad 17\text{-}11$$

where $AUC_{inhibited}/AUC_{normal}$ is the ratio of AUCs in the presence and absence of the inhibitor, and $F_{inhibited}/F_{normal}$ is the corresponding ratio of bioavailabilities. Figure 17-8 shows the AUC ratio as a function of Cu_I/K_I and fm assuming bioavailability remains unchanged, which is often, but not always so, as discussed subsequently. The impact of fm is clearly evident. If, for example, a dose adjustment becomes necessary when the AUC ratio increases beyond 50%, it is clear that this condition is met when $Cu_I/K_I = 0.5$ for a drug with $fm = 1$, is 0.8 when $fm = 0.75$, and is never met when $fm \leq 0.5$. Conversely, by rearrangement of Eq. 17-11, one can calculate the modification in dosing rate needed to maintain the AUC within the normal range

$$\frac{\left(Dose/\tau\right)_{inhibited}}{\left(Dose/\tau\right)_{normal}} = \frac{F_{normal}}{F_{inhibited}} \left[\frac{fm}{1 + \dfrac{Cu_I}{K_I}} + (1 - fm) \right] \qquad 17\text{-}12$$

For example, for the condition $fm = 0.75$ and $Cu_I/K_I = 2$, and again assuming bioavailability is unchanged, the dosing rate needed to maintain the normal AUC is 50% of the normal dosing rate. The other consideration is the dosing interval, bearing in mind that the decrease in clearance causes a corresponding prolongation in half-life. The normal practice would be to reduce the dose and maintain the dosing interval, but occasionally,

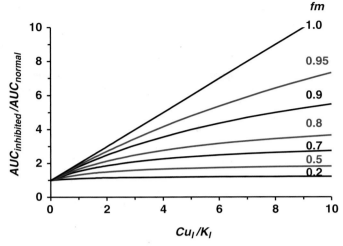

FIGURE 17-8. Prediction of the ratio of the *AUC* of a drug, following either a single dose or within a dosing interval at steady state, during the presence and absence of a reversible inhibitor as a function of the unbound inhibitor concentration, Cu_I relative to its K_I, for various values of *fm*, the fraction of the drug normally eliminated via the affected pathway. It is assumed that only one pathway of elimination is inhibited, that the inhibitor produces no change in the bioavailability of the drug, and that the unbound concentration of the inhibitor remains constant throughout the elimination of the drug. Notice that, for example, the condition of *AUC* ratio equals 2 is only met when *fm* >0.5, and then at lower Cu_I values the closer *fm* is to 1.

it may be more appropriate to make the adjustment by a mixture of some reduction in dose and a lengthening of the dosing interval, particularly for drugs normally given frequently. Examples of drugs that are substrates of either CYP3A4 or CYP2D6, for which oral *AUC* increases by at least fourfold when a strong inhibitor is coadministered, are listed in Table 17-5.

Much of the foregoing has centered on changes to exposure at steady state. But equally important is the temporal aspect of an interaction that has been mentioned when discussing the enoxacin–theophylline interaction but which can be more profound for drugs with *fm* ≈ 1. In this case, if inhibition causes a 10-fold reduction in clearance of the

TABLE 17-5	Substrates Showing at Least a Fourfold Increase in Oral *AUC* When Coadministered With a Strong Inhibitor	
CYP3A Substrates		**CYP2D6 Substrates***
Brecanavir	Perospirone	Atomoxetine
Buspirone	Quetiapine	Desipramine
Darunavir	Saquinavir	Dextromethorphan
Ebastine	Sildenafil	Metoprolol
Everolimus	Simvastatin	Nortriptyline
Felodipine	Tipranavir	Perphenazine
Lovastatin	Triazolam	Tolterodine
Midazolam	Vardenafil	
Nelfinavir	Voriconazole	

*Data in extensive metabolizers.

drug, there is a corresponding 10-fold increase in its half-life. Thus, a drug with normal half-life of 12 hr (0.5 day) becomes one with a 5-day half-life, so that even if this change occurred abruptly, it would take approximately 1 month to achieve the full 10-fold increase in the average concentration of the inhibited drug. In practice, it would take even longer, partly because it takes time for the inhibitor to reach its plateau and hence produce its maximum degree of inhibition on this regimen, and partly because as the inhibitor concentration rises in time to its plateau, so does the degree of inhibition. This, in turn, causes a continuous increase in the half-life of the inhibited drug and it is this continuous change that further prolongs the time to achieve the new plateau of the inhibited drug, as illustrated in Fig. 17-9. One consequence of this potentially insidious but progressive and potentially profound rise in inhibited drug concentration is that an adverse event, associated with the concentration reaching some critical value, may not occur for some time, perhaps several weeks, after the perpetrating drug has been added to the regimen of the patient, and neither patient nor prescriber may associate the cause of the toxicity with the comedication.

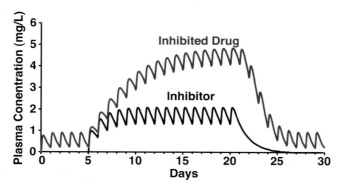

FIGURE 17-9. Inhibition can cause an insidious but profound increase over time in the plasma concentration of a drug when the inhibited pathway is normally the major route of elimination of the inhibited drug. The explanation lies in the progressive decrease in clearance, and hence prolongation in half-life of the inhibited drug, *colored line*, as the inhibitor, *black line*, rises toward its plateau. Initially short in the absence of the inhibitor, so that steady state is rapidly reached, the half-life of the inhibited drug can increase from a relatively few hours to several weeks, which in turn results in the rise of the concentration of the inhibited drug taking many weeks before the new, and much higher, plateau is reached. Toxicity associated with these higher concentrations may therefore not become apparent for some time after the inhibitor has been added, and may not be identified as the cause of the toxicity.

A last point here is also noteworthy. Patients may be receiving several moderate or weak competitive inhibitors of an enzyme. When each is administered alone the change in AUC of the inhibited drug may be considered too small to warrant a dose adjustment, but when multiple inhibitors are concurrently taken the net inhibition of the enzyme may be sufficiently great to perhaps warrant classifying the combination of inhibitors as a "strong inhibitor," necessitating a reduction in dose of the inhibited drug or seeking alternatives.

Route of Administration. To address the quantitative questions, and in particular make quantitative predictions, one outstanding question remains: What value should be used for Cu_I, the unbound inhibitor concentration? In vitro, the answer is clear; it is the unbound concentration at the enzyme (or transporter) site. However, in vivo this site cannot be sampled directly and a reasonable surrogate is needed. When dealing with events occurring in most organs of the body, the answer is still reasonably clear; it is the unbound systemic inhibitor concentration. This is less appropriate for events occurring in the liver during absorption of an inhibitor administered orally. Then the portal, and hence the hepatic blood, concentration perfusing the liver may be the appropriate measure because it can be very much higher than that in the systemic circulation, especially for inhibitors that are subject to a high first-pass hepatic extraction and have large volumes of distribution, a point considered in Chapter 7, *Absorption* (Eqs. 7-5 and 7-6) when discussing saturable oral absorption. Accordingly, the degree of inhibition can be much greater when the same dose of inhibitor is given orally than parenterally, with the impact of this difference expected to be greatest during the absorption phase of those drugs that are normally subjected to a high first-pass metabolic loss. Supportive data are provided in Table 17-6, which show that the increase in the *AUC* of orally administered lovastatin, a drug predominantly eliminated by CYP3A metabolism and subject to a high oral first-pass metabolic loss, is greater when the inhibitor diltiazem is given orally than intravenously, despite similar systemic exposures of diltiazem. What clouds an unambiguous assignment of this route effect of diltiazem solely to portal events is the unknown, but likely, significant contribution to increased systemic lovastatin exposure as a result of inhibition of its gut wall CYP3A-catalyzed metabolism by oral diltiazem.

TABLE 17-6	Impact of Route of Administration of Diltiazem on the Extent of Inhibition of Oral Lovastatin		
Route of Administration of Diltiazem	**Mean Diltiazem Concentration (μg/L)**	***AUC* of Lovastatin (μg-hr/L)**	**Lovastatin *AUC* Ratio (With Diltiazem/Alone)**
		Lovastatin Alone / **Lovastatin During Diltiazem Treatment**	
Intravenous*	73–140[‡]	64 (37)** / 81 (43)	1.27
Oral[†]	130 (58)	60 (25) / 214 (109)	3.57

*Single 20-mg oral dose of lovastatin given alone and during an i.v. protocol of diltiazem (20-mg loading dose with constant-rate input 10 mg/hr for 13 hr). (From: Masica AL, Azie NE, Brater DC, et al. Intravenous diltiazem and CYP3A-mediated metabolism. Br J Clin Pharmacol 2000;50:273–276.)
[†]Single 20-mg oral dose of lovastatin given alone and after 2 weeks of 120-mg diltiazem orally. (From: Azie NE, Brater DC, Becker PA, et al. The interaction of diltiazem with lovastatin and pravastatin. Clin Pharmacol Ther 1998;64:369–77.)
[‡]Range of mean diltiazem plasma concentration in subjects.
**Mean (standard deviation).

Notwithstanding this uncertainty, as a corollary to the route effect of the inhibitor, a route effect for inhibited drug is expected with a greater increase in systemic exposure when it is administered orally than parenterally, again particularly for drugs that are subject to a high first-pass loss. Evidence supporting this last expectation is demonstrated with the fluconazole–midazolam interaction. Displayed in Fig. 17-10 are midazolam data when given intravenously and orally with increasing oral doses of the inhibitor, fluconazole (100–400 mg). These data confirm the graded nature of such interactions, with a greater inhibitory effect seen at the higher doses of fluconazole for both routes of administration of midazolam. They also show an almost twofold greater increase in *AUC* following oral (5.6-fold higher following 400-mg fluconazole than control) than i.v. (twofold higher following 400-mg fluconazole than control) midazolam. Recall from Table 7-3 (page 193) that midazolam is subject about equally to gut wall and hepatic first-pass metabolic loss. Given both i.v. and oral midazolam for each of the doses of fluconazole administered, it is possible to partition the corresponding change in bioavailability, which increased from a control value of 24% to 63% when the 400-mg dose of fluconazole is

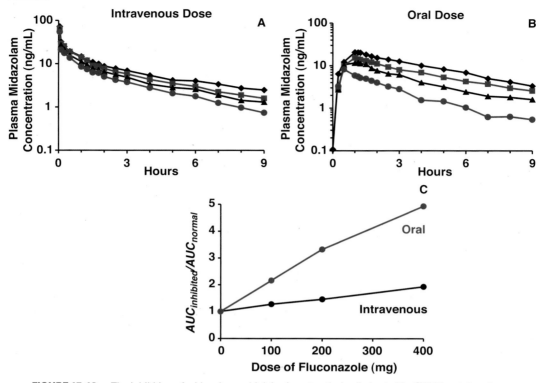

FIGURE 17-10. The inhibition of midazolam, which is almost entirely eliminated by CYP3A catalyzed metabolism, by fluconazole is graded as evidenced by the increase in mean plasma concentrations of midazolam following (**A**). intravenous (1 mg) and (**B**). oral (3 mg) administration to a panel of 12 healthy adults, alone (●) and on separate occasions with 100-mg (▲), 200-mg (■), and 400-mg (◆) fluconazole, each given as a single oral dose 2 hr prior to the midazolam administration. **C**: Plots of $AUC_{inhibited}/AUC_{normal}$ ratio against dose of fluconazole for oral and i.v. midazolam confirm the graded nature of the inhibition and also show that for any dose of fluconazole, the increase in AUC over control is greater following oral than i.v. midazolam administration. (From: Kharasch ED, Walker A, Hoffer C, Sheffels P. Sensitivity of intravenous and oral alfentanil and pupillary miosis as minimally invasive and noninvasive probes for hepatic and first-pass CYP3A activity. J Clin Pharmacol 2005;45:1187–1197.)

administered, to events occurring at these two sites, by noting that $F = F_G \cdot F_H$ and that an estimate of $F_H(= 1 - E_H)$ can be made from the corresponding i.v. data. Analysis indicates that F_H increased from 0.42 to 0.72 and F_G from 0.57 to 0.88. Almost complete inhibition of gut wall metabolism is not surprising given that the gut wall is exposed to very high concentrations of oral fluconazole. More generally, the expectation is that the impact of inhibition of gut wall first-pass loss on systemic exposure will be greatest for those drugs that are normally subject to a high extraction there, such as tacrolimus and atorvastatin, and least for those with minimal loss there, such as nifedipine (see Table 7-3 in Chapter 7, *Absorption*).

Drug interactions involving inhibition are not restricted just to those involving metabolism. Rosuvastatin (Crestor) is one of the newer potent statins. It is hydrophilic and largely eliminated unchanged in feces following biliary secretion. It is rapidly taken up by the liver on passage through this organ, where, like all statins, it acts to decrease cholesterol synthesis, and then is secreted into bile with relatively little appearing in the systemic circulation following oral administration, thereby minimizing the risk of systemic toxicity. It works effectively, and in common with other hydrophilic predominantly excreted statins, such as pravastatin, it is minimally subjected to metabolically mediated drug interactions. However,

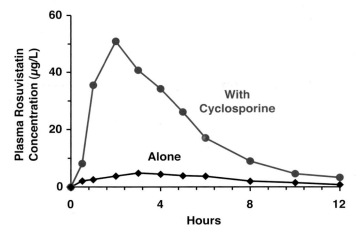

FIGURE 17-11. Cyclosporine inhibits the elimination of rosuvastatin, a drug primarily excreted unchanged in bile and urine. Shown are mean plasma rosuvastatin concentration–time plots within an interdosing interval at steady state in heart transplant recipients, on cyclosporine therapy to reduce the risk of organ rejection, after multiple dosing of 10-mg rosuvastatin once daily (●), and in healthy subjects receiving the same 10-mg multiple-dose regimen of rosuvastatin without cyclosporine (◆). (From: Simonson SG, Raza A, Martin PD, et al. Rosuvastatin pharmacokinetics in heart transplant recipients administered an antirejection regimen including cyclosporine. Clin Pharmacol Ther 2004;76:167–177.)

as shown in Fig. 17-11, cyclosporine caused, on average, an 11-fold increase in C_{max} and a sevenfold increase in AUC of rosuvastatin administered orally to heart transplantation patients, with even greater increases in some of the patients. The explanation lies primarily in cyclosporine inhibiting the hepatic transporter OATP1B1 (and perhaps other transporters) involved in the uptake of rosuvastatin, so that more escapes hepatic loss and enters into the systemic circulation. Inhibition by cyclosporine of biliary secretion of rosuvastatin and of intestinal efflux transporters that may be involved in absorption may also contribute to the increase in systemic exposure. Clearly, an i.v. arm in the study would have allowed the separation of changes in absorption and clearance processes.

Beneficial Interactions. As mentioned previously, advantage is taken of some drug interactions. A few elaborations are in order here. Penicillin–probenecid combination therapy is an example of the successful use of a drug interaction. Both of these acidic drugs are renally secreted by an anionic transport system. Probenecid competitively inhibits the renal secretion of penicillin, thereby substantially reducing its renal clearance, the major component of total clearance. Consequently, in the presence of probenecid, higher than usual and prolonged plasma concentrations of penicillin are achieved following a normal dosage regimen of the antibiotic. Of note is the lack of a major effect of penicillin on probenecid elimination. Although probenecid is also actively secreted into the kidney tubule, unlike penicillin, it is lipophilic and mostly reabsorbed. Consequently, the renal clearance of probenecid is low; metabolism is its major route of elimination.

Another example of a beneficial interaction is that between cilastatin and the antibiotic imipenem. Imipenem is metabolized extensively in the kidney by a dehydropeptidase, located at the brush border of the proximal tubular cell. Consequently, the urinary excretion of intact imipenem is low and often insufficient to guarantee effective treatment of urinary tract infections. To improve the efficacy of imipenem, it is marketed in combination with cilastatin, a dehydropeptidase inhibitor, which markedly increases the urinary excretion of unchanged imipenem (Fig. 17-12).

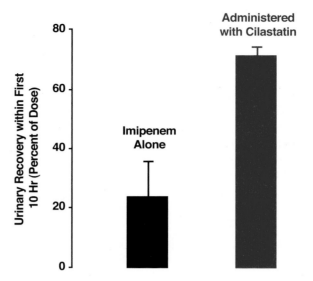

FIGURE 17-12. Cilastatin markedly increases the urinary excretion of the antibiotic imipenem by inhibiting the dehydropeptidase in the kidney responsible for its metabolism. The urinary recovery of imipenem is shown after a 500-mg i.v. bolus dose administered alone (*black*) and together with an i.v. bolus of 500-mg cilastatin (*color*). (From: Norby SR, Alestig K, Björnegärd B, et al. Urinary recovery of N-formimidoyl thienamycin (MK0187) as affected by coadministration of N-formimidoyl thienamycin dehydropeptidase inhibitors. Antimicrob Agents Chemother 1983;23:300–307.)

Mechanism-Based Inhibition. When a normal oral regimen of 500-mg clarithromycin twice daily is administered, the average plateau plasma concentration is approximately 0.7 mg/L. The fraction unbound in plasma is 0.25. In vitro, this macrolide antibiotic inhibits CYP3A4 with a K_I of 7 mg/L. Based of these data, which yields a Cu_I/K_I of 0.025, clarithromycin is not expected to be even a weak inhibitor of CYP3A4. However, as the data in Fig. 17-13 show it is a strong inhibitor that markedly increases the AUC of midazolam, a substrate of CYP3A4, whether midazolam is administered orally (sevenfold increase) or intravenously (2.7-fold increase). How can this be? One possibility is that the portal concentrations of clarithromycin perfusing the liver are much higher than those occurring systemically. But with absorption of this antibiotic relatively slow and clearance low, the additional contribution of absorbed drug to the rising recirculating systemic

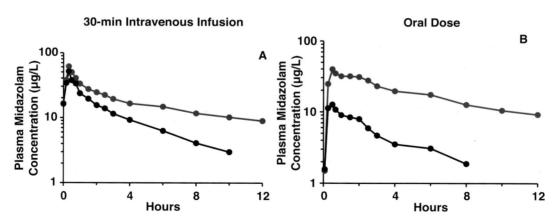

FIGURE 17-13. Clarithromycin irreversibly inactivates CYP3A, the enzyme responsible for the metabolism of midazolam. Shown are semilogarithmic plots of mean plasma concentration versus time of midazolam and $^{15}N_3$-midazolam, a stable isotope label, after simultaneous (**A**) i.v. (0.05-mg/kg midazolam over 30 min) and (**B**) oral (4-mg $^{15}N_3$-midazolam) administration to a group of 16 subjects alone (●) and on day 7 of a daily oral regimen of 500-mg clarithromycin twice daily (●). Clarithromycin causes a decrease in clearance and an increase in oral bioavailability of midazolam. (From: Gorski JC, Jones D, Haehner-Daniels BD, et al. The contribution of intestinal and hepatic CYP3A to the interaction between midazolam and clarithromycin. Clin Pharmacol Ther 1998;64:133–143.)

clarithromycin in the portal blood is modest, and fails to explain the magnitude of the interaction assuming reversible inhibition. The explanation lies in mechanism-based inhibition, whereby clarithromycin forms a metabolic intermediate complex with the heme moiety of CYP3A4, inactivating this enzyme. With the enzyme effectively consumed, its level in the liver falls, because its synthesis rate, which is unaffected, can no longer keep up with this additional rate of loss above that of the normal rate of degradation of CYP3A4. Accordingly, with less enzyme present, and with Vm directly proportional to the amount of enzyme, it follows that the associated intrinsic clearance of a substrate, in this case clarithomycin, falls. Two important questions remain to be addressed. First, how can a compound with a low Cu_I/K_I be a strong inhibitor? Second, how long does it take to restore the enzyme to the preclarithromycin level on removing this inhibitor?

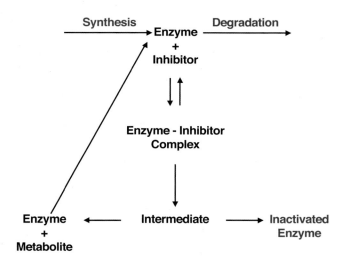

FIGURE 17-14. Scheme depicting mechanism-based inhibition. Drug complexes with enzyme to form a reactive intermediate part of which irreversibly reacts with, and inactivates, the enzyme and part is converted to a metabolite, liberating enzyme to reengage in the process. Normally, enzyme is in steady state with rate of degradation, with associated rate constant, matching the rate of synthesis, but the extra loss by the inhibitor causes a depletion in the level of enzyme.

To address these questions, consider the simple scheme depicted in Fig 17-14. As with conventional kinetics, the inhibitor first rapidly and reversibly binds to the enzyme to form an enzyme-inhibitor complex, which then produces a reactive intermediate, part of which reacts and consumes the enzyme and part forms a stable metabolite, liberating the enzyme to reengage in the process. In addition, the enzyme is turning over; that is, it is being continuously formed and degraded. Analysis of this scheme yields the following relationship for the formation clearance of the substrate in the presence and absence of the inhibitor

$$CL_{f,inhibited} = CL_{f,normal} \left[\cfrac{1}{1 + k_{inact} \cfrac{Cu_I}{K_I \cdot k_E}} \right] \qquad \text{17-13}$$

or, if fm is the fraction of drug normally eliminated by the affected pathway, then

$$CL_{inhibited} = CL_{normal} \left[\cfrac{fm}{1 + k_{inact} \cfrac{Cu_I}{K_I \cdot k_E}} + (1 - fm) \right] \qquad \text{17-14}$$

where k_{inact} is the rate constant that relates the maximum rate of inactivation of the enzyme by the inhibitor to the amount of active enzyme remaining, and k_E is the endogenous degradation rate constant, or fractional turnover rate, of the enzyme. It should be noted that inactivation of the enzyme only involves the inhibitor. Accordingly, Eq. 17-13 applies equally to all drugs that are substrates for the enzyme, whereas Eq. 17-14 additionally incorporates the drug-specific parameter, fm.

On comparing Eqs. 17-10 and 17-14, we see that the ratio Cu_I/K_I in Eq. 17-10 is replaced by $k_{inact} \dfrac{Cu_I}{K_I \cdot k_E}$ in Eq. 17-14. That is, k_{inact}/k_E acts as the modifier on Cu_I/K_I. Estimates for the k_E of CYP3A4 vary, but it is in the order of 0.23 day^{-1}, which corresponds to a half-life of approximately 3 days, although even longer estimates have been reported. Hence, this enzyme turns over, and so is replenished, very slowly. In contrast, inactivation of the enzyme by clarithromycin is relatively fast with k_{inact}, gained from in vitro studies of loss of enzyme activity with time on addition of clarithromycin, is 0.07 min^{-1}, so that $k_{inact}/k_E = 438$. That is, for midazolam ($fm \approx 1$), the reduction in clearance caused by the mechanism-based inhibition of CYP3A4 by clarithromycin is expected to be 11-fold ($1 + 438 \times 0.025$) rather than 1.025-fold ($1 + 0.025$) had clarithromycin only been a reversible inhibitor. This anticipated increase is somewhat higher but in the same order as observed in vivo (see Fig. 17-13). Also, because it is the enzyme that is effectively removed, a reduction in clearance, and an associated increase in systemic exposure, would occur with any other CYP3A4 substrate that a patient may be receiving.

Now to the question of time. In contrast to competitive inhibition, removal of the inhibitor, even instantly, does not lead to an immediate restoration of enzyme activity to the preinhibitor level in the case of mechanism-based inhibition. Rather, the time course of return is slow, governed by the normal half-life (or turnover time) of the enzyme. As discussed in Chapter 10, *Constant-Rate Regimens*, when discussing the turnover of endogenous compounds, the situation is analogous to going from a low plateau (in this case, caused by inactivation of the enzyme) to a higher one (once all inhibitor is removed) following a constant-rate infusion; it takes approximately 3.3 half-lives to return to normal activity, at least 2 weeks, and perhaps longer, for CYP3A4. This should be kept in mind when considering adjustment in dose of the inhibited substrate, or if other substrates are added to the regimen of a patient in whom the inhibitor is withdrawn.

Mechanism-based inhibitors are more common than was initially thought (see Table 17-5) and, as with reversible inhibitors, may be classified as strong, moderate, and weak inhibitors, except that, in addition to Cu_I/K_I, this classification also depends on k_E, a measure of the effectiveness of an inhibitor to inactivate the enzyme.

Before leaving this section on inhibition, several additional comments are warranted. First, the maximum exposure in genetically poor metabolizers when one of the other available pathways is inhibited, compared with extensive metabolizers under normal conditions on the same regimen, a measure of potential risk, can be very substantial, as the following calculation shows. Let CL_{EM}, CL_{PM}, be the clearances of a drug in extensive and poor metabolizers in the absence of the inhibitor, and $CL_{PM,inhibited}$ be the clearance in the poor metabolizers in the presence of the inhibitor. Furthermore, assume that the nonpolymorphic pathway subject to inhibition, CL_{NP}, and other unaffected pathways, CL_O, are the same in both groups, then

$$CL_{EM} = CL_{POLY} + CL_{NP} + CL_O \qquad \text{17-15}$$

$$CL_{PM} = CL_{NP} + CL_O \qquad \text{17-16}$$

and

$$CL_{PM,inhibited} = CL_O = (1 - fm_{POLY} - fm_{NP}) \cdot CL_{EM} \qquad \text{17-17}$$

where fm_{POLY}, fm_{NP} are the fractions of total clearance in extensive metabolizers associated with the polymorphic and nonpolymorphic metabolic pathways. It then follows that

$$\begin{array}{c}\text{Maximum} \\ \text{Exposure} \\ \text{Ratio}\end{array} = \frac{AUC_{PM,inhibited}}{AUC_{EM}} = \frac{1}{(1 - fm_{POLY} - fm_{NP})} \qquad \text{17-18}$$

from which it is seen that, the larger the value of fm_{POLY}, the greater is the AUC expected in poor metabolizers in the presence of the inhibitor compared with that in extensive

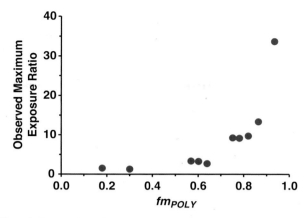

FIGURE 17-15. Plot of observed maximum exposure ratio in poor metabolizers for various drugs when coadministered with an inhibitor of a nonpolymorphic pathway versus the fraction of clearance in extensive metabolizers eliminated by the polymorphic pathway, fm_{POLY}. The substrate–inhibitor pairs on increasing fm_{POLY} values are citalopram–troleandomycin, diazepam–diltiazem, dolasteron–aprepitant, venlafaxine–ketoconazole, pimozide–clarithromycin, R-lansoprazole–clarithromycin, omeprazole–ketoconazole, S-lansoprazole–clarithromycin, omeprazole–troleandomycin, and omeprazole–clarithromycin. (From: Collins C, Levy R, Ragueneau-Majlessi I, Hachad H. Prediction of maximum exposure in poor metabolizers following inhibition of nonpolymorphic pathways. Curr Drug Metab 2006;7:295–299.)

metabolizers. Evidence supporting this analysis is shown in Fig. 17-15, in which it is seen that when fm_{POLY} reaches 0.75, exposure ratios in the order of 10 or more occur when one of the other pathways is strongly inhibited, often reason indeed to reduce the dose in poor metabolizers. Notice also that, in addition to fm_{POLY}, the critical factor determining the magnitude of the maximum exposure in poor metabolizers is the presence of other pathways of elimination not affected by the inhibitor.

Second is the general observation that there are far fewer important pharmacokinetically mediated drug interactions occurring extrahepatically. For example, despite the risk of increased brain exposure of many central nervous system (CNS) active P-glycoprotein (PgP) substrates resulting from inhibition of this efflux transporter, there are very few reports of significant CNS interactions, by drugs that in vitro studies clearly demonstrate are inhibitors of this transporter. However, they do exist. One example is the increase in cerebrospinal fluid exposure of ritonavir produced by orally administered ketoconazole, an inhibitor of PgP. Another example is the increased CNS depressive effect of loperamide produced by quinidine, another inhibitor of PgP. A metabolic interaction can be discounted, because loperamide is primarily eliminated by CYP3A oxidation, whereas quinidine at therapeutic doses is an inhibitor of CYP2D6. The reason for this relative paucity of systemically mediated clinically significant interactions is that for most drugs, therapeutic systemic concentrations are well below those needed to cause substantial inhibition of transporters and enzymes. Also, bear in mind that the site of inhibition of PgP is intracellular and with the high inherent barrier property of the cerebral capillaries, the concentration of a drug at the inhibitor site may be lower than exists systemically. For similar reasons, there are few significant drug interactions at the renal level, but again they do exist and are sometimes beneficial, such as the penicillin–probenecid interaction discussed previously, although effective doses of probenecid are at the gram level. Also, for the same reason, there is a tendency for fewer and often less severe drug interactions caused by parenterally than orally administered drugs. Lastly, drug interactions, occurring in the gut wall and liver during the absorption phase of reversible inhibitors, can sometimes be reduced by administering the drug and the inhibitor at different times of the day.

INDUCTION

A major cause of increased unbound clearance is induction of an enzyme, or more occasionally a transporter, when it influences elimination. Induction involves an increase in the rate of synthesis of the enzyme or transporter. Kinetic consequences of an increased clearance were discussed in Chapter 5, *Elimination*, and Chapter 7, *Absorption*. The implications of these changes on dosage requirements and the events that follow the addition or withdrawal of drug causing increased clearance are now presented.

In general, as with inhibition, dosage regimen adjustment is required only when the clearance of the affected pathway is or becomes a significant fraction of total drug clearance. Thus, a need to change the dose is anticipated if the clearance associated with a particular pathway, previously 20% of total clearance, were to increase sixfold, because total drug clearance is then doubled. No change in dose is anticipated, even if clearance associated with that pathway increases 20-fold, if this clearance contributes only 1% to total clearance. An exception arises when the metabolite formed is either the active species or is toxic, because its plasma concentration is then greatly increased.

The events depicted in Fig. 17-16 illustrate salient consequences of an increased clearance. In this illustration, a patient stabilized on one drug (Drug A) also receives another (Drug B) that doubles the clearance of Drug A. If the dosing rate of Drug A is not changed, then its concentration falls by one half, at a rate determined by the half-life of the drug *in the presence of Drug B* (Case I). The fall in concentration can be avoided by doubling the rate of administration of Drug A for as long as Drug B is given (Case II). However, a problem of excessive accumulation of Drug A exists if the higher dosing rate is maintained when Drug B is withdrawn. Because the half-life of Drug A is generally longer when given alone, especially for a drug of low extraction ratio, it follows that the time taken to reach a plateau is longer in the absence than presence of Drug B.

Two major assumptions were made in constructing the curves in Fig. 17-16, namely that the effect of Drug B is achieved instantly and remains constant as long as it is administered, and that the effect immediately disappears upon its withdrawal. In practice, both assumptions are invalid.

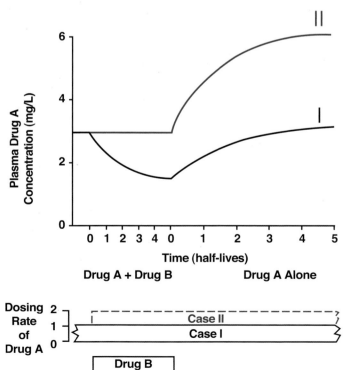

FIGURE 17-16. When a patient stabilized on Drug A also receives Drug B, a drug that increases the clearance of Drug A twofold, the plasma concentration of Drug A falls (*Case I*) unless the dosing rate is doubled (*Case II, colored*). The problem of excessive accumulation arises if administration of Drug A is not reduced to the previous rate when administration of Drug B is stopped. Note that the time to reach plateau is less in the presence, than in the absence, of Drug B and that the time scale in both the presence and absence of Drug B is expressed in half-lives of Drug A.

Enzyme induction was mentioned as the prime cause of increased metabolic clearance. However, a change in clearance is an indirect measure of the effect of an inducer; the direct effect is an increase in the synthesis rate of the drug-metabolizing enzyme. Accordingly, there is a delay between the direct effect and its reflection in the measured response, as amply discussed when considering turnover concepts in Chapter 10, *Constant-Rate Input.* Thus, even if the plasma concentration of the inducer were attained instantly and then maintained, the clearance of the affected drug would increase with time as the enzyme level rises from one plateau value to another. Similarly, there is a delay in the decrease in clearance of the affected drug on removing the inducer. The time delay depends, like other systems in the body, on the kinetics of both the drug and the enzyme involved.

When elimination of enzyme is a slower process than that of the drug, then changes in clearance of the affected drug are determined by the half-life of the enzyme. Clearance may continue to rise even though the concentration of the inducer is maintained relatively constant, until the enzyme has reached a new higher plateau. When, however, elimination of the inducer is the rate-limiting step, changes in the concentration of inducer are then reflected almost instantaneously by changes in the amount of enzyme and hence clearance of the affected drug. This last possibility may explain the effect of phenobarbital on the temporal changes in the plasma concentration of dicumarol and prothrombin time, a measure of its anticoagulant effect, in a patient chronically receiving dicumarol, an oral anticoagulant once prescribed as an alternative to warfarin (Fig. 17-17). Both the fall in the concentration and effect of this drug following phenobarbital treatment have been attributed to the barbiturate, inducing the enzymes responsible for dicumarol metabolism. It takes approximately 3 to 4 weeks for the plasma dicumarol both to fall to a minimum during phenobarbital administration and to return to the prebarbiturate value after phenobarbital is discontinued. Phenobarbital ($t_{1/2}$ of 4 days) also takes approximately the same period of time to reach a plateau in the body and to be eliminated. Thus, the observations are compatible with the hypothesis that the induced enzyme system responds relatively rapidly to changes in plasma phenobarbital concentration.

The data in Fig. 17-17 suggest that prothrombin time may be maintained at the prebarbiturate value by raising the dose of dicumarol during phenobarbital administration. An increased risk arises, however, if the dose of anticoagulant is not reduced when phenobarbital is discontinued. The plasma dicumarol concentration then rises insidiously, as

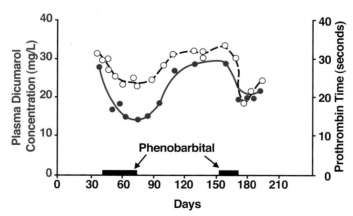

FIGURE 17-17.   Administration of phenobarbital (60 mg daily) to a patient receiving dicumarol chronically (75 mg daily) reduces, through induction, the plasma concentration of the anticoagulant (●) and prothrombin time (○), a measure of its effect on the concentration of the vitamin K_I-dependent clotting factors. The time course of the events is largely controlled by the kinetics of phenobarbital, half-life 4 days. (From: Cucinell SA, Conney AH, Sansur MS, Burns JJ. Lowering effect of phenobarbital on plasma levels of dicumarol and diphenylhydantoin. Clin Pharmacol Ther 1965;6:420–429.)

phenobarbital is slowly eliminated, and may go unnoticed for several weeks after discontinuing the barbiturate until, perhaps, a hemorrhagic crisis occurs.

Another dimension that influences the time course of changes in enzyme levels is that, as with most processes, induction is a graded effect, such that as the concentration of inducer changes so does the degree of induction, and hence clearance of the affected drug. The net effect is that the time to achieve a new plateau of enzyme content, and hence new clearance of induced drug, following initiation or withdrawal of a constant-rate regimen of inducer, will be longer than that expected had induction instantaneously reached the condition at plateau or ceased.

OTHER CAUSES OF ALTERED CLEARANCE

Unbound clearance can be altered in numerous ways other than inhibition or induction of metabolism and secretion. The lower hepatic clearance of lidocaine when given together with propranolol, a β-adrenergic blocking drug, is an example of a physiologically mediated pharmacokinetic interaction. Propranolol diminishes cardiac output and hence hepatic blood flow, which, in turn, reduces the clearance of lidocaine, a drug highly extracted by the liver. Presumably, because the degree of β-adrenergic blockade is a graded response, the interaction with lidocaine is dependent on the plasma concentration of propranolol.

Raising urine pH by giving acetazolamide or sodium bicarbonate increases the renal clearance of salicylic acid and other acids whose renal clearance is pH sensitive. Giving ammonium chloride or ascorbic acid to make the urine more acidic increases the renal clearance of pH-sensitive basic drugs. Some drugs increase the metabolic clearance of other drugs. They do so most commonly by inducing the drug-metabolizing enzymes, but they may also activate enzymes or retard enzyme degradation. Occasionally, like glucagon, they increase hepatic blood flow and thereby increase the hepatic clearance of drugs that are highly extracted by the liver.

MULTIFACETED INTERACTIONS

So far, emphasis has been on examining drug interactions involving alteration in one process. In practice, several processes may be altered and great care and attention are needed to ensure that the data are correctly interpreted, and placed into clinical perspective. Several examples follow.

WARFARIN–PHENYLBUTAZONE INTERACTION

Although the anti-inflammatory drug phenylbutazone is no longer used, its interaction with warfarin is well documented and offers some interesting lessons. The interaction has caused serious bleeding episodes, occasionally fatal. Warfarin is highly bound in plasma to albumin. Phenylbutazone, devoid of inherent anticoagulant activity, displaces warfarin. Consequently, displacement had been advocated as the primary mechanism for this interaction and sensitized the clinical community to be concerned about displacement interactions, a concern that still lingers.

Figure 17-18 shows the temporal effects of phenylbutazone administration on the plasma and unbound concentrations of warfarin in a subject who ingested 10-mg warfarin daily. The half-life of warfarin is approximately 2 days, and therefore, as anticipated, a steady state is reached within the first 12 days, when warfarin alone is administered. At this time, the warfarin plasma concentration is approximately 4 mg/L and only 0.5% ($Cu = 0.02$ mg/L) is unbound (i.e., $fu = 0.005$). Warfarin is completely absorbed, and its clearance, estimated by dividing the daily dosing rate by the steady-state plasma concentration, is 0.1 L/hr. Thus, warfarin is a highly bound drug with a low extraction ratio.

Phenylbutazone is also poorly cleared, is highly bound ($fu = 0.004$–0.010), and has a half-life (approximately 3 days), even longer than that of warfarin. Accordingly, when on

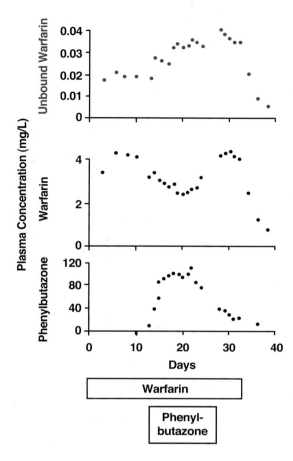

FIGURE 17-18. Warfarin–phenylbutazone interaction. A subject received 10-mg warfarin orally each day and 100-mg phenylbutazone 3 times a day on days 13 to 22. As the phenylbutazone concentration rose, bound warfarin was displaced, and the plasma warfarin concentration fell. The sustained elevation in the unbound warfarin during phenylbutazone administration implies inhibition of warfarin elimination. (From: Schary WL, Lewis RJ, Rowland M. Warfarin-phenylbutazone interaction in man: a long term multiple-dose study. Res Commun Chem Pathol Pharmacol 1975;10:633–672.)

day 13, the subject commences the formerly recommended dosage regimen of phenylbutazone, 100 mg 3 times a day, the plasma concentration of this drug rises and eventually reaches a plateau of approximately 100 mg/L, after approximately 10 days. During this period, the plasma warfarin concentration falls steadily in half, to 2 mg/L, and the value of fu for warfarin rises approximately threefold.

At this point, the events in plasma appear remarkably similar to those depicted in Fig. 17-4 for a pure displacement interaction. However, there is one important difference. The unbound warfarin concentration rises and remains elevated during phenylbutazone administration. Because the effect of warfarin is related to its unbound concentration, this sustained elevation is in accord with the observed sustained augmentation of the effect as long as phenylbutazone is coadministered. Examination of Eq. 17-3 indicates that to account for the elevated values of unbound drug, either the rate of entry of warfarin into the body is increased or the value of CL_{int} is decreased. As the dosage regimen of warfarin is unaltered and warfarin is fully bioavailable, CL_{int} must have decreased.

Warfarin is almost exclusively metabolized in the liver to either weakly active or inactive metabolites. Thus, a lower value for CL_{int} implies a decrease in the ability of the liver to metabolize warfarin. Analysis of several metabolites of warfarin in both plasma and urine subsequently confirmed that, indeed, phenylbutazone inhibits warfarin elimination, and it is this inhibition, and not displacement, that accounts for the clinical picture.

The interaction between phenylbutazone and warfarin is even more complex than portrayed above. Commercial warfarin is a racemate, and the S(−) isomer is five times more active than the R(+)-isomer. Phenylbutazone primarily inhibits the formation of 7-(S)-hydroxywarfarin, the major metabolite of the more active isomer. The lesson is clear: Drug interactions can be complex; careful observations are required to unravel the facts.

DIGOXIN–QUINIDINE INTERACTION

Although many patients with cardiovascular diseases have been comedicated with digoxin and the antiarrythmic agent quinidine over the past 50 years, it is only relatively recently that serious drug interactions have been identified with this combination, probably because such patients tend to experience a relatively high incidence of adverse events from various causes and identifying the specific contribution of each is difficult. The primary cause of the interaction is attributed to an increase in the plasma concentration of digoxin, a narrow therapeutic index drug. Table 17-7 summarizes the pharmacokinetics of digoxin in the absence and presence of quinidine. Quinidine alters all pri-

TABLE 17-7	Typical Pharmacokinetic Parameters of Digoxin in the Absence and Presence of Quinidine				
	Oral Bioavailability	Clearance (mL/min)	Renal Clearance (mL/min)	Volume of Distribution (L)	Fraction Unbound in Plasma
Alone	0.75	140	101	500	0.79
With quinidine*	0.85	72	51	240	0.79

*When the $C_{av,ss}$ of quinidine is 1 to 3 mg/L.

mary digoxin pharmacokinetic parameters, causing a marginal increase in oral bioavailability and a twofold decrease in (total) clearance (from 140–72 mL/min), renal clearance (from 101–51 mL/min), and volume of distribution (from 500–240 L). The twofold reduction in clearance dictates the need to reduce digoxin daily maintenance dose by an equal degree. When employed, the loading dose of digoxin also needs to be reduced by half given the twofold reduction in volume of distribution, if excessively high-plasma concentrations of digoxin during digitalization are to be avoided. But what are the mechanisms that explain these changes?

Digoxin is a large molecule (781 g/mol), minimally bound to plasma proteins ($fu =$ 0.79) but extensively distributed to tissues ($V = 500$ L). It is minimally metabolized, with 75% of its clearance associated with renal excretion. Initially, the mechanism associated with the change in each pharmacokinetic parameter was viewed separately. However, much may be explained by a common mechanism: inhibition by quinidine of transporters involved in digoxin pharmacokinetics. Digoxin is a substrate of the efflux transporter PgP, which is thought to be responsible for its normally incomplete systemic absorption. However, as the oral bioavailability of digoxin is already high, at 75%, there is little room for a large increase.

The renal clearance of digoxin, 101 mL/min, is close to glomerular filtration rate *(GFR)* (120 mL/min), and given its minimal plasma binding ($fu = 0.79$) and poor permeability characteristics, it had been long thought that digoxin was much like creatinine: filtered and neither secreted nor reabsorbed. The reduction by half by quinidine of digoxin renal clearance challenged this view. Quinidine has no effect on *GFR* but rather inhibits the tubular secretion of digoxin by PgP, which resides in the luminal brush border of the renal tubule. However, as a corollary, with $CL_R < fu \cdot GFR$, the only explanation is that digoxin must undergo tubular reabsorption. Substitution of fu, CL_R, and *GFR* into Eq. 5-18 of Chapter 5, *Elimination*, indicates that 46% of the filtered load must be reabsorbed. But, because in the absence of quinidine the CL_R of digoxin is close to *GFR*, it follows that normally its tubular secretion and reabsorption are roughly equal.

Digoxin nonrenal clearance $(CL − CL_R)$ is also reduced by quinidine, from 39 (140–101) to 21 (72–51) mL/min. The likely explanation is the same as for renal clearance; quinidine inhibits the hepatic secretion of digoxin by PgP into bile. We are left to explain the reduction in volume of distribution. With no change in *fu*, the cause must be a reduction in tissue distribution. Application of Eq. 4-26 of Chapter 4, *Membranes and Distribution,* ($V = V_P + V_{TW} \cdot fu/fu_T$) would suggest that quinidine either reduces the fraction unbound in tissues, fu_T, or restricts the aqueous space in tissue into which digoxin distributes, V_{TW}. Normally, one would be reasonably confident in the former explanation and reject the latter. However, another explanation has some merit. Being large and amphiphilic (having a hydrophobic polycyclic core and hydrophilic sugar chain), digoxin does not readily permeate membranes by passive diffusion. It is a substrate for the uptake transporter OATP1B3 and perhaps other uptake transporters. If uptake transport is a significant mechanism for tissue distribution of digoxin, and quinidine inhibits such processes so as to decrease the value of the uptake permeability-area product (P_{uptake}), the effect would that with less drug entering cells, the effective tissue-to-plasma concentration ratios (Kp), and hence the volume of distribution, of digoxin would be lower (see Eq. 4-29, Chapter 4, *Membranes and Distribution.* $V = V_P + V_{TW} \cdot \dfrac{P_{uptake}}{P_{efflux}} \cdot \dfrac{fu}{fu_T}$). Implicit in this explanation is a lower

unbound concentration in the affected tissues for a given amount in the body.

ATORVASTATIN–RIFAMPICIN INTERACTION

Atorvastatin, a potent statin, is extensively metabolized with little eliminated unchanged; some of the metabolites are active. Figure 17-19A shows the plasma concentration–time profiles of atorvastatin following administration of a single oral dose alone and during an i.v. infusion of rifampin, a macrolide antibiotic. A marked 10-fold increase in C_{max} and sevenfold increase in *AUC* are clearly evident, as is a pronounced shortening of the terminal half-life, from 8 to 3 hr, evident from a semilogarithmic plot of the data (Fig. 17-19B). Separate studies indicate that atorvastatin has a high clearance and a low oral bioavailability (14%) because of extensive first-pass metabolism, primarily by CYP3A. Analysis of the interaction data provide interesting findings. Oral clearance (*CL/F*) of atorvastatin is reduced ninefold from 6.8 to 0.88 mL/hr/kg, and to account for the shorter half-life in the presence of rifampin, *Vss/F* is reduced even

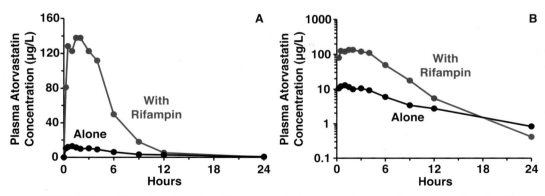

FIGURE 17-19. Rifampin, administered intravenously, increases the systemic exposure of orally administered atorvastatin, and shortens its half-life. **A.** Linear and (**B**) semilogarithmic plots of the mean plasma atorvastatin concentration time profiles in 11 subjects after a single oral dose of 40-mg atorvastatin with (●) and without (●) 600-mg rifampin given as intravenous 30-min infusion. The mechanism involves rifampin inhibiting the hepatic uptake transporter OATP1B1 and perhaps other uptake transport processes in this organ and other tissues. (From: Lau YY, HuangY, Frassetto L, Benet LZ. Effect of OATP1B transporter inhibition on the pharmacokinetics of atorvastatin in healthy volunteers. Clin Pharmacol Ther 2007;81:194–204.)

more, by 17-fold, from 66 L/kg to 3.8 L/kg. Furthermore, most of the area (and hence elimination) of systemically available atorvastatin occurs beyond t_{max}. The most plausible explanation of the *AUC* data is that rifampin decreases the clearance of atorvastatin and hence first-pass loss, with an associated increase in oral bioavailability. The temptation is to assign the mechanism as one of rifampin inhibiting the metabolism of atorvastatin. Certainly, rifampin is an inhibitor of CYP3A, but studies have shown that inhibition occurs only at much higher concentrations than obtained with rifampin in the current study. The mechanism lies elsewhere.

Atorvastatin is taken up into the liver by the uptake transporter OATP1B1, which rifampin inhibits. In doing so, rifampin moves the rate-limiting step for hepatic elimination of atorvastatin from metabolism to uptake. Clearance is reduced, now becoming sensitive to uptake, and oral bioavailability is increased. Reflect, clearance of an extensively metabolized drug is reduced as a result of inhibition of uptake transport into the eliminating organ; metabolism and transport are clearly intimately coupled. The reason behind the reduction in volume of distribution of atorvastatin by rifampin can be thought of as similar to that by which quinidine may reduce the volume of distribution of digoxin. Atorvastatin acts in the liver, which is a major organ of distribution for this drug. The reduction in its volume of distribution by rifampin is at least in part caused by inhibition of hepatic uptake. Also, inhibition of the distribution of this statin into other tissues cannot be discounted. Note that this strong interaction occurred following intravenously administered rifampin, emphasizing again that a systemically mediated interaction, although relatively uncommon, can and does occur. The magnitude of the interaction depends on the concentrations achieved, and hence on the dosage regimen and pharmacokinetics of the causative drug. In this case, the usual daily dose of rifampin, 600 mg, was administered on a single occasion. Lastly, there are many examples showing that rifampin is an inducer of drug metabolism, especially CYP3A4 (see also Fig. 17-5). Rifampin is a classic strong inducer. However, as also pointed out previously in this chapter, the full effect of enzyme induction takes time to develop, and only becomes apparent during multiple daily dosing of rifampin. Then, it is observed that both atorvastatin C_{max} and *AUC* fall to even lower values than seen when atorvastatin is administered alone, clearly more than offsetting the inhibitory effect of this macrolide antibiotic, at least at the metabolic and perhaps also at the transporter, level.

These multifaceted drug interactions illustrate the complexities that can, and do, occur, but at the same time, they help to shed light on the mechanisms responsible for the pharmacokinetic behavior of the affected drug. They also strongly emphasize the need to be cautious in the interpretation of drug interactions and in the extrapolation of such data to the clinical management of patients.

PHARMACODYNAMIC INTERACTIONS

It is mentioned at the beginning of this chapter how two or more drugs can interact pharmacodynamically, and that drug combinations are employed clinically to produce a greater beneficial response than can be achieved with any one component or less harm for a given desired response. Such drug combinations are often said to be clinically synergistic. The situation now considered, however, is one involving competition of two drugs for the same receptor, either both acting as agonists or antagonists, although administration of an agonist to offset an antagonist arises in drug therapy, and vice versa. For example, vitamin K is administered to restore the prothrombin time to within the normal therapeutic range in patients inadvertently over anticoagulated with warfarin. Recall from Chapter 3, *Kinetics Following an Intravenous Bolus Dose*, that the intensity of a graded response, *E*, can be related to concentration through the relationship

$$E = \frac{E_{max} \cdot C^{\gamma}}{C_{50}{}^{\gamma} + C^{\gamma}}$$

17-19

which, on dividing top and bottom by $C_{50}{}^{\gamma}$, the potency of the drug and rearrangement gives

$$\frac{E}{E_{max}} = \frac{\dfrac{C^{\gamma}}{C_{50}{}^{\gamma}}}{1 + \dfrac{C^{\gamma}}{C_{50}{}^{\gamma}}}$$

17-20

Now consider two full agonists, *A* and *B*, competing for the same target. Each can elicit the same maximum response, E_{max}, when administered alone. Assuming that the steepness factor, γ, is the same, then the fraction of the maximum response produced in the presence of the two drugs is

$$\frac{E}{E_{max}} = \frac{\dfrac{Cu_{A}{}^{\gamma}}{Cu_{50,A}{}^{\gamma}} + \dfrac{Cu_{B}{}^{\gamma}}{Cu_{50,B}{}^{\gamma}}}{1 + \dfrac{Cu_{A}{}^{\gamma}}{Cu_{50,A}{}^{\gamma}} + \dfrac{Cu_{B}{}^{\gamma}}{Cu_{50,B}{}^{\gamma}}}$$

17-21

where subscripts A and B denote the two drugs. The important feature of this relationship is that the presence of one drug effectively increases the C_{50} value of the other. Accordingly, as shown in Fig. 17-20, however, much of the concentration of Drug B is increased in the presence of Drug A; E_{max} cannot be exceeded. The closer the response achieved with drug alone is to E_{max}, the lower the impact on addition of the other.

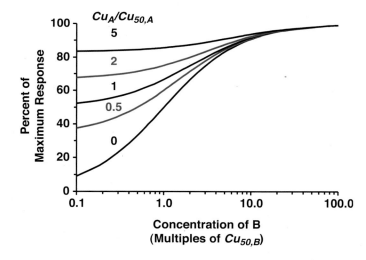

FIGURE 17-20. When two drugs, Drug A and Drug B, are full agonists (or antagonists) the effect of Drug B on Drug A depends on the percent of the maximum response achieved by Drug A in the absence of Drug B. The closer to E_{max} achieved with Drug A alone, the smaller the impact of adding Drug B.

Several additional points are worth noting. First, in principle, there is no distinction in the form of the relationship between the degree of inhibition of an enzyme or transporter and the concentrations of two competitive inhibitors, and that between the intensity of response and the concentrations of two agonists competing at a receptor site. The primary difference in practice is that with many pharmacokinetic interactions, the concentration of inhibited drug is often well below its Km (or K_T), so that it has minimal to no effect on the kinetics of the inhibitor, (i.e., the drug interaction is unidirectional). In contrast, with pharmacodynamic interactions, because most drugs only produce a measurable therapeutic effect above baseline when the concentration is at or above its C_{50}, each drug in the combination will affect the contribution to the total effect of the other. Second, drugs are invariably competing with one or more endogenous compounds for a target, so that in principle one could characterize the relationship between response and drug concentration if one also knew the pharmacodynamic parameters and concentration of the endogenous compound(s). Sometimes, however, the endogenous compound has not been identified, or even if it has been identified and its pharmacodynamic parameters determined, rarely is its concentration at the target site known. Part of the variability in response to a drug between and within individuals is likely to be a result of variability in the concentration of competing endogenous compound. Lastly, situations arise in which one or more of the metabolites of a drug are agonists or antagonists for the same target as the parent compound, an aspect considered in the next chapter, *Metabolite Kinetics and Response*.

One implicit property of Eq. 17-21 is that the drug combination is **additive**. But what does additivity mean in the context of pharmacodynamics when inherently, response is nonlinearly related to concentration? To address this question, imagine the simple case of two full agonists, that for each $\gamma = 1$, and that when given alone, Drug A produces 50% E_{max}, that is when $Cu_A = Cu_{50,A}$. Then, to increase the response to 75% E_{max} substitution into Eq. 17-16 shows that Cu_A must be increased to five times $Cu_{50,A}$. Alternatively, 75% E_{max} can be achieved by fixing Cu_A at $Cu_{50,A}$ and adding Drug B at a concentration of $2Cu_{50B}$. This is readily confirmed by appropriate substitution into Eq. 17-21. That is, Drugs A and B are equivalent when expressed as multiples of their respective potencies (Cu_{50}). The combination is additive in that the response is predictable knowing the potencies of each drug alone or, stated differently, the combination does not lead to any change in the potency of either drug.

One test for additivity is to fix response and vary the concentrations of the two drugs. It follows that if the combination is additive, then the sum of the equivalent concentrations (Cu divided by the respective C_{50} value) is also fixed, and therefore, a plot of the concentration of Drug A against the concentration of Drug B should be a straight line, as depicted in Fig. 17-21. The line of equal response is known as an *isobole*, and the graph is referred to as an **isobologram**. Observations may not fall on this line of additivity but instead fall either above the line, implying a less-than-additive effect, **antagonism**, or below the line, a greater-than-additive effect, or **synergism**. Antagonism can be thought of as one in which addition of Drug B to Drug A decreases the effective potency of Drug A, and synergism involves the converse. An example of synergism is that between midazolam and propofol in hypnosis used in the induction of anesthesia, and an example of antagonism is the decrease in cardiostimulant effect of

FIGURE 17-21. An isobologram comprises a plot of the combinations of the concentrations of two drugs, Drug A and Drug B, that produce a fixed response. When the line of equal responses, the isobole, is straight, the combination is additive. The combination is less-than-additive when the isobole curves above the line of additivity, and synergistic when it curves below the line of additivity.

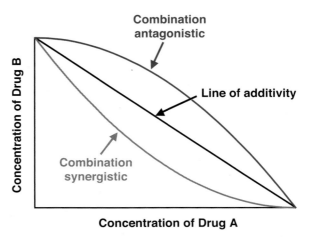

isoproterenol by β-blockers, such as propranolol. Although an isobologram is a useful means of detecting synergism or antagonism, it does not allow for an accurate assessment of the magnitude of the effect or the mechanism involved. For example, a drug combination may be synergistic either because one of the drugs modifies the receptor, thereby enhancing its interaction with the other drug, or because one drug inhibits the efflux of the other from the cell containing the receptor, thereby raising its internal concentration. Again, definitions are one thing, mechanisms involved and implications to drug therapy may well be another.

We have now explored various sources and causes of variability in drug response. We turn in the next chapter to the integration of this information and the underlying concepts to the initiation and maintenance of drug therapy.

KEY RELATIONSHIPS

$$t_{1/2,inhibited} = t_{1/2,normal} \cdot \frac{CL_{normal}}{CL_{inhibited}}$$

$$\frac{CL_{inhibited}}{CL_{normal}} = \frac{C_{ss,av,normal}}{C_{ss,av,inhibited}}$$

$$\text{Rate of metabolism} = \frac{CL_{int,f} \cdot Cu_{cell}}{1 + Cu_I/K_I} = \frac{fm \cdot CL_{int,f} \cdot Cu_{cell}}{1 + Cu_I/K_I}$$

$$CL_{inhibited} = CL_{normal} \left[\frac{fm}{1 + \dfrac{Cu_I}{K_I}} + (1 - fm) \right]$$

$$\frac{AUC_{inhibited}}{AUC_{normal}} = \frac{F_{inhibited}}{F_{normal}} \left[\frac{1}{\dfrac{fm}{1 + \dfrac{Cu_I}{K_I}} + (1 - fm)} \right]$$

$$\frac{(Dose/\tau)_{inhibited}}{(Dose/\tau)_{normal}} = \frac{F_{normal}}{F_{inhibited}} \left(\frac{fm}{1 + \dfrac{Cu_I}{K_I}} + (1 - fm) \right)$$

$$CL_{inhibited} = CL_{normal} \left[\frac{fm}{1 + k_{inact} \dfrac{Cu_I}{K_I \cdot k_E}} + (1 - fm) \right]$$

$$\begin{matrix} \text{Maximum} \\ \text{Exposure} \\ \text{Ratio} \end{matrix} = \frac{AUC_{PM,inhibited}}{AUC_{EM}} = \frac{1}{(1 - fm_{POLY} - fm_{NP})}$$

$$\frac{E}{E_{max}} = \frac{\dfrac{Cu_A{}^\gamma}{Cu_{50,A}{}^\gamma} + \dfrac{Cu_B{}^\gamma}{Cu_{50,B}{}^\gamma}}{1 + \dfrac{Cu_A{}^\gamma}{Cu_{50,A}{}^\gamma} + \dfrac{Cu_B{}^\gamma}{Cu_{50,B}{}^\gamma}}$$

STUDY PROBLEMS

(Answers to Study Problems are in Appendix J.)

1. Briefly comment on the accuracy of the following statements.

    a. Drug interactions are often detected when an interacting drug is initiated or withdrawn.

    b. Displacement of one drug by another occurs when the molar concentration of the "displacer" approaches that of the protein that binds the other drug.

    c. Displacement interactions are generally not *therapeutic drug interactions.*

    d. Of the various mechanisms of drug interaction, inhibition of metabolism is of primary therapeutic importance.

    e. Drug interactions are graded.

    f. Drug interactions at the transporter level are likely with class 1 compounds of the Biopharmaceutics Classification System.

2. The graphs below show the concentration–time curves following the method of administration given. Sketch the expected plasma concentration–time profile of each drug (low clearance, large volume of distribution) if administered again during the coadministration of another drug that is at steady state. The parameter given is altered twofold. Each graph should clearly indicate the consequence of a change in CL, V, and $t_{1/2}$ (or a combination).

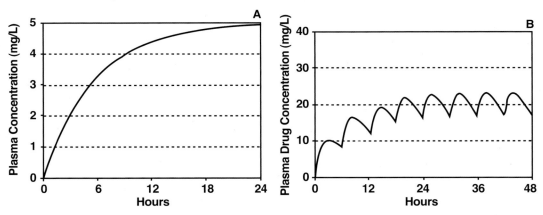

FIGURE 17-22. **A.** Constant-rate infusion (*fu* increased). **B.** Multiple oral doses (CL_{int} decreased).

3. Chlordiazepoxide, a benzodiazepine, was administered to six healthy volunteers (45 mg, i.v. bolus) in crossover fashion alone or in the fifth day of a daily 400-mg dose of ketoconazole, an antifungal agent. For the purpose of this problem, the drug has one-compartment model characteristics. Mean values of $C(0)$ and $t_{1/2}$ for chlordiazepoxide are shown in Table 17-8.

TABLE 17-8	**Pharmacokinetics of Chlordiazepoxide Alone and When Given With Ketoconazole**	
	Without Ketoconazole	**With Ketoconazole**
$C(0)$ (mg/L)	2.0	2.0
$t_{1/2}$ (hr)	23.9	43.4

From: Brown MW, Maldonado AL, Meredeith CG, et al. Effect of ketoconazole on hepatic oxidative drug metabolism. Clin Pharmacol Ther 1985;37:290–297.

a. (1) Prepare a semilogarithmic graph of the mean concentration–time profiles of chlordiazepoxide in the presence and absence of ketoconazole. Label both axes and identify both curves.

(2) Complete the following table:

	Without Ketoconazole	With Ketoconazole
V (L)		
CL (L/hr)		

b. Given that chlordiazepoxide is eliminated by biotransformation in the liver, what physiologic mechanism(s) (Q_H, fu, fu_T, CL_{int}) is responsible for the interaction of ketoconazole with chlordiazepoxide? Justify any assumptions that you make.

4. Drug A is given by infusion at a rate of 25 mg/hr to maintain a constant plasma concentration. The data in Table 17-9 are obtained in a subject who is infused at this rate in the absence and presence of Drug B (assume that it is at steady state when present).

TABLE 17-9 **Pharmacokinetic Data of a Drug Given Alone and in Presence of Another Drug**

	Data for Drug A			
Plateau Plasma Concentration of Drug B (mg/L)	Plateau Plasma Concentration (mg/L)	Urinary Excretion Rate at Steady State (mg/hr)	Fraction Unbound in Plasma	Half-life (hr)
0	10.0	15	0.1	12
20.0	6.7	4	0.3	8

Given this information and the observation that the creatinine clearance in this subject is 100 mL/min,

a. Determine if there is evidence for Drug A being secreted and/or reabsorbed in the kidneys.

b. Is the volume of distribution of Drug A affected by Drug B?

c. Determine the mechanism(s) by which Drug B interacts with Drug A.

d. Discuss the therapeutic implications of coadministering Drug A and Drug B.

5. Bergstrom et al. studied the pharmacokinetic interaction of the antidepressants fluoxetine and desipramine. Figure 17-23 and Table 17-10 summarize the observations following a single oral dose of desipramine (50 mg) alone and 3 hr after the eighth daily dose of fluoxetine (60 mg each). The concentration of fluoxetine during the time desipramine is quantified remains relatively constant (half-life of fluoxetine = 3–4 days after multiple doses). The value of fe for desipramine is about 0.03.

a. Given that the plasma-to-blood concentration ratio of desipramine is close to 1.0, that the drug is metabolized only in the liver, and that the "well-stirred" model of hepatic elimination applies, calculate the value of $fu \cdot CL_{int}$ in the presence and absence of fluoxetine.

b. Suggest one mechanism (combination of mechanisms is not acceptable) for the pharmacokinetic interaction observed. Document how you arrived at your conclusion.

c. Briefly explain why the factor by which half-life is altered is not the same as that of CL/F.

d. In the current study, a single dose of desipramine was administered on day 8 of daily administration of fluoxetine (half-life = 1.5 days). If administration of desipramine on day 8 had, instead, been the first dose of a once-daily multiple-dose regimen, would you expect the time for desipramine to achieve a steady state to be any different than had the subjects been first administered chronically desipramine to steady state and daily fluoxetine dosing then commenced, while maintaining the regimen of desipramine?

e. What implications do the observations of these authors have for the concurrent administration of these two antidepressants? Briefly discuss.

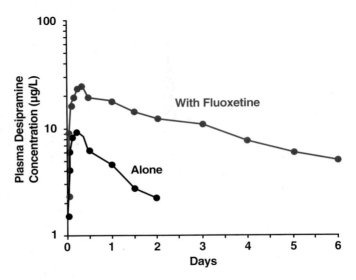

FIGURE 17-23. Mean plasma concentration of desipramine after a 50-mg oral dose given alone (●) and after 8 daily doses (60 mg each) of fluoxetine (●). (From: Bergstrom RF, Peyton AL, Lemberger L. Quantification and mechanism of the fluoxetine and tricyclic antidepressant interaction. Clin Pharmacol Ther 1992;51:239–248.)

TABLE 17-10	Pharmacokinetic Parameters and Measures (Mean, Standard Deviation) of Desipramine when Administered Orally as a Single 50-mg Dose Alone and after Eight Daily Doses of Fluoxetine	
Parameter/Measure	Given Alone (n = 6)	After Multiple Doses of 60 mg/day of Fluoxetine (n = 5)
$AUC(0\text{-}\infty)$ (μg · hr/L)	284 ± 244	2110 ± 900
C_{max} (μg/L)	9.4 ± 5.4	23.9 ± 5.6
t_{max} (hr)	5.3 ± 1.6	6.8 ± 1.1
$t_{1/2}$ (hr)	16.1 ± 5.2	63.8 ± 19.3
CL/F (L/hr)	289 ± 168	27.1 ± 10.3
V/F (L/kg)	77.1 ± 39.8	29.7 ± 7.7

6. Addition of the protease inhibitor ritonavir to the regimen of a patient on digoxin has produced severe digoxin toxicity. Ding et al. studied this interaction by administering a 0.5-mg i.v. bolus of digoxin to subjects alone and on day 3 of an 11-day oral

regimen of a 300-mg ritonavir twice daily, a therapeutic regimen. Table 17-11 summarizes their mean observations. The half-life of ritonavir, a known inhibitor of CYP3A4 and PgP, is 3 to 5 hr. The majority of digoxin, a substrate of PgP, is eliminated by a combination of renal and biliary excretion; its oral bioavailability is approximately 80%.

TABLE 17-11 **Pharmacokinetics of Digoxin Alone and During Ritonavir Administration**

Treatment	Clearance (mL/min)	Renal Clearance (mL/min)	Volume of Distribution (L)	Fraction Excreted Unchanged
Control	409	194	255	0.55
Ritonavir	238	126	451	0.59

From: Ding R, Tayrouz Y, Riedel K, et al. Substantial pharmacokinetic interaction between digoxin and ritonavir in healthy volunteers. Clin Pharmacol Ther 2004;76:73–84.

a. Why was digoxin given on day 3 of an 11-day regimen of ritonavir?

b. What is the likely mechanism by which ritonavir reduces the renal clearance of digoxin? Although not measured in the study, the value of fu of digoxin is close to 0.8, and independent of drug concentration.

c. Does ritonavir affect the nonrenal clearance of digoxin and if so, what is the likely mechanism?

d. Could the mechanism for reduction in renal clearance also be responsible for the increase in volume of distribution?

e. Why is the fraction of digoxin renally excreted not materially changed when coadministered with ritonavir?

f. What is your recommendation concerning the dosage regimen of digoxin if it is to be added onto the regimen of a patient stabilized on ritonavir?

g. On comparing the impact of ritonavir with that of quinidine, discussed in this chapter, what conclusions can be drawn on the likely role of transporters on the tissue distribution of digoxin?

7. Normal values for the pharmacokinetic parameters: clearance, fraction unbound in plasma, and fraction excreted unchanged are listed in Table 17-12 for Drugs A through G. Situations are presented that alter the kinetics of each of these drugs. On the right, indicate whether the value of each parameter would be observed to increase ($\uparrow$), decrease ($\downarrow$), or show little or no change ($\leftrightarrow$). Each drug is administered orally and has a volume of distribution greater than 50 L.

8. Tolbutamide, an oral hypoglycemic agent, has the following pharmacokinetic parameters in a 70-kg adult: $F = 1.0$, $V = 9$ L, $CL = 1.1$ L/hr, $fe = 0.03$. Elimination is almost exclusively via oxidation to hydroxytolbutamide.

a. Calculate the average plateau concentration and time to reach it when tolbutamide is administered in a regimen of 0.5 g orally twice daily.

b. Several drugs inhibit the metabolism of tolbutamide and cause excessive accumulation and hypoglycemic crises, unless the maintenance dose of tolbutamide is reduced. Given the following information about a competitive inhibitor: $F = 1.0$, $V = 13$ L, $CL = 0.6$ L/hr, $fu = 0.04$, $K_I = 0.6$ mg/L, calculate the following:

(1) The expected new average plateau plasma concentration of tolbutamide after the addition of a dosage regimen of 250 mg twice daily of the inhibitor to a patient previously stabilized on tolbutamide. The regimen of tolbutamide is continued unchanged.

(2) The time taken to reach this new plateau.

TABLE 17-12 Changes in Pharmacokinetic Parameters of Drugs A to G in Various Situations

Drug	Normal Values			Situations	Observations				
	Clearance* mL/min	Fraction* Unbound	Fraction Excreted Unchanged		Clearance*	Volume of Distribution†	Half-life	Fraction Excreted Unchanged	Oral Bioavailability
A	420	0.5	0.7	Simultaneous administration of a competitive inhibitor of renal secretion					
B (acid, CL_R pH sensitive)	200	0.1	1.0	Urine pH increased by another drug					
C	1200	0.5	0.99	Simultaneous administration of a competitive inhibitor of metabolism of Drug C					
D	1200	0.05	0.01	Simultaneous administration of a drug that displaces Drug D from plasma binding sites					
E	50	0.4	0.5	Simultaneous administration of a drug that displaces Drug E from tissue binding sites					
F	10	0.1	0.01	Simultaneous administration of a drug that displaces Drug F from plasma binding sites					
G	1300	0.7	0.95	Simultaneous administration for several days of an inducer of the enzymes that metabolizes Drug G					

*Based on measurement of drug concentration in blood.
†All drugs have $V_b > 50$ L.

(3) A practical regimen of tolbutamide that maintains a similar average preinhibitor plateau concentration, when coadministered in the presence of the inhibitor. Tolbutamide is available as a scored 500-mg tablet.

9. A drug has the following pharmacokinetic characteristics: $CL = 870$ mL/min, $t_{1/2} = 16$ hr, $fe = 0.01$, $F_{oral} = 0.15$. The low oral bioavailability is caused entirely by first-pass hepatic loss. The metabolites formed are inactive. The drug is likely to be given to patients receiving known enzyme inducers, and you have evidence to suspect that inducible enzymes are responsible for the metabolism of the drug under development. To provide some definitive data, you are asked to design a drug-interaction study in healthy volunteers. As a previous study showed that the kinetics of the test drug upon multiple dosing can be predicted from single dose administration, you decide on a single-dose study in the absence and presence of the potential inducer.

   a. Would you randomize the study with respect to the treatment sequence?
   b. Would you recommend giving the usual recommended dosage regimen of potential inducer?
   c. How long would you recommend administering the potential inducer before and after test drug administration?
   d. To ensure an adequate determination of the effects of induction, should they occur, would you recommend any change in the usual blood sampling times used to assess the pharmacokinetics of the test drug and if so, at what times and why. To assist, in answering this question, draw on the semilogarithmic plot in Fig. 17-24 the anticipated plasma concentration–time profile to show trends after induction following oral administration of 100 mg of the drug.

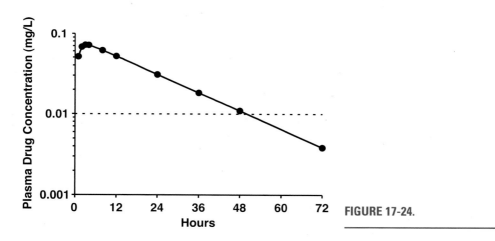

FIGURE 17-24.

   e. Which of the pharmacokinetic parameter(s) (F, V, CL, $t_{1/2}$, k) best reflects enzyme induction?

10. Diltiazem is thought to be a mechanism-based inhibitor of CYP3A4. It is extensively metabolized, partly via CYP3A4, to some active metabolites, and has a half-life in the range of 4 hr. What is your expectation of the pharmacokinetics of this drug with respect to dose and time dependency, and its effect on the pharmacokinetics of other drugs that are extensively metabolized by CYP3A4? Briefly discuss.

18

Initiating and Managing Therapy

OBJECTIVES

The reader will be able to:

- Suggest an approach for initiating a dosage regimen for an individual patient, given patient population pharmacokinetic and pharmacodynamic data and the individual's measurable characteristics.

- Describe why a pharmacokinetic or pharmacodynamic parameter in an individual patient is well known if the value in a typical population is known and its variability is small.

- Discuss why loading doses are sometimes given for drugs with half-lives in minutes and not given for drugs with half-lives in days.

- State why several sequential doses, instead of just one, are sometimes used as a loading dose.

- Explain why plasma concentration monitoring is useful for some low therapeutic index drugs but not others.

- Briefly discuss how tolerance to therapeutic and adverse effects can influence the chronic dosing of drugs.

- Discuss why adherence to the prescribed regimen is so important in drug therapy.

- Discuss why, for some drugs, dosage needs to be tapered downward gradually over time on discontinuing therapy.

- Describe how population information can be used to obtain initial estimates of an individual's pharmacokinetics.

- Upon evaluation of a pharmacokinetic problem observed during chronic drug therapy, ascribe the problem to a change in bioavailability, adherence, clearance, volume of distribution, or a combination of these values.

- Revise pharmacokinetic parameters of digoxin and vancomycin from measured plasma concentration data acquired under either steady-state or nonsteady-state conditions.

- Use the revised parameters (in the last objective) to calculate any modification in dosage required to ensure that the plasma concentration lies within the therapeutic window.

A s previously discussed, drugs are administered to achieve a therapeutic objective. Once this objective is defined, a drug and its dosage regimen are chosen for the patient. This choice is based on the assumption that the diagnosis is correct and with the expectation that the drug will be effective. Subsequently, drug therapy is often initiated and managed by one of two strategies shown schematically in Fig. 18-1.

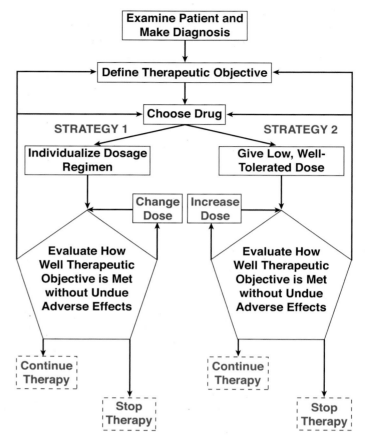

FIGURE 18-1. Scheme showing two strategies for initiating and managing drug therapy. The dashed line in strategy 1 indicates that changes in dosing rate may be carried out, but the main expectation is that the regimen has already been tailored to the needs of the individual patient. This is in contrast to strategy 2 in which the dosing rate starts low and is increased to find the patient's dosage requirement.

Management is usually, to one degree or another, accomplished by monitoring the incidence and intensity of therapeutic and adverse effects. In the first strategy, a "usual" dosage regimen anticipated for the patient is administered and adjusted only if the desired response is inadequate or an adverse response is excessive. In the second strategy, an individual's dosage requirements are established by initially giving a low dose and then titrating the dose upward based on assessment of therapeutic and/or adverse endpoints. Both strategies probably reach a similar optimal dosage regimen; only the method of getting there differs.

The first strategy is primarily based on population pharmacokinetics and pharmacodynamics, that is, on what is known about the general tendencies and variabilities in dosage–exposure (pharmacokinetics) and exposure–response (pharmacodynamics) relationships. This strategy also allows a degree of individualization of the regimen based on specific information about the individual patient. Most of the subsequent discussion revolves around this strategy. The second strategy, involving dose adjustment to measured effects, clearly is also a means of individualizing dosage and managing therapy.

This chapter examines pharmacokinetic and pharmacodynamic issues in the initiation (starting dose) and management (maintenance regimen) of drug therapy in both the patient population, in general, and the individual patient. It brings together, from previous chapters, many points presented there, often in other contexts.

ANTICIPATING SOURCES OF VARIABILITY

Choosing the right dose, loading dose and dosing rate, for patients with a given disease or condition is best accomplished when the sources of variability in the response to the drug are well understood and when there are good correlates between response and easily measured patient characteristics. First, consider the issue of the causes of variability.

Obviously, the desired therapeutic objective would be most efficiently achieved if the individual's dosage requirements could be established *before administering the drug*. In the absence of this information, one must often rely on knowledge from a typical patient population. In Chapters 12 to 17, we examined variability in drug kinetics and response. The question before us now is how to handle this information in treating individual patients.

PHARMACODYNAMIC VARIABILITY

In the pie chart of Fig. 18-2, the sources of pharmacodynamic variability of a hypothetical drug are indicated. For this drug, it is apparent that most of the variability in response is genetically related. Clearly, pharmacogenomic correlates of exposure and response could be very useful to guide therapy of this drug (e.g., trastuzumab). Such information would be useful to identify individuals who are unlikely to respond, and so would not be given the drug (e.g., trastuzumab), or who are likely to respond differently (have a different dosage requirement, exhibit a peculiar adverse event, or show an increase in the incidence of usual adverse events) to a given drug. As an example, recall, from Chapter 13, *Genetics*, the β-agonist albuterol in which response has been found to correlate with genotypic status. Knowing a patient's genotype may well help in selecting an appropriate dosage regimen for this individual.

Pharmacodynamic Variability

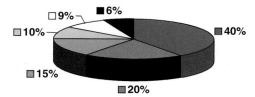

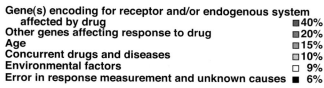

Gene(s) encoding for receptor and/or endogenous system affected by drug	▣ **40%**
Other genes affecting response to drug	▣ **20%**
Age	▣ **15%**
Concurrent drugs and diseases	▢ **10%**
Environmental factors	▢ **9%**
Error in response measurement and unknown causes	▪ **6%**

FIGURE 18-2. Schematic representation of the pharmacodynamic variability in drug response within the patient population. The variability occurs for various reasons. In this hypothetical analysis, six different categories causing the variability are identified along with the percent of the total variability associated with each category.

The data in the pie chart also suggest that one may be able to individualize dosage based on other factors, such as age, concurrent diseases, and environmental factors. The questions to be asked are how much of the variability can be captured by patient-specific information and whether or not major adjustment in the dosage or movement to another therapeutic procedure is needed.

PHARMACOKINETIC VARIABILITY

As discussed in several previous chapters, variability in dose–exposure relationships has an impact on the overall response to drugs. Again, one may be able to predict the dosage in an individual patient based on patient-specific information. The general approach is to move from population pharmacokinetic parameter estimates to those most likely to apply to the individual patient.

The first step is to identify the most variable parameters within the patient population. Variability in the various pharmacokinetic parameters within the patient population differs widely among drugs, as shown in Table 18-1 for several representative drugs. For some drugs, such as digoxin and propranolol, there is variability in absorption but for different reasons. With digoxin, the variability in absorption is caused primarily by differences in pharmaceutical formulation and efflux transport (involving P-glycopro-

TABLE 18-1	Degree of Variability in Oral Absorption and Disposition of Representative Drugs within the Target Patient Population			
Drug	**Bioavailability**	**Volume of Distribution**	**Clearance**	**Fraction Unbound**
Alendronate	++++*	++	++	+
Amiodarone	++	+++	++	++
Atorvastatin	+++	++	+++	+
Cyclosporine	++	+	++	+
Digoxin	+	++	+++	+
Ibuprofen	+	+	++	++
Nortriptyline	+++	++	+++	++
Phenytoin	+	+	++++	++
Propranolol	+++	+++	+++	+++
Salicylic Acid	+	+	++	++
Theophylline	+	+	+++	+
Trastuzumab	NA	+	+++	NA
Warfarin	+	+	++	+

NA, not applicable.

*Degree of variability: +, little; ++, moderate; +++, substantial; ++++, extensive.

tein) of the drug in the intestines, but with propranolol, it is caused by differences in the extent of first-pass hepatic metabolism. For other drugs, such as phenytoin, the only substantial source of variability is clearance. With others, the antiviral protease inhibitors and the statins included, significant variability exists in both absorption and disposition parameters.

The next step is to try to accommodate as much of the variability as possible with measurable characteristics. If the characteristic is discrete and independent, this can be achieved by partitioning the population into subpopulations. For example, as illustrated for clearance in Fig. 18-3, the discrete characteristics are hepatic disease and smoking (which are known to be important determinants of theophylline clearance). The population can be divided into four categories: (a) those who smoke and have no hepatic disease, (b) those who smoke and have hepatic disease, (c) those who have hepatic disease but do not smoke, and (d) those who neither have hepatic disease nor smoke. The frequency distribution for the entire population is determined from the relative size and shape of the distribution curve of each subpopulation. If, on the other hand, the measurable characteristic is continuous, such as age, weight, or renal function, it may be possible to find a functional relationship with one or more pharmacokinetic parameters, such as that seen between the renal clearance of ganciclovir, an antiviral agent, and creatinine clearance, a graded measure of renal function (Fig. 18-4). Clearly, the dosing rate of this drug should be reduced in patients with impaired renal function to avoid excessive adverse effects.

To envisage how the entire strategy would work, consider the data in Fig. 18-5 (page 532) for a drug, partly metabolized in the liver and partly excreted unchanged in the urine, for which population pharmacokinetic parameter values are: oral bioavailability, 0.73; volume of distribution, 83 L; renal clearance, 2.7 L/hr; and metabolic clearance, 14.1 L/hr. Depicted are four tablets, representing these four parameters. The size of each tablet is a measure of variability (coefficient of variation) of that parameter within the patient population. For this drug, oral bioavailability is the least

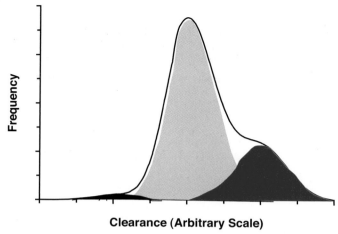

FIGURE 18-3. The frequency distribution of clearance of a drug within a total patient population (*heavy line*) is a function of the shapes of the frequency distributions within the various subpopulations that comprise the total patient population and the relative sizes of each of these subpopulations. In this simulation, the variables are smoking and hepatic disease, and the subpopulations are: those who neither have hepatic disease nor smoke (75%), the majority (*shaded gray*); those who smoke but have no hepatic disease (22.5%) (*shaded in red*); those who have hepatic disease but do not smoke (2%) (*shaded in black*); and those who both smoke and have hepatic disease (0.5%). The size of the last subpopulation is too small to be readily seen in this figure. The average values for clearance in the four subpopulations were set at 1, 1.5, 0.5, and 0.75 U, respectively, assuming that smoking increases clearance by induction and that clearance is reduced in hepatic disease.

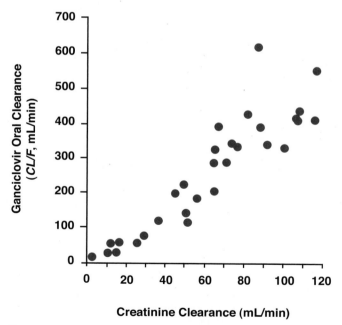

FIGURE 18-4. The apparent total body clearance (*Dose/AUC* or *CL/F*) of ganciclovir after oral administration of its prodrug, valganciclovir, increases linearly with creatinine clearance, a measure of renal function. Note that there is very little clearance when the renal function approaches zero (no creatinine clearance), indicating that this drug depends almost completely on renal excretion for its elimination. To maintain a comparable systemic exposure to the drug in patients with renal function impairment, the dosage of the drug needs to be decreased in proportion to the decrease in creatinine clearance. (From: Czock D, Scholle C, Rasche FM, et al. Pharmacokinetics of valganciclovir and ganciclovir in renal impairment. Clin Pharmacol Ther 2002;72:142–150.)

variable and hepatic clearance is the most variable. Stated differently, greatest confidence exists in assigning the population value of oral bioavailability to the patient; least confidence exists in assigning the population value of hepatic clearance to the patient. Moreover, as the population value for hepatic clearance is much greater than that for renal clearance, variability in total clearance within the population is also high.

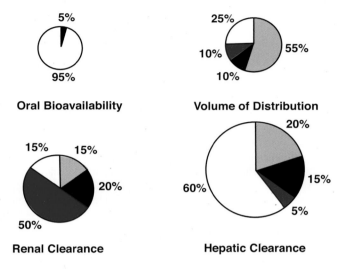

FIGURE 18-5. Schematic representation of variability in various pharmacokinetic parameters within a patient population. The size of each tablet is related to the degree of variability in the parameter. The portion of each tablet labeled with body weight (*gray*), age (*black*) or renal function (*colored*) reflects the fraction of total variability captured by each of these patient-specific measures.

Not unexpectedly, body weight accounts for most of the variability in volume of distribution and for some of the variability in hepatic clearance. Age, separated from its influence on body weight, accounts for some of the variability in hepatic clearance and, to a lesser extent, in volume of distribution. Renal function accounts for half of the variability in renal clearance. Surprisingly, perhaps, renal function helps to explain some of the variability in metabolic clearance and volume of distribution. Drug distribution and metabolism can be altered in patients with renal function impairment, because such patients manifest many systemic effects associated with this end-stage disease. Only 5% of the variability in oral bioavailability can be accounted for but, as mentioned, its value is small and acceptable. Correcting the population pharmacokinetic parameters for the patient's weight, age, and renal function should give reasonable individual estimates of F, V, and CL_R but little confidence in the estimate of CL_H and, hence, total clearance.

Genetics, concurrent disease(s), and associated concomitant medication undoubtedly play a role in determining CL_H, but the variability produced by them is not accounted for by the observed patient-specific information. Markers of genetic control of drug metabolism have been developed for some drugs that help to explain much of their inherited interindividual differences in metabolic clearance (Chapter 13, *Genetics*). An example (Fig. 18-6) is that of the antidepressant trimipramine. Like nortriptyline, this drug is primarily eliminated by CYP2D6-catalyzed metabolism. The patient population can be divided into four groups: (a) poor metabolizers (5%–10% of population), intermediate metabolizers (10%–15%), extensive metabolizers (65%–80%), and ultrarapid metabolizers (5%–10%). The last two groups are combined in the figure. The group to which an individual belongs can be determined by genotyping (pharmacogenomic test) or phenotyping. Phenotyping might involve a urine test of drug/metabolite ratio following a single dose of drug. The higher the ratio, the lower the amount of metabolite formed and the poorer the metabolic status of the individual, although renal function can affect the ratio thereby complicating the interpretation of this test.

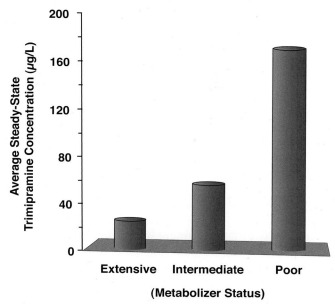

FIGURE 18-6. The daily maintenance dose of the antidepressant trimipramine depends on an individual's genotype. Without adjusting for genotype of CYP2D6, the average steady-state concentrations of trimipramine and its active metabolite, desmethyltrimipramine, vary greatly between the genotypes, identified here as extensive (including ultrarapid metabolizers), intermediate, and poor metabolizers. The concentrations are calculated from single-dose data for a regimen of 75 mg twice daily. The metabolite concentration (not shown) also goes up in the groups with intermediate and poor metabolism, a result of the demethylation reaction forming the metabolite (CYP2C19) not being affected by the genotype of CYP2D6, the enzyme responsible for hydroxylation of both trimipramine and desmethyltrimipramine. (From: Kirchheiner J, Müller G, Meinke I, et al. Effects of polymorphisms in CYP2D6, CYP2C9, and CYP2C19 on trimipramine pharmacokinetics. J Clin Psychopharmacol 2003;23:459–466.)

Another example is that of patients placed on thiopurine drugs (Chapter 13, *Genetics*) for which measurement of thiopurine S-methyltransferase activity can identify those patients likely to show severe adverse effects to drugs in this class, unless the normal dose is reduced accordingly. Pharmacogenomic information and its application in drug therapy are likely to become more common in the future. At the very least, knowledge of a patient's genotype can sensitize a clinician to a patient's needs before starting treatment. The clinician would then initiate therapy in this patient more cautiously, thereby reducing the risk of adverse events.

The pharmacokinetic approach presented previously for predicting an individual's optimal dosage regimen before administering a drug is based on the assumption that little interindividual variability in pharmacodynamics exists. This is, of course, frequently not so. Many times, the majority of variability in drug response within a patient population is of pharmacodynamic origin. Although knowing the mean pharmacokinetic parameters of the drug may help to explain the time course in response, quantifying pharmacokinetic variability then adds little to our ability to predict individual dosage. Nonetheless, the basic strategy still holds, namely, to determine the relative contribution of measurable characteristics, such as age and weight, to drug response within the patient population, and then to use the individual's characteristics to predict his or her therapeutic dosage regimen. Frequently, however, age, weight, and other measurable characteristics fail to account for much of the variability in pharmacodynamics. Then, there is little choice but to start the individual patient on a typical dosage regimen, which may be far from the individual's requirement, and to monitor and adjust the regimen based on the patient's response to the drug. When the drug has a low therapeutic index or when there is no urgency to starting therapy, it may be prudent to start with a low, generally safe dose and titrate up to the individual patient's need for the drug (strategy on right in Fig. 18-1). Let us now apply this information to initiating and managing drug therapy.

INITIATING THERAPY

The first dose given depends on the strategy used to treat a patient. There are situations in which the first dose needs to be smaller than the maintenance dose. For other drugs, a loading dose larger than the maintenance dose may be appropriate.

CHOOSING THE STARTING DOSE

Let us examine situations requiring a starting dose different from the maintenance dose and the determinants of its size. The argument was presented in Chapter 11, *Multiple-Dose Regimens*, that a priming or loading dose may be needed to rapidly achieve a therapeutic systemic exposure and, therefore, a therapeutic response. There are times when this strategy is appropriate and times when it is not.

When is a Loading Dose Needed? One consideration is the urgency of drug treatment. Recall from Table 10-1 (Chapter 10, *Constant-Rate Input*) that a loading dose is recommended for esmolol, a drug given by intravenous (i.v.) infusion to treat life-threatening supraventricular tachycardia. With a half-life of only 9 min, one would expect steady state to be reached in about 30 min; however, this is too long to wait in this emergency situation. By giving the loading dose at the time the infusion is started, an effective systemic concentration can be achieved within less than 5 min. The infusion thereafter maintains therapy. This strategy is relatively common to other drugs given by i.v. infusion (see Table 10-1).

When a loading dose is required, it may comprise the full therapeutic regimen. Consider the choice of an oral loading dose for the antimalarial, mefloquine hydrochloride. To treat patients with mild-to-moderate malaria caused by *Plasmodium vivax* or mefloquine-susceptible strains of *Plasmodium falciparum*, a loading dose of 1250 mg (five 250-mg tablets) is recommended. No maintenance dose is required because the drug has a 3-week half-life, a period of time sufficient to cure the patient. It is of interest to note in passing that the maintenance dose of mefloquine as a prophylaxis for the prevention of malaria is 250 mg once weekly, starting 1 week before going to areas where malaria is endemic and continuing for 4 weeks after returning from the area. The *accumulation* index of this drug on this regimen is 5 (Eq. 11-10 in Chapter 11, *Multiple-Dose Regimens*). Thus, the average amount of mefloquine in the body at steady state ($F \approx 1.0$) is about 1250 mg, the level found to be effective for treating an acute episode of malaria.

Adverse reactions often give rise to no loading dose being used or to the need to administer the loading dose over a period of time, but a short time relative to the drug's half-life. Another antimalarial drug serves as a good example of this situation. For treating an acute attack of chloroquine-sensitive malaria, chloroquine phosphate is given orally in a loading dose of 1000 mg initially, followed by 500 mg in 6 to 8 hr, and then 500 mg on each of 2 successive days for a total of 2500 mg. Again, this treatment completes therapy as the half-life of the drug is about 40 days. The reason for the divided loading dose is to reduce the occurrence of adverse effects (headache, drowsiness, visual disturbance, nausea, and vomiting, which, in the worst scenario, may lead to cardiovascular collapse, shock, and convulsions). These effects can occur within minutes of ingestion of a single 2500-mg loading dose.

The need for a loading dose is also a question of the kinetics of the pharmacodynamic response. Certainly, a loading dose is unnecessary for antidepressants, antihyperlipidemic agents, and agents used to treat and prevent osteoporosis. For these drugs, the therapeutic response takes from weeks to months to fully develop. Although a loading dose may shorten the time somewhat to achieve a therapeutic response, the major cause of the delay is in the response of the body to the drug. An example of a drug in this category is alendronate, an agent used to treat and prevent osteoporosis in postmenopausal women. As shown in Fig. 18-7, the increase in bone mineral density, a likely surrogate endpoint of the therapeutic use of the drug, namely, a reduction of bone fracturing, takes months, if not years, to fully develop.

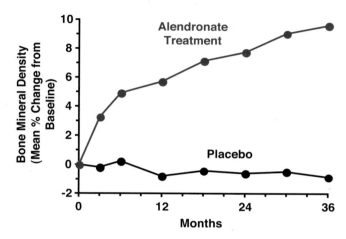

FIGURE 18-7. Time course of the change from baseline in bone mineral density following 10 mg of alendronate sodium daily in post-menopausal women with osteoporosis. Mean data for both treated (*colored*) and placebo (*black*) groups are shown. Note the time required for development of the effect, a surrogate of the desired reduction in frequency of bone fractures. (From: 2005 Physicians' Desk Reference. Montvale, NJ: Thomson PDR, 2005:2051.)

What Should the Loading Dose Be? A loading dose is a consideration for drugs with half-lives of 24 hr or more when they are administered in a convenient once-a-day or twice-a-day regimen. In these situations, the size of the loading dose may be anticipated from a pharmacokinetic perspective. The loading dose can be approximated from the amount accumulated in the body at plateau on chronic dosing and knowledge of the bioavailability. It might also be estimated from the window of concentrations associated with optimal therapy. As an example, consider the individual patient for whom data were presented in Fig. 18-5. As the ratio F/V strongly influences the peak plasma concentration after a single dose, reasonable confidence can be expected in estimating the patient's loading dose based on body weight, if required. This particularly applies to the administration of drugs to both very small and very large adults and to infants and children for whom the volume of distribution is expected to deviate extensively from that of a typical patient.

DOSE TITRATION

For those drugs that do not require an immediate response, a logical and safe procedure to initiate therapy is to titrate dosage in the individual. Dosage is adjusted until the desired therapeutic response is obtained without undue adverse effects. This procedure is recommended for several drugs. Flecainide acetate is an example of a drug dosed in this manner. For patients with paroxysmal supraventricular tachycardia, the recommendation is to start with 50 mg every 12 hr. Doses are then increased in 50-mg increments every 4 days until an optimal response is obtained. The 4-day interval between changing the dosing rate is based on the observation that at least 2 to 4 days is required to achieve a steady state of drug effect. This is not surprising from a pharmacokinetic point of view, because the half-life of the drug ranges from 12 to 27 hr in patients.

Another example is valproic acid, an agent used to treat complex partial seizures. When given alone, therapy is initiated with 10 to 15 mg/kg per day in divided doses.

The dosage is increased by 5 to 10 mg/kg per week until optimal control of seizures is achieved. Optimal clinical response is usually achieved with daily maintenance doses below 60 mg/kg per day. With terazosin, an agent used to symptomatically treat patients with an enlarged prostate and sometimes to treat hypertension, the recommendation is similar. The initial dose is 1 mg at bedtime. The nightly dose is increased in a stepwise fashion, based on blood pressure response, to 2 mg, then to 5 mg, then to 10 mg, or until the desired improvement in urine flow rate is achieved by relaxing the smooth muscles in the bladder neck. Daily doses of 10 mg are typically required. Accumulation of this drug is not very extensive on once-daily administration of a fixed regimen as the half-life is about 12 hr. Careful and slow upward titration of dosage reduces the incidence of severe postural hypotension and syncope and explains, in part, why weeks to months of treatment are often required to achieve the optimal response.

MANAGING THERAPY

For some drugs, there is a standard maintenance dosage regimen that works in almost all patients, with adjustments made for infants, children, and perhaps the elderly, especially those who are frail. For other drugs, therapy is frequently monitored and dosage is optimized by continual assessment of therapeutic or adverse effects, or both. For still a few others, measurement of plasma drug concentration is incorporated into the strategy for drug utilization. One of the key considerations that determines how therapy is managed is the therapeutic index of the drug.

LOW THERAPEUTIC INDEX

Recall from Chapter 9, *Therapeutic Window*, that a low therapeutic index drug is one for which the dosing rate required for a good therapeutic response is very close to that producing excessive adverse effects in an individual patient. To maintain a reasonably constant therapeutic response in the individual, the drug *must* show relatively little intrasubject variability in both its pharmacokinetics and pharmacodynamics. The dosing rate of such drugs needs to be individualized and the responses monitored more frequently than with high therapeutic index drugs. The degree of individualization and monitoring required depends on intersubject variability. As shown in Table 18-2, there may be less need for monitoring if intersubject variability is low in both the drug's pharmacokinetics and pharmacodynamics. If the interpatient pharmacodynamic variability is high and pharma-

TABLE 18-2	Interpatient Variability and Monitoring of a Low Therapeutic Index Drug	
Source of Interpatient Variability		**Monitoring**
Pharmacokinetics	**Pharmacodynamics**	
High	**High**	Full and continuous monitoring is required. If no good biomarkers or endpoints are available, the drug may not be useful.
Low	Low	Generally, there is less need for monitoring of the individual and the doses needed across the population are more similar.
Low	**High**	Assessment of therapeutic and/or adverse responses is essential. Little benefit is obtained by monitoring the plasma concentration of the drug.
High	Low	While monitoring of responses is important, concentration monitoring may be useful as well to aid in tailoring dosage to the individual patient.

cokinetic variability is low, then monitoring response is essential to establish the proper dose. If, on the other hand, the interpatient variability in response lies primarily in pharmacokinetics, which cannot be readily predicted from the patient's personal and clinical characteristics, then a strong case can be made to use plasma concentration monitoring as a strategy to aid in managing therapy with the drug, a subject discussed in greater depth toward the end of this chapter. For such drugs, a therapeutic window of concentrations determined for the patient population then applies to the individual patient. Plasma concentrations obtained at one or more appropriate times can then be used as a supplementary piece of information to guide the adjustment of dosage for the individual patient.

Warfarin and phenytoin, both low therapeutic index drugs, illustrate these principles. Recall that much of the interindividual variability in response to warfarin is in its pharmacodynamics (see Fig. 12-4). This results in a wide range of systemic exposures to the active drug (unbound S-warfarin concentration) giving the same response across the patient population. For this drug, monitoring the surrogate endpoint, clotting time, allows the dosage to be individualized. Monitoring of the plasma warfarin concentration provides little additional help in doing so. Phenytoin, on the other hand, has no nice surrogate endpoint of the clinical effect to guide therapy. Furthermore, from the data in Fig. 1-7, it is apparent that the drug exhibits a very large intersubject variability in its pharmacokinetics. How then can this drug be therapeutically useful? The answer lies in its intrapatient variability in both pharmacokinetics and pharmacodynamics and its intersubject variability in pharmacodynamics all being very low. The low intrasubject pharmacokinetic variability is seen in long-term studies in which a subject receives the drug orally for several weeks, as seen in Fig. 18-8. At a given daily dose, the steady-state concentration within the individual remains remarkably constant. The low intersubject variability in pharmacodynamics means that one can, using data from population studies, well define a window of concentrations where an individual's value should be. Concentration monitoring then becomes a useful tool to individualize therapy with this drug. The nonlinearity of phenytoin's disposition adds to the need to monitor its concentration, as previously discussed (Chapter 16, *Nonlinearities*).

An additional point needs to be made about how finely tuned an adjustment in dosage can be. In practice, one is frequently constrained by the products and dosage strengths commercially available. Often, the dose strengths of a given formulation differ

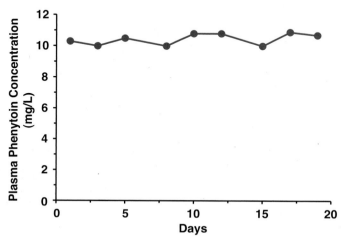

FIGURE 18-8. The average plasma phenytoin concentration remains remarkably constant during 20 days of oral administration of a fixed-dose regimen after steady state has been achieved in seven subjects, individually given daily doses ranging from 3.95 to 6.45 mg/kg. The implication is that the concentration within each individual remains relatively constant with time. (From: Wilder BJ, Serrano EE, Ramsey E, Buchanan RA. A method for shifting from oral to intramuscular diphenylhydantoin administration. Clin Pharmacol Ther 1974;16:507–513.)

by a factor of two. For example, pravastatin is available in 10-, 20-, 40-, and 80-mg tablets. Sometimes, a tablet is scored so that half of a tablet can be taken, but clearly, the ability to adjust doses is limited.

USE OF BIOMARKERS, SURROGATES, AND CLINICAL ENDPOINTS

Although preferable, it is not always possible to use a direct measure of the desired effect as a therapeutic endpoint. Sometimes, adverse effects are used as a dosing guide. Antineoplastics, such as 5-fluorouracil, and immunosuppressive agents, such as cyclosporine, are examples. Dosage is increased to levels at which the value of a biomarker of side effects or adverse effects approaches a limit (e.g., drop in blood cell count to a target range). In this sense, these are clearly low therapeutic index drugs.

Another example is again that of the antiepileptic drug, phenytoin. The therapeutic effect here is the nonoccurrence of seizures. Seizures may be infrequent, and as a result, delays and difficulties exist in assessing therapeutic success. Adverse effects that can be readily measured (e.g., nystagmus and ataxia) have therefore been used to assist in determining the upper limit of an epileptic patient's dosage requirement (see Fig. 9-6). As previously stated, plasma concentration monitoring is a supplementary approach to optimize phenytoin dosage; it offers an opportunity to avoid reaching severe adverse levels.

Another situation in which the therapeutic objective cannot readily be assessed is the prevention of thromboembolic complications with oral anticoagulants. In this case, an alternative, simple, and rapid laboratory test (i.e., the international normalized ratio test), which measures the tendency of blood to clot, is used as a surrogate measure of how well the therapeutic objective, prevention of thromboembolic complications, is achieved. Similarly, for antihypertensives, blood pressure is often considered a reasonable surrogate of clinical outcome (i.e., prevention of cardiovascular and renal disease associated with hypertension). For antihypercholesterolemic, hypoglycemic, and uricosuric agents, clinical laboratory tests of lipids and lipoproteins, blood glucose, and serum uric acid, respectively, are employed as biomarkers and surrogate endpoints. These and other examples of situations in which either biomarkers or surrogate endpoints are used to guide therapy are listed in Table 18-3.

Monitoring of therapeutic responses and toxicity is best accomplished when integrated with kinetic concepts. Half-life determines the time course of accumulation and hence the development of responses on starting drug therapy and on the waning of drug effect when drug administration is discontinued or reduced. The development or disappearance of response to many drugs may take even longer than predicted by half-life when pharmacodynamics is rate-limiting (see Chapter 8, *Response Following a Single Dose*). Tailoring an individual patient's dosage clearly requires integration of both kinetic and dynamic principles.

TOLERANCE

Another consideration in managing therapy is the build up of tolerance to a drug. As discussed in Chapter 11, *Multiple-Dose Regimens*, nitroglycerin, an antianginal agent with a 2- to 4-min half-life, is an example of a drug to which tolerance to the therapeutic response develops with continuous therapy. The use of transdermal patches to deliver the drug at a constant rate around the clock turned out to be unsuccessful because of the development of tolerance. The problem was, in large part, overcome by administering the patch only during the daytime, a time interval sufficient to allow for the subsidence of the tolerance to the therapeutic effect.

Tolerance can also develop to the adverse effects of a drug, as is the case with terazosin as mentioned previously. The drug, used to treat benign prostatic hyperplasia, produces hypotension. The adverse hypotensive effect can be kept under control by slowly increasing the dosing rate so that the therapeutic effect can be obtained without undue postural hypotension and syncope. How quickly the dosage can be titrated up to that needed chronically is primarily a function of the rapidity of the development of tolerance to the hypotensive effect.

TABLE 18-3	Examples of Monitoring Drug Therapy by the Effects Produced or by Alternative Tests			
Drug	**Condition**	**Observation Suggesting Increased Dosage**	**Observation Suggesting Holding or Decreasing Dosage**	**Severe Toxic Signs**
Group I. Drugs Monitored by Clinical Signs and Symptoms				
Salicylates	Rheumatoid arthritis or rheumatic fever	Inadequate reduction of inflammation and pain	Tinnitus, nausea, vomiting	Metabolic acidosis
Furosemide	Edema associated with congestive cardiac failure, cirrhosis, or renal disease	Excessive edema	Fluid and electrolyte imbalance associated with excessive dehydration	Severe hypotension, cardiac disturbances
Desipramine	Depression	Inadequate elevation of mood	Dry mouth, blurred vision, decreased effectiveness	Cardiac toxicity, orthostatic hypotension
Carbidopa/ levodopa	Parkinson's disease	Inadequate control of disease	Dyskinesia, blepharospasm	Involuntary movements, mental changes, depression
Thiopental	Induction of anesthesia	Insufficient anesthesia	Anesthesia too deep	Respiratory failure
Group II. Drugs Monitored by Tests in Vitro				
Warfarin	Thromboembolic disease	Prothrombin time too short	Prothrombin time too long	Hemorrhage
Cyclosporine	Organ transplantation	Signs of tissue rejection	Decreased renal function	Severe depression of renal function
L-Thyroxine	Hypothyroidism	Decreased unbound triiodothyronine (T_3) and thyroxine (T_4) in plasma	Elevated T_3 and T_4	Hyperthyroidism
Pravastatin	Hypercholesterolemia	Elevated cholesterol	Asymptomatic elevation of transaminases and creatine phosphokinase	Marked persistent rise in transaminases, myopathies
Uricosurics	Gout	Elevated serum uric acid	Decreased serum uric acid	Gastrointestinal irritation

DOSE STRENGTHS AND STRATIFICATION OF PATIENTS

Adjustment of either and initial dose or a maintenance dose to meet the requirements of an individual patient cannot be exact. As stated previously (Chapter 12, *Variability*, pages 333 and 352), solid dosage forms of drugs are commonly available in discrete dose strengths, which usually differ from each other by at least twofold. Simvastatin, for example, is available in 5-, 10-, 20-, 40-, and 80-mg tablets. Occasionally, the dose strengths are

TABLE 18-4	**Patterns of Nonadherence to Prescribed Dosage and Lack of Persistence in Taking Medications**

Nonadherence to Dosage Regimen (Daily Deviations)

    Change in time of day for taking dose.

    Omitting 1–3 doses per day.

    Taking extra doses to make up for missed doses.

Lack of Persistence in Taking Medication

    Discontinuing doses for periods of time (vacations, business trips, etc.).

    Completely stop taking drug.

From: Vrijens B, Voncze G, Kristanto P, et al. Adherence to prescribed antihypertensive drug treatments: longitudinal study of electronically compiled dosing histories. BMJ 2008;336:1114–1117; and Cramer JA, Roy A, Burrell A, et al. Medication compliance and persistence: terminology and definitions. Value in Health 2008;11:44–47.

closer together as is the case for the low therapeutic index drug warfarin, which comes in 1-, 2-, 2.5-, 5-, 7.5-, and 10-mg tablets. Obviously, dosage adjustment must be carried out consistent with the dose strengths available.

Similarly, there is a clinical tendency to stratify physiologic functions and disease severity that are, in reality, continuous. For example, patients with renal impairment are classified as having mild, moderate, or severe impairment or renal failure as in Fig. 15-5 (page 410) and Table 15-3 (page 415). Here too, a dosage regimen is often recommended for each group consistent with the dose strengths available.

ADHERENCE AND PERSISTENCE ISSUES

The most frequent patterns of nonadherence (Table 18-4) are failure to take drug at the times indicated, omitting an occasional dose, failure to take several consecutive doses, and occasional overdosing, particularly with once-daily dosing. Overdosing is often a result of "forgetfulness." "Did I take my medicine this morning or not?" Another form of nonadherence is discontinuance of drug therapy completely or for short periods (a few days to a week). The latter is sometimes called a "drug holiday." In these kinds of nonadherence, the primary issue is the lack of persistence in taking the medication.

Some drugs are forgiving, that is, nonadherence of the types in the first part of Table 12-3 may have little effect on therapy with the drug. This can occur when the dosing interval is small relative to the half-life, as is the case when using amiodarone, an antiarrhythmic agent with a half-life of 50 to 60 days, and phenobarbital, with a half-life of 4 days, to treat epilepsy. It also applies to drugs for which the response persists, relative to drug in the body, as is the case with the statins and the bisphosphonates, for which the recommended dosing frequency varies from once daily (e.g., alendronate) to once yearly (zoledronic acid). On the opposite extreme are drugs that are absolutely unforgiving, as is the case for a drug like esmolol for which the plasma drug concentration must be maintained. In this case, the drug is given by infusion, and the clinician, rather than the patient, must carefully and continuously monitor therapy.

Antimicrobials are frequently in the unforgiving category, as are the antiviral agents. Indeed, the replication, and hence potential mutation, rate of many viruses is much higher than that of bacteria so that the need to maintain an effective antiviral concentration throughout the dosing interval, to avoid emergence of resistance is paramount, a critical element in effective human immunodeficiency virus treatment. To achieve these objectives, adherence to the regimen for the duration of treatment is essential.

Consider now the kinetic impact of not taking an oral medication as directed.

Missed Dose(s). The lack of adherence to the prescribed manner of taking a drug is one of the sources, sometimes the major one, of variability in drug response. It is commonly believed that regimens of multiple (3–4) daily doses tend to produce greater frequencies of missed doses than those in which drug is taken once or twice daily. As shown in Fig. 18-9, such decreases in frequency (with corresponding increase in each dose to keep the same daily dose) may not improve therapy. Note that even when 3 doses are missed on the 3-times-a-day regimen (Fig. 18-9B) that the plasma concentration does not go as low as when one dose is missed on the once-a-day regimen (Fig. 18-9A). Clearly,

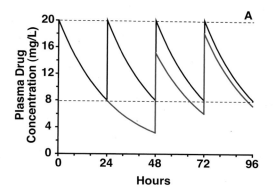
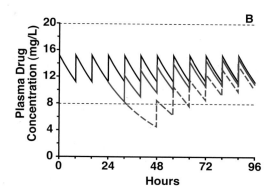
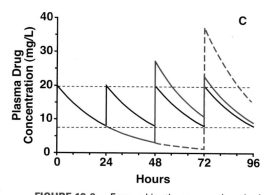
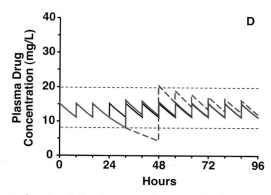

FIGURE 18-9.   From a kinetic perspective, the impact of a missed dose is greater the larger the dose and the less frequent the administration. Consider steady-state multidose conditions for a drug with a therapeutic window of 8 to 20 mg/L, a volume of distribution of 50 L, and a half-life of 18.2 hr. **A.** When a 600-mg dose is given once daily to maintain therapeutic concentrations (*black line*), a missed dose (*solid colored line*) results in a trough concentration of 3.2 mg/L, a value well below the lower limit of the therapeutic window. **B.** When a 200-mg dose is given every 8 hr (*solid black line*), the lowest concentration after a single missed dose (*colored line*) is 8.2 mg/L, a value within the therapeutic window. Even if 3 consecutive doses are missed (*dashed colored line*), the minimum concentration (5.0 mg/L) is still above that observed 24 hr after a single 600-mg dose is missed. **C.** When a patient attempts to make up for missed doses, the chances of adverse effects is increased, particularly on the once-a-day regimen. When a patient takes twice the daily dose at 48 hr, the peak concentration is increased (*solid colored line*), but not greatly. However, if the patient tries to make up for two missed doses (*dashed colored line*), that is, takes 3 times the normal dose, adverse effects become more likely. **D.** When the patient takes 2 doses at 32 hr after missing 1 dose on the 8-hr regimen (*solid red line*), the plasma concentration returns close to what would have been the case had no dose been missed. Even when 4 doses are taken at 48 hr after missing 3 consecutive doses, the peak plasma concentration is only 20.2 mg/L, a value just above the therapeutic window (*dashed colored line*). Note the difference in scales of concentration between the top and bottom panels.

an increase in the incidence of missed doses presumably occurring with an 8-hr regimen must be balanced against the benefits of giving the daily dose once only.

"Makeup" Dose(s). Another issue involving adherence is taking large doses to make up for missed doses. If one dose, or more, is missed, should the next dose be increased? Shown in Fig. 18-9C,D are situations in which missed doses are simply added to the dose taken at the next prescribed time. Again, note the greater risk associated with the once-daily regimen (Fig. 18-9C) compared to the 3-times-a-day regimen (Fig. 18-9D) with the "makeup" doses. This conclusion applies especially when a patient, who fails to take one or more consecutive doses, takes all the missed doses together to make up for drug not previously taken, as shown after 2 missed daily doses at 72 hr (Fig. 18-9C) and 3 missed 8-hr doses at 48 hr (Fig.18-9D).

Doubling up of Doses. Another adherence issue of clinical importance is the consequence of taking twice, or more, times the recommended dose at one time, either inadvertently (patient repeats a dose because he or she does not remember the dose already taken) or intentionally (if a little helps, more should be better). Figure 18-10 shows the consequence of doubling the dose. Clearly, a greater effect can be seen when the drug is given less frequently because of the larger dose given, particularly if adverse effects are related to the peak systemic exposure.

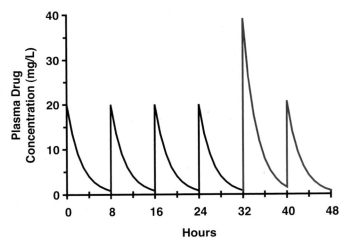

FIGURE 18-10. Another form of nonadherence to the prescribed regimen is when a patient takes more that one dose at essentially the same time. In this example, a patient takes two tablets instead of one at 32 hr, a consequence of forgetting that a dose was already taken or the patient does not feel well and believes that an additional dose may help. Note that the peak concentration of this drug, which has a 1.74-hr half-life, is nearly twice the usual peak concentration. When a drug is given infrequently compared to its half-life, the effect of taking multiple doses at once can be dangerous, particularly when the incidence and/or severity of adverse events increases sharply with higher C_{max} values.

The above simulations are generally based on a drug's pharmacokinetic properties. The therapeutic consequence of nonadherence to a drug also depends on the pharmacodynamics of a drug. All of the issues previously discussed regarding drug response, for example, the pertinent region of the exposure–response curve, the presence of a delay in the response relative to the systemic exposure, and the therapeutic index of the drug, apply here as well. They should be considered when evaluating nonadherence. When critical, patient education and motivation are essential to obtain effective therapy. This has been shown to be the case for antitubercular therapy and for protease inhibitors used in treating acquired immune deficiency syndrome (AIDS). Low drug concentrations increase the emergence of resistant strains of the bacillus and the virus, respectively. For many other drugs, such as the statins, omeprazole and alendronate, used in lowering cholesterol levels, gastroesophageal reflux disease, and osteoporosis, respectively, adherence to the prescribed manner of taking the medication is, perhaps, not so critical.

DISCONTINUING THERAPY

On stopping administration, the plasma concentration of a drug declines as governed by its pharmacokinetics. The speed of decline in response and the consequences of stopping vary. They are often dependent on the dynamics of the affected system as well. For many drugs, administration can be stopped abruptly without appreciable immediate safety concerns. This is the case with antibiotics, antihistamines, and nonsteroidal anti-inflammatory agents. However, for some others, sudden discontinuation of therapy can have serious consequences. This often occurs because the chronic exposure to drug causes a resetting in the level of one or more important body constituents, and if the drug is withdrawn too rapidly, particularly if it has a short half-life so that it is rapidly eliminated, an acute disequilibrium occurs within the body with potential adverse effects. One example is the increased β-receptor sensitivity noticed with the sudden withdrawal of β-blocking drugs, with sometimes fatal consequences. Another is the adverse effects, such as rapid weight loss, fatigue, and joint pain seen on sudden withdrawal of oral corticosteroids, especially following chronic high-dose therapy. In such cases, it is important to gradually reduce the daily dose, thereby allowing the body to adjust to the change in systemic exposure. The rate of reduction and duration of tapering dosage can vary, from days to weeks or months, depending on the kinetics of the drug and the dynamics of the affected system.

TARGET CONCENTRATION STRATEGY

We return in the final part of this chapter to the concept and application of **target concentration strategy**, where pharmacokinetics plays a critical role. This strategy is useful as an adjunct in initiating and monitoring drug therapy when a number of criteria listed subsequently are satisfied.

CRITERIA FOR MONITORING PLASMA DRUG CONCENTRATIONS

Some of the criteria are absolute in nature, others are relative. Most of them, however, must be met for the strategy to be routinely effective.

Good Concentration–Response Relationship. The plasma concentration of a drug must correlate quantitatively with either the intensity or probability of therapeutic or toxic effects across the patient population. Even a strong relationship between concentration and effect may be insufficient grounds for plasma concentration monitoring if the therapeutic effect itself, or a good surrogate of it, is easily monitored, which is often the case. The strategy becomes particularly attractive when a therapeutic endpoint is difficult to quantify, as with the nonoccurrence of epileptic seizures. The strategy is most pertinent when the objective is to maintain a therapeutic effect, and achieving this result requires the maintenance of the systemic exposure within a limited range (Chapter 10, *Constant-Rate Input,* and Chapter 11, *Multiple-Dose Regimens*) or when the likelihood of toxicity can be predicted from the concentration.

High Probability of Therapeutic Failure. Target concentration strategy is also indicated when there is a high probability of encountering a therapeutic failure (i.e., either a lack of effect or an occurrence of undue toxicity). A therapeutic failure is most likely to arise if the drug has a low therapeutic index and a great intersubject variability in its pharmacokinetics or if the patient is at particular risk because of genetic factors (Chapter 13, *Genetics*), concurrent disease (Chapter 15, *Disease*), or multiple drug therapy (Chapter 17,

TABLE 18-5	Information Pertinent to the Plasma Concentration Monitoring of Selected Drugs				
Drug	**Concurrent Disease States**	**Plasma Protein Binding**	**Concurrent Drug Therapy**	**Active Metabolites**	**Other Pertinent Information**
Cyclosporine	Autoimmune diseases	Extensively bound to lipoproteins and blood cells	Phenobarbital, rifampin, erythromycin, ketoconazole	Some metabolites have activity	Renal toxicity is major concern
Digoxin	Renal disease, congestive cardiac failure, thyroid disease	*	Diuretics	*	Distribution characteristics
Gentamicin	Renal disease	*	Some penicillins	*	Composed of three isomers
Nortriptyline	Alcoholic hepatic disease	Extensively bound to α_1-acid glycoprotein	Quinidine, fluoxetine, carbamazepine	10-Hydroxynor-tryptyline	Polymorphic hydroxylation
Phenytoin	Renal disease, chronic hepatic disease	Extensively bound to albumin	Valproic acid, carbamazepine, cimetidine	*	Saturable metabolism
Theophylline	Pneumonia, chronic obstructive pulmonary disease, congestive cardiac failure, hepatic cirrhosis, acute pulmonary edema	Moderately bound to albumin	Enoxacin, erythromycin, phenobarbital	*	Available in many dosage and salt forms

*Therapeutically unimportant.

Drug Interactions). A higher frequency of therapeutic failures is also anticipated when either nonadherence or erratic absorption is likely. Examples of drugs for which target concentration strategy has been found to be clinically helpful, together with general information pertinent to their monitoring, are listed in Table 18-5.

When a Problem Arises. For some drugs, the strategy is applied only when a problem arises. The problem may be a lack of response at usual or even higher dosages as a result of one or more of the following conditions: nonadherence, poor bioavailability, unusually rapid elimination, or a pharmacodynamic resistance to the drug. Measurement of the plasma concentration permits distinction to be made among the causes of the problem. Similarly, the cause of a toxic or unusual response at customary or lower dosages may be ascertained.

Population Pharmacokinetic Information Available. Efficient use of the strategy requires prior knowledge of the pharmacokinetic parameters of the drug, the conditions in which these parameters and the target concentrations are likely to be altered, and if altered, the extent of the changes. The last two requirements are relative in that, by monitoring the concentration, adjustments in dosage can be made for altered pharmacokinetics.

Reliable Assay. A sensitive, accurate, and specific assay for the drug must be readily available. In addition, to be useful, the results should be available before the next therapeutic decision is to be made. Often, the half-life of the drug is a useful index of this "turn-around" time because it is the time frame in which accumulation on multiple dosing and disappearance on discontinuing a drug occurs.

CONCENTRATION MONITORING

At a minimum, the plasma concentration serves as an additional piece of information to guide and assess drug therapy. It can also help to distinguish between pharmacokinetic and pharmacodynamic causes of either a lack of response or an excessive response.

When Is It Useful? Monitoring of plasma concentrations may be useful when a drug has a low therapeutic index and pharmacokinetics accounts for much of the interpatient variability in its response (see Table 18-4). Concentration monitoring is especially helpful when there are only poor endpoints/biomarkers to assess response, as is the case for cyclosporine, sirolimus, and other agents used in organ transplantation.

The Target Concentration. The target concentration initially chosen is the value or range of values with the greatest probability of therapeutic success (Table 9-1), keeping in mind that higher concentrations may be appropriate when the patient's condition is severe and the converse when the condition is mild. If altered plasma protein binding is anticipated, such as in uremia, after surgery, or when displacing drugs are coadministered, then the target total concentration should be adjusted to attain the same therapeutically important unbound concentration.

In contrast to many endogenous substances, which remain relatively constant, drug concentrations can vary greatly with time. The time of sampling and an appropriate kinetic model are therefore essential to interpret measured concentration(s). Several kinds of information are needed to evaluate a measured plasma concentration efficiently. A history of drug administration, which includes doses and times of dosing, is mandatory as are the times of sampling.

Frequency of Monitoring. Frequency of monitoring is a function of the presumed change in the factors that influence drug response. For example, the plasma concentration of sirolimus, an immunosuppressive agent, needs to be monitored for approximately only 7 to 14 days after changing dosage because of its 3-day half-life. More frequent monitoring may be indicated for this and other drugs when a patient's health is rapidly deteriorating or when therapy with coadministered drugs is altered. For example, weekly monitoring of plasma phenytoin concentrations may be helpful in treating an epileptic patient, when treatment with other drugs, which are inhibitors or inducers of phenytoin metabolism, are changed or withdrawn.

PERTINENT INFORMATION NEEDED

Several kinds of information, given in Table 18-6 are needed to evaluate a measured plasma concentration efficiently. Specific patient population pharmacokinetic information is essential. Population pharmacokinetic information for two drugs, digoxin and vancomycin, is given in Table 18-7 (page 547). These two drugs are used throughout the remainder of this chapter as examples of the application of the principles of plasma drug concentration monitoring.

EVALUATION PROCEDURE

Using the dosing history and the time(s) of sampling, judgment is needed on whether the measured value(s) is a good estimate of the maximum, average, or minimum concentration at steady state on a fixed regimen or of a nonsteady-state concentration(s) obtained either shortly after starting dosing or following an erratic schedule. Having established the

TABLE 18-6 Data Collection

History of Drug Administration

  Drug, dose, dosage forms, routes of administration, times of administration, adherence, inpatient or
  outpatient

Time of Sampling (relative to previous dose)

Present and Previous (if any) Plasma Drug Concentrations

Clinical Status of Patient

  Weight, age, gender, condition being treated, smoking, ethnicity, concurrent disease states (especially
  cardiovascular, hepatic, and renal diseases)

Laboratory Data

  Renal function (serum creatinine, creatinine clearance)

  Hepatic function (prothrombin time, serum albumin, serum bilirubin)

  Protein binding (albumin, total plasma proteins)

Concurrent Drug Therapy

  Interacting drugs

  Assay interferences

Active Metabolites

Assay Method (reproducibility, sensitivity, and specificity)

Usual Pharmacokinetic Parameters Associated With Type of Patient in Question

  Bioavailability, absorption rate constant, volume of distribution, unbound fraction in plasma, total
  clearance, renal clearance

---

conditions and an appropriate kinetic model, a generally recommended procedure to evaluate one or more concentrations is as follows:

1. Estimate the likely values of the pharmacokinetic parameters (F, CL, V, and hence $t_{1/2}$) in the patient based on population parameters, taking into account the patient's age, weight, renal function, concurrent diseases, drug therapy, dosage form, route of administration, and any other information about the patient known to affect the kinetics of the drug. A major intent here is to identify the subpopulation to which the patient belongs (Chapters 13–17).

2. Using the appropriate kinetic model and the parameter values above, estimate the plasma concentration(s) expected at the time(s) of sampling, taking into account the dosing history of the patient.

3. Compare the observed and expected concentrations. If they are in agreement, then one's confidence in knowing the parameters in the patient is increased. A clinical decision to modify the dosage in the patient depends on the concentration observed and on several other factors including, most importantly, the current response(s) of the patient.

4. If observed and expected concentrations are judged to be different, then one may wish to revise the pharmacokinetic parameter estimates. Here, it is necessary to weigh how much confidence one has in the initial parameter estimates from previous population studies relative to that in the estimates obtained from the measured plasma concentration(s).

Differences in observed and expected concentrations suggest several possibilities. For example, the patient's kinetics may differ from that expected, he or she may have been nonadherent, the sampling times may not have been noted correctly, or an assay problem may have occurred.

TABLE 18-7 **Usual Dosage Regimens and Patient Population Pharmacokinetic Parameters of Digoxin and Vancomycin**

Usual Dosage Regimen	Digoxin		Vancomycin	
	Murphy*	Winter[†]	Murphy*	Winter[†]
	Loading Dose*	Maintenance Dose*		
Infants and Children				
<2 years	38–63 μg/kg*	13–15 μg/kg*	10–15 mg/kg/6 hr	
2–10 years	25–44 μg/kg*	10–13 μg/kg*	Infused over 60 min	
>10 years	10–15 μg/kg*	4–13 μg/kg*		
Adults (16–65 years)	10–15 μg/kg in divided doses*	0.25–0.5 mg/day*	15 mg/kg/12 hr	10–15 mg/kg/12 hr
Elderly (>65 years)	1–1.5 mg in divided doses*	0.25 mg/day*	10–15 mg/kg/ 12–24 hr	Adjust to renal function
Renal Disease—Adult	0.5 mg in divided doses*	For CL_{cr} <20mL/min: – 0.125mg/day*		
Pharmacokinetic Parameter Values				
Bioavailability				
Intravenous	100%	100%	100%	100%
Oral—Tablets	75%	70%	<5%	<5%
Capsules	95%	100%		
Elixir	80%	80%		
Fraction excreted Unchanged	0.70		0.95	0.95
Fraction Unbound	0.75		0.45–0.70	
Clearance				
Infants (1 month–1 year)	11 L/hr/m²		3.47 ± 0.83 L/hr/ 1.73 m²	$CL = CL_{cr}$
Children (1–16 years)	8 L /hr/m²		8.45 ± 0.85 L/hr/ 1.73 m²	$CL = CL_{cr}$
Adults (16–65 years)	‡	**	0.073 ± 0.025 L/ hr/kg	$CL = CL_{cr}$
Elderly (>65 years)	‡	**	0.053 ± 0.003 L/ hr/kg	$CL = CL_{cr}$
Volume of Distribution				
Infants (1 month–1 year)	16 ± 2 L/kg		0.69 ± 0.17 L/kg	
Children (1–16 years)	16 ± 0.8 L/kg		0.70 ± 0.12 L/kg	
Adults (16–65 years)	6.7 ± 1.4 L/kg	††	0.62 ± 0.15 L/kg	‡‡
Elderly (>65 years)	6.7 ± 1.4 L/kg	††	0.76 ± 0.06 L/kg	‡‡
Renal Disease–Adult		††		‡‡

(continued)

TABLE 18-7	Usual Dosage Regimens and Patient Population Pharmacokinetic Parameters of Digoxin and Vancomycin *(continued)*

Half-life

Infants (1 month–1 year)	18 ± 9 hr		4.1 hr	
Children (1–16 years)	36 ± 14 hr		2.6 hr	
Adults (16–65 years)	36 ± 8 hr	2 days	7.0 ± 1.5 hr	5–10 hr
Elderly (>65 years)			12.1 ± 0.8 hr	
Renal Disease–Adult		Up to 4–6 days		Up to 7 days

Therapeutic Concentrations

Peak	—	—	Not applicable	40–50 mg/L
Trough	0.8–2 μg/L	0.5–2 μg/L CHF:0.5–1 μg/L	5–15 mg/L, 5–20 mg/L (when no other nephrotoxins are present.)	5–15 mg/L

---

*Murphy JE, ed. Clinical Pharmacokinetics Pocket Reference. 2nd ed. Bethesda, MD: American Society of Health-System Pharmacists, Inc.; 2001.

†Winter ME. Basic Clinical Pharmacokinetics. 4th ed. Philadelphia: Lippincott Williams and Wilkins; 2003.

‡CHF (congestive heart failure) absent: CL (mL/min) = 1.3 × CL_{cr} + 41. CHF present: CL (mL/min) = 1.3 × CL_{cr} + 20

**Non-CHF patients: CL (mL/min) = 0.8 × Wt. (in kg) + CL_{cr} (in mL/min); Patients with CHF: CL (mL/min) = 0.33 × Wt. (kg) + 0.9 × CL_{cr} (mL/min)

†† V (L/70 kg) = 226 + $\dfrac{298 \times CL_{cr} \text{ (in mL/min)}}{29 + CL_{cr} \text{ (in mL/min)}}$

‡‡ V (L) = 0.17 × Wt (kg) + 0.22 × Total Body Water (in kg) + 15

The major decision is how much to rely on the measured concentration relative to information known about patients such as the one being treated. Such decisions are beyond the scope of this chapter but are very important in concentration monitoring. For the purpose of this chapter, the concentrations, dosing histories, sampling times, and assay procedures are considered to be accurate. The next step is then how to determine the pharmacokinetic parameters in the patient.

The model used for predicting the concentration(s) must be appropriate for determining the individual's parameter values. For example, if intravenously infused to steady state, the expected concentration is determined from $C_{ss} = R_{inf}/CL$. Rearranging, clearance can be estimated from $CL = R_{inf}/C_{ss}$.

5. A recommendation for dosage adjustment or patient education (nonadherence) may be appropriate. In addition, comments to the clinician could aid in the interpretation of the drug concentration. Such comments include the need to adjust the therapeutic window when altered protein binding is expected and when a change in time of sampling is appropriate.

DOSING SCENARIOS

As previously stated, Chapter 10, *Constant-Rate Input*, and Chapter 11, *Multiple-Dose Regimens*, contain the basic concepts and key relationships needed for evaluating concentrations obtained during constant-rate and multiple-dose regimens. These key relationships are now supplemented with additional ones useful for evaluating three scenarios. These are: when nonadherence is suspected (one or more doses is missed); when a patient is on a 4-times-a-day regimen in which the intervals are not equal, for example: 9 A.M., 1 P.M., 5 P.M., 9 P.M. (subsequently called a "9-1-5-9" regimen and common to hospital settings); and when the doses vary and the dosing intervals are erratic. Emphasis here is on step 2 (evaluation procedure), particularly on determining the appropriate kinetic model for estimating concentration(s) at time(s) of sampling.

For digoxin, the systemic absorption is assumed to be much more rapid than its elimination (i.e., the i.v. bolus model approximation), with correction for incomplete systemic absorption, applies. The same model is used to evaluate the vancomycin scenarios. Unless otherwise noted, dosing and sampling times are subsequently based on the 24-hr clock.

Missed Dose(s). Although it would seem that missed doses would greatly complicate the evaluation of a measured concentration, it is not necessarily so. Figure 18-11 shows a fixed-dose, fixed-interval multiple-dose regimen of digoxin in which one dose is missed. To account for the missed dose, one needs to subtract the concentration expected at the time of sampling had only the missed dose been given from that expected if no dose was missed. This correction is based on the principle of additivity of concentrations from each dose at all times. In this example, a concentration is measured at time, t, within the dosing interval. The concentration expected at steady state with no missed dose is

$$C(t)_{ss} = F \cdot \frac{Dose}{V} \left(\frac{e^{-k \cdot t}}{1 - e^{-k \cdot \tau}} \right)$$

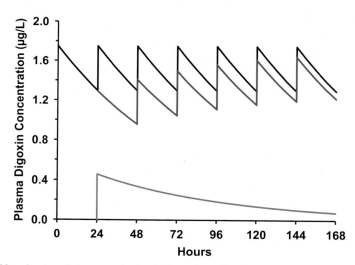

FIGURE 18-11. A missed dose results in the lowering of the fluctuating concentrations from the steady-state values. The degree of this lowering is equivalent to the concentration remaining from the missed dose. The expected concentration at any time following the missed dose (*colored line*) can then be estimated by the difference between the value expected with no missed dose (*black line*) and the concentration expected at that time had only the missed dose been given (*gray line*). The parameters used in the figure are those expected in the patient in the digoxin example case history given just after Eq. 18-2.

The concentration expected at the time of the missed dose (t, missed dose) after giving only a single dose is

$$C_{ss} (t, \text{missed dose}) = \frac{F \cdot Dose}{V} \cdot e^{-k \cdot t}$$

The concentration expected in the therapeutic setting is then

$$C_{ss} (t) = \frac{F \cdot Dose}{V} \cdot \left[\frac{e^{-k \cdot t}}{1 - e^{-k \cdot \tau}} - e^{-k \cdot t} \right] \qquad 18\text{-}1$$

The concentration expected when two consecutive doses are missed, the second one at time t_2, is

$$C_{ss}(t_2) = \frac{F \cdot Dose}{V} \cdot \left[\frac{e^{-k \cdot t_2}}{1 - e^{-k \cdot \tau}} - e^{-k \cdot t_1} - e^{-k \cdot t_2} \right]$$

18-2

where t_1 and t_2 are the times since the first and second should have been given.

For an example, consider a typical patient (60 years old, 70 kg, $CL_{cr} = 75$ mL/min) who misses 2 doses while on a digoxin regimen of 0.25-mg tablets once daily for the treatment of congestive heart failure. From the information in Table 18-7, the following pharmacokinetic parameters are obtained:

$$F = 0.8$$

$$V (L) = 226 + \frac{298 \times 75}{29 + 75} = 441 \ L$$

$$CL \ (\text{mL/min}) = 0.33 \times 70 + 0.9 \times 75 = 91 \ \text{mL/min or } 5.46 \ \text{L/hr}$$

$$k = \frac{CL}{V} = \frac{5.46 \ L/h}{441 \ L} = 0.0123 \ hr^{-1} \ or \ 0.3 \ day^{-1}$$

The concentration expected following the two consecutive missed doses 24 hr after a daily dose of 0.25 mg in the typical patient who has missed doses at 24 and 48 hr before sampling is:

$$C_{ss}(t_2) = 0.8 \times \frac{250 \ \mu g}{441 \ L} \cdot \left[\frac{e^{-0.0123 \times 48}}{1 - e^{-0.0123 \times 24}} - e^{-0.0123 \times 24} \ e^{-0.0123 \times 48} \right] = 0.39 \ \mu g/L,$$

a value below the therapeutic range, 0.8–2.0 µg/L.

9-13-17-21 Regimen. In institutional settings, many drugs are given in regimens similar to the one portrayed in Fig. 18-12. Such regimens have a 24-hr repetitive or

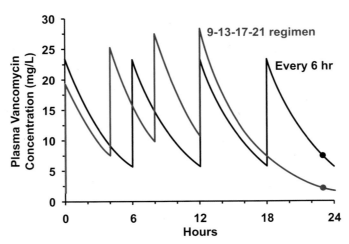

FIGURE 18-12. The plasma vancomycin concentration varies extensively at steady-state (24-hr repeating pattern) with a "9-13-17-21" type of regimen of 250 mg in an average 4-year-old child (*colored line*). In this example, the concentration, 1.6 mg/L, at the time of the morning dose (9:00 = "zero" time) would be ineffective (desired trough concentration = 5–15 mg/L). A twofold or threefold increase in the dose to overcome this low trough value, however, may cause toxicity, particularly during the evening hours after the dose at 21:00. The parameter values used are those given in the vancomycin case history. The expectation when 250 mg is given to the child every 6 hr (*black line*) is also provided.

regular cycle, even though the dosing intervals within the day are unequal. The expected concentration at any time during the day can be viewed simply as the sum of the steady-state concentrations resulting from each of the 4 daily doses. When given once daily, the first dose of the day is expected to yield a concentration, $C(t_1)$, at steady state, given by

$$C_{ss}(t_1) = \frac{F \cdot Dose}{V} \cdot \left(\frac{e^{-k \cdot t_1}}{1 - e^{-k \cdot \tau}} \right)$$

where t_1 is the time during the day between giving the dose and sampling the blood. The concentration resulting from giving only the second dose on a daily regimen is

$$C_{ss}(t_2) = \frac{F \cdot Dose}{V} \cdot \left(\frac{e^{-k \cdot t_2}}{1 - e^{-k \cdot \tau}} \right)$$

where t_2 is the time between the administration of the second dose and the time of blood sampling, and so on. Thus, the concentration expected on such a regimen is

$$C_{ss}(t_2) = \frac{F \cdot Dose}{V} \cdot \left(\frac{e^{-k \cdot t_1} + e^{-k \cdot t_2} + e^{-k \cdot t_3} + e^{-k \cdot t_4}}{1 - e^{-k \cdot \tau}} \right) \qquad \text{18-3}$$

where τ is 24 hr, the dosing interval in each of the once daily regimens.

To demonstrate the use of this relationship, consider the administration of vancomycin to a 20-kg, 5-year-old boy with a creatinine clearance of 55 mL/min and in whom the expected pharmacokinetic parameters are estimated to be as follows:

$$F = 1.0$$

$$V = 0.7 \, L/kg \times 20 \, kg = 14 \, L$$

$$CL = 8.45 \, L/hr \times \left(\frac{20}{70} \right)^{0.75} = 3.3 \, L/hr$$

If determined from $CL = CL_{cr}$, the value of CL would be 55 mL/min or 3.3 L/hr, so that

$$k = \frac{CL}{V} = \frac{3.3 \, L/hr}{14 \, L} = 0.24 \, hr^{-1}$$

The recommended dosage regimen for the child is 10 to 15 mg/kg every 6 hr. The child was in the hospital and was given a dose of 250 mg on a 9-13-17-21 regimen. A blood sample was obtained at 8:00 on the third day, 1 hr before the next dose was given. Estimate the concentrations expected at 8:00 (a) if the regimen of every 6 hr (9-15-21-3) had been used and (b) when the previous regimen was used in the child.

Regimen: 250 mg every 6 hr:

$$C_{ss}(8{:}00) = \frac{F \cdot Dose}{V} \cdot \left(\frac{e^{-k \cdot t}}{1 - e^{-k \cdot \tau}} \right) =$$

$$1.0 \times \frac{250 \, mg}{14 \, L} \cdot \left(\frac{e^{-0.24 \times 5}}{1 - e^{-0.24 \times 6}} \right) = 7.1 \, mg/L$$

Regimen at 9-13-17-21 hr:

$$C_{ss}(8{:}00) = \frac{F \cdot Dose}{V} \cdot \left(\frac{e^{-k \cdot t_1} + e^{-k \cdot t_2} + e^{-k \cdot t_3} + e^{-k \cdot t_4}}{1 - e^{-k \cdot \tau}} \right) =$$

$$1.0 \cdot \frac{250 \, mg}{14 \, L} \cdot \left(\frac{e^{-0.24 \times 23} + e^{-0.24 \times 19} + e^{-0.24 \times 15} + e^{-0.24 \times 11}}{1 - e^{-0.24 \times 24}} \right) = 2.03 \, mg/L$$

The therapeutic plasma concentration of vancomycin is 5 to 15 mg/L. Note that the 9-13-17-21 regimen is expected to result in a concentration at 8:00 A.M. of only 2 mg/L, a systemic exposure to the drug that is most likely to be insufficient.

Dose and Interval Unequal. The situation in which neither dose nor interval have any degree of regularity is frequently observed in therapeutic monitoring. In this situation, one can simply sum up drug that remains from previous doses with the realization that doses given more than four patient half-lives ago can be disregarded, since so little drug remains in the body from each of them. The plasma concentration expected after four doses, for example, is

$$C = \frac{F}{V} \cdot (Dose_1 \cdot e^{-k \cdot t_1} + Dose_2 \cdot e^{-k \cdot t_2} + Dose_3 \cdot e^{-k \cdot t_3} + Dose_4 \cdot e^{-k \cdot t_4}) \qquad 18\text{-}4$$

where $Dose_1$, $Dose_2$, $Dose_3$, and $Dose_4$ represent the doses taken at times t_1, t_2, t_3, and t_4 before sampling.

As an example of this situation, consider a 68-kg, 60-year-old male patient, with atrial fibrillation, whose dosing history of i.v. vancomycin therapy is as follows:

Date	Time	Dose (mg)	Blood Sampling Time and Plasma Concentration
22 February	9:00	500	
22 February	17:00	1000	
22 February	24:00	1000	
23 February	8:00	500	13:00 (34 mg/L)

This patient has reduced renal function (deduced from a serum creatinine of 2.2 mg/dL). The following are the calculated values for the key pharmacokinetic parameters:

$$F = 1.0$$

$$CL = CL_{cr} = \frac{(140 - 60)\,68}{72 \times 2.2} = 34 \ mL/min \ (or \ 2.06 \ L/hr)$$

$$V = 0.62 \ L/kg \times 68 \ kg = 42.2 \ L$$

$$k = \frac{CL}{V} = \frac{2.06 \ L/hr}{42.2 \ L} = 0.049 \ hr^{-1}$$

Does the observed concentration differ greatly from that expected in this patient?
Calculation of the expected concentration:

$$C\,(13{:}00) = \frac{F}{V} \cdot (Dose_1 \cdot e^{-k \cdot t_1} + Dose_2 \cdot e^{-k \cdot t_2} + Dose_3 \cdot e^{-k \cdot t_3} + Dose_4 \cdot e^{-k \cdot t_4}) =$$

$$\frac{1.0}{42.2 \ L} \times (500 \cdot e^{-0.049 \times 28} + 1000 \cdot e^{-0.049 \times 20} + 1000 \cdot e^{-0.049 \times 13}$$
$$+ 500 \cdot e^{-0.049 \times 5}) = 33.7 \ mg/L$$

The two values are similar, indicating consistency with the expected pharmacokinetics of the drug in this patient, but the dosage needs to be reduced.

Confidence in Estimates. Evaluation of a plasma concentration requires knowing whether clearance or volume of distribution is the more variable and appreciating on which of these two parameters the concentration is more dependent. The latter may be considered from the events depicted in Fig. 18-13 during the infusion of a drug in three separate situations. In Case A, the values of the clearance and volume parameters are those anticipated, the average values. In the other two situations, the half-life is three times longer than the average value, in Case B due to a threefold reduction in clearance and in Case C due to a threefold increase in volume of distribution.

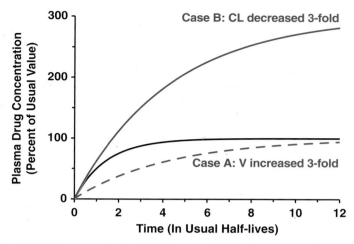

FIGURE 18-13. Following a constant-rate infusion, monitoring the concentration at one usual half-life does little to distinguish between a patient with average values of clearance and volume of distribution (*black line*) and one with a threefold reduction in clearance and an average volume of distribution (*colored line*). Distinguishing between these patients, without producing undue toxicity, is probably best done by monitoring at four usual half-lives. Although a threefold increase in volume of distribution (*colored dashed line*) is readily detected at one usual half-life, this observation provides little information on the final plateau concentration to be achieved.

With little drug having been eliminated, an early concentration is primarily a function of infusion rate and volume of distribution. Accordingly, there is little virtue in taking a sample before the usual half-life to estimate the dosage requirements needed to achieve therapeutic concentrations. A steady-state concentration depends only on the rate of administration and the value of clearance (Chapter 10, *Constant-Rate Input*). Accordingly, sampling when this condition is met provides the most confidence in estimating dosing rate requirements.

Sampling of blood between the time of initiating an infusion and steady state can lead to inconclusive information. At two usual half-lives, the observation of the concentration expected, Case A, does not mean that *CL* and *V* have the expected values. They may both differ and fortuitously give the expected concentration. The lower-than-expected concentration at two usual half-lives, Case C, could be a result of either an increased clearance or an increased volume, as shown. In contrast, the observation at this time of a concentration equal to or above the expected steady-state value, Case B, is a clear indication that clearance is less than usual. Indeed, the greater this difference, the lower is the probable value of clearance and the greater the need to reduce the rate of administration to avoid toxicity.

In the region of 2 to 6 half-lives (within the patient), a major consideration in interpreting a single observation is whether clearance or volume of distribution is the more variable. For example, clearance (in units of L/hr/kg) of vancomycin varies more (larger coefficient of variation), particularly if age and disease state are factored in, than volume of distribution (L/kg). Thus, by fixing volume of distribution, estimates of the clearance of vancomycin made from nonsteady-state values obtained within this time span are more accurate than would otherwise be the case. Furthermore, to ensure that the estimated pharmacokinetic parameters are not outlandish advantage is generally taken of conditioning the limited observations in an individual patient to the existing body of population pharmacokinetic data, with the view that any parameter estimate well outside the 95% population bounds is seriously questioned, and alternative explanations, such as incorrect assay or declared time of blood sampling, before reaching a final decision, need to be explored. Moreover, subsequent blood samples are often taken from the patient during the course of therapy and used to update and refine their parameter estimates.

Although the preceding concepts regarding estimates of parameters were developed for administration by infusion, they generally apply to all forms and schedules of drug administration intended to produce a plateau concentration.

CHANGES IN THERAPY

To this point in the chapter, drug therapy has been generally assumed to be initiated and managed in the absence of other drugs and other disease conditions. In practice, a drug is commonly initiated when one or more other drugs are being administered for the same or other conditions. These other drugs and diseases or conditions must be integrated into the evaluation of the individualization process. The pharmacokinetic and pharmacodynamic principles are the same, but an adaptation to the specific therapeutic setting must be made.

Other common scenarios are those in which one or more of the other drugs that a patient is concurrently taking is adjusted in its dosage or withdrawn, or a new medication is added. In all of these and similar situations, drug interactions should be considered, not only in terms of the magnitude of the potential effect of the interaction, but also in terms of the timeframe for drug accumulation and elimination and the rapidity of gain and loss of drug response. In addition, for drugs prescribed for treatment of chronic disease, the degree of severity of the disease or condition may change with time, requiring an adjustment in the dosage, as is often the case for drugs used in chronic treatment (e.g., in treating Parkinson's disease or hypertension).

With these final comments on changes in therapy, it is fitting to end this section on individualization of drug therapy. It is hoped that, armed with these principles, the reader will be in a better position to ensure the optimal administration of drugs for the benefit of patients taking them. Four additional selected topics on *Distribution Kinetics* (Chapter 19), *Metabolites and Drug Response* (Chapter 20), *Protein Drugs* (Chapter 21), and *Prediction of Human Kinetics from In Vitro and Preclinical Data* (Chapter 22) follow this chapter for those who wish to expand their knowledge in these areas.

KEY RELATIONSHIPS

$$C_{ss}(t) = \frac{F \cdot Dose}{V} \cdot \left[\frac{e^{-k \cdot t}}{1 - e^{-k \cdot \tau}} - e^{-k \cdot t} \right]$$

$$C_{ss}(t_2) = \frac{F \cdot Dose}{V} \cdot \left[\frac{e^{-k \cdot t_2}}{1 - e^{-k \cdot \tau}} - e^{-k \cdot t_1} - e^{-k \cdot t_2} \right]$$

$$C_{ss}(t_2) = \frac{F \cdot Dose}{V} \cdot \left(\frac{e^{-k \cdot t_1} + e^{-k \cdot t_2} + e^{-k \cdot t_3} + e^{-k \cdot t_4}}{1 - e^{-k \cdot \tau}} \right)$$

$$C = \frac{F}{V} \cdot (Dose_1 \cdot e^{-k \cdot t_1} + Dose_2 \cdot e^{-k \cdot t_2} + Dose_3 \cdot e^{-k \cdot t_3} + Dose_4 \cdot e^{-k \cdot t_4})$$

STUDY PROBLEMS

(Answers to Study Problems are in Appendix J.)

1. a. Briefly describe the two basic strategies most widely used to determine the optimal regimen of a drug with a low-to-intermediate therapeutic index for the treatment of an individual patient, and give examples of each.

   b. Briefly discuss why tailoring a dosage regimen of a drug to an individual patient should be considered before initiating therapy.

   c. List and briefly describe the criteria for performing drug concentration monitoring and applying target concentration strategy.

2. a. State why several sequential doses, instead of just one, are sometimes used as the loading dose.

   b. Discuss why loading doses are sometimes given for drugs with half-lives in minutes.
   c. Briefly comment on why loading doses are sometimes not used for drugs with long (>24-hr) half-lives.

3. Explain why plasma concentration monitoring is useful for some low therapeutic index drugs but not for others.

4. Give one example each of how tolerance to therapeutic and adverse effects can influence how drugs are administered.

5. Define nonadherence and give examples of it. Also, state why adherence is such an important issue in drug therapy.

6. Give two classes of drugs for which a slow decrease in dosing rate is needed when discontinuation of drug therapy is desired.

7. Meloxicam (Mobic MW = 351.4 g/mol) is a nonsteroidal anti-inflammatory agent. It is typically given in a regimen of 7.5 mg once daily, but the dosage may be increased to 15 mg daily. It is 99.4% bound to plasma albumin (0.6 mM) at a plasma concentration of 1 mg/L. It has a volume of distribution of 10 L, a half-life of 20 hr, and an oral bioavailability of 0.9.

   a. Draw on Fig. 18-14 the amount of meloxicam in the body with time on an oral regimen of one 7.5-mg tablet once daily. Assume that the drug is very rapidly, but incompletely, absorbed (model of multiple i.v. bolus doses). Be sure to show the salient features (steady state and peak and trough values on approach to steady state) of drug accumulation.

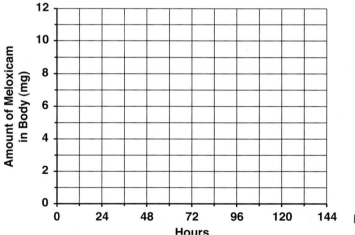

FIGURE 18-14.

   b. Also draw on the graph (use a dashed line) the amount in the body with time (0–144 hr) had the third and fourth doses both been skipped (not taken). The fifth and sixth doses were taken.
   c. Estimate the average steady-state plasma concentration of meloxicam on a 7.5-mg daily regimen.
   d. Only 0.2% of an i.v. dose of meloxicam is excreted unchanged in the urine. Would you expect the drug to be:
   (1) Filtered and the amount reabsorbed to be equal to the amount secreted?
   (2) Filtered and secreted?
   (3) Extensively reabsorbed in the renal tubule?
   Explain your answer.

8. DK, a 62-kg, 85-year-old man with a hospital-acquired staphylococcal infection, is currently receiving 500 mg of vancomycin intravenously (1-hr infusion) at 8:00 and 20:00 daily. Mr. DK has a serum creatinine of 2.1 mg/dL. On his third day of treatment, plasma vancomycin concentrations of 38 mg/L and 26 mg/L were measured at 9:30 and 19:50.

   a. Calculate the patient's creatinine clearance.

   b. Estimate the expected "peak" and "trough" concentrations of vancomycin, using a model of multiple short-term infusions.

   c. Compare the observed and expected concentrations and discuss whether the dosage should be changed. If you suggest a change, provide the details of the new regimen.

9. Piroxicam, a nonsteroidal anti-inflammatory drug, has a half-life of 50 hr and is given orally once daily. The drug accumulates extensively on chronic administration and the anti-inflammatory effect takes many days to fully develop, as expected. Loading doses are not usually recommended because of gastrointestinal adverse effects. Figure 18-15 below shows the typical plasma concentration–time profile under steady-state conditions following administration of a 20-mg capsule at bedtime daily. The drug is rapidly (peaks in 1–2 hr) and completely ($F = 1$) absorbed. The volume of distribution is 10 L. The figure is based on a one-compartment model of multiple i.v. bolus doses. The simulated peak and trough plasma concentrations are 7.07 and 5.07 mg/L, respectively.

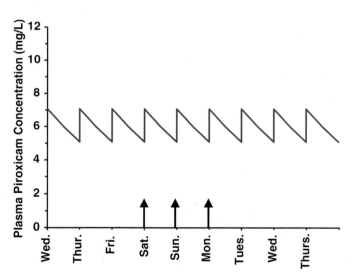

FIGURE 18-15.

A patient with osteoarthritis goes on a "drug holiday" (see arrows) because he forgot to take his medicine (piroxicam) with him over a 3-day Memorial Day weekend trip (Saturday through Monday). After his return late on Memorial Day (Monday), he decided to take the 3 doses he missed (Saturday, Sunday, and Monday morning's doses) on Tuesday morning (total of three 20-mg tablets).

   a. Sketch on the same figure the expected concentration–time curve for the patient. The times (7:00 A.M.) of the missed doses are indicated by arrows. Show values every 24 hr during and after the Memorial Day weekend (peak and troughs on Tuesday and Wednesday). Use the space on the side of the figure for calculations.

   b. Also sketch on the same figure the expected concentration–time profile on Tuesday and Wednesday had the patient simply resumed the 20-mg once daily dosing on Tuesday morning.

10. DH, a 53-year-old, 82-kg female patient with congestive cardiac failure for the past 3 years, was admitted on April 16 to hospital at 16:00 because of a worsening of her congestive heart failure symptoms. Her admission history indicated that she had taken her digoxin tablet (0.25 mg) that morning at the usual time (8:00–9:00), but had failed to take a tablet on the previous day (April 15). A plasma sample (blood withdrawn at 17:00) was obtained to see if the symptoms were consistent with nonadherence. A plasma digoxin concentration of 0.9 µg/L and a serum creatinine of 0.9 mg/dL were reported.

    a. Estimate the creatinine clearance in the patient.
    b. Calculate the expected values of F, CL, V, k, and $t_{1/2}$ in this patient.
    c. Estimate the digoxin concentration at the time of sampling.
    d. Compare the observed and expected concentrations.

11. Consider the situation of an arthritic male patient regularly taking 500 mg of an immediate-release naproxen product twice daily, morning and evening ($\tau = 12$ hr). Assume a one-compartment model of multiple i.v. bolus doses ($F = 1$) for this problem.

The patient goes on a "drug holiday," as he forgot to take his medicine with him over a 3-day Labor Day weekend fishing trip (Saturday through Monday). He returned home late on Labor Day (Monday). Tuesday morning he decided to take all 6 of the doses he missed (twice daily at 8:00 and 20:00 on Saturday, Sunday, and Monday, a total of six 500-mg tablets). The half-life of naproxen is 15 hr. The graph begins ($t = 0$) at 20:00 on Thursday. Show calculations below and be sure to identify each of the four conditions.

    a. Determine the amount of naproxen in the body with time on the 500-mg twice-daily regimen at steady state within one dosing interval. You only need to calculate the peak and trough values. Put these values on Fig. 18-16 by drawing the expected steady-state amount–time profile over the 144 hr.

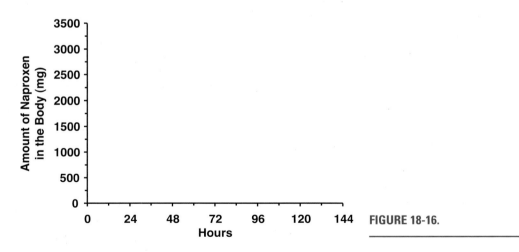

FIGURE 18-16.

    b. Draw on the figure the amount of naproxen in the body from the time the first dose was missed until 8:00 on Tuesday when the makeup dose was taken. Show calculations.
    c. Draw on the figure the amount of naproxen in the body from the time the makeup dose of six 500-mg tablets was taken on Tuesday morning to the end of the graph. He resumed taking 500 mg every 12 hr on Tuesday evening.
    d. Also draw on Fig. 18-16 the amount of naproxen in the body with time had the regular regimen of 1 tablet twice daily been simply resumed on Tuesday morning (no makeup doses).

Supplemental Topics

Distribution Kinetics

The reader will be able to:

- State why the one-compartment model is sometimes inadequate to describe kinetic events within the body.

- Compare the sum of two exponentials with the compartment model for representing plasma concentration data showing distribution kinetics.

- Estimate clearance and the half-life of the phase associated with most of elimination given plasma concentration–time data of a drug showing distribution kinetics.

- Define and estimate the distribution parameters: initial dilution volume (V_1), volume during the terminal phase (V), and volume of distribution at steady state (V_{ss}).

- Describe the impact of distribution kinetics on the interpretation of plasma concentration–time data following administration of a single dose.

- Explain the influence of distribution kinetics and duration of administration on the time courses of concentration in plasma and amount in tissue during and after stopping a constant-rate infusion.

- Describe how distribution kinetics influences the fluctuations of plasma and tissue levels with time during a multiple-dose regimen.

- Describe how distribution kinetics impacts the design of an oral multiple-dose regimen, when the effect wears off during the distribution phase of the drug.

- Explain how distribution kinetics can influence the interpretation of plasma concentration–time data and terminal half-life when clearance is altered.

- Describe the influence of distribution kinetics on the relationship between onset, duration, and intensity of response with time following single and multiple doses.

P ortraying the body as a single compartment is appropriate for establishing the fundamental principles of pharmacokinetics but is an inaccurate representation of events that follow drug administration. A basic assumption of the concept of a one-compartment representation of distribution is that equilibration of drug between tissues and blood occurs spontaneously. In reality, distribution takes time. The time required depends on tissue perfusion, permeability characteristics of tissue membranes for drug, and its partitioning between tissues and blood (Chapter 4, *Membranes and Distribution*). Ignoring distribution kinetics is reasonable as long as the error incurred is acceptable. This error becomes unacceptable when the one-compartment representation fails to explain adequately observations following drug administration; there is a danger of significant misinterpretation of the observations; and major discrepancies occur in the calculation of drug dosage. Such situations are most likely to arise when either sub-stantial amounts are eliminated or response wears off before distribution equilibrium is achieved. This chapter deals with the pharmacokinetic consequence of distribution kinetics together with some aspects of pharmacodynamics not covered elsewhere in the book.

EVIDENCE OF DISTRIBUTION KINETICS

Evidence of distribution kinetics is usually inferred from an early rapid decline in plasma (blood) concentration following an intravenous (i.v.) bolus dose, when little drug has been eliminated, and from the rapid onset and decline in the pharmacologic effect of some drugs during this early phase. Data in Fig. 19-1 (same as Fig. 4-11, repeated here in the con-text of distribution kinetics), which show the concentration of thiopental in various tissues after an i.v. bolus dose of this preoperative general anesthetic to a dog, provide direct evi-dence of distribution kinetics. Thiopental is a small, highly lipid-soluble drug for which dis-tribution into essentially all tissues is perfusion rate-limited. The results seen with this drug are therefore typical of those observed with many other small lipophilic drugs.

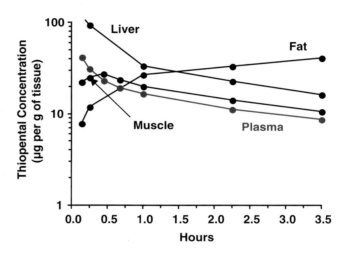

FIGURE 19-1. Semilogarithmic plot of the concentration of thiopental in various tissues (*black lines*) and plasma (*colored line*) following an i.v. bolus dose of 25 mg/kg to a dog. Note the early rise and fall of thiopental in the well-perfused tissues (e.g., liver) and in lean muscle tissue. After 3 hr, much of the drug remaining in the body is in adipose tissue. (From: Brodie BB, Bernstein E, Mark L. The role of body fat in limiting the duration of action of thiopental. J Pharmacol Exp Ther 1952;105:421–426.)

Notice that thiopental in liver, a highly perfused organ, reaches distribution equilib-rium with that in plasma by 5 min (the first observation), and thereafter, the decline in liver parallels with that in plasma. The same holds true in other highly perfused tissues, including brain and kidneys.

Redistribution of thiopental from well-perfused tissues to less well-perfused tissues, such as muscle and fat, primarily accounts for the subsequent decline in plasma concen-tration over the next 3 hr; less than 20% of the dose is eliminated during this period. As a result of a combination of poor perfusion and high partitioning, even by 3 hr distribu-tion equilibrium in adipose tissue has not been established. Analysis of the situation indi-cates that this does not occur for several more hours, at which time the majority of thiopental remaining is in fat. Recall that the greater the partition of a drug into fat, or into any tissue, the longer is the time required to achieve distribution equilibrium (Chapter 4, *Membranes and Distribution*). However, only if the apparent volume of distri-bution of a tissue ($K_p \cdot V_T$) is a major fraction of the total volume of distribution does up-take into that tissue substantially affect events within plasma. With thiopental, which has an adipose-to-plasma partition coefficient of 10, fat (0.12 L/kg) constitutes approxi-mately 40% of the total (apparent) volume of distribution (2.3 L/kg). Accordingly, the plasma concentration of thiopental not only falls markedly, but distribution takes many hours. For other drugs, distribution throughout the body may be faster or even take longer if partitioning into tissues is much less or more extensive than for thiopental. Certain aspects of distribution kinetics have been discussed in Chapter 4, *Membranes and Distribution*, Chapter 5, *Elimination*, and Chapter 10, *Constant-Rate Input*. What follows is a quantitative consideration starting with events following a single dose and finishing with events following infusion and multiple doses.

INTRAVENOUS BOLUS DOSE

PRESENTATION OF DATA

Sum of Exponential Terms. The early rapid and subsequent slower decline in the plasma concentration of aspirin in an individual subject following a 650-mg i.v. bolus dose (Fig. 19-2) is typical of many drugs. Had no samples been taken during the first 20 min, the terminal linear decline of the plasma concentration when plotted on semilogarithmic graph paper would have been characterized by a monoexponential equation, and one-compartment disposition characteristics would have been applied to aspirin. Recall that the monoexponential equation is $C(0)e^{-k \cdot t}$, where k is the rate constant with an associated half-life, given by $0.693/k$, and $C(0)$ is the anticipated initial plasma drug concentration, given as the intercept on the plasma concentration axis when the line is extrapolated back to time zero. For aspirin, k is 0.050 min^{-1}, the corresponding half-life is 14 min, and $C(0)$ is 33 mg/L. Going further, the volume of distribution ($C[0]$) is 20 L and clearance ($k \cdot V$) is 0.98 L/min.

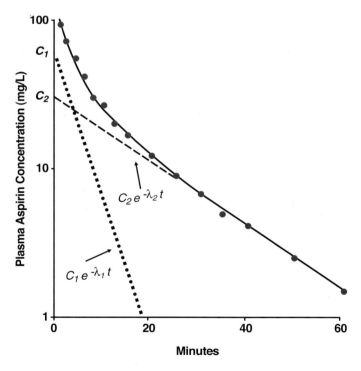

FIGURE 19-2. When displayed semilogarithmically, the fall in the plasma concentration of aspirin is initially rapid but then slows after an i.v. bolus dose of 650 mg to a subject. The decline in concentration (——) can be characterized by the sum of two exponential terms: $C_1 \cdot e^{-\lambda_1 \cdot t}$ (●●●●) and $C_2 \cdot e^{-\lambda_2 \cdot t}$ (– – –). (From: Rowland M, Riegelman S. Pharmacokinetics of acetylsalicylic acid and salicylic acid after intravenous administration in man. J Pharm Sci 1968;57: 1313–1319.)

Notice that the early plasma concentrations are higher than those anticipated by back extrapolation of the terminal slope and that the earlier the time, the greater is the difference. When the difference at each sample time is plotted on the same graph, all the difference values fall on another straight line, which can be characterized by a monoexponential equation, $B(0)e^{-\alpha \cdot t}$, where α is the decay rate constant and $B(0)$ is the corresponding zero-time intercept. For aspirin, $\alpha = 0.23$ min^{-1}, $t_{1/2} = 3.0$ min, and $B(0) = 67$ mg/L.

Because all the plasma concentrations at the later times can be fitted by one equation, $C(0)e^{-k \cdot t}$, and because at the earlier times, all the difference values can be fitted by another equation, $B(0)e^{-\alpha \cdot t}$, it follows that the entire plasma drug concentration (C) versus time data can be fitted by the *sum* of these two exponential terms. That is

$$C = B(0)e^{-\alpha \cdot t} + C(0)e^{-k \cdot t}$$ 19-1

For example, the biexponential equation $C = 67e^{-0.23t} + 33e^{-0.050t}$, for which t is time in minutes and $B(0)$ and $C(0)$ are in mg/L, adequately describes the decline in the plasma aspirin concentration following a 650-mg bolus dose. Sometimes, when using this difference procedure, known commonly as the **method of residuals**, a sum of three and occasionally four exponential terms is required to fit adequately the observed concentration–time data. Because the principles in approaching such data are the same as those used to analyze and interpret events described by a biexponential equation, only the simpler case is considered further in this book.

To facilitate the discussion, a more uniform set of symbols is needed. Rather than using the different symbols α and k, the general symbol λ is used to denote the exponential coefficient. Thus, Eq. 19-1 can be rewritten as

$$C = C_1 e^{-\lambda_1 \cdot t} + C_2 e^{-\lambda_2 \cdot t}$$ 19-2

where the subscripts 1 and 2 refer to the first and second exponential terms respectively, and C_1 and C_2 refer to the corresponding zero-time intercepts, or coefficients. By convention, the exponential terms are arranged in decreasing order of λ. For example, in the case of aspirin, $C_1 = 67$ mg/L, $\lambda_1 = 0.23$ min^{-1}, $C_2 = 33$ mg/L, and $\lambda_2 = 0.050$ min^{-1}.

With aspirin, two exponential terms and hence two phases are seen when plasma concentration–time data are displayed on a semilogarithmic plot. Commonly, the last phase is called the **terminal phase**. With aspirin and many other drugs, it is a correct description. Sometimes, however, there is an additional, still slower phase, indicating that distribution equilibrium has not been achieved with all tissues. The terminal phase may sometimes be missed, because the assay procedure employed insufficiently sensitive to measure the drug concentration at these later times. This certainly was the case with aminoglycosides and some other drugs in the past, although it is less of a problem today with the availability of more sensitive instrumentation. In the subsequent discussion, the observed terminal phase is assumed to be correctly designated.

At time zero the anticipated plasma concentration is, by reference to Eq. 19-2, equal to the sum of the coefficients, $C_1 + C_2$. At that time, the amount in the body is the dose. Hence, by definition, the volume into which drug appears to distribute initially, the initial dilution volume, V_1, is given by

$$V_1 = \frac{Dose}{C_1 + C_2}$$ 19-3

For aspirin, the anticipated initial concentration is 100 (= 67 + 33) mg/L, so that the initial dilution volume of aspirin is 6.5 L.

It is important to realize that the time for concentration to fall by one half is only equal to a half-life during the terminal phase. Before then, the plasma concentration falls in half in a period of less than one terminal half-life but more than one initial half-life. This is clearly evident on comparing the fall in plasma aspirin concentration in the earlier moments with the decline of the first exponential term.

A Compartmental Model. Although for many situations in pharmacokinetics the desired information can be obtained directly from modification of Eq. 19-2, it is sometimes conceptually helpful to represent disposition pictorially, as was done in Chapter 3, *Kinetics Following an Intravenous Bolus Dose*, and Chapter 10, *Constant-Rate Input*, to explain some events following bolus doses and infusions. One such common representation, depicted in Fig. 19-3, is the two-compartment model. Compartment 1, the initial dilution volume

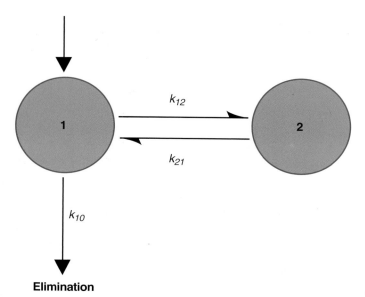

FIGURE 19-3. A two-compartment model of the body. Drug is administered into and eliminated from compartment 1 and distributes between compartments 1 and 2. The rate constants for the processes are indicated.

mentioned previously, is also frequently called the central compartment because drug is administered into and distributed from it. As mentioned, the initial dilution volume of aspirin is 6.5 L; for many other drugs, particularly basic compounds, it is much larger. These values are clearly greater than the plasma volume, 3 L, and therefore this initial dilution volume must be composed of spaces in addition to plasma into which drug distributes extremely rapidly. These spaces must be in well-perfused tissues, such as the lungs and generally liver and kidneys, the major eliminating organs. Elimination is therefore usually depicted as occurring *directly* and *exclusively* from the central compartment. Drug distributes between this central compartment and a peripheral compartment, made up of tissues into which drug distributes more slowly.

Several points are worth mentioning here. First, the model is defined by the data. The number of compartments or pools required equals the number of exponential terms needed to describe the plasma concentration–time data. Thus, a three-compartment model is needed when the data are best fitted by a triexponential equation. Next, the model depicted in Fig. 19-3, or any other model for which drug elimination is portrayed as occurring exclusively from the central compartment, is not unique. Three two-compartment models can adequately describe a biexponential plasma concentration decay curve: the one depicted in Fig. 19-3, one with elimination occurring from both compartments, and one with loss occurring exclusively from the peripheral compartment. No distinction between these three possibilities can be made from plasma concentration–time data alone, and although the model depicted in Fig. 19-3 is the most favored one, based on physiologic considerations such as the initial dilution volume exceeding the plasma volume, elimination can sometimes occur in tissues of the peripheral compartment. Sometimes, the liver (or kidneys) is not part of the central compartment. For example, the initial dilution volume of many very large protein drugs is only 3 L, the plasma volume (see Chapter 21, *Protein Drugs*). Last, drug distribution within a compartment is not homogenous. Although the concentrations of drug within and among such tissues usually vary enormously, tissues are lumped together into a compartment because the times to achieve distribution equilibrium in each tissue are similar.

In Fig. 19-3, movement of drug between compartments can be characterized by transfer rate constants, where k_{12} denotes the rate constant associated with movement of drug from compartment 1 to compartment 2, and k_{21} is the rate constant associated with the reverse process. The rate constant k_{10}, associated with elimination, is related to clearance ($k_{10} = CL/V_1$), and can be further partitioned into a renal (k_{1e}) and nonrenal component. The unit of all rate constants is reciprocal time.

Rate equations can be written for movement of amounts between the compartments and for drug elimination. Following an i.v. bolus dose these equations are:

Rate of change of amount of drug in compartment 1 $= -k_{12} \cdot A_1 - k_{10} \cdot A_1 + k_{21} \cdot A_2$ ⠀⠀19-4

| | Rate of movement from compartment 1 to compartment 2 | Rate of elimination | Rate of movement from compartment 2 to compartment 1 |

Rate of change of amount of drug in compartment 2 $= k_{12} \cdot A_1 - k_{21} \cdot A_2$ ⠀⠀19-5

| | Rate of movement from compartment 1 to compartment 2 | Rate of movement from compartment 2 to compartment 1 |

where A_1 and A_2 are the amounts of drug in compartments 1 and 2, respectively. Integration of these rate equations provides a biexponential equation, of the same form as Eq. 19-2, for the decline of drug from plasma, except that the coefficients and exponents are recast in terms of the parameters defining the compartmental model. Equivalent relationships between the biexponential and two-compartment models are listed in Table 19-1.

Although expressing data in terms of a compartmental model and associated parameters may appear to give greater insight into the data, caution should be exercised in doing so. Remember that the compartmental model chosen is often not unique, and one can rarely assign a physical or physiologic meaning to the value of any of the rate constants. Accordingly, much of the subsequent discussion is related to describing drug disposition by the sum of exponentials. However, pharmacokinetic observations are discussed in terms of the compartmental model when this procedure facilitates general understanding. It is also useful when assigning variability within the population of a pharmacokinetic parameter, such as renal clearance ($k_{2e} \cdot V_2$ within the compartmental model), to say renal function. Recall, these two are directly related (as discussed in Chapter 15, *Disease*). In contrast as can be seen from the interrelationships in Table 19-1, a change in renal clearance and hence clearance ($V_1 \cdot k_{10}$) impacts on all the parameters of a biexponential equation making it is virtually impossible to correlate renal function with these parameters. Lastly, when describing nonlinear pharmacokinetics, the use of exponential equations (which assume linearity) is inappropriate. Here, compartmental models are the appropriate choice, in which any parameter of the model can be expressed as a nonlinear function of the concentration or amount of drug in the associated compartment, such as clearance expressed as a function of plasma concentration using the full Michaelis-Menten equation. Recall also that pharmacodynamics is generally nonlinear, so compartment models are frequently applied to such data.

PHARMACOKINETIC PARAMETERS

Clearance. Elimination occurs at all times. Just as plasma concentration is highest immediately following an i.v. bolus dose, so is rate of elimination ($CL \cdot C$). Subsequently, both plasma concentration and corresponding rate of elimination fall rapidly. To calculate the amount eliminated in a small unit of time, dt, recall that

$$\text{Amount eliminated during interval } dt = \text{Clearance} \cdot C \cdot dt \qquad 19\text{-}6$$

where $C \cdot dt$ is the corresponding small area under the plasma concentration–time curve within the interval dt. The total amount eliminated, the dose administered, is

TABLE 19-1   Equivalent Relationships between the Biexponential and Two-Compartment Models*

Measures	Sum of Exponentials	Two-Compartment Model
Plasma concentration (C)	$C_1 e^{-\lambda_1 t} + C_2 e^{-\lambda_2 t}$	$\left[\dfrac{Dose}{V_1} \cdot \dfrac{(k_{21} - \lambda_1)}{(\lambda_2 - \lambda_1)} \right] e^{-\lambda_1 t} + \left[\dfrac{Dose}{V_1} \cdot \dfrac{(k_{21} - \lambda_2)}{(\lambda_1 - \lambda_2)} \right] e^{-\lambda_2 t}$
	λ_1	$\dfrac{1}{2} \left[(k_{12} + k_{21} + k_{10}) + \sqrt{(k_{12} + k_{21} + k_{10})^2 - 4k_{21}k_{10}} \right]$
	λ_2	$\dfrac{1}{2} \left[(k_{12} + k_{21} + k_{10}) - \sqrt{(k_{12} + k_{21} + k_{10})^2 - 4k_{21}k_{10}} \right]$
	$\lambda_1 + \lambda_2$	$k_{12} + k_{21} + k_{10}$
	$\lambda_1 \cdot \lambda_2$	$k_{21} \cdot k_{10}$
Initial concentration	$C_1 + C_2$	$Dose/V_1$
Parameters		
Initial dilution volume (V_1)	$Dose/(C_1 + C_2)$	V_1
Clearance (CL)	$Dose / \left(\dfrac{C_1}{\lambda_1} + \dfrac{C_2}{\lambda_2} \right)$	$V_1 \cdot k_{10}$
Volume of distribution (V)	CL/λ_2	$V_1 \cdot k_{10}/\lambda_2$
Volume of distribution at steady state (V_{ss})	$\dfrac{Dose \left[\dfrac{C_1}{\lambda_1^2} + \dfrac{C_2}{\lambda_2^2} \right]}{\left[\dfrac{C_1}{\lambda_1} + \dfrac{C_2}{\lambda_2} \right]^2}$	$V_1 \cdot (1 + k_{12}/k_{21})$

*Assuming elimination takes place from the initial dilution volume only.

the sum of all the small amounts eliminated from time zero to time infinity. Therefore,

$$Dose = Clearance \cdot AUC \qquad \text{19-7}$$

where AUC is the *total* area under the plasma drug concentration–time curve. Accordingly, as with the simpler one-compartment model, clearance (CL) is most readily estimated by dividing dose by AUC. The area may be determined from the trapezoidal rule (Appendix A, *Assessment of AUC*) or, more conveniently, by realizing that the total area underlying each exponential term is the zero-time intercept divided by its corresponding exponential coefficient. Thus, the total area corresponding to Eq. 19-2 is given by

$$AUC = \underbrace{\frac{C_1}{\lambda_1}}_{\substack{\text{Area associated} \\ \text{with initial term}}} + \underbrace{\frac{C_2}{\lambda_2}}_{\substack{\text{Area associated} \\ \text{with last term}}} \qquad \text{19-8}$$

When inserting the appropriate values for the aspirin example into Eq. 19-8, the value of AUC associated with the 650-mg dose is 951 mg-min/L, so that the total clearance of aspirin in the individual is 683 mL/min. Notice that clearance is considerably smaller than the value calculated assuming a one-compartment model, 985 mL/min. The latter is an overestimate of the true value, because more drug is eliminated during the attainment of distribution equilibrium than accounted for by the last term. If instead of the first phase a later phase is missed, the error in estimating clearance is large only if the missed area is a major fraction of the total area. Obviously, given the ease of estimating total area and provided that blood sampling times are adequate, the true value for clearance should always be calculated.

Volume of Distribution. One purpose of a volume term is to relate plasma concentration to amount in the body. The initial dilution volume fulfills this purpose initially. Subsequently, however, as drug distributes into the slowly equilibrating tissues, the plasma concentration declines more rapidly than does the amount in the body (A). Accordingly, as illustrated in Fig. 19-4, the effective volume of distribution (A/C) increases with time until distribution equilibrium between drug in plasma and all tissues is achieved; this occurs during the terminal phase. Only then does decline in all tissues parallel that in plasma and is proportionality between plasma concentration and amount in body achieved.

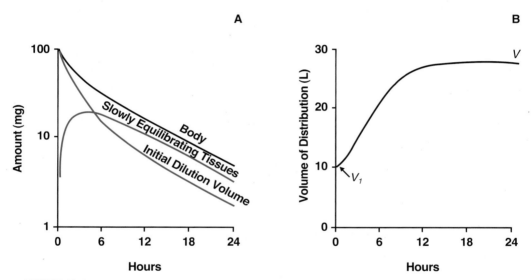

FIGURE 19-4.   Several events occur following a single i.v. bolus dose. **A.** Loss of drug from the initial dilution volume, of which plasma is a part, is a result of both elimination from the body and distribution into the more slowly equilibrating tissues. The fall in amount of drug in the body is therefore initially less than the fall in the amount in the initial dilution volume. Only when distribution equilibrium has been achieved do the amounts in the initial dilution volume and in plasma decline in parallel (*same slope*) with that in the body. **B.** Reflecting these events, the apparent volume of distribution (A/C), which just after giving the dose equals the initial dilution volume (V_1), increases with time approaching a limiting value (V), which occurs when distribution equilibrium is achieved.

The volume of distribution during the terminal phase (V) can be calculated as follows. During this phase, the concentration is given by $C_2 \cdot e^{-\lambda_2 \cdot t}$ (see Fig. 19-2), and correspondingly,

$$\begin{array}{l} \textit{Amount of drug} \\ \textit{in body during} \\ \textit{terminal phase} \end{array} = V \cdot C = V \cdot C_2 \cdot e^{-\lambda_2 \cdot t} \qquad\qquad 19\text{-}9$$

Hence, extrapolating back to time zero, $V \cdot C_2$ must be the amount needed to give a plasma concentration of C_2, had drug spontaneously distributed into the volume, V. The amount, $V \cdot C_2$, remains to be calculated. When placed into the body, the amount, $V \cdot C_2$, is eventually matched by an equal amount eliminated. As the amount remaining to be eliminated is the product of clearance and area, and as C_2/λ_2 is the associated area, it follows that

$$V \cdot C_2 \quad = \quad CL \cdot \frac{C_2}{\lambda_2} \qquad\qquad 19\text{-}10$$

Amount   Amount remaining
in Body   to be eliminated

or

$$V \quad = \quad \frac{CL}{\lambda_2} \qquad\qquad 19\text{-}11$$

Volume of   Total Clearance
Distribution   Terminal exponential
coefficient

Returning to the example of aspirin, $CL = 683$ mL/min and $\lambda_2 = 0.050$ min^{-1}; therefore, its volume of distribution is 13.7 L. That is, if during the terminal phase the plasma concentration is 10 mg/L, then the amount in the body is 137 mg. Because 65 mg (10 mg/L $\times$ 6.5 L) are in the initial dilution volume, the remaining 71 mg must be in the tissues with which aspirin slowly equilibrates.

A comparison of Eq. 19-11 with the one that has been used in all previous chapters to define the volume of distribution ($V = CL/k$) shows them to be the same, recognizing the equivalence of k and λ_2, the terminal exponential coefficient.

The ratio V_1/V gives an estimate of the degree of error in predicting the initial plasma concentration using a one-compartment model. For example, for aspirin, with values for V_1 and V of 6.5 and 13.7 L, respectively, the error in predicting initial concentrations from the plasma concentration–time data during the terminal phase can be relatively large. The error can be even larger when predicting conditions beyond the measured final phase if a still slower one exists. This last error is only of concern if there is an appreciable accumulation of drug in this phase during chronic administration, a point considered subsequently in this chapter.

DISTRIBUTION KINETICS AND ELIMINATION

During the initial rapidly declining phase, more elimination occurs than would have been expected had distribution been spontaneous. Additional elimination is a result of the particularly high concentrations of drug presented to organs of elimination during this period. For many drugs this increased elimination is small, and, with respect to elimination, viewing the body as a single compartment is adequate. For other drugs, the additional elimination represents a major fraction of the administered dose, and approximating the kinetics with a one-compartment model is inappropriate. Area considerations are a basis for making this decision.

Recall from Eq. 19-9 that elimination associated with the concentrations defined by the terminal exponential term, $C_2 \cdot e^{-\lambda_2 \cdot t}$, gives an amount equal to $CL \cdot C_2/\lambda_2$. Expressing this amount as a fraction, f_2, of the administered dose and utilizing the relationship in Eq. 19-8 gives

$$\textit{Fraction of elimination associated with} \atop \textit{last exponential term} \quad = f_2 = \frac{C_2/\lambda_2}{AUC} \qquad 19\text{-}12$$

The remaining fraction, f_1, must therefore have been eliminated as a result of concentrations above those expected had spontaneous distribution occurred (i.e., those concentrations defined by $C_1 \cdot e^{-\lambda_1 \cdot t}$).

Applying Eq. 19-12 to the case of aspirin, elimination of 69% of the dose is associated with the terminal slope; therefore, the remaining 31% must be associated with plasma concentrations above those expected had spontaneous distribution occurred. Although distribution kinetics cannot be ignored, the majority of aspirin elimination is clearly associated with events defined by the terminal phase, which has a half-life of 14 min. Based on the same reason, the terminal half-life is the elimination half-life for most drugs. This is because distribution is much faster than elimination. There are some drugs, however, for which the calculated value of f_2 is low because elimination is much faster than distribution. Gentamicin is an example. As mentioned in Chapter 3, *Kinetics Following an Intravenous Bolus Dose*, over 98% of an i.v. bolus dose is eliminated before distribution equilibrium within the body has been achieved. In this case, the reason lies in a permeability-limited distribution of gentamicin into certain tissues. Clearly, for gentamicin and similar drugs, the appropriate half-life (biexponential model) defining elimination after a bolus dose is $0.693/\lambda_1$.

A MATHEMATICAL AID

For all but the mathematically inclined, analysis and prediction of plasma concentration–time data for a drug that displays multiexponential disposition characteristics are difficult. A useful mathematical aid to facilitate such analyses and predictions is to imagine that each exponential term arises from the independent administration of a different drug having one-compartment characteristics, and that the sum of their individual concentrations is the observed one. For example, imagine that a biexponential equation, $C = C_1 e^{-\lambda_1 \cdot t} + C_2 e^{-\lambda_2 \cdot t}$, arises from administration of two hypothetical drugs, Drug 1 and Drug 2; Drug 1 produces the curve $C_1 e^{-\lambda_1 \cdot t}$, and Drug 2 produces the curve $C_2 e^{-\lambda_2 \cdot t}$. Furthermore, assume that each hypothetical drug has the same clearance, CL. Therefore, because the two drugs have different rate constants, λ_1 and λ_2, they have different volumes of distribution, which are given by CL/λ_1 and CL/λ_2, respectively. To complete the analysis, the doses of the hypothetical drugs are needed. These are obtained from area considerations as follows. Because dose is the product of clearance and area, the respective doses are $CL \cdot (C_1/\lambda_1)$ and $CL \cdot (C_2/\lambda_2)$. Furthermore, because $CL \cdot (C_1/\lambda_1 + C_2/\lambda_2)$ equals the total dose administered, it follows from Eq. 19-12 that $f_1 \cdot Dose$ and $f_2 \cdot Dose$ are the corresponding doses. Hence, the total observed concentration is given by

$$C = f_1 \cdot \frac{Dose}{CL} \cdot \lambda_1 \cdot e^{-\lambda_1 t} + f_2 \cdot \frac{Dose}{CL} \cdot \lambda_2 \cdot e^{-\lambda_2 \cdot t} \qquad 19\text{-}13$$

Although the above equation is a device that cannot, for example, predict events in slowly equilibrating tissues, it readily permits calculation of events in plasma under various circumstances, as subsequently shown.

AN EXTRAVASCULAR DOSE

Often, absorption is slower than distribution, so approximating the body as a single compartment after an extravascular dose is reasonable. Occasionally, it is not, as illustrated with digoxin in Fig. 19-5. Following oral administration, digoxin is absorbed before much distribution has occurred, and consequently, the distribution phase is still evident beyond the peak concentration. The therapeutic implication of this observation is discussed in Chapter 8, *Response Following a Single Dose*. In contrast to digoxin, many drugs equilibrate rapidly with highly perfused tissues such as heart and brain; then, plasma concentration correlates positively with response at all but the earliest times.

The distribution phase tends to disappear when the absorption process is slower than distribution. This principle is demonstrated by the simulation in Fig. 19-6 for digoxin. The drug is given orally, and systemic absorption is assumed to be first order. The figure contains a model that incorporates first-order absorption and disposition (two-compartment

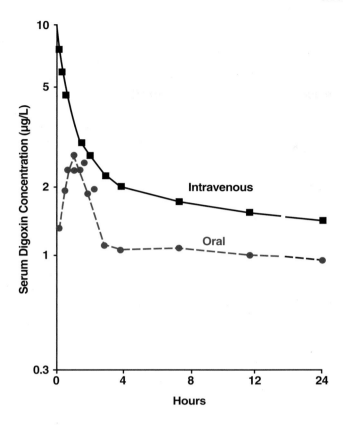

FIGURE 19-5. Depicted is a semilogarithmic plot of the mean concentration of digoxin following 0.5 mg administered orally (two 0.25-mg tablets, *colored circles*) and i.v. (*black squares*) to four volunteers. Because absorption is much faster than distribution, a biphasic curve is still seen after attainment of the peak concentration following the oral dose. (From: Huffman DH, Azarnoff D. Absorption of orally given digoxin preparations. JAMA 1972;222:957–960. Copyright 1972, American Medical Association.)

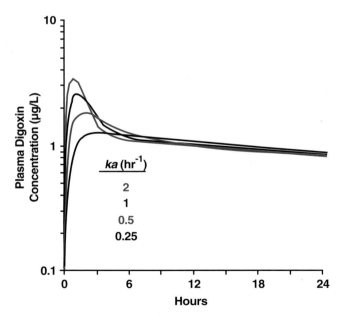

FIGURE 19-6. A simulation of the effect of the speed of absorption on the concentration–time profile of digoxin. A distribution nose is observed for digoxin (Fig. 19-5) with the conventional dosage form, because its absorption is relatively fast compared with the distribution and elimination of the compound. A two-compartment model of digoxin disposition with first-order absorption, as shown, is used in the simulation. Note that when the absorption rate constant is sufficiently small (about 0.5 hr^{-1} for this drug), the distribution nose disappears. The values of the absorption rate constants are given in the legend.

model) that applies to an i.v. bolus. Several values for the absorption rate constant are simulated. Note that the distribution nose (Fig. 19-6) is almost gone when the absorption rate constant is about 0.5 hr^{-1} (half-life = 1.4 hr), a slower rate of absorption than is typically observed for immediate-release digoxin tablets. Also, note that the terminal half-life does not increase with ka, because absorption never becomes rate-limiting (terminal half-life is 44 hr). The effect of slowing absorption becomes even more apparent when the concentration is plotted on a linear scale with time.

As with the simple one-compartment model, as long as rate of elimination = $CL \cdot C$ bioavailability is given by $F = CL \cdot AUC/Dose$, and relative bioavailability is estimated by comparison of AUC values following various formulations or routes of administration, correcting for dose differences.

CONSTANT-RATE INFUSION

SHORT-TERM INFUSION

Midazolam is an effective i.v. sedative. However, if it is administered too rapidly, there is a significant risk of severe centrally mediated respiratory depression and respiratory arrest, associated with the very high arterial and hence brain concentrations for this highly permeable drug in the early moments, before much drug has had time to distribute to the less well-perfused tissues. The solution is to deliver the dose as a short-term constant-rate infusion, rather than as a distinct bolus, thereby lowering the C_{max}. How substantial the lowering of the C_{max}, and hence risk, can be even with only a modest extension in the duration of administration is demonstrated in Fig. 19-7 for a drug with pharmacokinetics similar to that of midazolam. Thus, for the same total dose (2 mg), the C_{max} is decreased from 16 µg/L to 4 µg/L when the duration of infusion is extended from 1 to 10 min, during which time the fraction of the administered eliminated from the body is minimal, and seen by all the curves converging to a common concentration by 20 min since the start of the infusion, so that essentially one may consider that a bolus dose is in the body at the end of the infusion.

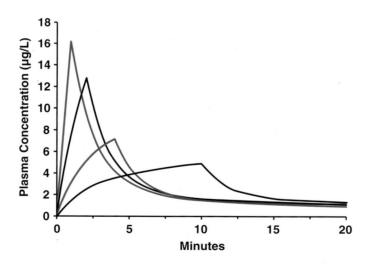

FIGURE 19-7. Even when the desire is for rapid onset of effect, it is safer to administer a drug by short-term infusion than as an i.v. bolus. Shown are changes in the duration of infusion, for the same total dose (2 mg), on C_{max}. Notice, just modest changes in the duration, from 1 to 10 min, profoundly lowers the C_{max} and potential risk. During this period, little drug is lost from the body, evident by the concentrations associated with each curve converging to a common value by 20 min since the start of the infusion. Data are for a drug with disposition kinetics similar to that of midazolam.

    This practice of giving a short-term infusion during the distribution phase of a drug is the norm when the intention is to give a bolus dose, because this minimizes risk while still achieving effective systemic concentrations of a drug with only a minor delay in the onset of action.

LONG-TERM INFUSION

Some drugs are infused long term relative to the pharmacokinetics of the drug, with the intention of achieving and maintaining a constant plasma concentration, and hence therapeutic effect, for a given period of time. The case of propofol was considered in Chapter 10, *Constant-Rate Regimens.* Fig. 19-8 illustrates the anticipated effect of distribution kinetics on the plasma concentration, for a drug in general, on stopping a constant-rate infusion at various times during approach to plateau. At early times, a pronounced distribution phase is seen on stopping an infusion, because distribution equilibrium has yet to be achieved between drug in blood and that in many tissues. With a more prolonged infusion, more drug enters the tissues. The tendency of drug to move from blood to tissues is then much reduced, and the distribution phase appears much shallower on stopping the infusion. Even at plateau, however, some distribution may still be seen on stopping the infusion. At plateau, the rates of drug entry in and out of the tissues are

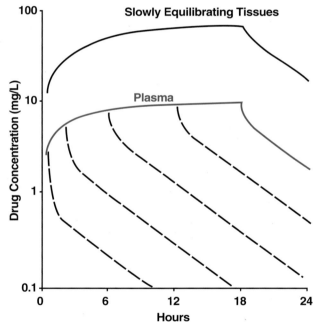

FIGURE 19-8.   Events in plasma (*colored line*) and in slowly equilibrating tissues (*top curve*) during and after stopping a constant-rate 18-hr infusion. As concentration in the slowly equilibrating tissues rises during the infusion, the net tendency of drug to enter these tissues decreases. Consequently, on stopping the infusion, the distribution phase in plasma ($---$) appears shallower the more prolonged the infusion. For simplicity, only the decline in tissue concentration when the infusion is stopped at plateau is shown. Equation 19-27 describes the plasma concentration during an infusion. At the end of an infusion of duration τ, the concentration, $C(\tau)$, is therefore $Css \cdot (f_1 \cdot (1 - e^{-\lambda_1 \cdot \tau}) + f_2 \cdot (1 - e^{-\lambda_2 \cdot \tau}))$. Furthermore, on stopping the infusion, the plasma concentration is given by $Css \cdot (f_1 \cdot (1 - e^{-\lambda_1 \cdot \tau}) \cdot e^{-\lambda \cdot t_{post}} + f_2 \cdot (1 - e^{-\lambda_2 \cdot \tau}) \cdot e^{-\lambda_2 \cdot \tau_{post}})$, where t_{post} is the time after stopping the infusion. The last equation can be derived using the mathematical aid (Eq. 19-13), recognizing, for example, that $(f_1 \cdot Css \cdot (1 - e^{-\lambda_1 \cdot \tau})$ is the concentration at the end of the infusion associated with the first phase, and $e^{-\lambda_1 \cdot t_{post}}$ is the corresponding fraction remaining at time t_{post}.

equal. On stopping the infusion, elimination of drug from plasma, along with the fall in plasma concentration, creates a gradient for return of drug from tissues. Initially, the rate of elimination from plasma exceeds the rate of return from the tissues, and the plasma concentration falls rapidly. Eventually, however, the rate of return from the tissues limits the rate of elimination from plasma. The body then acts, once again, as a single compartment; plasma concentration and amount in the tissues, and hence amount in the body as a whole, fall with a half-life equal to that seen during the terminal phase following an i.v. bolus dose.

The actual events seen after stopping an infusion at steady state depend largely on the kinetics of distribution. If distribution from tissues is slow relative to elimination from plasma, the plasma concentration falls substantially before the terminal phase is reached. Conversely, distribution may be so fast that, on stopping the infusion, drug in tissue and plasma stay in virtual equilibrium; then only the terminal monoexponential decay is seen. The latter situation contrasts with events that would be seen following an i.v. bolus dose; a biexponential curve is invariably seen if blood is sampled early enough. As a guiding principle, a frank biphasic curve, on stopping an infusion at steady state is seen when most of drug in plasma (and rapidly equilibrating tissues) is eliminated before distribution equilibrium is achieved.

Returning to events during infusion, two basic questions remain: What controls the plateau concentration? and How long does it take to reach plateau?

Events at Plateau. The plateau plasma concentration is reached when rate of drug elimination matches rate of infusion, R_{inf}. The plasma concentration, C_{ss}, is therefore readily given by the familiar equation,

$$C_{ss} = \frac{R_{inf}}{CL} \qquad\qquad \text{19-14}$$

Thus, as long as clearance is accurately determined, the rate of infusion needed to produce a given steady-state concentration can be calculated. Conversely, clearance can be determined from the infusion rate and the concentration at steady state.

Although the volume of distribution, V, usefully relates amount in body to plasma concentration during the terminal phase, its value is influenced by elimination. As seen in Fig. 19-9, the faster a drug is eliminated relative to distribution, the greater is the ratio of drug in slowly equilibrating tissues to that in plasma during the terminal phase and, correspondingly, the larger is the apparent volume of distribution. A need, therefore, exists to define a volume term to reflect distribution only. This volume term applies to steady state when drug is infused at a constant rate. This volume term, **volume distribution at steady state**, V_{ss}, is defined by

$$V_{ss} = \frac{Amount\ in\ body\ at\ steady\ state}{Plasma\ concentration\ at\ steady\ state} \qquad\qquad \text{19-15}$$

Conceptualization of this volume may be helped by considering the two-compartment model depicted in Fig. 19-3. At steady state, the rates at which drug enters and leaves the slowly equilibrating tissues are exactly matched. It then follows that the amount in the slowly equilibrating compartment at steady state, $A_{2,ss}$, of the two-compartment model is given by

$$A_{2,ss} = \frac{k_{12}}{k_{21}} \cdot A_{1,ss} \qquad\qquad \text{19-16}$$

The amount in the body at steady state, A_{ss}, is the sum of $A_{1,ss}$ and $A_{2,ss}$. Therefore,

$$A_{ss} = \left(1 + \frac{k_{12}}{k_{21}}\right) \cdot A_{1,ss} \qquad\qquad \text{19-17}$$

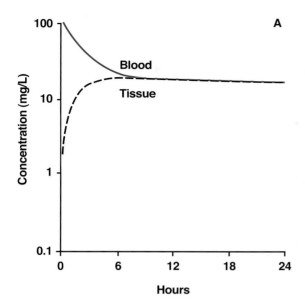

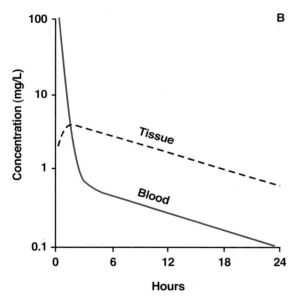

FIGURE 19-9. Elimination influences volume of distribution during the terminal phase. To appreciate this statement, consider the distribution of a drug between blood (volume, V_B, 5 L) and a tissue (volume, V_T, 20 L). Furthermore, let $K_p = 1$, so that the concentrations in each compartment at equilibrium are equal if no elimination occurs (**A**). The volume of distribution at equilibrium is then 25 L. With elimination of drug, the concentration in the tissue (− − −) lags behind that in blood (——) during the terminal phase, thereby giving rise to a higher apparent value of K_p, $K_{p,app}$ (**B**). Consequently, the apparent volume of distribution ($V_B + K_{p,app} \cdot V_T$) is increased above that expected under true equilibrium conditions, $V_B + K_P \cdot V_T$.

Finally, as $A_{1,ss} = V_1 \cdot C_{ss}$ and $A_{ss} = V_{ss} \cdot C_{ss}$, it follows that

$$V_{ss} = \left(1 + \frac{k_{12}}{k_{21}}\right) \cdot V_1$$ 19-18

Volume of
distribution
at steady state

In practice, as amount in the body cannot be determined physically, V_{ss} is usually calculated from the disposition parameters (C_1, λ_1, C_2, and λ_2) following i.v. bolus administration (see Table 19-1). The rationale, based on the concept of mean residence time, *MRT*, is as follows. Recall (Chapter 3, *Kinetics Following an Intravenous Bolus Dose*), *MRT* is the mean time molecules remain in the body when all are placed there at the same time (i.e., following an i.v. bolus). Consider now a system at steady state, achieved by means of a constant-rate infusion, R_{inf}, with $R_{inf} = CL \cdot C_{ss}$. Then, during a subsequent period of infusion of duration equal to *MRT*, by definition on average all the molecules in the body (mass, $A_{ss} = V_{ss} \cdot C_{ss}$) have been replaced by an equal number of new molecules. Accordingly,

$$\begin{matrix} \text{Amount delivered} \\ \text{in } MRT \end{matrix} = R_{inf} \cdot MRT = CL \cdot C_{ss} \cdot MRT = A_{ss} = V_{ss} \cdot C_{ss} \qquad \text{19-19}$$

from which it is seen that

$$V_{ss} = MRT \cdot CL \qquad \text{19-20}$$

Now *MRT* is obtained experimental following an i.v. bolus from the relationship (Appendix H, *Mean Residence Time*)

$$MRT = \frac{AUMC}{AUC} \qquad \text{19-21}$$

where $AUMC = \int_0^\infty t \cdot C \cdot dt$, the area under the first moment curve, which for a biexponential i.v. disposition curve *AUMC*, is given by

$$AUMC = \frac{C_1}{\lambda_1^2} + \frac{C_2}{\lambda_2^2} \qquad \text{19-22}$$

Accordingly, substituting *Dose/AUC* for *CL* and Eq. 19-21 into Eq. 19-20

$$V_{ss} = Dose \frac{AUMC}{AUC^2} \qquad \text{19-23}$$

which, on substituting Eq. 19-22 for *AUMC*, yields

$$V_{ss} = Dose \frac{\left(\dfrac{C_1}{\lambda_1^{\;2}} + \dfrac{C_2}{\lambda_2^{\;2}} \right)}{\left(\dfrac{C_1}{\lambda_1} + \dfrac{C_2}{\lambda_2} \right)^2} \qquad \text{19-24}$$

The value of V_{ss} can also be calculated from data obtained after an i.v. infusion. Here, to obtain the correct value of *MRT* due regard needs to be taken to correct the observed ratio $AUMC/AUC^2$ by the mean time to input the drug, which is half the duration of the infusion (i.e., $\tau/2$) (see Appendix H, *Mean Residence Time*). Accordingly, V_{ss} is given by

$$V_{ss} = CL \cdot \left(\frac{AUMC}{AUC^2} - \frac{\tau}{2} \right) \qquad \text{19-25}$$

The value of V_{ss} lies between the initial dilution volume, V_1, and the volume of distribution during the terminal phase, *V*. In general, the difference between the values of V_{ss} and *V* is small. Much depends on the disposition kinetics of the drug. The difference is larger, the greater the extent of elimination before distribution equilibrium is achieved. To appreciate this last point, consider three drugs, aspirin, salicylic acid, and gentamicin. The disposition kinetics, normalized to a 100-mg i.v. bolus dose for a 70-kg subject, are aspirin, $C = 9.7\, e^{-13.8t} + 5.1\, e^{-3.0t}$; salicylic acid, $C = 10.2\, e^{-2.8t} + 8.7\, e^{-0.23t}$; gentamicin, $C = 7.1\, e^{-0.42t} + 0.05\, e^{-0.015t}$, where *C* is in milligrams per liter and time in hours. Substitution of these parameter values to the respective equations listed in Table 19-1 yields: for aspirin, $V = 13.6$ L, $V_{ss} = 10.4$ L, $V_1 = 6.8$ L; for salicylic acid, $V = 10.5$ L, $V_{ss} = 10.2$ L, $V_1 = 5.3$ L; and for gentamicin, $V = 345$ L, $V_{ss} = 56$ L, $V_1 = 14$ L. Notice that for aspirin and salicylic acid, the values of V_{ss} are very similar; they are both acids, predominantly bound to albumin and nothing else in the body, and accordingly have small volumes of distribution. The greater value of *V* relative to V_{ss} for aspirin arises because appreciable elimination ($CL = 41$ L/hr) occurs before distribution equilibrium is achieved compared with that for salicylic acid ($CL = 2.4$ L/hr). Finally, for gentamicin, *V* is much larger than V_{ss}, because most of the administered drug is eliminated before distribution equilibrium is attained. In such circumstances, estimating V_{ss} is worthwhile if, for any reason, disposition kinetics were altered and one wishes to assign the change to altered distribution or elimination, or to both.

Another view of distribution at steady state is to consider the ratio of amount in body (A_{ss}) to amount in the initial dilution volume ($A_{1,ss}$). The ratio, V_{ss}/V_1, is obtained from $\left[\dfrac{A_{ss}}{V_{ss}} = \dfrac{A_{1,ss}}{V_1}\right]$. For aspirin and salicylic acid, this ratio is approximately 1.5 and 1.9, respectively, indicating that these drugs are equally distributed between the initial dilution volume and the rest of the body. For gentamicin, the ratio is 4, indicating that at steady state more of this antibiotic resides outside, than inside, the initial dilution volume.

Finally, a connection needs to be made between V_{ss} and the volume of distribution used to consider the influence of plasma and tissue binding on distribution (e.g., $V = V_P + V_T \cdot fu/fu_T$) (Chapter 4, *Membranes and Distribution*). They are essentially the same. The term V_{ss} applies to a model in which no net elimination occurs and distribution equilibrium (steady state) has been achieved (Fig. 19-9A). In practice, elimination always occurs and confounds the estimation of a purely distributional volume term; V_{ss}, and not V (during the terminal phase), is the closest estimate of it.

Turnover of Endogenous Substances. A particular application of an i.v. bolus dose is the estimation MRT and V_{ss} of endogenous substances. These substances, such as drugs, show distribution kinetics within the body. This distribution is not apparent from the plasma concentration measurement of the endogenous compound under the usual steady-state conditions, but becomes so when a *tracer* dose of the compound, in an isotopically labeled form, is administered. In the analysis of the tracer data, two major assumptions are often made. First, the disposition of the tracer is identical to that of the endogenous substance. Second, both input (formation) and elimination occur in the initial dilution volume. Unlike for most drugs, these restrictions are more problematic for body constituents that are often formed and destroyed in tissues and that do not equilibrate rapidly between such tissues and plasma.

To illustrate the use of a tracer to determine V_{ss} and turnover parameters of an endogenous substance, consider the following biexponential equation, which summarizes the experimental observations after a 10-MBq i.v. bolus dose of a radiolabelled tracer.

$$C^* = 1.2\,e^{-1.2t} + 0.2\,e^{-0.01t}$$

where C^* is the plasma concentration in units of megaBecquerel (MBq) per liter and t is in minutes. One Becquerel equals one disintegration per second. The AUC is 21 MBq-min/L (1.2/1.2 + 0.2/0.01) and $AUMC$ is 2001 MBq-min^2/L (1.2/1.2^2 + 0.2/0.01^2). Accordingly, the MRT (Eq. 19-21) is 95 min, and V_{ss} (Eq. 19-23) is 45 L.

Calculation of turnover rate requires knowledge of the concentration of the endogenous substance, for example, 9 mg/L. The amount in the body (pool size) is then 9 mg/L × 45 L = 405 mg, and from turnover time, turnover rate (A_{ss}/MRT) is 4.3 mg/min, and fractional turnover rate is 0.01 min^{-1}. The turnover of this substance is now quantified.

Time to Reach Plateau. Recall that for practical purposes, plateau is said to be reached when the concentration is 90% of C_{ss}. Because of distribution kinetics, the time to reach plateau differs between plasma and tissue.

Events in Plasma. The terminal half-life of the antihypertensive agent nicardipine is approximately 12 hr. Therefore, one would normally expect 50% of the plateau plasma concentration to be reached by 12 hr during a constant-rate infusion. Instead, it takes only 1 hr (Fig. 19-10). Also, 90% of the plateau is reached by approximately 15 hr instead of the expected 40 hr (3.3 · $t_{1/2}$).

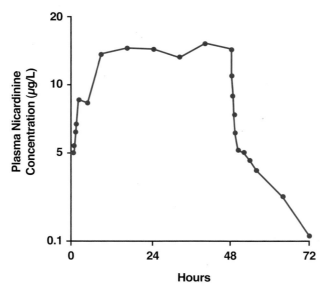

FIGURE 19-10. By approximately 1 hr into a 48-hr constant-rate i.v. infusion of nicardipine (0.5 mg/hr), the plasma concentration has risen to 50% of the plateau value (14 μg/L) despite a terminal half-life of 12 hr. This rapid approach to plateau is a result of events in plasma being primarily controlled by an initial phase, with a half-life of 20 min, during which time significant elimination occurs following a bolus dose. The data are the means of 37 patients with mild-to-moderate hypertension. (From: Cook E, Clifton GG, Bienvenu G, et al. Pharmacokinetics, pharmacodynamics and minimum effective clinical dose of intravenous nicardipine. Clin Pharmacol Ther 1990;47:706–718.)

This difference arises because nicardipine's disposition kinetics is biphasic, with substantial elimination occurring during the first phase, which has a half-life of approximately only 20 min. The result is a rapidly rising initial curve followed by a much slower approach to plateau.

The importance of not only the half-lives but also the relative rates of distribution and elimination on the approach of the plasma concentration to plateau can be appreciated by the events depicted in Fig. 19-11, for which the values of λ_1 and λ_2 are fixed and the fractional term associated with the terminal phase, f_2, is varied between 0.01 and 1. When $f_2 = 1$, drug distributes spontaneously relative to elimination; the body appears as a single compartment and, as expected, all the drug is eliminated during the terminal phase. In this case, it takes 1 terminal half-life ($0.693/\lambda_2$) and 3.3 such half-lives to reach 50% and 90% of the plateau, respectively. However, at lower values of f_2, more drug is correspondingly eliminated before distribution equilibrium is established. As a result, the time to achieve (e.g., 50% of the plateau) occurs earlier until, when $f_2 = 0$; the time required is the half-life of the first phase, $0.693/\lambda_1$. The body once again acts as a single compartment, but with a smaller volume of distribution, V_1. For most drugs, f_2 exceeds 0.8, and so the terminal half-life primarily determines the time to reach plateau. For nicardipine, significant elimination occurs before distribution equilibrium is achieved and hence the observation in Fig. 19-10. For gentamicin, with f_2 close to 0, it is the half-life of the first phase, usually 2 to 4 hr, that primarily determines the time for this aminoglycoside to reach plateau in plasma.

Another view of events in plasma relates to the expanding volume of distribution on approach to distribution equilibrium (see Fig. 19-4). A plateau is reached when the rates of infusion and elimination are equal. When distribution into the tissue is slow, the effective volume of distribution remains close to the initial dilution volume, V_1, for

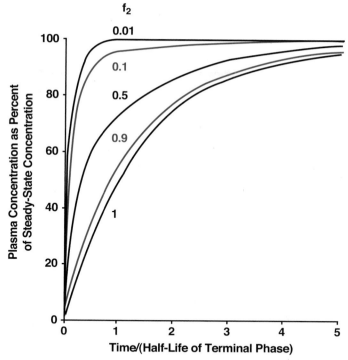

FIGURE 19-11. During a constant-rate i.v. infusion, approach to plateau in plasma, for a drug that displays biexponential disposition kinetics, is determined by the relative rates of distribution and elimination. In this example, the two exponential coefficients λ_1 and λ_2 are kept constant (with $\lambda_1 = 10\,\lambda_2$), and the fractional elimination term associated with the terminal phase, f_2, is varied from 0.01 to 1. When drug distributes rapidly compared with elimination (f_2 approaches 1), the terminal half-life controls the time to approach plateau. When f_2 is very low (e.g., 0.01), implying elimination occurs much faster than distribution, the approach to plateau is determined primarily by λ_1. Included for reference is the expected curve when the drug exhibits one-compartment characteristics ($f_2 = 1$), in which case 50% and 90% of the plateau are reached by 1 and 3.3 terminal half-lives, respectively. Note that time is expressed in units of terminal half-life.

some time, so that for a given rate of input the plasma concentration rises much faster than if distribution into tissue is rapid. Therefore, as rate of elimination $= CL \cdot C$, it follows that, for a given clearance value, the approach to plateau in plasma (and other tissues comprising the initial dilution space) occurs earlier, the slower the distribution to tissues.

The plasma concentration at any time on approach to plateau can be calculated using concepts presented in Fig. 19-11. Remember for a drug with one-compartment characteristics, the concentration at any time during an infusion is given by $R_{inf}(1 - e^{-kt})/CL$. For a drug that exhibits biexponential disposition characteristics, the corresponding equation is

$$C = f_1 \cdot \frac{R_{inf}}{CL} \cdot (1 - e^{-\lambda_1 t}) + f_2 \cdot \frac{R_{inf}}{CL} \cdot (1 - e^{-\lambda_2 t}) \qquad \text{19-26}$$

As $C_{ss} = R_{inf}/CL$, the concentration during the infusion, C, relative to the concentration at plateau is

$$\frac{C}{C_{ss}} = f_1 \cdot (1 - e^{-\lambda_1 t}) + f_2 \cdot (1 - e^{-\lambda_2 t}) \qquad \text{19-27}$$

These relationships follow by imagining that total concentration is the sum derived from two hypothetical drugs, each with the same clearance value, infused at rates $f_1 \cdot R_{inf}$ and $f_2 \cdot R_{inf}$, respectively. Equations 19-25 and 19-26 emphasize the importance of f_2 (and hence C_1 and C_2) as well as λ_1 and λ_2 in determining the events in plasma following a constant-rate infusion. Equation 19-26 also permits ready calculation of the percent of plateau reached at any time. For example, if the half-lives associated with the first and terminal exponential terms are 1 and 12 hr, respectively, and $f_2 = 0.5$, then at 6 hr, the concentration is 64% of plateau. The converse (i.e., the time required to reach a certain percent of plateau) cannot be calculated directly, because there are two exponential terms containing the unknown, time. The time can be determined by iteration (i.e., by substituting different times into Eq. 19-26 until C = the given fixed percent of C_{ss}). In the example mentioned, the time to reach 50% of plateau is 2.75 hr.

Events in Peripheral Tissue. As illustrated in Fig. 19-12, the time to achieve plateau in slowly equilibrating tissues is primarily determined by the terminal half-life, irrespective of the time required to achieve plateau in plasma. To appreciate this point, consider events in terms of the two-compartment model depicted in Fig. 19-3. When distribution occurs rapidly, drug in tissue for most of the time is virtually at equilibrium with drug in plasma. That is,

$$\underset{\substack{\text{Rate drug} \\ \text{leaves tissue}}}{k_{21} \cdot A_2} \quad \approx \quad \underset{\substack{\text{Rate drug} \\ \text{enters tissue}}}{k_{12} \cdot A_1} \qquad \text{19-28}$$

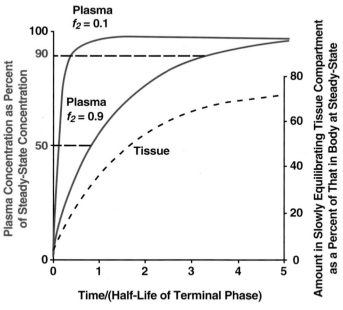

FIGURE 19-12. Shown are events in plasma and slowly equilibrating tissue for two drugs that both display biexponential disposition kinetics. They have the same values for each of the exponential coefficients (λ_1 and λ_2) but differ in the contribution of each phase to elimination, signified by the value of f_2. For one drug $f_2 = 0.1$, for the other $f_2 = 0.9$. Despite differences seen in plasma (*colored curves*), reproduced from Fig. 19-11, the approach to plateau in the slowly equilibrating tissue (————) during a constant-rate i.v. infusion is primarily controlled by the terminal half-life, which is the same for both drugs. Note that time is expressed in terminal half-lives. The horizontal dashed lines correspond to 50% and 90% of the plateau plasma concentration.

and therefore,

$$A_2 \approx \frac{k_{12}}{k_{21}} \cdot A_1 \qquad\qquad 19\text{-}29$$

which shows that the amount in tissue parallels that in plasma. When, however, distribution is slow relative to elimination, the concentration in plasma approaches its plateau before much drug has entered the slowly equilibrating tissue. The situation is then analogous to a constant-rate input into a compartment from which loss occurs. Accumulation is determined by the elimination half-life, which in this case is associated with k_{21}, the exit rate constant from the slowly equilibrating tissue. In reality, the situation is somewhat more complex because of the reversible movement of drug between plasma and tissue. Nonetheless, under these circumstances, the constant for transfer out of the slowly equilibrating tissue is a major determinant of the terminal rate constant, λ_2.

Bolus Plus Infusion. Recall that eptifibatide is used intravenously to treat acute coronary syndrome in emergency settings (Chapter 10, *Constant-Rate Input*). A bolus is given to rapidly achieve an effective concentration, followed by a constant-rate infusion to maintain a therapeutic concentration. Otherwise, with a half-life of 2.5 hr, it will take too long (4–6 hr) to achieve adequate concentrations with an infusion alone. When considered previously, this drug was assumed to display one-compartment characteristics. However, as seen in Fig. 19-13, it clearly displays distribution kinetics. Thus, although the infusion eventually achieves the desired objective, initially it cannot match the fall in plasma concentration associated with distribution into the tissues, potentially leading to a period of ineffective concentrations, as was the case for propofol discussed in Chapter 10, *Constant-Rate Input*. A larger bolus dose would overcome the problem but would also increase the likelihood of toxicity because of the initially higher concentrations. The recommended solution is to give an equal-size supplemental bolus 10 min after the first one. Notice that this still raises the concentration higher than either the

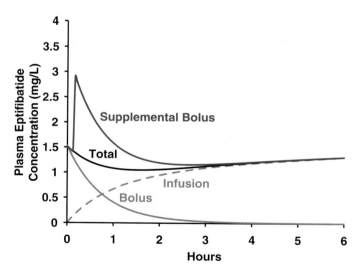

FIGURE 19-13. Although a bolus ($V_1 \cdot C_d$) of 180 μg/kg is given to initially achieve a desired plasma eptifibatide concentration of 1.5 mg/L, C_d, constant infusion at a rate (2 μg/kg/min) required to maintain this value at steady state (rate $= CL \cdot C_d$) fails to do so in the early moments, owing to distribution kinetics. Note that the observed plasma concentration (———) is the sum of that associated with the bolus (———) (Eq. 19-2) and with the constant-rate infusion (— — —) (Eq. 19-26). A 180-μg/kg supplemental bolus at 10 min overcomes the deficiency (———). (From: Gilchrist IC, O'Shea JC, Kosoglou T, et al. Pharmacodynamics and pharmacokinetics of higher-dose, double-bolus eptifibatide in percutaneous coronary intervention. Circulation 2001;104:406–411.)

initial or steady-state concentrations, but is not considered excessive. If there was concern, smaller supplemental boluses could be given at various times after the initial bolus to compensate for this period of potential deficiency. In general, a more elegant solution lies in giving a supplemental, exponentially declining infusion. The object of the supplemental infusion is to match the net rate of movement into tissue. This rate is highest initially, when no drug is in tissue. However, as the tissue concentration rises toward plateau, the net movement into tissue progressively declines. Finally, returning to eptifibatide, approximately 50% is excreted unchanged. Consequently, the recommended infusion rate is half of normal for patient with poor renal function but, with no evidence of altered distribution in this condition, the loading of the patient, as expected, remains unchanged.

MULTIPLE DOSING AND REGIMEN DESIGN

The impact of distribution kinetics on events during multiple dosing and on the design of a multiple-dose regimen depends on disposition characteristics of the drug and, when given extravascularly, on absorption kinetics. This is illustrated by the data in Fig. 19-14, obtained following an 8-hourly intramuscular (i.m.) regimen of gentamicin administered to a patient for the treatment of a serious infection for 8 days. Absorption is very much faster than distribution. Seen are large fluctuations in plasma concentration resulting from this regimen and a long terminal half-life on stopping therapy. Common with other aminoglycosides, gentamicin is polar and while it distributes rapidly into the extracellular water space, approximate volume of 15 L, it enters cells very slowly. Accordingly, although gentamicin has a long terminal half-life, 87 hr in this patient, the majority of a dose is eliminated by 8 hr, associated with the 4-hr half-life of the first phase in the patient. As a reasonable approximation, the terminal phase can be ignored with respect to events in plasma. The reason for this approximation is borne out by the observed rapid establishment of a plateau in plasma and by the continuance of large fluctuations in concentration, a result expected for a drug with a half-life of 4 hr when it is given every 8 hr. Associated with this regimen, however, is a slow but continual accumulation of drug in the slowly equilibrating tissues, where it takes approximately 12 days (3.3 terminal half-lives) to reach plateau. However, at plateau, accumulation is so extensive that more gentamicin exists in these tissues than, on average, in the rapidly equilibrating pool. Furthermore, little fluctuation of drug occurs in the slowly equilibrating pool because of slow distribution.

Accumulation, both time course and extent thereof, are clearly dependent on site of measurement. For gentamicin, little accumulation occurs in plasma, and a plateau is reached soon after initiating therapy. In contrast, extensive accumulation occurs in the slowly equilibrating tissues, where it takes much longer to attain plateau. In Chapter 11, *Multiple Dose Regimens* (Eq. 11-10), based on consideration of the minimum amount of drug after the first dose and at plateau, a proposed index of accumulation was $1/(1 - e^{-k \cdot \tau})$. As a reasonable approximation, this index can also be employed here using the appropriate exponential coefficient. For example, for gentamicin in plasma ($\lambda_1 = 0.17$ hr^{-1}; $t_{1/2} = 4$ hr) with $\tau = 8$ hr, the accumulation index associated with the first term, which primarily reflects drug in plasma is only 1.35, whereas that associated with the last term ($\lambda_2 = 0.008$ hr^{-1}), which reflects drug in the slowly equilibrating pool, is as much as 16.

The events on stopping gentamicin administration are predictable. The plasma concentration falls rapidly for the first 2 days, with a half-life controlled by the first phase. Eventually, however, elimination of drug from plasma is rate-limited by return from the slowly equilibrating tissues. Except for the high degree of fluctuation, the events seen in plasma with gentamicin are those expected following a constant-rate infusion for any drug with a low value of f_2 (see Fig. 19-12).

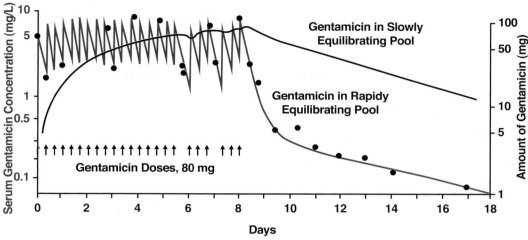

FIGURE 19-14. Depicted are semilogarithmic plots of the levels of gentamicin in the body occurring during and after i.m. administration, 80 mg, almost every 8 hr (*times indicated by arrows*) to a patient for just over 8 days. The biphasic decline in serum concentration (●) when administration was stopped was fitted by a model that assumes that gentamicin distributes between a slowly equilibrating compartment and a rapidly equilibrating compartment from which elimination, entirely by renal excretion, occurs (see Fig. 19-3). The lines are the predicted concentrations (*colored line, left-hand ordinate*), the amount in the rapidly equilibrating compartment (*colored line, right-hand ordinate*), a value obtained by multiplying the serum concentration by the estimated initial dilution volume, and the predicted amount in the slowly equilibrating compartment (*black line, right-hand ordinate*). Little accumulation and large fluctuations of drug occur in plasma and the rest of the rapidly equilibrating pool. In contrast, gentamicin slowly, but extensively, accumulates in the slowly equilibrating pool during drug administration, with little fluctuation within a dosing interval; disappearance of drug from the slowly equilibrating tissues is also slow on stopping gentamicin. During administration, the concentration in plasma after the Nth dose can be calculated from the formula

$$C = \frac{D_M}{V_1} \left\{ f_1 \left[\frac{1 - e^{-N\lambda_1\tau}}{1 - e^{-\lambda_1\tau}} \right] e^{-\lambda_1 t} + f_2 \left[\frac{1 - e^{-N\lambda_2\tau}}{1 - e^{-\lambda_2\tau}} \right] e^{-\lambda_2 t} \right\}$$

where D_M is the maintenance dose given every τ, t is the time since the last dose, and V_1 is the initial dilution volume. This equation can be derived using the multiple-dosing equation (Appendix I), assuming instantaneous absorption, and the mathematical aid (Eq. 19-13). (From: Schentag JJ, Jusko WJ. Renal clearance and tissue accumulation of gentamicin. Clin Pharmacol Ther 1977;22:364–370. Reproduced with permission of C.V. Mosby.)

Significant clinical implications arise from the distribution kinetics of gentamicin. Most organisms, against which gentamicin is used, reside in the rapidly equilibrating extracellular space, and so frequent administration is needed to maintain an adequate antimicrobial concentration. Unfortunately, ototoxicity and nephrotoxicity, associated with the accumulation of drug at slowly equilibrating sites within the ears and kidneys, can eventually occur. Accumulation cannot be avoided if an effective plasma concentration is to be maintained. To minimize the problem, a prudent practice is to limit the total duration of gentamicin administration whenever possible. Monitoring the plasma concentration may also help. Of the measures in plasma, the trough value is the most sensitive indicator of the rising concentration in the slowly equilibrating tissues, although as illustrated in Fig. 19-14, even this measurement is not that sensitive. Nonetheless, monitoring of trough concentrations is of value, particularly if the concentration continues to rise, indicating a greater-than-expected rise in the slowly equilibrating pool with a corresponding increase in the potential for toxicity.

ABSORPTION KINETICS

The importance of the initial events, and associated half-life, in determining the dosing frequency of gentamicin is driven by the need to maintain effective extracellular concentrations. For many other drugs, the concern in the initial phase is to keep the C_{max} below a level producing adverse events, such as central nervous system or cardiovascular toxicity. Both of these limitations are particularly pertinent to those drugs that are perfusion rate-limited in their distribution to the active site, as drug at the active site quickly equilibrates with that in plasma. The speed of absorption, rather than the terminal half-life, is then critical in determining the degree of fluctuation in exposure at the active site, and hence the choice of the dosing interval that minimizes the risk of an adverse effect. Slowing the kinetics of absorption, even relatively modestly, can profoundly blunt having a high C_{max} even at plateau on chronic dosing, without materially affecting the trough concentration when pronounced distribution kinetics prevail, as shown in Fig. 19-15A, and can permit a significant prolongation of the dosing interval. For example, in the case of the drug depicted in Fig. 19-15, despite it having a terminal half-life of 29.7 hr, during which time the majority of drug is eliminated, an increase in the absorption half-life by just 1 hr, from 0.5 to 1.5 hr, enables the dosing interval that ensures that the plasma concentration stays within the therapeutic window (set between 1 and 2 mg/L) to be increased from approximately 12 to 24 hr (Fig. 19-5B).

Obviously, frequent dosing relative to the terminal half-life, such as in the case of gentamicin, does not preclude extensive accumulation of drug in the rest of the body, especially in the slowly equilibrating tissues, although the fluctuation there is relatively insensitive to variation in absorption kinetics. Accumulation in the tissue compartment is a concern if activity resides there. Clearly, the important issue is the location of the sites of action and toxicity.

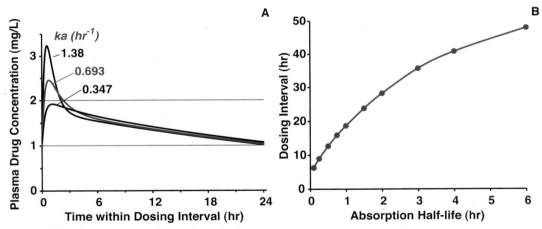

FIGURE 19-15. Changes in the absorption kinetics of a drug can profoundly influence the dosing interval that ensures effectiveness while minimizing risk, when the response directly tracks plasma concentration. **A.** Depicted are plasma concentration–time profiles of a drug within an interdosing interval at steady state administered once daily when the absorption rate constant is decreased from 1.386 to 0.347 hr^{-1} (corresponding to an increase in absorption half-life of 0.5–2hr), for a drug with the following disposition kinetics: $C'_1 = 0.9162$, $C'_2 = 0.0838$, $\lambda_1 = 3.2$ hr^{-1}, $\lambda_2 = 0.0233$ hr^{-1}, $f_2 = 0.926$, terminal half-life = 29.7 hr. Notice that despite 92.6% of the elimination of the drug being associated with the long terminal phase, even a small change in absorption half-life has a marked effect on the degree of fluctuation in the plasma concentration and whether it remains within the therapeutic window, here set between 1 and 2 mg/L. **B.** Same drug as in A. Plot shows that despite the long terminal half-life of the drug (29.7 hr), a relatively small change in absorption half-life markedly prolongs the dosing interval that ensures that the ratio $C_{max,ss}/C_{min,ss}$ stays within a factor of 2, the therapeutic window for this drug.

FREQUENCY OF DOSING

When events wear off during the distribution phase of the drug, another approach in reducing the chance of an adverse effect is reduction in the dose along with a shortening of the dosing interval, while maintaining the same average dosing rate. This would narrow the degree of fluctuation in plasma concentration around the average at plateau and thereby better maintain a therapeutic systemic exposure. Again, as with consideration of the impact of absorption kinetics, the primary factors controlling the size of the dose and dosing interval is the kinetics of distribution between target site and plasma and the therapeutic window of the drug, rather than the terminal half-life of the drug.

UTILITY OF VOLUME TERMS

A comment needs to be made about the application of volume terms to multiple dosing when distribution kinetics prevails. The purpose of a volume term is to relate plasma concentration to amount in the body. To appreciate the issues involved, consider the events at steady state. Following a constant-rate infusion, V_{ss} is the appropriate volume term to relate plasma concentration to amount in the body. With multiple dosing, a true steady state does not apply throughout a dosing interval; the plasma concentration fluctuates around a steady-state value, creating a concentration gradient between plasma and tissues. However, as illustrated in Fig. 19-16, as long as the fluctuation in plasma concentration is small, the condition is sufficiently close to the true steady state that V_{ss} can still be applied

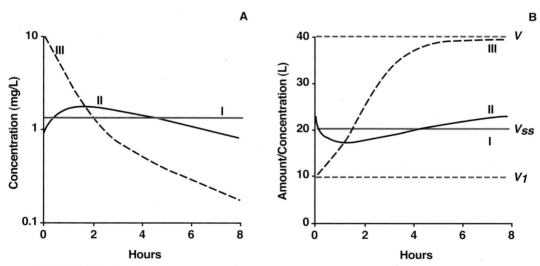

FIGURE 19-16. The utility of the volume terms V and V_{ss} for calculating amount in the body from plasma concentration within a dosing interval at steady state, during a multiple-dose regimen, depends on the degree of departure from the true steady state. Shown are the logarithm of the plasma concentration (**A**) and the ratio of amount in body to plasma concentration (**B**) within a dosing interval at steady state for three situations (*I, II, III*). Also shown in *B* are the values for V, V_{ss}, and V_1. In *Case I*, a constant-rate infusion, V_{ss} applies throughout the equivalent of an 8-hr dosing interval at steady state. In *Case II*, input is first order and sufficiently slow that the fluctuation in plasma concentration is small. Here, the use of V_{ss} to calculate amount in body is still reasonable. In *Case III*, bolus dose administration, the deviation from steady state is now too large to render V_{ss} of use. Distribution equilibrium is virtually achieved, however, toward the end of the dosing interval. Then, V can be used to calculate the amount in the body. At earlier times, the volume needed to estimate amount in the body is changing rapidly. Calculations have been made using the following parameter values: Disposition kinetics (single 100-mg i.v. bolus dose); $C(mg/L) = 9e^{-1.386t} + 1e^{-0.231t}$ (t in hours). Input kinetics: *Case I*, constant rate of infusion of 12.5 mg/hr; *Case II*, input half-life of 4 hr, $F = 1$; *Cases II* and *III*, 100-mg doses, 8-hr dosing interval.

to estimate amount in the body. This condition exists when input into the body is slow, relative to disposition kinetics, or when the dosing interval is short relative to the time to achieve distribution equilibrium. As one moves away from this condition, either with use of more rapid input (extreme being an i.v. bolus) or by widening the dosing interval, the deviation from the true steady state increases so that V_{ss} has less application. If the dosing interval is long enough so that distribution equilibrium is achieved, then V becomes the appropriate volume term to use but, clearly, only during the terminal phase. The problem is exaggerated when distribution equilibrium is not achieved within the dosing interval, such as the case with gentamicin (see Fig. 19-12). Then, the ratio of amount in body to plasma concentration is continually changing, and neither volume term, V or V_{ss}, is very useful. Frequently, however, distribution is sufficiently rapid to allow one-compartment disposition characteristics to apply on multiple dosing at steady state. Then, V and V_{ss} are almost equal, and either can be used to gain a reasonable estimate of amount in the body.

ALTERED CLEARANCE

When discussing the use of gentamicin in patients with renal insufficiency, the terminal phase is ignored in adjusting dosing regimens to achieve therapeutic concentrations. The reason for this approach is illustrated in Fig. 19-17. Only the initial half-life is altered

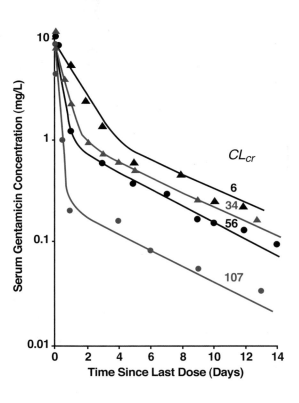

FIGURE 19-17. Semilogarithmic plot of the decline in the serum concentration of gentamicin in four patients with different degrees of renal function, as assessed by creatinine clearance, CL_{cr}, after stopping gentamicin administration. Notice that renal function impairment primarily affects the half-life of the first phase and the depth of the decline in concentration before the terminal phase is reached. (From: Schentag JJ, Jusko WJ, Plaut ME, et al. Tissue persistence of gentamicin in man. JAMA 1977;238:327–329. Copyright 1977, American Medical Association.)

among patients with varying degrees of renal insufficiency; the terminal half-life is virtually unaffected. The observation may be rationalized in the following manner. When renal function is unimpaired, gentamicin in the rapidly equilibrating pool is mostly eliminated before distribution equilibrium is either achieved after administration of a bolus dose (Fig. 19-18) or reestablished on stopping administration after chronic dosing (see Fig. 19-14). Under these circumstances, elimination may be viewed as occurring from volume V_1 with a clearance, CL. Hence, the rate constant for decline in the rapidly equilibrating pool (including plasma) approaches CL/V_1, with a corresponding half-life of $0.693 \cdot V_1/CL$. Reduction in clearance is then reflected by an almost proportional increase in half-life of the first phase. In contrast, during the terminal phase, loss of drug from plasma (and the rapidly equilibrating pool) is controlled by return from the slowly equilibrating tissues and not by its clearance from plasma. Accordingly, the terminal half-life is unchanged. However, with a reduction in clearance, distribution equilibrium takes somewhat longer to be established and, because less drug is eliminated by then, the concentration of gentamicin in plasma is higher compared with that in a patient with unimpaired renal function (see Figs. 19-17 and 19-18). Ultimately, if renal function is sufficiently low, the terminal half-life is sensitive to renal function. Then, the first phase primarily reflects distribution, as shown in Fig. 19-18.

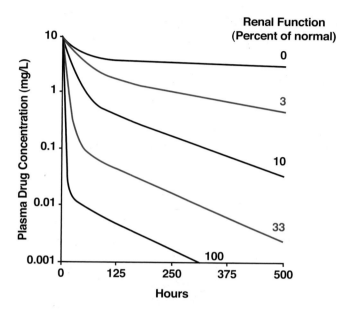

FIGURE 19-18. Semilogarithmic plots of the simulated decline in the plasma concentration after i.v. bolus administration of a drug, with disposition characteristics similar to gentamicin, for different degrees of renal function from 0% to 100% of normal. Notice that renal function primarily affects the half-life of the first phase and the depth of decline in concentration before the terminal phase is reached, until renal function is very low. When renal function is very low, the initial decline is determined primarily by distribution, and the impairment is reflected by changes in the terminal half-life.

To appreciate the last point, consider administration of a bolus dose of drug to a patient with no renal function. Drug in plasma would still decline initially with a half-life determined solely by distribution. Between this extreme and unimpaired renal function is a range over which the terminal half-life changes noticeably with renal function. For gentamicin, calculation shows this to occur when renal function is less than 7% of normal. Then, albeit slowly for gentamicin, distribution is achieved before much drug is eliminated, the condition that normally prevails for most drugs. Now, return to a point made previously about V and V_{ss}. As renal function diminishes, so does the value of V. This is a result of less drug being eliminated before distribution equilibrium is achieved. In contrast, the value of V_{ss} remains unchanged.

With gentamicin, concern exists for excessive accumulation in the slowly equilibrating tissues during chronic dosing, particularly in patients with renal insufficiency. However, provided that dosing rate has been adjusted to compensate for diminished renal function, the risk of toxicity in patients with renal insufficiency should be no greater than in those with unimpaired renal function. This conclusion is based on consideration of events at plateau. The amount in the slowly equilibrating tissues at steady state is the difference between the amount in the body ($V_{ss} \cdot C_{ss}$) and that in the rapidly equilibrating pool ($V_1 \cdot C_{ss}$). That is,

$$\begin{array}{l} \textit{Amount in slowly equilibrating} \\ \textit{tissues at steady state} \end{array} = (V_{SS} - V_1) \cdot C_{SS} \qquad 19\text{-}30$$

From this last relationship, it is seen that provided dosing rate is adjusted to maintain a given steady-state plasma concentration, the amount in the slowly equilibrating tissues is unaltered because both V_1 and V_{ss} are purely distribution terms that, at least for gentamicin, are unaltered by renal insufficiency.

CHANGES IN CONCENTRATION AND HALF-LIFE

A comment is needed here about changes in plasma concentration and half-life. Consider the following three questions. What is the time needed for the plasma concentration to fall by one half following an i.v. bolus dose? How long does it take to reach 50% of plateau following a constant-rate infusion? What is the dosing interval needed to ensure that the maximum and minimum plasma concentrations at plateau differ twofold following a fixed-dose multiple i.v. bolus regimen? When disposition kinetics is characterized by a one-compartment model, the answers to all three questions are simple and the same—the (elimination) half-life. It should be apparent, however, from what has been discussed in this chapter, that the answers cannot be directly inferred from the terminal half-life when distribution kinetics is evident. Then, terminal half-life, or indeed any half-life, ceases to have simple application. The answers no longer lie just in the half-life value of an exponential term, but rather in all the parameters that define the entire pharmacokinetic model (e.g., C_1, λ_1, C_2, λ_2). Knowing these parameters, the time to achieve any concentration can be calculated during and following drug administration, and hence help in the design of an appropriate dosing regimen.

DRUG REDISTRIBUTION

An important consideration in evaluating the potential use of hemodialysis in patients with end-stage renal disease, and in the treatment of an overdose, discussed in Chapter 15, *Disease*, is drug redistribution. For certain drugs, the procedure may remove drug more readily from the plasma than it can be replaced from tissue stores, thereby resulting in a rebound of the plasma drug concentration when the procedure is stopped. Two primary mechanisms account for this slow return—slow diffusion through cell membranes and limited vascular perfusion of the tissues in which drug is stored.

Lithium (Fig. 19-19) is an example of a drug that exhibits postdialysis rebound because of slow diffusion from cells. Dialysis clearance adds substantially to the total body clearance

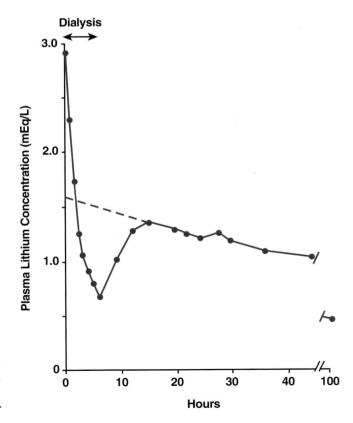

FIGURE 19-19. During 6.5 hr of hemodialysis (*arrow*) of a patient poisoned with lithium, the plasma concentration of lithium (●) dropped dramatically; however, on discontinuing dialysis the plasma concentration rose with redistribution of drug from tissue cells to plasma, so that only about one half of the lithium initially in the body was removed by dialysis. A rough estimate of fraction lost can be obtained by extrapolating (----) the terminal curve back to the time dialysis was started. A semilogarithmic plot should be used for the extrapolation in those situations in which the postdialysis concentration declines linearly on such a plot. (From: Amdisen A, Skjoldborg H. Haemodialysis for lithium poisoning. Lancet 1969;2:213.)

(virtually all renal clearance) of this drug in patients with end-stage renal disease. Lithium disappears rapidly from plasma during dialysis, and a large fraction in the body is expected to be removed into the dialysate. The slow return from tissue stores, however, limits the total amount removed and produces a rebound in the plasma concentration on stopping dialysis treatment. In this case, assessment of the actual fraction of the initial amount of drug in the body removed by dialysis is relatively simple, because virtually all the drug eliminated by the body is excreted into the urine. The fraction is the amount recovered in the dialysate divided by the sum of the amounts in the dialysate and the urine during the dialysis period.

PHARMACODYNAMIC CONSIDERATIONS

Various aspects of the influence of distribution kinetics on pharmacologic response following single and multiple dosing have been considered in previous chapters (Chapter 5, *Elimination*, and Chapter 10, *Constant-Rate Input*). We now explore the situation further considering the onset, duration, and intensity relationships for those drugs that distribute relatively slowly into tissues. A two-compartment model is emphasized.

SINGLE BOLUS DOSE

Consider the situation in which the site of action is in a rapidly equilibrating, and hence well-perfused tissue and in which drug at the site of action immediately produces an effect. The peak effect is then seen almost immediately after an i.v. bolus dose, and thereafter, the effect is directly related to the plasma concentration. Typical plasma concentration–time curves observed after various bolus doses are shown in Fig. 19-20A; the curves only become

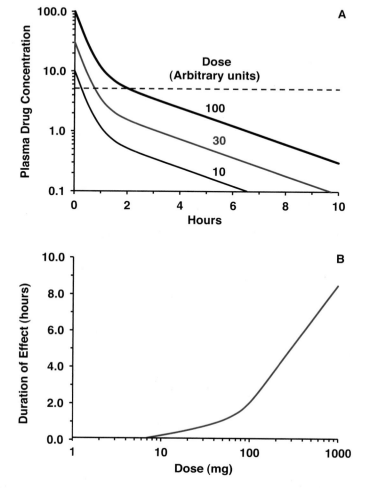

FIGURE 19-20. Duration of effect increases linearly with the logarithm of dose only when the effect wears off well into the terminal phase of a drug for which the site of action is in a rapidly equilibrating tissue. When the effect wears off during the distribution phase, because either the dose is small or substantial response still exists at the predetermined end point, duration of effect increases disproportionally for small increases in dose. Shown are semilogarithmic plots of simulated plasma concentration–time profiles for different i.v. bolus doses of a drug that displays pronounced multiexponential disposition kinetics (**A**), and the corresponding duration of response-versus-log dose plot for a predetermined endpoint (----) corresponding to a given degree of maximal response (**B**).

linear on this semilogarithmic plot when distribution equilibrium is achieved in all tissues. If dose is small (here less than 10 units), plasma concentration falls to the minimum effective value, and response wears off, during the distribution phase. One example previously considered is thiopental. Another is diazepam. Despite being slowly eliminated with a half-life of 1 to 2 days, when administered as an i.v. bolus for the treatment of a prolonged epileptic seizure, the duration of effect is only in the order of 20 to 30 min. This drug readily and rapidly distributes into brain, and the effect wears off because plasma and brain concentrations rapidly decline as it redistributes into the less well-perfused tissues. Returning to the general case, as seen in Fig. 19-20B, on increasing dose, duration of effect increases disproportionally with the logarithm of dose. It takes disproportionally longer to reach the minimum effective concentration as a result of a slowing in the decline of plasma concentration with time. Only when the effect wears off well into the terminal phase is duration of effect proportional to the logarithm of dose, as seen with all doses of a drug that exhibits one-compartment characteristics (Chapter 8, *Response Following a Single Dose*).

Supporting these general expectations are the times of recovery to 50% (T50) of normal muscle twitch after i.v. injection of bolus doses (between 4 and 16 mg/m^2) of the neuromuscular blocking agent d-tubocurarine (Fig. 19-21A). The plasma concentration–time profile displays pronounced distribution kinetics; it takes an hour before the plasma concentration reaches the terminal exponential phase (Fig. 19-21B). Relative to this time frame, drug equilibrates quite rapidly between plasma and neuromuscular junction, the site of action. The recovery time increases proportionally with the logarithm of the dose when the duration of effect is well in excess of 1 hr. This condition is met only at the highest doses of d-tubocurarine. At lower doses, the duration of effect is seen to increase disproportionally with the logarithm of dose.

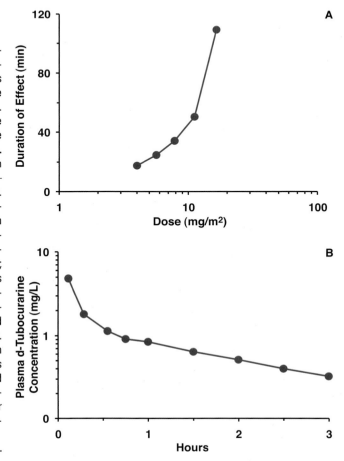

FIGURE 19-21. **A.** Relationship between the median duration of response (T_{50}) and size of the bolus dose (*log scale*) of d-tubocurarine given i.v. to a group of subjects. T_{50} indicates 50% recovery of muscle twitch (a measure of the degree of return of muscle function). **B.** Semilogarithmic plot of estimated mean plasma d-tubocurarine concentration–time profile following a 0.5-mg/kg i.v. bolus dose of drug to a group of 10 subjects. (**A** from: Gibaldi M, Levy G, Hayton W. Kinetics of elimination and neuromuscular blocking effect of d-tubocurarine in man. Anesthesiology 1972; 36:213–218. Original data from: Walts LF, Dillon JB. Duration of action of d-tubocurarine and gallamine. Anesthesiology 1968;29:498–504. Reproduced with permission of J.B. Lippincott. **B** from: Sheiner LB, Stanski DR, Vozeh S, Miller RD, Harm J. Simultaneous modeling of pharmacokinetics and pharmacodynamics: application to d-tubocurarine. Clin Pharmacol Ther 1979;25:358–371. Reproduced with permission of Nature Publishing Group.)

MULTIPLE DOSING

First, consider the common situation in which a fixed dose is given at fixed time intervals. Specifically, consider the data in Fig. 19-22 showing the plasma drug concentration and response during and after stopping an oral 5-mg nightly 28-day regimen of donepezil (Aricept), a highly selective acetylcholinesterase inhibitor, used in the treatment of patients with Alzheimer disease. Notice, as expected, the rise of the trough concentrations to

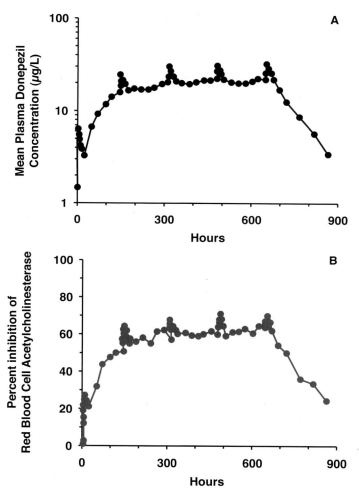

FIGURE 19-22. **A.** Semilogarithmic plot of the mean plasma drug concentration during and after stopping an oral 5-mg evening 28-day regimen of donepezil, a highly selective acetylcholinesterase inhibitor, used in the treatment of patients with Alzheimer's disease. Full plasma kinetic profiles (multiple-time points) were obtained on days 1, 7, 14, 21, and 28. All other points are trough concentrations (obtained just before the next dose). **B.** Linear plot of response, red blood cell acetylcholinesterase inhibition, with time determined at the same sampling times as blood. The data are the mean of 14 subjects. Notice evidence of distribution kinetics during a dosing interval even at plateau because of absorption being faster than distribution. Response shows a similar trend although with a much lower degree of relative fluctuation within a dosing interval owing to response being in the region of 30% to 70% of the maximum response, when response is proportional to the logarithm of the plasma concentration. Notice also that on stopping administration whereas plasma concentration declines logarithmically, as expected, response declines linearly. (From: Tiseo PJ, Rogers SL, Friedhoff LT. Pharmacokinetic and pharmacodynamic profile of donepezil HCl following evening administration. Br J Clin Pharmacol 1998;46[Suppl 1]:13–18.)

plateau reflects extensive accumulation of this drug resulting from the relatively frequent (daily) dosing compared with the long elimination half-life of this drug (3 days), which is also readily seen on stopping administration. However, with absorption occurring faster than distribution, a distinct distribution phase occurs within each dosing interval, even at plateau, as evident on those days of extensive blood sampling. The impact of distribution kinetics on response during such multiple dosing depends on the temporal relationship between response and plasma concentration. In the case of donepezil, the measured effect, red blood cell acetylcholinesterase inhibition, correlates directly with plasma drug concentration without hysterisis. Accordingly, response is also seen to rise and fall within a dosing interval despite the slow accumulation, and hence limited fluctuation, of drug in the body (Fig. 19-22B). However, the percent change in response is much less than in plasma concentration because for much of the time response lies between 30% and 70% of the maximum response, a region in which response is proportional to the logarithm of the plasma concentration, as shown more clearly in Fig. 19-23. Notice also that with response lying predominantly in this region of the concentration–response curve for much of the time on stopping administration, as expected, response declines linearly. Obviously, had the concentration been mostly in the lower part of the concentration–response curve, then during dosing, response would have been expected to fluctuate almost as much as plasma concentration within each dosing interval. In contrast, any hysteresis between response and plasma concentration would further reduce the degree of fluctuation in response.

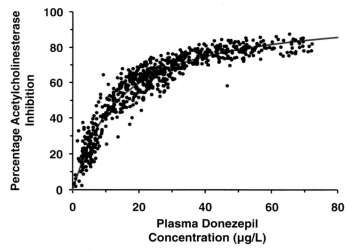

FIGURE 19-23. Plot of the relationship between response and plasma concentration for donepezil, a highly selective inhibitor of acetylcholinesterase. The data are taken from those shown in Fig. 19-22. Notice the absence of any hysterisis and that the relationship is characterized by a simple E_{max} model ($\gamma = 1$; ——). (From: Tiseo PJ, Rogers SL, Friedhoff LT. Pharmacokinetic and pharmacodynamic profile of donepezil HCl following evening administration. Br J Clin Pharmacol 1998;46[Suppl 1]:13–18.)

Major differences between rapidly and slowly equilibrating sites of action are apparent on administering a drug on a fixed-dose, fixed-interval regimen, as illustrated in Fig. 19-24. When drug at the effect site equilibrates rapidly, response follows the plasma concentration with minimal delay. When, however, equilibration is slow, it may take several doses before the maximal response is seen, even though the plasma concentration is at virtual steady state. In addition, on stopping administration, response wears off slowly and may remain noticeable long after the plasma concentration falls below detection. In the absence of such insight, there may be a temptation to mistakenly classify the drug as one that acts long after drug has been eliminated.

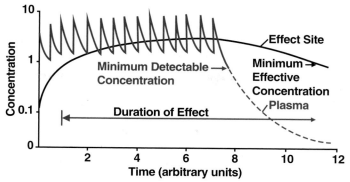

FIGURE 19-24. When distribution to and from a tissue where the drug acts is slow relative to elimination, drug in the tissue accumulates slowly on multiple dosing. This delays the onset of effect, even when the drug is given intravenously. After discontinuing drug administration, the plasma concentration may quickly fall below the detectable limit, but the concentration at the site of action may persist for some time. The dashed line represents the time course of the plasma concentration below the detection limit. (From: Gibaldi M, Levy G, Weintraub H. Drug distribution and pharmacologic effects. Clin Pharmacol Ther 1971;12:734–742. Reproduced with permission of Nature Publishing Group.)

Instead of fixing the dose and dosing interval, a safer approach to avoid excessively high concentrations is to give the same dose each time the effect reaches a predetermined value (e.g., just when the effect wears off). This approach can be used when there is a good biomarker to determine the response to the drug. It is common for drugs used in anesthesia, but is not practical for most situations. Before discussing the impact of distribution kinetics under these circumstances, first consider the events when the kinetics of the drug is adequately characterized by a one-compartment model (Fig. 19-25). With

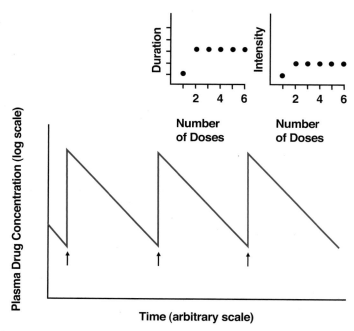

FIGURE 19-25. For a drug that displays one-compartment disposition kinetics, both the duration and the intensity of a graded response increase with the second, but not with subsequent bolus doses when each dose is given, indicated by an arrow, at the time the effect (or concentration) reaches a predetermined level.

this approach, an increase in duration and, if the response is graded, an increase in intensity is expected with the second dose. The reason is readily apparent. Immediately after giving the second dose, the amount in the body is not the dose, but *Dose + Amin*, where *Amin* is the minimum amount needed in the body. How much intensity or duration of effect increases, therefore, depends on the relative magnitude of *Dose* and *Amin*. If *Amin* is small relative to *Dose*, very little remains from the first dose when the second one is given, and little increase in response, or duration of effect, is expected. In contrast, large increases in both response and duration are expected when the response from the first dose wears off before much drug is lost. No further increase in intensity or duration of effect is anticipated with third or subsequent doses, because the amount in the body always returns to the same value, *Amin*, before the next dose is given. Stated differently, from the second dose onward, during each dosing interval, the amount lost equals the dose given.

Figure 19-26 depicts the events expected following the same dosing strategy just considered, except that the effect reaches the predetermined value during the distribution phase of the drug. Again, the second dose produces a higher concentration in plasma and all tissues of the body and a correspondingly more intense response and longer

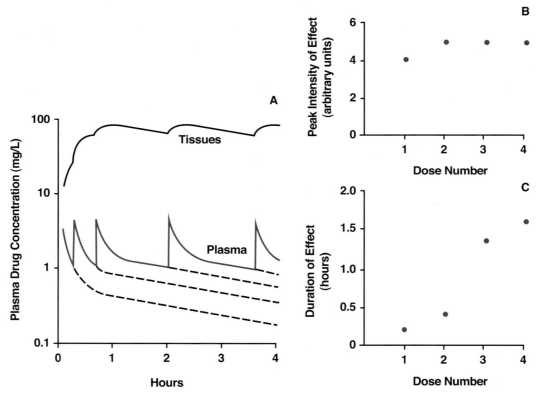

FIGURE 19-26. **A.** When the same dose size is administered repeatedly each time the response wears off and the response is directly related to the plasma concentration, the duration of response (time above a predetermined value following each successive dose) increases for a drug showing distribution kinetics. The increase in duration is explained by accrual of drug in tissues. This reduces the tendency for net movement from plasma into tissue and slows the decline of plasma concentration on repetitive dosing (*colored line*). Also shown is the plasma concentration expected had the successive doses not been given (– – –). **B.** Note that the peak intensity of response is expected to increase only with the second dose. **C.** In contrast to duration of effect, notice how duration increases dramatically when the time the response wears off moves into the terminal phase of the concentration–time curve (*graph A*).

duration of response than achieved after the first dose. However, on administering the third and successive doses, differences emerge from that expected for a drug displaying one-compartment characteristics (see Fig. 19-25). On repeated administration, drug in the slowly equilibrating tissues rises and the tendency to distribute out from blood and other rapidly equilibrating tissues diminishes. Accordingly, the duration of effect becomes progressively longer until, within a dosing interval, the amount eliminated from the body equals the dose administered. Only then are the concentrations of drug in all tissues the same at the beginning as at the end of the dosing interval. In contrast to duration, intensity of response does not increase beyond the second dose, because the concentration at the site of action just before the next dose is always the same.

The events shown in Fig. 19-27 with thiopental, for which response closely relates to plasma concentration, are illustrative of dosing to a minimum effect. Following repetitive i.v. dosing, the plasma concentration declines more slowly and the effect lasts longer after the second and third doses, even though these doses were smaller than the first to prevent too great a response. The data with thiopental also indicate that the brain is a rapidly equilibrating site, with a minimal delay in response. In addition, these data do not support a common suggestion that tolerance to the hypnotic effect of thiopental occurs acutely. If tolerance had occurred, the sensitivity to thiopental would have decreased; it would have been expressed as a higher C_{50} value. However, no such increase in C_{50} value with time is observed.

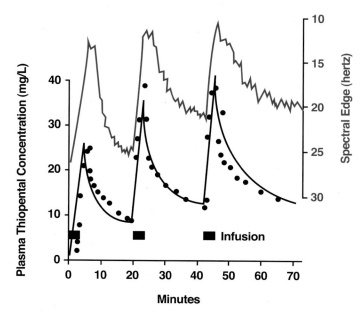

FIGURE 19-27. Both plasma concentration of thiopental (●) and spectral edge (*jagged colored line*), an electroencephalographic measure of anesthetic effect, were monitored in a subject who received three successive short-term i.v. infusions of thiopental. The tendency for concentration to fall in plasma and in rapidly equilibrating tissues such as the brain diminishes, and response is prolonged, on the second and third doses, associated with the rise of drug concentration in slowly equilibrating tissues. To minimize the increase in maximal effect, above that produced with the first dose (8.4 mg/kg), the sizes of the two successive doses were reduced (to 5.7 mg/kg). The solid line close to the plasma concentration values is the predicted concentration after fitting a biexponential disposition model to the plasma concentration–time data. Because thiopental produces a diminution in the spectral edge, the spectral edge scale is inverted for clarity. (From: Hudson RJ, Stanski DR, Saidman LJ, Meathe E. A model for studying depth of anesthesia and acute tolerance to thiopental. Anesthesiology 1985;59:301–308. Reproduced with permission of J.B. Lippincott.)

KEY RELATIONSHIPS

$$C = C_1 e^{-\lambda_1 \cdot t} + C_2 e^{-\lambda_2 \cdot t}$$

$$V_1 = \frac{Dose}{C_1 + C_2}$$

$$Dose = Clearance \cdot AUC$$

$$V = \frac{CL}{\lambda_2}$$

$$\begin{array}{c} \textit{Fraction of elimination associated} \\ \textit{with last exponential term} \end{array} = f_2 = \frac{C_2/\lambda_2}{AUC}$$

$$V_{ss} = \left(1 + \frac{k_{12}}{k_{21}}\right) \cdot V_1$$

$$V_{ss} = MRT \cdot CL$$

$$V_{ss} = Dose \frac{AUMC}{AUC^2}$$

$$V_{ss} = Dose \frac{\left(\dfrac{C_1}{\lambda_1^2} + \dfrac{C_2}{\lambda_1^2}\right)}{\left(\dfrac{C_1}{\lambda_1} + \dfrac{C_2}{\lambda_2}\right)^2}$$

$$\frac{C}{C_{ss}} = f_1 \cdot (1 - e^{-\lambda_1 \cdot t}) + f_2 \cdot (1 - e^{-\lambda_2 \cdot t})$$

STUDY PROBLEMS

(Answers to Study Problems are in Appendix J.)

1. Define the following terms: initial dilution volume, volume of distribution during the terminal phase, and volume of distribution at steady state.

2. Comment on the following statements:

   a. All drugs are expected to exhibit distribution kinetics.

   b. For most drugs, it is reasonable to represent the disposition kinetics by a compartmental model, with elimination occurring exclusively from the central compartment.

   c. Following an i.v. bolus dose, essentially the entire dose is eliminated from the body by 5 terminal plasma half-lives.

3. A single 30-mg i.v. dose of irbesartan (Avapro), a potent, long-acting angiotensin II receptor (AT_1) antagonist for treating hypertension, was given to a patient. The concentration–time profile in this subject is shown in Table 19-2 and displayed

TABLE 19-2	Irbesartan Plasma Concentration with Time in an Individual Subject after a 30-mg Intravenous Dose												
Time (hr)	0.5	1	1.5	2	3	4	6	8	12	16	24	36	48
Plasma irbesartan concentration (ng/mL)	4211	1793	808	405	168	122	101	88	67	51	30	13	6

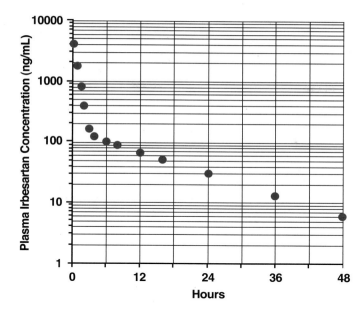

FIGURE 19-28.

semilogarithmically in Fig. 19-28. This problem was adapted from data in Vachharajani NH, Shyu WC, Chando TJ, et al. Oral bioavailability and disposition chacteristics of irbesartan, an angiotensin antagonist, in healthy volunteers. J Clin Pharmacol 1998;38:702–707.

a. Using the method of residuals, estimate the values (and units) of the parameters C_1, C_2, λ_1, λ_2 of the following biexponential equation: $C = C_1 e^{-\lambda_1 \cdot t} + C_2 e^{-\lambda_2 \cdot t}$.

b. Calculate the clearance of the drug.

c. Estimate the values for V_1 and V.

d. From the biexponential equation, predict the plasma concentrations at 45 min, 5 hr, and 11 hr after the bolus dose.

e. Had another 30-mg dose of irbesartan been administered 6 hr after the first, what is the plasma concentration 6 hr later?

f. What fraction of the dose has been eliminated associated with the initial exponential phase?

g. What is the elimination half-life of the drug?

h. The oral bioavailability of irbesartan is 0.8. What average plasma irbesartan concentration would you expect at steady state when 150 mg is given orally once daily, a common oral regimen?

4. Hamilton et al. (reference in Table 19-3) assessed the effect of acetylator phenotype on the disposition kinetics of amrinone, a positive inotropic agent with vasodilatory properties. The acetylator status was determined for the subjects with isoniazid. Each subject then received a 75-mg bolus dose intravenously (infused over 10 min). Table 19-3 lists the plasma concentration–time data in two subjects, one slow and one fast acetylator, both of equal weight. The drug is metabolized (probably in the liver) and is excreted unchanged.

a. Display semilogarithmic plots of both sets of data and determine the values of the parameters of the biexponential equations that fit each set of data: C_1, λ_1, C_2, and λ_2, using the method of residuals.

b. From the parameter values obtained in *a*, calculate *CL*, V_1, *V*, *MRT*, and V_{ss} for each subject. Which of these parameters show(s) major differences between the slow and fast acetylator phenotypes?

c. Is the assumption that the liver and kidneys are part of the initial dilution volume reasonable?

	Plasma Concentration (mg/L)	
Time (hr)	**Slow Acetylator**	**Fast Acetylator**
0.16	1.30	1.20
0.25	1.03	0.93
0.33	0.89	0.76
0.5	0.72	0.54
0.67	0.64	0.42
1	0.59	0.31
2	0.52	0.19
3	0.47	0.13
4	0.42	ND
8	0.27	ND
12	0.17	ND
15	0.12	ND

TABLE 19-3   Plasma Concentrations of Amrinone in Slow and Fast Acetylators

ND, below detection limit of assay.
From: Hamilton RA, Kowalsky SF, Wright EM, et al. Effect of acetylator phenotype on amrinone pharmacokinetics. Clin Pharmaocol Ther 1986;40:615–619.

   d. Had data only been available from 1 hr onward so that only the terminal phase is evident, what values for *V* and *CL* would be calculated? Compare and comment on these values for the slow and fast acetylators with those obtained in *b*.
   e. For each subject, what fraction of the dose eliminated is associated with the second exponential term.
   f. Is it reasonable to conclude, for both subjects, that the terminal half-life principally determines the time to reach a plateau in plasma following a constant-rate infusion?

5. In Fig. 20-9 (Chapter 20, *Metabolites and Drug Response*), the plasma concentrations of the benzodiazepine halazepam are shown during and following an oral dosage regimen of 40 mg of the drug every 8 hr for 14 days.

   a. Why is the plasma concentration of halazepam fluctuating markedly even at steady state?
   b. Can the terminal half-life of halazepam be determined well during administration of the dosage regimen?

6. A moderately polar drug is eliminated entirely by renal excretion. Following a 50-mg i.v. bolus dose to a 68-kg healthy subject, the plasma concentration was observed to decline biexponentially: C (mg/L) $= 2.71 \, e^{-0.19t} + 0.034 \, e^{-0.00095t}$, where t is in hours. The fraction of the drug in plasma unbound is 0.37 and is independent of drug concentration over the range seen in plasma.

   a. Given that elimination occurs only from the initial dilution volume (central compartment), calculate the following pharmacokinetic parameters: V_1, CL, V, V_{ss}.
   b. Comment on the mechanism of renal excretion of the drug and the appropriateness of the assumption that elimination occurs only from the central compartment.
   c. Comment on the large difference between V and V_{ss}.
   d. Calculate the fractions of the dose eliminated that are associated with each exponential term, and comment on the question, "What is the half-life of the drug?"

e. The drug is given by a constant-rate infusion.

1. Using an iterative procedure, calculate how long it takes for the plasma concentration to reach 50% and 90% of the steady-state value. Comment on the statement, "It takes 1 half-life to reach 50% of plateau and 3.3 half-lives to reach plateau."

2. Comment on why a pronounced biexponential curve is still seen during the postinfusion decline of the plasma concentration after steady state has been reached.

3. Would you expect to have detected a biexponential curve on stopping the infusion at steady state had the disposition kinetics of the drug following a 50-mg bolus dose been defined by the equation $C(t) = 0.56e^{-0.19t} + 0.14e^{-0.0095t}$ (t in hours). That is, the same biexponential coefficients (and half-lives), such as the drug discussed previously, but different coefficients.

7. Briefly discuss the uses and limitations of exponential equations versus compartmental models to represent disposition kinetics of drugs in the context of:

a. Predicting the events following a constant-rate infusion.

b. Accounting for variability among individuals in terms of covariates such as body weight and renal function.

8. The fractions of drug normally excreted unchanged after i.v. administration of both the neuromuscular-blocking agents d-tubocurarine and pancuronium are similar at approximately 0.65. However, as seen in Fig 19-29, the effect of compromised renal function on the disposition kinetics of these drugs is different. For pancuronium, the terminal half-life is prolonged, whereas for d-tubocurarine the terminal half-life is unchanged. Briefly discuss the reason for the difference in the effect of renal dysfunction on these two drugs.

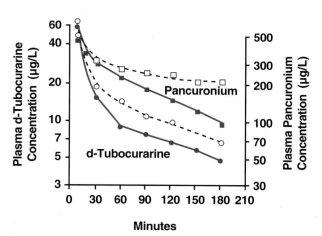

FIGURE 19-29. The disposition kinetics of d-tubocurarine (○,●) and pancuronium (□,■) in patients with normal (*colored lines*) and impaired renal function (——). (From: Miller RD. Pharmacokinetics of muscle relaxants and their antagonists. In: Pry-Roberts C, Hug CC, eds. Pharmacokinetics of Anesthesia. Oxford: Blackwell Scientific Publications Limited; 1984:255).

9. A continuous infusion of the anesthetic agent propofol has been widely used for sedation of critically ill patients in the intensive care unit. Figure 19-30 from the 2003 *Physicians' Desk Reference* shows the concentration–time profile on infusing 1.0 mg/kg per hour for 5 hr after coronary artery bypass surgery. The solid bar represents the duration of the infusion.

Figure 19-31 from the 2004 *Physicians' Desk Reference* illustrates the fall in plasma propofol concentration following intensive care unit sedation infusions of various durations. Briefly discuss why the duration of anesthesia after stopping an infusion is prolonged the longer the infusion of propofol. You may wish to review the material previously presented on propofol on pages 272 and 273.

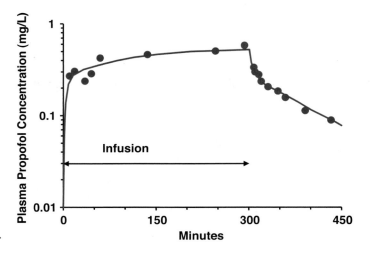

FIGURE 19-30.

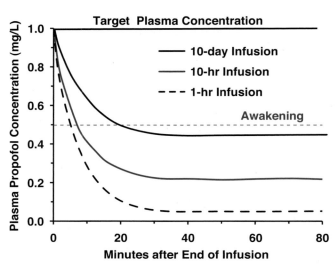

FIGURE 19-31.

10. Listed in Table 19-4 are the disposition kinetic parameters of three i.v. anaesthetic drugs such as alfentanil, fentanyl, and sufentanil. Notice that each requires the sum of three exponential terms to describe adequately the kinetics after single i.v. bolus doses.

One of the critical factors in the use of these drugs is the time taken for the plasma concentration to fall on stopping administration. Generally, the shorter the time, the quicker a patient recovers, a desirable characteristic.

The subsequent equations describe the plasma concentration at the end of an infusion of duration τ, $C(\tau)$, and the fraction of that concentration at time t_{post} after stopping the infusion: $C(\tau) = C_{ss} \cdot [f_1(1 - e^{-\lambda_1 \tau}) + f_2(1 - e^{-\lambda_2 \tau}) + f_3(1 - e^{-\lambda_3 \tau})]$.

Fraction of $C(\tau)$ at

$$t_{post} = [f_1(1 - e^{-\lambda_1 \tau}) \, e^{-\lambda_1 t_{post}} + f_2(1 - e^{-\lambda_2 \tau}) \, e^{-\lambda_2 t_{post}} + f_3(1 - e^{-\lambda_3 \tau}) \, e^{-\lambda_3 t_{post}}]/C(\tau),$$

where

$$f_1 = \frac{\dfrac{C'_1}{\lambda_1}}{\left(\dfrac{C'_1}{\lambda_1} + \dfrac{C'_2}{\lambda_2} + \dfrac{C'_3}{\lambda_3}\right)}, \quad f_2 = \frac{\dfrac{C'_2}{\lambda_2}}{\left(\dfrac{C'_1}{\lambda_1} + \dfrac{C'_2}{\lambda_2} + \dfrac{C'_3}{\lambda_3}\right)} \quad \text{and } f_3 = 1 - f_1 - f_2$$

TABLE 19-4	**Disposition Kinetic Parameters of Three Intravenous Anesthetic Drugs**		
Drug parameters	**Alfentanil**	**Fentanyl**	**Sufentanil**
$C_1'^{,*}$	0.83	0.90	0.84
$\lambda_1 (min^{-1})$	1.03	0.67	0.48
C_2'	0.12	0.08	0.15
$\lambda_2 (min^{-1})$	0.052	0.037	0.030
C_3'	0.050	0.020	0.010
$\lambda_3 (min^{-1})$	0.0062	0.0015	0.0012
Terminal half-life (min)	111	462	577

$*C_1' = C_1/(C_1 + C_2 + C_3); C_2' = C_2/(C_1 + C_2 + C_3); C_3' = 1 - C_1' - C_2'$
From: Hughes MA, Glass PSA, Jacobs JR. Context-sensitive half-time in multicompartment pharmacokinetic models for i.v. anesthetic drugs. Anesthesiology 1992;76:334–341.

C_1', C_2', and C_3' are defined in the footnote of Table 19-4. These equations are expansions of those given in the legend to Fig. 19-8, which apply when the disposition kinetics are described by a biexponential equation.

a. Calculate the values of f_1, f_2, and hence f_3 for alfentanil, fentanyl, and sufentanil.
b. Calculate the fraction of the final concentration for each drug at the following times after stopping an infusion of 1-hr duration ($\tau = 60$ min).
   Alfentanil $t_{post} = 24.5$ min
   Fentanyl $t_{post} = 15.6$ min
   Sufentanil $t_{post} = 14.8$ min
c. Given that the patient awakens when the plasma concentration falls by 50% after stopping the 1-hr infusion, by reference to your answer to *b*, comment on the utility of the terminal half-life (see Table 19-4) in predicting duration of action of the three i.v. anesthetic drugs.
d. Would the ranking be any different if the plasma concentration had to fall by 50% after stopping an infusion at steady state before the patient awakens? (Hint: In answering this question, you need to determine, by iteration, the value of t_{post} in each of the above equations that gives a fraction of the steady-state concentration of 0.5).
e. Comment on the impact of the duration of infusion when attempting to rank the duration of action of these three drugs on stopping administration.

11. Table 19-5 lists the duration of effect achieved with the neuromuscular-blocking agent pancuronium following administration of a 0.02 mg/kg i.v. dose each time the response returned to 10% of maximal effect. Assume that drug at the site of action rapidly equilibrates with drug in plasma.

   a. Suggest why the duration of effect progressively increases each time a dose is administered.
   b. Will the duration of effect continue to increase if drug administration continues to be administered in the same manner?

TABLE 19-5	**Neuromuscular Blocking Effect of Successive Doses* of Pancuronium**			
Dose number	1	2	3	4
Duration of effect (min)[†]	14	20	36	>54

* 0.02 mg/kg i.v.
[†]Time to recover 90% of normal function.
From: Gibaldi M, Levy G, Weintraub H. Commentary. Drug distribution and pharmacologic effects. Clin Pharmacol Ther 1971;12(5):734–742; original data from: Norman J, Katz RL, Seed RF. The neuromuscular blocking action of pancuronium in man during anaesthesia. Br J Anaesth 1970;42(8):702–710.

12. The concentration–time profile of testosterone (Fig. 19-32) in an elderly man with coronary artery disease after infusion of 300 μg (dissolved in 0.3 mL of 95% alcohol and diluted into 50 mL of normal saline). For the purpose of this problem, assume that a true i.v. bolus had been administered. The concentration of the exogenously administered drug was obtained by subtracting the essentially constant baseline (3.6 μg/L or 360 ng/dL, the common units of serum testosterone) from the measured value.

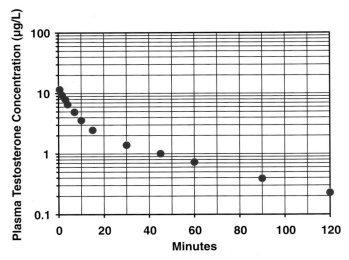

FIGURE 19-32. Serum testosterone concentration with time in an individual patient with coronary artery disease. (From: White CM, Ferraro-Borgida MJ, Moyna NM, et al. The pharmacokinetics of intravenous testosterone in elderly men with coronary artery disease. J Clin Pharmacol 1998;38:792–797.)

a. Determine the *approximate* values (C_1, λ_1, C_2, λ_2) of the biexponential equation ($C = C_1 e^{-\lambda_1 t} + C_2 e^{-\lambda_2 t}$) that describes the concentration–time profile of the exogenously administered drug.

b. Does the rate constant of the first or the second term more closely relate to the elimination half-life of testosterone? State how you come to your conclusion.

c. Calculate the clearance of testosterone in this individual.

d. In the individual mentioned, the baseline testosterone serum concentration was 3.6 μg/L. Estimate the daily rate of production (mg/day) of endogenous testosterone in this individual.

Metabolites and Drug Response

OBJECTIVES

The reader will be able to:

- State the pharmacokinetic parameters that influence the area under the metabolite concentration-time curve after a single dose and the average plasma metabolite concentration and amount of metabolite in the body following a multiple-dose regimen.

- Determine if elimination of a metabolite is rate-limited by its formation after a single intravenous (i.v.) dose of drug.

- Determine if total clearance of a metabolite is less than that of its parent drug, given plasma concentration-time data for both drug and metabolite following i.v. drug administration.

- Describe the consequence of hepatic extraction on plasma metabolite concentrations following oral administration of both high and low hepatic extraction ratio drugs.

- State the pharmacokinetic parameters that control the concentration of metabolite at plateau following administration of drug as either a constant-rate i.v. infusion or an oral multiple-dose regimen.

- Describe why elimination half-life of metabolite, and not the half-life of the drug, is the determinant of accrual of metabolite, when a constant amount of drug is initiated (loading dose) and maintained (with constant-rate infusion) in the body.

- Describe why elimination half-life of the slowest step, drug elimination or metabolite elimination, controls accrual of metabolite following drug administration either by constant-rate i.v. infusion or an oral multiple-dose regimen.

- Calculate the average plateau concentration of metabolite following an oral multiple-dose drug regimen, given the dosing interval and the area under the curve (*AUC*) of the metabolite after a single dose of the drug.

- Discuss the need to adjust the maintenance dosing rate of a drug in a patient with end-stage renal disease when all the activity (desired and adverse) resides with the metabolite under the following scenarios:

  - The formation of the metabolite is the major pathway for drug elimination.

  - The formation of the metabolite is a minor route of drug elimination. The major route is renal excretion.

  - The formation of the metabolite is a minor route of drug elimination, but the metabolite is almost exclusively eliminated by renal excretion.

- Explain why the half-life of a drug, which is renally excreted unchanged to only a small extent and undergoes interconversion with a metabolite, can increase substantially in patients with renal function impairment.

- Calculate the apparent fraction of drug converted to a metabolite using *AUC* measurements of drug and metabolite after separate i.v. doses of each.
- Describe the potential influence of an active metabolite to the total response following drug administration when the metabolite is a competitive agonist with parent drug.
- Discuss the kinetic consequences of nonlinearities in the formation or elimination of a metabolite.

CONTRIBUTION OF METABOLITES TO DRUG RESPONSE

T he reason for our interest and concern with metabolites can be summed up in five words: action, toxicity, inhibition, induction, and displacement. All too often, metabolites are thought of as weakly active or inactive waste products. For many, this is so, but as seen in Table 20-1, for many others it is not. Sometimes, the agent administered is an inert prodrug, which depends on metabolism for activation. Examples are enalapril, which is hydrolyzed to enalaprilat, an active angiotensin-converting enzyme inhibitor, and prazepam, which is metabolized to the active benzodiazepine desmethyldiazepam. Some metabolites have pharmacologic properties in common with the parent drug and augment its effect. Some metabolites have a different pharmacologic profile and may even be the cause of toxicity; whereas others are inactive but may, by acting as inhibitors, prolong or enhance the response to a drug or, as inducers, reduce the response. Still, others may affect the disposition of a drug by competing for plasma and tissue-binding sites or inhibit secretion or reabsorption in the renal tubule. It is not sufficient, however, to know that a metabolite possesses any or all of these properties. Unless a sufficient concentration exists to substantially exert any of these effects, the presence of a metabolite is of little therapeutic concern.

TABLE 20-1	**Representative Therapeutically Important Metabolites**		
Compound Administered	**Metabolite**	**Compound Administered**	**Metabolite**
Acetylsalicylic acid	Salicylic Acid	Isosorbide dinitrate	Isosorbide-5-mononitrate
Amiodarone	Desethylamiodarone	Lidocaine	Desethyllidocaine
Amitriptyline	Nortriptyline	Meperidine	Normeperidine
Carbamazepine	Carbamazepine-10, 11-epoxide	Morphine	Morphine-6-glucuronide
Cefotaxime	Desacetylcefotaxime	Pentoxifylline	5-hydroxypentoxifylline
Chlordiazepoxide	Desmethylchlordiazepoxide	Prazepam	Desmethyldiazepam
Chlorpromazine	7-hydroxychlorpromazine	Prednisone	Prednisone
Codeine	Morphine	Primidone	Phenobarbital
Diazepam	Desmethyldiazepam	Propranolol	4-Hydroxypropranolol
Diltiazem	Desacetyldiltiazem	Quinidine	3-Hydroxyquinidine
Enalapril	Enalaprilat	Sulindac	Sulindac sulfide
Encainide	O-desmethylencainide	Verapamil	Norverapamil
Fluoxetine	Norfluoxetine	Zidovudine	Zidovudine triphosphate
Imipramine	Desipramine		

This chapter examines the factors that influence the kinetics of metabolites in the body and the consequences that ensue, including some aspects of pharmacodynamics. The pathways involved and the sites of drug metabolism are discussed in Chapter 5, *Elimination.* For purposes of clarity, unless otherwise stated, it is assumed that the body acts as a single compartment for both drug and metabolites, that all kinetic processes are first order, and that no change in plasma protein binding of either drug or metabolite occurs.

Information about a metabolite is usually obtained following drug administration. Although this information is arguably the most relevant to drug therapy, situations do arise that require more specific information on the pharmacokinetics and activity of the metabolite. Then, the metabolite must be administered separately. This chapter, however, emphasizes the pharmacokinetics and pharmacodynamics of metabolites after drug administration.

SINGLE DOSE OF DRUG

RATE-LIMITING STEP

To appreciate the factors influencing the amount of metabolite in the body, $A(m)$, with time following a single i.v. dose of drug, consider the scheme:

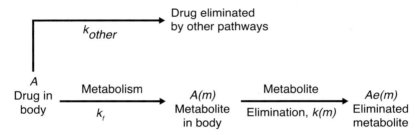

in which a fraction of drug in the body is converted to a metabolite that, in turn, is eliminated. The two steps, formation and elimination of metabolite, are characterized by the respective first-order rate constants k_f and $k(m)$. The overall elimination rate constant of drug (k) is the sum of k_f and k_{other}, the rate constant for other routes of drug elimination. Also, at any time

$$\begin{array}{c} \text{Rate of change of} \\ \text{amount of metabolite} \\ \text{in body} \end{array} = \underset{\substack{\text{Rate of} \\ \text{formation}}}{k_f \cdot A} - \underset{\substack{\text{Rate of} \\ \text{elimination}}}{k(m) \cdot A(m)} \qquad 20\text{-}1$$

Strictly speaking, $k_f \cdot A$ refers to rate of entry of metabolite into the systemic circulation. It may not be its rate of formation. Sometimes, a metabolite formed within an organ is further metabolized while there, so that only a fraction of the formed metabolite is released from the organ into the bloodstream. This is referred to as **sequential metabolism** during passage through an organ. A metabolite formed within the liver may also be excreted into the feces via the bile. For simplicity, in the subsequent discussion, only the case in which all of the metabolite formed reaches the systemic circulation is considered.

In the scheme above, either drug or metabolite elimination can rate limit the elimination of metabolite; the rate-limiting step has the smaller rate constant. Figure 20-1, displaying two semilogarithmic plots of the amounts of drug and metabolite in the body against time following a single dose of drug, shows the consequence of a rate limitation in each step.

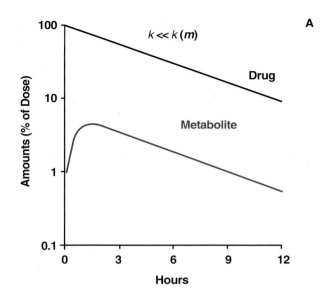

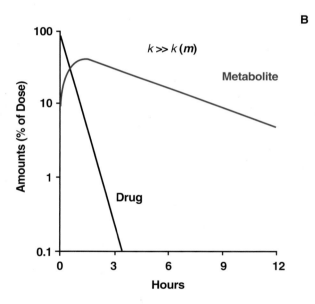

FIGURE 20-1. Consequences of a rate limitation shown in semilogarithmic plots of drug and metabolite. **A.** When the elimination rate constant of the drug is smaller than that of metabolite, $k \ll k(m)$, metabolite (*colored line*) declines in parallel with the drug (*black line*). **B.** Conversely, when the elimination-rate constant of metabolite is smaller than that of drug, $k \ll k(m)$, metabolite (*colored line*) declines more slowly than drug (*black line*). In the former case (*A*), decline of metabolite is governed by elimination of drug and, in the latter case (*B*), by its own elimination. The graphs are simulated using k_f, k_{other}, and $k(m)$ values of 0.2, 0, and 2 hr^{-1}, respectively, in the former case, and 2, 0, and 0.2 hr^{-1}, respectively in the latter.

A rate limitation in drug elimination, the most common situation, has several consequences (Fig. 20-1A). First, the half-life of the metabolite appears to be the same as that of the drug, but it is much longer than that seen when administered separately. Second, there is always more drug than metabolite in the body. Last, *metabolite elimination is formation rate-limited* (i.e., metabolite is cleared so rapidly that during its decline phase, whatever is formed is almost immediately eliminated). Approximately, therefore

$$\underbrace{k(m) \cdot A(m)}_{\substack{\text{Elimination rate} \\ \text{of metabolite}}} \approx \underbrace{k_f \cdot A}_{\substack{\text{Formation rate} \\ \text{of metabolite}}} \qquad \text{20-2}$$

and on rearranging,

$$\underset{\substack{\text{Amount of metabolite} \\ \text{in body}}}{} \approx \frac{k_f}{A} \cdot \underset{\substack{\text{Amount in drug} \\ \text{in body}}}{} \qquad \text{20-3}$$

In this case, the metabolite declines with the same half-life as the drug. Obviously, throughout the decline phase, the rate of elimination of metabolite exceeds that of its formation; otherwise, the amount of metabolite would not decline. But the difference in the rates is small.

A metabolite accrues substantially in the body only when its elimination is the slower step. That is, the half-life of metabolite is longer than that of the drug. When this occurs, most of the drug is eliminated by the time the metabolite peaks; decline of metabolite is subsequently controlled by its elimination half-life.

In Eqs. 20-1 to 20-3, $k(m)$ refers to the rate constant for metabolite elimination. Just how many pathways are involved in metabolite elimination is not important. What is important is to know whether drug or metabolite elimination is the rate-limiting step. In any sequence, substances formed beyond the rate-limiting step decline with the half-life of this slowest step. To emphasize this point consider the following scheme:

$$
A \xrightarrow[0.3]{\overset{0.03}{\nearrow} C \quad 0.2} B \xrightarrow{1.5} E \xrightarrow[8.2]{\overset{2.2}{\nearrow} F} G \xrightarrow{0.05} H \xrightarrow{0.5} I \xrightarrow{2.0} J
$$

in which A refers to the drug, B, E, G, H, and I refer to sequentially formed metabolites, J is the excreted metabolite I, and the number above each arrow is the value of the respective rate constant in hr^{-1}.

Question: What is the rate-limiting step in the entire sequence?
Answer: Elimination of metabolite G, terminal elimination half-life $(t_{1/2}) = 0.693/0.05 =$ 13.9 hr.
Question: What are the terminal half-lives for decay of A, B, E, H, and I from the body following administration of drug?
Answer: Elimination of A rate-limits decline of B and E, $t_{1/2} = 0.693/(0.03 + 0.2 + 0.3)$ = 1.31 hr for all three components. Elimination of G rate-limits terminal decline of H and I, $t_{1/2} = 0.693/0.05$ $hr^{-1} = 13.9$ hr.

Occasionally, the half-lives of drug and metabolite are comparable, and then neither step is rate-limiting. However, metabolite declines somewhat more slowly than anticipated from its half-life, because some drug remains to sustain the level of metabolite throughout its elimination.

PLASMA CONCENTRATION

The preceding discussion, helpful in realizing the importance of rate-limiting steps, deals with amounts of drug and metabolite in the body. However, plasma concentrations are measured and are of greater interest. Furthermore, in most cases, a metabolite has not been cleared for human use by regulatory authorities to permit determination of its volume of distribution, and therefore, its amount in the body. However, much can be gained from clearance concepts, as illustrated in several examples.

The first example concerns methylprednisolone. Owing to its low solubility, formulation of an i.v. preparation is difficult. Yet, clinical situations (e.g., treatment of shock) sometimes demand rapid input of this steroid. One solution has been to administer the water-soluble hemisuccinate ester, which is rapidly hydrolyzed to methylprednisolone by esterases within the body. Shown in Fig. 20-2 are the plasma concentrations of both the hemisuccinate and methylprednisolone following an i.v. bolus dose of the ester. It is readily apparent that the hemisuccinate is so rapidly hydrolyzed to steroid that elimination of methylprednisolone in its decline phase is not rate-limited by its formation.

These data also permit the conclusion to be drawn that the clearance of methylprednisolone (metabolite), $CL(m)$, is much lower than that of its hemisuccinate. The argument is as follows:

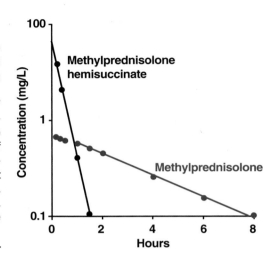

FIGURE 20-2. Displayed semilogarithmically are the plasma concentrations of methylprednisolone (●) and its water-soluble hemisuccinate ester (●) following an i.v. bolus injection of 80 mg of the ester; mean of 11 subjects. The decline of methylprednisolone ($t_{1/2} = 2.7$ hr) is rate-limited by its disposition, not by the disposition of its hemisuccinate ester ($t_{1/2} = 0.25$ hr). The clearance of methylprednisolone is lower than that of its hemisuccinate, a conclusion drawn from the observation (seen on a corresponding linear plot) that the AUC of methylprednisolone is the larger of the two. (From: Derendorf H, Mollmann H, Rohdeward P, et al. Kinetics of methylprednisolone and its hemisuccinate ester. Clin Pharmacol Ther 1985;37:502–507.)

At any time,

$$\begin{array}{c} \textit{Rate of change of} \\ \textit{amount of metabolite} \\ \textit{in body} \end{array} = \underbrace{CL_f \cdot C}_{\substack{\text{Rate of} \\ \text{formation}}} - \underbrace{CL(m) \cdot C(m)}_{\substack{\text{Rate of} \\ \text{elimination}}} \qquad \text{20-4}$$

where CL_f is the clearance associated with the hydrolysis of the hemisuccinate ester to methylprednisolone, sometimes referred to as the *formation clearance*, $CL(m)$ is the total clearance of this metabolite, and C and $C(m)$ are the respective plasma concentrations of drug and metabolite.

Integrating the foregoing equation after a single i.v. dose of drug gives the amount of metabolite in the body with time. Because no methylprednisolone is present in the body initially or at infinity, it follows, upon integrating Eq. 20-4 between these time limits, that

$$\frac{AUC(m)}{AUC} = \frac{CL_f}{CL(m)} \qquad \text{20-5}$$

where $AUC(m)$ and AUC are the total areas under the metabolite and drug concentration-time profiles, respectively. Substituting $fm \cdot CL$ for CL_f, where fm is the fraction of an i.v. dose of drug converted to systemically available metabolite, the following relationship is obtained:

$$\frac{AUC(m)}{AUC} = fm \cdot \frac{\textit{Clearance of drug}}{\textit{Clearance of metabolite}} \qquad \text{20-6}$$

Returning to Fig. 20-2, the data suggest that the area for methylprednisolone ($AUC[m]$) is greater than that for the administered ester (AUC). Calculation confirms this; the respective areas are 3.9 and 2.1 mg-hr/L. Accordingly, because the value of fm cannot exceed unity, the clearance of methylprednisolone must be less than that of its ester. If the ratio of areas had been less than 1, then the ratio of the total clearance values cannot be assessed unless the value of fm is known. Had fm been smaller than the ratio of areas, the ratio of clearances could have been greater than one. Because no knowledge of the amount of drug in the body is necessary to arrive at the above conclusions, this area method of interpreting metabolite data can be extremely useful, especially in cases of drug poisoning in which the amounts ingested and absorbed are frequently unknown.

The second example deals with propranolol. Based on the data in Fig. 20-3, obtained after giving propranolol intravenously, the drug has the following characteristics: total clearance, 1.1 L/min; volume of distribution, 380 L; and elimination half-life, 4 hr. Other data suggest that almost the entire dose is metabolized in the liver. Metabolites of propranolol include one or more glucuronides and naphthoxylactic acid, which was measured specifically in this study. What can be learned from the data displayed semilogarithmically in Fig. 20-3?

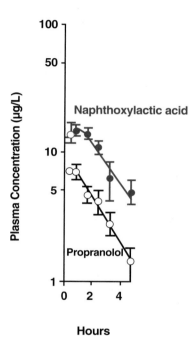

FIGURE 20-3. Semilogarithmic plot of the plasma concentrations of propranolol (○) and of one of its metabolites, naphthoxylactic acid (●), (mean ± SEM) after a single i.v. dose of 3.7-mg propranolol to three subjects. Note that the elevated metabolite concentration declines in parallel with parent drug because of a lower total clearance and a smaller volume of distribution of naphthoxylactic acid compared with propranolol. For a strict comparison, the naphthoxylactic acid should be expressed in propranolol equivalents, but the difference in their molecular weights (260 and 284 g/mol, respectively) is small. (From: Walle T, Conradi EC, Walle K, et al. Naphthoxylactic acid after single and long-term doses of propranolol. Clin Pharmacol Ther 1979;26:548–554. Reproduced with permission of Mosby CV.)

From considerations of areas of drug and metabolite, one must conclude that the clearance of naphthoxylactic acid is much lower than that of propranolol. However, the parallel decay of metabolite and drug indicates that elimination of this metabolite is rate-limited by its formation. Hence, the elimination half-life of this more polar metabolite must be shorter, and amount in the body always lower than that of the parent drug (see Fig. 20-1A).

The only explanation consistent with these observations is that volume of distribution of metabolite, $V(m)$, must be smaller than that of parent drug by a factor even greater than the ratio of clearance values. This conclusion follows from a comparison of the elimination-rate constants for metabolite and drug:

$$\frac{k(m)}{k} = \frac{\dfrac{CL(m)}{CL}}{\dfrac{V(m)}{V}} \qquad\qquad 20\text{-}7$$

For $k(m)/k$ to be greater than 1, the ratio $V(m)/V$ must be smaller than $CL(m)/CL$. Confirming this conclusion is a concentration of metabolite much higher than that of the parent drug (see Fig. 20-3), despite a much lower amount of metabolite in the body when elimination of metabolite is formation rate-limited (see Fig. 20-1A). The findings with propranolol are quite commonly encountered, particularly with basic drugs that are converted to acidic metabolites. The volumes of distribution of basic drugs are often in excess of 100 L (1.4 L/kg), whereas those of their acidic metabolites are closer to 10 to 20 L (0.14–0.30 L/kg). These metabolites not only are more polar and tend to bind less to tissue constituents than the parent drug, but also are bound more strongly to albumin, thereby further restricting their tissue distribution.

Kinetically, giving an i.v. bolus of drug and measuring the plasma metabolite concentration is similar to giving an oral dose of drug and measuring its plasma concentration. In both situations, the appearance and disappearance of species (metabolite in one case, drug in the other) are monitored after placing a bolus dose in the preceding compartment; thus,

Formation and elimination of metabolite after i.v. bolus of drug

$$A \xrightarrow{\ k_f\ } A(m) \xrightarrow{\ k(m)\ }$$

A		$A(m)$	
Drug	Metabolism	Metabolite	Elimination
in body		in body	of metabolite

Absorption and elimination of drug after a single oral dose

$$Aa \xrightarrow{\ ka\ } A \xrightarrow{\ k\ }$$

Aa		A	
Drug at	Absorption	Drug	Elimination
absorption site		in body	of drug

Recall from Chapter 6, *Kinetics Following an Extravascular Dose,* that the peak plasma concentration of a drug given extravascularly reflects the balance between rates of drug absorption and elimination. Correspondingly, the 1.5 to 2 hr required for naphthoxylactic acid to reach a peak in Fig. 20-3 reflects the balance between its rates of formation and elimination.

The last example concerns tolbutamide, an effective oral hypoglycemic agent. This drug is extensively metabolized to hydroxytolbutamide, which, although active, is therapeutically unimportant. As seen in Fig. 20-4, the concentrations of hydroxytolbutamide are so low that they never augment the effect of tolbutamide. One possible explanation

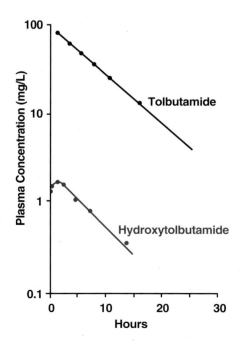

FIGURE 20-4. A subject receives a 1-g i.v. bolus of tolbutamide. The concentration of tolbutamide in plasma falls with a half-life of 4 hr. Although oxidation to hydroxytolbutamide is almost obligatory for tolbutamide elimination, the plasma concentration of this metabolite is always very low, owing to its extremely high clearance. As a consequence, because the volumes of distribution are similar (0.15–0.30 L/kg), $k(m) \gg k$, oxidation of tolbutamide rate-limits hydroxytolbutamide elimination. (From: Matin SB, Rowland M. Determination of tolbutamide and metabolites in biological fluids. Anal Letters 1973;6:865–876.)

for the low concentration of metabolite is that little is formed. However, in the case of tolbutamide, based on urinary recovery, almost all the drug is converted to hydroxytolbutamide. That is, *fm* is close to 1. Accordingly, the 20-fold ratio of drug and metabolite areas reflects a corresponding ratio in total clearance values, with that of hydroxytolbutamide being the much higher of the two.

IMPACT OF HEPATIC EXTRACTION

Ingesting drugs that are cleared by the liver is like taking a mixture of drug and metabolite. The reason, as mentioned in Chapter 2, *Fundamental Concepts and Terminology*, is that all ingested drug must pass through the liver before entering the general circulation. The composition of the mixture leaving the liver depends on the hepatic extraction ratio of the drug. When the extraction ratio is high, metabolism during absorption is extensive, and the situation comes close to that of administering just metabolite. Table 20-2 lists some drugs undergoing extensive first-pass hepatic elimination and forming active metabolites. Caution must be taken against attempting to relate plasma drug concentration alone to effect following oral administration of such drugs.

TABLE 20-2	Representative Drugs Undergoing First-Pass Hepatic Extraction and Having Active Metabolites		
Drug	**Active Metabolite***	**Drug**	**Active Metabolite***
Alprenolol	4-Hydroxyalprenolol	Imipramine	Desipramine
Amitriptyline	Nortriptyline	Isosorbide dinitrate	Isosorbide-5-mononitrate
Buspirone	1-Pyrimidinylpiperazine	Meperidine	Normeperidine
Codeine	Morphine	Metaprolol	α-Hydroxymetoprolol
Desipramine	10-Hydroxydesipramine	Morphine	Morphine-6-glucuronide
Dextropropoxyphene	Norpropoxyphene	Naloxone	6-β-Hydroxynaloxone
Dihydroergotamine	8-Hydroxydilhydroergotamine	Pentoxifylline	5-Hydroxypentoxifylline
Diltiazem	Descetyldiltiazem	Propranolol	4-Hydroxypropranolol
Doxepin	Desmethyldoxepin	Quinidine	3(S)-Hydroxyquinidine
Encainide	O-Desmethylencainide	Verapamil	Norverapamil

*For some drugs, more than one active metabolite is formed.

To appreciate the impact of first passage of drug through the liver on the plasma concentration of metabolite, consider the data in Fig. 20-5 obtained following oral administration of propranolol. Compared with the situation following an i.v. dose (see Fig. 20-3), the naphthoxylactic acid-to-propranolol concentration ratio is much higher, and the metabolite concentration peaks as early as the parent drug. These observations are understood by examining the following scheme:

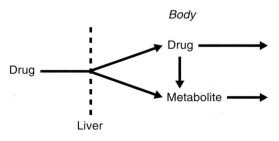

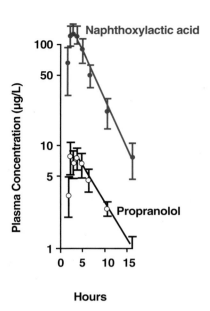

FIGURE 20-5. Semilogarithmic plot of the plasma concentrations of propranolol (○) and naphthoxylactic acid (●), (mean ± SEM) after a single 20-mg oral dose of propranolol to five subjects. As a consequence of extensive hepatic metabolism, only a small fraction of the dose is absorbed intact. The remainder appears as metabolites, such as naphthoxylactic acid, which reaches a peak value at the same time as propranolol, 1.5 to 2 hr after drug administration. For a strict comparison, the naphthoxylactic acid should be expressed in propranolol equivalents, but the difference in their molecular weights (260 and 284 g/mol, respectively) is small. (From: Walle T, Conradi EC, Walle K, et al. Naphthoxylactic acid after single and long-term doses of propranolol. Clin Pharmacol Ther 1979;26:548–554. Reproduced with permission of Mosby CV.)

As anticipated from its high hepatic clearance and confirmed by comparing AUC values after oral and i.v. administration with correction for differences in dose, only 21% of an oral dose of propranolol filters past the liver; most of the dose enters the body directly as metabolites. The small fraction of propranolol absorbed systemically is then handled like an i.v. dose of the drug. Thus, the observed concentration of each metabolite is the sum of the amounts derived from the two sources (Fig. 20-6).

The therapeutic implications of the preceding discussion depend on the activities of drug and metabolite. A shorter onset and a more intense response may occur when giving a compound orally, rather than parenterally, if the compound is a prodrug, is rapidly absorbed, and undergoes extensive first-pass conversion to an active metabolite. Furthermore, a low bioavailability of prodrug does not mean a poor therapeutic effect following chronic oral administration. On the other hand, if only the administered compound is active, a larger oral than parenteral dose is required to achieve and maintain an

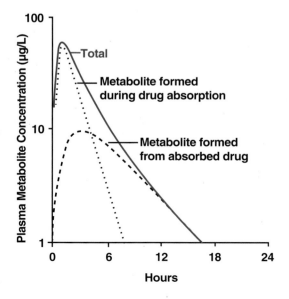

FIGURE 20-6. Following an oral dose of drug, the observed plasma concentration of metabolite (——) is the sum of metabolite from two sources: that formed during the systemic absorption of drug (···) and that formed from absorbed drug (---). Note that on this semilogarithmic plot, the decline of metabolite formed during absorption is determined by the elimination half-life of the metabolite, whereas decay of metabolite formed from the absorbed drug is determined by the half-life of the drug, the rate-limiting step here. If the hepatic extraction ratio of the drug is high, then most of the dose is converted to metabolite during the absorption of drug, and the decline phase appears biphasic. In this simulation, drug and metabolite have half-lives of 3.5 and 1.1 hr, respectively, and 90% is converted to metabolite during drug absorption.

equivalent therapeutic response. The situation with propranolol appears to lie somewhere between these two extremes. Following a single oral dose, the pharmacologic effect is maximal at the peak propranolol concentration, but for a given plasma concentration of propranolol, the response seen after an oral dose is greater than that observed following an i.v. dose. The explanation appears to be the presence of a significant concentration of one or more pharmacologically active metabolites, formed on the first pass through the liver. Certainly, one identified metabolite, 4-hydroxypropranolol, is as active as propranolol.

In Table 7-2 of Chapter 7, *Absorption* , examples of drugs stated to be partially metabolized within the gastrointestinal tract are given. For some, evidence favoring this site of metabolism is the failure to detect a metabolite when drug is given parenterally, yet significant concentrations of this metabolite are measured after oral drug administration. Were metabolism to occur primarily within the liver and renal excretion of drug were to be minimal, then the fraction of the dose converted to the metabolite should be independent of the route of drug administration. Thus, given that ingested drug entirely traverses the gastrointestinal wall and that hepatic metabolism is the only route of elimination, drug, whether given orally or parenterally, is equally and fully available to the liver for metabolism. The oral bioavailability of the drug may be low if its hepatic extraction ratio is high, but the fraction of dose converted to a metabolite must be independent of the route of drug administration. The data in Fig. 20-7 support this last point. Morphine is highly and almost exclusively cleared by the liver. Using *AUC* as a measure of the amount of material entering the body, the oral bioavailability of morphine is low (21%), but the amount of the active metabolite, morphine-6-glucuronide, formed is the same when comparing results after oral and i.v. drug administration. Likewise, the equality of areas of naphthoxylactic acid following oral and i.v. administration of propranolol (see Figs. 20-3 and 20-5), appropriately correcting for differences in dose administered, supports the formation of this metabolite, primarily if not totally, in the liver. The finding does not support formation in the gastrointestinal tract.

An exception to the rule above arises when one, or more, of several conditions is present. For example, the drug may undergo extensive renal excretion (fe high) as well as extensive first-pass metabolism. Here, the $AUC(m)$ values may differ following oral and i.v. drug administration, but the major effect may be on the ratio of AUC values for the drug itself. Alternatively, extensive metabolism in the gut wall or gut lumen as well as other sites in the body may result in differences in the ratio of $AUC(m)$ values. Such has been observed for example for isoproterenol, a drug formerly used for treating asthma. The data in Table 20-3 show large differences in the composition of metabolites recovered in the urine following oral and i.v. administration. The conjugates are extensively formed in the gut wall during first pass, giving rise to a very different route-dependent pattern of drug metabolism, which although not determined in the study will reflect a route dependence in corresponding $AUCs$. Contributing to the large differences seen is the metabolism of the drug in extrahepatic sites, particularly adrenergic nerve endings. The extrahepatic metabolism is primarily due to catechol-O-methyl transferase and monoamine oxidase.

CONSTANT-RATE DRUG INFUSION

In Chapter 10, *Constant-Rate Input*, the kinetics of a constant-rate i.v. infusion was examined. Recall that infusion rate and clearance determine the plateau concentration and that half-life alone determines the time to approach plateau. These concepts can be extended to metabolites. The essential features can be understood by expanding the previous scheme for drug disposition after a single dose to include a constant-rate i.v. input of drug.

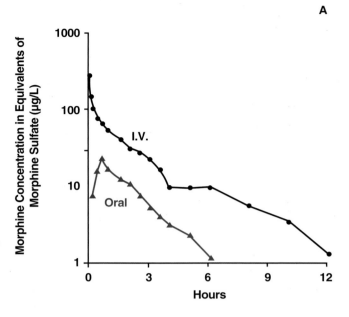

A

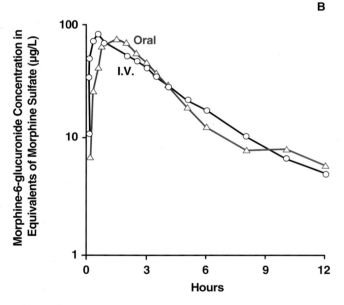

B

FIGURE 20-7. Subjects received morphine sulfate orally (11.7 mg, *colored lines*) and intravenously (5 mg, *black lines*) on separate occasions. Plasma concentrations of drug (▲, oral; ●, i.v.) **(A)** and an active metabolite, morphine-6-glucuronide (△, oral; ○, i.v.) **(B)** were measured. Average data in 10 subjects are shown; concentrations of drug **(A)** and metabolite **(B)** are normalized to a 10-mg dose of morphine sulfate. The oral bioavailability of morphine is low ($F = 0.20$). Even so, the same amount of metabolite enters the circulation, as judged by the equality of $AUC(m)$ associated with the metabolite following the two routes of morphine administration, implying the cause of the low bioavailability is a result of extensive first-pass hepatic metabolism. (From: Osbourne R, Joel S, Trew, D, Slevin M. Morphine and metabolite behavior after different routes of morphine administration. Demonstration of the importance of the active metabolite morphine-6-glucuronide. Clin Pharmacol Ther 1990;47:12–19.)

	Recovery (% of dose)			
Route	Isoproterenol	Isoproterenol Conjugate	O-Methyl Isoproterenol	O-Methyl Isoproterenol Conjugate
i.v.	62.2	0	13.0	24.8
Oral	6.3	62.0	5.6	1.3

TABLE 20-3 **Percent Urinary Recovery Following Administration of Isoproterenol**

From: Dollery CT, Davies DS, Conolly ME. Differences in the metabolism of drugs depending upon their routes of administration. Ann NY Acad Sci 1971;179:108–114.

THE PLATEAU

As with a bolus dose, Eq. 20-1 applies at any time during drug infusion,

$$\begin{matrix} \textit{Rate of change of} \\ \textit{amount of metabolite} \\ \textit{in body} \end{matrix} = \underset{\substack{\textit{Rate of} \\ \textit{formation}}}{k_f \cdot A} - \underset{\substack{\textit{Rate of} \\ \textit{elimination}}}{k(m) \cdot A(m)}$$

Expressing the equation in terms of plasma concentrations

$$\begin{matrix} \textit{Rate of change of} \\ \textit{amount of metabolite} \\ \textit{in body} \end{matrix} = CL_f \cdot C - CL(m) \cdot C(m) \qquad \text{20-8}$$

When steady state is reached for both drug and metabolite, the rates of infusion and drug elimination are equal and so are the rates of metabolite formation and elimination. Equations 20-8 and 20-9 then simplify to

$$\begin{matrix} \textit{Amount of metabolite} \\ \textit{in body at steady state} \end{matrix} = \frac{k_f}{k(m)} \cdot A_{ss} \qquad \text{20-9}$$

and

$$\begin{matrix} \textit{Metabolite concentration} \\ \textit{in plasma at steady state} \end{matrix} = \frac{CL_f}{CL(m)} \cdot C_{ss} \qquad \text{20-10}$$

As fm is the fraction of an i.v. dose of a drug converted to the systemically available metabolite, the term $fm \cdot R_{inf}$ must be equal to the rate of metabolite formation at the plateau, namely $k_f \cdot A_{ss}$ or $CL_f \cdot C_{ss}$. So,

$$\begin{matrix} \textit{Amount of metabolite} \\ \textit{in body at steady state} \end{matrix} = \frac{fm \cdot R_{inf}}{k(m)} \qquad \text{20-11}$$

and

$$\begin{matrix} \textit{Concentration of metabolite} \\ \textit{at steady state} \end{matrix} = \frac{fm \cdot R_{inf}}{CL(m)} \qquad \text{20-12}$$

Suppose, for example, that a drug is infused at 5 mg/hr, fm is 0.5, $k(m)$ is 0.1 hr^{-1}, and $CL(m)$ is 1.0 L/hr. Then,

$$\begin{matrix} \textit{Amount of metabolite} \\ \textit{in body at plateau} \end{matrix} = \frac{0.5 \times 5 \ mg/hr}{0.1 \ hr^{-1}} = 25 \ mg$$

$$\begin{matrix} \textit{Plasma concentration of} \\ \textit{metabolite at plateau} \end{matrix} = \frac{0.5 \times 5 \ mg/hr}{1.0 \ L/hr} = 2.5 \ mg/L$$

TIME TO PLATEAU

Bolus Plus Infusion. The time required for a metabolite to reach plateau depends on whether a bolus of drug is given at the start of the constant-rate drug infusion. If a bolus is given and the infusion maintains that amount of drug in the body, resulting in a constant drug concentration, then the approach of the metabolite toward plateau depends only on its half-life. This point becomes apparent when one realizes that at constant drug concentration, metabolite is formed at a constant rate, $fm \cdot R_{inf}$. As this is analogous to giving a constant-rate infusion of metabolite, it follows (from Chapter 10,

Constant-Rate Input) that the approach to plateau is governed *solely* by the metabolite's half-life. Thus, 50% and 90% of the plateau are reached in 1 and 3.3 metabolite half-lives, respectively. Hence, metabolites with short half-lives reach plateau quickly, and the converse.

Infusion Alone. If no bolus is given, the situation is more complicated. The time for a metabolite to reach plateau can be governed primarily by either the drug's or metabolite's half-life, *whichever is the longer*. To appreciate this point, consider two situations, both shown in Fig. 20-8. In the more prevalent situation, Case A, the drug has the longer half-life. As expected, the amount of drug in the body reaches plateau in approximately 3.3 drug half-lives. The amount of metabolite and, hence, the rate of metabolite elimination also rises. However, because elimination of the metabolite is a much faster process than that of the drug ($k(m) \gg k$), the rate of metabolite elimination soon becomes limited by and approximately equal to its rate of formation. Metabolite is then at virtual steady state with respect to, and cannot rise any faster than, drug. This follows, because under this condition (Eq. 20-3)

$$\begin{array}{c} Amount\ of\ metabolite \\ in\ body \end{array} \approx \frac{k_f}{k(m)} \cdot A \approx \frac{fm \cdot k}{k(m)} \cdot A$$

(i.e., the amount of metabolite in the body proportionally reflects and is only a small fraction of the amount of drug in the body). Therefore, the metabolite reaches plateau within approximately four drug half-lives.

In Case B, the drug is eliminated faster than the metabolite ($k \gg k[m]$). Now, drug reaches steady state before the level of the metabolite has barely risen. From then on, the rate of metabolite formation is constant and, as observed previously when a bolus is given to achieve a constant concentration of drug, accumulation of metabolite to plateau is

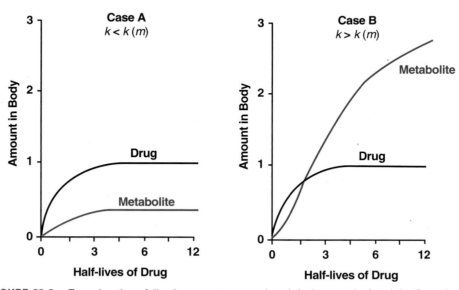

FIGURE 20-8. Two situations following constant-rate drug infusion are depicted. In *Case A*, the more usual situation, the metabolite half-life is shorter than that of the drug. Throughout most of drug accumulation, metabolite elimination is formation rate-limited; therefore, the approach to the metabolite plateau is determined by the half-life of the drug. In the less common situation, *Case B*, the half-life of drug is less than that of metabolite. Drug is at steady state well before metabolite. Approach of the metabolite to plateau is now determined by its half-life.

controlled by its half-life. Examples of Cases A and B are the oxidation of tolbutamide to hydroxytolbutamide and the hydrolysis of methylprednisolone hemisuccinate to methylprednisolone, respectively.

POSTINFUSION

As should now be anticipated, on stopping an infusion, the decline of metabolite is governed by the longer half-life (i.e., drug or metabolite). For example, on stopping a tolbutamide infusion, hydroxytolbutamide would decline by one half each tolbutamide half-life, whereas methylprednisolone's decline would be determined by its half-life after stopping an infusion of its hemisuccinate ester.

MULTIPLE-DOSE DRUG REGIMEN

The concepts that apply to metabolite following administration of drug as a single dose or a constant-rate infusion can readily be extended to the most common situation of a multiple-dose oral drug regimen. As with infusion of drug, accumulation of metabolite to plateau depends as much on its half-life as on that of the parent drug. For example (Fig. 20-9), accumulation of N-desalkylhalazepam, a metabolite of the benzodiazepine halazepam, lags behind parent compound during drug administration and falls more slowly after administration is stopped. Both observations occur because this metabolite has a longer half-life than that of the parent drug. In addition, the plateau concentration of N-desalkylhalazepam is higher than that of halazepam, signifying that the metabolite has the lower clearance. Fluctuations in the plasma concentrations of both drug and metabolite are the only noticeable differences expected between an infusion and a multiple-dose regimen. The degree of fluctuation depends on the dosing frequency and half-lives of drug absorption, drug elimination, and metabolite elimination.

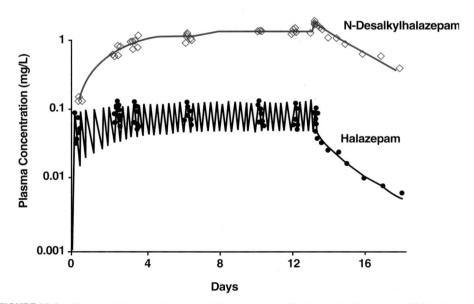

FIGURE 20-9. Because it has the longer half-life, the metabolite N-desalkylhalazepam (◇) both accumulates more extensively and falls more slowly than its parent drug, halazepam (•), during and after stopping the ingestion of 10-mg halazepam every 8 hr for 13 consecutive days. The metabolite also has a lower clearance, indicated by its higher plateau concentration, and because of a longer half-life, undergoes less fluctuation compared with parent drug. (From: Chung M, Hilbert JM, Gural RP. Multiple-dose halazepam kinetics. Clin Pharmacol Ther 1984;35:838–842. Reproduced with permission of Mosby CV.)

PREDICTION FROM SINGLE-DOSE DATA

The concentration of metabolite during an oral multiple-dose drug regimen can readily be calculated from the plasma metabolite concentration-time profile after a single oral dose of drug, using the principle of superposition. The approach is analogous to that taken for drug alone (Chapter 11, *Multiple-Dose Regimens*). The metabolite concentration at any time into the multiple-dose regimen of drug administration is obtained by adding the metabolite concentrations expected from each of the previous doses; there is no need to know any pharmacokinetic parameter of either drug or metabolite. For example, if four oral doses of drug are given at 0, 12, 24, and 36 hr, then the concentration of metabolite expected at 48 hr after the first dose is equal to the sum of the metabolite concentrations at 48, 36, 24, and 12 hr after a single dose of drug. The average concentration of metabolite at plateau can also be readily calculated from *AUC* considerations. The area under the metabolite concentration-time curve after a single dose of drug, $AUC(m)_{single}$, is given by

$$AUC(m)_{single} = \frac{Amount\ available}{CL(m)} = \frac{F(m) \cdot Dose}{CL(m)} \qquad 20\text{-}13$$

where $F(m)$ is the fraction of the administered oral dose of drug that enters the general circulation as metabolite. At plateau, within the dosing interval τ, the amount formed ($F_m \cdot Dose$) is matched by the amount eliminated ($CL(m) \cdot C(m)_{av,ss}$) so that the average metabolite concentration, $C(m)_{av,ss}$, is

$$C(m)_{av,ss} = \frac{F(m) \cdot Dose}{\tau \cdot CL(m)} \qquad 20\text{-}14$$

Substituting Eq. 20-13 into Eq. 20-14 gives

$$C(m)_{av,ss} = \frac{AUC(m)_{single}}{\tau} \qquad 20\text{-}15$$

For example, if the $AUC(m)_{single}$ is 120 mg-hr/L after a 100-mg dose of drug, then the expected plateau metabolite concentration is 10 mg/L when this dose is given every 12 hr. Obviously, if the observed average plateau metabolite concentration differs from that expected, then either $F(m)$, clearance of metabolite, or both, have been altered during chronic drug administration.

VARIABILITY

As with parent drug, the pharmacokinetics of a metabolite varies widely in the patient population. With additional variability in clearance of metabolite formation, this often means that interpatient variability in metabolite concentration can be even greater than that seen with parent drug. Sources of variability in metabolite kinetics are the same as those affecting parent drug and include genetics, age, disease, and interacting drugs. Differences exist among patients in both clearance and volume of distribution of metabolite and as with a drug itself, preferably all parameters should be related to the unbound species, when considering the contribution of metabolites to observed activity.

Concern about metabolites is greatest when they contribute significantly to therapeutic response or toxicity. Frequently, the concentration of metabolite is too low to produce an effect, because only a small fraction of a dose is converted to a particular metabolite, and the clearance of the metabolite is higher than that of the drug. Situations can arise,

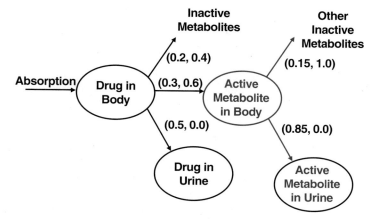

FIGURE 20-10. Model for absorption and disposition of a hypothetical drug and disposition of its active metabolite (*colored*). The first number in parentheses refers to the fraction of drug or metabolite that is normally by the pathway shown with an arrow. The second number refers to the same fraction when there is no renal function.

however, in which metabolites reach concentrations high enough to be of concern. This occurs particularly in patients with renal insufficiency, because many metabolites are relatively polar and are primarily excreted unchanged. For example, the clearance of morphine-6-glucuronide, an active metabolite of morphine, is reduced in patients with renal impairment.

Prediction of the total activity of drug and dosage adjustment needed in patients with renal insufficiency is therefore more complex than usual. There are ways of treating such situations. The most useful is by the steady-state approach. To illustrate the use of this approach, consider the scheme in Fig. 20-10, which shows the input and disposition of a drug and its active metabolite. Table 20-4 lists average values for several pharmacokinetic parameters of this drug and its active metabolite in the typical patient with unimpaired renal function. In this example, both drug and active metabolite are equipotent and equitoxic in terms of plasma concentration (with each activity additive). The average rate of drug administration is 10 mg/hr.

At steady state, the plasma drug concentration may be calculated from average rate of absorption and total clearance,

$$C_{av,ss} = \frac{0.8 \times 10 \ mg/hr}{30 \ L/hr} = 0.27 \ mg/L$$

TABLE 20-4	Average Pharmacokinetic Parameters of a Drug and Its Active Metabolite	
Parameter	**Drug**	**Active Metabolite**
Total clearance	30 L/hr	10 L/hr*
Renal clearance	15 L/hr	8.5 L/hr
Fraction excreted unchanged	0.5	0.85*
Oral bioavailability	0.8	0.3†

*Obtained following administration of metabolite.
†Fraction of drug converted to active metabolite.

The rate of formation of the active metabolite is 0.3 times the rate of input of the drug; therefore,

$$C(m)_{av,ss} = \frac{0.3 \times 0.8 \times 10 \; mg/hr}{10 \; L/hr} = 0.24 \; mg/L$$

In an anuric patient, who has essentially no renal function, total clearance is extrarenal clearance. For this drug, extrarenal clearance is 15 L/hr; for metabolite, it is 1.5 L/hr. Therefore, the predicted steady-state concentration of drug in the anuric patient, $C(d)_{av,ss}$, is

$$C(d)_{av,ss} = \frac{0.8 \times 10 \; mg/hr}{15 \; L/hr} = 0.53 \; mg/L$$

Because 0.6 of the total elimination, $CL_f / (CL - CL_R)$ or 9 L/hr / (30 − 15) L/hr, goes to the active metabolite in the anuric patient, the steady-state concentration of metabolite, $C(m,d)_{av,ss}$, is

$$C(m,d)_{av,ss} = \frac{0.6 \times 0.8 \times 10 \; mg/hr}{1.5 \; L/hr} = 3.2 \; mg/L$$

Note that the average drug concentration is twice as great in the anuric patient, whereas the active metabolite concentration is increased 13 times. With drug and active metabolite equipotent and additive in their activities, the rate of administration in the anuric patient should be (0.27 + 0.24)/(0.53 + 3.2) or 0.14 that of normal. Thus, the anuric patient would require only 1.4 mg/hr. This example illustrates clearly that although a metabolite may make a relatively minor contribution to the total activity in patients with normal renal function, in an anuric patient, it may be primarily responsible for activity.

Let us expand further on this issue of contribution of metabolite to activity and dosage-regimen adjustment in patients with renal impairment. In the last example, for drug normally $fe = 0.5$, $fm = 0.3$, and $fe(m) = 0.85$, and in the anephric patient $fm = 0.6$, because of the renal excretion pathway being no longer available to parent drug. Consider now two additional scenarios. The first is one in which almost all the drug is converted to the metabolite (fm approaches 1), which is then eliminated via pathways other than renal excretion ($fe[m]$ approaches 0). Then, as renal impairment has no impact on either fraction of drug converted to metabolite or metabolite clearance, no change in either drug or metabolite concentration is anticipated, and accordingly, no change in dosage regimen of the drug is warranted. The second is that in which a minor fraction of drug is normally excreted unchanged or converted to metabolite, but elimination of metabolite is exclusively via renal excretion. Obviously then, although renal impairment will not materially change the clearance of drug or the fraction of drug converted to metabolite, metabolite clearance is profoundly reduced (now dependent on minor non-renal pathways) and the concentration of metabolite increases profoundly in functionally anephric patients. Then, if active, the much higher concentration of the metabolite may be enough to necessitate a decrease in drug dosing rate to avoid adverse effects.

NONLINEAR METABOLITE FORMATION OR ELIMINATION

Nonlinear formation or elimination of a metabolite is of therapeutic interest when it accounts for some or all of either the therapeutic response, or toxicity, or both. The consequences of such nonlinearities depend on the cause and the site of occurrence. The general tendencies for changes in steady-state concentrations following chronic dosing are the same as those for AUC after a single dose. Here, however, the compound (drug or metabolite) with capacity-limited metabolism may not reach steady state if it is formed at a rate that exceeds its Vm.

Dose dependence is expected in the degree of autoinduction for drugs that undergo this behavior. Such is observed with carbamazepine. As shown in Fig. 20-11A, the

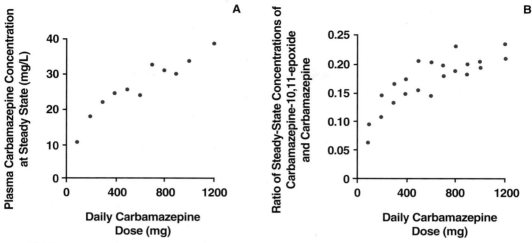

FIGURE 20-11. **A.** The steady-state concentration of carbamazepine fails to increase in direct proportion to the daily dose, evidence of nonlinear kinetics. **B.** The ratio of the concentrations of the metabolite, carbamazepine-10,11-epoxide, and carbamazepine increase with daily dose. These observations indicate that either the clearance of formation increases or the clearance of elimination of the epoxide decreases at higher dosing rates. The former, a consequence of dose-dependent autoinduction of metabolite formation, is the explanation. Each point in both graphs is the mean of data from 77 patients. (From: Kudriakova T, Sirotsa LA, Rozova GI, et al. Autoinduction and steady-state pharmacokinetics of carbamazepine and its major metabolites. Br J Clin Pharmacol 1992;33:611–615.)

steady-state concentration of carbamazepine fails to increase in direct proportion to daily dose ($C_{av,ss}/(D/\tau)$ decreases). Furthermore, the ratio of the steady-state concentrations of the metabolite carbamazepine-10, 11-epoxide, and carbamazepine increase with dose (Fig. 20-11B). These results demonstrate nonlinearity in the formation of the metabolite. The directions of the changes suggest that formation clearance of the epoxide is increased.

ADDITIONAL CONSIDERATIONS

Four other aspects of metabolite kinetics warrant consideration. One is response, another is interconversion between metabolite and drug, and the other two are the use of metabolite data to quantify metabolite clearance and to identify possible causes of a change in pharmacokinetics.

RESPONSE

When all activity or toxicity resides with a particular metabolite, relating response to metabolite concentration is relatively straightforward. The problem is more difficult when both drug and metabolite contribute to activity or toxicity. Occasionally, it may be possible to relate the response to a linear combination of the plasma concentrations of drug and metabolite as was done in the last section. However, the relationship between response and concentration is more complicated when, for example, drug and metabolite act as competitive agonists or antagonists. Then, if the response produced by the drug alone approaches the maximum, E_{max}, the response changes little with increases in the concentration of a metabolite, and vice versa. More generally, response can be related to drug and metabolite using an equation of the form of Eq. 17-21 in Chapter 17, *Drug Interactions.* Although, such an approach is unlikely to be used clinically, measurement of an active metabolite concentration can help to explain an observation and account for variability in drug response. Accordingly, such measurements can serve as useful semiquantitative guides to therapy.

INTERCONVERSION

Among the list of therapeutically important metabolites in Table 20-1 are some that are enzymatically converted back to the administered drug substance; they include prednisolone, the metabolite of prednisone, and sulindac sulfide, the metabolite of sulindac. Both drugs are prescribed as anti-inflammatory agents, but in each case the activity resides with the metabolite. These and other examples of drug-metabolite pairs that undergo interconversion are listed in Table 20-5. A group of notable examples is the extensively metabolized statins, which include lovastatin, simvastatin, and atorvastatin, in which the interconversion is between the inactive lactone and the associated active open acid.

Figure 20-12 illustrates some common features of interconversion. Shown are the plasma concentrations of prednisolone and prednisone after administration of single doses of each steroid on separate occasions. Notice, irrespective of which is administered,

TABLE 20-5	**Representative Drug–Metabolite Pairs Undergoing Interconversion**		
Drug	**Metabolite***	**Compound That Predominates at Equilibrium in Plasma**	**Comment**
Canrenone[†]	Canrenoate	Canrenone	Canrenoate is inactive.
Clofibric acid[‡]	Glucuronide	Clofibric acid	In renal impairment, glucuronide excretion is reduced; this causes reduced apparent clearance of clofibric acid.
Cortisol	Cortisone	Cortisol	Cortisone is inactive.
Dapsone	Monoacetyldapsone	Dapsone	Acetylation shows polymorphism; metabolite is less active.
Haloperidol	Reduced haloperidol	Haloperidol	Haloperidol is reduced by a carbonyl reductase; the reduced form is oxidized by CPY2D6.
Lovastatin**	Open-acid	Open-acid	The liver is the target organ; lovastatin, given orally, is extensively converted to metabolites during the first pass through the liver.
Methylprednisolone	Methylprednisolone	Methylprednisone	Methylprednisolone is inactive.
Prednisone[††]	Prednisolone	Prednisolone	Prednisone is inactive.
Sulindac	Sulindac sulfide	Sulindac sulfide[‡‡]	Sulindac (a sulfoxide) is inactive and therefore acts as prodrug for sulindac sulfide.
Vitamin K	Vitamin K-epoxide	Vitamin K	Epoxide is inactive; oral anticoagulants work by blocking reduction of epoxide back to vitamin K, which is needed for blood clotting.

*Definition of drug and metabolite are somewhat arbitrary; the term drug tends to be reserved for the administered compound.
[†]Canrenone, an active aldosterone antagonist, is the major metabolite of spironolactone.
[‡]Clofibric acid is administered orally as the inactive ethyl ester, which is rapidly hydrolyzed during adsorption.
**Lovastatin, a lactone, is hydrolyzed to the ring-opened acid.
[††]Commercially available as a drug substance.
[‡‡]Situation complicated by enterohepatic cycling of sulindac and sulindac sulfide.

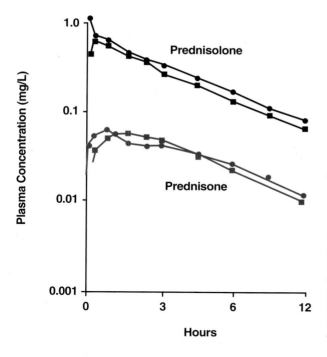

FIGURE 20-12. Once equilibrium is established, the concentrations of prednisone (*in color*) and prednisolone (*in black*) in plasma are independent of which compound is administered. Data are obtained after a single oral dose of 50-mg prednisone (*squares*) and an i.v. dose of prednisolone (*circles*), as prednisolone succinate (40 mg), to a subject on separate occasions. Prednisolone succinate, not shown, is hydrolyzed very rapidly to prednisolone. (From: Rose JQ, Yurchak AM, Jusko WJ, et al. Bioavailability and disposition of prednisolone tablets. Biopharm Drug Disp 1980;1:247–258. Reprinted by permission of John Wiley & Sons, Ltd.)

both steroids are present in plasma. Also, the ratio of prednisolone to prednisone rapidly reaches a fixed value of 10:1, after which time the steroids decline in parallel on a semi-logarithmic plot. How quickly the equilibrium is established and where the ratio lies depend not only on the kinetics of interconversion, but also on the irreversible loss of each species from the body, as can be visualized in the scheme below.

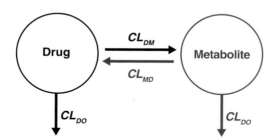

Each pathway is characterized by an associated clearance, and each species may differ in its volume of distribution. The terminal half-life of the interconverted pair is a hybrid of all these parameters. This scheme resembles the two-compartment distribution model discussed in Fig. 19-3 of Chapter 19, *Distribution Kinetics*, except the two compartments now represent drug and metabolite. The difference between the two models is that with interconversion, loss can also occur from the "peripheral" (metabolite) compartment. If no such loss occurs then, viewed from drug in plasma, the metabolite acts as a storage site, and as such is effectively a component of drug distribution, because under these circumstances, no drug is irreversibly lost via this pathway.

The therapeutic importance of interconversion varies with drug and circumstance. For example, interconversion between sulindac and its sulfide helps to moderate and sustain the concentration of active sulfide. In contrast, interconversion between the antileprotic drug dapsone and its less active metabolite monoacetyldapsone has no therapeutic relevance; the equilibrium is always strongly toward dapsone, which is primarily eliminated via pathways other than *N*-acetylation. Normally, interconversion between clofibric acid

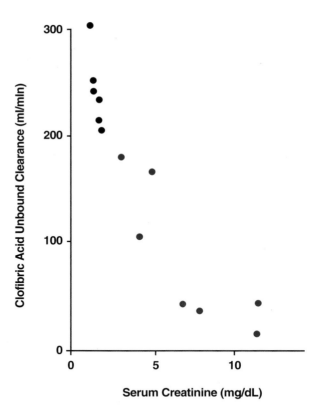

FIGURE 20-13. Unbound clearance of clofibric acid in patients with unimpaired (●) and compromised (●) renal function is shown. Although little clofibric acid is excreted unchanged (*fe* = 0.06–0.1) when renal function is normal, the unbound clearance of clofibric acid decreases markedly with an increase in serum creatinine, an inverse measure of renal function. The apparent dependence of clofibric acid's unbound clearance on a patient's renal function is explained by its interconversion to a polar glucuronide, the clearance of which depends on renal function. (From: Gugler P, Kurten JW, Jensen CJ, et al. Clofibrate disposition in renal failure and acute and chronic liver disease. Euro J Clin Pharmacol 1979;15:341–347.)

(derived from the rapid hydrolysis of the administered ethyl ester, clofibrate) and its inactive glucuronide is not of concern; the glucuronide is renally excreted so rapidly that glucuronidation can be regarded as a pathway of irreversible loss of clofibric acid. Consequently, because only 6% of clofibric acid is usually excreted unchanged and all the activity resides with clofibric acid, no change in its pharmacokinetics is anticipated in patients with renal insufficiency. However, as shown in Fig. 20-13, the unbound clearance of clofibric acid is markedly reduced (and its half-life is prolonged) as renal function decreases. The explanation lies in reduced renal clearance of the glucuronide, which then accumulates and is hydrolyzed back to the parent acid; effectively, a major route of elimination of clofibric acid is increasingly blocked. To what extent the observation with clofibric acid applies to other drugs that depend heavily on glucuronidation for elimination is not known, but does appear to be seen mostly with acidic drugs, like clofibric acid, that form ester glucuronides. These include ciprofibrate and some arylpropionic nonsteroidal anti-inflammatory drugs, such as ketoprofen. Many other drugs form more stable ether glucuronides, which are not interconverted.

ESTIMATION OF METABOLITE FORMATION

From Plasma Metabolite Concentration. The amount of administered dose of drug converted to systemically available metabolite can be calculated if metabolite clearance $CL(m)$ is known, because this amount equals the amount of metabolite eliminated, $CL(m) \cdot AUC(m)$. To gain an estimate of $CL(m)$, the metabolite needs to be given intravenously. In the general case, the ratio $CL(m) \cdot AUC(m)/Dose$ gives the fraction of administered drug available systemically as metabolite. This ratio may be low (e.g., if a drug is given orally) and it has a low bioavailability due to incomplete dissolution. An estimate of the importance of a particular metabolic pathway to the elimination of a drug can be made in the special case in which metabolite data are available following i.v. administration of both drug and metabolite on separate occasions. Such

TABLE 20-6	**Pharmacokinetic Parameters and *AUC* After Intravenous Administration of Isosorbide-5-Mononitrate and Isosorbide Dinitrate on Separate Occasions**	
	After Isosorbide-5-Mononitrate	**After Isosorbide Dinitrate**
AUC (mg-hr/L)	0.60	0.37
CL (L/hr)	8.3	—
Half-life (hr)	4.2	4.3

From: Straehl P, Galeazzi RL, Soliva M. Isosorbide 5-mononitrate and isosorbide-2-mononitrate kinetics after intravenous and oral dosing. Clin Pharmacol Ther 1984;36:485–492; and Straehl P, Galeazzi RL. Isosorbide dinitrate bioavailability, kinetics, and metabolism. Clin Pharmacol Ther 1985;38:140–149.

data for isosorbide-5-mononitrate are listed in Table 20-6. Isosorbide-5-mononitrate is one of the active metabolites of isosorbide dinitrate, an antianginal drug. The amount of metabolite formed following a 5-mg i.v. dose of parent drug $CL(m) \cdot AUC(m)$ is 8.3 L/hr $\times$ 0.37 mg-hr/L, that is, 3.07-mg or 3.8-mg drug equivalents after correcting for differences in molecular weight (dinitrate, 236 g/mol: 5-mononitrate, 191 g/mol). Clearly, with 3.8 mg of a 5-mg dose converted to this metabolite, the formation of the 5-mononitrate is a major route of elimination of isosorbide dinitrate.

From Metabolite Excretion. Many metabolites are polar and eliminated almost exclusively by renal excretion. The elimination (excretion) of these metabolites in the terminal phase is frequently formation rate-limited, either because they have a much higher clearance, smaller volume of distribution, or both, compared with parent drug. Recall, for a metabolite almost completely excreted unchanged, when formation is rate-limiting, as a reasonable approximation during the terminal phase,

$$\frac{\text{Rate of metabolite}}{\text{excretion}} \approx \underset{\substack{\text{Rate of metabolite}\\\text{formation}}}{CL_f \cdot C} \qquad \text{20-16}$$

Thus, by measuring the rates of excretion of metabolite and the corresponding plasma drug concentration, clearance associated with formation of metabolite may be estimated. Note that when Eq. 20-16 applies, the fall in metabolite excretion rate is determined by, and can be used to estimate, the half-life of the drug. Equation 20-16 is most accurate under steady-state conditions.

DETECTION OF CHANGES IN PHARMACOKINETICS

Comparison of drug and metabolite areas is helpful in identifying the organ of drug metabolism (i.e., gastrointestinal tract, liver) when drug is administered by different routes (see section on *Impact of Hepatic Extraction*). Area analysis can also be used to examine possible causes of a change in the pharmacokinetics of a drug or metabolite. Suppose, for example, that when given orally, the plasma concentration of a drug of low clearance is reduced on Occasion B compared with the value on Occasion A. Possible explanations are reduced oral bioavailability, increased clearance, or both. Examination of drug data alone might give a clue, but the situation is helped considerably by simultaneous use of metabolite data.

The following example is that of a single dose of drug. An analogous analysis can be extended to steady-state conditions. Following a single dose, the area ratios for drug are

$$\text{Occasion A: } F_A \cdot Dose = CL_A \cdot AUC_A \qquad \text{20-17}$$

$$\text{Occasion B: } F_B \cdot Dose = CL_B \cdot AUC_B \qquad \text{20-18}$$

and for metabolite the corresponding equations are

$$\text{Occasion A: } fm_A \cdot F_A \cdot Dose = CL(m)_A \cdot AUC(m)_A \qquad \text{20-19}$$

$$\text{Occasion B: } fm_B \cdot F_B \cdot Dose = CL(m)_B \cdot AUC(m)_B \qquad \text{20-20}$$

When the same dose is given on both occasions,

$$\frac{AUC_B}{AUC_A} = \frac{F_B}{F_A} \cdot \frac{CL_A}{CL_B} \qquad \text{20-21}$$

$$\frac{AUC(m)_B}{AUC(m)_A} = \frac{F_B \cdot fm_B}{F_A \cdot fm_A} \cdot \frac{CL(m)_A}{CL(m)_B} \qquad \text{20-22}$$

and since $fm \cdot CL = CL_f$, then

$$\left[\frac{AUC(m)}{AUC}\right]_A = \frac{CL_{f,A}}{CL(m)_A} \qquad \text{20-23}$$

$$\left[\frac{AUC(m)}{AUC}\right]_B = \frac{CL_{f,B}}{CL(m)_B} \qquad \text{20-24}$$

Now consider the various possibilities.

Possibility 1. Reduced bioavailability that is caused by incomplete dissolution of drug $(F_B < F_A)$. If this is so, as clearance terms of neither drug nor metabolite are altered, it follows from Eqs. 20-23 and 20-24 that

Expectation:

$$\frac{AUC_B}{AUC_A} = \frac{AUC(m)_B}{AUC(m)_A}$$

That is, the ratios of areas of drug and metabolite should be equal and less than 1. Of course, the reason could also be due to the patient's failing to take the dose as instructed, an adherence problem.

Possibility 2. Increased clearance of drug $(CL_B > CL_A)$. If this is the reason for the decreased drug concentration, then the expected outcome for the metabolite depends on the mechanism responsible for the increase in drug clearance namely, decreased binding of drug, enzyme induction, or increased renal clearance, and also depends on the extraction ratios of drug and metabolite. Given a low extraction ratio, the expectation is the following:

a. Decreased drug binding ($fu \uparrow$).

If this occurs, CL_f is increased but fm is unaltered, because clearances by all pathways of drug elimination are equally affected. As neither bioavailability nor metabolite clearance is altered,

Expectation:

$$\frac{AUC(m)_A}{AUC(m)_B} = 1$$

$$\left[\frac{AUC(m)}{AUC}\right]_B > \left[\frac{AUC(m)}{AUC}\right]_A$$

b. Enzyme Induction.

If this occurs, CL_f may or may not change depending on which metabolic pathway is induced. Remember, there is often more than one enzyme responsible for drug metabolism, and all are not equally susceptible to induction by a given inducing agent.

1. Formation of metabolite induced.

Since CL_f is increased, it follows that

Expectation:

$$\left[\frac{AUC(m)}{AUC}\right]_B > \left[\frac{AUC(m)}{AUC}\right]_A$$

Whether the metabolite area ratio changes depends on whether the metabolite is the only pathway of drug elimination. If it is, then, since $fm = 1$ and cannot increase further, no change in the metabolite area ratio is expected. Otherwise,

Expectation:

$$\frac{AUC(m)_A}{AUC(m)_B} > 1$$

2. Another metabolic pathway induced.

Since CL_f is not changed but fm is decreased (as CL is increased), it follows that

Expectation:

$$\frac{AUC(m)_A}{AUC(m)_B} > 1$$

$$\left[\frac{AUC(m)}{AUC}\right]_B = \left[\frac{AUC(m)}{AUC}\right]_A$$

c. Increased renal clearance of drug (CL_R ↑).

The outcome in terms of the metabolite is the same as that predicted for case *b2*, because CL_f is unaltered and fm is decreased.

Expectation:

$$\frac{AUC(m)_A}{AUC(m)_B} > 1$$

$$\left[\frac{AUC(m)}{AUC}\right]_B = \left[\frac{AUC(m)}{AUC}\right]_A$$

From the above analyses, it is apparent that metabolite data may help to narrow the number of likely reasons for reduced plasma concentrations of a drug. Giving drug intravenously would have resolved the issue, but it is not always possible or practical to do so. Measurement of protein binding and of drug in urine would certainly have helped distinguish between the various possibilities. Of course, it is possible that both bioavailability and clearance of both drug and metabolite had changed. Such changes complicate the interpretation. Notwithstanding such complications, it is often possible to make reasonable conclusions as to the likely cause of a change in drug pharmacokinetics from combined drug and metabolite data.

KEY RELATIONSHIPS

$$\begin{array}{ccc} \text{Rate of change of} \\ \text{amount of metabolite} \end{array} = \underset{\substack{\text{Rate of} \\ \text{formation}}}{k_f \cdot A} - \underset{\substack{\text{Rate of} \\ \text{elimination}}}{k(m) \cdot A(m)}$$

$$\begin{array}{c} \textit{Rate of change of} \\ \textit{amount of metabolite} \end{array} = \underset{\substack{\text{Rate of} \\ \text{formation}}}{CL_f \cdot C} - \underset{\substack{\text{Rate of} \\ \text{elimination}}}{CL(m) \cdot C(m)}$$

$$\frac{AUC(m)}{AUC} = \frac{CL_f}{CL(m)}$$

$$\frac{AUC(m)}{AUC} = fm \cdot \frac{\textit{Clearance of drug}}{\textit{Clearance of metabolite}}$$

$$\frac{k(m)}{k} = \frac{CL(m)}{CL} \bigg/ \frac{V(m)}{V}$$

$$\begin{array}{c} \textit{Amount of metabolite} \\ \textit{in body at steady state} \end{array} = \frac{k_f}{k(m)} \cdot A_{ss}$$

$$\begin{array}{c} \textit{Metabolite concentration} \\ \textit{in plasma at steady state} \end{array} = \frac{CL_f}{CL} \cdot C_{ss}$$

$$\begin{array}{c} \textit{Concentration of metabolite} \\ \textit{at steady state} \end{array} = \frac{fm \cdot R_{inf}}{CL(m)}$$

$$C(m)_{av,ss} = \frac{AUC(m)_{single}}{\tau}$$

STUDY PROBLEMS

(Answers to Study Problems are in Appendix J.)

1. Which (if any) of the explanations offered below are consistent with the following statement? An increase in the ratio of $AUC(m)/AUC$ suggests that any of the following could have happened.

   a. Induction of the metabolite formation pathway.
   b. Reduction of the volume of distribution of the metabolite.
   c. Increase in dose of drug absorbed.
   d. Reduction in clearance of an alternative pathway of elimination of drug.

2. Eichelbaum et al. (Eichelbaum M, Tomson T, Tybring G, et al. Autoinduction and steady-state pharmacokinetics of carbamazepine and its major metabolites. Clin Pharmacokinet 1985;10:80–90) found that the terminal half-lives of carbamazepine and its trans-diol metabolite were equal, approximately 30 hr, following oral administration of carbamazepine. Do the data suggest the possibility of a rate-limiting step in the process, and if so, where does it lie?

3. Elson et al. (Elson J, Strong JM, Lee WK, et al. Antiarrhythmic potency of N-acetylprocainamide. Clin Pharmacol Ther 1975;17:134–140) determined the ratio of plasma concentrations of active metabolite, N-acetylprocainamide, and procainamide in patients on long-term procainamide therapy. Figure 20-14 is a histogram of the results of 33 patients; there is considerable variation. Given, as is likely, that these values are reasonable estimates of the ratio at plateau, comment on which pharmacokinetic parameters of drug and metabolite contribute to the observed variability in the ratio.

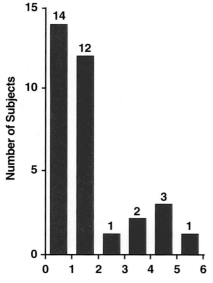

N-Acetylprocainamide/Procainamide Plasma Concentration Ratio

FIGURE 20-14.

4. Glycine conjugation, with the formation of salicyluric acid, is one of the major pathways for the elimination of salicylic acid in humans. Salicylic acid is cleared slowly from the body, whereas salicyluric acid is cleared so rapidly and completely into urine that the plasma concentration of this metabolite is very low. Discuss why measuring salicyluric acid in the urine could be successfully used to assess its rate of formation.

5. As discussed in this chapter, isosorbide dinitrate is extensively metabolized to the 2- and 5-mononitrates. Table 20-7 lists the mean pharmacokinetic data for isosorbide-2-mononitrate following independent i.v. administration of isosorbide dinitrate and the 2-mononitrate, each 5 mg, to a panel of volunteers. (Molecular weights: dinitrate, 236 g/mol; 2-mononitrate, 191 g/mol).

TABLE 20-7 Mean Pharmacokinetic Data for Isosorbide-2-Mononitrate

Isosorbide-2-mononitrate Parameters	After i.v. Isosorbide 2-mononitrate*	After i.v. Isosorbide Dinitrate[†]
AUC (mg-hr/L)	0.22	0.044
CL (L/hr)	23.0	–
Half-life (hr)	1.93	1.82

*From: Straehl P, Galeazzi RL, Soliva M. Isosorbide 5-mononitrate and isosorbide-2-mononitrate kinetics after intravenous and oral dosing. Clin Pharmacol Ther 1984;36:485–492.
[†]From: Straehl P, Galeazzi RL. Isosorbide dinitrate bioavailability, kinetics and metabolism. Clin Pharmacol Ther 1985;38:140–149.

a. Calculate the fraction of isosorbide dinitrate metabolized to the 2-mononitrate.
b. What assumptions have you made in your calculation in a.?
c. By reference to the corresponding data for the 5-mononitrate provided in this chapter, what percentage of i.v.-administered isosorbide dinitrate is eliminated by denitration?

6. Shown in Fig. 20-15 are semilogarithmic plots of the mean ($\pm$SD) plasma concentration of propranolol ($\bigcirc$) and its active metabolite, 4-hydroxypropranolol ($\bullet$), after oral administration of propranolol (80 mg) to six healthy subjects. Discuss why the plasma concentration of 4-hydroxypropranolol peaks earlier and initially declines more rapidly than that of propranolol.

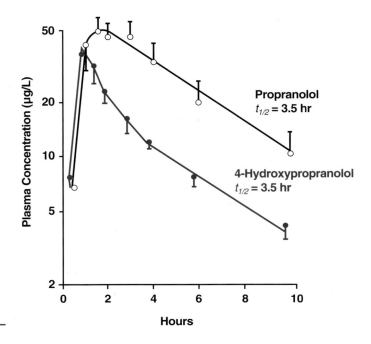

FIGURE 20-15.

7. Predict the general tendencies (clockwise, counterclockwise, or no hysteresis) for the observed relationship between response and plasma *drug* concentration after a single oral dose of a drug as a consequence of each of the following conditions. See Problem 5 of Chapter 8, *Response Following a Single Dose*, for complementary information on conditions producing hysteresis. Elimination occurs solely by hepatic metabolism.

  a. Activity resides solely with a metabolite. Low-clearance drug with metabolite elimination rate-limiting the decline of the metabolite concentration in terminal phase.
  b. Activity resides solely with a metabolite. High first-pass metabolism of drug with drug elimination rate-limiting the decline of metabolite concentration in terminal phase.

8. Osborne et al. (Osborne R, Joel S, Trew D, et al. Morphine and metabolite behavior after different routes of morphine-6-glucuronide. Clin Pharmacol Ther 1990;47:12–19) studied the pharmacokinetics of the analgesic morphine and its two glucuronide metabolites, the active morphine-6-glucuronide, and the inactive morphine-3-glucuronide. Table 20-8 lists mean ($\pm$ SD) and AUC and C_{max} data obtained following administration of morphine sulphate as an i.v. bolus (5 mg), oral tablet (11.7 mg), and sublingual tablet (11.7 mg) to 10 healthy volunteers. Molecular weight of morphine is 285.3 g/mol; morphine sulphate, 669 g/mol, contains 85.3% morphine base.

  a. Calculate the bioavailability of morphine following oral administration.
  b. Given that the plasma-to-blood concentration ratio of morphine is 0.45 and that 8% of an i.v. dose is excreted unchanged in urine, do the i.v. data for morphine itself suggest that its low oral bioavailability is due to a substantial first-pass hepatic loss?
  c. Do the data for both glucuronides support the concept that the liver is the primary site of formation of these metabolites?

TABLE 20-8	Mean ($\pm$SD) *AUC* and C_{max} Data* for Morphine and Its Glucuronides Following Administration of Morphine by Different Routes			

Species		Route		
		i.v. Bolus	Oral	Sublingual
Morphine	*AUC* (nmol-hr/L)	229 $\pm$ 37	43 $\pm$ 13	48 $\pm$ 10
	C_{max} (nmol/L)	273 $\pm$ 65	21 $\pm$ 7.7	19 $\pm$ 4.5
Morphine-6-glucuronide	*AUC* (nmol-hr/L)	313 $\pm$ 87	371 $\pm$ 159	298 $\pm$ 159
	C_{max} (nmol/L)	80 $\pm$ 15	84 $\pm$ 26	74 $\pm$ 19
Morphine-3-glucuronide	*AUC* (nmol-hr/L)	1765 $\pm$ 300	2180 $\pm$ 808	1664 $\pm$ 485
	C_{max} (nmol/L)	407 $\pm$ 100	440 $\pm$ 125	386 $\pm$ 81

*All data are normalized to a 10-mg dose of morphine base.

d. One reason for the use of sublingual tablets, in general, is to increase the systemic bioavailability of a drug that exhibits a high first-pass hepatic loss, because blood perfusing the buccal cavity drains directly into the superior vena cava. Do the data in Table 20-8 support this rationale for morphine?

e. Comment briefly regarding what extent the estimation of oral bioavailability of morphine may be used to guide any difference in dosage requirements of morphine given orally and intravenously.

f. Suggest why the C_{max} for morphine-3-glucuronide is greater than that of morphine, after i.v. morphine administration.

g. Independently, Osbourne et al. (Osbourne R, Thompson P, Joel S, et al. The analgesic activity of morphine-6-glucuronide. Br J Clin Pharmacol 1992;34:130–138) studied the pharmacokinetics of morphine-6-glucuronide after i.v. administration of this glucuronide to cancer patients. Given that the clearance found, 5.8 L/hr, applies to the volunteers who participated in the study that generated the data in Table 20-8, calculate the fraction of orally administered morphine converted to the 6-glucuronide.

h. The values of *fe* for morphine and morphine-6-glucuronide are 0.1 and 1, respectively.

(1) Briefly discuss the expected impact of renal function impairment on the ratio of average plateau concentrations of morphine and morphine-6-glucuronide, following multiple oral dosing of morphine.

(2) Using the data in Table 20-8 gained in subjects with normal renal function, calculate the expected dosage regimen of oral morphine required in a patient with renal function of 0.20 compared with that of a patient with normal renal function, assuming that both patients require the same degree of analgesia for relief of pain. Although there is some uncertainty about the relative potency of morphine-6-glucuronide, given that as with morphine this metabolite acts centrally and hence must access the brain, assume for calculation purposes that based on plasma concentrations morphine-6-glucuronide has 10% of the activity of morphine. Keep also in mind that an appreciable fraction of morphine-6-glucuronide is formed during absorption of oral morphine.

CHAPTER 21

Protein Drugs

OBJECTIVES

The reader will be able to:

- Discuss the breadth of polypeptide and protein drugs available commercially.
- State why protein drugs must generally be given parenterally.
- Compare the distribution of protein drugs within the body with that of small conventional nonprotein drugs.
- Contrast the renal and hepatic handlings of protein drugs with those of small conventional nonprotein drugs.
- State why the systemic absorption of large protein drugs is often slow and incomplete after intramuscular (i.m.) and subcutaneous (s.c.) administration.
- Describe why the lymphatic system plays a major role in the systemic absorption of protein drugs given intramuscularly or subcutaneously.
- List the primary factors affecting the rate and extent of systemic absorption of protein drugs from i.m. and s.c. sites of administration.
- Discuss the effects of renal disease on the elimination of protein drugs with molecular weights (MW) below about 30,000 g/mol.
- State why the disposition of many protein drugs is nonlinear.
- Give one example each of a pharmacokinetic and a pharmacodynamic rate-limited response seen with protein drugs.
- Discuss how nonlinear pharmacodynamics and nonlinear pharmacokinetics of protein drugs, especially antibodies, often have a mechanism in common.

PEPTIDE, POLYPEPTIDE, AND PROTEIN DRUGS

Peptide, polypeptide, and protein drugs are taking an ever larger role in the armamentarium of agents to prevent, diagnose, and treat disease. In recent years, many of the new chemical entities have been in this category. But what are peptide, polypeptide, and protein drugs?

Terminology for these drugs is not well defined, but all contain multiple amino acids that are linked via peptide bonds. They are all therefore peptides. Some have restricted the word polypeptides to peptides with 20 to 50 amino acids, with 50 as the cutoff for defining when a polypeptide becomes a protein; but there is no "official" definition. Some use a MW of 5000 g/mol as the cutoff for where proteins begin. Subsequently in this chapter, "protein" is used as an all-encompassing term for all compounds containing two or more amino acids. Antibodies are examples of proteins at the upper end of the spectrum of size with about 1300 amino acids. However, some proteins, like the largest of the lipoproteins, have more than 15,000.

There are many types of protein drugs on the market today. Table 21-1 lists examples of nonantibody protein drugs by therapeutic class. The table demonstrates a wide range of molecular sizes and activities of the drugs in this category.

TABLE 21-1 Examples of Polypeptide and Protein (Nonantibody) Therapeutic Agents*

Therapeutic Class	Polypeptide/Protein	Molecular Weight (g/mol)	Comments
Adrenocorticotropic hormone	Cosyntropin	2934	Synthetic polypeptide; test for adrenal function.
Adrenohypophyseal hormones and hypothalamic-releasing hormones	Chorionic gonadotropin	36,700	Fertility medication in lieu of luteinizing hormone.
	Menotropin	-	Contains follicle-stimulating hormone and luteinizing hormone; used in treatment of fertility problems.
	Sermorelin	3358	Synthetic human growth hormone–releasing hormone.
	Gonadotropin-releasing hormone	1182	Luteinizing-hormone–releasing hormone.
	Somatropin	22,124	Human growth hormone.
Agents affecting calcification and bone turnover	Calcitonin-Salmon	3432	Used to treat osteoporosis.
Agents for control of gastric acidity and treatment of peptic ulcer	Pentagastrin	768	Polypeptide that has effects like gastrin; namely, stimulates secretion of gastric acid, pepsin, and intrinsic factor.
Agents that cause contraction of the uterus	Oxytocin	940	Used during pregnancy to induce labor.
Agents to treat congestive heart failure (acutely decompensated)	Neseritide	3464	Given by intravenous bolus plus infusion.
Agents to treat rheumatoid arthritis	Anakinra	17,258	Given subcutaneously.
	Abatacept	>150,000	Fusion protein of IgG1 and CTLA-4.
Agents to treat specific genetic disorders	Agalsidase beta	100,000	Enzyme used to treat Fabry's disease.
	Alglucosidase	105,338	Enzyme used to treat Pompey's disease.
	Laronidase	83,000	Enzyme for treating Hurler and Hurler-Schele forms of mucopolysaccharidosis.

TABLE 21-1 **Examples of Polypeptide and Protein (Nonantibody) Therapeutic Agents** (*continued*)

Therapeutic Class	Polypeptide/Protein	Molecular Weight (g/mol)	Comments
	Imiglucerase	60,430	Enzyme for treatment of type I Gaucher disease.
Agents to treat human immuno-deficiency virus (HIV)	Enfuvirtide	4492	Used in combination with other drugs for the treatment of patients with HIV infections.
Agents used for acromegaly and carcinoid syndrome	Octreotide	1019	Mimics the effects of natural somastatin.
	Pegvisomant	~47,000	Highly selective growth hormone receptor antagonist.
Agents used in cystic fibrosis	Dornase alpha	37,000	Synthetic version of naturally occurring deoxyribonuclease, an enzyme that cleaves DNA.
Anticoagulant	Lepirudin	6980	Used in patients who have developed heparin-induced thrombocytopenia.
Antifungal agents	Anidulafungin	1140	Used to treat *Candida* infections (intra-abdominal abscess, peritonitis, and esophageal infection).
Antiplatelet drug used to prevent blood clotting	Eptifibatide	832	Cyclic heptapeptide used during acute coronary syndrome or during percutaneous coronary intervention.
Antiviral agents and modifiers	Interferon alfacon-1	19,434	Commonly taken to treat hepatitis C viral infections.
	Interferon Alpha-2b (pegylated)	20,027	Commonly taken with ribavirin to treat hepatitis C.
	Interferon Beta-1b	~31,000	Used to treat multiple sclerosis.
Débriding agents	Collagenase	112,023	Enzyme that breaks the peptide bound in collagen.
	Fibrinolysin	13,800	Enzyme (inactivates fibrin) combined with deoxyribo-nuclease (destroys DNA) to enhance wound cleaning and healing.
	Papain	23,000	Commonly used to treat skin wounds.
Digestive enzymes	Pancrelipase	-	Contains pancreatic enzymes (lipases, amylases, and proteases) in an enteric-coated dosage form.

(continued)

TABLE 21-1 **Examples of Polypeptide and Protein (Nonantibody) Therapeutic Agents (*continued*)**

Therapeutic Class	Polypeptide/Protein	Molecular Weight (g/mol)	Comments
Drugs affecting renal function	Vasopressin	1084	Used to treat diabetes insipidus.
Hematopoietic agents	Aldesleukin	15,300	Used to treat metastatic renal cell carcinoma and melanoma.
	Epoietin alfa	30,400	Stimulate the body to produce red blood cells; used in anemic conditions, especially chronic kidney disease and chemotherapy.
	Filgrastim	18,800	Decrease the incidence of infection in patients with nonmyeloid malignancies and who are receiving anticancer drugs.
	Interleukin-11	19,000	Used to prevent low platelet counts and to reduce the need for blood transfusions following cancer treatments.
Immunomodulators	Cyclosporine	1203	May be used to treat several diseases including rheumatoid arthritis, psoriasis, nephrotic syndrome, and Crohn's disease.
Insulin and related agents	Glucagon	3483	Treatment of severe hypoglycemia.
	Insulin	5808 (natural hormone)	Treatment of diabetes mellitus; insulin comes in many forms and variations.
Oncolytic agents	Asparaginase	~175,000	Treatment of acute lymphocytic leukemia.
	Leuprolide	1209	Palliative treatment of advanced prostate cancer and treatment of anemia caused by uterine leiomyomas.
Parathyroid hormone	Teriparatide	4118	Synthetic polypeptide of the active part of the parathyroid hormone.
Thrombolytic and related agents	Alteplase	59,042	Used to break up and dissolve blood clots after acute heart attack or pulmonary embolism.
	Antihemophilic factor (Factor VIII)	~200,000	Used to treat or prevent bleeding in patients with hemophilia A.

TABLE 21-1   **Examples of Polypeptide and Protein (Nonantibody) Therapeutic Agents** (*continued*)

Therapeutic Class	Polypeptide/Protein	Molecular Weight (g/mol)	Comments
	Antithrombin III	58,000	Thromboembolism associated with hereditary antithrombin III deficiency.
	Aprotinin	6512	Protease inhibitor that modulates the systemic inflammatory response associated with cardiopulmonary bypass surgery.
	Clotting Factor IX	~55,000	Therapy of factor IX deficiency, hemophilia B, or Christmas disease.
	Clotting Factor VIIa	~50,000	Treating or preventing bleeding in patients with hemophilia A or B, acquired hemophilia, or congenital factor VII deficiency.
	Urokinase	32,400	Enzyme which breaks up and dissolves blood clots.
Tuberculostatic agent	Viomycin	686	Used in combination with other antitubercular drugs.

*Only selected drugs are listed.
From: 2008 Physicians' Desk Reference. Montvale, NJ; PDR: 2008.

A major effort has been underway in the last decade or two to develop monoclonal antibody drugs. There are five classes of endogenous antibodies. The antibodies used as drugs belong to the immunoglobulin G (IgG) class. This group of antibodies accounts for the majority (75%–80%) of naturally occurring antibodies in the body. Collectively, they are the second most common protein in plasma (5–13 g/L); albumin is first (35–50 g/L). The general structure of IgG molecules is shown in Fig. 21-1. They are heterodimeric molecules, approximately 150,000 g/mol in size, and are composed (Fig. 21-1B) of two different kinds of polypeptide chains, heavy (~50,000 g/mol) and light (~25,000 g/mol). There are two kinds of light chains, kappa (κ) and lambda (λ). Upon cleavage with the enzyme papain, the fragment–antigen binding (Fab) portion of the molecule can be separated from the Fc (fragment crystalline) portion (Fig. 21-1C). The Fab fragments contain the variable amino acid domains responsible for antibody specificity. There are literally millions of specific molecules that come under the general name IgG.

Monoclonal antibodies (mab), monospecific antibodies that are identical because they are produced by immune cells of a single type and all these cells are clones of a single parent cell, are named by the World Health Organization International Nonproprietary Name and the *United States Adopted Names* by a common scheme. The prefix is variable for specifying the antibody. The suffix (mab) identifies the drug as a monoclonal antibody. Infixes identifying the target system and the source of the antibody, in that order, are listed in Table 21-2. Thus, the drug adalimumab is a

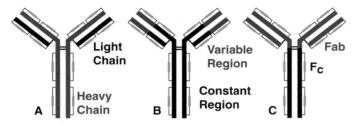

FIGURE 21-1. Antibody drugs structurally are forms of IgG. **A.** IgG consists of two heavy chains (*colored*, ~50,000 g/mol and 440 amino acids each) and two light chains (*black*, ~25,000 g/mol and 220 amino acids each). **B.** The variable portions of the heavy and light chains (*colored*, about 110–130 amino acids each) provide the specificity to the molecule. **C.** When split by papain, IgG forms two molecules of Fab (*colored*, fragment–antigen binding, 53,000 g/mol) and Fc (*black*, fragment crystalline). F(ab)$_2$ (93,000 g/mol), the fragment formed when Fc is stripped from the rest of the molecule, is also formed. The small grey boxes denote disulfide bonds that help hold the molecule together.

TABLE 21-2	Nomenclature of Monoclonal Antibodies: Target and Source Infixes

	Target				Source
-o(s)	Bone	-me(l)	Melanoma	-u-	Human
-vi(r)	Viral	-ma(r)	Mammary tumor	-o-	Mouse
-ba(c)	Bacterial	-go(t)	Testicular tumor	-a-	Rat
-li(m)	Immune system	-go(v)	Ovarian tumor	-e-	Hamster
-le(s)	Infectious lesions	-pr(o)	Prostate tumor	-i-	Primate
-ci(r)	Cardiovascular	-tu(m)	Misc. tumor	-xi-	Chimeric
-mu(l)	Musculoskeletal	-neu(r)	Nervous system	-zu-	Humanized
-ki(n)	Interleukin as target	-tox(a)	Toxin as target	-axo-	Rat/murine hybrid
-co(l)	Colonic tumor	-fu(ng)	Fungal	-xizu-	Chimeric + humanized

monoclonal antibody (-mab) of human origin (-u-), acting on the immune system (-li[m]-). To further demonstrate the naming of these drugs, selected monoclonal antibody drugs are classified in Table 21-3 based on their source, which include murine, chimeric (fusion protein), humanized, and human technologies. Also included are their therapeutic uses, their half-lives, dosing intervals, and routes of administration. Table 21-4 lists polyclonal antibodies, derived from different immune cells. Tables 21-1, 21-3, and 21-4, although quite long, are exemplary, not exhaustive. They do, however, clearly demonstrate the wide range of agents available in the category of *protein drugs.*

It is virtually impossible to summarize the pharmacokinetic and pharmacodynamic properties of protein drugs for the category as a whole because of the wide range of compounds and activities involved. In this chapter, the general differences in the kinetic behavior of protein drugs relative to that observed with small molecules is emphasized. The kinetic and dynamic behaviors of antibody drugs are also compared to those of other protein drugs.

Type	Antibody (Brand Name)	Therapeutic Use	Half-life (hr)	Administration (Dosing Interval)
Murine Monoclonal Antibodies				
	Muromomab-CD3 (Orthoclone OKT3)	Transplant rejection.	-	i.v. (daily)
	Tositumomab (Bexxar)	Non-Hodgkin's lymphoma.	67	Given in two steps: dosimetric and therapeutic
Chimeric Monoclonal Antibodies				
	Abciximab (ReoPro) (Fab fragment)	Percutaneous coronary intervention.	30 min, Platelet-bound longer	i.v. infusion (up to 12 hr)
	Basiliximab (Simulect)	Transplant rejection.	228	i.v. (single dose)
	Cetuximab (Erbitux)	Squamous cell carcinoma of the head and neck and colorectal cancer.	97	i.v. (weekly)
	Infliximab (Remicade)	Rheumatoid arthritis.	204	i.v. (every 8 weeks)
	Rituximab (Rituxan, Mabthera)	Non-Hodgkin's lymphoma.	76	i.v. (once weekly)
Humanized Monoclonal Antibodies				
	Alemtuzumab (Campath)	Chronic lymphocytic leukemia.	144	i.v. (3 times per week)
	Bevacizumab (Avastin)	Colorectal cancer and lung cancer.	480	i.v. (every 3 weeks)
	Efalizumab (Raptiva)	Plaque psoriasis.	600	s.c. (weekly)
	Gemtuzumab ozogamicin (Mylotarg)	Acute myelogenous leukemia.	-	i.v.
	Omalizumab (Xolair)	Allergy-related asthma.	624	s.c. (every 2–4 weeks)
	Palivizumab (Synagis)	Respiratory syncytial virus infection in children.	480	i.m. (monthly)
	Ranibizumab (Lucentis)	Macular degeneration.	216	Intravitreal injection (monthly)
	Trastuzumab (Herceptin)	Breast cancer.	~200	i.v. (once weekly)
Human Monoclonal Antibodies				
	Adalimumab (Humira)	Autoimmune inflammatory disorders.	336	s.c. (every other week)
	Panitumumab (Vectibix)	Colorectal cancer.	180	i.v. (every 2 weeks)

TABLE 21-4 FDA-Approved Polyclonal Immune Globulins and Antibody Fragments

Crotalidae immune Fab	Pertussis immune globulin
Digoxin immune Fab	Rabies immune globulin
Hepatitis B immune globulin	Rho(D) immune globulin
Intravenous gamma globulin	Tetanus immune globulin
Lymphocyte antithymocyte immune globulin	Vaccinia immune globulin
Normal immune globulin	Varicella-zoster immune globulin

COMPARISON OF THE PHARMACOKINETICS OF PROTEIN DRUGS WITH THAT OF CONVENTIONAL NONPROTEIN DRUGS

As with small conventional drugs, the processes of absorption, distribution, excretion, and metabolism of protein drugs are of interest kinetically. Differences in these processes between the two kinds of drugs are subsequently examined. But first, let us consider the purity of the drugs themselves.

In Chapter 2, *Fundamental Concepts and Terminology*, we spent some time discussing chemical purity and analytic specificity and their importance in pharmacokinetic evaluations. Although these issues have received extensive attention for drugs that are small molecules, this has not been as easy to do with protein drugs. With protein drugs, one often uses the term *heterogeneity* to refer to the fact that the *drug* is not a pure substance but rather a mixture of substances. When MW of a protein drug is given, as in Table 21-1, it often refers to an average for the active components. In addition, the analysis of proteins in plasma or other biologic fluids is often based on immunoassays, which show some cross-reactivity with similar proteins. What is being measured is always of concern. With these caveats in mind, let us examine the general pharmacokinetic differences between protein drugs and small conventional ones.

ABSORPTION

In contrast to small conventional drugs, systemic absorption is a major problem with protein drugs. These kinds of drugs generally cannot be taken orally because of their instability in the gastrointestinal tract and great difficulty in permeating the intestinal epithelium. By this route, they are, simply put, a source of amino acids for protein synthesis within the body. As a consequence, their oral bioavailabilities are usually extremely low and erratic. They generally must be given parenterally. However, even when given subcutaneously or intramuscularly, common routes of their administration, their systemic bioavailabilities are often low and variable, an area explored further later in the chapter. To circumvent the lack of absorption after oral administration, some proteins are only used locally or are given for their systemic effect by less conventional methods as shown in Table 21-5. In the case of the leuprolide acetate polymeric matrix formulations and its implant, as discussed in Chapter 7, *Absorption*, the intent is not just systemic delivery, but to prolong its systemic input. Indeed, considerable effort has been, and will continue to be, placed on developing pharmaceutical systems to improve systemic delivery of protein drugs.

DISTRIBUTION

With few exceptions, protein drugs are hydrophilic molecules that have difficulty entering cells of the body. They therefore tend to have volumes of distribution that lie between that of plasma (0.04 L/kg) and the extracellular space (0.23 L/kg), as shown in Table 21-6 for both nonantibody and antibody proteins. For those that enter the extracellular matrix of tissues, they often do so slowly, particularly large ones, because they have difficulty permeating the blood capillary endothelium (as discussed later in this chapter). One exception to this generalization of a small volume of distribution is the immunosuppressive drug, cyclosporine (not in Table 21-6), a cyclic undecapeptide with a MW of 1202 g/mol and a volume of distribution of 3 to 5 L/kg. This unusual peptide, having no charge at physiologic pH, is highly lipophilic with an n-octanol/water partition coefficient of about 1000 and a high affinity for tissues, especially adipose tissue.

Many protein drugs that are endogenous substances have carrier proteins within the body that may improve their stability as well as aid in the delivery to the site of action at a higher rate than would occur if there were no such binding. Examples of such protein

TABLE 21-5 **Examples of Less Conventional Sites and Methods of Administration for Local and Systemic Delivery of Protein Drugs**

Polypeptide/Protein	Therapeutic Use	Site And Method of Administration
Local		
Bacitracin and polymyxin B (anti-infective agents)	Superficial ocular and skin infections	Application of ointment.
Dornase alfa (recombinant human deoxyribonuclease)	Cystic fibrosis	Inhalation using nebulizer to help clear lungs.
Gladase (papain, a proteolytic enzyme, plus urea)	Removal of necrotic tissue	Topical; ointment applied directly to wound.
Pancrelipase powder (lipase, protease, and amylase—digestive enzymes)	Cystic fibrosis (local intestinal effect)	Taken orally with meals. Enteric-coated particles in dosage form.
Thrombin, topical	To stop local bleeding that cannot be readily stopped with surgery	Topical; applied to area of slow, but persistent, bleeding.
Systemic		
Calcitonin-salmon (thyroid hormone that acts primarily on bone)	Postmenopausal osteoporosis	Nasal spray; the relative bioavailability (compared to i.m dose) is 3%.
Desmopressin (synthetic form of antidiuretic hormone)	Primary nocturnal enuresis and diabetes insipidus	Intranasal; administered through a soft, flexible, plastic rhinal tube; also in a nasal spray.
Leuprolide acetate (naturally occurring GnRH)	Advanced prostatic cancer	Polymeric matrix formulations of the drug, formulated to last 1, 3, 4, and 6 months.
		Implant; inserted subcutaneously on inner side of upper arm; product constantly releases 120 μg/day and is replaced once yearly.

drugs with carrier proteins are given in Table 21-7 (page 643). Some carriers also help to stabilize the protein. An example is that of human growth hormone, Table 21-8 (page 643). When given with human growth hormone–binding protein, clearance of the drug and its volume of distribution are greatly reduced in the rat, an animal that has neither the human binding protein nor human growth hormone.

Binding sometimes occurs within the extracellular space or on cell membranes of tissues. As with small drugs, the volume of distribution of a protein depends on the relative binding within tissues and plasma, as well as the aqueous space into which the protein gains access. Furthermore, for large proteins, the steady-state unbound concentration of protein in interstitial fluid is much lower than that in blood. This is different from our expectation for most small molecule drugs, where in many cases diffusion is the primary mechanism responsible for drug distribution. Protein concentrations are lower in the interstitial fluid and vary from tissue to tissue because of differences in the efficiency of convective uptake, capillary permeability, lymph flow, and tissue metabolism.

In many cases, it may be impossible to infer accurate distribution information from plasma data alone. Common methods applied for analysis of *Vss* and *V* assume that all elimination occurs at sites that are in rapid equilibrium with plasma. This assumption is

TABLE 21-6 **Volumes of Distribution of Selected Nonantibody Proteins, Antibodies, and Antibody Fragments**

Protein	V_1 (L/kg)*	V_{ss} (L/kg)[†]
Nonantibody Proteins		
r-Activated factor VII	-	0.08
h-Albumin	0.06	0.11
Bivalirudin	-	0.20
rh-Factor VIII	-	0.07
rh-Follicle-stimulating hormone	0.06	0.16
GnRH	-	0.22
r-Hirudin	-	0.20
Human tumor necrosis factor binding protein-1	0.06	0.14
rh-Insulin-like growth factor	-	0.23
rh-Interleukin-10	-	0.06
rh-Interleukin-2	0.06	0.11
Pegylated-r-interleukin-2	0.03	0.05
rh-Soluble CD4	0.07	0.10
r-Superoxide dismutase	-	0.10
Tenecteplase	0.07	0.12
Antibodies and Antibody Fragments[‡]		
Adalimumab	-	0.067–0.086
Alefacept	-	0.094
Alemtuzumab	-	0.18
Basiliximab	-	0.12
Bevacizumab	-	0.043
Cetuximab	-	0.05–0.07
Digoxin immune Fab	-	0.086
Etanercept**	-	0.15
Omalizumab	-	0.05
Trastuzumab	-	0.043

h, human; r, recombinant.
*Initial dilution space.
[†]Volume at steady state.
[‡]From: 2008 Physicians' Desk Reference. Montvale, NJ: PDR; 2008.
**Fusion protein of tissue necrosis factor and Fc portion of IgG1.

TABLE 21-7	Representative Protein Drugs that Bind to Other Proteins (Carrier Proteins) in Plasma

Cyclosporine	Interferon
Deoxyribonuclease I	Interleukin-2
Growth Hormone	Nartogastrim
Insulin-like Growth Factor-I	Nerve Growth Factor
Insulin-like Growth Factor-II	Tissue Plasminogen Activator

TABLE 21-8	h-Growth Hormone in Rat

	Clearance (mL/min-kg)	V_{ss} (mL/kg)
Complexed* h-Growth Hormone	2.3 ± 0.2	71 ± 33
Unbound h-Growth Hormone[†]	14.0 ± 2.2	256 ± 39

*Complexed with human growth hormone–binding protein.
[†]Human growth hormone ≈ 22,000 g/mol.
From: Baumann G, Amburn, KD, Buchanan TA. The effect of circulating growth hormone-binding protein on metabolic clearance, distribution, and degradation of human growth hormone. J Clin Endocrinol Metab 1987;64:657–660.

valid in most cases for small molecules, as most elimination occurs in the liver and kidney, organs that are very highly perfused. Many proteins, however, may be eliminated from sites that are poorly perfused, and application of mammillary models (Chapter 19, *Distribution Kinetics*) may lead to significant underestimations of the actual extent of drug distribution.

RENAL EXCRETION

No matter the size, protein drugs, which are usually highly hydrophilic, generally have low renal clearances (when defined as rate of urinary excretion relative to the plasma concentration). However, this does not mean that many are not extensively eliminated in the kidneys. The low renal clearance of protein drugs arises from one of two properties: their size, proteins larger than about 60,000 g/mol are not materially filtered, or from their metabolism (or degradation) in the proximal tubule after their filtration. Because of extensive metabolism of smaller proteins, it is better to use the terms **renal handling** or **renal processing**, instead of renal excretion to describe the elimination of protein drugs in the kidneys.

The key to understanding the loss of protein drugs in the kidneys, as viewed from plasma, is glomerular filtration. Although 60,000 g/mol has been given as a rough cut-off for filtration, molecular size is not the only factor determining the extent of filtration. Table 21-9 lists the glomerular sieving coefficients (concentration in glomerular filtrate relative to that unbound in plasma) of selected proteins. It is apparent from the data for horseradish peroxidases that charge also plays a role. This is reinforced by studies with dextrans (branched polysaccharides made with glucose molecules) prepared with and without charges on them (Fig. 21-2). Anionic dextrans undergo filtration much less readily than cationic ones at the same molecular size, measured here by effective molecular radius (crudely, MW = $[1.14 \times \text{molecular radius}]^3$). Albumin, a protein with a MW of 69,000 g/mol, has a negative charge and thus has a sieving coefficient

TABLE 21-9	Glomerular Sieving Coefficients of Selected Proteins*	
Protein	Size (g/mol)	Glomerular Sieving Coefficient
Insulin	6000	0.89
Bovine parathyroid hormone	9000	0.69
Lysozyme	14,600	0.75
Myoglobin	16,900	0.75
Growth hormone	22,000	0.65
Superoxide dismutase	32,000	0.33[†]
Horseradish peroxidases	40,000 (anionic)	0.007
	(neutral)	0.06
	(cationic)	0.34
Bence-Jones (λ-L chain)	44,000	0.085
Albumin	69,000	0.001[‡]

*From: Maack T, Johnson V, Kau ST, et al. Renal filtration, transport, and metabolism of low-molecular-weight proteins: a review. Kidney Int 1979;16:251–290.
[†]From: Tsao C, Green P, Odlind B, Brater C. Pharmacokinetics of recombinant human superoxide dismutase in healthy volunteers. Clin Pharmacol Ther 1991;50:713–720.
[‡]From: Oaken DE, Cotes SC, Mende CW. Micropuncture study of tubular transport of albumin in rats with aminonucleoside nephrosis. Kidney Int 1972;1:3–11.

FIGURE 21-2. Glomerular sieving coefficients of dextran derivatives reflect the influence of size and charge of molecules. Cationic molecules tend to be much more readily filtered than neutral ones which, in turn, are more readily filtered than anionic ones. Added is a value for albumin (▲), a molecule with a net negative 52 charges at physiologic pH. (From: Arendshorst WJ, Navar LG. Renal circulation and glomerular hemodynamics. In: Schrier RW, ed. Diseases of the Kidney and Urinary Tract. 8th ed. Philadelphia: Lippincott Williams & Wilkins; 2006.)

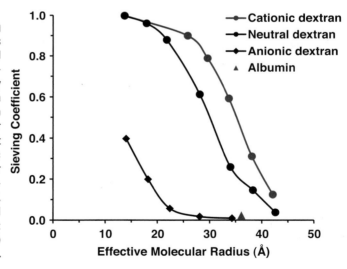

less than that expected had it been neutral or cationic in nature. Shape of the molecule and rigidity also play a role as does binding to other proteins within plasma. Those proteins that are bound to large carrier proteins have reduced glomerular filtration as one would expect.

As shown in Fig. 21-3, low MW proteins are often extensively metabolized by enzymes located in the brush border of the lumen, whereas higher MW proteins are transported into the proximal tubular cells by endocytosis and metabolized (degraded) there by lysosomal enzymes. Generally, catabolism of proteins continues until the constituent amino acids are formed, although some are only partially degraded. For small proteins that are metabolized on the brush border, the amino acids and fragments are largely conserved by trans-

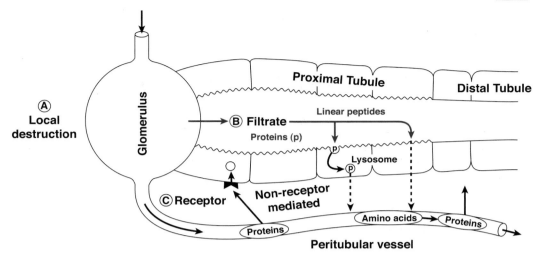

FIGURE 21-3. Pathways of protein elimination in the kidney. **A.** Local degradation by the glomerulus represents a minor site of elimination for small peptide hormones such as angiotensin, bradykinin, atrial natriuretic peptide, and possibly calcitonin. **B.** Glomerular filtration and tubular absorption is the major route for proteins and peptides. Proteins and complex peptides require internalization prior to degradation. Small linear peptides are hydrolyzed at the luminal membrane. **C.** Postglomerular peritubular elimination constitutes an important though lesser route of elimination for some protein hormones. Their basolateral uptake is largely receptor mediated and is followed by intracellular degradation. (From: Rabkin R, Dahl DO. Renal uptake and disposal of proteins and peptides. In: Audus KL, Raub TJ, eds. Biological Barriers to Protein Delivery. New York: Plenum Press; 1993.)

porters that reabsorb them back into the vasculature. Some peptides and small proteins undergo postglomerular and peritubular transport and metabolism. This is analogous to secretion of small molecules, but little or none of the protein drug may appear in the urine. Although quantitative information is often lacking, for many protein drugs with a molecular size less than 30,000 g/mol, the kidney is *a*, if not *the*, major organ of elimination.

METABOLISM

Proteins are metabolized by proteolytic enzymes, which ultimately break the substances down to their constituent amino acids. These enzymes are ubiquitous, some within cells, some on cell surfaces, and some in extracellular fluids in essentially all tissues of the body. Virtually all protein drugs are eliminated by metabolism; exceptions appear to be restricted to a few small peptides, which are primarily eliminated by renal excretion. In general, however, metabolism predominates, but where the metabolism occurs varies from one protein to another. Size of the molecule is particularly important. Indeed, two issues seem to be overriding in determining the location and the rate of metabolism of proteins, namely, substrate specificity/reactivity, and accessibility to the metabolizing enzymes. Glycosylation, addition of glycan (carbohydrate) to a protein and pegylation, attaching one or more chains of polyethylene glycol, usually increase the half-life of a protein by either making it a poorer substrate for proteolysis or decreasing its access to the metabolizing enzymes, or both. Certainly, they have the potential to reduce glomerular filtration and renal metabolism of those polypeptides and proteins that become larger than about 30,000 g/mol. Provided that activity is retained, this procedure has therefore become a common one to try to improve therapy with certain protein drugs.

For antibody drugs, being very large, there is no glomerular filtration in the kidneys, and the liver appears to not contribute much to their metabolism either. The majority of antibody elimination occurs following fluid-phase endocytosis, by cells at sites throughout the body, followed by intracellular catabolism. As mentioned previously, generally, the clearances of antibodies are extremely low when only this process is involved in elimination. This relative stability may be caused, at least in part, by binding to the Brambell receptor (FcRn), which protects the antibody by preventing its uptake and degradation by the acidic lysosomes within the cell. The complex is eventually returned to the cell surface, where it rapidly dissociates to liberate the antibody.

PHARMACODYNAMICS

PHARMACODYNAMICS OF NONANTIBODY PROTEIN DRUGS

Nonantibody proteins have a wide range of pharmacologic effects (see Tables 21-1 and 21-3). They act as hormones, enzymes, replacement proteins (lacking in certain genetic disorders), anticoagulants, immunomodulators, antitubercular agents, and antibiotics, to name a few. Needless to say, there are many potential models for the pharmacodynamics of this class of drugs. The models that are most likely to be successful and useful in understanding and rationalizing the dosage regimen of protein drugs are those that are mechanistically based (i.e., those that incorporate the physiologic and biochemical processes involved). An interesting example of a mechanistic model is shown in Fig. 21-4 for a neutrophil inhibitory factor, UK-279,276 (a 257 amino acids, 41,000 g/mol recombinant glycoprotein) with an intended indication of treatment of stroke.

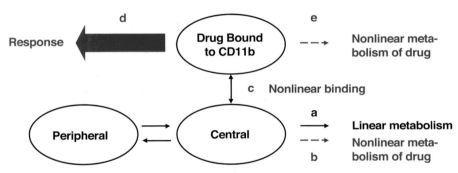

FIGURE 21-4. A schematic pharmacokinetic/pharmacodynamic model for UK-279,276, a recombinant neutrophil inhibitory factor, which distributes reversibly between central and peripheral compartments. The drug is eliminated from the body by three mechanisms: a linear metabolic pathway (**a**), a nonlinear metabolic pathway (**[b]** *colored*), and a pathway that relates to the site of action, namely, binding to the integrin, CD11b/CD18 (identified as CD11b) on the surface of the neutrophil cell. Nonlinear binding at this site (**[c]**, *colored*) leads to the nonlinear pharmacodynamic response (**[d]**, *colored*); it also is associated with another nonlinear pathway of elimination of the drug (**[e]**, *colored*), presumably by endocytosis of the bound drug. These processes result in the pharmacokinetics and pharmacodynamics of the drug being intimately linked. (From: Marshall S, Macintyre F, James I, Krams M, Jonsson NE. Role of mechanistically-based pharmacokinetic/pharmacodynamic models in drug development: a case study of a therapeutic protein. Clin Pharmacokinet 2006;45:177–197.)

UK-279,276 is a selective antagonist of CD11b, an integrin located on the surface of neutrophils and certain other cell types. The binding of UK-279,276 to CD11b blocks several neutrophil adhesion–dependent functions, for example, the infiltration of activated neutrophils to the site of an infarction. Its pharmacokinetics comprises saturable binding to the active site, and metabolism by both linear and nonlinear processes. One initially confusing aspect was the clear difference in the model needed to characterize the pharmacokinetics in patients compared to healthy volunteers, which was subsequently traced to the binding to CD11b. Namely, binding to this receptor relates not only to the drug's pharmacodynamic action, but also to its pharmacokinetics, in that once bound the complex is internalized by endocytosis and eliminated. Stroke or trauma markedly increases the number of circulating neutrophils and, as a result, a much greater fraction of drug in the body is bound to this receptor, which is evidenced in its kinetics by a more pronounced nonlinearity and more rapid elimination, at below saturating concentrations, in patients than in healthy volunteers.

PHARMACODYNAMICS OF ANTIBODY DRUGS

Because of the high degree of specificity of antibodies, they can be developed to do specific tasks. They, too, show nonlinear pharmacokinetics, which, again, is often linked to their pharmacodynamics by a similar type of mechanism as seen with UK-279,276. At high doses, the binding approaches saturation and the elimination of the drug is slower than that seen when a larger percentage of the drug in the body is bound to the receptor. The longer half-life and a more fully occupied receptor at higher doses over increasingly longer time spans suggest that higher doses may be therapeutically preferred. Such receptor target–mediated nonlinear kinetics is much more common with protein drugs than with small MW ones.

In general, the pharmacodynamics of antibodies (monoclonal, polyclonal, fragments, and fusion proteins) can be divided into four categories as shown in Table 21-10. Let us examine the actions of one drug in each of the categories listed.

TABLE 21-10 Therapeutic Uses of Antibodies, Antibody Fragments, and Fusion Proteins	
Purpose	**Examples—Indication**
Immunotoxicotherapeutic Agents	
To prevent or reverse toxicities associated with venoms, toxins, drugs, or endogenous compounds	Adalimumab—rheumatoid arthritis and psoriatic arthritis. Crotalidae polyvalent immune Fab—to treat snake bites. Digoxin immune Fab—detoxify patients on digoxin.
Agents that Destroy Target Cells	
To destroy target cells, such as lymphocytes, cancer cells, and bacteria either by opsonizing target cells for destruction by the immune system or as a targeting vector for delivery of cytotoxic agent	Alemtuzumab—B-cell chronic lymphocytic leukemia in patients treated with alkylating agents. Muromonab—to treat acute allograft rejection in transplant patients. Rituximab—CD20-positive, non-Hodgkin lymphoma.
Agents that Alter Cell Function	
To alter cell function, such as platelet aggregation, allograft rejection, and leukocyte adhesion	Abciximab—to prevent cardiac ischemic complications. Daclizumab—to prevent organ rejection in patients who receive renal transplants. It is used in combination with other agents. Efalizumab—to treat moderate-to-severe plaque psoriasis.
Antibody-Directed Drug Delivery	
To improve the specific delivery of active drug to the site of action	Gemtuzumab ozogamicin—treatment of patients with CD33 positive acute myeloid leukemia. Indium-111 Capromab pendetide—The drug is indicated as a diagnostic imaging agent in newly diagnosed patients with biopsy-proven prostate cancer. It is thought to be clinically localized after standard diagnostic evaluation in patients who are at high risk for pelvic lymph node and in postprostatectomy patients with a rising prostate-specific antigen (PSA) and a negative or equivocal standard metastatic evaluation in whom there is a high clinical suspicion of occult metastatic disease.

From: Lobo ED, Hansen RJ, Balthasar JP. Minireview. Antibody pharmacokinetics and pharmacodynamics. J Pharm Sci 2004; 93:2645–2668.

Immunotoxicotherapeutic Agents.   Digoxin immune Fab is a preparation of digoxin-immune Fab immunoglobulin fragments obtained from the blood of sheep. The sheep are immunized with a digoxin derivative, digoxin dicarboxymethoxylamine, which is coupled to keyhole limpet hemocyanin. The final product is obtained by isolating the immunoglobulin fraction, digesting it with papain, and isolating the digoxin-specific Fab fragments by affinity chromatography. The fragments have a MW of about 46,000 g/mol. Figure 21-5 shows the time course of the concentrations of unbound digoxin (*fu* is about 0.8 normally) and digoxin-fragment complex with time in a patient intoxicated with digoxin. Typical therapeutic concentrations of digoxin are 1 to 2.5 μM (0.8–2 μg/L). Note that the concentration of unbound digoxin dramatically decreases when the protein drug is given and then slowly rises and then falls with time. The total concentration, including that bound to the immunoglobulin fragment, dramatically increases as drug is pulled out of the tissues as the association constant is in the range of 10^9 to 10^{10} M^{-1}, a value much greater than that of digoxin for its sodium pump receptor. With time the fragment is eliminated by the kidney and the reticuloendothelial system. The key effect of this protein drug is to rapidly decrease the unbound digoxin level to stop the intoxication. Each vial of the product binds the equivalent of 0.5 mg of digoxin.

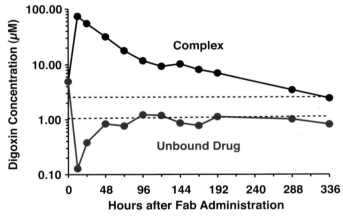

FIGURE 21-5.   Semilogarithmic plot of the concentration of unbound (●) and total (including that bound to the antibody, ●) digoxin with time immediately before and after the i.v. administration (30 min for each vial, equivalent to 0.5 mg) of the digoxin Fab antibody in an individual intoxicated subject. The usual therapeutic window of digoxin is shown by the dashed lines. The drug clearly moves out of the tissues onto the antibody in plasma with a decrease in the unbound concentration in plasma and throughout the body. (From: Ujhelyi MR, Robert S, Cummings DM, et al. Influence of digoxin immune Fab therapy and renal dysfunction on the disposition of total and free digoxin. Ann Int Med 1993;119:273–277.)

Agents that Destroy Target Cells.   Alemtuzumab binds to CD52, a nonmodulating glycoprotein antigen (21,000–28,000 g/mol) that is present on the surface of essentially all B and T lymphocytes, a majority of monocytes, macrophages, and a few other cell types. The proposed mechanism of action is antibody-dependent lysis of leukemic cells following cell surface binding. The drug is indicated for the treatment of B-cell chronic lymphocytic leukemia in patients who have been treated with alkylating agents and who have failed fludarabine therapy.

Agents that Alter Cell Function.   Efalizumab is an immunosuppressive recombinant humanized IgG1 kappa isotype monoclonal antibody that binds to human CD11a (1). At a dose of 1 mg/kg weekly by the s.c. route, it reduces expression of CD11a on circulating T lymphocytes to approximately 15% to 25% of predose values and reduces free CD11a binding sites to a mean of less than 5% of predose values. These pharmacodynamic effects were seen 1 to 2 days after the first dose and are maintained with weekly dosing. Following discontinuation, CD11a expression returned to a mean of 74% of baseline at 5 weeks and stayed at comparable levels at 8 and 13 weeks. Following discontinuation, free CD11a binding sites returned to a mean of 86% of baseline at 8 weeks and stayed at comparable levels at 13 weeks.

Antibody-Directed Drug Delivery. Gemtuzumab ozogamicin is a chemotherapy agent composed of a recombinant humanized IgG4, kappa antibody conjugated with a cytotoxic antitumor antibiotic, calicheamicin, isolated from fermentation of a bacterium, *Micromonospora echinospora* subsp. *calichensis.* The antibody portion of the drug binds specifically to the CD33 antigen, a sialic acid–dependent adhesion protein found on the surface of leukemic blasts and immature normal cells of myelomonocytic lineage, but not on normal hematopoietic stem cells. This antigen is expressed on the surface of leukemic blasts in more than 80% of patients with acute myeloid leukemia. Binding of the anti-CD33 antibody portion of the drug with the CD33 antigen results in the formation of a complex that is internalized. Upon internalization, the calicheamicin derivative is released inside the lysosomes of the myeloid cell. The released calicheamicin derivative binds to DNA in the minor groove resulting in DNA double-strand breaks and cell death.

PHARMACOKINETIC AND PHARMACODYNAMIC RATE LIMITATIONS

Pharmacodynamic principles previously learned from small nonprotein molecules apply to protein drugs as well, for example, those involving rate-limiting steps. The kinetics of the development and decline of a measured response can be rate-limited by either the pharmacokinetics or pharmacodynamics of the drug, as previously presented in Chapter 8, *Response Following a Single Dose* . An example of a peptide drug for which pharmacokinetics is rate limiting is eptifibatide, used to prevent blood clotting in acute coronary syndrome and in certain medical procedures. The drug acts by preventing platelet aggregation. The effect is immediate. The development and maintenance of the effect in vivo depends on the pharmacokinetics of the drug. With a half-life of about 2 hr, it may take several hours of a constant rate infusion to develop the full desired effect. Consequently, a bolus dose is recommended. Discontinuance of drug effect depends on how quickly the drug leaves the body. Response here is clearly pharmacokinetically driven.

Leuprolide acetate, a gonadotropin-releasing hormone (GnRH) agonist, is used to palliatively treat advanced prostate cancer. This peptide has a half-life of 3 hr, yet its effect on testosterone levels takes days to develop, as shown in Fig. 21-6 for a depot formulation that releases drug for 3 months after a s.c. injection. The plasma concentration of leuprolide is also shown in the figure. The drug initially increases but thereafter decreases pituitary secretion of the gonadotropins, luteinizing hormone, and follicle-stimulating hormone. The net result is that when administered to men, the levels of testosterone, an endogenous hormone with a 1-hr half-life, initially rise and then fall to levels even below castration values. The kinetics of measured response in this case is pharmacodynamically driven. It is the dynamics of the pituitary hormones and the complexities of the decrease in testosterone production that determine how quickly the effect develops.

Another example of pharmacodynamics rate-limiting the response to a protein drug was presented in Chapter 11, *Multiple-Dose Regimens,* Fig. 11-17, in which the hematocrit increased for about 70 days when erythropoietin (half-life 6 hr) was administered in a multiple-dose regimen. The increase in the measured response with time here is caused by the slow turnover of erythrocytes in blood. The full impact of the increase in the rate of erythrocyte production is not evident until the cells initially formed during drug treatment reach their lifespan, at which time the rate of cell death then equals the rate of cell production.

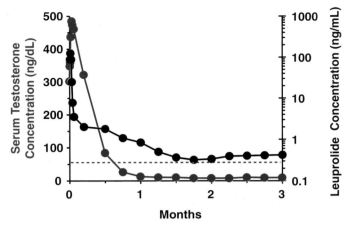

FIGURE 21-6. The serum testosterone concentration (*colored*) increases and then falls to levels below castration values (50 μg/dL, *dashed colored line*) in male patients given a single i.m. dose (22.5 mg) of leuprolide acetate in a depot formulation designed to release the drug systemically for at least 3 months (leuprolide concentration in black). By causing stimulation of the pituitary GnRH receptors, the drug initially causes stimulation but thereafter, through feedback, decreases pituitary secretion of the gonadotropins, luteinizing hormone, and follicle-stimulating hormone. Note that it takes about 2 weeks to bring the testosterone concentration below the castration level, in spite of the fact that the half-life of testosterone is only 1 hr. (From: 2008 Physicians' Desk Reference. Montvale, NJ: PDR; 2008:2832.)

INTRAVENOUS ADMINISTRATION

Intravenous (i.v.) administration (short-term or constant-rate infusion) is the most pharmacokinetically reliable mode of administration of protein drugs, but it is less convenient for both patients and caregivers than the s.c. or i.m. routes. Because the half-life of many nonantibody protein drugs is quite short (minutes to a few hours), a short dosing interval or a constant-rate infusion is often needed for maintenance of therapy when given intravenously as, for example, is the case for eptifibatide (Chapter 10, *Constant-Rate Input*). Most antibodies, on the other hand, have half-lives of 5 to 30 days, and consequently those with the longer half-lives can be given relatively infrequently (e.g., once weekly, every other week, or occasionally once a month). When given as a single i.v. dose, care must be taken to administer most protein drugs slowly over 10 min to an hour or more, depending on the drug, to prevent adverse effects associated with rapid administration.

SUBCUTANEOUS AND INTRAMUSCULAR ADMINISTRATION

In contrast to small molecules, size, polarity, and charge are important for s.c. and i.m. administration of proteins and large polypeptide drugs, because their transport across many membranes is hindered. Most of the pharmacokinetic and pharmacodynamic information on these kinds of drugs has been obtained following s.c. and i.m. administration. The general differences in the systemic absorption of small molecules and protein drugs are summarized in Table 21-11.

LARGE PROTEINS AND LYMPHATIC TRANSPORT

Following administration by these routes, protein drugs reach the systemic circulation by two parallel mechanisms: (a) diffusion through the interstitial fluids and transport across blood capillaries and (b) convective flow of the interstitial fluids into lymphatic

TABLE 21-11	Systemic Absorption of Protein Drugs Compared to Conventional Small Molecule Drugs following Subcutaneous and Intramuscular Injections

Conventional Drugs	Protein Drugs*
• Rapidly enter systemic circulation through blood capillaries (polarity and charge do not matter)	• Larger molecules (>15,000–20,000 g/mol) primarily reach systemic circulation via lymphatics
• Systemic absorption usually almost complete ($F \approx 1.0$)	• Subject to proteolysis during interstitial and lymphatic transit. First-pass loss is sometimes extensive

*Porter CJ, Charman SA. Minireview. Lymphatic transport of proteins after subcutaneous administration. J Pharm Sci 2000;89:297–310.

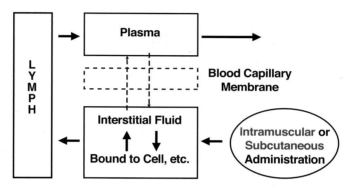

FIGURE 21-7. After i.m. or s.c. administration of a drug in solution, a drug can reach the systemic circulation via the blood capillaries or the lymphatic system. Size is the primary determinant. The capillary membrane becomes less permeable to larger molecules regardless of their lipophilicity. A large molecule, by default, then moves into the lymphatic capillaries and reaches the systemic circulation via the lymphatic vessels. This is a slow process, but not as slow as its movement across blood capillaries, so that the concentration in lymph fluid tends to be lower than in plasma.

capillaries into lymphatic channels, as shown schematically in Fig. 21-7. Molecular size is of primary importance for passage across the capillary endothelium. This is a result of greatly decreased capillary permeability as the size of the molecule is increased.

Capillary Permeability. In several animal and human models, it is apparent (Fig. 21-8) that permeability drops off dramatically with increasing molecular size, particularly in the 5000 to 60,000 g/mol size range. Interestingly, in these models, permeability does not appear to drop to zero, even for molecules that approach 1,000,000 g/mol in size.

In general, polypeptides/proteins of less than approximately 5000 g/mol in size primarily reach the systemic circulation via the blood capillaries. Because proteins of greater than about 20,000 g/mol are less able to traverse the capillary membranes, they, by default, primarily reach the systemic circulation via the lymphatic system. Some drug, of course, moves across the capillary membrane, just at a slower rate.

A schematic representation of the lymphatic system is shown in Fig. 21-9. Interstitial fluid enters the lymphatic system via lymphatic capillaries; the fluid (lymph) within the lymphatic vessels returns to the blood via the thoracic duct and the right lymphatic duct. Systemic circulating protein will then enter tissues throughout the body, but because impedance at the capillary membrane is greater than for entry into the lymphatic vessels for large proteins, such as the size of albumin, their concentration in tissue lymph is lower than in plasma. Furthermore, their concentrations in the interstitial fluids vary throughout the body. This is primarily a function of both differences in capillary permeability and the density of lymphatic capillaries.

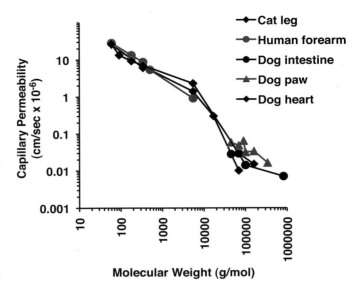

FIGURE 21-8. Capillary permeability to lipid-insoluble molecules, including proteins, in selected animal models (*see legend*). Note the dramatic decrease in permeability for molecules between 5000 and 60,000 g/mol in all the model systems shown. (From: Renkin EM. Multiple pathways of capillary permeability. Circ Res 1977;41: 735–743.)

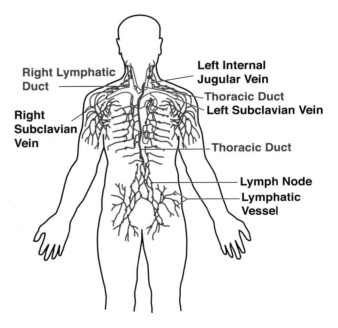

FIGURE 21-9. A sketch of the lymphatic system. Note that drug in the interstitial fluids of s.c. or muscular tissue, placed there by injection, moves through the lymphatic vessels and one or several lymph nodes before reaching the systemic circulation. Lymph returns drug to the bloodstream from a portion of the right side of the body via the right lymphatic duct and from the tissues of the rest of the body via the thoracic duct. These ducts empty into the right and left subclavian veins, respectively.

Molecular Size. The importance of molecular size is demonstrated in Fig. 21-10, which shows the increasing percentage of an injected dose recovered in lymph as a function of MW following s.c. administration in sheep. Note that more than 50% of the injected dose is recovered in the lymph for compounds with a MW above about 16,000 g/mol. Recent studies have indicated some uncertainty about the significance of lymphatic versus capillary absorption of proteins following i.m. and s.c administration, but there is no question that macromolecules reach the systemic circulation slowly and that molecular size is of paramount importance.

RATE AND EXTENT OF SYSTEMIC ABSORPTION

Lymph flow is very slow (movement of interstitial fluid into lymphatic vessels is roughly 500 times and return of lymph to blood 5000 times slower than cardiac output, 5 L/min)

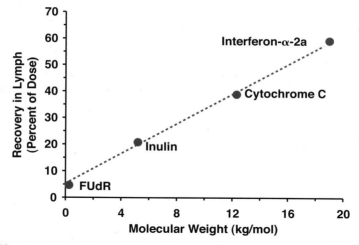

FIGURE 21-10. Correlation between MW and the cumulative recovery (mean ± SD) of recombinant interferon alpha-2a (19,000 g/mol), cytochrome C (12,300 g/mol), inulin (5200 g/mol) and 5-fluorouracil deoxyribotide (246 g/mol) in the efferent lymph from the right popliteal lymph node following s.c. administration into the lower part of right hind leg of sheep. (From: Supersaxo A, Hein WR, Steffen H. Effect of molecular weight on the lymphatic absorption of water-soluble compounds following subcutaneous administration. Pharm Res 1990;7:167–169.)

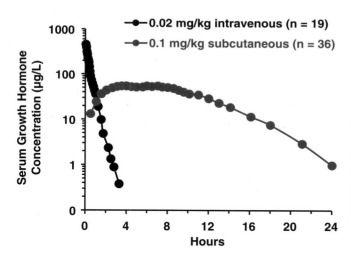

FIGURE 21-11. Mean growth hormone concentrations in healthy adult males following the administration of 0.1 mg/kg subcutaneously (*colored circles*) and 0.02 mg/kg intravenously (*black circles*). (From: 2008 Physicians' Desk Reference. Montvale, NJ: PDR; 2008:1212.)

and causes absorption from nonvascular parenteral sites to continue for many hours, as shown in Fig. 21-11 for somatropin (Nutropin), human growth hormone obtained by recombinant DNA (rDNA) technology and used for the treatment of growth failure. This drug (MW = 22,125 g/mol) has a half-life of 2.1 hr after i.v. administration of a single dose, but following s.c. administration, the plasma concentration is prolonged for at least 24 hr, with a rate of decline indicating continuing input even at this time. Elimination of this protein drug after s.c. administration is clearly absorption rate limited. It is also clear that some absorption must begin almost immediately, probably via the blood capillaries.

Subcutaneous and i.m. routes thus offer the advantage of providing prolonged input for short half-life proteins that are more than 5000 to 10,000 g/mol in size. This often permits less frequent administration than would be required by the i.v. route. However, one

TABLE 21-12 Representative Bioavailability Values and Times to Reach the Peak Plasma Concentration following Subcutaneous Administration of Various Nonantibody Protein Drugs in Humans

Protein	Approximate Monomeric Molecular Weight (kg/mol)	Bioavailability	Time of Peak Concentration (hr)
Insulin*	5.6	0.84	1–2
Insulin-like growth factor I	7.6	1.00	7
Interleukin-2	15.5	0.3–0.8	2–4
Interleukin-10[†]	18.7	0.42	4–6
Interleukin-11	19	0.65	2–3
Tumor necrosis factor-α	17.4	<0.1	2
Granulocyte macrophage colony–stimulating factor[‡]	15.5–19.5	0.5	3
Human growth hormone	22	0.5–0.8	5–8
Interferon-α	19.5	>0.8	6–8
Interferon-γ[‡]	20–25	0.3–0.7	6–13
Follicle-stimulating factor[†‡]	36	0.66	0.5
Erythropoietin[‡]	34–39	0.2–0.36	13–18

*Normally present as a hexamer.
[†]Normally present as a dimer.
[‡]May be glycosylated.
From: Porter CJ, Charman SA. Lymphatic transport of proteins after subcutaneous administration. J Pharm Sci 2000;89:297–310.

must take into account that nonvascular parenteral administration often results in reduced and more variable systemic bioavailability, as shown in Table 21-12.

The speed of absorption, after both i.m. and s.c. administration and for both small molecules and macromolecules, has been shown to be highly dependent on the site of injection, local temperature, and rubbing at the injection site, which increases movement of drug into both the vasculature and the lymphatic system, in addition to molecular size. Table 21-16 in the "Study Problems" at the end of the chapter illustrates differences in rate of absorption of growth hormone when it is subcutaneously administered in the thigh and the abdomen.

For all routes of administration, consideration should be given to both the particular properties of the site of administration and the drug itself. For example, when given nasally, a relatively permeable site with low proteolytic activity, some of the dose is systemically absorbed. However, it is often not retained there long enough for absorption to be complete (*F* is often just a few percent). Nonetheless, the factors influencing absorption from such less conventional sites are in common with those (e.g., blood flow, charge, molecular size, permeability, polarity) generally influencing absorption from oral, i.m., and s.c. sites of administration.

Generally, most antibody drugs are given by short-term i.v. infusion (see Table 21-3) as excessive adverse events occur when they are given too rapidly. After s.c. or i.m. administration, the systemic absorption of antibody drugs is even slower than that of nonantibody drugs (Table 21-13). The peak time observed is typically about 2 to 8 days, partly a result of very slow systemic input through the lymphatic system and partly because of the very long half-life of these drugs. The slow systemic absorption may, in large part, be a result of very slow diffusion of the large molecule within the interstitial fluid. The interstitial space is not a simple aqueous cavity; there are proteins that give structure to it. One might view the space like gelatin through which large protein molecules diffuse more slowly than through simple water, because of impedance causes by the interaction of the protein with the polymeric network of the extracellular matrix.

TABLE 21-13	Bioavailability of Selected Monoclonal Antibody Drugs after Subcutaneous and Intramuscular Administration of a Single Dose*				
Antibody	**Molecular Weight (kg/mol)**	**Bioavailability**	**Route of Administration**	**Peak Time (Days)**	**Terminal Half-life (Days)**
Adalimumab	148	0.64	s.c.	5.5	30
Alefacept	91.4	0.80	i.m. and i.v.	3.2[†]	11
Efalizumab	150	0.50	s.c.	-	17
Omalizumab	149	0.62	s.c.	7.5	26
Palivizumab	148	-	i.m.	2.0	20 (Pediatric)

*From: 2008 Physicians' Desk Reference. Montvale, NJ: PDR; 2008.
[†]From: Sweetser MT, Woodworth J, Swan S, Ticho B. Results of a randomized open-label crossover study of the bioequivalence of subcutaneous versus intramuscular administration of alefacept. Dermatol Online J 2006;30:12(3):1.

CONCURRENT DISEASE STATES

The effect of disease on the pharmacokinetics and pharmacodynamics of protein drugs has received much less attention than that for small conventional drugs. Most is known about the impact of renal disease. In addition, it is known that capillary endothelial permeability increases dramatically with local inflammation, allowing ready access of proteins, and even (white) cells, into the interstitial space of inflamed tissue sites and many solid tumors.

RENAL DISEASE

The clearance of those protein drugs that are primarily eliminated by the kidneys, as expected, decreases with a decrease in renal function. This is demonstrated in Fig. 21-12 by the observations for anakinra (Kineret), an interleukin-1 receptor antagonist (17,258 g/mol) used to treat rheumatoid arthritis, following s.c. administration of single doses. There is some nonrenal elimination of the drug, but in patients with normal

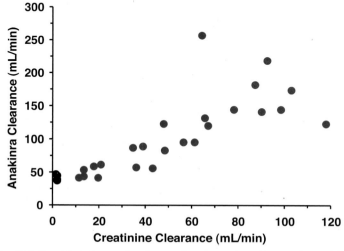

FIGURE 21-12. Relationship between the plasma clearance of anakinra and creatinine clearance in a population of subjects with varying degrees of renal function. The drug is given intravenously in a single dose of 1 mg/kg. Those subjects with end-stage renal disease are identified with the black circles and their clearances are placed on the graph at a creatinine clearance of 2 mL/min. (From: Yang BB, Baughman S, Sullivan JT. Pharmacokinetics of anakinra in subjects with different levels of renal function. Clin Pharmacol Ther 2003;74:85–94.)

TABLE 21-14 | **Area under the Curve, Peak Concentration, and Half-life of Anakinra in Healthy Subjects and Patients with Varying Degrees of Renal Function Impairment**

	Group I (Normal Renal Function)	Group II (Mildly Impaired Renal Function)	Group III (Moderately Impaired Renal Function)	Group IV (Severely Impaired Renal Function)	Group V (End-Stage Renal Disease)
Creatinine Clearance (mL/min)	95 (87–117)*	65 (57–78)	41 (35–48)	16 (12–21)	ND[†]
Cmax (mg/L)	0.77 ± 0.12[‡]	0.98 ± 0.25	1.32 ± 0.48	1.67 ± 0.43	2.17 ± 0.72
AUC (mg-hr/L)	10.2 ± 2,1	13.0 ± 3.94	21.1 ± 5.9	33.1 ± 5.3	39.4 ± 4.34
Half-life (hr)	5.24 ± 0.45	4.48 ± 1.27	5.24 ± 1.02	7.15 ± 1.73	9.71 ± 3.44

*Mean and range.
[†]Not determined.
[‡]Mean ± SD.
From: Yang BB, Baughman S, Sullivan, JT. Pharmacokinetics of anakinra in subjects with different levels of renal function. Clin Pharmacol Ther 2003;74:85–94.

renal function, its contribution is small. Again, recall that renal elimination for most protein drugs that are eliminated in the kidneys means metabolism. The drug is filtered and then metabolized by the tubular cells.

Table 21-14 lists the average peak concentration, area under the curve (*AUC*), and terminal half-life of anakinra in each of the groups studied. Note that the half-life hardly changes except in the two most severe renal dysfunction groups. This is a result of the terminal decline being rate limited by absorption from the s.c. site in at least the first two groups with the most renal function. The half-life after an i.v. dose is only 2.6 hr. The elimination half-life must exceed that of the absorption half-life before any change is expected in the terminal decline, which occurs only in the two most severe renal dysfunction groups. The terminal half-life actually increases from 2.6 to 9.7 hr, a factor of change (3.7) comparable to that for the increase in *AUC* or decrease in *Dose/AUC* (3.8).

Another generalization that can be made is that as antibodies and other very large proteins are not appreciably filtered at the glomerulus, their kinetics is therefore generally not materially affected by renal disease. However, antibody fragments, including Fab, appear to be primarily eliminated by the kidney in man in that creatinine clearance and Fab clearance are highly correlated.

HEPATIC DISEASE

There is insufficient information to make generalizations here. Some proteins are eliminated in the liver, at least in part, but others are primarily eliminated in other tissues and organs. As there is no good correlate of hepatic function, even when metabolism is primarily in the liver, one is not able to predict the effect of hepatic disease (especially cirrhosis) quantitatively. Because antibody drugs are not appreciably eliminated in the liver, one generally does not expect their kinetics to be altered in patients with hepatic disease. However, the liver is the site of formation of many endogenous proteins, such as albumin, clotting factors, and many enzymes, whose synthesis rates are reduced in hepatic disease, resulting in lower serum concentrations.

NONLINEARITIES

Nonlinear kinetic behavior is quite common to both nonantibody and antibody protein drugs. An example of the former is recombinant human granulocyte colony–stimulating

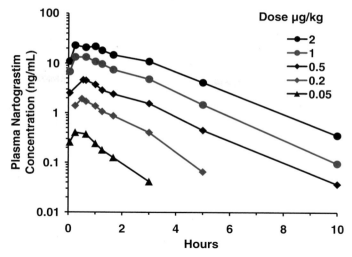

FIGURE 21-13. Plasma concentration–time profiles for recombinant human granulocyte colony–stimulating factor (nartograstim) after i.v. administration of various doses to humans. The volunteers received 30-min i.v. infusions (see legend for doses). Each point represents the mean of 4 to 6 subjects. Note that the half-life increases with the dose administered. (From: Kuwabara T, Kato M, Kobayashi S, Suzuki H, Sugiyama Y. Nonlinear pharmacokinetics of a recombinant human granulocyte colony-stimulating factor derivative [nartograstim]: species differences among rats, monkeys and humans. J Pharmacol Exp Ther 1994;271:1535–1543.)

factor (Fig. 21-13). After 30-min i.v. infusions to humans, the drug shows clear evidence of nonlinearity. The *AUC* and slopes of the decline in the plasma concentration are disproportionately increased at higher doses. An example of the latter is the observation after various doses of efalizumab (Fig. 21-14). Nonlinearity is particularly common to antibody drugs, as previously mentioned, primarily because of their saturable binding to cell surfaces, the mechanism involved in their elimination.

Because nonlinearity is common to many protein drugs, the concepts of clearance and half-life must be viewed in a guarded manner. The values given often only apply to the specific dose and conditions of a drug's administration.

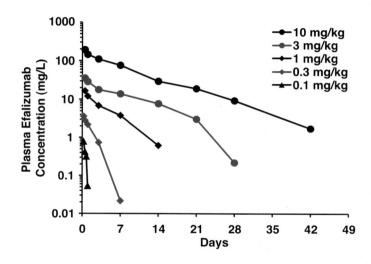

FIGURE 21-14. Plasma concentration–time curves of efalizumab following single i.v. doses of 0.1, 0.3, 1, 3, and 10 mg/kg in psoriasis patients. Note that the larger the dose the longer it takes to eliminate 50%. (From: Joshi A, Bauer R, Kuebler P, et al. An overview of the pharmacokinetics and pharmacodynamics of efalizumab: a monoclonal antibody approved for use in psoriasis. J Clin Pharmacol 2006; 46:10–20.)

IMMUNOGENIC RESPONSES

The use of protein drugs of human origin is an ideal to minimize the risk of immuno-genic responses. However, even antibodies and other therapeutic protein drugs of human origin, but especially those of animal origin, have the potential to elicit an im-mune response that causes the formation of endogenous antibodies that are directed against the therapeutic protein. Several factors appear to be important in producing the immune response. Included are the method and route of administration (occurrence in the order: s.c > i.m. > i.v.), the degree of aggregation of the therapeutic product, and the similarity of the administered protein to that of the endogenous one. An immuno-genic response often takes some time to develop as shown in Fig. 21-15 for the develop-ment of antibodies to tetanus toxoid in cynomolgus monkeys. Note that the antibody titer develops in about 200 hr and peaks in about 400 hr. However, in general, immuno-genicity is insufficiently understood to be able to predict its occurrence.

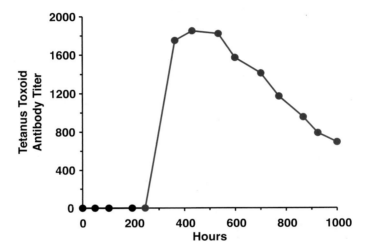

FIGURE 21-15. Endogenous antibody titer following i.m. administration of the immunogenic pro-tein(s) in tetanus toxoid in cynomolgus monkeys. Measurable antibody was detected about 200 hr fol-lowing administration of the toxoid. Peak concentrations occurred at about 400 to 500 hr. (From: Gobburu JV, Tenhoor C, Rogge MC, et al. Pharmacokinetics/dynamics of 5c8, a monoclonal antibody to CD154 [CD40 ligand] suppression of an immune response in monkeys. J Pharmacol Exp Ther 1998;286:925–930.)

FUTURE OF THE AREA

In spite of the challenges (purity of drug, preparation of quantity needed, specificity/sensitivity of assays, nonlinearities, immunogenic response), considerable progress has been made in developing many very useful and promising protein drugs to treat diseases, many of which have never been amenable to treatment before. This chapter has pre-sented many of the fundamental pharmacokinetic and pharmacodynamic concepts and principles known to date. We are certain, that many new ones will be forthcoming as this area develops in the future.

STUDY PROBLEMS

(Answers to Study Problems are in Appendix J.)

1. State why protein drugs must generally be given parenterally and provide two examples of situations in which protein drugs are not given by injection to achieve the therapeutic objective.

2. Discuss the primary factors determining the rate and extent of systemic absorption of protein drugs following their i.m. or s.c. administration.

3. Kampf et al. studied the pharmacokinetics of recombinant human erythropoietin, a glycosylated protein (MW = 34,000 g/mol) used to increase red blood cell formation patients with end-stage renal disease, after single i.v. and s.c. administrations of 40 U/kg on separate occasions. Table 21-15 lists the salient findings of these studies. The mean weight of the patients was 60 kg.

   a. Determine the clearance and volume of distribution of this drug.
   b. Calculate the bioavailability of erythropoietin after s.c. administration in these patients. How might you explain your answer?
   c. The maximum concentration observed was much lower and the terminal decline phase much slower after the s.c. dose than after the i.v. dose. How do you explain these observations?

TABLE 21-15 Mean *AUC*, Maximum Plasma Concentration, and Terminal Half-life of Erythropoietin in End-Stage Renal Disease Patients following Intravenous and Subcutaneous Administration

Administration	*AUC* (U-hr/L)	Maximum Concentration (U/L)	Time of Maximum Concentration	Terminal Half-life (hr)
i.v.	3010	417	5 min*	6.7
s.c.	1372	40.5	12 hr	16.1

*Time of first sample.
From: Kampf D, Echardt KU, Fischer HC, et al. Pharmacokinetics of recombinant human erythropoietin in dialysis patients after single and multiple subcutaneous administration. Nephron 1992;61:393–398.

4. Beshyah et al. examined the effect of s.c. injection site on the absorption of human growth hormone. Table 21-16 lists the mean serum concentrations in 11 subjects observed during the first 12 hr after the administration of 4 IU (international units) of biosynthetic human growth hormone. The drug was injected, on separate occasions, into a lifted fold of skin on the anterior thigh and a lower quadrant of the abdomen.

   a. Display the data on a semilogarithmic plot. Is there information in these data, gleaned from the graphical analysis, to suggest whether absorption or disposition of growth hormone rate-limits the terminal decline? Briefly discuss.
   b. Many proteins given subcutaneously or intramuscularly are partially degraded within the lymphatic system before reaching the systemic circulation. Calculate the relative bioavailability of the drug after s.c. injection into the thigh (relative to abdomen).

TABLE 21-16 Mean Serum Concentrations of Growth Hormone for 12 hr following Subcutaneous Injection of 4 IU in the Abdomen and Thigh

Time (hr):	0	1	2	3	4	5	6	7	8	9	10	11	12
Injection Site						Serum Concentration (milliunits/L)							
Abdomen	<2	33	56	94	85	75	74	51	31	25	21	15	10
Thigh	<2	16	28	27	39	29	30	25	22	21	16	14	12

From: Beshyah SA, Anyaoku V, Niththyananthan R, et al. The effect of subcutaneous injection site on absorption of human growth hormone: abdomen versus thigh. Clin Endocrinol (Oxf) 1991;35:409–412.

   c. The clearance of growth hormone has been reported in the literature to average about 5 L/hr. Roughly estimate the bioavailability of the drug following abdominal s.c. injection.

5. Examination of the data in Fig. 10-16 (Chapter 10, *Constant-Rate Input*) indicates that the normal (basal) plasma concentration of erythropoietin is 10 U/L. A semilogarithmic plot (see Fig. 10-16B) of the difference between the erythropoietin concentration after the dose of epoetin alfa and the basal value (10 units/L), taken as the average over the period of study following the placebo (not shown) yields the following values for exogenous epoetin alfa after a single i.v. dose ($V = 4$ L/70 kg; $CL = 0.5$ L/hr per 70 kg), calculate the following parameters for endogenous erythropoietin, assuming that epoetin alfa kinetically behaves identically to erythropoietin.

   a. Turnover rate
   b. Turnover time
   c. Fractional turnover rate

6. Table 21-17 lists the half-lives and urinary recoveries of hirudin, an antithrombotic protein (6964 g/mol), in healthy individuals and in patients with renal function impairment.

TABLE 21-17 **Half-life and Fraction Excreted Unchanged of Hirudin in Healthy Volunteers, and in Patients: (a) with Preterminal Renal Insufficiency, (b) on Chronic Dialysis, or (c) Having Undergone Bilateral Nephrectomy***

	Creatinine Clearance (mL/min)	Half-life (hr)	Percent Excreted Unchanged
Healthy volunteers (previous studies)	>60	$1.7 \pm 1.5^{\dagger}$	38 ± 10
Preterminal renal insufficiency (N = 4)	14 ± 5	24 ± 11	39 ± 8
Chronically dialyzed (N = 3)	<10	33 ± 7	-
Bilateral nephrectomy (N = 2)	-	168 and 316	-

*From: Nowak G, Bucha E, Göock TH Thieler H, Markwardt F. Pharmacology of r-hirudin in renal impairment. Thromb Res 1992;66:707–715.
†From: Vanholder R, Camez A, Veys N, et al. Pharmacokinetics of recombinant hirudin in hemodialyzed end-stage renal failure patients. Thromb Haemost 1997;77:650–655.

   a. Why does the half-life change so much in patients with renal function impairment for a drug that is only about 40% excreted unchanged in healthy individuals?
   b. How do you reconcile that the fraction (of an i.v. dose) excreted unchanged appears to be about the same in healthy subjects and in renal disease patients with creatinine clearances of greater than 60 mL/min and 14 mL/min, respectively, when the half-life increases from about 1.7 to 24 hr?
   c. Speculate on the reason that the half-life is 33 ± 7 hr in patients on chronic dialysis (creatinine clearances less than 10 mL/min), but 168 and 316 hr in two patients who have been bilaterally nephrectomized.

7. Gonadotropin-releasing hormone (GnRH) has been studied in normal subjects and in patients with liver disease and chronic renal failure. Table 12-18 lists the total body clearance values and half-lives of the drug and serum creatinine values of the individual subjects and patients in the study. GnRH is located in plasma, not in blood cells.

   a. Does hepatic disease seem to have much of an effect on the disposition of GnRH? Briefly discuss.
   b. Approximately what is the renal clearance of GnRH?
   c. Is there evidence that GnRH undergoes secretion into the renal tubule?

TABLE 21-18	Total Body Clearance and Half-life of Gonadotropin-Releasing Hormone and Serum Creatinine Values in Normal Subjects, Patients with Chronic Renal Failure, and Patients with Hepatic Disease		

Total Body Clearance (mL/min, mean $\pm$ SE)	Half-life (Minutes, Mean, and Range)	Serum Creatinine (mg/dL, Mean, and Range)
Normal Subjects		
1640 $\pm$ 60	6.6 (5.5–8)	1.0 (0.8–1.2)
Chronic Renal Failure		
631 $\pm$ 63	14 (12–16.5)	12 (9–15)
Hepatic Disease		
1487 $\pm$ 113	7.0 (6–8.5)	0.8 (0.4–1.1)

From: Pimstone B, Epstein S, Hamilton SM, LeRoith D, Hendricks S. Metabolic clearance and plasma disappearance time of exogenous gonadotropin releasing hormone in normal subjects and in patients with liver disease and chronic renal failure. J Clin Endocrinol Metab 1977;44:356–360.

8. Figure 21-16 shows the mean anakinra concentration–time profiles after a single 70 mg/70-kg i.v. dose to subjects with normal renal function and to patients with end-stage renal disease on hemodialysis (HD). The AUC values, half-lives, and initial dilution volumes (V_I) are listed in Table 21-19.

   a. Determine the apparent volume of distribution during the terminal decline in both groups.
   b. State why the extent of the initial drop in the concentration for the patients with renal disease is much less than that for the healthy patients.

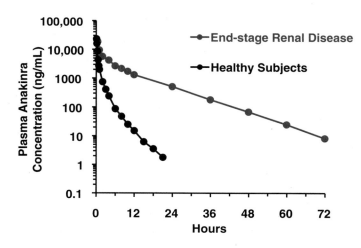

FIGURE 21-16. Plasma concentration of anakinra after i.v. administration of 1 mg/kg to healthy subjects (*black line*, n = 12) and to subjects with end-stage renal disease who are undergoing hemodialysis (*red line*, n = 10). (From: Yang BB, Baughman S, Sullivan, JT. Pharmacokinetics of anakinra in subjects with different levels of renal function. Clin Pharmacol Ther 2003;74:85–94.)

TABLE 21-19	Area Under the Curve, Half-life, and Initial Dilution Volume of Anakinra in Subjects with Normal Renal Function and in Patients on Hemodialysis	

	Subjects with Normal Renal Function	Patients on HD
AUC (mg-hr/L)	9.5 $\pm$ 1.43	63.7 $\pm$ 9.6
Half-life (hr)	2.64 $\pm$ 0.28	7.15 $\pm$ 1.20
Initial dilution volume (L)	3.32 $\pm$ 0.62	2.95 $\pm$ 1.08

   c. Explain why the half-life increased 2.7-fold for the patients on HD and relative to the value in the healthy subjects, but the *AUC* increased 6.7-fold.

 9. Explain how nonlinear pharmacodynamics and nonlinear pharmacokinetics of protein drugs, especially antibodies, often have a mechanism in common.

10. The turnover of albumin has been studied using tracer techniques (Sterling KJ. The turnover rate of serum albumin in man as measured by ^{131}I-tagged albumin. J Clin Invest 1951;30:1228–1237). In one of the subjects, who received 6.75 MBq of ^{131}I-labeled albumin intravenously, the concentration of radioactivity was observed to decline according to the following relationship (1 Bq = 1 disintegration per second [dps]):

$$C(megaBecquerels/L) = 1.5\ e^{-1.4t} + 1.2\ e^{-0.06t}$$

where *t* is in days.

Knowing that the plasma albumin concentration was 42 g/L in this 51-kg subject and making the assumption that both labeled and unlabeled albumin show the same kinetic behavior (observed to be a good approximation using other techniques), calculate the following:

   a. The turnover time and fractional turnover rate of albumin.
   b. The amounts of albumin in intravascular (initial dilution volume) and extravascular fluids.
   c. The synthesis rate of albumin.
   d. Does the data allow one to say where degradation of albumin is occurring?

11. van Griensven et al. (van Griensven JM, Koster RW, Burggraaf J, et al. Effects of liver blood flow on the pharmacokinetics of tissue-type plasminogen activator (alteplase) during thrombolysis in patients with acute myocardial infarction. Clin Pharmacol Ther 1998;63:39–47) have shown that the plasma clearance of tissue-type plasminogen activator (t-PA) correlates with the clearance of indocyanine green, a marker of hepatic blood flow, in patients with acute myocardial infarction. The average (± S.D.) values of clearance for t-PA activity and indocyanine green were 470 ± 138 and 585 ± 144 mL/min, respectively.

   a. From these data alone, would you conclude that the drug is eliminated by the liver?
   b. Discuss the reason for the relationship between the clearances of the two substances.
   c. Both of these substances are restricted to plasma (a typical value for the plasma–blood concentration ratio is 2), indocyanine green because of extensive binding to albumin and t-PA because of its size (59,042 g/mol) and polarity. Using the mean values of clearance, estimate the hepatic extraction ratio for t-PA. Assume that the clearance of indocyanine is a good measure of hepatic plasma flow.
   d. Discuss the implications of these findings for the use of t-PA in patients with acute myocardial infarction.

Prediction and Refinement of Human Kinetics from In Vitro, Preclinical, and Early Clinical Data

OBJECTIVES

The reader will be able to:

- Define the following terms: allometry, equivalent time, microdosing, whole-body physiologically based modeling.

- Define allometry and give an example of its application in drug development.

- Appreciate the use and limitations of allometric scaling in predicting the absorption and disposition kinetics of drugs in humans from animal data.

- Discuss the strategy commonly used for predicting clearance in humans from a combination of in vitro and animal data, together with a model of hepatic clearance.

- Discuss the purpose and development of whole-body physiologically based pharmacokinetic models.

- Discuss how simulation using physiologically based pharmacokinetic models can be useful in evaluating drug interactions.

- Discuss what is meant by "simulation of virtual patient populations."

P revious chapters emphasize an understanding of the physiologic concepts underlying the determinants of pharmacokinetics and their integration with kinetic principles. They show how such knowledge applies to the interpretation of observed concentration–time data, a deductive approach, and, ultimately, to drug therapy. Much of this last chapter takes a more synthetic approach. It is devoted to the prediction of human pharmacokinetics for a specific drug based on various pieces of information acquired prior to its administration to humans. It can also be extremely useful at various stages in the selection and evaluation of a new molecular entity. Examples include anticipating whether the new compound is likely to have the appropriate pharmacokinetic properties for the intended therapeutic application, helping to optimally plan a clinical trial to address specific questions, and helping to address various aspects in the labeling instruction for the use of a new medicine, such as whether there is a need to modify the dosage when a patient is on concurrent medication. These and other examples are explored in this chapter.

ALLOMETRY AND DISPOSITION KINETICS

ORIGIN

Since the days of Galileo, and perhaps before, there has been a quest to understand the relationship between size and function. The longer the nail, the thicker it needs to be, to avoid being bent when hammered into the wall; elephants need thicker legs than humans to stand, otherwise, they would not be able to support their weight. This interest in scale extends to the relationship between body size and physiologic parameters. The subject has come to be known as **allometry**, or the study of relationship between the size of the body and its component parts and functions.

The easiest measure of body size is body weight. Figure 22-1 shows the relationship between various properties (heart weight, glomerular filtration rate, cardiac output, daily heat production) and body weight among mammals, that is, animals, including humans,

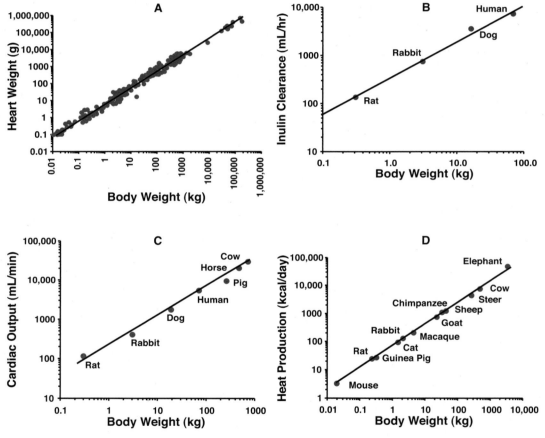

FIGURE 22-1. Allometric relationships between body weight of mammals and (**A**) heart weight, for 104 species spanning the weight range from mouse to blue whale, exponential coefficient $b = 0.98$; (**B**) inulin clearance, a measure of glomerular filtration rate, $b = 0.74$; (**C**) cardiac output, $b = 0.78$; and (**D**) heat production, $b = 0.75$. Note that the data are displayed as log–log plots, and that the slope of the line is approximately 1 for heart weight and 0.75 for the three measures of body function. (From: Prothero J. Heart weight as a function of body weight in mammals. Growth 1979;43:139–150 [heart weight]; Aldolph, EF. Quantitative relationships in physiological constituents of mammals. Science 1949;109:579–585 [inulin clearance]; Holt JP, Rhode EH, Kines J. Venticular volumes and body weight in mammals. Am J Physiol 1968;215:704–715 [cardiac output]; McMahon, T. Size and Shape in Biology: Elastic criteria impose limits on biological proportions, and consequently on metabolic rates. Science 1973;179:1201–1204 [heat production].)

that suckle their young and maintain their internal body temperature regardless of their environment. These animals include, in increasing order of weight, mouse, rat, guinea pig, cat, dog, rabbit, monkey, and man and extend to larger mammals, such as cow and elephant. There are several points to note. First, the data are displayed as log–log plots. This is needed to allow data for all mammals to be displayed on one graph, given that the average body weight ranges from 0.02 kg for a mouse to 70 kg for a human adult to 3400 kg for an elephant. Second, for each property Y, such as glomerular filtration rate, the relationship across the species can be described by a straight line, given by

$$log\ Y = log\ a + b \cdot log\ W \qquad\qquad 22\text{-}1$$

where **a** and **b** are constants, and W is body weight. Or, taking antilogs,

$$Y = aW^b \qquad\qquad 22\text{-}2$$

Second, examination of the relationships in Fig. 22-1 indicates that the value of b, the exponential coefficient, lies between about 0.75 and 1. It has a value of about 1, for example, when relating heart weight, and the weight of many other tissues and organs, with body weight. In particular, skeletal muscle weight, needed for posture and locomotion, is a relatively constant 45% of body weight among mammals. In contrast, the exponential coefficient b is about 0.75 when relating glomerular filtration rate, cardiac function, heat production, and many other physiologic functions to body weight. Notice also that although the range 0.75 to 1 appears narrow, as shown in Fig. 22-2, the predicted value of a property varies greatly across this range in moving from mouse to human, given the 3500-fold difference in body weight. For example, if the value for a 20-g mouse is 1, substitution

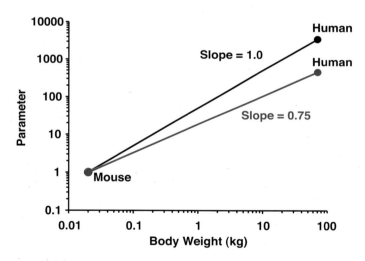

FIGURE 22-2. Although exponents of 0.75 and 1 on relating a physiologic parameter to body weight do not appear to differ greatly, when applied across animal species that differ greatly in body weight, in this case from 0.02 kg (mouse) to 70 kg (human), the differences in the projected parameter values become large. The value of the parameter is arbitrarily set at 1 for mouse.

into Eq. 22-2 indicates that it is predicted to be 3500 in an adult human using $b = 1$ ($1 \times (70000/20)^1$), but only 455 ($1 \times (70000/20)^{0.75}$) using $b = 0.75$, a 7.7-fold difference. Another property for which b is approximately 0.75 is body surface area, as shown in Fig. 22-3, which is the reason why physiologic functions are often said to vary in direct proportion to body surface area, both across and within species. For example, recall that when considering creatinine clearance, or glomerular filtration rate, in Chapter 14, *Age, Weight, and Gender*, and Chapter 15, *Disease*, values are expressed per 1.73 m^2, which is the average body surface area of a 70-kg adult. The rationale for b being in the order of 0.75 when a property correlates with surface area is as follows. Assuming that the body is a sphere of radius r, its surface area and volume (which relates to weight through specific density) are $4\pi r^2$ and $4\pi r^3/3$, respectively. On taking the logarithm of each, we see that, with respect

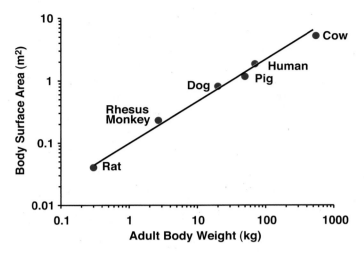

FIGURE 22-3. Allometric relationship between body surface area of mammals and typical adult body weight for each species. The exponent is close to two thirds (0.67). The body surface area for the typical adult was obtained from the allometric relationship for a range of body weights within each respective species. (From: Calder, WA III. Size, Function, and Life History. Harvard University Press, Cambridge; 1984.)

to r, surface area varies by a factor of 2, whereas volume (and weight) varies by a factor of 3. Hence, for a sphere, a plot of log (surface area) against log (weight) would have a slope of two thirds or 0.67. In reality, we are not spherical, and functions are not directly proportional to body surface area, and a value for b in the order of 0.75 is more appropriate. Furthermore, given the inherent biological variability across species, in practice the experimental data often do not allow a ready distinction between values of 0.67 and 0.75.

APPLICATION TO DRUGS

An obvious extension of these general physiologic and anatomic observations is their application to scaling pharmacokinetic parameters, specifically those of drug disposition, across species. Noting that body composition varies relatively little from one mammalian species to another, the expectation is that, as with muscle mass, volume of distribution should vary in direct proportion to body weight (i.e., $b = 1$), whereas for drug clearance, being a measure of functional activity, like cardiac output and glomerular filtration rate, the value of b is expected to be about 0.75. Evidence supporting these expectations is provided in Fig. 22-4 for the chemotherapeutic agent, cyclophosphamide, for which the esti-

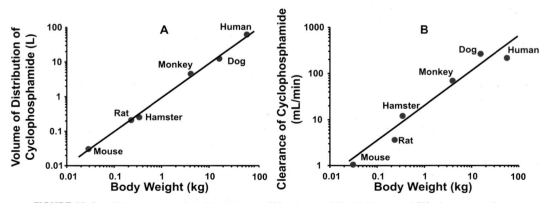

FIGURE 22-4. Allometric relationship between (**A**) volume of distribution, and (**B**) clearance of cyclophosphamide and body weight among mammals. The exponents are 0.985 and 0.754, respectively. Note the differences in the scales of the y-axes of the two graphs. (From: Boxenbaum, H. Interspecies scaling, allometry, physiological time, and the ground plan of pharmacokinetics. J Pharmacokin Biopharm 1982;10:201–228.)

mated values of b for volume of distribution and clearance are 0.985 and 0.754, which for practical purposes are 1 and 0.75, respectively. Notice that no assumption has been made regarding the nature of processes governing the distribution or elimination of the compound. Indeed, these allometric relationships have been found to apply not only to small molecules such as cyclophosphamide but also equally to large therapeutic proteins too, although most attention for proteins is on clearance (Fig. 22-5), because proteins tend to be restricted to the vascular space, or at most the extracellular space, both of which are similar on a L/kg basis among mammals, although discrepancies would be expected when target-mediated disposition occurs involving a specific human target.

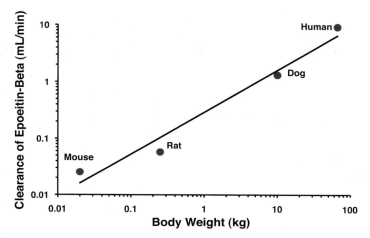

FIGURE 22-5. Allometric relationship between clearance of epoetin-β, a therapeutic protein, and body weight among mammals. The exponent is 0.775. (From: Bleul H, Hoffmann R, Kaufmann B, et al. Kinetics of subcutaneous versus i.v. epoetin-beta in dogs, rats and mice. Pharmacology 1996;52:329–338 [animal data]; Halstenson CE, Macres M, Katz AS, et al. Comparative pharmacokinetics and pharmacodynamics of epoetin alfa and epoetin beta. Clin Pharmacol Ther 1991;50:702–712 [human data].)

Now consider the application of these ideas to methotrexate. Shown in Fig. 22-6A is a semilogarithmic plot of plasma methotrexate concentration with time following either its intravenous (i.v.) or intraperitoneal (i.p.) administration of different doses to various mammals, including humans. The equations describing the data among the species are similar in form but vary in both intercept and slope, giving the impression that data are species specific. However, all the data can be brought together by applying allometric relationships. Assume for simplicity that the data for each species can be described by a one-compartment model, characterized by the general equation

$$C = \frac{Dose}{V} e^{-\frac{CL}{V}t} \qquad 22\text{-}3$$

which, on dividing by dose/body weight ($Dose/W$), gives

$$\frac{C}{Dose/W} = \frac{1}{V/W} e^{-\frac{CL}{V}t} \qquad 22\text{-}4$$

Now, assuming that the observations for cyclophosphamide apply equally to methotrexate, then

$$V = a_1 W^1 \qquad 22\text{-}5$$

$$CL = a_2 W^{0.75} \qquad 22\text{-}6$$

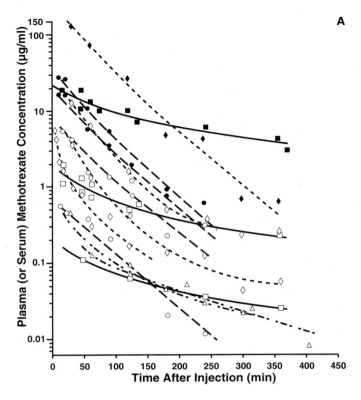

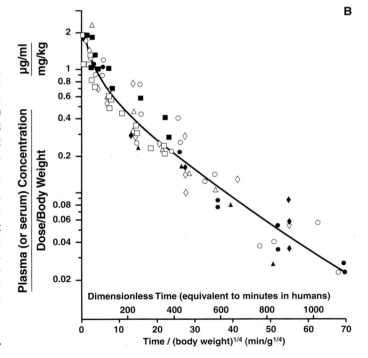

FIGURE 22-6. **A.** Plasma concentration of methotrexate after i.v. or i.p. injection. Mouse -----; rat –––; monkey ––––; dog ----; human ——. Observations: mouse ◇ (i.v. 3 mg/kg; i.p. 4.5, 45, 450 mg/kg), rhesus monkey ▲ (i.v. 0.3 mg/kg), beagle dog △ (i.v. 0.2 mg/kg), adult patients ■ (i.v. 0.1, 1, 10 mg/kg). **B.** Plot of plasma concentrations in graph A normalized to dose per kg versus time raised to the 0.25 power. The plot has become known as the Dedrick plot after the author who first proposed it. (From: Dedrick RL, Bischoff KB, Zaharko DS. Interspecies correlation of plasma concentration history of methotrexate (NSC-740). Cancer Chemotherap Rep Part 1 1970;54:95–101.)

where a_1 and a_2 are coefficients with values specific to methotrexate. It remains to evaluate CL/V

$$\frac{CL}{V} = \frac{a_2}{a_1} \cdot \frac{W^{0.75}}{W^1} = a_3 W^{(0.75-1)} = a_3 W^{-0.25} = \frac{a_3}{W^{0.25}} \qquad 22\text{-}7$$

where a_3, the ratio of a_2 and a_1, is also specific to methotrexate. Finally, substitution of Eqs. 22-5 and 22-7 into Eq. 22-4 yields

$$\frac{C}{Dose/W} = \frac{1}{a_1} e^{-\frac{a_3 \cdot t}{W^{0.25}}} \qquad 22\text{-}8$$

Hence, it is expected that when the plasma concentration for each species is divided by the corresponding dose per kilogram body weight and time is divided by $W^{0.25}$, data for all species should fall on the same curve, which is the case for methotrexate (Fig. 22-6B). Dividing chronologic time by $W^{0.25}$ has been called **equivalent time** in that it tends to bring events in all mammals within a common time scale. It is similar in concept to expressing temporal events in a mammal in terms of its life span, recognizing that generally the smaller the mammal the shorter is its life span. Thus, a mouse lives for only 2 years, a dog for 15 years, and so on. A month in the life of a mouse is, therefore, approximately the same as 7 months in the life of a dog. It is also apparent from Eq. 22-7, that as $t_{1/2} = 0.693 \cdot V/CL$, the $t_{1/2}$ of a drug is shorter in smaller than larger animal species, although the increase with size is relatively small as it is predicted to vary in direct proportion to $W^{0.25}$. For example, if the half-life of a drug is 2 hr in a mouse, it is 9.5 hr in a 10-kg dog $(2 \times (10{,}000g/20g)^{0.25})$; that is, a 500-fold increase in body weight is predicted to result in only a 4.75-fold increase in half-life. The data for ceftizoxime, a drug predominantly renally excreted unchanged, support this expectation, with the half-life increasing from 13 min in a mouse to 65 min in a dog, and close to 80 min in humans (Fig 22-7).

Recall that a similar approach of relating V to body weight and clearance to body surface area or $W^{0.75}$ was adopted when scaling kinetic data obtained in adults to those in

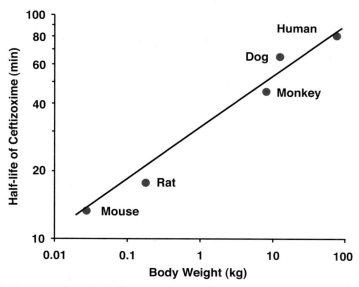

FIGURE 22-7. Log–log plot of half-life versus body weight for ceftizoxime. The solid circles represent the values reported in the literature for each species. The solid line is the best fit line for animals, excluding humans. The predicted antibiotic half-life in humans is read off the linear regression line at 70 kg. (From: Mordenti J. Forecasting cephalosporin and monobactam antibiotic half-lives in humans from data collected in laboratory animals. Antimicrob Agents Chemother 1985;27:887–891.)

children (Chapter 14, *Age, Weight, and Gender*). Also, adjustment of dosing rate of many chemotherapeutic agents across the patient population is made on a body surface area basis. This approach is similar to observations in animals that show that for many such drugs, particularly the alkylating agents, when administered chronically, toxicity in the form of neutropenia was seen at similar plasma concentrations across species and that the dosing rate needed to achieve a steady-state concentration was directly proportional to body surface area. As $C_{SS} = R_{inf}/CL$, it was therefore inferred that CL scales in direct proportion to body surface area rather than to body weight. Obviously, this adjustment is only warranted if surface area explains variability in clearance better than body weight (Chapter 14, *Age, Weight, and Gender*).

DEVIATION FROM EXPECTATION

The allometric approach appears to offer a means of using animal data, which is often collected as part of the initial examination of a potentially useful compound, to predict the likely disposition kinetics in humans, and hence help select compounds having desired characteristics. For example, predicting half-lives of 40 min and 12 hr for two different compounds in humans may favor selection of the latter if the aim of therapy is to maintain a relatively constant concentration over extended periods. However, simple allometry of the type applied so far often fails to provide an accurate prediction of events in humans; this is not too surprising as the assumption that the only difference among mammals is size, which is certainly not the case, is rather simplistic. Indeed, if the allometric approach always applied, it could be argued that the pharmacokinetics of a drug needs to be determined in only one animal species to predict human pharmacokinetics. One clue to a potential problem with this approach is when the observed value of b is very different from that expected based on body size alone. For example, the allometric exponent for clearance of saruplase, a high–molecular-weight thrombolytic agent, is 1.28 based on animal data. The resulting prediction in humans is 2100 mL/min, far from the observed value of 530 mL/min, indicating that one or more of the processes responsible for elimination of this compound, in one or more of the animal species, are substantially different from that in humans, making prediction problematic. But, why does allometry work with methotrexate and some other drugs, and not with others.

One reason for a likely successful application of allometry is when the organ extraction ratio of the compound is high in all species, as then blood clearance approaches organ blood flow, which scales well across species with an exponential coefficient of 0.75. Another is when renal excretion is the predominant route of elimination, because, as illustrated with fluconazole (Fig. 22-8), renal clearance generally scales well allometrically, again with

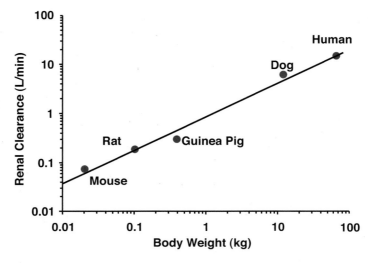

FIGURE 22-8. Allometric plot of renal clearance of fluconazole in mammals versus body weight. The exponent of the line is 0.67. (From: Jezequel SG. Fluconazole: interspecies scaling and allometric relationships of pharmacokinetic properties. J Pharm Pharmacol 1994;46: 196–199.)

a value for b on the order of 0.75. Indeed, renal clearance tends to correlate well with glomerular filtration rate, even for renally secreted drugs and, as mentioned previously, filtration scales well across species. The allometric approach, which as applied is largely empirical, fails, however, when one or more of the underlying assumptions do not hold.

CORRECTING FOR PROTEIN BINDING

Given that the values of CL and V may depend on the fraction unbound in plasma, fu, implicit in the allometric approach based on total plasma data is that fu is relatively constant across species. This is often the case, but as shown in Fig. 22-9, not always so, with fu sometimes varying across species by as much as 10-fold and occasionally even more. Correcting for fu would then be reasonable, certainly for drugs with a volume of distribution greater than 0.5 L/kg ($V \approx V_{TW} \cdot fu/fu_T$) and for predominantly metabolized drugs of low clearance ($CL = fu \cdot CL_{int}$). Theoretically, if most of the variability lies in fu_T rather than fu then clearly scaling unbound volume of distribution ($Vu \approx V_{TW/fu_T}$) allometrically would not materially improve prediction. In practice, fu_T tends not to vary so much across species probably because drugs generally bind to many tissue components, and the composition of tissues, such as a muscle, is very similar across species. In contrast, binding in plasma is often predominantly at a specific site to a single protein, for example, albumin, which differs structurally among mammalian species. However, sometimes, correction for fu does not substantially improve the prediction, especially for hepatic clearance of relatively stable compounds having a low extraction ratio, owing to significant species differences in drug metabolism and transport processes, caused by qualitative and quantitative differences in the enzymes and transporters involved. Then, increasingly, reliance is placed on the use of in vitro humanized systems.

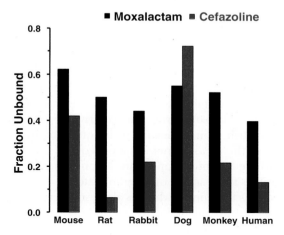

FIGURE 22-9. The degree of variation in the fraction unbound in plasma across species depends on the drug. Often, as seen with moxalactam (■), it varies little across species. Sometimes, however, the variation can be very large as seen with cefazoline (■) where the fraction unbound ranges between 0.07 in rat and 0.7 in dog. For both drugs the primary binding protein is albumin. (From: Sacher G. Relation of lifespan to brain weight and body weight in mammals. In: GEW Wolstenholme, M O'Connor [Eds.]. CIBA Foundation Colloquia on Aging. London: Churchill; 1959.)

MICRODOSING

Another essentially empirical approach in vivo, referred to as **microdosing**, uses man himself as the model. Its appeal is greatest for compounds that exhibit linearity over the therapeutic dose range. It involves the administration of a minute dose, termed a microdose, intended not to produce any pharmacologic response, followed by linear scaling of the resultant pharmacokinetic data to pharmacologic doses. An example of this approach is illustrated with midazolam in Fig. 22-10. The advantage of this approach is that because the risk of producing harm with such a low dose is extremely small, the compound can be given to humans with minimal animal and in vitro safety data, thereby providing an early signal as to the likely pharmacokinetics of the compound at higher doses. Clearly, not all compounds exhibit linear pharmacokinetics at therapeutic doses, as discussed in Chapter

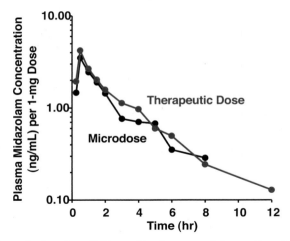

FIGURE 22-10. An oral microdose (100 μg, *black*) successfully predicts the pharmacokinetics following a therapeutic oral dose of midazolam (7.5 mg, *colored*), as evidenced by the virtual super-position of the plasma concentration–time profiles when normalized to a common 1-mg dose. Data are geometric means of observations in 6 subjects receiving the two 75-fold different doses on separate occasions. (From: Lappin G, Kuhnz W, Jochemsen R, et al. Use of microdosing to predict pharmacokinetics at the therapeutic dose: experience with five drugs. Clin Pharmacol Ther 2006;80:203–215.)

16, *Nonlinearities,* and Chapter 21, *Protein Drugs,* but many do. These include particularly extremely potent drugs for which the C_{50} is well below that causing saturation of any of the pharmacokinetic processes ($C_{50} << Km, K_T,$ or K), or ones with rates of administration much smaller than $Vm,$ or $Tm,$ such as glucuronidation and some transport processes, or ones that distribute extensively, binding to many tissue components throughout the body, such as many basic compounds, so that the bound concentration is much less than $n \cdot Pt,$ A critical factor in the application of the approach, which used to be a severe limitation, but is often no longer the case, is the availability of a suitable extremely sensitive analytical technique capable of measuring minute concentrations of a drug, particularly one having a low oral bioavailability or a large volume of distribution. One such technique is accelerated mass spectrometry, which, because it allows the measurement of atoms of ^{14}C (a rare element in nature), enables investigation into the fate of not only parent compound, but also all drug-related material in plasma, as well as the fraction of an administered dose of ^{14}C-labeled drug excreted in urine and feces. This technique, which is also used in carbon dating of fossils, is so sensitive that the amount of radiolabeled drug needed to be administered is well below that producing safety concerns.

PREDICTION OF CLEARANCE

Other approaches to the prediction of human pharmacokinetics center on a basic understanding of the qualitative and quantitative features of the individual processes controlling pharmacokinetic events, the basis of much of this book. Several of these processes are subsequently considered. Various approaches to date have been taken to predict hepatic clearance of small molecules in humans. A common strategy is shown schematically in Fig 22-11. It utilizes two familiar features: one is additivity of clearance; the other is the application of the well-stirred model of hepatic clearance (although other models could be employed) to integrate intrinsic clearance, protein binding, and blood flow (Chapter 5, *Elimination*).

The first step is to estimate hepatic intrinsic metabolic clearance in vitro, $CL_{H,int,m,in\ vitro}$ by incubating drug with either liver microsomes or hepatocytes derived from human liver,

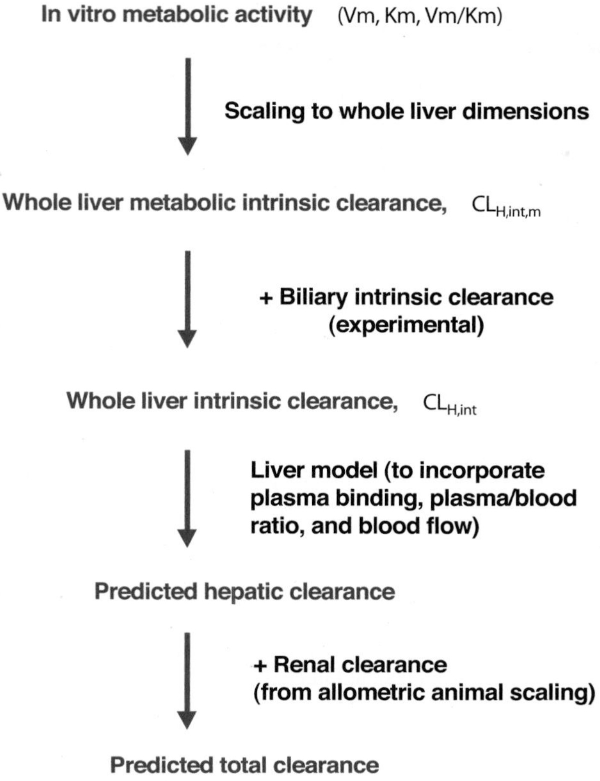

In vitro metabolic activity   (Vm, Km, Vm/Km)

↓ Scaling to whole liver dimensions

Whole liver metabolic intrinsic clearance, $CL_{H,int,m}$

↓ **+ Biliary intrinsic clearance (experimental)**

Whole liver intrinsic clearance, $CL_{H,int}$

↓ **Liver model (to incorporate plasma binding, plasma/blood ratio, and blood flow)**

Predicted hepatic clearance

↓ **+ Renal clearance (from allometric animal scaling)**

Predicted total clearance

FIGURE 22-11. Schematic diagram of an approach to estimate hepatic metabolic clearance from in vitro metabolic data. When coupled with scaled renal (and, when significant, biliary) clearance, total human in vivo clearance in humans is predicted.

or with individual human expressed enzymes, and follow either depletion of drug or formation of metabolite(s) that allow calculation of *Vm* and *Km*, or simply the ratio *Vm/Km*, when operating below saturation. Literally, in vitro means in glass (or more generally to measurements made outside the body), in contrast to in vivo, within the body. To predict the whole liver metabolic clearance, $CL_{H,int,m}$, it is necessary to scale $CL_{H,int,m,in\ vitro}$ by multiplying this value by the ratio of the total amount of microsomal protein, number of hepatocytes, or amount of enzyme in the in vitro system, depending on the system chosen, to the corresponding amount in the whole liver. Attention also needs to be given to differences in the activity of the specific enzymes in the various in vitro systems compared to that in vivo, and to correcting for binding of drug within the systems, given that events are driven by unbound drug. For drugs that are extensively metabolized in the liver, with minimal biliary secretion, then $CL_{H,int,m}$ can be approximated to $CL_{H,int}$, the whole liver intrinsic clearance. Otherwise, one needs to add to the metabolic term the estimated intrinsic clearance due to biliary secretion, usually obtained from allometric scaling, in much the same way that renal clearance is scaled. Together with fu_b, and hepatic blood flow, $CL_{H,int}$ is then used to predict the in vivo hepatic clearance, $CL_{b,H}$

$$CL_{b,H} = Q_H \left[\frac{fu_b \cdot CL_{H,\ int}}{Q_H + fu_b \cdot CL_{H,\ int}} \right]$$

22-9

This approach has been quite successful in predicting hepatic clearance in humans, particularly for the many compounds that are extensively metabolized by CYP enzymes, the most studied drug-metabolizing enzymes, as seen for example in Fig. 22-12. Complications can arise, however, including the presence of hepatic processes in vivo not fully expressed in vitro, such as glucuronidation and cytosolic mixed-function oxidation, those involving transporters, and when membrane permeability becomes the rate-limiting process in hepatic elimination. However, quantitative information relating to

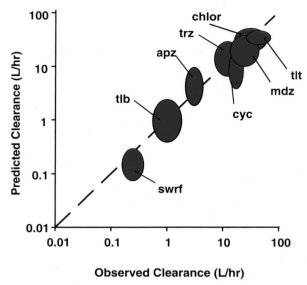

FIGURE 22-12. Log–log plot showing a generally good accord between predicted and observed clearance in humans, including interindividual variability, for eight drugs predominantly eliminated by CYP enzymes. Prediction using the well-stirred model of hepatic elimination is based on a combination of physiologic, biochemical, and demographic data together with drug-specific human data, including in vitro metabolic microsomal activity and plasma and microsomal binding. The ellipses delineate the 90% confidence intervals for both predictions and observations; the *broken line* is the line of identity. *Apz*, alprazolam; *chlor*, chlorzoxazone; *cyc*, cyclosporine; *mdz*, midazolam; *swarf*, S-warfarin; *tlb*, tolbutamide; *tlt*, tolterodine; *trz*, triazolam. (From: Howgate EM, Rowland-Yeo K, Proctor NJ, Tucker GT, Rostami-Hodjegan A. Prediction of in vivo drug clearance from in vitro data. 1: impact of individual variability. Xenobiotica 2006;36:473–497.)

these processes is becoming increasingly available. Extrahepatic metabolism, for example by lung, also complicates prediction of metabolic clearance although for most drugs this is relatively uncommon or is of minor significance. Like many in vivo predictions from in vitro data, success is not universal, and great care needs to be taken to ensure optimal application of the approach. Finally, addition of renal clearance, gained from allometry (there currently being no reliable in vitro predictive method), to hepatic clearance gives the predicted total clearance.

PREDICTION OF DISTRIBUTION

Of all the kinetic processes, allometry has been most successful in predicting volume of distribution in humans. Yet, this approach has shed little light on the factors controlling the distribution of drugs among organs of the body, a topic extensively discussed in Chapter 4, *Membranes and Distribution.* Recall, organs differ greatly in their affinity for drugs, depending on the structural and physicochemical properties of the drug and the constituents within an organ, such as neutral lipids and both neutral and acidic phospholipids. As the type and percentage of these constituents within an organ, such as the heart and skeletal muscle, often do not differ markedly among mammals, animal organ drug distribution (*Kp*) data are often assumed to apply to man, correcting for any differences in plasma protein binding. An additional factor for some drugs is the role of transporters. As these factors are becoming better understood, so is the ability to predict the likely distribution of a compound based on in vitro and in silico (within silicon or using a computer) approaches. Factors involved in the prediction of drug distribution are shown schematically in Fig. 22-13.

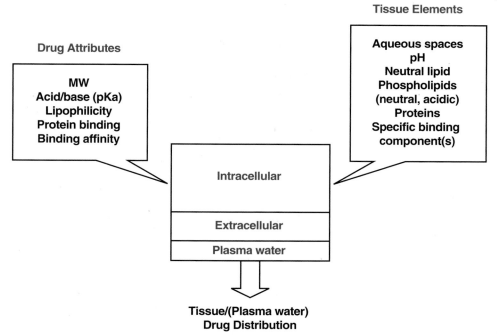

FIGURE 22-13. Scheme depicting the elements used in the prediction of distribution of a drug in individual tissues based on a combination of structural and physicochemical properties of the drug and the structure and composition of the tissue.

PREDICTION OF ABSORPTION

Absorption is much less dependent on body size than volume of distribution or clearance, and hence is less scalable allometrically. This is especially true for bioavailability. For example, finding that oral bioavailability of a drug is 50% in rat and 11% in dog, does little to help predict with any confidence the oral bioavailability in humans, although knowing that it is 100% in all animal species tested gives some confidence that it is very likely to be the same in humans. Absorption, and in particular, gastrointestinal absorption, is a complex process with many physiologic variables, including diet, superimposed onto which are numerous formulation variables. An approach to predict oral bioavailability is to consider the events occurring within the gastrointestinal tract, namely, those within the lumen, across the gut wall, and through the liver, as sequential, so that the overall bioavailability is the product of the fractions escaping loss at each of these sites, that is, $F = F_F \cdot F_G \cdot F_H$ (Chapter 7, *Absorption*).

An experimental approach to the prediction of the extent of intestinal absorption, F_G, relies on reference to a calibration curve. It applies particularly to drugs administered in solution, or which dissolve so rapidly within the stomach that they enter the small intestine in solution, and which are stable within the gastrointestinal fluids and intestinal wall ($F_F = 1$). In one such method, reference of its permeability across the small intestine, gained from human in situ intubation studies, is made to a calibration curve of intestinal permeability (obtained in a similar manner) against extent of intestinal absorption for a series of compounds whose extent of intestinal absorption in human is already known, an approach discussed in Chapter 7, *Absorption* (see Fig. 7-3). Alternatively, permeability assessed in a suitable human intestinal cell line may be used, but again some form of calibration to in vivo absorption human data is required (Fig. 22-14). For drugs that are subject to uptake or efflux transporters and intestinal

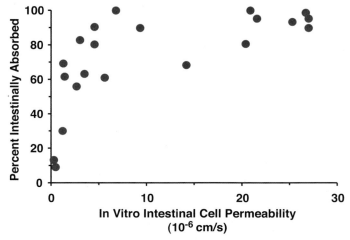

FIGURE 22-14. Correlation between in vitro permeability in a human intestinal cell line and extent of intestinal absorption for a series of compounds. (From: Usansky HH, Sinko PJ. Estimating human drug oral absorption kinetics from Caco-2 permeability using an absorption–disposition model: model development and evaluation and derivation of analytical solutions for *ka* and *Fa*. J Pharmacol Exp Ther 2005;314:391–399.)

metabolism, these processes need to be factored in to correctly predict F_G, as does the stability of the drug in gastric and intestinal fluids for susceptible compounds.

When dealing with solids or suspensions, or modified-release dosage forms, various approaches have been taken to predict F_F, the fraction released and available to permeate the intestinal wall. The important factors were discussed in Chapter 7, *Absorption*, and depicted graphically in Fig. 7-8. These include the dose relative to the solubility of the drug in solution in the gastrointestinal fluids, the salt form and its solubility, the particle size distribution (which changes as drug dissolves), and other formulation and manufacturing variables. One common approach is to use in vitro dissolution data, gained by placing the solid material in simulated gastric and intestinal fluids under stirring and pH conditions that mimic those occurring in the gastrointestinal tract, and operating under sink conditions that mimic those in vivo as dissolved drug is absorbed. An additional factor to be taken into account is the transit times of such materials in the stomach and small and large intestine.

The simpler approaches consider the gastrointestinal tract as comprising just two components, the stomach and intestine. To accommodate the known heterogeneity along the gastrointestinal tract, the more realistic ones divide it into a series of seven or more segments, starting with the stomach and ending with the rectum, each with their assigned individual characteristics (dimensions, fluid flow rate and pH, transit time, luminal contents, permeability, transporter, and enzymatic activities). As drug moves through each segment, some is absorbed, some is metabolized or degraded, while the remainder leaves to enter the next segment, and so forth, as depicted in Fig. 22-15. Summing the rate of absorption from all segments over time automatically provides the extent of intestinal absorption.

Finally, the component escaping hepatic first-pass loss, F_H is predicted from Eq. 22-9 (i.e., $1 - CL_{b,H}/Q_H$), although due regard needs to be taken of the situation in which the rate of portal absorption is fast enough that it approaches the maximum rate of hepatic metabolism, thereby saturating hepatic elimination resulting in a higher oral bioavailability than predicted assuming nonsaturable conditions. An example of the successful application of this modeling approach to prediction of the plasma concentration–time profile following administration of a solid dosage form is depicted in Fig. 22-16. Given the complexity, and associated uncertainties involved, perhaps unsurprisingly not all predictions are successful. Nonetheless, the application of realistic models of gastrointestinal

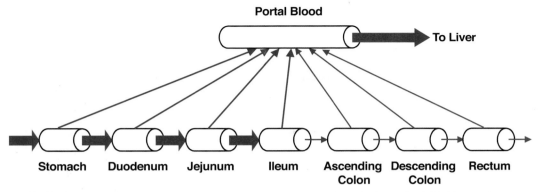

FIGURE 22-15. Model of intestinal drug absorption. The gastrointestinal tract is divided into various anatomical regions, here seven, from stomach to rectum. As drug moves sequentially through each region, some is absorbed into the mesenteric blood to enter the portal blood, some may be metabolized, and the remainder enters the next region. This results in a declining flux and delays in absorption of drug on movement along the intestinal tract. The thickness of the arrows (*colored*) denotes the magnitude of the flux relative to the concentration within a given region. For many drugs, despite a short sojourn of about 3 hr, absorption is predominantly from the small intestine, particularly the ileum where they reside the longest before entering the large intestine.

absorption allows an exploration of the critical factors likely to influence the rate and extent of systemic absorption of a drug from various formulations and under various conditions. The approach can also be extended to other sites of absorption, such as the lungs, muscle, subcutaneous tissues, and skin. The important consideration is that the models need to be physiologic and of sufficient detail to allow reasonable prediction over a wide range of conditions.

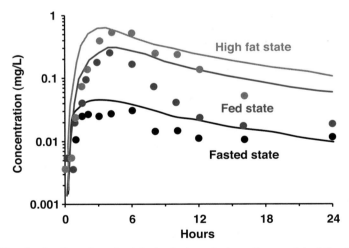

FIGURE 22-16. Application of a physiologically based absorption model of the type shown in Fig. 22-16 successfully predicts the influence of food on the absorption of a sparingly soluble compound. Shown are the observed mean and predicted plasma concentration–time profiles following oral administration of 400 mg of a solid formulation of the compound to 18 subjects when fasted (observed ●, predicted ———), fed with an average fat content meal (observed ●, predicted ———) and when fed with a high fat meal (observed ●, predicted ———). An important element of the prediction was the use of physiologically relevant simulated gastric and intestinal media in the assessment of in vitro dissolution data used in the predictions. (From: Jones H, Parrott N, Ohlenbusch G, et al. Predicting pharmacokinetic food effects using biorelevant solubility media and physiologically based modeling. Clin Pharmacokinet 2006;45:1213–1226.)

WHOLE-BODY PHYSIOLOGIC MODELS

As mentioned, a limitation of the allometric approach is that scaling simply for body size is essentially empiric. There is no direct or ready way of integrating human specific data, such as that gained from in vitro hepatocyte (metabolism) or intestinal (absorption) systems, into the scaled animal plasma data to better predict human profiles, when it is found that scaling for body size alone fails. The problem is that the allometric approach uses the description of the observed data in animals rather than starting with the underlying processes that on integration yield the predicted data. A different and more mechanistic approach is needed to address this deficiency. The approach adopted for prediction of oral absorption and for hepatic clearance (i.e., a physiologic model of the liver) offers a way forward. Namely, to represent organs of the body as separate entities, each of which can be characterized to the degree of complexity desired, arranged anatomically and linked together via the circulating blood. The result is a full **whole-body physiologic model** portrayed for example in Fig. 22-17,

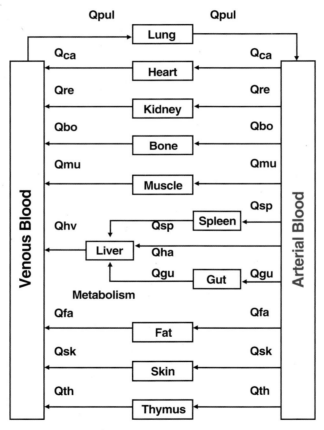

FIGURE 22-17.   Whole-body physiologic model comprising organs connected to each other via the recirculating vasculature. Q denotes the blood flow rate to a tissue. Q_{CA} is cardiac output: flows to organs are denoted by the first two letters of the organ name, except *ha* and *hv*, which are the flows in the hepatic artery and the hepatic vein, respectively. Some organs such as the gastrointestinal tract and the liver are in series, whereas most tissues are in parallel with drug entering via the arterial supply and leaving via the vein. Because of the connectivity of organs, the temporal profile of drug in any organ, and in blood, is dependent to varying extents on the events occurring in all other organs. The degree of complexity needed to characterize any organ depends on the intended application of model. For some applications, where extensive detail is not required, the full model is reduced by grouping together organs with similar kinetic parameters. The extreme example is the situation in which all organs of the body are lumped together, the one-compartment body model applied throughout much of the book.

which is an expansion of the more simplified figure presented in Chapter 2, *Fundamental Concepts and Terminology* (Fig. 2-4). It is apparent from this model that the observed plasma concentration–time profile of a drug is a consequence of two major processes: the single-pass events as drug moves through each organ of the body (with elimination in some of them) and recirculation, primarily via the vasculature. Predicting the concentration–time profile in plasma, and in any tissue, therefore requires an understanding of events occurring throughout the body. We have dealt with organs involved in absorption and elimination. It remains to deal with tissue distribution. Much is covered in Chapter 4, *Membranes and Distribution*, where both the rate and extent of tissue distribution were considered. Two additional points are noteworthy here. First, because of the different time constants for distribution of drug among organs and their anatomical relationships to each other, the resulting plasma concentration–time profiles of drugs are complex. Accordingly, characterizing a plasma concentration–time profile by a simple monoexponential or even a biexponential equation is a gross oversimplification of reality, although this simplification is often adequate for many clinical purposes. Second, the kinetic behavior of a drug in some organs is similar to that in others. They have similar values of the distribution rate constant, k_T (Chapter 4, *Membranes and Distribution*), and such organs can often be combined or lumped into groups such as those that are relatively rapidly equilibrating and those that are more slowly equilibrating.

Understanding the factors controlling the processes of the body opens the way to predicting mechanistically the pharmacokinetics of drugs in human based on a combination of physiologic and anatomic information coupled with in vitro or in silico drug data, an example of which is illustrated for cyclosporine in Fig. 22-18. In this example, reasonably good agreement was seen between prediction and observation. However, where deviations between predictions and observations are seen, parameters of the physiologic model can

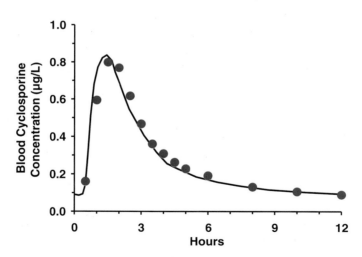

FIGURE 22-18. Measured (●) and predicted (*solid line*) blood cyclosporine concentration–time profile within a dosing interval at steady state in renal transplant patients receiving 1.5 mg/kg twice daily. Measured data are the mean observations in 18 patients. The predictions were generated with the whole body physiologic model depicted in Fig. 22-17, using a combination of anatomical, physiologic, and drug-specific information, including in vitro drug metabolism, intestinal permeability, binding within blood, and dissolution data together with animal tissue distribution data. (From: Kawai R, Matthew D, Tanaka C, Rowland M. Physiologically based pharmacokinetics of cyclosporine A: extension to tissue distribution kinetics in rats and scale-up to human. J Pharmacol Exp Ther 1998;287:457–468; clinical data from: Müeller E, Kovarik J, van Bree J, et al. Pharmacokinetics and tolerability of a microemulsion formulation of cyclosporine in renal allograft recipients—a concentration-controlled comparison with the commercial formulation. Transplantation 1994;57:1178–1182.)

be refined. The potential therefore exists of having a mechanistic model able to predict confidently the likely pharmacokinetic profile of the drug in the much wider patient population studied in the larger clinical trials and in the ultimate patient population.

PREDICTING PHARMACODYNAMICS

The concepts underpinning the prediction of human pharmacokinetic events can be extended to prediction of pharmacodynamics, with some similarities and some distinctions. In all cases, activity needs to be related to unbound drug. Also, in some cases, such as antimicrobial agents and antibiotics, the target is a microorganism and the activity is essentially independent of the host, so that once this information is obtained, often in vitro, all that is needed is to know or be able to predict is the pharmacokinetics of the compound to ensure adequate exposure in humans, although complications do arise when aiming to treat brain infections, owing to the blood-brain barrier, or infections involving the development of avascular areas, when diffusion can become a severe limitation. However, for the majority of other classes of compounds, due consideration needs to be taken of the generally complex pharmacodynamic events occurring within the body.

Recall that response comprises two major components, one is the interaction of the drug with the primary target and the other is the cascade of events between occupation of the target site and the observed response. The former can often be usefully studied in vitro, although as with pharmacokinetics it is important to correlate in vitro with in vivo data, as shown for some benzodiazepines in Fig. 22-19. In contrast, generally, the biologic response to a target stimulus requires an integrated system, which can only be fully assessed in vivo. Accordingly, such studies need to be undertaken in animals. Even then, although many target systems are conserved across species and similar primary responses directly associated with the mechanism of action can be demonstrated in healthy subjects, there are situations for which this does not translate into a clinical benefit. This occurs because the intended disease or condition, such as depression and many chronic diseases, for which there may be no true animal counterpart, is unresponsive to the drug.

As discussed in Chapter 2, *Fundemental Concepts and Terminology*, and Chapter 8, *Response Following a Single Dose*, various models may be used to characterize the relationship

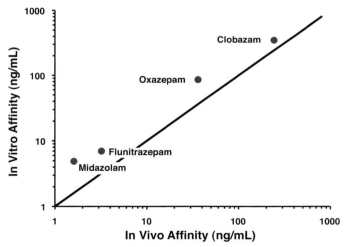

FIGURE 22-19. Receptor affinity of four benzodiazepines estimated both in vitro, using a receptor preparation (y-axis), and in vivo, based on analysis of plasma concentration–electroencephalographic effect relationships (x-axis). The solid line is the line of identity. (From: Tuk B, van Oostenbruggen MF, Herben VM, et al. Characterization of the pharmacodynamic interaction between parent drug and active metabolite in vivo: midazolam and alpha-OH-midazolam. J Pharmacol Exp Ther 1999;289:1067–1074.)

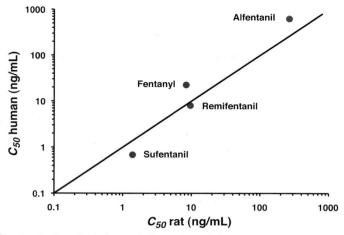

FIGURE 22-20. Synthetic opioids have similar unbound C_{50} values in rats and humans based on analysis of the electroencephalographic effect produced by these drugs. The line is the line of unity. (From: Cox EH, Langemeijer MWE, Gubbens-Stibbe JM, et al. The comparative pharmacodynamics of remifentanil and its metabolite, GR90291, in a rat EEG model. Anesthesiology 1999;90:535–544.)

between drug concentration and response. Often, they are empiric, such as the sigmoid E_{max} model, although, as with pharmacokinetics, the more biologically relevant a model, the more informative and predictive it tends to be. For some pharmacodynamic systems the unbound C_{50} value of a drug is similar across species, as is evident for the four opioids shown in Fig. 22-20. In other cases, differences are seen which may be accommodated based on in vitro target data. However, affinity and potency do not scale allometrically. What does need to be scaled, however, are the time constants of the biological system between the test animal and human, keeping in mind that the dynamics and turnover of most biological systems tend to be faster in smaller than larger mammals. Illustrative data for flesinoxan are provided in Figs. 22-21 and 22-22. Flesinoxan is an agent that both

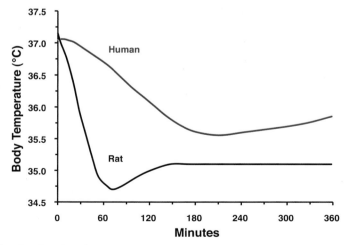

FIGURE 22-21. Predicted median body temperature–time relationship in humans following a 5-mg i.v. infusion of flesinoxan based on allometrically scaled parameters determined in the rat. Notice the much delayed and dampened response in humans due primarily to the slower time constants of the pharmacodynamic system in humans than in the rat. (From: Zuideveld KP, Van der Graaf PH, Peletier LA, Danhof M. Allometric scaling of pharmacodynamic responses: application to 5-HT$_{1A}$ receptor mediated responses from rat to man. Pharm Res 2007;24:2031–2039.)

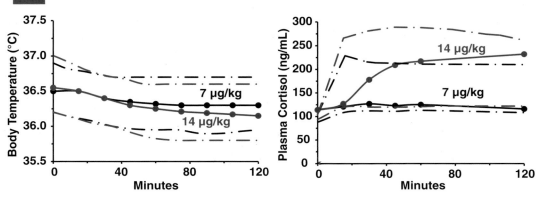

FIGURE 22-22. Observed median times (*solid circles and lines*) and 90% prediction intervals (*dashed lines*) for (**A**) hypothermic response and (**B**) cortisol response, following i.v. administration of 7 (*black*) and 14 (*colored*) μg/kg flesinoxan to 11 subjects. The predictions are based on allometrically scaled parameters determined in rat. Cortisol data have been corrected for placebo response. (From: Zuideveld KP, Van der Graaf PH, Peletier LA, Danhof M. Allometric scaling of pharmacodynamic responses: application to 5-Ht1A receptor mediated responses from rat to man. Pharm Res 2007;24:2031–2039; clinical data from: Seletti B, Benkelfat C, Blier P, Annable L, Gilbert F, de Montigny C. Serotonin 1A receptor activation by flesinoxan in humans: body temperature and neuroendocrine responses. Neuropsychopharmacology 1995;13:93–104.)

lowers body temperature, by lowering the set point control within the brain, and raises plasma cortisol concentration, by increasing cortisol production. The pharmacokinetics and pharmacodynamics of both response systems in rat were modeled and used to predict events in humans. To do so, the time constants of the pharmacodynamic systems were scaled allometrically using an exponential coefficient (b) of -0.25, that is, a rate constant k in rat was scaled by $k/W^{0.25}$ to obtain a value for humans, a process analogous to that found appropriate for scaling half-life (and k) of some drugs. The impact of these differences in magnitude of the time constants on the anticipated temporal profile of hypothermic response between rat and humans is shown in Fig. 22-21, whereas the comparison of the model predictions with observed responses at two doses of flesinoxan in humans, given in Fig. 22-22, indicate a good accord between the two.

Although the biologic time constants are independent of the drug, once this component of the model is established, it is possible to simulate the impact of changes in the pharmacokinetics of a compound, operating by the same mechanism on the target, on the temporal response in man, and assess under what circumstances pharmacokinetics or pharmacodynamics rate limits response with time. Furthermore, once understood, it should be possible to predict the changes in pharmacodynamics as a function of age, genetics, and disease, in a similar manner to that taken to predict changes in pharmacokinetics.

MOVING TO VIRTUAL PATIENT POPULATIONS

There is virtually no end to the number of pharmacokinetic studies required to cover all the possibilities that can, and often do, arise within a patient population in clinical practice. Reflect for a moment on some of these factors: age, disease, genetics, gender, concomitant drugs, herbal preparations, diet, dosage form, and smoking. These factors, each alone and more frequently in combination, produce a virtual limitless array of individual pharmacokinetic profiles, so that no two individuals are likely to have identical profiles. Indeed, the case can be made that even for an individual the pharmacokinetic profile of a drug is constantly changing from time to time, sometimes subtlety, sometimes more profoundly. These arguments, of course, also extend to pharmacodynamics. Yet, there are many circumstances in which we might want to generate the likely range of profiles in a particular patient population prior to performing specific studies, or indeed make predictions for situations that we have not and may never specifically study. Consider, for example, the following situation.

A drug is under development for the treatment of diabetes mellitus. Based on a combination of in vitro data and observations in various early relatively small clinical studies, primarily in young adults, the drug is known to have good oral bioavailability and to be eliminated predominantly by CYP3A4 metabolism (mean $fm = 0.87$), with some renal excretion. The kinetics of the drug appears to be linear over a fairly wide dose range. The two major metabolites are essentially inactive, as both are less potent and present at much lower unbound plasma concentrations than the parent compound. Multiple dosing studies demonstrate that efficacy is best correlated with AUC (0–24 hr) at plateau, and that the therapeutic window lies in the range of 1 to 5 mg-hr/L. Based on this information, together with that on the pharmacokinetics of the drug in the typical patient population and knowing that CYP3A4 activity in any patient cannot currently be reliably predicted, the decision is made to market three dose strengths, namely, 5, 10, and 20 mg and to recommend that patients be started with 5 mg and titrated upward based on response.

Included in the intended target population are elderly patients, some of whom are expected to concurrently receive another drug that is used for treatment of hypertension, a relatively common comorbidity. The antihypertensive drug is a known moderately effective reversible inhibitor of CYP3A4. Of primary concern are those patients who would be at particular risk from the combination of the two drugs. Although we could just include such patients in subsequent larger clinical trials and monitor them carefully, it would be preferable to make this assessment of risk prior to commencing such studies. Indeed, given the known very large interpatient variability in CYP3A4 activity, it is not clear that the number of patients in this subgroup would be large enough to ensure that those at greatest risk are captured to allow adequate recommendations for this situation expected in the wider population once the drug is marketed. A specific drug interaction study in a more robust group, such as young adults, may be, and often is, undertaken to gain some idea of the likely magnitude of the interaction, but again such a study does not address the critical question. Here, as in so many cases, advantage can be taken of the large body of prior knowledge regarding how many processes, including those affecting drug absorption, metabolism, and excretion, change with advancing years or other factors. These changes often can be adequately described as continuous functions. Also, knowing the relative importance of CYP3A4 to the elimination of the drug, and how this enzyme normally varies in the typical patient population, coupled with the age dependencies, it is possible to generate plasma concentration–time profiles in many hundreds or even thousands of virtual patients receiving the drug (at a reduced daily dose to prevent excessive response to the drug), by randomly sampling from the distribution of possible values for each of the parameters, and if appropriate how they covary. This is illustrated in Fig. 22-23A, which shows the 5% to 95% prediction interval in plasma concentration of drug at plateau expected in the elderly (>74 years old) patient population receiving 10 mg orally once a day. The finding that concentrations observed occasionally from patients in this group are contained essentially within these prediction intervals gives some credence to the assumptions underlying the predictions.

As the inhibitor is already marketed, much is known about its pharmacokinetics, including that in the elderly patient population. Such information allows prediction, through simulation, of the envelope of plasma inhibitor concentration–time profiles expected in this population, supported in this case by prior data (Fig. 22-23B). Knowing its inhibition constant, K_I, for CYP3A4, it is therefore possible to generate, using a competitive inhibitor model, the expected 5% to 95% prediction interval of the exposure profiles of the drug of interest in elderly patients concurrently orally taking 5-mg doses of the

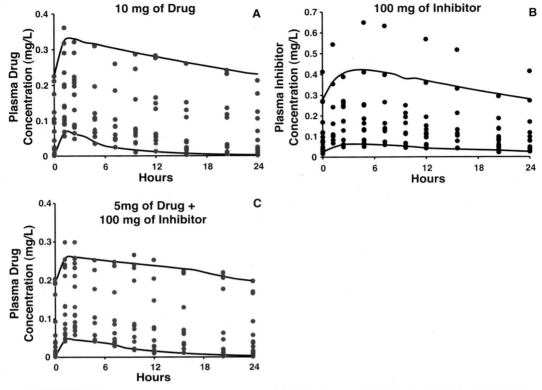

FIGURE 22-23. Strategy for assessing, through simulation, the possible inclusion in clinical trials of elderly patients concurrently receiving a moderately strong inhibitor of CYP3A4 for a drug, under development, that is primarily eliminated by this enzyme. **A.** The black continuous lines are the 5% and 95% prediction interval for the plasma concentration of drug at plateau in elderly patients, following a 10-mg oral once-daily regimen. These prediction intervals were obtained through simulation of thousands of virtual patients, based on the pharmacokinetics of the drug in young adults, and how physiological functions, including CYP3A4 activity, progress with advancing age. The observations (*solid circle, colored*) are those subsequently obtained in a random selection of elderly patients on the regimen. Location of the majority of the observations within the prediction intervals increases one's confidence in the underlying assumptions made in the simulation. **B.** As in A, except this graph applies to the concentration–time profile of the inhibitor at plateau following an oral regimen of 100 mg of this compound daily. Notice the large interindividual variability. **C.** As in A, except this graph applies to the concentration–time profile of the drug at plateau following a regimen of 5 mg of the drug and 100 mg of the inhibitor once daily in elderly patients. Similarity of these prediction intervals with those obtained in A was the basis of deciding that elderly patients receiving the inhibitor could be included in clinical trials. Subsequent observations in such patients (*solid circles, colored*) confirmed the reasonableness of this decision. (From: Moshen Aarabi, Simcyp Ltd, Sheffield, UK.)

drug and 100-mg doses of the inhibitor chronically, as shown in Fig. 22-23C. Halving the dose was considered because it was noted that the mean plateau I/K_I ratio for the 100-mg regimen of the inhibitor is approximately two.

Collectively, the foregoing provides the sort of quantitative information needed to address the original question of the likely risk. Based on these simulations, coupled with the therapeutic window of the drug, it is concluded that elderly patients receiving the inhibitor can safely be treated with the drug provided they are started on 2.5 mg. This in turn implies that this additional dose strength needs to be available, by either scoring the 5-mg tablet, so it can be broken, or producing a specific 2.5-mg tablet. For complete-

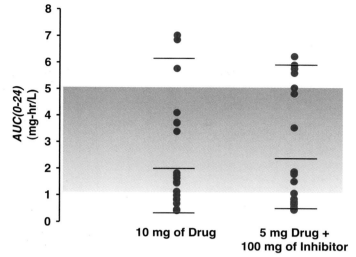

FIGURE 22-24. Shown are *AUC* (0–24 hr) values at plateau for the drug considered in Fig. 22-23 in elderly patients receiving 10 mg once daily alone (*left*) or 5 mg once daily when coadministered with the inhibitor (*right*). The respective three horizontal lines in ascending order are the 5% prediction, the mean, and the 95% interval obtained through simulations of thousands of virtual patients. Also shown are values derived from observed plasma concentrations (●) as well as the therapeutic window of this drug (*shaded area*, 1–5 mg-hr/L). Clearly, several dose strengths are needed because no one dose can keep the *AUC* (0–24 hr) within the therapeutic window for all patients.

ness, as a check, subsequently, we might randomly take occasional blood samples in some elderly patients receiving the inhibitor during clinical trials, as in this example. Agreement with predictions (see Figs. 22-23C and 22-24) gives further confidence to the recommended strategy. It should be readily apparent that this approach can be extended to situations in which patients are on different doses of the inhibitor, or to more complex situations, such as patients on multiple potentially interacting drugs, as commonly occurs in the elderly, as well as including other factors.

This concludes the section on specialized topics, the final part of the book. We hope that these chapters have provided further insights useful in optimizing the therapeutic use of drugs.

KEY RELATIONSHIPS

$$log\ Y = log\ a + b \cdot log\ W$$

$$Y = aW^b$$

$$\frac{C}{Dose/W} = \frac{1}{a_1} e^{-\frac{a_3 \cdot t}{W^{0.25}}}$$

$$CL_{b,H} = Q_H \left[\frac{fu \cdot CL_{H,int}/R}{Q_H + fu \cdot CL_{H,int}/R} \right]$$

Assessment of *AUC*

Several methods exist for measuring the area under the concentration–time curve (*AUC*). One method, discussed here, is the simple numeric estimation of area by the **trapezoidal rule**. The advantage of this method is that it only requires a simple extension of a table of experimental data. Other methods involve either greater numeric complexity or fitting of an equation to the observations and then calculating the area by integrating the fitted equation.

Consider the concentration–time data, first two columns of Table A-1, obtained following oral administration of 50 mg of a drug. What is the total *AUC*?

TABLE A-1	Calculation of Total *AUC* Using the Trapezoidal Rule			
Time (hr)	Concentration (mg/L)	Time Interval (hr)	Average Concentration (mg/L)	Area (mg-hr/L)
0	0	—	—	—
1	7	1	3.5	3.5
2	10	1	8.5	8.5
3	5	1	7.5	7.5
4	2.5	1	3.75	3.75
5	1.25	1	1.88	1.88
6	0.6	1	0.93	0.93
7	0.2	1	0.4	0.4
8	0	1	0.1	0.1
			Total Area = 26.60	

Figure A-1 is a plot of the concentration against time after drug administration. If a perpendicular line is drawn from the concentration at 1 hr (7 mg/L) down to the time axis, then the area bounded between zero time and 1 hr is a trapezoid with an area given by the product of average concentration and time interval. The average concentration is obtained by adding the concentrations at the beginning and end of the time interval and

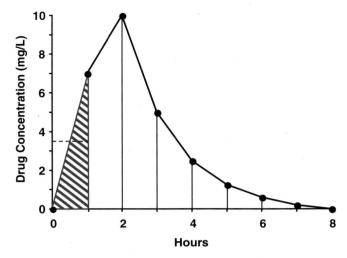

FIGURE A-1. Plasma concentration–time profile. The *AUC* (*shaded colored region*) is the average concentration (*dashed line*) within the interval times the interval itself (0–1 hr).

dividing by 2. Since, in the first interval, the respective concentrations are 0 and 7 mg/L and the time interval is 1 hr, it follows that:

$$AUC_1 \qquad = \qquad \frac{0+7}{2}\ mg/L \qquad \times \qquad 1\ hr$$

Area of trapezoid within   Average concentration   First time
the first time interval   over the first interval   interval

or

$$AUC_1 = 3.5\ mg\text{-}hr/L$$

In this example, the concentration at zero time is 0. Had the drug been given as an intravenous (i.v.) bolus, the concentration at zero time might have been the extrapolated value, $C(0)$.

The area under each time interval can be obtained in an analogous manner to that outlined previously. The total *AUC* over all times is then simply given by

Total AUC = Sum of the individual areas

Usually, *total AUC* means the area under the curve from zero time to infinity. In practice, infinite time is taken as the time beyond which the area is insignificant.

The calculations used to obtain the *AUC*, displayed in Fig. A-1, are shown in Table A-1. In this example, the total *AUC* is 26.6 mg-hr/L.

SPECIAL CASE

AN INTRAVENOUS BOLUS

When a drug is given as an i.v. bolus and the decline in plasma concentration is monoexponential, total *AUC* is calculated most rapidly be dividing the extrapolated zero-time concentration, $C(0)$, by elimination rate constant, k. For example, if $C(0)$ is 200 mg/L and k is 0.1 hr^{-1}, then the total *AUC* is 1000 mg-hr/L.

Proof: The total AUC is given by

$$Total\ AUC = \int_0^\infty C \cdot dt \qquad \text{A-1}$$

But $C = C(0) \cdot e^{-k \cdot t}$, and since $C(0)$ is a constant, it follows that

$$Total\ AUC = C(0) \cdot \int_0^\infty e^{-k \cdot t} \cdot dt \qquad \text{A-2}$$

which, on integrating between time zero and infinity, yields

$$Total\ AUC = \frac{C(0)}{-k} \cdot [e^{-k \cdot t}]_0^\infty = \frac{C(0)}{-k} [0 - 1] = \frac{C(0)}{k} \qquad \text{A-3}$$

WHEN DECLINE IS LOGARITHMIC

The numeric method used to calculate AUC by the trapezoidal rule assumes a linear relationship between observations. Frequently, especially during the decline of drug concentration, the fall is exponential. Then a more accurate method for calculating area during the decline, the **log trapezoidal rule**, can be used, as follows.

Consider, for example, two consecutive observations $C(t_i)$ and $C(t_{i+1})$ at times t_i and t_{i+1}, respectively. These observations are related to each other by

$$C(t_{i+1}) = C(t_1) \cdot e^{-k_i \cdot \Delta t_i} \qquad \text{A-4}$$

where k_i is the rate constant that permits the concentration to fall exponentially from $C(t_i)$ to $C(t_{i+1})$ in the time interval $t_{i+1} - t_i$, that is Δt_i. The value of k_i is given by taking the logarithm on both sides of Eq. A-4 and rearranging, so that

$$k_i = \frac{ln\ [C(t_i)/C(t_{i+1})]}{\Delta t_i} \qquad \text{A-5}$$

Now the AUC during the time interval Δt_i, AUC_i, is the difference between the total areas from t_i to ∞ and from t_{i+1} to ∞, respectively. It therefore follows from events after an i.v. dose that

$$AUC_i = \frac{C(t_i) - C(t_{i+1})}{k_i} \qquad \text{A-6}$$

and, by appropriately substituting for k_i in Eq. A-6, one obtains

$$AUC_i = \frac{[C(t_i) - C(t_{i+1})] \cdot \Delta t_i}{ln\left(\dfrac{C(t_1)}{C(t_{i+1})}\right)} \qquad \text{A-7}$$

This calculation is then repeated for all observations that lie beyond the peak concentration.

In practice, a large discrepancy arises between the method above and that using the (linear) trapezoidal rule only when consecutive observations differ by more than twofold.

STUDY PROBLEMS

(Answers to Study Problems are in Appendix J.)

1. Table A-2 lists the plasma concentrations of zileuton (Zyflo), a drug used in the treatment of asthma, following a 600-mg oral dose. (Adapted from Wong SL, Awni WM,

TABLE A-2	Plasma Concentration of Zileuton with Time After a Single 600-mg Oral Dose

Time (hr)	0	0.5	1	1.5	2	3	4
Concentration (mg/L)	0	2.14	2.95	3.25	3.27	2.68	2.15
Time (hr)	6	8	10	12	14	24	
Concentration (mg/L)	1.12	0.611	0.321	0.180	0.101	0.011	

Cavanaugh JH, et al. The pharmacokinetics of single oral doses of zileuton 200 to 800 mg, its enantiomers, and its metabolites, in normal healthy volunteers. Clin Pharmacokinet 1995;29[suppl 2]:9–21.)

Using the trapezoidal rule, determine the AUC from 0 to 24 hr after the single 600-mg oral dose. Remember that the area of each trapezoid formed by the successive concentrations is the product of the average concentration ($[C(t) + C(t-1)]/2$) and the time interval between them ($[t] - [t-1]$). The total area is the sum of the areas of each of the successive trapezoids.

Ionization and the pH Partition Hypothesis

Most drugs are weak acids or weak bases. In solution, they exist as an equilibrium between un-ionized and ionized forms. When two aqueous phases of different pH are separated by a lipophilic membrane, there is a tendency for the compounds to concentrate on the side with greater ionization. The un-ionized form is assumed to be sufficiently lipophilic to traverse membranes. If it is not, theory predicts that there is no transfer, regardless of pH. The ratio of ionized and un-ionized forms is controlled by both the pH and the pKa of the drug according to the Henderson-Hasselbalch equation. Thus, for acids,

$$pH = pKa + log_{10}\left(\frac{Ionized\ concentration}{Un\text{-}ionized\ concentration}\right) \qquad \text{B-1}$$

and for bases,

$$pH = pKa + log_{10}\left(\frac{Un\text{-}ionized\ concentration}{Ionized\ concentration}\right) \qquad \text{B-2}$$

As log_{10} (1) = 0, the pKa of a compound is the pH at which the un-ionized and ionized concentrations are equal. The pKa is a characteristic of the drug (Fig. B-1, page 692). Consider, for example, the anticoagulant warfarin. Warfarin is an acid with pKa 4.8; that is, equimolar concentrations of un-ionized and ionized drug exist in solution at pH 4.8. Stated differently, 50% of the drug is un-ionized at this pH. At 1 pH unit higher (5.8), the ratio is 10 to 1 in favor of the ionized drug, that is, 10 of 11 total parts or 91% of the drug now exists in the ionized form, and only 9% is un-ionized. At 1 pH unit lower than the pKa (3.8), the percentages in the ionized and un-ionized forms are 9 and 91, the converse of those at pH 5.8.

Figure B-2 (page 693) shows changes in the percent ionized with pH for acids and bases of different pKa values. The pH range 1.0 to 8.0 encompasses values seen in the gastrointestinal tract and the renal tubule. Several considerations are in order and are exemplified by transport across the gastrointestinal barrier. First, very weak acids, such as phenytoin and many barbiturates, whose pKa values are greater than 7.5, are essentially un-ionized at all pH values. For these acids, drug transport should be rapid and independent of pH, provided the un-ionized form is permeable and in solution. Second, the fraction un-ionized changes dramatically only for acids with pKa values between 3.0 and 7.5. For these compounds, a change in rate of transport with pH is expected and has been observed. Third, although transport of still stronger acids—those with pKa values less than 2.5—should theoretically also depend on pH, in practice, the fraction un-ionized is so low that transport across the gut membranes may be slow even under the most acidic conditions.

As originally proposed, the pH partition hypothesis relates to events at equilibrium, with the assumption that this condition is reached when the un-ionized concentrations

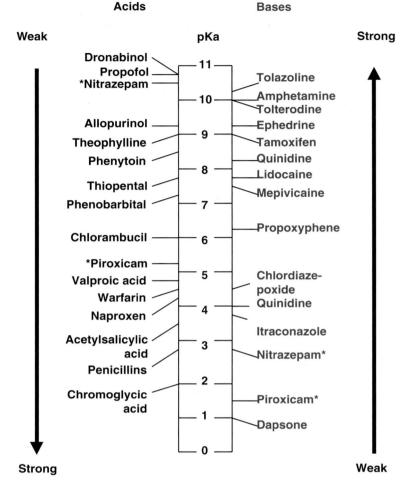

FIGURE B-1. The pKa values of acidic and basic drugs vary widely. Drugs marked with an asterisk are amphoteric; they have both acidic and basic functional groups.

on both sides of the membrane are equal. Yet, it has been applied most widely to predict the influence of pH on the *rates* of absorption and distribution. The likely influence of pH on a rate process depends, however, on where the rate limitation lies. Only if the limitation is in permeability is an effect of pH on rate expected. If the limitation is in perfusion, the problem is not one of movement of drug through membranes and, therefore, any variation in pH is unlikely to have much effect on the rate process. Where the equilibrium lies, however, is independent of what process rate-limits the approach toward equilibrium. Accordingly, the distribution of an ionizable drug across a membrane at equilibrium when the membrane is permeable only to un-ionized drug tends to be affected by differences in pH across the membrane.

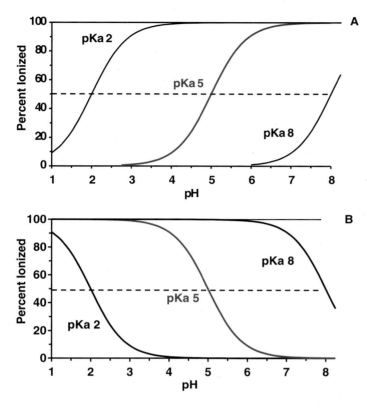

FIGURE B-2. A. Weak acids with pKa values greater than 8.0 are predominantly (*below dashed line*) un-ionized at all pH values between 1.0 and 8.0. Profound changes in the fraction ionized occur with pH for an acid whose pKa value lies within the range of 2.0 to 8.0. Although the fraction ionized of even stronger acids may increase with pH, the absolute value remains high at most pH values shown. **B.** For weak bases, the trends are the converse of those for weak acids. Ionization decreases toward higher pH values.

STUDY PROBLEMS

(Answers to Study Problems are in Appendix J.)

1. Phenobarbital, a weak acid, has a pKa of 7.2.

   Calculate the percent ionized: (a) in blood (pH 7.4) and (b) in urine at (pH 6.2). The percent ionized is:

   $$\frac{Ionized\ concentration \times 100}{Ionized\ concentration\ +\ Un\text{-}ionized\ concentration} \qquad \text{B-3}$$

   or

   $$\left(\frac{\dfrac{Ionized\ concentration}{Un\text{-}ionized\ concentration}}{\dfrac{Ionized\ concentration}{Un\text{-}ionized\ concentration} + 1}\right) \times 100 \qquad \text{B-4}$$

2. Itraconazole, a weak base, has a pKa of 3.8. Calculate the percent ionized: (a) in the stomach (pH 1.8) and (b) in the blood (pH 7.4).

Distribution of Drugs Extensively Bound to Plasma Proteins

The distribution of the plasma protein to which a drug binds is a major determinant of the distribution of a drug with a small (<0.2 L/kg) volume of distribution. This gives rise to kinetic consequences that are different from those expected for a drug with a large volume of distribution when binding to the plasma protein is altered.

Using albumin as a prototypic binding protein, the body can be represented as having three aqueous compartments, as shown in Fig. C-1. The amount of drug in plasma is the product of volume of plasma and plasma drug concentration. The amount of drug in extracellular fluids outside plasma is the product of the aqueous volume of this space and the average concentration within it. The amount outside the extracellular space (in or on cells or bound to connective elements) is accounted for by the product of the aqueous volume into which drug distributes outside the extracellular fluids and the average concentration in this compartment.

	Extracellular Space	**Intracellular Space**
Intravascular	**Extravascular**	
(V_P)	(V_E)	(V_R)
Drug Bound to Intravascular Plasma Proteins	Drug Bound to Extravascular Plasma Proteins	Drug Bound to Cellular Components
Unbound	Unbound	Unbound

FIGURE C-1. Drug distributes among plasma (volume = V_P), the extracellular fluids outside plasma (volume = V_E), add the remainder of the body water (volume = V_R). Equilibrium is achieved when unbound concentrations in all three spaces are the same. The bound concentrations in the three spaces are functions of the affinities of drug for the substances in these spaces to which the drug binds. Throughout the extracellular fluids (V_P and V_E), drug is bound to the same protein(s).

Using the symbols defined in Table C-1,

$$
\underset{\substack{\text{Amount} \\ \text{in body}}}{V \cdot C} = \underset{\substack{\text{Amount} \\ \text{in plasma}}}{V_P \cdot C} + \underset{\substack{\text{Amount in} \\ \text{extracellular} \\ \text{fluids outside plasma}}}{V_E \cdot C_E} + \underset{\substack{\text{Amount in} \\ \text{the remainder} \\ \text{of the body}}}{V_R \cdot C_R} \tag{C-1}
$$

Defining fu_R as Cu/C_R, fu as Cu/C, and Cb_E in Eq. C-2 as the average concentration of bound drug in the extracellular space outside plasma and dividing by C yields

$$
V = V_P + V_E \cdot fu \cdot \frac{(Cu + Cb_E)}{Cu} + V_R \cdot \frac{fu}{fu_R} \tag{C-2}
$$

To be useful, it is necessary to solve for Cb_E in Eq. C-2. This is accomplished as follows.

For a given protein with one class of binding sites, the law of mass action gives

$$
Ka = \frac{Cb_P}{Cu \cdot (P)_P} = \frac{Cb_E}{Cu_E \cdot (P)_E} \tag{C-3}
$$

where Cb_P and Cb_E are the bound drug concentrations and $(P)_P$ and $(P)_E$ are the concentrations of unoccupied protein binding sites in plasma and in other extracellular fluids, all expressed in equivalent units, respectively, and Ka is the association or affinity constant between drug and protein. If unbound drug concentrations are identical in both fluids $(Cu_E = Cu)$, then

$$
\frac{Cb_P}{(P)_P} = \frac{Cb_E}{(P)_E} \tag{C-4}
$$

TABLE C-1	Symbols and Their Definitions

Symbol	Definition
C	Total concentration of drug in plasma
Cb_P	Concentration of bound drug in plasma
Cb_E	Average concentration of bound drug in extracellular fluids outside plasma
Cb_R	Average concentration of drug bound outside the extracellular fluids
C_E	Average total concentration of drug in extracellular fluids outside plasma
C_R	Average total concentration of drug outside the extracellular fluids
Cu	Concentration of unbound drug in plasma and presumably, throughout aqueous spaces into which drug distributes
fu	Fraction unbound to protein in plasma, Cu/C
fu_R	Fraction unbound outside the extracellular fluids, Cu/C_R
Ka	Association or affinity constant between drug and protein
$(P)_P$	Concentration of available binding sites on protein in plasma
$(P)_E$	Average concentration of available binding sites on plasma protein in extracellular fluids outside plasma
$R_{E/I}$	Ratio of the total binding sites (or amount of protein) in the extracellular fluids outside plasma to the total binding sites in plasma
V	Apparent volume of distribution of drug
V_{bw}	Volume of total body water, average value = 42 L/70 kg
V_P	Plasma volume, average value = 3 L/70 kg
V_E	Extracellular fluid volume, average value = 12 L/70 kg
V_R	Aqueous volume outside extracellular fluids into which drug distributes

Also,

$$(Pt)_P = (P)_P + Cb_P \qquad \text{C-5}$$

and

$$(Pt)_E = (P)_E + Cb_E \qquad \text{C-6}$$

where $(Pt)_P$ and $(Pt)_E$ are the average total concentrations of binding sites in plasma and in other extracellular fluids, respectively. It follows from Eq. C-4 that $(Pt)_P/(P)_P = \dfrac{(Pt)_E}{(P)_E}$ (obtained by dividing Eq. C-5 by $(P)_P$ and Eq. C-6 by $(P)_E$). Consequently,

$$Cb_E = Cb_P \cdot \frac{(Pt)_E}{(Pt)_P} \qquad \text{C-7}$$

or

$$Cb_E = Cb_P \cdot R_{E.I} \cdot \frac{V_P}{V_E} \qquad \text{C-8}$$

where $R_{E/I}$ is the ratio of total number of binding sites, or amount of protein, in extracellular fluids outside plasma (extravascular) to that in plasma (intravascular). This relationship, Eq. C-8, can also be shown to be valid when two more classes of binding sites exist on a protein or when saturation is approached. Substituting Eq. C-8 into Eq. C-2 gives

$$V = V_P + fu \cdot \left[\frac{V_E \cdot Cu + Cb_P \cdot V_P \cdot R_{E/I}}{Cu} \right] + \frac{V_R \cdot fu}{fu_R} \qquad \text{C-9}$$

However, since by dividing by C,

$$\frac{Cb_P}{Cu} = (1 - fu)/fu \qquad \text{C-10}$$

then

$$V = V_P (1 + R_{E/I}) + (V_E - V_P \cdot R_{E/I}) \cdot fu + \frac{V_R \cdot fu}{fu_R} \qquad \text{C-11}$$

The volume of the extracellular fluids outside plasma is, on average, 12 L and the plasma volume is 3 L in a normal 70-kg human. Furthermore, as about 60% of the total body albumin is usually found outside plasma (Table 4-5), its extravascular/intravascular distribution ratio, $R_{E/I}$, is approximately 1.5. Using these typical values, Eq. C-11 becomes

$$V = 7.5 + 7.5 \cdot fu + V_R \cdot \frac{fu}{fu_R} \qquad \text{C-12}$$

or

$$V = 7.5 + \left[7.5 + \frac{V_R}{fu_R} \right] \cdot fu \qquad \text{C-13}$$

These last two equations show that if a drug is distributed only in the extracellular fluids, for example, if it cannot enter the cells ($V_R = 0$), the smallest apparent volume of distribution it can have is

$$V = 7.5 + 7.5 \cdot fu \qquad \text{C-14}$$

Thus, at distribution equilibrium, the observed apparent volume of distribution cannot be less that 7.5 L, the volume of distribution of albumin, no matter how tightly the drug is bound to albumin. For a drug that is restricted to the extracellular fluids only ($V_R = 0$) and is not plasma protein bound ($fu = 1$), the apparent volume of distribution is limited to the value of the total extacellular fluid volume, 15 L. Furthermore, it is apparent from Eqs. C-13 and C-14 that the volume of distribution varies linearly with fu whether drug is bound in tissue (fu_R less than 1; $V_R = 27$ L) or restricted to extracellular space ($V_R = 0$).

As $Vu \cdot Cu = V \cdot C$, the volume of distribution based on unbound drug, Vu, by definition is V/fu. Thus, from Eq. C-12

$$Vu = \frac{7.5}{fu} + 7.5 + \frac{V_R}{fu_R} \qquad \text{C-15}$$

Note that the smallest value of Vu possible is 15 L, a value expected for a drug that is neither bound to plasma proteins ($fu = 1$) nor to tissue components ($fu_R = 1$) and does not enter cells. If it does readily enter cells ($V_R = 27$ L), but does not bind anywhere, the unbound volume is that of total body water, 42 L (0.60 L/kg). Increased binding (fu decreased) to plasma proteins increases the unbound volume of distribution. In contrast, increased binding to plasma proteins decreases the volume of distribution based on the total drug concentration in plasma (Eqs. C-12 through C-14). These changes in V and Vu with fraction unbound are shown in Fig. C-2 for three drugs with normal fu values of 0.01, 0.05, and 0.1.

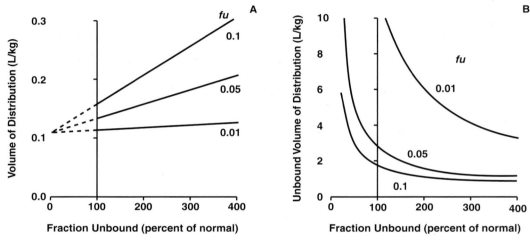

FIGURE C-2. An increase in fraction unbound in plasma, expressed here as percent of the normal value, has only a minor effect on (total) volume of distribution **(A)**, but dramatically decreases unbound volume of distribution **(B)** for three hypothetical drugs. These drugs bind only to albumin ($fu_R = 1$), distribution throughout body water, and have normal fractions unbound in plasma of 0.1, 0.05, and 0.01. Note that with this model (Eq. C-13), the (total) volume of distribution approaches a limiting value of 0.11 L/kg, the apparent volume of distribution of the binding protein, albumin, as fu approaches zero. On the other hand, the unbound volume of distribution (Eq. C-15) approaches a large value as fu approaches zero.

DISTRIBUTION IN BODY

The model expressed by Eq. C-11 and schematically shown in Fig. C-1 can be used to analyze the distribution of a drug in the body. Relationships, listed in Table C-2, for the fractions of total drug in body that are in the three compartments in the form of total, unbound, and bound drug are derived as follows:

The fraction of drug in plasma is simply

$$\text{Fraction in plasma} = \frac{V_P}{V} \qquad \text{C-16}$$

and that outside plasma is

$$\text{Fraction outside plasma} = \frac{V - V_P}{V} \qquad \text{C-17}$$

TABLE C-2	Relationships and Their Approximations for Analyzing the Distribution of Drugs Bound to Albumin

Fraction of Drug in Body	Relationships	Approximation*
In plasma	V_P/V	$3/V$
Unbound in body water	$\dfrac{V_{bw} \cdot fu}{V}$	$\dfrac{42 \cdot fu}{V}$
Unbound in extracellular fluids	$\dfrac{(V_P + V_E) \cdot fu}{V}$	$\dfrac{15 \cdot fu}{V}$
In extracellular fluids	$\dfrac{V_P(1 + R_{E/I}) + fu(V_E - V_P \cdot R_{E/I})}{V}$	$\dfrac{1.5(1 + fu)}{V}$
Outside extracellular fluids	$\dfrac{V - V_P(1 + R_{E/I}) - fu(V_E) - V_P \cdot R_{E/I})}{V}$	$\dfrac{V - 7.5(1 + fu)}{V}$
Bound to proteins in plasma	$\dfrac{V_P \cdot (1 - fu)}{V}$	$\dfrac{3(1 - fu)}{V}$
Bound to extracellular proteins	$\dfrac{V_P}{V}(1 - fu)(1 + R_{E/I})$	$\dfrac{7.5(1 - fu)}{V}$
Bound outside the extracellular fluids	$\dfrac{V - V_{bw} \cdot fu - V_P(1 + fu)(1 + R_{E/I})}{V}$	$\dfrac{V - 35 \cdot fu - 75}{V}$

*Applies to drugs that bind to albumin and distribute throughout total body water; approximations of V_P, V_E, and V_R are 3, 12, and 27 L, respectively, and $R_{E/I} = 1.5$.

The fraction of drug in the body unbound in the total body water, V_{bw}, is

$$\frac{(V_P + V_E + V_R)\,Cu}{V \cdot C} = \frac{V_{bw} \cdot fu}{V} \qquad \text{C-18}$$

and that

$$Fraction\ unbound\ in\ extracellular\ fluids = \frac{(V_P + V_E)}{V} \cdot fu \qquad \text{C-19}$$

Since

$$\begin{array}{ccccccc} \text{Amount bound to} \\ \text{extracellular} & = & V \cdot C & - & (V_P + V_E) \cdot Cu & - & V_R \cdot C_R \\ \text{protein} \end{array} \qquad \text{C-20}$$

$$\begin{array}{ccc} \text{Amount in} & \text{Amount unbound in} & \text{Amount in} \\ \text{body} & \text{extracellular fluids} & \text{remainder of body} \end{array}$$

it follows that

$$\begin{array}{c} \textit{Fraction of drug in body} \\ \textit{bound to extracellular protein} \end{array} = \frac{V \cdot C - (V_P + V_E)Cu - V_R \cdot C_R}{V \cdot C} \qquad \text{C-21}$$

Knowing that $V_R \cdot C_R = \dfrac{V_R \cdot fu \cdot C}{fu_R}$, solving Eq. C-1 for $V_R \cdot C_R$, and substituting these

relationships and Eq. C-9 into Eq. C-21 gives

$$\begin{array}{c} \textit{Fraction bound to} \\ \textit{extracellular protein} \end{array} = \frac{V_P(1 - fu)(1 + R_{E/I})}{V} \qquad \text{C-22}$$

The fraction of drug bound outside the extracellular fluids is 1 minus the sum of the fractions of drug in the total body water (Eq. C-18) and bound to extracellular proteins (Eq. C-22). That is,

$$\frac{\text{Fraction bound outside}}{\text{extracellular fluids}} = \frac{V - V_{bw} \cdot fu - V_P(1 - fu)(1 + R_{E/I})}{V} \qquad \text{C-23}$$

Similar relationships for the fractions inside and outside the extracellular fluids can be derived; these too are listed in Table C-2.

The relationships summarized in Table C-2 have a potential utility in identifying, analyzing, and predicting alterations in the apparent volume of distribution of any drug when there is an alteration either in the unbound fraction in plasma or in the unbound fraction outside the extracellular fluids, or when there is a change in the extravascular/intravascular distribution ratio of the binding protein as occurs, for example, in severe burns, after surgery or trauma, in the nephritic syndrome, and in pregnancy.

DISTRIBUTION OF PROTEIN

When virtually all the drug in the body is bound to a single plasma protein, the apparent volume of distribution of the drug is identical with the apparent volume of distribution of that binding protein. In this situation, Eq. C-11 simplifies to

$$V = V_P(1 + R_{E/I}) \qquad \text{C-24}$$

If V_P is known or is measured, the value of $R_{E/I}$ can be calculated.

The principles above for distribution of drug and its binding protein may also be applied to other plasma proteins. α_1-Acid glycoprotein, the protein that binds many basic drugs, appears to have an extravascular/intravascular distribution ratio that is the inverse of that of albumin, that is, its value of $R_{E/I}$ is about 0.7 rather than 1.5.

STUDY PROBLEMS

(Answers to Study Problems are in Appendix J.)

1. a. Given the information in Table C-3, complete Table C-4 by replacing the dashes with values.
   b. For which one of the drugs in Table C-3 would a twofold increase in the fraction unbound in plasma give the greatest percent change in the apparent volume of distribution?

TABLE C-3	**Distribution Parameters of Selected Drugs**		
	Volume of Distribution*		
Drug	**(L/kg)**	**L**	**Fraction Unbound in Plasma**
Nafcillin	0.35	24.5	0.11
Naproxen	0.16	11.2	0.003
Nitrazepam	1.90	133.0	0.13

*For this problem, assume that the unbound form of each drug distributes evenly throughout total body water and that albumin is the only protein to which each drug binds in plasma, a reasonable approximation for these drugs. The extravascular/intravascular distribution of albumin is 1.5.

From: Benet LZ, Williams RL. Appendix II. In: Gilman AG, Rall TW, Nies AS, Taylor P. The Pharmacological Basis of Therapeutics. 8th ed. New York: Macmillan; 1993.

| TABLE C-4 | Analysis of the Distribution of Nafcillin, Naproxen, and Nitrazepam* |

Percent of Drug in Body that is . . .	Nafcillin	Naproxen	Nitrazepam
In plasma	12	27	—
Unbound		—	4
In extracellular fluids	34	—	—
Outside extracellular fluids	—	33	94
Bound to protein in plasma	11	27	2
Bound intracellularly (in or on tissue cells Including blood cells)	54	32	—

*For a 70-kg person.

2. The information contained in Table C-5 summarizes the effect of acute viral hepatitis on the disposition of tolbutamide, a drug that is eliminated almost exclusively by hepatic metabolism. Explain the apparent differences in tolbutamide disposition between these two groups. What is the cause of the shorter half-life in the subjects with acute viral hepatitis?

| TABLE C-5 | Effect of Acute Viral Hepatitis on Tolbutamide Disposition |

Subjects	Half-life (hr)	Volume of Distribution (L/kg)	Clearance (mL/hr per kg)	Fraction of Drug in Plasma Unbound
Healthy	5.8	0.15	18	0.06
Acute viral hepatitis	4.0	0.15	26	0.10

From: Williams RL, Blaschke TF, Meffin PJ, et al. Influence of acute viral hepatitis on disposition and plasma binding of tolbutamide. Clin Pharmacol Ther 1977;21:301–309.

D

Plasma-to-Blood Concentration Ratio

The interrelationships among extraction ratio, blood flow, and blood clearance of drugs require measurement of drug concentration in whole blood. Because plasma is the usual site of measurement, knowledge of how plasma concentration and blood concentration are related can be useful. The ratio of the concentrations at equilibrium is the key measure of this relationship.

The plasma-to-blood concentration ratio depends on plasma protein binding, partitioning into blood cells, and the volume occupied by blood cells. This dependence is, perhaps, most readily appreciated from mass–balance considerations, as follows:

$$C_b \cdot V_B \quad = \quad C \cdot V_P \quad + \quad C_{BC} \cdot V_{BC}$$

Amount in blood	Amount in plasma	Amount in blood cells	D-1

Where
C_b = blood concentration of drug
V_B = blood volume
C = plasma concentration of drug
V_P = plasma volume
C_{BC} = blood cell concentration of drug
V_{BC} = volume occupied by blood cells

The ratio of concentration in blood cells, C_{BC}, to that unbound in plasma, Cu, is a measure of the affinity of blood cells for drug. Using Kp_{BC} for this ratio and since $Cu = fu \cdot C$,

$$C_{bc} = Kp_{BC} \cdot Cu = Kp_{BC} \cdot fu \cdot C \qquad \text{D-2}$$

The volume occupied by blood cells is a function of hematocrit, H, and blood volume, that is,

$$V_{BC} = H \cdot V_B \qquad \text{D-3}$$

The plasma volume is related to hematocrit by

$$V_P = (1 - H)V_B \qquad \text{D-4}$$

Substituting Eqs. D-2 to D-4 into Eq. D-1,

$$C_b \cdot V_B = (1 - H) V_B \cdot C + fu \cdot Kp_{BC} \cdot H \cdot V_B \cdot C \qquad \text{D-5}$$

Finally, dividing by $V_B \cdot C_b$, and rearranging,

$$\frac{C}{C_b} = \frac{1}{1 + H[fu \cdot Kp_{BC} - 1]} \qquad \text{D-6}$$

This relationship clearly shows how the ratio of concentrations, plasma/blood, varies with hematocrit, plasma protein binding, and affinity of drug for blood cells. The ratio can be calculated if these parameters are known. The correlation is useful in situations in which plasma protein binding is variable, such as for certain drugs in uremia, in hypoalbuminemic and hyperalbuminemic states and in displacement interactions.

Note that the blood-to-plasma concentration ratio (C_b/C), the reciprocal of Eq. D-6, is

$$\frac{C_b}{C} = 1 + H \cdot [fu \cdot Kp_{BC} - 1] \qquad \text{D-7}$$

If hematocrit and affinity are constant, a plot of this ratio against fu gives a straight line with an intercept of $1 - H$ and a slope of $H \cdot Kp_{BC}$.

On rearranging Eq. D-6 or Eq. D-7 to solve for Kp_{BC}, a useful means of determining affinity of blood cells for the drug is obtained, namely,

$$Kp_{BC} = \frac{H - 1 + (C_b/C)}{fu \cdot H} \qquad \text{D-8}$$

Determination of Kp_{BC} requires measurement of hematocrit, concentration ratio, and fraction of drug in plasma unbound to proteins.

STUDY PROBLEMS

(Answers to Study Problems are in Appendix J.)

1. The ratio of concentrations (plasma/blood) of a given drug averages about 0.425 in a typical patient who has a hematocrit of 0.45 and a fraction unbound in plasma of 0.1.

   a. Calculate the ratio of the concentration in blood cells to that unbound in plasma (p).
   b. Hematocrit is decreased to 0.27 in an anemic patient, but serum concentration of albumin, the protein to which this drug binds, remains normal (4.3 g/dL). Calculate the expected plasma-to-blood ratio in this patient, given that p is unchanged.
   c. Predict the ratio of plasma-to-blood concentrations in a patient with the nephrotic syndrome in whom the hematocrit is normal but the fraction unbound in plasma is increased to 0.32, a secondary consequence of the loss of plasma proteins into urine.

Well-Stirred Model of Hepatic Clearance

MODEL I: RAPID EQUILIBRATION BETWEEN DRUG IN BLOOD AND LIVER

This is a steady-state model in which distribution equilibrium is maintained between drug in blood and in the liver, and the only reason for a drop in concentration across the organ is elimination. It is assumed that all three aqueous spaces within the liver (blood [*b*], interstitial space [*is*], and intracellular space [*cell*]) are well-mixed, each providing uniform, albeit potentially different, concentrations of drug within them. Furthermore, distribution occurs by passive diffusion, and the liver acts as one compartment with unbound drug in the blood, leaving the liver in equilibrium with, and equal to, that unbound within the liver.

Consider events occurring across the organ:

$$V_H \frac{dC_H}{dt} = Q_H \cdot C_{b,in} - Q_H \cdot C_{b,out} - CL_{int} \cdot Cu_{cell} \qquad \text{E-1}$$

$$\underbrace{\phantom{V_H \frac{dC_H}{dt}}}_{\substack{\text{Rate of change} \\ \text{of amount of} \\ \text{drug in liver}}} \quad \underbrace{\phantom{Q_H \cdot C_{b,in}}}_{\text{Rate in}} \quad \underbrace{\phantom{Q_H \cdot C_{b,out}}}_{\substack{\text{Rate of} \\ \text{return to} \\ \text{body}}} \quad \underbrace{\phantom{CL_{int} \cdot Cu_{cell}}}_{\substack{\text{Rate of} \\ \text{elimination}}}$$

where the liver, of volume V_H and the total liver concentration C_H, is perfused with blood at flow rate Q_H with entering and leaving concentrations $C_{b,in}$, $C_{b,out}$ respectively. Within the hepatocyte, CL_{int} is the intrinsic clearance and Cu_{cell} is the unbound intracellular concentration.

Now

$$Cu_{cell} = Cu_{out} = fu_b \cdot C_{b,out} \qquad \text{E-2}$$

where fu_b is the ratio of unbound concentration in plasma to the whole blood concentration. Substituting Eq. E-2 into Eq. E-1, and collecting terms yields

$$V_H \frac{dC_H}{dt} = Q_H \cdot C_{b,in} - (Q_H + fu_b \cdot CL_{int}) C_{b,out} \qquad \text{E-3}$$

Furthermore, recognizing that at steady state $dC_H/dt = 0$, it follows that

$$\frac{C_{b,out}}{C_{b,in}} = \frac{Q_H}{Q_H + fu_b \cdot CL_{int}} \qquad \text{E-4}$$

Now, given that the extraction ratio is

$$E_H = 1 - \frac{C_{b,out}}{C_{b,in}} \qquad \text{E-5}$$

it can be seen by substituting Eq. E-4 into Eq. E-5, rearranging, and collecting terms, that

$$E_H = \frac{fu_b \cdot CL_{int}}{Q_H + fu_b \cdot CL_{int}} \qquad \text{E-6}$$

And since, by definition of the terms,

$$CL_{b,H} = Q_H \cdot E_H \qquad \text{E-7}$$

it follows that

$$CL_{b,H} = Q_H \left[\frac{fu_b \cdot CL_{int}}{Q_H + fu_b \cdot CL_{int}} \right] \qquad \text{E-8}$$

MODEL II: ADDITION OF PERMEABILITY CONSIDERATIONS

This is an extension of model I. Although there is still no barrier for drug movement between perfusing blood and the interstitial space, a permeability barrier now exists at the level of the hepatocyte.

Consider events within the hepatic cell:

$$V_{cell} \frac{dC_{cell}}{dt} = P_{in} \cdot SA \cdot Cu_{is} - P_{out} \cdot SA \cdot Cu_{cell} - CL_{int} \cdot Cu_{cell} \qquad \text{E-9}$$

where V_{cell} is the volume of the cell, C_{cell} is the total cellular drug concentration, Cu_{is} is the unbound concentration of drug in the interstitial space and in the blood leaving the liver, and $P_{in} \cdot SA$, $P_{out} \cdot SA$ are the uptake and efflux permeability-surface area (SA) products of the cell membrane to unbound drug between the interstitial and intracellular spaces (with units of flow). When uptake and efflux of drug occur by passive diffusion, then $P_{in} = P_{out}$. However, when active transporters are involved, it is likely that $P_{in} \neq P_{out}$.

Now, at steady state $dC_{cell}/dt = 0$, so that

$$Cu_{cell} = \frac{P_{in} \cdot SA \cdot Cu_{is}}{P_{out} \cdot SA + CL_{int}} = \rho \cdot Cu_{is} \qquad \text{E-10}$$

where $\rho = P_{in} \cdot SA/(P_{out} \cdot SA + CL_{int})$. From Eq. E-10, the meaning of ρ is clear; it is the ratio of the intracellular to extracellular unbound concentrations. Note that P_{in}, P_{out}, and CL_{int} all influence the rate of drug elimination for a given unbound extracellular concentration.

Furthermore,

$$Cu_{is} = Cu_{out} = fu_b \cdot C_{b,out} \qquad \text{E-11}$$

Hence, on substituting Eqs. E-10 and E-11 into Eq. E-9, recognizing that, at steady state, $V_{cell} \dfrac{dC_{cell}}{dt} = 0$ and then following through as for model I, it follows that

$$E_H = \frac{fu_b \cdot \rho \cdot CL_{int}}{Q_H + fu_b \cdot \rho \cdot CL_{int}} \qquad \text{E-12}$$

And

$$CL_{b,H} = Q_H \left[\frac{fu_b \cdot \rho \cdot CL_{int}}{Q_H + fu_b \cdot \rho \cdot CL_{int}} \right] \qquad \text{E-13}$$

Now, generally, basolateral permeability is very high (i.e., P_{in}, $P_{out} >> CL_{int}$) in which case, when distribution occurs only by passive diffusion ($P_{in} = P_{out}$), $\rho \approx 1$ and Eqs. E-12 and E-13 reduce to those of model I. At the other extreme, when basolateral permeability is much lower than intrinsic clearance (P_{in}, $P_{out} << CL_{int}$), for passive diffusion $\rho = P_{in} \cdot SA/CL_{int}$ which, on substitution into Eq. E-13, yields

$$CL_{b,H} = Q_H \left[\frac{fu_b \cdot P_{in} \cdot SA}{Q_H + fu_b \cdot P_{in} \cdot SA} \right] \qquad \text{E-14}$$

Now, we see that clearance is dependent on permeability and insensitive to intrinsic clearance. Furthermore, this condition is most likely to arise with large or polar molecules. In such cases, permeability is much lower than blood flow ($P_{in} << Q_H$), in which case Eq. E-14 reduces to

$$CL_{b,H} = fu_b \cdot P_{in} \qquad \text{E-15}$$

That is, clearance now is rate limited by the permeability of the hepatocyte to drug. Changes in permeability, because, for example, of disease or other drugs competing with an uptake transporter, will result in corresponding changes in observed hepatic clearance.

EVENTS AFTER ORAL DOSE

If loss of oral bioavailability is solely because of hepatic extraction on first pass through liver, it then follows from Eq. E-13 that,

$$Oral\ Bioavailability\ F = 1 - E_H = \frac{Q_H}{Q_H + fu_b \cdot \rho \cdot CL_{int}} \qquad \text{E-16}$$

But after a single oral dose

$$F \cdot Dose = CL \cdot AUC_{po} \qquad \text{E-17}$$

Substituting Eq. E-16 for F, and Eq. E-13 for CL, into Eq. E-17 for a drug exclusively cleared by the liver gives

$$\frac{Q_H \cdot Dose}{Q_H + fu_b \cdot \rho \cdot CL_{int}} = \frac{Q_H \cdot fu_b \cdot \rho \cdot CL_{int}}{Q_H + fu_b \cdot \rho \cdot CL_{int}} \cdot AUC_{po} \qquad \text{E-18}$$

so that

$$AUC_{po} = \frac{Dose}{fu_b \cdot \rho \cdot CL_{int}} \qquad \text{E-19}$$

Also on multiple oral dosing of a fixed-dose, fixed-dosing–interval regimen of such a drug

$$AUC_{ss,po} = \frac{F \cdot Dose}{CL} = \frac{Dose}{fu_b \cdot \rho \cdot CL_{int}} \qquad \text{E-20}$$

Thus, changes in permeability, in addition to protein binding and intrinsic clearance, can influence the AUC versus dose relationship after an oral dose.

STUDY PROBLEMS

(Answers to Study Problems are in Appendix J.)

1. The hepatic clearance of a drug is 2.7 L/min, $fu = 0.05$ and its plasma-to-blood concentration ratio (R) is 0.17. Given that hepatic blood flow is 1.35 L/min, distribution of the drug into the liver is perfusion rate limited, and the well-stirred model applies, calculate the following parameters:

a. Hepatic extraction ratio
b. Intrinsic clearance
c. Comment on the value of intrinsic clearance relative to hepatic blood flow.

2. This question should only be attempted after completion of Chapter 11, *Multiple-Dose Regimens.*

For a drug entirely eliminated by the liver, with hepatic extraction being the only cause of loss of oral bioavailability, prove that when clearance is uptake permeability rate-limited, the unbound plateau concentration during oral multiple dosing is given by

$$Cu_{av,ss} = \frac{Dose}{PS_{influx} \cdot \tau}$$

Absorption Kinetics

W hen absorption and elimination are first-order and a one-compartment model applies, the concentration–time profile is a function of the difference between two exponential terms. In this situation, a graphic procedure called **method of residuals** can be used to determine the absorption half-life. To show this method, consider the plasma data in Table F-1, obtained following a 100-mg oral dose of a drug. The data are plotted in Fig. F-1. The half-life, estimated from the linear portion of the decline phase, is 5 hr, a value also obtained following intravenous administration.

TABLE F-1	Plasma Concentration–Time Data following Oral Administration of a 100-mg Dose of a Drug		
	Observation	**Treatment of Data**	
Time (hr)	**Plasma Concentration** C **(mg/L)**	**Extrapolated Plasma Concentration** $\overleftarrow{C}$ **(mg/L)**	**Difference in Concentrations** $(\overleftarrow{C} - C)$**(mg/L)**
1	0.38	1.90	1.52
2	0.73	1.65	0.92
3	0.91	1.40	0.49
4	0.97	1.23	0.26
5	0.97	1.07	0.10
6	0.92	0.95	0.03
8	0.71	0.71	—
10	0.53	0.53	—
12	0.40	0.40	—
14	0.30	0.30	—

METHOD OF RESIDUALS

The method is as follows: (a) The terminal log linear portion of the decline is back extrapolated to time zero. (b) Letting $\overleftarrow{C}$ denote the plasma concentration along this extrapolated line, the observed plasma concentration (C) at each time point is then subtracted from the corresponding value on the extrapolated line. These calculations are shown in Table F-1. (c) The residuals ($\overleftarrow{C} - C$) are plotted against time on the same semilogarithmic graph paper (Fig. F-1). If, as in this example, the residual plot is a straight line, then absorption is a first-order process. The absorption half-life, taken as the time

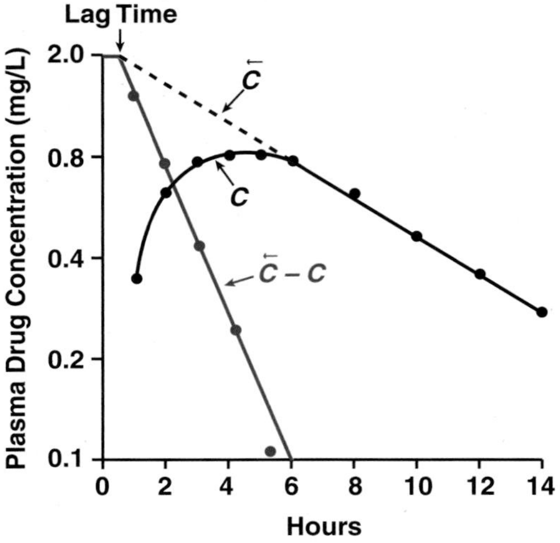

FIGURE F-1. By the method of residuals, an estimate can be made of both the absorption half-life (from the slope of *colored line*) and the lag time (noted by the *arrow*) following extravascular administration. Data from Table F-1.

for the residual value to diminish by one half, is 1.3 hr. The corresponding absorption rate constant, *ka*, is 0.693/1.3 hr or 0.53 hr^{-1}.

Let us examine the underlying basis of the method of residuals. At any time, the plasma concentration following extravascular administration (obtained by simultaneous integration of Eqs. 6-2 and 6-3 in Chapter 6, *Kinetics Following an Extravascular Dose*, and realizing that $C = A/V$ and the amount absorbed is $F \cdot Dose$) is given by

$$C = \left(\frac{F \cdot Dose \cdot ka}{V(ka - k)}\right)(e^{-k \cdot t} - e^{-ka \cdot t}) \qquad \text{F-1}$$

The reader is encouraged to prove the derivation of Eq. F-1, using a standard calculus book.

When (as is most frequently the case) absorption is more rapid than elimination ($ka > k$), the value of $ka \cdot t$ is greater than $k \cdot t$ and hence $e^{-ka \cdot t}$ approaches zero more rapidly than does $e^{-k \cdot t}$. At some point past the peak plasma concentration, $e^{-ka \cdot t}$ becomes essentially zero, absorption is over and the extrapolated line is given by

$$\overleftarrow{C} = \left(\frac{F \cdot Dose \cdot ka}{V(ka - k)}\right) \cdot e^{-k \cdot t} \qquad \text{F-2}$$

Subtracting C from $\overleftarrow{C}$ therefore yields

$$\overleftarrow{C} - C = \left(\frac{F \cdot Dose \cdot ka}{V(ka - k)}\right)e^{-ka \cdot t} \qquad \text{F-3}$$

And taking natural logarithms

$$ln(\overleftarrow{C} - C) = ln\left(\frac{F \cdot Dose \cdot ka}{V(ka - k)}\right)e^{-ka \cdot t} \qquad \text{F-4}$$

Hence, if absorption is a first-order process, a semilogarithmic plot of the residual value against time yields a straight line with a slope of $-ka$. When this residual line is not log linear, absorption is not a simple first-order process, and other methods, such as the Wagner-Nelson method (Appendix G, *Wagner-Nelson Method*), are needed to calculate how absorption varies with time.

LAG TIME

Examination of Eqs. F-2 and F-3 suggests a simple graphic method for estimating lag time, that is, the time between administration and start of absorption. By definition, absorption begins when the extrapolated and residual curves intersect. This must be so since only at time $t = 0$, when $e^{-ka \cdot t} = e^{-k \cdot t} = 1$, are the values of the two equations the same and equal to $(F \cdot Dose \cdot ka)/[V(ka - k)]$. As shown in Fig. F-1, the lag time in this example is approximately 30 min.

EVENTS AT THE PEAK

The **peak concentration**, C_{max}, and the time of its occurrence, t_{max}, also called **peak time**, are often important factors influencing drug therapy. Together, they can sometimes provide sufficient information on the speed of drug absorption for a given dose of drug. However, both C_{max} and t_{max} are also influenced by the disposition kinetics of the drug, and questions sometimes arise concerning the impact of changes in absorption and disposition on these values. The answers to such questions are most readily provided by solving Eq. F-1 for the condition at the peak. It is seen that if t_{max} is known, C_{max} can be calculated. The value of t_{max} is determined as follows. At that time, rate of absorption is matched by rate of elimination, and hence, rate of change of plasma concentration is zero, that is, $dC/dt = 0$. So, to determine t_{max}, we must first determine dC/dt, which by differentiation of Eq. F-1 is

$$\frac{dC}{dt} = \frac{F \cdot Dose \cdot ka}{V(ka - k)}(-k \cdot e^{-k \cdot t} + ka \cdot e^{-ka \cdot t}) \qquad \text{F-5}$$

At t_{max} when $dC/dt = 0$, it follows from Eq. F-5 that

$$t_{max} = \frac{ln\left(\frac{ka}{k}\right)}{(ka - k)} \qquad \text{F-6}$$

Equation F-6 clearly shows that only the rate constants for absorption and elimination influence t_{max}. Thus, for a given value of k, t_{max} can be calculated for various values of ka. Note, however, that if t_{max} and k are known, ka can be determined only by substituting values for ka into the right-hand side of Eq. F-6 until the calculated t_{max} equals the observed value. Finally, when there is a lag time, C_{max} occurs at $t_{max} + t_{lag}$.

STUDY PROBLEMS

(Answers to Study Problems are in Appendix J.)

1. The following plasma concentrations (Table F-2) were observed in a patient who took a 100-mg tablet of a drug.
   a. Prepare a semilogarithmic plot of the data and determine the rate constants for absorption and elimination.
   b. Estimate when absorption begins.
   c. Given that absorption is complete (100%), calculate:
      (1) clearance
      (2) volume of distribution
2. The absorption kinetics of a drug, known to be acid labile, was studied in two groups: group A, patients with normal gastric function; group B, patients with achlorhydria (a condition in which little or no acid is secreted into the stomach). Each group received

TABLE F-2	Plasma Concentration with Time Following a Single 100-mg Oral Dose of a Drug									
Time (hr)	0.25	0.5	1	2	3	4	6	8	10	12
Plasma concentration (mg/L)	1.6	2.7	3.7	3.5	2.7	2.0	1.02	0.49	0.26	0.12

the same dose of drug. Analysis of the plasma concentration–time curves yielded the following estimates: group A, $F = 0.30$, $ka = 1.5 \text{ hr}^{-1}$; group B, $F = 0.90$, $ka = 0.39$ hr^{-1}. The investigators proposed that the longer half-life for absorption in patients with achlorhydria was caused by a slower gastric emptying in this group. Suggest an alternative proposal that is consistent with all the observations.

G

Wagner-Nelson Method

general procedure for assessing absorption kinetics of a drug is the **Wagner-Nelson method**. It can be used when a one-compartment model of the body applies, but a modified form is also useful for models with two or more compartments. The only requirement is that linear disposition kinetics apply. It is one of several methods of **deconvolution** for assessing drug input. It is based on the concept that the observation after an extravascular dose must be a **convolution** of both the input and disposition of a drug. If one knows the disposition function (obtained after an intravenous [i.v.] bolus), then, by deconvolution, the input function can be obtained. For now, let us examine the basic elements of the Wagner-Nelson method, which is applicable even when no i.v. data are available.

At any time, the amount absorbed is given by the familiar mass–balance equation

$$
\underset{\text{Amount absorbed}}{A_{ab}} = \underset{\text{Amount in body}}{A} + \underset{\text{Amount eliminated}}{A_{el}} \qquad \text{G-1}
$$

Now, $A = V \cdot C$ and $A_{el} = CL \cdot \int_0^t C \cdot dt$, which on substitution into Eq. G-1 gives

$$
A_{ab} = V \cdot C + CL \cdot \int_0^t C \cdot dt \qquad \text{G-2}
$$

Hence, if CL and V are known from i.v. data, changes in A_{ab} with time can then be calculated. The value rises until absorption stops. Then, $A_{ab} = F \cdot Dose = CL \cdot AUC$, allowing bioavailability to be determined. Notice that no assumption is made regarding the nature of the absorption process; it may be simple or complex. Indeed, the calculated absorption–time profile can be analyzed further to characterize the absorption process.

Often, no i.v. dosage form is available, and then Eq. G-2 must be modified to allow assessment of absorption kinetics. This is accomplished by noting that $CL = k \cdot V$, so that division of Eq. G-2 by V yields

$$
\frac{A_{ab}}{V} = C + k \cdot \int_0^t C \cdot dt \qquad \text{G-3}
$$

Thus, knowing the elimination rate constant, k, the ratio A_{ab}/V can be determined from the plasma concentration–time data, with AUC to each time estimated by the appropriate numeric method (Appendix A, *Assessment of AUC*).

Ultimately, the value calculated using Eq. G-3 reaches an upper limit, signifying that absorption has stopped. This limiting value is therefore $F \cdot Dose/V$, which also equals $k \cdot \int_0^\infty Cdt$, as $F \cdot Dose = CL \cdot \int_0^\infty Cdt$. Accordingly, the fraction of bioavailable dose that is absorbed with time can be estimated; it is given by

$$
\begin{array}{c}
\textit{Fraction of} \\
\textit{bioavailable} \\
\textit{drug absorbed}
\end{array} = \frac{C + k \cdot \int_0^t Cdt}{k \cdot \int_0^\infty Cdt} = \frac{\dfrac{C}{k} + \int_0^t Cdt}{\int_0^\infty Cdt} \qquad \text{G-4}
$$

TABLE G-1	Estimation of Cumulative Amount of Bioavailable Drug Absorbed with Time

Observation		Treatment of Data			
Time (hr)	Plasma Drug Concentration C (mg/L)	AUC (mg-hr/L)	$k \cdot AUC$ (mg/L)	$C + k \cdot AUC$ [Aab/V] (mg/L)	Fraction of Bioavailable Drug Absorbed
0	0	0	0	0	0
0.5	0.18	0.045	0.006	0.19	0.095
1	0.35	0.178	0.025	0.38	0.19
2	0.66	0.683	0.096	0.75	0.38
3	0.91	1.468	0.210	1.12	0.56
4	1.12	2.483	0.350	1.47	0.78
5	1.27	3.678	0.520	1.79	0.90
6	1.28	4.953	0.693	1.97	0.99
8	0.99	7.223	1.011	2.00	1.00
10	0.75	8.963	1.254	2.00	1.00
12	0.57	10.283	1.439	2.01	1.00
15	0.38	11.708	1.638	2.01	1.00
24	0.11	13.912	1.946	2.05	1.00

To illustrate the method, consider the concentration–time data listed in the first two columns of Table G-1 and displayed semilogarithmically in Fig. G-1 following the oral administration of a 100-mg dose of drug. First, k is estimated from the declining concentration–time data; it is 0.14 hr^{-1} ($t_{1/2} = 5$ hr). Next, the AUC to each time point is calculated; the values, calculated using the trapezoidal rule, are also listed in Table G-1 (third column). The product $k \cdot \int_0^t Cdt$ is then calculated and added to the plasma concentration to yield Aab/V. For example, the value of $k \cdot AUC$ at the first sampling time of 1 hr is 0.14 $hr^{-1} \times$ 0.045 mg-hr/L or 0.006 mg/L, which when added to 0.18 mg/L gives 0.186 or 0.19 mg/L for Aab/V. The values of Aab/V with time are listed in Table G-1 (penultimate column) and displayed in Fig. G-2. They show that absorption proceeds almost lin-

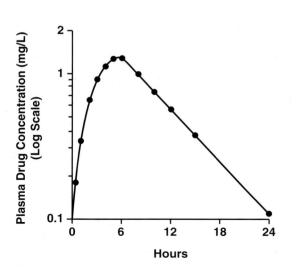

FIGURE G-1.

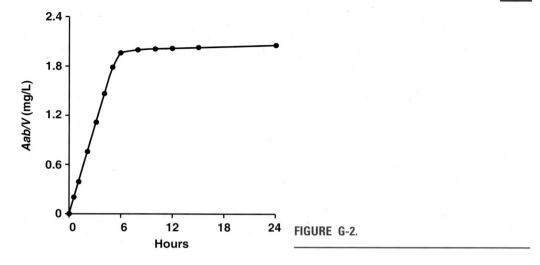

FIGURE G-2.

early with time for much of the absorption process, but absorption stops abruptly at about 6 hr, suggesting that absorption may be close to zero order. Furthermore, statements can be made about the fraction of the bioavailable drug that is absorbed at various times (also shown in Table G-1 [last column]).

Finally, a word of caution is needed here. Critical to the method is an accurate estimate of k. Problems arise when the decline of plasma concentration is absorption rate-limited. Then, no reliable estimate of k can be made. The problem often arises when evaluating modified-release products. A possible solution is to use an estimate of k in the subject, obtained following administration of a rapid-release dosage form on a separate occasion. The assumptions, often reasonable, are that the decline in plasma concentration is now limited by elimination and that the disposition kinetics (both V and CL) in the subject do not vary significantly from one occasion to another.

STUDY PROBLEMS

(Answers to Study Problems are in Appendix J.)

1. A 500-mg modified-release oral formulation was tested against a solution (500 mg) of a drug in 18 healthy volunteers. A previous study demonstrated that the drug is rapidly and completely absorbed when given in solution. Subjects took a single dose of each formulation on a fasted stomach on separate occasions.

   Plasma drug concentration–time data following oral ingestion of the modified-release product are listed in Table G-2 for one subject. Following administration of the oral solution, the AUC and half-life of the drug in the subject were 86.6 mg-hr/L and 5 hr, respectively.

   a. Using the Wagner-Nelson method, complete Table G-2 by calculating Aab/V with time, following administration of the modified-release dosage form. In your calculation, use the half-life obtained in this subject following administration of the solution.
   b. What assumption have you made in applying the Wagner-Nelson method?
   c. What is the bioavailability of the drug in the subject from the modified-release product relative to that from the oral solution.
   d. By an appropriate graphical analysis of the absorption data, ascertain whether absorption of drug from modified-release product in vivo is first-order, and if so, the half-life of the absorption process.

TABLE G-2	Plasma Concentration and *AUC* Data following a 500-mg Modified-Release Product		
Time (hr)	Plasma Concentration (mg/L)	Area (mg-hr/L)	*Aab/V* (mg/L)
0	0.00	0.00	
0.5	0.76	0.19	
1	1.42	0.73	
2	2.48	2.68	
3	3.24	5.54	
4	3.75	6.03	
6	4.27	17.05	
8	4.31	25.63	
10	4.09	34.03	
12	3.72	41.84	
18	2.46	60.38	
24	1.45	72.11	
36	0.43	83.39	
48	0.11	86.63	

2. In problem 4, Chapter 10, *Constant-Rate Input*, plasma concentration–time data are provided during and following a 24-hr i.v. constant-rate infusion and a rectal delivery device of droperidol.

a. Given a half-life of 1.9 hr estimated from the declining concentration after stopping the i.v. infusion, apply the Wagner-Nelson method to the plasma concentration–time data to calculate the absorption kinetics of droperidol following administration of the rectal device.

b. The device is intended to deliver the drug at a constant rate for 15 hr. Do the absorption kinetics in vivo meet this expectation?

Mean Residence Time

 dose of drug comprises many millions of molecules. For example, even a dose as small as 1 mg of a drug with a molecular weight of 300 g/mol contains close to 2×10^{18} molecules (10^{-3} g/$300 \times 6.023 \times 10^{23}$ [Avogadro's number]). On administration, these drug molecules each spend a different time within the body. Some are eliminated rapidly; others stay for a long time. A few may remain for a lifetime. The result is a distribution of residence times that can be characterized by a mean value.

The **mean residence time** (*MRT*) is the average time the molecules introduced reside within the body, that is,

$$MRT = \sum_{i=1}^{N} t_j/N \qquad \text{H-1}$$

where t_j is the residence time of the *jth* molecule (time between its input and its elimination from the body). Individual molecules cannot be counted, of course, but groups of them can. Letting n_1 be the number of molecules remaining in the body for a time of t_1, and n_2 be the number remaining for time t_2, then the mean time of the two groups becomes

$$\frac{(t_1 \cdot n_1) + (t_2 \cdot n_2)}{n_1 + n_2} \qquad \text{H-2}$$

Extending this concept to account for all molecules administered, the *MRT* becomes

$$MRT = \frac{\sum_{i=1}^{m} t_i \cdot n_i}{\sum_{i=1}^{m} n_i} = \frac{\sum_{i=1}^{m} t_i \cdot n_i}{N} \qquad \text{H-3}$$

where n_i is the number of molecules in the *i*th group; t_i is their average time in the body; m is the number of groups; and the denominator N is the total number of molecules introduced.

The *MRT* is determined more readily after an intravenous (i.v.) bolus dose than after any other mode of drug administration. Here, all the molecules of the dose start their residence in the body at the same time; thus, for each group, t_i is the time between drug administration and elimination. When the number of molecules eliminated in each group (dn) approaches a relatively small value, the *MRT* can be expressed in integral notation.

$$MRT = \frac{\int_0^N t \cdot dn}{N} \qquad \text{H-4}$$

The limits correspond to the number of molecules eliminated at zero and infinite times. None of the molecules has been eliminated at time zero; at infinite time, all have been eliminated. The number of molecules eliminated by all pathways can be expressed in terms of the amounts eliminated, $Ael = n \cdot$ (molecular weight)/(Avogadro's number).

$$MRT = \frac{\int_0^{Ael_\infty} t \cdot dAel}{Ael_\infty} \qquad \text{H-5}$$

The denominator of Eq. H-5 is the dose of drug administered. Integration of Eq. H-5, by parts, leads to

$$MRT = \frac{\int_0^\infty (Dose - Ael)\, dt}{Dose} = \frac{\int_0^\infty A \cdot dt}{Dose} \qquad \text{H-6}$$

where A is the amount of drug remaining in the body and Ael is the amount eliminated up to a given time t.

The MRT after an i.v. bolus dose can be estimated from either urinary excretion or plasma drug concentration data as follows.

EXCRETION DATA

When the fraction excreted unchanged, fe remains constant with time, the amount of drug excreted unchanged in the urine, Ae, equals $fe \cdot Dose$. On substituting these values into Eq. H-6, it is apparent that MRT can be determined from urinary excretion data using the relationship.

$$MRT = \frac{\int_0^\infty (Ae_\infty - Ae(t))\, dt}{Ae_\infty} \qquad \text{H-7}$$

Figure H-1 shows the cumulative amount excreted unchanged, $Ae(t)$, at various times and the amount ultimately excreted unchanged, Ae_∞. The area between these curves (shaded), the area under the amount remaining to be excreted curve, is the numerator in Eq. H-7. For a given amount excreted unchanged, it is apparent that this area and, therefore, the MRT are increased when drug remains longer in the body.

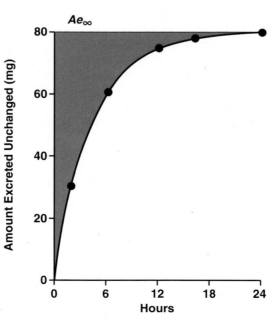

FIGURE H-1. The difference between amount excreted unchanged (*solid line*) and amount ultimately excreted (*dashed line*) is the amount remaining to be excreted. The area under the amount-remaining-to-be-excreted versus time curve (*shaded*), relative to total amount excreted (Eq. H-7 in text), is a measure of mean residence time of a substance in the body. Data from Table H-1.

PLASMA CONCENTRATION DATA

When clearance is constant with time, the rate of elimination is proportional to the plasma concentration, that is, $dAel/dt = CL \cdot C$. Substituting $CL \cdot C \cdot dt$ for $dAel$ and $CL \cdot \int_0^\infty C \cdot dt$ for Ael_∞ into Eq. H-5 gives

$$MRT = \frac{\int_0^\infty t \cdot C \cdot dt}{\int_0^\infty C \cdot dt} \qquad \text{H-8}$$

The product $t \cdot C$ is called the *first-moment* of the concentration, because concentration is multiplied by time raised to the power of 1. Therefore, the numerator is called the area under the (first)-moment versus time curve ($AUMC$), whereas the denominator is the area under the plasma concentration–time curve (AUC). The time course of both the plasma concentration and its first-moment are shown in Fig. H-2.

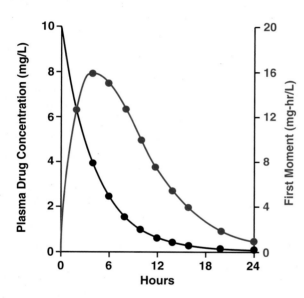

FIGURE H-2. After an i.v. bolus dose, the plasma concentration (*black*) declines with time. The first-moment (*colored*), product of time and concentration, rises to a peak and declines with time. The area beyond the last sampling time is much greater for the first-moment time curve than for the concentration–time curve. Data from Table H-1.

The *MRT* concept is equally applicable to measurement of the turnover of an endogenous substance, using a tracer, and determination of the mean time a drug resides in the body. As example, let us examine the measured *MRT* after an i.v. bolus dose of a drug from both the urinary and plasma data contained in Table H-1. The value of *AUC* can be estimated as shown in Appendix A, *Assessment of AUC*. The value of *AUMC* is calculated from the first-moment (column 3) in a manner similar to that of *AUC*, but the extrapolated area after the last point (C_{last} at t_{last}) is different. In this case, the area remaining following exponential decline can be shown to be

$$\int_{t_{last}}^\infty t \cdot C \cdot dt = \frac{C_{last} \cdot t_{last}}{\lambda_z} + \frac{C_{last}}{\lambda_z^2} \qquad \text{H-9}$$

where λ_z is the rate constant of the terminal decay of the plasma drug concentration. When the entire concentration–time profile can be described by a sum of exponentials, the area under the first-moment curve can be determined directly from the coefficients and exponential coefficients defining the equation. For example, if $C = C_1 e^{-\lambda_1 t} + C_2 e^{-\lambda_2 t}$, then

$$AUMC = \frac{C_1}{\lambda_1^2} + \frac{C_2}{\lambda_2^2} \qquad \text{H-10}$$

In the example considered, the calculated *AUC*, *AUMC*, and area under the amount remaining to be excreted versus time curve are 44.2 mg-hr/L, 17.7 mg-hr²/L, and 340 mg-hr,

---

TABLE H-1 Plasma Concentration–Time and Urinary Excretion–Time Data following an Intravenous Bolus Dose of a Drug

Time (hr)	Plasma Drug Concentration (mg/L)	First-Moment of Plasma Concentration (mg-hr/L)	Cumulative Amount Excreted (mg)	Amount Remaining to be Excreted (mg)
0	10*	0	0	80†
2	6.3	12.6	30	50
4	4.0	16.0	48	32
6	2.5	15.0	60	20
8	1.6	12.8	67	13
10	1.0	10.0	72	8
12	0.63	7.6	75	5
14	0.39	5.5	—	—
16	0.25	4.0	78	2
20	0.10	2.0	—	—
24	0.04	0.96	80	0

*Estimated by extrapolation on a semilogarithmic plot to zero time.
†The cumulative amount excreted at infinite time.

respectively. The areas remaining under the first two curves after the last time point are 0.17 mg-hr/L and 4.9 mg-hr^2/L respectively. Figures H-1 and H-2 contain the data from Table H-1. The calculated *MRT* values from Eqs. H-7 (urinary data) and H-8 (plasma data) are then 4.25 hr and 4.0 hr, respectively. The simulated value is 4.3 hr. The differences in the estimates arise from approximations introduced by the use of the trapezoidal rule to calculate area.

The *MRT*, calculated by either Eq. H-7 or Eq. H-8, is a measure of the average time a substance spends in the body after an i.v. bolus dose. When a drug is given by a constant-rate i.v. infusion or by an extravascular route, the drug spends additional time in the syringe or at the site of administration (e.g., gastrointestinal tract [oral], muscle [intramuscular (i.m.)] or subcutaneous tissues [s.c.]). The observed time, estimated from Eq. H-7 or Eq. H-8, is then the sum of the mean times at these sites and in the body. Table H-2

TABLE H-2 Mean Residence Times for Selected Models* of Drug Input

Mode of Administration	Model†	Mean Input Time	Observed Mean Residence Time
Single i.v. bolus dose	$\triangledown \xrightarrow{k}$	0	$1/k$
Constant-rate i.v. infusion	$R_{inf} \rightarrow \bigcirc \xrightarrow{k}$	$t_{inf}/2$‡	$1/k + t_{inf}/2$
Single extravascular dose	$\triangledown \xrightarrow{ka} \bigcirc \xrightarrow{k}$	$1/ka$	$1/k + 1/ka$

*Disposition is assumed to be first-order from a one-compartment model.
†The symbol $\triangledown$ denotes an i.v. bolus input.
‡t_{inf} is the duration of constant-rate i.v. infusion.

shows the mean input times (*MIT*) and observed mean total residence times for three common modes of drug input.

Following extravascular administration of a drug solution, the observed total *MRT* is the sum of the *MRT* in the body and the *mean absorption time*. The mean absorption time can be determined from the difference between the *MRT* values (calculated from Eq. H-7 or Eq. H-8), after extravascular and i.v. bolus doses given on separate occasions. After giving a solid dosage form, the *MIT* includes time for disintegration, deaggregation, dissolution, and absorption from solution. Gastric emptying, intestinal motility, and other physiologic and physicochemical factors influence the mean absorption time as well.

STUDY PROBLEMS

(Answers to Study Problems are in Appendix J.)

1. Using the definition of *MRT* in Eq. H-8 and an equation from the time-course of plasma concentration after an i.v. bolus dose, prove mathematically that the observed *MRT* given in Table H-2 for this route of administration is correct for a one-compartment model.

2. Prove that the mean time that a drug is in a syringe during a constant-rate i.v. infusion is equal to $t_{inf}/2$, where t_{inf} is the duration of the infusion.

3. The observed mean total residence times in an individual subject, calculated from plasma concentration–time data (Eq. H-8) following an i.v. bolus dose, an i.v. infusion, and an oral dose, on separate occasions, were 8, 10, and 12 hr, respectively.

   a. Given a constant-rate input, determine the duration of the infusion.
   b. Given a first-order input, determine the absorption half-life.

4. Using Eq. F-1 of Appendix F, *Absorption Kinetics*, and Eq. H-8 of this appendix, prove mathematically that the value of *AUMC/AUC* after an extravascular dose depends on neither dose nor bioavailability.

5. In study problem 5, Chapter 10, *Constant-Rate Input*, plasma concentration–time data are provided during and following a 24-hr i.v. constant-rate infusion and a rectal delivery device of droperidol.

   a. From the i.v. infusion data, calculate the ratio of *AUMC/AUC* and, hence, *MRT* of droperidol. (Note: The extrapolated *AUMC* beyond the last concentration measurement is given by Eq. H-9).
   b. How does your estimate of *MRT* compare with that calculated from $1.44 \cdot t_{1/2}$, where $t_{1/2}$ (1.9 hr) is the half-life after stopping the infusion, and what conclusion do you draw from the comparison?
   c. Calculate the ratio *AUMC/AUC* associated with the rectal delivery device and, hence, the *MIT*.
   d. Assessed in vitro, the mean release time of the rectal delivery device is 9 hr. If this time is also applied in vivo, what is the mean absorption time of droperidol from solution in the rectum, once released from the device? For this calculation, release and subsequent transfer across the rectal epithelium are taken to be sequential processes.

Amount of Drug in Body on Accumulation to Plateau

 ccumulation of drug in the body is addressed here for multiple intravenous (i.v.) doses of fixed size and dosing interval.

ACCUMULATION

Consider the situation in which a dose of drug is given as an i.v. bolus every dosing interval, τ. Recall that after each dose, the fraction remaining in the body at time, t, is e^{-kt}. The fraction of drug remaining at the end of a dosing interval τ, therefore is $e^{-k\tau}$. When time is equal to 2τ, the fraction remaining is $e^{-2k\tau}$. The amount of drug in the body following multiple doses is simply the sum of amounts remaining from each of the previous doses. The amount in the body just after the next dose is shown in Table I-1 for four successive equal doses given every τ.

| TABLE I-1 | Drug in Body Just After Each of Four Successive Doses |

	Amount Remaining in Body from Each Dose			
Time	1st Dose	2nd Dose	3rd Dose	4th Dose
0	Dose			
τ	$Dose \cdot e^{-k\tau}$	Dose		
2τ	$Dose \cdot e^{-2k\tau}$	$Dose \cdot e^{-k\tau}$	Dose	
3τ	$Dose \cdot e^{-3k\tau}$	$Dose \cdot e^{-2k\tau}$	$Dose \cdot e^{-k\tau}$	Dose

It is apparent from the table that the maximum amount of drug in the body just after the fourth dose, $A_{max,4}$, is the fourth dose plus the sum of the amounts remaining from each of three previous doses (sum of terms in the last row of Table I-1). That is, letting $r = e^{-k\tau}$,

$$A_{max,4} = Dose(1 + r + r^2 + r^3) \tag{I-1}$$

Just after the nth dose, the amount in the body is

$$A_{max,N} = Dose(1 + r + r^2 + r^3 ... + r^{N-2} + r^{N-1}) \tag{I-2}$$

Multiplying by r,

$$A_{max,N} \cdot r = Dose(r + r^2 + r^3 + r^4 ... + r^{N-1} + r^N) \tag{I-3}$$

Subtracting Eq. I-3 from Eq. I-2,

$$A_{max,N} \cdot (1 - r) = Dose\,(1 - r^N) \qquad\qquad \text{I-4}$$

Therefore,

$$A_{max,N} = Dose\, \frac{(1 - r^N)}{(1-r)} \qquad\qquad \text{I-5}$$

As r equals $e^{-k\tau}$, and $N \cdot \tau$ is the time elapsed, the value of r^N is $e^{-k \cdot N \cdot t}$. Hence,

$$A_{max,N} = Dose\, \frac{(1 - e^{-k \cdot N \cdot \tau})}{(1 - e^{-k \cdot \tau})} \qquad\qquad \text{I-6}$$

At the end of the dosing interval, it follows that the minimum amount in the body after the nth dose, $A_{min,N}$, is

$$A_{min,N} = A_{max,N} \cdot r = Dose\, \frac{(1 - r^N) \cdot r}{(1 - r)} \qquad\qquad \text{I-7}$$

or

$$A_{min,N} = A_{max,N} \cdot e^{-k \cdot \tau} = Dose\, \frac{(1 - e^{-k \cdot N \cdot \tau}) \cdot e^{-k \cdot \tau}}{(1 - e^{-k \cdot \tau})} \qquad\qquad \text{I-8}$$

STEADY STATE

As the number of doses, N, increases, the value of r^N ($e^{-k \cdot N \cdot \tau}$) approaches zero, because r is always a value less than 1. The maximum and minimum amounts of drug in the body during an interval approach upper limits. Then, the amount lost in each interval equals the amount gained, the dose. For this reason, drug in the body is then said to be at *steady state* or *at plateau.* Here, the maximum, $A_{max,ss}$, and the minimum, $A_{min,ss}$, are readily obtained by letting $r^N = 0$ in Eqs. I-5 and I-7, respectively.

$$A_{max,ss} = \frac{Dose}{1-r} = \frac{Dose}{1 - e^{-k \cdot \tau}} \qquad\qquad \text{I-9}$$

$$A_{min,ss} = \frac{Dose \cdot r}{1 - r} = \frac{Dose \cdot e^{-k \cdot \tau}}{1 - e^{-k \cdot \tau}} = A_{max,ss} - Dose \qquad\qquad \text{I-10}$$

STUDY PROBLEM

(Answers to Study Problems are in Appendix J.)

1. The amount of diazepam remaining (A) in the body with time after a single i.v. dose in an individual subject is summarized by the equation,

$$A(mg) = 10 \cdot e^{-0.5t}$$

where t is in days.

a. Complete the second column (1st Dose) of Table I-2, which has the same format as Table I-1, by calculating the amount of diazepam remaining in the body from the first dose at 1, 2, and 3 days, respectively.

	Amount of Diazepam (mg) in Body From Each Daily Dose			
TABLE I-2 **Diazepam in the Body Just After Each of Four Successive Daily 10-mg Doses**				
Time*	**First Dose**	**Second Dose**	**Third Dose**	**Fourth Dose**
0	10			
τ	_____	10		
2τ	_____	_____	10	
3τ	_____	_____	_____	10

*τ, 1 day.

b. A second 10-mg dose is given at $\tau = 1$. The amount remaining at 2τ and 3τ are therefore equal to $Dose \cdot e^{-k\tau}$ and $Dose \cdot e^{-2k\tau}$, respectively. Calculate these values and place them in Table I-2. Also, calculate the amount remaining at time τ after the third dose.

c. Calculate the maximum ($A_{max,ss}$) and minimum ($A_{min,ss}$) amounts of diazepam in the body at steady state.

Answers to Study Problems

CHAPTER 1. THERAPEUTIC RELEVANCE

(*No Study Problems*)

CHAPTER 2. FUNDAMENTAL CONCEPTS AND TERMINOLOGY

1. **The terms are defined in the text, where the word or phrase is emboldened, in the following order:** local administration, metabolites, prodrug, intravascular administration, extravascular administration, parenteral administration, compartment, systemic absorption, first-pass loss, intestinal absorption, bioavailability, disposition, distribution, enterohepatic cycling, elimination, excretion, metabolism, metabolic interconversion, up-or-down regulation, agonist, antagonist, full agonist, full antagonist, partial agonist, partial antagonist, clinical response, surrogate endpoint, biomarker, safety biomarker, graded response, quantal response, all-or-none response, endogenous, exogenous, baseline, placebo, disease progression, steepness factor, cumulative frequency, potency, specificity, maximum effect, turnover, turnover rate, pool size, fractional turnover rate, turnover time.

2. a. **Plasma;** b. **Whole blood;** c. **Same;** d. **Plasma.**

3. a. **Absorption or disposition, or both, can be different for R- and S-isomers.** Measurement of the sum of the two isomers can therefore give erroneous information following administration of a racemic mixture. The overall kinetic profile is then not that of either isomer. The difference in the kinetics becomes particularly important in therapy when the isomers have different pharmacologic or toxic activities.
   b. **Yes.** They appear to have the same half-lives, but very different systemic exposures, so their dispositions are the same, but their bioavailabilities are different. First-pass metabolism might explain the differences in systemic bioavailability.

4. a. **Correct.** It is possible, although uncommon, that the drug forms an unstable metabolite, which during storage of the urine sample is converted back to parent drug before the assay is performed. The statement is generally correct.
   b. **Correct.** At the maximum, the net rate of change of drug in the body is zero. Thereafter, the rate of elimination exceeds that of absorption, so that the amount of drug in the body declines.
   c. **Correct.** The rate of absorption is now zero. Thereafter, the only reason for the decline of drug in the body is elimination. Under these conditions, the rate of change of drug in the body is the rate of elimination.

d. **Incorrect.** The drug may have been degraded in the stomach because of low pH, metabolized by the digestive enzymes in the intestine, or metabolized by the microflora in the colon. All of the breakdown products may then have been systemically absorbed and excreted in the urine. In the extreme case, none of the drug may have been systemically absorbed, but the radioactivity would still be recovered quantitatively in the urine.

e. **Incorrect.** The route of elimination of this drug is the formation of the glucuronide. The glucuronide is then secreted into the bile and subsequently excreted into the feces.

f. **Incorrect.** The rate of change of drug in the body is zero at the peak time. Here, the rates of absorption and elimination are equal.

5. Enterohepatic cycling refers to the process of drug leaving the body by secretion into the bile and being reabsorbed from the gastrointestinal tract back into the body. When the cycling is complete, no drug is eliminated from the body via the feces. However, when the cycling is not complete, for example, when drug is decomposed in the gut lumen, metabolized in the gut wall, or excreted in the feces, then some of the drug that was secreted into the bile undergoes elimination. In some cases, none of the drug secreted into the bile may be recycled.

6. a. **Correct.** In the equation, $E = E_{max} \cdot C^\gamma/(C_{50}^\gamma + C^\gamma)$, it is apparent that when $C = C_{50}$, then $E = E_{max}/2$, irrespective of the value of γ.

b. **Correct.** In this region, where E is approximately equal to $(E_{max}/C_{50}^\gamma) \cdot C^\gamma$, its value is directly proportional to C only if $\gamma = 1.0$.

c. **Correct.** The concentration always decreases with time. Thus, a complete *hysteresis* loop is not possible.

d. **Correct.** Without a placebo response, it is virtually impossible to quantify drug response.

7. a. **Graded.** The heart rate clearly increases with drug concentration.

b. $E_{max} = $ **30 beats/min**; $C_{50} = $ **0.3 μmol/L**; $\gamma = 1$. Response appears to approach a limit of 30 beats/min, and the concentration (C_{50}) at which the response is one half of E_{max} is 0.3 μmol/L. The slope can be estimated from the concentrations being approximately 1/10 and 10 times the value of C_{50}, respectively at values of 0.1 and 0.9 for E/E_{max}. The data appear to show this relationship, although the best fit of the model using statistics may occur with a γ slightly greater than 1. The line shown in Fig. 2-20 has a γ of 1.0.

8. $C_{20} = $ **5.7 mg/L** and $C_{80} = $ **17.4 mg/L.** On rearrangement of Eq. 2-4 in the text

$$C = C_{50} \cdot \left[\frac{Effect}{1 - Effect} \right]^{1/\gamma}$$

where *Effect* is the response expressed as a fraction of its maximum value. For $\gamma = 2.5$ and $C_{50} = 10$ mg/L, C_{20} (*Effect* = 0.2) = 5.7 mg/L, and C_{80} (*Effect* = 0.8) = 17.4 mg/L.

9. a. **The response is quantal.** Although serum alanine aminotransferase (ALT) is a continuous measure, such that changes in ALT may vary with drug exposure in a graded manner, this measure has been made quantal by defining hepatic toxicity as occurring when the ALT value is threefold or more greater than the normal value. One then examines for the likelihood or incidence of this occurring against drug exposure.

b. Many adverse outcomes take time to develop and require reasonably prolonged exposure to the drug. This appears to be the case in this example. Under these circumstances, the incidence of the harmful effect depends not so much on the drug concentration at any particular time but on the overall exposure to the drug, which is best reflected by area under the curve (*AUC*).

10. a. **21.9 g/day.** The turnover rate of albumin equals the amount in the body at steady state divided by the turnover time (the average time albumin spends in the body), $R_t = \dfrac{A_{ss}}{t_t} = \dfrac{350\ g}{16\ days}$.

b. **0.0625 day^{-1}.** The fractional turnover rate is the reciprocal of the turnover time, $k_t = 1/t_t = 1/16$ days. Therefore, 6.25% of the albumin in the body is replaced every day.

CHAPTER 3. KINETICS FOLLOWING AN INTRAVENOUS BOLUS DOSE

1. **Clearance**—The proportionality term between rate of elimination of drug from the body and plasma drug concentration, with units of flow per unit time (e.g., mL/min or L/hr).

   Compartmental model—A model in which the body is characterized by one or more spaces into which drug appears kinetically to be distributed.

   Disposition kinetics—The kinetic events occurring within the body following an intravenous (i.v.) bolus dose of drug.

   Elimination half-life—The time taken for 50% of the drug to be eliminated from the body following an i.v. bolus dose, usually assessed from the terminal slope of a semilogarithmic plot of the plasma concentration–time profile.

   Elimination rate constant—The fractional rate of elimination of a drug with units of reciprocal time (e.g. hr^{-1} or min^{-1}).

   Extraction ratio—The fraction of drug entering that is eliminated on single passage through an organ. It is the ratio of rate of elimination to rate of presentation of drug to an eliminating organ.

   First-order process—A process in which the rate is directly proportional to the amount of compound present.

   Fraction excreted unchanged—The fraction of an i.v. dose that is excreted unchanged in urine.

   Fraction in plasma unbound—The fraction of drug in plasma that is unbound; given by the ratio of the unbound concentration to total concentration of drug in plasma.

   Fractional rate of elimination—Rate of elimination expressed relative to the amount of drug in the body.

   Half-life—Time for the concentration or amount of drug to fall by one half.

   Mean residence time—Average time that a drug remains in the body following an i.v. bolus dose.

   Monoexponential equation—An equation in which the decline in plasma concentration or amount of drug with time is characterized by a single exponential term.

   Renal clearance—The proportionality term between rate of renal excretion of drug from the body and plasma drug concentration, with units of flow per unit time (e.g., mL/min or L/hr).

   Terminal phase—The final linear decline phase of a semilogarithmic plot of the plasma concentration–time profile.

   Volume of distribution—The apparent volume into which a drug distributes in the body at equilibrium, or the volume of plasma needed to account for the amount of drug in the body at equilibrium.

2. a. **Correct.** $k = 0.693/t_{1/2} = 0.693/4$ hr $= 0.173$ hr^{-1}.

   b. **Incorrect.** 16 hr is 4 half-lives; in 4 half-lives, 0.925 $(1 - 1/2 \times 1/2 \times 1/2 \times 1/2)$, or 92.5%, has been eliminated from the body; 87.5% is eliminated in 3 half-lives.

   c. **Correct.** It takes 2 half-lives to eliminate 37.5 mg following a 50-mg bolus dose; it takes 1 half-life to eliminate 50 mg following a 100-mg dose.

   d. **Incorrect.** By 12 hr (3 $t_{1/2}$), only 87.5% of Ae_∞ is excreted; to gain a good estimate of Ae_∞, all urine should be collected for 5 half-lives (i.e., up to approximately 24 hr).

   e. **Generally correct.** For many drugs, within the therapeutic dose range, the pharmacokinetic parameters do not change with dose. Occasionally, one or more of the parameters do, as discussed further in Chapter 16, *Nonlinearities.*

3. a. **Fraction remaining = 0.71.** $k = 0.693/6$ hr $= 0.1155$ hr^{-1}. Hence, fraction remaining in 3 hr $= e^{-kt} = e^{-0.1155 hr^{-1} \times 3 hr} = 0.71$.

   b. $t_{1/2} = 1.6$ **hr.** Fraction remaining at 4 hr $= 0.18 = e^{-k \times 4hr}$. Taking antilogarithms and rearranging gives $k = 0.43$ hr^{-1}, $t_{1/2} = 0.693/0.43$ hr$^{-1} = 1.6$ hr.

4. a. **Rate of elimination = 15 mg/hr.**

$$Rate\ of\ Elimination = CL \cdot C = 0.5\ L/hr \times 30\ mg/L = 15\ mg/hr$$

   b. **Half-life = 12.5 hr.**

$$Half\text{-}life = \frac{0.693\ V}{CL} = \frac{0.693 \times 9\ L}{0.5\ L/hr} = 12.5\ hr$$

   c. **Amount in body = 540 mg.**

$$Amount\ in\ Body = V \cdot C = 9\ L \times 60\ mg/L = 540\ mg$$

   d. **Plasma concentration = 40 mg/L.**

$$\frac{Plasma}{Concentration} = \frac{Dose}{V}e^{-k \cdot t} = \frac{700\ mg}{9\ L}e^{-\frac{0.693 \times 12\ hr}{12.5\ hr}} = 40\ mg/L$$

5.

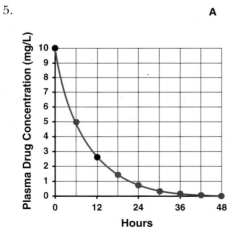

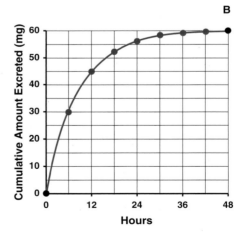

FIGURE J3-P5.

Notes: a. **Plasma data:** Two half-lives have elapsed during the 10 hr for the concentration to fall from 10 to 2.5 mg/L. Hence, the half-life is 5 hr, which allows the concentration to be calculated at all other times.

   b. **Urine data.** In 1 half-life (5 hr), the cumulative amount excreted is 0.5 Ae_∞ or 30 mg. At 2 half-lives (1 hr), it is 0.75 Ae_∞, or 45 mg, and so on.

6. a. **77.2%.** The fraction eliminated by 3 hr = *AUC (0 to 3 hr) / AUC (0,∞)* = 5.1 mg-hr/L)/(22.4 mg-hr/L) = 0.228 or 22.8%. Hence, the percent remaining in the body as drug at 3 hr is 77.2%.

   b. CL = **2.2 L/hr.** $CL = Dose/AUC$ = 50 mg/22.4 mg-hr/L.

   c. CL_R = **0.49 L/hr.** $CL_R = Ae_\infty/AUC$ = 11 mg/22.4 hr/L.

   d. *fe* = **0.22.** *fe = Ae∞/Dose* = 11 *mg*/50 *mg*. Alternatively, *fe = CL_R / CL* = 0.49 *L/hr/* 2.2 *L/hr*.

7. a. V = **14 L.** $V = Dose/C(0)$ = 100 mg/7.14/L.

   b. $t_{1/2}$ = **13.6 hr.** $t_{1/2}$ = 0.693 / k = 0.693 / 0.051 hr⁻¹.

   c. **Total AUC = 140 mg-L/hr.** $AUC = C(0)/k$ = (7.14 mg/L)/0.051 hr⁻¹.

   d. **Total clearance, CL = 0.714 L/hr.** $CL = Dose/AUC$ = (100 mg)/(140 mg-hr/L). Alternatively, $CL = k \cdot V$ = 0.051 hr⁻¹ ×14 L.

   e. C = **19.8 mg/L.** $C = (Dose / V)e^{-kt}$ = (250 mg/14 L)e⁻(0.051 hr⁻¹×70 min/60 min).

8. a. **0.0144 hr⁻¹.**

$$k = \frac{0.693}{t_{1/2}} = \frac{0.693}{48\ hr} = 0.0144\ hr^{-1}$$

   b. **0.105 mg/L.**

$$C = \frac{Dose}{V}e^{-k \cdot t} = \frac{10\ mg}{80\ L}e^{-0.0144\ hr^{-1} \times 12\ hr}$$

   c. **50%.**
   The half-life is 48 hr. Therefore, 50% remains in body at 48 hr.

   d. **1.15 L/hr.**

$$CL = k \cdot V = 0.0144\ hr^{-1} \times 80\ L.$$

   e. **0.864 mg/hr.**
   Initial rate of elimination = $k \cdot Dose$ = 0.0144 hr⁻¹ × 60 mg.

   f. **8.70 mg-hr/L.**

$$AUC = \frac{Dose}{CL} = \frac{10\ mg}{1.15\ L/hr}$$

   g. **0.89 mg.**

$$A = Dose \cdot e^{-k \cdot t} = 10\ mg \cdot e^{-0.0144 hr^{-1} \times 168 hr}$$
$$1\ week = 7 \times 24\ hr = 168\ hr.$$

9. a. **See Fig. J3-P9.**

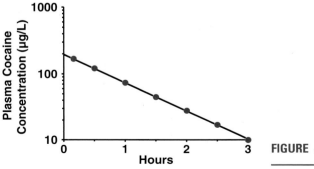

FIGURE J3-P9.

   b. **Half-life = 0.7 hr.**

   c. **Using the relationship $AUC = C(0)/k$, AUC = 0.200 mg-hr/L.** Using the trapezoidal rule and remembering that at zero time the concentration is *C(0)* (0.2 mg/L), and that the area beyond the last data point, *C(3 hr)* is *C(3 hr)/k*, the

AUC is 0.204 mg-hr/L. The slightly higher value using the trapezoidal rule arises because, at any time, the concentration along the straight line connecting two data points is always greater than the corresponding concentration on the declining exponential curve. A closer correspondence between $C(0)/k$ and AUC calculated numerically is obtained by using the log linear trapezoid approximation (Appendix A, *Assessment of AUC*).

d. **Clearance = 147 L/hr.** $CL = Dose/AUC = 33$ mg $\times$ (304 g/mol/340 g/mol)/0.200 mg-hr/L.

e. **Volume of distribution = 1.96 L/kg.** $V = CL/k = 147$ L/hr/1 hr^{-1} = 147 L/75 kg.

10. a. **Clearance is 4 L/hr.**

$$CL = \frac{Dose}{AUC} = \frac{500\ mg}{125\ mg\text{-}hr/L} = 4\ L/hr$$

b. **Yes, the initial rapidly declining phase is the distribution phase.**
This conclusion is based on area considerations. The fraction of the dose eliminated within the first 30 min is given by

$$\frac{Fraction\ eliminated\ in\ first\ 30\ min}{Fraction\ totally\ eliminated} = \frac{CL \cdot AUC\ (0,t)}{CL \cdot AUC\ (0,\infty)} = \frac{AUC\ (0,t)}{AUC\ (0,\infty)}$$

$$= \frac{13.1\ mg\text{-}hr/L}{125\ mg\text{-}hr/L} = 0.105$$

Thus, with only 10.5% eliminated, it is reasonable to describe the first phase as the distribution phase of this drug.

c. **Eighty percent of the dose has left the plasma by 5 min predominantly due to distribution into tissues.** Knowing that the plasma volume is 3 L, at a plasma concentration of 33 mg/L, 99 mg must be there. The remainder of the 500-mg dose, 401 mg, or 80% must therefore have left the plasma, and have almost exclusively distributed out into tissues, because even by 30 min only 10.5 % of the theophylline dose has been eliminated, so that by 5 min the fraction of theophylline eliminated must be minimal.

d. **Renal clearance = 0.4 L/hr.**

$$CL_R = fe \cdot CL = 0.1 \times 4\ L/hr = 0.4\ L/hr$$

e. **Half-life = 5 hr.**
The time for the plasma concentration to decrease by a factor of 2 in the terminal part of Fig. 3-11 is about 5 hr.

f. **Volume of distribution is 29 L.**

$$\begin{matrix} Volume\ of \\ Distribution \end{matrix} = \frac{CL}{k} = 1.44 \cdot CL \cdot t_{1/2} = 1.44 \times 4\ L/hr \times 5\ hr = 29\ L$$

CHAPTER 4. MEMBRANES AND DISTRIBUTION

1. a. **Active transport**—Transport through membranes facilitated by an energy source that permits movement of drug against a concentration gradient.

   Extravasation—Movement of substrates out of the vasculature into the tissues.
   Paracellular transport—Movement of a compound across membranes by way of passages between the cells.
   Passive facilitated transport—Passage of a compound through membranes by an equilibrating transporter that facilitates bidirectional movement but does not change the equilibrium conditions.

Permeability—Measure of the ability of a compound to cross membranes. A highly permeable substance passes across membranes quickly and the converse.

Transcellular transport—Passage of a compound through cells.

Transporter—A system that facilitates movement of a substance across a membrane.

b. **Apparent volume of distribution**—Parameter that relates the amount in the body to the plasma concentration.

Fraction unbound—Ratio of unbound and total concentrations in plasma.

Tissue-to-blood equilibrium distribution ratio—Ratio of concentrations in tissue and whole blood when there is no net transfer of drugs to or from the tissue. It is best determined under steady-state conditions.

Perfusion and permeability rate-limitations in drug distribution—Conditions in which the rate of distribution to a tissue from blood, or the converse, is limited by the flow of blood and the ability to cross cell membranes, respectively.

2. **Hydrophilic**—A water-(hydro) loving (philic) property. Generally, a hydrophilic substance is readily soluble in water.

Hydrophobic—A water-(hydro) hating or fearing (phobic) property. Substances with this property are poorly soluble in water but dissolve in organic solvents.

Lipophilic—A fat- (lipo) loving (philic) property. A substance with this property is generally highly soluble in organic solvents and relatively insoluble in water.

Lipophobic—A fat-hating property. Generally, a lipophobic substance is readily soluble in water.

3. a. **Not accurate.** The ratio starts at zero and rises with time. The ratio at steady state depends on the tissue-to-blood equilibrium partition ratio.

b. **Not accurate.** Permeability and surface area are two different measures. The net rate of penetration depends on permeability, surface area, and the difference in concentrations across a membrane.

c. **Not accurate.** Diffusion continues; however, the rates in both directions are the same at equilibrium. The total concentrations on the two sides may be different at equilibrium if there is binding on either side or an active transporter is involved.

d. **Not accurate.** Carrier-mediated transport occurs for both equilibrating and concentrating transporters. The latter require an energy source.

e. **Not accurate.** Binding to proteins affects the distribution–equilibrium ratio of concentrations, but does not change the permeability of the diffusible form, the unbound drug.

4. a. **0.1 mg/L.** $C = \dfrac{A}{V} = \dfrac{30\ mg}{300\ L}$

b. **60 mg.** $A = V \cdot C = 300\ L \times 0.2\ mg/L$

c. (1) **1%.** $\dfrac{V_P \cdot C}{V \cdot C} = \dfrac{V_P}{V} = \dfrac{3}{300}\ (\times\ 100\ for\ percent)$

(2) **99%.** $\dfrac{V - V_P}{V} = \dfrac{300 - 3}{300}\ (\times\ 100\ for\ percent)$

5. Both influx and efflux transporters influence absorption of some compounds from the intestinal tract. Influx transporters aid in the absorption of some compounds (e.g., the antibiotic amoxicillin, B vitamins, and vitamin C), whereas efflux transporters tend to reduce the absorption of others (e.g., the immunosuppressive agent cyclosporine, used to prevent organ transportation, and saquinavir, a protease inhibitor used in the treatment of acquired immune deficiency syndrome [AIDS]). Transporters are important in drug distribution, particularly in the central nervous

system. Efflux transporters, such as P-glycoprotein (PgP), reduce brain exposure to some substances such as the newer antihistamines, thereby reducing the sedative properties of these agents, as well as the reasonably hydrophilic β-adrenergic blocking agent, atenolol, used in the treatment of hypertension. Transporters are also extensively involved in drug elimination in the kidneys (secretion [e.g., p-aminohippuric acid] and active reabsorption [e.g., vitamin C]) and in the liver (biliary excretion, e.g., pravastatin).

6. a. **False.** Equilibrium is reached when the net flux of compound across a membrane is zero. This condition can be achieved with both equilibrating and concentrating transporters. The principal difference between equilibrating and concentrating transporters, which are both facilitative transporters, is that the concentrating transporters are capable of producing a much higher concentration of the diffusible form of the drug on one side of the membrane, at equilibrium. Equilibrating transporters facilitate the rate of achievement of equilibrium, but do not change the concentration of the diffusible form of the drug on both sides of the membrane at equilibrium.

   b. **True.** Had the initial rate of movement into a tissue increased in direct proportion to tissue blood flow rate, reflecting the ease in which the compound distributes into the tissues, then distribution would have been limited by blood flow, a perfusion rate-limitation. The failure to do so indicated that distribution is limited by the barrier property of the tissue, a permeability rate-limitation.

   c. **True.** Molecular size, lipophilicity (and permeability) of the drug, and blood flow in the intestine are assumed to be the same, as "all other factors are the same." The weak acid is almost completely un-ionized at pH 6.4, whereas the weak base is extensively ionized, thereby slowing its absorption.

7. **By extensively adsorbing the compound, thereby effectively taking it out of solution, activated charcoal can reduce oral drug absorption if administered concurrently or shortly after the drug.** This is particularly true for lipophilic drugs that are tightly adsorbed onto the activated charcoal that has high capacity owing to a very high surface area per gram. **Ingestion of activated charcoal can also help detoxify patients who have already systemically absorbed a drug, because the charcoal in the gastrointestinal tract then causes the intestinal lumen to act as a sink, pulling drug out of the body.** This process is generally fairly slow, but is much faster when drugs undergo extensive enterohepatic cycling. For maximum effect in this latter case, the charcoal should be present in the small intestine at the time the gallbladder empties (with food).

8. **The permeability decreases disproportionally as the molecular weight is increased.** With molecular weights of 100, 200, 400, and 800 g/mol, the permeabilities (for drug with an n-octanol/water partition coefficient of 2.0) are roughly $10^{-5.5}$, $10^{-6.0}$, $10^{-7.3}$, and $10^{-9.7}$ cm/sec. Notice that permeability decreases 20-fold for a molecular weight of 400 g/mol compared with that of 200 g/mol and 200-fold on going from 400 g/mol to 800 g/mol. Also notice that the eightfold increase in molecular size (100 to 800 g/mol) had as much effect as a millionfold (10^6) increase in the n-octanol/water partition coefficient (log values on x-axis) for compounds of any given size (e.g., 800 g/mol).

9. **Times (min); lungs, 0.07; kidneys, 0.7; heart, 3.5; liver, 13; and skin, 347.**

   Calculated from: $\dfrac{\textit{Time to reach 50\%}}{\textit{of equilibrium}} = t_{1/2} = \dfrac{0.693 \cdot K_P}{Q/V_T}$

10. **a and b.**

    a. If the drug were not bound to plasma protein, it would distribute into an apparent volume at least that of the extracellular space, 16 L.

b. For a drug bound to albumin, the smallest volume possible is 7.5 L/70 kg. There is, therefore, no evidence of tissue binding.

c. See (a) above.

11. a. **0.0172.**

$$\frac{fu'}{fu} \approx \frac{P_t}{P_t'} = \frac{43}{12.5} = 3.44 \qquad fu' = \frac{P_t}{P_t'} \cdot fu = 3.44 \times 0.005$$

b. **14 L.**

Given under control conditions, $V = 9.4$ L and $fu = 0.005$. Hence, by substitution into Eq. 4-30, $fu_R = 0.0725$. Accordingly, in patients with nephrotic syndrome, and using $fu'(0.0172)$ from "a" above,

$$V' = 7.5 + \left(7.5 + \frac{27}{fu_R}\right)fu' = 7.5 + \left(7.5 + \frac{27}{0.0725}\right) \times 0.0172$$

c. **Yes.** The shortening of half-life is expected from the minor increase in V compared to the large increase in CL.

12. a. **True.** From Eq. 4-13, it is apparent that the volume of distribution must be greater than 75 L as the term for the product of the volume of the liver (1.16 L) and the liver-to-blood partition ratio (50) alone is 80 L.

b. **True.** Poorly perfused tissues come into distribution equilibrium slowly, especially when the equilibrium partition ratio is high. This drug has a large apparent volume of distribution; for distribution equilibrium to be essentially achieved in 30 min, the drug must primarily go (high K_P) to well-perfused tissues.

CHAPTER 5. ELIMINATION

1. **Blood clearance**—The proportionality term between rate of elimination of a compound from the body and its whole blood concentration, with units of flow per unit time (e.g., mL/min or L/hr). Also defined as, the volume of blood effectively cleared completely of compound per unit time.

Enterohepatic cycle—The cycle completed when a compound on entering the liver is secreted into the bile, which enters the small intestine, only to be returned to the liver on absorption from the intestine.

Filtration clearance—The proportionality term between rate of glomerular filtration of a compound and its plasma concentration with units of flow per unit time (e.g., mL/min or L/hr). It is the product of the fraction of compound in plasma unbound and the glomerular filtration rate.

Glomerular filtration rate—Volume of plasma water filtered through the glomerulus of the kidney per unit time, with units of flow per unit time (e.g., mL/min or L/hr).

Hepatic acinus—The physiologic unit of the liver.

Hepatic clearance—The proportionality term between rate of hepatic elimination (metabolism plus biliary excretion) of drug and plasma drug concentration, with units of flow per unit time (e.g., mL/min or L/hr). It is also defined as the volume of plasma effectively cleared completely of drug by the liver per unit time.

Intrinsic clearance—The proportionality term between rate of elimination of drug from an organ and unbound drug concentration at the site of elimination within the organ (model parameter), with units of flow per unit time (e.g., mL/min or L/hr).

Perfusion rate-limited elimination—The condition in which the rate of elimination of compound from an organ is limited by the rate of delivery, perfusion, of blood to it.

Plasma-to-blood concentration ratio—The ratio of the concentration of a compound in plasma to that in whole blood; it has no units.

Unbound clearance—The proportionality term between the rate of elimination of compound from the body and its unbound concentration in plasma, with units of flow per unit time.

2.

| | **TABLE J5-P2** | **Selected Pharmacokinetic Parameters of Drugs A to D** | | | | | |

Drug	Fraction Unbound		Hepatic Clearance (L/hr) Based on Concentration in:			Concentration Ratio (Plasma/ Blood)	Hepatic Extraction Ratio
	Blood fu_b	Plasma fu	Blood CL_b	Plasma CL	Plasma Water CLu	C/C_b	E_H
A	0.15	0.2	1.2	1.6	8.0	0.75	0.015
B	0.0067	0.3	2.0	90	300	0.022	0.025
C	0.0074	0.02	72	194.4	9720	0.37	0.9
D	0.16	0.1	0.8	0.5	5	1.6	0.01

Missing numbers were calculated from the relationships:

$$fu = fu_b / \frac{C}{C_b} \qquad CLu = fu \cdot CL$$

$$CL = CL_b / \frac{C}{C_b} \qquad CLu = fu_b \cdot CL_b$$

$$E_H = \frac{CL_{b,H}}{Q_{b,H}}$$

3. a. **Generally, a high plasma clearance is seen because the drug has a high clearance by one or more organs.** However, there are exceptions. One case is when the drug has a very high affinity for blood cells, as seen for Drug C in problem 2. Then, the plasma-to-blood concentration ratio can be very low, and the important blood clearance is then much lower than plasma clearance. Another situation is where a drug is eliminated by many organs of the body, for example, by hydrolysis by esterases, which are ubiquitous, and the individual organ clearances, and corresponding extraction ratios, are low.

b. **This statement is incorrect.** Intrinsic clearance (CL_{int}) is a property of the eliminating organ (without consideration of blood flow or plasma binding), and relates rate of elimination to the unbound concentration of drug at the site(s) of elimination. Unbound clearance (CLu) relates rate of elimination to the unbound plasma concentration in the systemic circulation. By definition, the relationships $CL = fu \cdot CLu$ and $CL_b = fu_b \cdot CLu$ always hold. When organ extraction ratio is low then because $CL = fu \cdot CL_{int}$, it follows that $CLu = CL_{int}$. However, when extraction ratio is very high, $CL_b \approx Q$, and therefore, $CLu = CL_b/fu_b \approx Q/(fu \cdot C/C_B)$. Now, $C/C_B = 1/(1 + H[fu \cdot Kp_{BC} - 1])$ (see Appendix D, *Plasma-to-Blood Concentration Ratio*), so that $fu \cdot C/C_B = fu/(1 + H[fu \cdot Kp_{BC} - 1])$. Thus, as Q, H, and Kp_{BC} (the ratio of blood cell to unbound drug concentration ratio) are fixed, it is seen that CLu is not equal to CL_{int} and varies with fu.

c. **Generally, clearance is an additive property, as discussed within the text of the chapter.** This arises because the major organs of elimination, liver and kidneys, are in parallel and are exposed to a common arterial blood concentration. An exception is when the organs of elimination are in series. Then, the second organ receives the venous output from the first, and if the first is a high—extraction ratio organ, the concentration entering the second organ will be much lower than the systemic concentration perfusing the first organ. Examples are gut and liver, and the lungs with the rest of the body. The gut may be an eliminating organ for some drugs, but the contribution to systemic clearance is generally low, because only 10% of intestinal blood flow perfuses the intestinal epithelium where the enzymes and efflux transporters reside. Occasionally, lung is an eliminating organ for drugs. Then, the arterial concentration will be less than the mixed venous concentration entering the lung. As most determinations of clearance are made following i.v. administration, the assumption that all of the drug has reached the systemic circulation via the arterial blood no longer holds, and the ratio *Dose/AUC* can be very high and exceed hepatic blood flow, or even cardiac output, when the pulmonary extraction ratio is high. This is unlikely given the very high perfusion and low-to-negligible drug metabolic activity of the lungs.

d. **Generally, organ clearance is rate-limited either by perfusion, when extraction ratio is high, or by enzymatic, excretory, or transport processes, when extraction ratio is low.** In the case of renal clearance, clearance may also be limited by *GFR* (for drugs that are not secreted), although *GFR* tends to be relatively stable. More generally, another potential rate-limiting step, particularly for polar compounds undergoing hepatic elimination, is uptake permeability, as appears to be the case for pravastatin.

e. **This statement is partially true.** Had biliary secreted drug not been reabsorbed from the intestines to complete the enterohepatic cycle, either directly or through a metabolite, it would be a pathway for elimination and add to total clearance. Enterohepatic cycling itself is simply a component of distribution.

4. a.

TABLE J5-P4   Changes in Hepatic Handling of Selected Drugs

Drug	Hepatic Extraction Ratio	Hepatic Blood Flow	Unbound Fraction in Blood	Intrinsic Clearance	(Plasma) Clearance
A.	High	↑	↔	↔	↑
B.	Low	↔	↓	↔	↓
C.	Low	↔	↔	↑	↑
D.	High	↔	↔	↑	↔
E.	Low	↔	↑	↔	↑
F.	High	↔	↓	↔	↔
G.	Low	↓	↔	↔	↔
H.	High	↓	↔	↔	↓

↑, increase; ↔, little or no change; ↓, decrease.

b. **Drug A, $t_{1/2}$ ↓.**
A change in hepatic blood flow has no effect on V. Hence, as CL↑, it follows that $t_{1/2}$ ↓.
Drug C, $t_{1/2}$ ↓.
A change in intrinsic clearance has no effect on V. Hence, as intrinsic clearance is increased, so must CL ($CL = fu \cdot CL_{int}$ for low extraction ratio drug). It follows that $t_{1/2}$ ↓.

5. a. **A low–extraction ratio drug.**
Even based on a plasma clearance of 4.2 L/hr, the conclusion would be that tacrolimus has a low hepatic extraction ratio. But with a plasma-to-blood ratio of 0.03, resulting in a very low blood clearance of only 0.126 L/hr, there can be no doubt as to the low–extraction ratio status of this drug.

b. **Extensive uptake into blood cells.**
With such extensive binding to plasma proteins (fraction bound 0.99) one would have anticipated that most of the drug in blood would have been located in plasma, whereas the plasma-to-blood concentration ratio of only 0.03 indicates that the vast majority of tacrolimus in blood resides in the blood cells. This can only occur because the affinity of blood cells (particular erythrocytes) for tacrolimus is very much greater than that to plasma proteins, or that transporters concentrate drug in the cells.

c. **Clearance would increase, and half-life shorten, with induction.** With tacrolimus being a drug of very low extraction ratio, induction of CYP3A4, by increasing hepatocellular metabolic activity, is expected to increase clearance, since $CL = fu \cdot CL_{int}$. And, as induction is not expected to cause any change in drug distribution, and hence in V, it follows that half-life will decrease, since $t_{1/2} = 0.693V/CL$.

6. **Phenytoin (CL_R of 0.15 mL/min $< fu \cdot GFR$, 12 mL/min) is filtered and extensively reabsorbed.** It is close to the expectation of equilibrium ($fu \cdot$ urine flow $= 0.1 \times$ 1–2 mL/min) if compound is not ionized (with a pKa of 8.3, it is effectively not).

Cefonicid (CL_R of 20 mL/min $> fu \cdot GFR$ of 2.4 mL/min) is filtered and secreted. Reabsorption cannot be discounted, although like cephalosporins, in general, cefonicid should be relatively polar so that significant passive reabsorption is unlikely to occur.

Digoxin (CL_R of 100 mL/min $= fu \cdot GFR$) is either filtered and neither secreted nor reabsorbed, or that secretion and reabsorption occurs but occur to an approximately equal extent. Additional information is needed to distinguish between these two possibilities, as discussed further when considering the quinidine–digoxin interaction (Chapter 17, *Drug Interactions*).

7. a. **Nicotine must be a base**, as renal clearance increases with increasing acidity, reflecting lower tubular reabsorption associated with a declining fraction of drug unionized at lower pH values.

b. **Yes.** pH sensitivity for nonpolar bases is expected in the pKa range 7 to 12, and nicotine has a pKa of 8.3.

c. **Under alkaline urine conditions.** With a renal clearance of only 39 mL/min, and knowing it is minimally bound in plasma, nicotine must be extensively reabsorbed as its renal clearance is 562 mL/min under acidic conditions, when reabsorption is the least, pointing to extensive secretion of nicotine. With extensive reabsorption, renal clearance should become more sensitive to urine flow.

d. **When metabolism is substantially inhibited or impaired.** Despite the marked pH sensitivity of nicotine, under normal circumstances nonrenal (hepatic) clearance is so high (1150 mL/min) that it dominates so that clearance and hence half-life only changes modestly with acidification of urine. For renal clearance to dominate, metabolic clearance would have to be drastically reduced. This may occur in the presence of a strong metabolic inhibitor, in severe hepatic cirrhosis, or if metabolism became saturated.

8. a. **Theophylline is a low–extraction ratio drug.** CL is 4 L/hr, and even in the extreme case that the plasma blood concentration ratio is 2, implying none entered the blood cells, CL_b cannot exceed 8 L/hr, which is considerable less than either hepatic or renal blood flow.

   b. **Yes, there is definitely net reabsorption.** $CL_R = 0.4$ L/hr ($fe \cdot CL$), which is less than filtration clearance ($fu \cdot GFR = 0.1 \times 7.5$ L/hr $= 0.75$ L/hr).

   c. (1) i. **The fraction of theophylline in the body unbound is 0.87.**

$$\frac{Fraction}{unbound} = \frac{Amount\ of\ body\ unbound}{Total\ amount\ in\ body} = \frac{Cu \times 42\ L}{C \times V} = \frac{fu \times 42\ L}{V}$$

$$= \frac{0.6 \times 42\ L}{29\ L} = 0.87$$

   Hence, 87% of theophylline in the body is unbound at equilibrium.

   ii. **Unbound concentration = 10.4 mg/L.**

$$Cu = \frac{fraction\ unbound\ in\ body \times Dose}{42\ L} = \frac{0.87 \times 500\ mg}{42\ L} = 10.4\ mg/L$$

   (2) i. **Volume of distribution is 16 L, when $fu = 0.3$.**

$$V = Vp + \frac{fu \cdot V_{TW}}{fu_T}$$

   With only fu changing, it is possible to predict the volume of distribution for a given value of fu. The approach is as follows. Upon rearrangement, one obtains

$$\frac{V_{TW}}{fu_T} = \frac{V - Vp}{fu}$$

   where V_{TW} is the aqueous volume outside of plasma into which drug distributes at equilibrium. As theophylline distributes into all body water spaces, volume 42 L, and the plasma volume $Vp = 3$ L, it follows $V_{TW} = 39$ L. Therefore, as $V = 29$ L when $fu = 0.6$, it follows that

$$\frac{V_{TW}}{fu_T} = \frac{29\ L - 3\ L}{0.6} = 43.3\ L$$

   Substituting this ratio back into the equation for V, and for an fu of 0.3,

$$V = Vp + \frac{fu \cdot V_{TW}}{fu_T} = 3\ L + 0.3 \times 43.3 = 16\ L$$

   ii. **Unbound concentration = 9.4 mg/L. The unbound concentration of theophylline is relatively insensitive to changes in the fraction unbound in plasma.**

$$\frac{Fraction}{unbound} = \frac{Amount\ in\ body\ unbound}{Total\ amount\ in\ body} = \frac{fu \times 42\ L}{V} = \frac{0.3 \times 42\ L}{16\ L} = 0.79$$

   Hence,

$$Cu = \frac{fraction\ unbound\ in\ body \times Dose}{42\ L} = \frac{0.79 \times 500\ mg}{42\ L} = 9.4\ mg/L$$

   Thus, for a twofold decrease in fu, despite the expected similar fold decrease in V (from 29–16 L), the fraction of theophylline in the body unbound decreases by only about 9%. In practical terms, this means that for 500 mg in the body, the unbound concentration would only decrease from 10.3 mg/L (0.87×500 mg/42 L) to 9.4 mg/L (0.79×500 mg/42 L), a small drop, and of little clinical value. This example stresses the importance of focusing attention in drug therapy on the pharmacologically active unbound drug, especially when, as here, there are significant changes in the fraction of drug unbound in plasma. Basing conclusions on the total plasma concentration under these circumstances can be highly misleading. *Note:* Although the conclusion that Cu will minimally change with a change in fu could be have been readily answered knowing that 87% of drug in the body is unbound when $fu = 0.6$, in making quantitative decisions, it is important to go through the formal analysis, as the magnitude of change is not always so apparent.

9. a. **With inhibition, a 2.5-fold reduction in clearance and 2.5-fold increase in half-life.** Meperidine is a drug of intermediate hepatic extraction ratio. Its blood clearance is 700 mL/min, or 42 L/hr. Correcting for the 7% renally excreted, $E_H = CL_{b,H} \cdot (1 - fe)/Q_H = 42$ L/hr $(1 - 0.07)/80$ L/hr $= 0.49$.

The impact of a fivefold reduction of hepatocellular activity (CL_{int}, and hence $fu_b \cdot CL_{int}$) on $CL_{b,H}$ is calculated as follows. Upon rearranging the well-stirred model

$$CL_{b,H} = Q_H \cdot \left[\frac{fu_b \cdot CL_{int}}{Q_H + fu_b \cdot CL_{int}} \right]$$

yielding

$$fu_b \cdot CL_{int} = Q_H \cdot \left[\frac{1 - E_H}{E_H} \right]$$

so that $fu_b \cdot CL_{int} = 80 \times (1 - 0.49/0.49) = 83$ L/hr. On reduction by fivefold, $fu_b \cdot CL_{int} = 16.7$ L/hr, which on substitution back gives $CL_{b,H} = 13.8$ L/hr. Adding this value to renal blood clearance, 2.94 L/hr (0.07×42 L/hr), gives $CL_b = 16.7$ L/hr, a 2.5-fold (42 L/hr/16.7 L/hr) reduction in $CL_{b,H}$, much less than the decrease in $fu_b \cdot CL_{int}$. Half-life will therefore also increase by 2.5-fold.

b. **With induction, a 1.65-fold increase in clearance and 1.65-fold reduction in half-life.** Induction increases $fu_b \cdot CL_{int}$ by fivefold, to 415 L/hr (5×83 L/hr), which on substitution yields $CL_{b,H} = 67$ L/hr and $CL_b = 69.4$ L/hr, a 1.65-fold (69.4/42) increase in clearance, and a corresponding 1.65-fold shortening of half-life. Overall, the expected impact of inhibition and induction on CL_b of meperidine is less severe than changes occurring at the enzymatic level, and somewhat less for induction than inhibition, both in relative and absolute terms, as clearance approaches hepatic blood flow.

10. a. **Fraction unbound: propranolol 0.056, disopyramide 0.187.**

$$fu = \frac{1}{1 + Ka \cdot P_t}$$

Under control conditions, $P_t = 18$ μM, so that for propranolol ($fu = 0.1$) $Ka = 0.5$ μM^{-1}, and for disopyramide ($fu = 0.3$) $Ka = 0.128$ μM^{-1}. Accordingly, when $P_t = 34$ μM, propranolol $fu = 0.056$, disopyramide $fu = 0.187$.

b. **Propranolol half-life = 1.94 hr, disopyramide half-life = 7.3 hr.**
Propranolol.
   Clearance. This drug has a high blood clearance, ($CL_b = CL \cdot (blood / plasma)$) $= 60 \times 1.1 = 66$ L/hr, essentially all by hepatic elimination, given that $fe = 0.02$. Hence, its clearance is insensitive to changes in fu, certainly over the narrow twofold range (from 0.1 to 0.056).

Volume of distribution. Under control conditions $V = 300$ L, $V = Vp + V_T \cdot fu / fu_T$, Vp can be ignored, and defining V' and fu' as the new volume of distribution and fraction unbound respective, it follows that $V' = V \cdot fu' / fu$, which on substitution gives $V' = 300$ L $\times (0.056/0.1) = 168$ L.

Half-life. Accordingly, the $t_{1/2}$ on Day 5 after surgery is 0.693×168 L$/60$ L/hr $= 1.94$ hr. Hence, compared with the control value (3.5 hr), the elevation of α_1-acid glycoprotein by surgery is expected to cause a shortening in the $t_{1/2}$ of propranolol.

Disopyramide.

Clearance. This is a low-clearance compound; its blood clearance 3.15 L/hr (3.5 L/hr $\times 0.9$ [plasma/blood ratio]) is low, and given that $fe = 0.46$, $CL_{b,H}$ and $CL_{b,R}$ are 1.70 L/hr and 1.5 L/hr, both low relative to their respective organ blood flows. Hence, for this drug, $CL = fu \cdot CL_{int}$, so that after surgery $CL = (0.178/0.30) \times 3.5$ L/hr $= 2.18$ L/hr.

Volume of distribution. Based on the same procedure applied to propranolol, for disopyramide $V' = (0.187/0.30) \times 35$ L $= 23$ L.

Half-life. Accordingly, the $t_{1/2}$ on Day 5 after surgery is 0.693×23 L$/2.18$ L/hr $= 7.3$ hr. Hence, compared with the control value (7.3 hr), it is apparent that the elevation of α_1-acid glycoprotein by surgery is expected to produce little or no change in the $t_{1/2}$ of disopyramide.

c. **The data with propranolol and disopyramide do not support the statement, "The half-life of a drug can be increased by increasing the extent of plasma protein binding."** In these examples, half-life either remains unchanged (the case of a low-clearance compound with a moderate-to-large volume of distribution) or shortens (the case of a high-clearance compound with a moderate-to-large volume of distribution) when fu decreases. Further examination will show that the only case in which half-life becomes longer is that of a low-clearance compound with a small volume of distribution. For such a drug, V tends to remain unchanged with changes in fu, so with CL ($fu \cdot CL_{int}$) decreasing, half-life increases with a decrease in fu.

11. **Either hepatic uptake or biliary efflux could rate-limit the hepatic clearance of fexofenadine. Distinguishing between these two possibilities is difficult because it requires a means of independently affecting OATP1B1 and PgP and observing the change, if any, in the clearance and renal clearance, and hence by difference the hepatic clearance. One way would be to coadminister inhibitors of each process, but the problem in practice is that inhibitors of transporters often lack specificity rendering interpretation difficult.**

Fexofenadine is a low-clearance compound, $CL_b = 15$ L/hr, hence $CL_{b,H}$ must be low, and therefore is rate-limited by uptake or elimination, which is primarily by biliary excretion as the compound is minimally metabolized. Being polar, it is likely that its hepatic uptake could be dependent to some extent on OATP1B1.

12. a. (1) **Propranolol.** Only for this drug are the pKa in the correct range and its unionized form nonpolar, enabling tubular reabsorption to occur.

(2) **Amoxicillin.** CL_R ($0.693 \cdot fe \cdot V/t_{1/2}$) $= 12.5$ L/hr; the CL_R values of the other drugs are very much lower.

(3) **Amoxicillin.** Being polar, it will have great difficulty crossing the placenta into the fetus.

(4) **Cyclosporine.** It has the lowest Cu: $Cu = Dose/Vu = Dose \times fu/V = 0.024$ mg/L. The corresponding values for amoxicillin and propranolol are 2.8 and 0.028 mg/L, respectively.

(5) **Amoxicillin.** It has the lowest clearance ($CL = 0.693 \times V/t_{1/2} = 22.3$ L/hr).

b. (1) **Show little change**—because the clearance of propranolol (almost exclusively metabolic with negligible renal excretion), 63 L/hr, is comparable to hepatic blood flow (80 L/hr), signifying that it is likely to be a high extraction ratio drug, and hence relatively insensitive to changes in plasma protein binding.

(2) **Alkalinization**—Propranolol is expected to show the greatest sensitivity of CL_R to changes in urine pH. Cyclosporine being neither an acid nor a base is unaffected by changes in pH. Amoxicillin is not expected to show pH sensitivity either; it is polar and unlikely to be reabsorbed. Propranolol is a lipophilic amine for which tubular reabsorption is likely to be more extensive at higher pH values, at which the fraction un-ionized is greater.

(3) **Is not**—because amoxicillin would have to have a volume of distribution of 15 L and be unbound in plasma.

(4) **Decrease**—because V is reasonably large. Then, $V \simeq fu \cdot V_{TW} / fu_T$. In plasma, cyclosporine is primarily associated with lipoproteins, the concentration of which varies with diet and disease.

(5) **99.2%**—because this is the percent of propranolol outside plasma $[(V - V_p)/V]$.

c. (1) **Propranolol.** Fraction remaining $= e^{-k \cdot t}$, $k = 0.693/t_{\frac{1}{2}} = 0.173$ hr^{-1}, $t = 12$, $e^{-k \cdot t} = 0.125$. Or, 12.5% remains after 3 $t_{1/2}$, so that $t_{1/2} = 12/3 = 4$ hr.

(2) **Amoxicillin.** It has the lowest CL and hence highest AUC for a given dose.

(3) **Amoxicillin.** $C = Dose \cdot e^{-k \cdot t}/V$ at 6 hr is 0.034 mg/L, 0.098 mg/L, and 0.24 mg/L for amoxicillin, propranolol, and cyclosporine, respectively.

(4) **Cyclosporine.** $AUC(0 - t)/AUC(0 - \infty)$ is the fraction of the dose lost by time t, $1 - e^{-kt}$. The respective values at 3 hr for amoxicillin, propranolol, and cyclosporine are 0.90, 0.41, and 0.33.

CHAPTER 6. KINETICS FOLLOWING AN EXTRAVASCULAR DOSE

1. **Any six of the following: buccal, inhalation, intramuscular, intranasal, oral, rectal, subcutaneous, sublingual, transdermal.**

2. **c and d.**

   a. The slower the absorption process, the *lower* is the peak plasma concentration after a single oral dose.

   b. In some situations, there may be an increase in bioavailability and a shortening of the peak time ($ka \uparrow$), but they do not necessarily go together. For example, the bioavailability may be increased in hepatic disease for a drug extensively metabolized during the first pass through the liver, but the rate constant associated with drug reaching the liver may not be affected.

3. **See Fig. J6-P3.**

4. a. **From AUC analysis, $F = 0.76$; $F_{rel} = 0.95$.**

   From Ae_∞ analysis, $F = 0.83$; $F_{rel} = 0.95$.

   Plasma

   $$F = \frac{[AUC/Dose]_{oral}}{[AUC/Dose]_{i.v.}} = \frac{[(10.9\ mg\text{-}hr/L)/1000\ mg]}{[(13.1\ mg\text{-}hr/L)/500\ mg]}$$

   $$F_{rel} = \frac{[AUC/Dose]_2}{[AUC/Dose]_1} = \frac{[(19.9\ mg\text{-}hr/L)/1000\ mg]}{[(20.9\ mg\text{-}hr/L)/1000\ mg]}$$

   Urine

   $$F = \frac{[Ae_\infty/Dose]_{oral}}{[Ae_\infty/Dose]_{i.v.}} = \frac{(554\ mg/1000\ mg)}{(332\ mg/500\ mg)}$$

   $$F_{rel} = \frac{[Ae_\infty/Dose]_2}{[Ae_\infty/Dose]_1} = \frac{(554\ mg/1000\ mg)}{(589\ mg/500\ mg)}$$

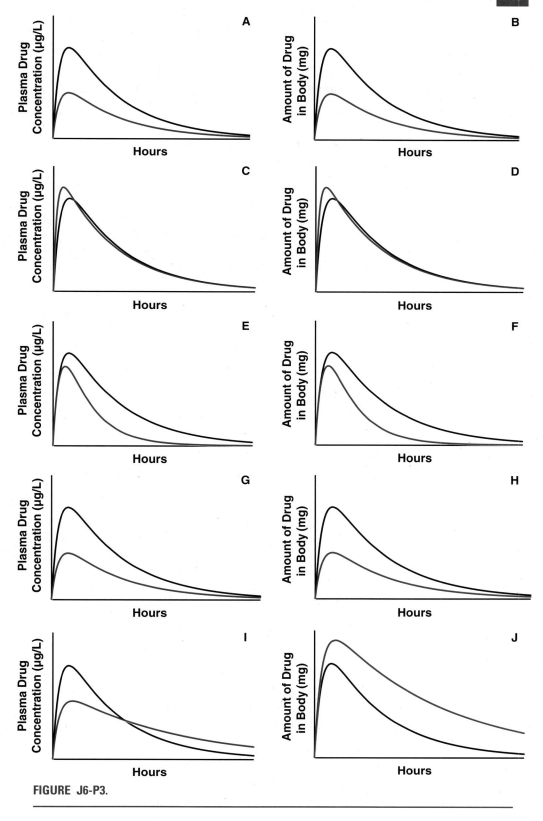

FIGURE J6-P3.

Assumptions made are:
1. *CL* and *fe* do not vary between treatments.
2. Estimates of *AUC* and *Ae∞* are accurate (e.g., no missed urine collections, correct extrapolations to infinity).

b. **Yes.** Time interval of 48 hr is adequate to ensure a good estimate of *Ae∞*. With half-life of about 2.7 hr, 48 hr corresponds to 18 half-lives. The high percent of the dose excreted unchanged (*fe* = 332 mg/500 mg = 0.66) indicates that urine analysis is appropriate for assessment of bioavailability of procainamide.

c. **CL_R values ($Ae_∞/AUC$) are 25, 28, and 28 L/hr for the i.v. formulation 1 and formulation 2 treatments, respectively.** The differences among them are small and probably insignificant (only mean data are shown).

5. a. **A delayed esophageal transit profoundly affects the rapidity, but not the extent, of absorption of acetaminophen.** The peak concentration is much lower (delayed transit group, 3.9 mg/L; normal transit group, 6.3 mg/L) and delayed (90 versus 40 min), but the *AUC* values (990 versus 999 mg-hr/L) are comparable. *AUC* remaining after last time point is calculated from C_{last}/k; $k = 0.0048$ min^{-1} for both groups.

b. **Drug disposition is the rate-limiting step.** Displayed semilogarithmically, the declines in the plasma concentration for the two groups are parallel. The slopes would probably be different if absorption had been the rate-limiting step.

c. **Yes.** To ensure rapid absorption, acetaminophen should be taken while upright with plenty of water.

6. a. **16.7 hr.** Estimated from slope of semilogarithmic plot of data following i.v. administration (not shown). $k = 0.0415$ hr^{-1}.

b. **$AUC_{i.v.}$ = 217 mg-hr/L; AUC_{oral} = 191 mg-hr/L.** Estimated by trapezoidal rule up to 48 hr, with extrapolation given by $C(48)/k$.

c. **CL = 2.3 L/hr; V = 55 L.** $CL = Dose/AUC_{i.v.}$ = 500 mg/217 mg-hr/L. $V = CL/k$ = 2.3 L/hr/0.0415 hr^{-1}.

d. **F = 0.88.** $F = (AUC/Dose)_{oral}/(AUC/Dose)_{i.v.}$

e. **CL_R = 1.86 L/hr.** $CL_R = fe \cdot CL = 0.81 \times 2.3$ L/hr.

7. a. **Absorption rate-limits griseofulvin elimination for 24 to 40 hr.** This time corresponds to the normal transit time of food in the gut. Thereafter, unabsorbed drug is expelled from the gut, and the plasma concentration of griseofulvin then falls parallel to that following the i.v. dose.

b. **Griseofulvin is incompletely absorbed in this patient.** A cursory examination of the data from plots on regular graph paper indicate that, based on *AUC* corrected for dose, griseofulvin is poorly bioavailable (*F* approximately 0.4). Griseofulvin, sparingly soluble in water (10 mg/L), is difficult to dissolve.

8. a. (1) **F = 0.994 from plasma data.**

For 3-mg/kg doses:

$$F = \frac{AUC\,(0-\infty)_{s.c.}}{AUC\,(0-\infty)_{i.v.}} = \frac{17.8\ \mu g\text{-}hr/mL}{17.9\ \mu g\text{-}hr/mL} = 0.994$$

(2) **F = 1.038 from urine data.**

$$F = \frac{Ae\,(\infty)_{s.c.}}{Ae\,(\infty)_{i.v.}} = \frac{2.47\ mg/kg}{2.38\ mg/kg} = 1.038$$

b. (1) **$F = <0.055$ from plasma data.**

For 10-mg/kg dose:

$$F = \frac{AUC\,(0-\infty)_{p.o.}}{AUC\,(0-\infty)_{i.v.}} = \frac{<3.5\ \mu g\text{-}hr/mL}{64.2\ \mu g\text{-}hr/mL} = <0.055$$

(2) **$F = 0.023$ from urine data.**

$$F = \frac{Ae\,(\infty)_{p.o.}}{Ae\,(\infty)_{i.v.}} = \frac{0.24\ mg/kg}{10.5\ mg/kg} = 0.023$$

c. *Dose*   *fe**

   1 mg/kg   0.92

   3 mg/kg   0.79 $*fe = \dfrac{Ae\,(\infty)}{Dose}$ *for each dose.*

   10 mg/kg   1.05

9. a. **Absorption.** The elimination half-life (11.6 hr) is associated with a rate constant of $0.06\ hr^{-1}$. This value is the smaller of the two exponential coefficients in the equation obtained after oral administration. Therefore, the absorption half-life is 1.4 hr $(0.693/0.5\ hr^{-1})$.

   b. **See Fig. J6-P9.**

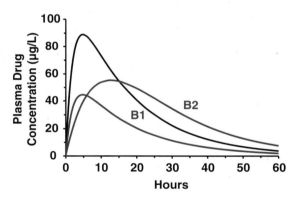

FIGURE J6-P9.

c. **2.9 hr.** $t_{max} = \dfrac{\ln(ka/k)}{ka - k} = \dfrac{\ln\,(0.5/0.06)}{0.5 - 0.06} = 2.9\ hr$

10.

TABLE J6-P10	90% and 95% Confidence Intervals in Five Separate Studies		

Study Interval*	90% Confidence Interval*	95% Confidence Interval*	Conclusions that Apply
101	0.72–0.94	0.70–0.96	b, d
102	0.86–1.20	0.83–1.23	a, f
103	1.07–1.23	1.05–1.25	a, d
104	1.28–1.46	1.26–1.48	c, d
105	0.78–1.11	0.75–1.14	b, f

*Confidence interval in the ratio of test/reference values of *AUC* after antilog transformation.

CHAPTER 7. ABSORPTION

1. **Five of the following or any other reasonable explanation(s):**

   Examples of reasons for low and variable oral bioavailability.

   a. Lack of complete release of drug from dosage form in a region of the intestine where there is insufficient permeability to allow absorption to occur.
   b. Decomposition of drug in stomach (low pH).
   c. Enzymatic digestion within gastrointestinal tract.
   d. Drug is too water soluble to be absorbed across lipophilic gastrointestinal membranes and too large to readily penetrate by the paracellular route.
   e. Metabolism of drug in gut wall.
   f. Extensive extraction of drug during first pass through the liver.
   g. Decomposition of drug by microflora in large intestine.
   h. Formation of virtually insoluble complexes with materials within the gastrointestinal lumen.
   i. Effect of food, other drugs, gastrointestinal disease, and abnormalities.

2. a. **True.** Small lipophilic drugs in solution are very rapidly absorbed across the small intestine, relative to that in the stomach. When these drugs are given orally, their absorption is generally rate-limited by their movement from the stomach into the small intestine.
   b. **False.** When intestinal absorption is rate-limited by permeability, absorption kinetics, and hence, the plasma concentration–time profile, may be relatively insensitive to changes in dissolution kinetics. For rapidly dissolving products of such drugs, most of the drug has dissolved before appreciable absorption has occurred.
   c. **False.** Polar drugs primarily traverse membranes via the paracellular pathway; they have great problems traversing relatively lipophilic cell membranes, unless transported by a carrier.
   d. **True.** The time in the stomach is, however, highly variable.

3. **Saturable first-pass occurs by capacity-limited metabolism during first pass of orally administered drug through the intestines and liver.** It can occur without apparent saturable elimination after an equivalent i.v. dose, because the concentration entering the intestines or the liver early on after the oral dose greatly exceeds that after the i.v. dose. Factors favoring this separation of saturable effects include rapid absorption (large ka) and a large volume of distribution.

4. **Systemic absorption after i.m. administration may be faster or slower than that after oral administration.** Which route shows faster systemic absorption depends on many factors including the site of intramuscular administration, precipitation at the intramuscular injection site, gastric emptying time, the intestinal permeability of the drug, and so on.

5. a. **Small intestine.** Based on comparison of AUC as a measure of the amount absorbed, little drug is absorbed from the large intestine (ascending and descending colon). And, absorption of drugs from the stomach is much slower than from the small intestine.
   b. **Duodenum.** Jejunal delivery results in only 26% absorption compared with gastric delivery ($AUC_{duodenal}/AUC_{gastric}$ = 0.38 mg-hr/L/1.48 mg-hr/L). As drugs are poorly absorbed across the gastric epithelium, and the duodenum separates the stomach from the jejunum, the duodenum is likely to be a primary site of absorption for ciprofloxacin.
   c. **Poor.** For dosage forms that readily empty from the stomach (e.g., those comprising small multipelleted units), within 6 hr of administration the dosage form

would be in the large intestine where, because of poor absorption characteristics, rate control from the delivery system is likely to be lost. A possible solution is to use a large controlled-release nondisintegrating product, which, when taken on a full stomach, is retained there (although retention is highly variable) and delivers drug continuously to the more permeable small intestine. In addition, it would be important for release of drug from the delivery system to be independent of such factors as pH, stirring rate, and electrolyte composition, which can vary markedly in the stomach.

6. See Fig. J7-P6.

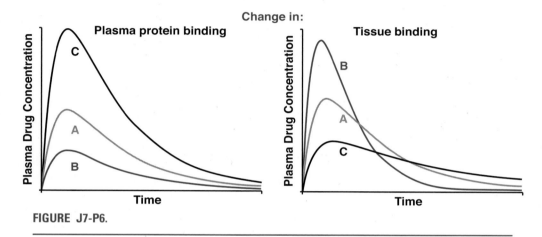

FIGURE J7-P6.

7. a.

	Before	After
$CL = \dfrac{Dose_{i.v.}}{AUC_{i.v.}}$	$\dfrac{800}{1207} = 0.66$ (L/min)	$\dfrac{800}{1405} = 57$ (L/min)
$F = \dfrac{AUC_{p.o.}}{AUC_{i.v.}}$	$\dfrac{142}{1207} = 0.12$	$\dfrac{716}{1405} = 0.51$

b. **The blood clearance is 1.1 L/hr ($CL \cdot C/C_b$). This value indicates the probability of a high first-pass loss.** Inhibition of metabolism of 6-mercaptopurine increases bioavailability with only a small decease in clearance because of its high extraction ratio.

8. **Yes.** The high-protein meal, which causes an increased portal blood flow, produces a 70% increase in oral bioavailability. This is accompanied by a 38% increase in clearance and an insignificant change in AUC after an oral dose. Propranolol is a drug with a high hepatic extraction ratio ($CL_b = 1.1$ L/min). For such a drug, an increase in hepatic blood flow is expected to produce an increase in both bioavailability and clearance. The observation of different extents of increase may be explained by the increased blood flow being primarily restricted to early times when the food given is digested and absorbed. Absorption of drug occurs during this period, while elimination of absorbed drug ($t_{1/2} \approx 3.6$ hr, data not given) occurs predominantly thereafter. The small change in AUC is a consequence of similar changes in both CL_b and F.

9. For all situations, eating a meal (especially one with high fat content) slows gastric emptying compared with that occurring on a fasted stomach.

a. Being water soluble and given as an immediate-release tablet, the drug would be expected to dissolve rapidly in the stomach, effectively becoming a solution. A slowed gastric emptying rate would then slow the rate of delivery of drug to the small intestine, where absorption occurs. The extent may not be affected because food has no material effect on small intestinal transit time. However, when immediate response is desired, the product should be taken on a fasted stomach. Acetaminophen is an example of a drug in this category.

b. For a sparingly soluble compound, dissolution may not only rate-limit absorption but also affect the extent of oral absorption if dissolution is not complete by the time the compound has entered the large intestine. By slowing gastric emptying, facilitating gastric mixing, and increasing the content of the stomach, food prolongs and increases the chance for dissolution of the compound within the stomach and slowly releases drug to the small intestine, where absorption is favored. Itraconazole is an example in this category.

c. Large (>7 mm), single, nondisintegrating entities tend to be retained in the stomach as long as food is there. Only on a fasted stomach is a large entity ejected from the stomach relatively quickly, the action of housekeeping waves. Therefore, delivery of a single enteric-coated product into the small intestine, where removal of the enteric coating and absorption occurs, is significantly delayed. The time of leaving the stomach is highly variable. Once the enteric coating is removed, however, subsequent release and absorption of the compound should be the same, regardless of food. If, however, the release of drug is delayed after reaching the small intestine, the extent may be reduced as well. Delayed-release capsules of erythromycin, an anti-infective agent, or didanosine, a drug used to treat HIV, are examples. For these products, the enteric coating is on the small pellets contained in the capsule. This allows the pellets to enter the small intestine after the capsule disintegrates, so that there is no great delay in drug absorption. If taken with food, the drug is slowed somewhat as seen with small pellets in Fig. 7-10.

The slowdown is not as extensive as that observed with aspirin contained in enteric-coated whole tablets; the enteric coating around the entire tablet is to prevent gastric irritation rather than decomposition. Here, the time drug absorption starts is greatly delayed and highly variable.

10. a. $F_{oral} = 0.13$ **(plasma); 0.12 (urine).**

$$\text{Plasma} \qquad\qquad\qquad \text{Urine}$$

$$F_{oral} = \frac{AUC_{oral}}{AUC_{i.v.}} = \frac{0.25}{1.93} \qquad\qquad \frac{Ae_\infty(oral)}{Ae_\infty(i.v.)} = \frac{1.22}{10.5}$$

b. $F_H = 0.15$. **Yes, first-pass loss appears to account for the low bioavailability.**

$$fe = \frac{Ae_\infty}{Dose_{i.v.}} = \frac{10.5\ mg}{100\ mg} = 0.105 \qquad CL = \frac{Dose_{i.v.}}{AUC_{i.v.}} = \frac{100\ mg}{1.93\ mg\text{-}hr/L} = 51.8\ L/hr$$

$$F_H = 1 - E_H = 1 - \frac{(1 - 0.105)\times 51.8\ L/hr \times 1.5}{81\ L/hr} = 0.15$$

CHAPTER 8. RESPONSE FOLLOWING A SINGLE DOSE

1. **Effect compartment**—A compartment for the site of action that is needed to account for the time to distribute drug to that site from plasma.

Direct response—One in which response rises and falls in time with plasma concentration without hysteresis.

Hysteresis—The lack of concordance of the plasma concentration–response relationship when the concentration rises with that when it falls after drug administration.

Hysteresis can occur following extravascular administration or when input is not instantaneous.

Pharmacokinetic rate-limited response—One in which changes in measured response with time are limited by the kinetics of the drug, rather than the dynamics of the affected system, following its administration.

Time delay—The lag in response with time relative to that in plasma drug concentration.

2. a. **T. A hysteresis loop is not possible because after an i.v. bolus dose, the plasma concentration always decreases with time.** Clearly, it is also not possible even if the effect had been due to a metabolite, and not the drug. A plot of response against an ever declining drug concentration would rise and fall but no hysteresis would be evident, even through the metabolite concentration rises and then falls after drug administration.

   b. **F. Response declines linearly, not exponentially, with time within the region between 80% and 20% maximum response.** This occurs because in this region, the intensity of response is proportional to the logarithm of the plasma concentration, but as the plasma concentration is declining exponentially with time, it follows that the logarithm of the concentration declines linearly with time.

   c. **F. A quantal response, involving an event that is either present or absent, cannot be related to concentration of drug.** Rather, it is the frequency, or the cumulative frequency, of the event that is related.

   d. **F.** Considering even the simplest pharmacokinetic model ($C = D / V \cdot e^{-kt}$), for a given endpoint, with an associated concentration, C_{min}, the duration of t_d is proportional to log Dose:

$$t_d = \frac{1}{k} \cdot ln\left[\frac{Dose}{V \cdot C_{min}}\right]$$

   e. **T.** Before distribution equilibrium is achieved, interpretation of plasma concentrations is complicated by temporal aspects.

3. a. **Correct.** There is a clear relationship between response and the exposure giving the minimal response. Pharmacokinetics encompasses those processes that determine the concentration–time profile, and hence, the duration of response under these circumstances.

   b. **No.** Clearly not true if the duration of effect is already less than 1 half-life.

   c. **Correct.** No qualification is necessary.

4. $E_{max} = 25$ mm Hg, $C_{50} = 0.15$ mg/L, and $\gamma = 0.6$.

The graph appears to be leveling off at about 25 mm Hg, the E_{max} value. The concentration at which the response is 50% of E_{max} (12.5 mm Hg) occurs at about 0.15 mg/L. The value of γ can be estimated from any point on the line and the C_{50} value. Using a response of 5 mm Hg at a concentration of 0.015 mg/L and the C_{50} value,

$$5 = \frac{25 \times 0.015^{\gamma}}{0.15^{\gamma} + 0.015^{\gamma}} \qquad \text{or} \qquad 0.2 = \frac{0.015^{\gamma}}{0.15^{\gamma} + 0.015^{\gamma}}$$

Collecting terms

$$\frac{0.15^{\gamma}}{0.015^{\gamma}} = 4$$

which on taking logs gives

$$\gamma \cdot \log 10 = \log 4, \text{ so that } \gamma = \frac{\log 4}{\log 10} = 0.6$$

5. a. **Counterclockwise.**

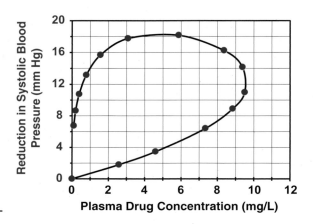

FIGURE J8-P5.

b. Possible explanations include:
- Formation of an active metabolite.
- Delay in equilibration of drug at active site with drug in plasma.
- Occurrence of sequential time-delaying events between binding to receptor and eliciting response.

6. Examples in which changes in response with time are rate-limited by the kinetics of the drug include the decrease in exercise tachycardia produced by propranolol, the relief of pain with naproxen, the sedative hypnotic activity of benzodiazepine, and muscle paralysis produced by neuromuscular-blocking agents. Another example, not discussed in this chapter, is anesthesia induced by volatile anesthetics and opioids. Examples in which changes in response with time are rate-limited by the dynamics of the affected system are the lowering of body temperature with ibuprofen, the lowering of the plasma prothrombin complex by acenocoumalone, and the return of the blood leukocyte count following paclitaxel administration. Another example, not discussed in the chapter, is that of the thiazide diuretics. These drugs, which help remove sodium and lower blood pressure, are eliminated rapidly from the body, primarily by renal excretion. On initiating therapy with these drugs, however, blood pressure takes a reasonably long time to fall, owing to the various homeostatic control mechanisms. Likewise, blood pressure rises very slowly on withdrawing these agents after chronic treatment.

7. $C_{20} = 5.7$ mg/L and $C_{80} = 17.4$ mg/L. On rearrangement of Eq. 2-4:

$$C = C_{50} \cdot \left[\frac{Effect}{1 - Effect} \right]^{1/\gamma}$$

where *Effect* is expressed as a function of the maximum response. For $\gamma = 2.5$ and $C_{50} = 10$ mg/L, $C_{20} = 5.7$ mg/L, and $C_{80} = 17.4$ mg/L.

8. a. **The apparent half-life of propranolol is 2.3 hr**.
   This value is calculated from the plot of intensity of effect versus time. This shows a linear decline with time, as expected when response lies within the region of 80% to 20% of the maximum response, with a slope $(-m \cdot k) = -3.5\%$/hr. Given that the slope of the plot of the intensity of response against the logarithm of plasma propranolol concentration $(m) = +11.5\%$, it follows that k, the apparent elimination rate constant of propranolol, must be equal to 0.3 hr^{-1}. Hence, the corresponding half-life $(0.693/k)$ is 2.3 hr. The half-life is apparent in the sense that it is assumed that only propranolol is active, and ignores the possibility that some of its metabolites may contribute to the observed response.

b. **The minimum amount of propranolol needed in the body is 6 mg.**
   After a 20-mg dose, the effect remains above 15% for 4 hr (see Fig. 8-24). Hence,

$$A_{min} = Dose \cdot e^{-k \cdot t_D} = 20\ mg \times e^{-0.3hr^{-1} \times 4hr} = 6\ mg$$

c. **6.3 and 8.2 hr.**
   After a 20-mg dose, the effect remains above 15% for 4 hr (see Fig. 8-24).
   (1) After a 40-mg dose, a doubling of the dose, the duration of effect is expected to increase by one half-life, 2.3 hr (for a total of 6.3 hr).
   (2) The duration is expected to increase an extra 4.2 hr, as the duration of effect following 70 mg is:

$$t_D = \frac{\ln (Dose/A_{min})}{k} = \frac{\ln (70\ mg/6\ mg)}{0.3\ hr^{-1}} = 8.2\ hr$$

9. a. $t_D = 11.4$ hr. $C_{min} \cdot V = 32$ mg; substitute into Eq. 8-11.
   b. t_D after 200 mg = **18.3 hr** (11.4 hr + half-life).
   c. **(1) 22.8 hr and (2) 8.9 hr.**
   d. **Doubling the dose increases the duration of effect by one half-life, 6.9 hr.** The effect of doubling the half-life depends on the mechanism of the change. A decreased clearance leads to a doubling of the duration of effect, whereas in this example, duration is decreased when the cause of the increased half-life is a doubling of the volume of distribution.

10. a. Table J8-P10 summarizes the data for the synthesis rate and plasma concentration of S.

   The synthesis rate was calculated from the relationship:

$$R_{syn} = \frac{dA_s}{dt} + k_s \cdot A_s$$

   which for a small time interval, Δt, is approximated by

$$R_{syn} = \frac{\Delta A_s}{\Delta t} + k_s \cdot A_{s,av}$$

   where R_{syn} is the average rate of synthesis over Δt; $\Delta A_s/\Delta t$ is the average rate of change of A_s and $A_{s,av}$ is the average value of A_s, over Δt. Its value is approximated by $A_{s,av} = [A_s(t_i) + A_s(t_i + 1)]/2$ and occurs at the midpoint time, $t_{mid} = [t_i + t_{i+1}]/2$, where t_i and t_{i+1} are the ith and $(i + 1)^{th}$ times.
   Estimation of k_s. The first 50% fall of A_s is the same whether 100 or 200 mg of drug was injected. Hence, during this time, inhibition of synthesis must be almost complete ($R_{syn} = 0$), then

$$\frac{dA_s}{dt} = -k_s \cdot A_s$$

   Hence, k_s is estimated from the slope of the initial straight line when A_s values are plotted on a logarithmic scale against time.

TABLE J8-P10	**Synthesis Rate and Plasma Concentration of Substance S with Time Following Drug Administration**													
Midpoint Time (hr)	1	3	5	7	9	11	14	20	27	33	42	54	66	78
Synthesis Rate (%/hr)	0.62	1.13	1.41	1.54	1.75	2.20	2.85	4.38	6.05	9.47	12.2	14.9	16.3	16.8
Plasma Concentration of S (% of Control)	86	62.5	46.5	35.5	28.0	23.3	20.3	21.8	28.3	40	60	80	92	97.5

Answer, $k_s = 0.170$ hr^{-1} ($t_{\frac{1}{2}} = 4.1$ hr), therefore, $R_{syn,0} = k_s \cdot A_s = 17\%$ hr^{-1}. Direct effect, percent inhibition of synthesis, is given by $100 \cdot (1 - R_{syn}/R_{syn,0})$. Figure J8-P10 is a plot of the direct effect versus the log of the plasma drug concentration.

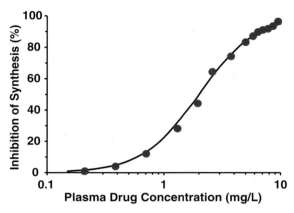

FIGURE J8-P10.

b. $C_{50} = 2$ mg/L; $\gamma = 1.8$. **The line with these parameters is shown in black.**
C_{50} is concentration at which the synthesis is 50% of normal (8.5% of normal amount/hr). The value of γ is obtained by substituting an effect–concentration data pair into the equation.

$$\frac{E}{E_{max}} = \frac{C^{\gamma}}{C_{50}{}^{\gamma} + C^{\gamma}}$$

where E/E_{max} is one minus the synthesis rate as a fraction of the normal value, a measure of the degree of inhibition of synthesis. Using a concentration of 5 mg/L and an E/E_{max} of 0.84, the value of γ is about 1.8.

CHAPTER 9: THERAPEUTIC WINDOW

1. **Dosage regimen**—A systematic manner of administration of a drug intended for the treatment or amelioration of a disease or condition.

   Therapeutic index—The degree of separation *within an individual* between a regimen of a drug that is beneficial and tolerable and one that is limited by the adverse effects produced. The therapeutic index is low when the degree of separation between these two regimens is small.

   Therapeutic utility—The difference in weighted probabilities between the desired and adverse effects for a given drug exposure. It is a measure of the likelihood of the net benefit of a drug.

   Therapeutic utility curve—The relationship between the therapeutic utility and the exposure of the body to a drug, usually the plasma concentration.

   Therapeutic window—The range of exposures to a drug associated with successful therapy. Usually systemic exposure is used, but dose or dosing rate is commonly used in general terms.

2. The major factors determining the dosage regimens of drugs are: pharmacokinetics, pharmacodynamics, the clinical state of the patient population, including the disease or condition to be treated, other concurrently administered drugs, and individual patient factors such as genetics, age, body weight, and concomitant diseases.

3. Response, both desired and adverse, is often better correlated with drug exposure than dose for several reasons. First, although changes in response can be correlated

with plasma concentration over time following a single dose of drug, these cannot be correlated with a single value, dose. Second, even following chronic dosing, response is often better correlated with plasma concentration than dose owing to large variability in pharmacokinetics within the patient population, thereby resulting in a wide variation in drug exposure for the same maintenance dose. However, as discussed in the text, there are exceptions.

4. **See Table 9-1.** Situations that limit the upper bound of the therapeutic window include: when adverse effects are an extension of the pharmacology of the drug (e.g., warfarin); when effectiveness reaches a peak and then diminishes at higher concentrations (e.g., tricyclic antidepressants); when there is a limiting off-target toxicity (e.g., renal toxicity with gentamicin).

5. One potential benefit of using drug combinations to treat a specific disease is that, because the dose of each drug in the combination needed to produce a given therapeutic effect is often lower than that needed for any individual drug if used alone, and adverse effect profiles tend to be drug specific, the therapeutic window of the combination tends to be wider than that of any of the drugs within the combination. Also, combining drugs that attack the disease or condition by different mechanisms can enhance efficacy beyond that that can be achieved with any one drug. An example of the former is the use of a combination of low doses of a thiazide diuretic, an angiotensin-converting enzyme (ACE) inhibitor, and a β-adrenergic blocking drug to treat of hypertension. The use of drug combinations to treat HIV infections, AIDS, and tuberculosis are examples of the latter.

6. Examples, given in the chapter, of situations in which complexity exists when attempting to correlate response with systemic drug exposure include the development of tolerance to a drug; when metabolites contribute significantly to drug response; when single-dose therapy is totally effective; and when response is a function of both dose and duration of treatment.

7. a.

TABLE J9-P7	Impact of Weighting of Beneficial and Adverse Effects on the Therapeutic Utility of a Drug			
Column	A	B	C	D
Plasma Drug Concentration (mg/L)	Probability of Efficacy (percent)	Probability of Adverse Response (percent)	Therapeutic Utility When Weighting Efficacy +1	Therapeutic Utility When Weighting Efficacy +0.6
0	2.5	1.5	1.0	0
0.5	7.4	1.5	5.9	2.9
1.0	20.1	1.9	18.2	10.2
1.5	35.7	3.2	32.5	18.2
2.0	51.7	5.1	46.6	25.9
2.5	65.8	14.9	50.9	24.6
3.0	76.3	33.3	43.0	12.5
3.5	82.9	53.6	29.3	−3.9
4.0	86.0	64.6	21.4	−13.0
4.5	87.5	69.0	18.5	−16.5
5.0	90.1	70.9	19.2	−16.8

b. With weighting efficacy by +1 and adverse response by −1 and setting the minimum desired probability of therapeutic utility at 20%, the therapeutic window is 1.1 to 4.1 mg/L, (Fig. J9-P7, black line) and the probability of patients being effectively treated within this window ranges from 20 to 87%. On down weighting efficacy to +0.6, while maintaining the other conditions, the therapeutic window narrows considerably, from 1.7 to 2.7 mg/L (Fig. J9-P7, colored line), and by reference to Table 9-2, it is seen that the probability of effective treatment, now ranging from 35.7% to around 73%. Clearly, the acceptable therapeutic window depends on the relative weightings of desired and undesired response, which varies with the therapeutic indication and often on the therapeutic profile of alternative treatments.

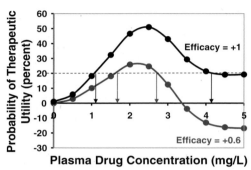

FIGURE J9-P7.

CHAPTER 10. CONSTANT-RATE INPUT

1. **b.**
   a. The approach to plateau depends on half-life. The higher the rate of infusion, the higher is the plateau concentration.
   b. By definition of CL, concentrations must be the same if R_{inf} is the same ($R_{inf} = CL \cdot C_{ss}$).
   c. Only if the volumes of distribution of the dugs are also the same. Otherwise, the half-lives are different.
   d. It can if the elimination rate constants (CL/V) are the same. The amount at steady state is R_{inf}/k.

2. **3.5 and 35 min.** At plateau, infusion rate $R_{inf} = k \cdot A_{ss}$ or $t_{1/2}$ is given by $0.693 \cdot A_{ss}/R_{inf}$. For succinylcholine, $A_{ss} = 20$ mg, so that when $R_{inf} = 0.4$ mg/min, $t_{1/2} = 35$ min and when $R_{inf} = 4$ mg/min, $t_{1/2} = 3.5$ min. The wide range in the half-life of succinylcholine arises from differences in the amount and type of pseudocholinesterase, the enzyme responsible for succinylcholine hydrolysis and inactivation. The longer half-life is only rarely encountered.

3. **See Fig J10-P3.**

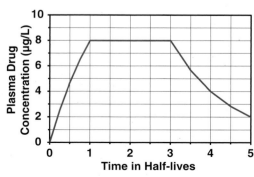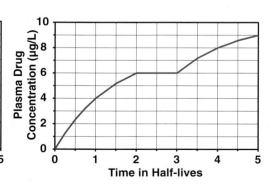

FIGURE J10-P3.

4. a. $CL = 1.2$ **L/min;** $t_{1/2} = 1.6$ **hr;** $V = 164$ **L;** $MRT = 137$ **min.** $CL = R_{inf}/C_{ss}$. The half-life is estimated from the slope of a semilogarithmic plot of the declining plasma concentration observed on stopping the infusion. The volume of distribution is obtained by dividing clearance by the elimination rate constant $(0.693/t_{1/2})$. $MRT = 1/k = V/CL$.

   b. **Yes.** Half the plateau value, 10.5 μg/L, should be reached by 1.6 hr, and 14.5 μg/L should be reached by 2 hr. More precisely, using the equation $C = C_{ss}$ $(1 - e^{-kt})$, the expected values at 1, 2, 4, and 6 hr are 7.4, 12, 17, and 19.6 μg/L, which are in reasonably close agreement with the observed values.

   c. **Plasma concentrations expected are 14.8 (1 hr), 24 (2 hr), and 42 μg/L (plateau).** Doubling the infusion rate results in a doubling of the concentration at all times.

   d. **Loading dose = 6.9 mg.** $Dose = V \cdot C(0) = 164$ L $\times$ 42 μg/L.

5. a. $t_{1/2} = 19$ **hr.** Estimated from semilogarithmic plot (not shown) of the plasma concentration against time after stopping i.v. infusion.

   b. $MRT = 2.74$ **hr.** $MRT = 1/k = 1.44 \, t_{1/2}$.

   c. $F = 0.50$. Calculated from AUC considerations.
   $AUC_{i.v.} = AUC(0-30 \text{ hr}) + C(30 \text{ hr})/k = 69.6 + 1.0 = 70.6$ μg-hr/L
   $AUC_{rectal} = AUC(0-30 \text{ hr}) + C(30 \text{ hr})/k = 34.9 + 0.3 = 35.1$ μg-hr/L
   where AUC (0–30 hr) is estimated using the trapezoidal approximation (Appendix A, *Assessment of AUC*).

$$F = (AUC/Dose)_{rectal}/(AUC/Dose)_{i.v.} = \frac{((35.1 \, \mu g/L)/3 \, mg)}{((70.6 \, \mu g/L)/3 \, mg)}$$

   d. $CL = 42$ **L/hr.** $CL = Dose/AUC_{i.v.} = 3000$ μg/70.6 μg-hr/L.

   e. $V = 116$ **L.** $V = CL \times MRT = 42$ L/hr $\times$ 2.74 hr.

6. a. **12.8 μg/hr.** Over the interval 12 to 24 hr, the plasma concentration is essentially constant, average value 1.53 μg/L, signifying the attainment of plateau. At plateau, rate of absorption = rate of elimination, therefore,

$$\textit{Rate of absorption} = CL \cdot C_{ss}$$
$$= 8.4 \, L/hr \times 1.53 \, \mu g/L$$

   b. **330 μg.** The amount absorbed equals the amount eliminated, that is,

$$\textit{Amount absorbed} = CL \cdot AUC$$
$$\textit{Amount absorbed} = 8.4 \, L/hr \times 39.3 \, \mu g\text{-}hr/L$$

   c. **No.** There is an apparent lag time (~2 hr) in the appearance of drug in the systemic circulation, a common observation with transdermal devices.

TIME (hr)	0	1	2	4	6	8	∞
Concentration (mg/L)							
Expected*	0	0.33	0.59	0.97	1.2	1.35	1.6
Observed	0	0	0.05	0.8	1.1	1.5	1.6

*$C = C_{ss}(1 - e^{-kt})$.

7. a. $CL = 2.5$ **L/hr** $V = 21.6$ **L** $t_{1/2} = 6$ **hr.**

   Clearance

   The concentration at 6 hr is at 1 half-life (see *half-life* below). The steady-state concentration then must be 20 mg/L (2 × 10 mg/L). Therefore,

$$CL = \frac{R_{inf}}{C_{ss}} = \frac{300 \, mg/ \, 6 \, hr}{20 \, mg/ \, L} = 2.5 \, L/hr$$

Volume of distribution

$$V = \frac{CL}{k} = \frac{CL \cdot t_{1/2}}{0.693} = \frac{2.5 \ L/hr \times 6 \ hr}{0.693} = 21.6 \ L$$

Half-life

From the decline after 24 hr, the half-life appears to be about 6 hr. Also, from 6 to 12 hr (no drug infused) the concentration drops in half, another proof of the 6-hr half life.

b. $R_{inf} (0 - 6) = 50$ mg/hr $R_{inf} (12 - 24) = 12.5$ mg/hr.

$$R_{inf} \ (0 - 6) = \frac{300 \ mg}{6 \ hr} = 50 \ mg/hr$$

Because the plasma concentration did not change between 12 and 14 hr, the rates of infusion and elimination must have been equal, that is,

$$R_{inf} (12 - 24) = CL \cdot C_{ss} = 2.5 \ L/hr \times 5 \ mg/L = 12.5 \ mg/hr$$

The value might also be obtained from the C_{ss} of 20 mg/L attained on 50 mg/hr. Therefore, 5 mg/L would be the C_{ss} that would be attained on 12.5 mg/hr.

$$R_{inf_1} = CL \cdot C_{ss_1} \qquad R_{inf_2} = CL \cdot C_{ss_2}$$

or

$$\frac{R_{inf_2}}{R_{inf_1}} = \frac{C_{ss_2}}{C_{ss_1}}$$

c. **See Fig. J10-P7.**

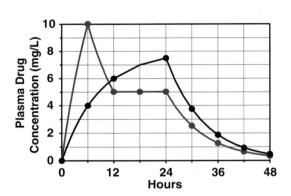

FIGURE J10-P7.

8. a. $CL = 2.0$ **L/min.**

$$1 \ ng/mL = 1 \ \mu g/L$$

$$CL = \frac{R_{inf}}{C_{ss}} = \frac{(0.25 \ \mu g/kg \times 66 \ kg) \ per \ min}{8.25 \ \mu g/L}$$

b. $V = 14.4$ **L.**

$$V = \frac{CL}{k} = \frac{CL \cdot t_{1/2}}{0.693} = \frac{2.0 \ L/min \times 5 \ min}{0.693} = 14.4 \ L$$

c. **Yes.** The drug gains access to most of the extracellular fluids. Since it is virtually unbound in plasma, it can not be bound in tissue or distribute extensively into intracellular fluids and still have a 14.4-L volume of distribution. The drug must be essentially evenly distributed throughout the extracellular fluids.

d. **Yes.** For a drug with a 5-min half-life, 15 min is long enough to virtually (87.5%) achieve the new steady state and to obtain the effect one would expect on continuing to infuse at that rate. Because of the urgency of the situation, however, waiting longer than 15 min to adjust the infusion rate to that needed by the patient is, perhaps, not warranted.

e. $CL_R = $ **80 mL/min. There is no evidence that the drug is either secreted or reabsorbed in the kidneys.**

$$CL_R = fe \cdot CL = 0.04 \times 2\ L/min = 0.08\ L/min\ or\ 80\ mL/min$$

$$\frac{CL_R}{fu \cdot GFR} = \frac{80}{0.8 \times 100} = 1.0$$

9. a. k_t **(urea) = 0.10 hr^{-1};** k_t **(creatinine) = 0.17 hr^{-1}.**

$$k_t = \frac{CL \cdot C}{V \cdot C} = \frac{CL}{V}$$

$$k_t\ (urea) = \frac{4.2\ L/hr}{42\ L} = 0.1\ hr^{-1}$$

$$k_t\ (creatinine) = \frac{7.2\ L/hr}{42\ L} = 0.17\ hr^{-1}$$

b. **Urea = 20 hr; creatinine = 11.8 hr.** For both compounds, the time required is twice the turnover time. In an anephric patient with no elimination of either compound, the rate of increase in plasma concentration ($\Delta C/\Delta t$) is R_t/V. The total increase (ΔC) over time Δt or $\frac{(CL \cdot C_{ss} \cdot \Delta t)}{V}$. Thus,

$$\Delta t = \frac{\Delta C \cdot V}{CL \cdot C_{ss}} = \frac{\Delta C}{C_{ss}} \cdot \frac{1}{k_t}$$

For urea,   For creatinine,

$$\Delta t = \frac{30\ mg/100\ mL}{15\ mg/100\ mL} \times \frac{1}{0.1\ hr^{-1}} \qquad \Delta t = \frac{2\ mg/100\ mL}{1\ mg/100\ mL} \times \frac{1}{0.17\ hr^{-1}}$$

c. **15.1 g.** Amount excreted in 1 day ($CL_R \cdot C_{ss} \cdot \Delta t$)

$$= \frac{4.2\ L}{hr} \times \frac{24\ hr}{day} \times \frac{150\ mg}{L} \times 1\ day$$

10. **2.8 days.** The enzyme activity (concentration) will increase to a new steady state three times its normal value. The doubling of the concentration (half-way between 1 and 3) will occur at 1 half-life or 0.693 × turnover time (0.693 × 4 days).

11. a. $CL_b = $ **77 L/hr;** $CL = $ **154 L/hr;** $Vu = $ **24,000 L;** $V_b = $ **120 L.**

Blood clearance

$$CL_b = Q_H \cdot E_H = 81\ L/hr \times 0.95 = 77\ L/hr$$

Plasma clearance

$$fu \cdot C = fu_b \cdot C_b \qquad \frac{C_b}{C} = \frac{fu}{fu_b} = \frac{0.01}{0.005} = 2$$

$$CL = CL_b \cdot \frac{C_b}{C} = 77\ L/hr \times 2 = 154\ L/hr$$

Volume of distribution (plasma)

$$Vu = \frac{V}{fu} = \frac{240\ L}{0.01} = 24,000\ L \qquad V_b = \frac{V \cdot C}{C_b} = \frac{240\ L}{2} = 120\ L$$

b. **Yes.** fu_T **(usual)** $= V_T \times 0.000042$.
   fu_T **(uremia)** $= V_T \times 0.00021$
   The value of fu_T **is increased fivefold.**

$$V = V_P + V_T \cdot \frac{fu}{fu_T}$$

Rearranging

$$fu_T = \frac{V_T \cdot fu}{(V - V_P)}$$

Usual value	In uremia

$$fu_T = \frac{V_T \times 0.01}{(240 - 3)} \qquad fu_T = \frac{V_T \times 0.03}{(143 - 3)}$$

$$fu_T\ (usual) = V_T \times 0.000042 \qquad fu_T\ (uremia) = V_T \times 0.00021$$

c. **Ratio of** Cu_{ss} **(presence/absence of other drug) = about 3.**
   The drug has a high extraction ratio (CL_b approaches blood flow). Under this condition, little or no change in CL_b is expected with a change in fu_b. The unbound concentration however, depends on the input rate, and fu_b.

$$CLu \cdot Cu = CL_b \cdot C_b \qquad CLu \cdot fu_b = CL_b$$

$$Cu_{ss} = \frac{R_{inf}}{CLu}$$

Therefore,

$$Cu_{ss} = \frac{R_{inf} \cdot fu_b}{CL_b}$$

fu_b triples, but CL_b should remain nearly the same.

CHAPTER 11. MULTIPLE-DOSE REGIMENS

1. **Drug accumulation**—The build up of drug in the body associated with repetitive administration due to some drug always remaining from previous doses.

   Accumulation index—Ratio of the amount at steady state, such as maximum or minimum, compared with the corresponding value after the first dose, following a regimen of fixed-dose and fixed-dosing interval.

   Average level at plateau—The average amount of drug in the body, or the average plasma concentration, at steady state after a regimen of fixed-dose and fixed-dosing interval.

   Loading dose—A dose, or a series of doses, given initially to rapidly attain the desired plasma concentration or amount of drug in the body. Sometimes it is called a priming dose.

   Maintenance dose—The dose needed to ensure maintenance of drug response, which is often achieved by maintaining a given exposure at steady state.

Modified-release product—A dosage form designed to slow or delay the release of drug compared with that produced with an immediate release dosage form.

Plateau—The condition in which there is no change in the profile of drug in the body from one dosing interval to another. It is also known as the steady-state condition and is usually associated with a regimen of fixed-dose and fixed-dosing interval.

Relative fluctuation—The difference between the maximum and minimum plasma concentrations compared with the average plasma concentration within a dosing interval at plateau following a regimen of fixed-dose and fixed-dosing interval.

Trough concentration—The lowest plasma concentration within a dosing interval of a regimen. It is usually the value just before the next dose is given.

2. a. **True.** The process of accumulation always occurs on multiple dosing, as some drug always remains in the body from the first dose when the second and subsequent doses are given.

b. **False.** The less frequently a drug is given, the lower its extent of accumulation.
c. **False.** The time to reach plateau depends on the elimination half-life.
d. **Only true if $F = 1$.**
e. **False.** $C_{av,ss}$ is independent of volume of distribution.
f. **False.** $C_{av,ss}$ is independent of the absorption kinetics, unless absorption becomes so protracted as to affect bioavailability.

3. a. (1) $A_{max,ss} = 100$ **mg;** $A_{min,ss} = 68$ **mg.**

$$k = \frac{CL}{V} \qquad A_{max,ss} = \frac{F \cdot Dose}{(1 - e^{-k\tau})} \qquad A_{min,ss} = A_{max,ss}\, e^{-k\cdot\tau}$$

(2) **Accumulation ratio = 3.1.**

$$R_{ac} = \frac{1}{(1 - e^{-k\tau})}$$

(3) $C_{min,ss} = 0.24$ **mg/L.**

(4) **Time to reach 50% of plateau is 1.8 days ($t_{1/2}$).**

b. **See table below.**

TABLE J11-P3 **Maximum and Minimum Amounts of Chlorthalidone in the Body When 50 mg is Taken Once Daily**

Dose	1	2	3	3	5	6	7	∞
$A_{max,N}$ (mg)*	32	54	69	79	85	90	93	100
$A_{min,N}$ (mg)†	22	37	47	53	58	61	63	68

$$^*A_{max,N}\,(mg) = \frac{F \cdot Dose(1 - e^{-Nk\tau})}{(1 - e^{-k\tau})}$$

$$^\dagger A_{min,N} = A_{max,N} \cdot e^{-k\tau}$$

c. **Axes of the sketch of the data in the above table should be scaled as follows: Amount to 100 mg ($A_{max,ss}$) and time to at least 7 days (5 half-lives).**
d. **Loading dose = 150 mg ($A_{max,ss}/F$).**

4. **Three 100-mg tablets every 8 hr comes the closest. There are several possibilities, no single solution. All of the regimens explored below may suffice if the drug is given as a modified-release product.**

Maintenance Design

$$t_{1/2} = \frac{0.693 \cdot V}{CL} = 8.7 \ hr$$

$$t_{max} = 1.44 \cdot t_{1/2} \cdot log \ (C_{max}/C_{max}) = 8.7 \ hr$$

$$D_{max} = \frac{V}{F} \ (C_{max} - C_{min}) = \begin{array}{c} 5 \ mg/kg \ or \ 300 \ mg \\ of \ theophylline \end{array}$$

$$Dosing \ rate = \frac{D_{max}}{\tau_{max}} = \begin{array}{c} 34 \ mg/hr, \ 204 \ mg/6 \ hr, \\ 272 \ mg/8 \ hr, \ 408 \ mg/12 \ hr \end{array}$$

TABLE J11-P4 Possible Maintenance Regimens

Regimen	$C_{max,ss}$*	$C_{min,ss}$†	Comment
One 200-mg tablet every 6 hr‡	14.9	9.2	Under
Two 200-mg tablets every 8 hr	24	12.7	Over
Three 100-mg tablets every 8 hr	18	9.5	Under
Two 200-mg tablets every 12 hr	18.4	7.1	Under

$$*C_{max,ss} = \frac{F \cdot D}{V(1 - e^{-k\tau})}$$

$$†C_{min,ss} = C_{max,ss} e^{-k\tau}$$

‡One 200-mg tablet = 170-mg theophylline.

Loading dose

$$D_L = \frac{V}{F} \cdot C_{max,ss} = \frac{30}{1} \times 15 \ mg/L = 450 \ mg$$

That is, approximately three tablets of 170 mg of theophylline (200 mg of amino-phylline).

5. a. **Oral maintenance dosing rate = 6.2 mg/hr.**

$$Dose_{single} = \frac{CL}{F} \cdot AUC_{single} \qquad \frac{D_M}{\tau} = \frac{CL}{F} \cdot C_{av,ss}$$

$$\frac{D_M}{\tau} = Dose_{single} \cdot \frac{C_{av,ss}}{AUC_{single}} = 50 \ mg \times \frac{10 \ mg/L}{80.6 \ mg\text{-}hr/L} = 6.2 \ mg/hr$$

b. (1) **Maintenance dose = 75 mg** (12 hr × 6.2 mg/hr).

(2) **At plateau, the trough plasma concentration at 12 hr is 5.4 mg/L.** The trough concentration at plateau is the sum of the concentrations at 12, 24, 36, 48 hr, etc., after a single dose of 75 mg. Concentrations associated with a 75-mg oral dose are 1.5 times those obtained with a 50-mg oral dose. At plateau, one can ignore contributions from doses that are given more than 5 half-lives previously, that is, five times 8 hr, or 40 hr. Hence,

$$C_{ss}(12 \ hr) = 1.5 \ [C(12) + C(24) + C(36) + C(48)]$$

$$= 1.5 \ [2.8 + 0.6 + 0.14 + 0.03]$$

Note: Although helpful, it is not essential to know the half-life of the drug. One includes concentration values until they become insignificant, which can be judged directly from the concentration–time curve following the single oral dose. Also, either absorption or disposition can rate-limit the terminal decline. There is no need to determine F, CL, V, k, or ka to solve this problem.

6. a. **70 mg.** Situation analogous to a constant-rate infusion. Amount in formulation = $k \cdot A_{ss} \cdot \Delta t$, where Δt is time desired to maintain A_{ss}. Amount = $(0.693/4 \text{ hr}) \times 50$ mg $\times$ 8 hr.

   b. **Immediately.** Loading dose (50 mg) + sustaining dose (70 mg, released over 8 hr).

   c. **Total dose for day 1 = 260 mg; total dose for day 2 = 210 mg.**

   d.

TABLE J11-P6 **Amount in Body (mg)**									
Time (hr)	0	4	8	12	16	20	24	28	32	36
Regimen										
Every 4 hr	0	25	63	81	91	95	98	99	99.5	100
Every 8 hr	0	25	38	44	47	49	49	50	50	50
Every 12 hr	0	25	38	19	34	42	21	36	43	22

7. a. **Release from the modified-release product.** This conclusion follows from the terminal half-life following this product (5.5 hr) being much longer than after the immediate-release product (2.2 hr.)

   b. **Yes.** The time taken to reach plateau is essentially determined by the half-life associated with the terminal decline phase. For the immediate-release product ($t_{1/2} = 2.2$ hr), a plateau is expected to be reached by 3.3 $t_{1/2}$ or 7.3 hr, that is, by the second dose of the 8-hourly regimen. For the modified-release product ($t_{1/2} = 5.5$ hr), a plateau should be reached by 18 hr. That is, by the third dose of the 12-hourly regimen. In the multiple-dose study, both preparations were administered for 7 days.

   c. **Yes, very close.**

   For immediate-release (IR) product: 40 mg every 8 hr.

$$AUC_{ss}(0\text{–}24)_{expected} = 3 \times AUC(single)_{40\ mg} = 3 \times 0.57\ mg\text{-}hr/L$$

$$= 1.71\ mg\text{-}hr/L$$

$$AUC_{ss}(0\text{–}24)_{observed} = 1.57\ mg\text{-}hr/L$$

   For modified-release product:

$$AUC_{ss}(0\text{–}24)_{expected} = 2 \times AUC(single)\ 60\ mg = 2 \times 0.88\ mg\text{-}hr/L$$

$$= 1.76\text{-}hr/L$$

$$AUC(0\text{–}24\ hr)_{observed} = 1.57\ mg\text{-}hr/L$$

   d. **Following single dose, $F_{rel} = 1.03$; on multiple dosing, $F_{rel} = 0.91$.**
   Single dose

$$f_{rel} = \frac{[AUC/Dose]_{MR}}{[AUC/Dose]_{IR}} = \frac{[0.88\ mg\text{-}hr/L/60\ mg]}{[0.57\ mg\text{-}hr/L/40\ mg]} = 1.03$$

   Multiple dosing

$$f_{rel} = \frac{[AUC_{SS}/Dose]_{MR}}{[AUC_{SS}/Dose]_{IR}} = \frac{[1.57\ mg\text{-}hr/L/120\ mg]}{[0.72\ mg\text{-}hr/L/20\ mg]} = 0.91$$

e. **Yes.** Generally, t_{max} after multiple dosing is shorter than after single-dose administration. This arises because, with accumulation, the condition when rate of elimination equals rate of absorption is met earlier with multiple dosing. In the specific case of adinazolam, the t_{max} values following single doses of the IR and MR products are 1.0 and 2.5 hr, respectively, which are already short relative to the multiple-dosing intervals of 8 hr, respectively, for these products. Hence, following multiple dosing, the durations over which the plasma concentration are expected to decline are at least 7 hr for the IR and MR products, respectively. These times are at least 3 expected terminal half-lives for the IR product and close to 2 expected terminal half-lives for MR product. Obviously, for the MR product, it would be better to determine the half-life after stopping administration. Clearly, difficulties in estimating the terminal half-life within the dosing interval would be expected had the MR product been given 8 hourly.

f. **Degree of accumulation is 1.27 for the IR product and 1.78 for the MR product.**

$$Degree\ of\ accumulation = \frac{AUC\ (0 - \tau)_{ss}}{AUC\ (0 - \tau)_{single}}$$

For both IR and MR products, information provided concerns the AUC over 24 hr at plateau ($AUC[(0–24\ hr]_{ss}$), that is, over three dosing intervals for IR product and two dosing intervals for the MR product. Hence,

for IR product,

$$Degree\ of\ accumulation = \frac{(1.72\ mg\text{-}hr/L)/3}{0.45\ mg\text{-}hr/L}$$

for MR product,

$$Degree\ of\ accumulation = \frac{(1.57\ mg\text{-}hr/L)/2}{0.44\ mg\text{-}hr/L}$$

8. a. **Average steady-state concentrations: acetaminophen = 7.14 mg/L; ibuprofen = 13.3 mg/L; naproxen = 72.0 mg/L.**

Equation	Acetaminophen	Ibuprofen	Naproxen
$C_{av,ss} = \dfrac{F \cdot Dose}{CL \cdot \tau}$	$\dfrac{0.9 \times 1000\ mg}{21\ L/hr \times 6\ hr} = 7.14$	$\dfrac{0.7 \times 400\ mg}{3.5\ L/hr \times 6\ hr} = 13.3$	$\dfrac{0.95 \times 500\ mg}{0.55\ L/hr \times 12\ hr} = 72\,(mg/L)$

Note that despite the longer dosing interval and the relatively modest maintenance dose, the $C_{av,ss}$ of naproxen is much higher than that of the other two drugs because of its much lower clearance.

b. **Ibuprofen reaches plateau the fastest.** The time to reach a plateau depends only on the half-life; the shorter the half-life, the sooner the plateau is reached. The half-lives of the three drugs are:

Equation	Acetaminophen	Ibuprofen	Naproxen
$t_{1/2} = \dfrac{0.693 \cdot V}{CL}$	$\dfrac{0.693 \times 67\ L}{21\ L/hr} = 2.21$	$\dfrac{0.693 \times 10\ L}{3.5\ L/hr} = 1.98$	$\dfrac{0.693 \times 11\ L}{0.55\ L/hr} = 14\,(hr)$

Note that in practice, the difference in the half-lives of acetaminophen and ibuprofen is inconsequential. For both drugs, the plateau is effectively achieved by the time the second dose is given, 6 hr after the first one. With naproxen, there is a case for giving a loading dose if the full therapeutic effect is needed as soon as possible; otherwise, it would take about 2 days to reach plateau. Increased gastric irritation is an argument for not doing so.

c. **Naproxen accumulates the most extensively, even though its dosing interval is the longest.**

	Equation	Acetaminophen	Ibuprofen	Naproxen
Accumulation Ratio	$\dfrac{1}{(1 - e^{-kt})}$	$\dfrac{1}{\left(1 - e^{-\frac{21\,L/hr\,\times\,6\,hr}{67\,L}}\right)}$ $= 1.18$	$\dfrac{1}{\left(1 - e^{-\frac{3.5\,L/hr\,\times\,6\,hr}{10\,L}}\right)}$ $= 1.14$	$\dfrac{1}{\left(1 - e^{-\frac{0.55\,L/hr\,\times\,12\,hr}{11\,L}}\right)}$ $= 2.22$

Notice that the greatest degree of accumulation occurs with naproxen, because it is given more frequently relative to its half-life than the other two drugs.

d. **The maximum concentrations at plateau are ibuprofen = 31.9 mg/L, naproxen = 95.7 mg/L.**

	Equation	Ibuprofen	Naproxen
$C_{max,ss}$ (mg/L)	$\dfrac{F \cdot Dose}{V \cdot (1 - e^{-k \cdot \tau})}$	$\dfrac{0.7 \times 400\,mg}{10 \times \left(1 - e^{-\frac{3.5\,L/hr\,\times\,6\,hr}{10}}\right)} = 31.9$	$\dfrac{0.95 \times 500\,mg}{11 \times \left(1 - e^{-\frac{0.55\,L/hr\,\times\,12\,hr}{11}}\right)} = 95.7$

e. **The minimum concentrations at plateau are ibuprofen = 3.91 mg/L, naproxen = 52.5 mg/L.**

	Equation	Ibuprofen	Naproxen
$C_{min,ss}$ (mg/L)	$C_{max,ss}\,e^{-k \cdot \tau}$	$31.9 \times e^{-\frac{3.5\,L/hr\,\times\,6\,hr}{10\,L}} = 3.91$	$95.7 \times e^{-\frac{0.55\,L/hr\,\times\,12\,hr}{11\,L}} = 52.5$

f. **Relative fluctuations are ibuprofen = 2.1, naproxen = 0.6.**

	Equation	Ibuprofen	Naproxen
Relative Fluctuation	$\dfrac{C_{max,ss} - C_{min,ss}}{C_{av,ss}}$	$\dfrac{31.9 - 3.91}{13.3} = 2.1$	$\dfrac{95.7 - 52.5}{72} = 0.60$

Note: The fluctuation of naproxen concentration is much less than that of ibuprofen, even though it is given every 12 hr compared with every 6 hr. This is primarily a function of the disproportionately longer half-life of naproxen.

9. This is often the case, but not always so, such as when tolerance to the beneficial effect occurs.

10. a. **No. But relative to elimination, yes.**

The plasma concentrations of the enantiomers after a single dose peak at 18 and 30 hr, indicating that absorption continues for some time. However, relative to the respective half-lives of 128 and 409 hr, the peak concentrations are indeed rapidly achieved.

b. **Both V and CL increase for (+)-MQ relative to those of (−)-MQ.**

The following discussion applies to the single-dose data. A difference in C_{max} (0.36 mg/L for (−)-MQ versus 0.12 mg/L for (+)-MQ) primarily reflects a difference in V/F. If F is not changed, then V is greater for (+)-MQ.

The difference in $AUC(0–\infty)$ (i.e., 20 mg-hr/L for $(+)$MQ and 190 mg-hr/L for $(-)$-MQ) reflects a difference in CL/F $(Dose/AUC)$. If F is unchanged, then CL is almost 10-fold greater for $(+)$-MQ.

c. $C_{max,ss} = 1.45$ mg/L.

$$C_{max,ss} = \frac{C_{max,1}}{1 - e^{-k\tau}} = \frac{0.36}{1 - e^{-\frac{0.693}{409} \times 168}}$$

$$k = \frac{0.693}{409\ hr} \qquad \tau = 24\ hr/day \times 7\ days = 168\ hr$$

The observation was 1.42 mg/L, an almost identical value.

d. **Yes, but not for individuals with half-lives greater than about 4 weeks (672 hr).**

The $(-)$-MQ isomer has an average half-life of 430 hr on multiple dosing. Thirteen weeks is 2184 hr (168 hr/week $\times$ 13) or about 5.1 half-lives (2184 hr/439 hr). However, its standard deviation is 255 hr. Therefore, some individuals may have much longer half-lives. If 2184 hr is 3.32 half-lives, the corresponding half-life is 657 hr. For those individuals with half-lives of this value or higher, steady state is not yet achieved.

e. **Accumulation ratio = 4.0.**

$$Accumulation\ Ratio = \frac{1}{1 - e^{-k\tau}} = \frac{1}{1 - e^{-\frac{0.693 \times 168}{409}}} = 4.0$$

f. **Relative fluctuation of steady state: $(+)$-MQ = 0.83; $(-)$-MQ = 0.35.**

$$Relative\ fluctuation = \frac{C_{max,ss} - C_{min,ss}}{C_{av,ss}}$$

For $(+)$-MQ,

$$Relative\ fluctuation = \frac{0.26 - 0.11}{0.18}$$

For $(-)$MQ,

$$Relative\ fluctuation = \frac{0.42 - 1.01}{0.17}$$

The difference in the values is explained by $(+)$-MQ having a much shorter half-life ($\sim$173 hr) than $(-)$-MQ ($\sim$430 hr), therefore showing greater fluctuation on the once-weekly regimen.

g. **Yes. For both treatment and prevention.**

The accumulation ratio for once-weekly dosing was 4 (part e above). Thus, a loading dose of four or five tablets seems reasonable to rapidly achieve the steady-state level normally achieved on once-a-week dosing. The half-life is so long that the single large loading dose comprises the dosage regimen. If a patient does not respond to the drug in 48 to 72 hr, an alternative therapy should be considered.

The requirement of 2 to 3 weekly doses before going to an endemic area allows some accumulation to occur before being exposed to the parasite. Three weeks is 504 hr (3 $\times$ 168 hr); this is well over one average half-life. Thus, the plasma concentration is now more than 50% of the steady-state value.

11. **Minimum oral maintenance dose = 220 mg.**
    The renal clearance of ampicillin is 128 mL/min (CL_R = fe · CL = 0.8 × 160 mL/min). The plasma ampicillin concentration when the urine concentration is 50 mg/L is therefore 0.39 mg/L.

$$C = \frac{(Urine\ flow) \cdot (Urine\ drug\ concentration)}{CL_R} = \frac{1\ mL/min \times 50\ mg/L}{128\ mL/min}$$

The steady-state trough plasma concentration must be 0.39 mg/L. The maintenance dose required to achieve this value is 220 mg.

$$C_{min,ss} = \frac{F \cdot Dose}{V} \cdot \frac{e^{-k\tau}}{(1 - e^{-k\tau})}$$

Rearranging,

$$Dose = \frac{C_{min,ss} \cdot V (1 - e^{-k\tau})}{F \cdot e^{-k\tau}} = 220\ mg$$

$$k = 0.48\ hr^{-1};\ \tau = 6\ hr;\ V = 20\ L;\ and\ F = 0.6$$

12. **Pharmacodynamics, rather than pharmacokinetics, drives the choice of a dosage regimen when the therapeutic effect is obtained when the response is near E_{max}; response develops or declines slowly relative to systemic exposure due to sluggish nature of affected system within the body; tolerance develops to adverse effects of drug.**

CHAPTER 12. VARIABILITY

1. **Adherence**—The keeping by the patient to the prescribed dosage regimen. It includes the dose, the interval between doses, and the duration of treatment.

   Coefficient of variation—The ratio of the standard deviation of a measure to its mean. It is a dimensionless value that allows comparison of the degree of variability of quantities that are often of different dimensions, such as body weight and drug clearance. It is often expressed as a percent.

   Intrapatient variability—Variability in a parameter value or a measure observed within an individual patient when assessed repeatedly. A related term is interoccasional variability, which is the variability in a parameter or measure from one occasion to another, for example, following administration of drug on two occasions.

   Persistence—The continued adherence of a patient to the prescribed dosage regimen for the duration of treatment, be that a week, a month, or a lifetime.

   Population pharmacokinetics—Study of the central tendency (mean) and the variability in the pharmacokinetic measures and model parameters of a drug within the population, particularly within the population for which the drug is intended.

2. **Six major sources of variability in drug response are genetics, age, body weight, disease, concurrent drugs, and nonadherence to a regimen.** The relative importance of each of depends on the drug, the response, and the patient population being treated. Genetics is often the most important, but least understood, of these sources of variability, and only recently has knowledge and technology become available that promises to help predict likely outcomes from genomic information. In addition, there is sometimes a significant degree of covariance between these sources. For example, during early development to adulthood, much of the influence of age on pharmacokinetic parameters can be explained by body size.

3. Understanding, and in particular quantifying, variability in drug response is very important in the optimization of drug administration for the individual patient. There is a view that one dose fits all, but as our understanding of variability in drug response and the relative contribution of pharmacokinetics and pharmacodynamics as well as important factors influencing such variability improves, it is clear that often there is a need to adjust the dosage regimen of many drugs to the individual. One important distinction to be made is between *inter*individual and *intra*individual variability. Large interindividual variability in pharmacokinetics and pharmacodynamics is often reflected in a range of dose strengths being made available for a drug. Large intraindividual variability would make stabilization of drug therapy for an individual patient difficult, unless the therapeutic index of the drug was very wide. Fortunately, in most cases intraindividual variability is much smaller than interindividual variability.

4. **Low therapeutic index drugs, for which the therapeutic dose is close to the dose giving undue adverse events, have a low intrasubject variability in both pharmacokinetics and pharmacodynamics, but intersubject variability in either pharmacokinetics or pharmacodynamics, or both, may be high and is accommodated by the availability of different dose strengths.**

    When the intersubject variability is high in pharmacokinetics, plasma drug concentration monitoring may be of value (e.g., phenytoin). When intersubject variability in pharmacodynamics is high, drug administration is possible only if there is a good measure of drug response (e.g., blood pressure).

5. a. Answers provided in Table J12-P5.

TABLE J12-P5	Unbound Steady-State Concentration, Clearance, and Volume of Distribution of a Drug in Five Subjects				
Subject	1	2	3	4	5
Cu_{ss} (mg/L)	0.25	0.24	**0.27**	**0.24**	0.28
CL (L/hr)	**8**	12.5	6.7	13.3	**8.7**
V (L)	**7.8**	34.3	**16.4**	57.6	35.2

    b. (1) Volume of distribution is the most variable and Cu_{ss} the least variable because these have the largest and smallest coefficient of variability, respectively.
    (2) As V is much more variable than fu and depends on both fu and fu_T, tissue binding (fu_T) appears to be the major source of variability in V.
    c. Therapeutically, unbound concentration is more important than total plasma concentration. As such, given that the unbound concentration is very similar among the patients, they can all receive the same of infusion (assuming that the interindividual variability in pharmacodynamics is small). If the decision is to give a loading dose to achieve the same unbound concentration, the dose needed differs by a factor of 2 among the patients (which can be seen by calculating dose, from the relationship: $Dose = V \cdot C = V \cdot Cu/fu$, and noting that $Vu = V/fu$ ranges from 161–360 L). Clearly, different conclusions would have been reached had the calculation erroneous been based on the total plasma concentration.

6. **Wide differences in hepatic metabolic activity.** Alprenolol is highly cleared by the liver. Accordingly, differences in hepatic enzyme activity do not produce much variability in clearance, which is perfusion rate-limited; but these small differences in clearance may cause wide differences in bioavailability ($F_H = 1 - E_H$).

7. a. **There is the danger of not being able to define a clear dose–response relationship.** The fourfold range in dose is less than the fivefold range in clearance, so that some

patients of low clearance receiving the low-dose regimen will have similar average plasma concentrations to those of high clearance receiving the high-dose regimen, thereby potentially introducing considerable variability in the dose–response relationship. One solution is to use very large numbers of patients in each group.

b. **If feasible in clinical practice, a more efficient design, requiring fewer patients to test for a dose–response relationship, involves exposing each patient to two, and preferably all three, doses strengths of the drug.** Refer to the heading "Defining the Dose–Response Relationship" in this chapter for further discussion.

8. **Although the underlying effect, sedation, is graded, the clinical response adopted is all-or-none; the patient either met the desired criterion used (e.g., lack of gag response to gastroscope insertion) or he/she did not.** The curve reflects the distribution of the relationship between the measured propofol concentration and the desired event within the patient population. The difference in steepness of the probability of the desired event against plasma propofol concentration reflects differences in interpatient variability; the shallower the curve, the greater is the interpatient variability. If all patients were identical in their response–concentration relationship, the probability of the desired event curve would be a straight vertical line from 0% to 100% at that concentration that produces the all-or-none effect. The difference in C_{50} values among the three measured desired events reflects differences in average potency among the patients studied. However, the differences are not large. More important is the fraction of the patient group in whom the desired endpoint is met. Notice that although some of the patients needed a lower concentration of propofol to avoid the gag response to gastroscope insertion than the other two desired endpoints, much higher concentrations were needed for other patients, and even at the highest concentration, some patients still had a gag response, whereas all patients responded favorably in relation to response to verbal command and to lack of a somatic response to gastroscope insertion.

CHAPTER 13. GENETICS

1. **Allele**—One of the two alternate forms each occupying corresponding positions on paired chromosomes, one inherited from the male and the other the female.

   Genotype—The internally coded, inheritable information of a living organism, contained within the DNA. It is the "blueprint" or set of instructions for all components within a living organism.

   Genetic polymorphism—The occurrence of distinguishable differences in a given characteristic under genetic control, defined clinically as occurring with a frequency of at least 1% within the population.

   Haplotype—A set of nearby single-nucleotide polymorphisms (SNPs) on the same chromosome, inherited as a block rather than a single SNP, which determines phenotypic behavior.

   Heterozygous—An individual possessing a pair of different alleles for a gene.

   Pharmacogenomics—The application of genomic information to the identification of drug targets and to an understanding of the genetic causes of variability in drug response.

   Phenotype—Anything that is part of the observable structure, function, or behavior of a living organism, such as their weight, metabolic function, and physical appearance.

2. **Pharmacodynamic sources of variability can be distinguished from pharmacokinetic sources in drug response by measuring drug (and metabolite, if important) exposure**

(usually in plasma) and response in the patient population receiving the drug. Preferably, concentration and response should be determined in the same patient, but this is not always possible or appropriate, for example, because the taking of a blood sample, with its associated trauma, may influence the response itself. Also, preferably, any pharmacodynamic relationship should be based on unbound drug concentration, particularly in situations where plasma protein binding is known to be variable within the patient population.

Examples of inherited variability in pharmacokinetics include clearance of nortriptyline caused by polymorphism of CYP2D6; clearance of S-warfarin caused by polymorphism of CYP2C9, and clearance of azathioprine caused by polymorphism of thiopurine S-methyltransferase. In each of these cases, the drug can be any substrate for which its elimination is predominantly mediated by the respective enzyme.

Examples of inherited variability in pharmacodynamics include response to trastuzumab (Herceptin) in the treatment of primary breast cancer caused by polymorphism of the HER 2 proto-oncogene; FEV_1 (forced expiratory volume in 1 sec) to β-adrenergic agonists, such as albuterol, caused by polymorphism of the receptor; development of cough in some patients on ACE inhibitors caused by polymorphism in the bradykinin B2 receptor. Other examples are provided in the chapter.

3. **An inherited source of variability in a pharmacokinetic parameter is suggested by a polymodal distribution of the parameter value within the population and by comparative studies between identical and nonidentical twins.** It is characterized by familial studies and by correlation studies with genotypic status and with other drugs that are known to exhibit genetically determined polymorphism in their pharmacokinetics.

4. **The optimal dosage regimen of the drug may vary among different ethnic groups.** The frequency of slow acetylators varies being relatively high in whites and blacks, and low in Japanese and Chinese. The therapeutic implication depends on whether activity and toxicity resides in drug, in the *N*-acetylated metabolite, or both. The implication is clear. Due regard to ethnicity should be taken in the prescribing of drugs worldwide. That said, within any ethnic group, there is often substantial interindividual variability, and knowing genotypic status and other factors may be very important when treating the individual patient.

5. The poor correlation of atenolol pharmacokinetics with CYP2D6 genotype status is expected; atenolol is primarily excreted unchanged. The strong correlations seen with metoprolol and timolol indicate that they are predominantly eliminated either via a major metabolic pathway or via several pathways that involve CYP2D6. Propranolol is predominantly metabolized; the weak correlation with this compound suggest that the major metabolic pathways involved (e.g., formation of naphthoxylactic acid, Chapter 20, *Metabolites and Drug Response*) are not eliminated by CYP2D6-catalyzed metabolism. Note that metoprolol and propranolol are high hepatic clearance compounds (the plasma-to-blood concentration ratio of both is close to 1), so that the clearances of both are less sensitive to an underlying variation is intrinsic hepatocellular clearance than had they been low–extraction ratio compounds.

6. a. **Encainide, dextromethorphan.** See Table 13-1 for additional examples.

   b. (1) Normally, flecainide is predominantly excreted unchanged, so that variation in the formation of the metabolite via CYP2D6 has little effect on total clearance, and hence, dosage requirements. In patients with severe renal impairment, however, little drug is excreted unchanged, and formation of the metabolite is the major route of drug elimination. Under such circumstances, genetic polymorphism is of increasingly therapeutic importance.

(2) The minor metabolite of dapsone is *N*-acetyldapsone, a less active antitubercular compound than dapsone. In contrast, although a minor metabolite, most of the analgesic activity associated with codeine administration is caused by morphine. Under such circumstances, genetic polymorphism of CYP2D6 is of considerable therapeutic importance.

(3) Quinidine is a specific inhibitor of CYP2D6, effectively converting extensive metabolizers to poor metabolizer status. For drugs for which genetic polymorphism involving CYP2D6 normally has a therapeutic implication, coadministration of quinidine is likely to produce a clinically significant drug interaction in extensive metabolizers.

c. Unlike CYP2D6, for example, which is not inducible, CYP3A4 is a highly inducible enzyme, so that even if there is genetic polymorphism in this enzyme its activity is dominated by environmental factors.

7. **Frequencies of slow and fast oxidizers are 2.25% and 97.75%, respectively.** Frequency of allele associated with slow oxidation (p) = 0.15; frequency of allele associated with fast oxidation (q) = 0.85. Hence, the frequency of homozygous slow oxidizers (p^2) is 0.0225; whereas 0.9775 ($2pq + q^2$) is the frequency of heterozygous and homozygous fast oxidizers.

CHAPTER 14. AGE, WEIGHT, AND GENDER

1. a. **False.** Oral bioavailability is independent of body weight; there is no rational basis to consider otherwise.

   b. **True.** Volume of distribution (V) per kilogram of body weight tends to be independent of body weight. An exception concerns distribution of polar compounds in the obese, where volume of distribution correlates better with ideal body weight than total body weight.

   c. **True.** In children beyond 1 year of age, CL tends to vary in direct proportion to body surface area (or $Wt^{0.75}$). As age increases, so does body weight, and as surface area/body weight decreases with increasing size, so does CL/body weight.

   d. **False.** Renal function tends to decrease by approximately 1% per year beyond 20 years of age.

   e. **False.** The half-life tends to be the shortest in the 1-year-old child.

2. a. **Issues are listed below.**

   Pharmacodynamic issues

   (1) What is the response–systemic exposure (Cu) relationship in the 1-month-old infant relative to an adult?

   (2) Does response vary with age in a 1-month-old infant?

   Pharmacokinetic issues

   (1) Are the changes in metabolism the same as those for a renally excreted drug?

   (2) How rapidly does renal clearance and metabolic clearance change with time about 1 month of age?

   (3) Is plasma protein binding altered in a 1-month-old child relative to that in an adult?

   (4) How variable are pharmacokinetic parameter values at this age?

   b. (1) **The daily dose needed to produce a given INR clearly decreases with age regardless of genetic makeup or gender.** Genetics also clearly plays a role in determining the daily dose required. Gender appears to be of minor importance. The dose in females is consistently lower in all genetic group classifications. As females in this age range (Fig. 14-6) are smaller by about the same percentage as the dose is lower, the dose per kilogram is about the same.

(2) **No.** There is no information to rule out this idea. Information on the change in metabolism with age, genetics, and gender is needed. Information on the genetic component at a given average age was provided in Fig. 13-4 in which genetic control of metabolism was shown to play a major role in determining dosage requirements. Further information is needed on the changes in metabolism with age and gender. The tendency for drugs, in general, is for metabolism to decrease with age, and therefore, there is no strong support for a conclusion that pharmacodynamics changes extensively with age or gender.

3. a. **No.** As a first approximation, the volume of distribution normalized for body weight (L/kg) is expected to be independent of body weight and age. The observed values are 18, 15, and 10 L/kg for children, young adults, and elderly adults, respectively. Possible explanations include variations in plasma protein and tissue binding with age.

   b. **Yes, for the elderly; no, for children.** First, consider the adults. Assuming a 1% per year decline in clearance, the expected clearance in a 69-year-old adult is reasonably close to the observed clearance, 50 L/hr. Second, consider the data in children. The observed clearance (93 L/hr) is much higher than that expected (65 L/hr). Assuming a 1% decline in clearance beyond 20 years,

   Expected clearance in a 20-year-old $= 1.14 \times CL(\text{32-year-old}) = 1.14 \times 98 \; L/hr$

   $$Expected\;child's\;clearance = \left(\frac{Wt_{child}}{Wt_{20-year-old}} \right)^{0.75} \cdot CL_{20-year-old}$$

   $$= \left(\frac{32 \; kg}{70 \; kg} \right)^{0.75} \times 112 \; L/hr = 65 \; L/hr$$

   There is no obvious explanation for the observation (93 L/hr) to be higher than that expected in children.

4. **7.0 mg/day.** By application of Eq. 14-5 in text,

   $$Child's\;maintenance\;dosage = 1.5 \times \left[\frac{10 \; kg}{70 \; kg} \right]^{0.75} \times 20 \; mg/day$$

   Because of an expected shorter half-life in the child than in adults, consideration should be given to administering one half the daily dose (3.5 mg) every 12 hr.

5. a. **165 mg (11 mg/kg) daily in divided doses.** Because the half-life is shorter in the child, a regimen of 80 mg every 12 hr or 50 mg every 8 hr is indicated. Calculation made using Eq. 14-6. *Note:* The age of the adult patient population was not given. If, as is likely, those adults with severe infections requiring gentamicin are older; then assuming a mean age of 60 years, as was done, seems reasonable.

   b. **107 mg (1.7 mg/kg) gentamicin administered intramuscularly every 12 hr, or 214 mg (3.4 mg/kg) administered every 24 hr.** The half-life is longer in the elderly patient compared with the typical patient. Calculation made using Eq. 14-6.

   Note: There is a relatively small difference in the maintenance dosing rate (mg/12 hr) between the 4-year-old child in part "a" and in this elderly patient, despite the large difference in body weight.

   c. **7 mg (or 2.8 mg/kg) every 24 hr.**
   From the relationship $CL_{cr} \; (mL/hr) = 0.0045 \; e^{+ \; 0.16 \times \text{age (in weeks)}}$ for premature neonates and for conceptional age of 36 weeks,

   $$CL_{cr} = 0.0045 \; e^{+0.16 \times 36} = 1.5 \; mL/min$$

To maintain the same average plasma concentration as a typical adult,

$$Dosage\ rate\ in\ infant = \frac{1.5\ mL/min}{75\ mL/min} \times Adult\ dosing\ rate$$

$$= 0.02 \times \frac{350\ mg}{day}$$

Note: Because of a longer half-life in the premature infant, a dosing interval of 24 hr or more may be more appropriate (same daily dose). Consideration should also be given to a loading dose (e.g., 3–5 mg/kg, a usual initial dose in adults).

6. a. **The observations, in broad agreement with the expectations for a drug primarily excreted, suggest that biliary excretion follows a trend with age similar to that of renal function.** The low clearance per square meter of body surface area in the neonate and the elder reflects depressed excretory function at both extremes of life. Between 1 and 20 years, clearance per square meter is expected to be relatively constant; data in this age range are too few to draw a firm conclusion.

   b. **The half-life should be shortest at around 1 to 2 years of age, and should be greater than the minimum by a factor of 2 to 3 at the extremes of age.** This conclusion is based on the relationship $t_{1/2} = 0.693\ V/CL$; volume of distribution does not vary much on a weight basis, but clearance per square meter of body surface area is at a maximum around 1 year of age. As clearance per square meter varies by a factor of 3 (Fig. 14-7), so should half-life.

   c. **Dosing rate needs to be reduced in neonates and in patients older than 70 years of age, even when correcting for weight.** Because of a longer half-life, dosing less frequently than in the typical adult patient should be considered at these ages.

7. a. **Much depends on the therapeutic window of the drug.** For felodipine, it is relatively narrow, and it would seem appropriate to consider adjusting dose for age. It is noted, however, that hypertensive patients are generally middle aged or older and with only a modest increase in $AUC(0–12\ hr)_{ss}$, between those in the age groups 40 and 59 and 60 and 80 years, dose adjustment for age might not be needed. An increase in the usual adult dose might be appropriate if felodopine is used to treat young adults with hypertension.

   b. **There is no trend for a change in the volume of distribution with age.** The estimated mean values of $V (= 1.44 \cdot CL \cdot t_{1/2})$ are 17, 15, and 15 L/kg for the age groups 20 to 39, 40 to 59, and 60 to 80 years, respectively. Given the inherent interpatient variability of this, and other pharmacokinetic parameters, the changes in V with age are not significant.

   c. **F = 0.14, 0.16, 0.14 for the age groups 20 to 39, 40 to 59, and 60 to 80 years, respectively.** At steady state: $F \cdot Dose = CL \cdot AUC_{ss,\tau}$. Note that $CL \cdot AUC_{ss,\tau}$ has been normalized to a 10-mg twice-daily regimen.

$$F_{20–39\ years} = \frac{(0.82\ L/min \times 60\ min/hr) \times 0.028\ mg\text{-}hr/L}{10\ mg}$$

$$F_{40–59\ years} = \frac{(0.64\ L/min \times 60\ min/hr) \times 0.041\ mg\text{-}hr/L}{10\ mg}$$

$$F_{60–80\ years} = \frac{(0.45\ L/min \times 60\ min/hr) \times 0.052\ mg\text{-}hr/L}{10\ mg}$$

   d. **First-pass hepatic loss.** The clearance of felodipine is high, and with little excreted unchanged in urine, the most likely explanation for the low bioavailability in all age groups is first-pass metabolic loss.

e. **Clearance.** $AUC(0 - \tau)_{ss} = F \cdot Dose/CL$. Although F does not change with age, the decrease in CL explains the increase in $AUC(0 - \tau)_{ss}$ with advancing age.

f. **A decrease in hepatic blood flow with increasing age.** For drugs for which a low oral bioavailability is caused by first-pass hepatic loss, $F \approx 1 - F_H = 1 - CL_{b,H}/Q_H$. For F not to change, the ratio of $CL_{b,H}/Q_H$ must remain constant. But, as CL (a reflector of $CL_{b,H}$) decreases with increasing age, Q_H would also need to decrease in parallel for F_H to remain constant.

8. a. **Differences among theophylline, digoxin, and diazepam can be explained by differences in the partitioning of these drugs into fat.** Obese adult patients primarily differ from normal patients in having a much greater addition of fat; the body water space is essentially unchanged. Both theophylline and digoxin are poorly lipophilic and so, for these drugs, volume of distribution does not increase with the increase in body fat. In contrast, diazepam is lipophilic, and so its volume of distribution increases in the obese patient, both on absolute and weight-corrected bases.

b. **The information has relevance to the loading dose and the degree of fluctuation in plasma concentration on chronic dosing, but not to the maintenance dose requirement, which depends on clearance.** No weight correction in the loading dose is needed for either digoxin or theophylline. Diazepam is administered intravenously over 1 to 4 min as a sedative, for relief of muscle spasm and as an anticonvulsant. Under these circumstances, because fat is poorly perfused, there may be little difference in the initial concentrations in plasma and in highly perfused tissue, such as the brain, in obese patients compared with normal-weight patients. Accordingly, there may be little need to adjust the i.v. dose of diazepam in the obese patient. A loading dose is not used with oral diazepam regimens. However, associated with the larger volume of distribution is a longer half-life of diazepam in the obese patient. Even so, because the half-life of diazepam in normal-weight patients is already long ($\sim$40 hr), there should be no need to adjust the usual recommended dosing regimen of diazepam in obese patients, although there may be less fluctuation in the plasma concentration at plateau.

9. a.

	Recommended Daily Dose (mg)	Predicted Daily Dose (mg)
Adult (15 years and older)	10 mg	10 mg
Child (6–14 years)	5 mg	**5.7 mg**
Child (2–5 years)	4 mg	**3.3 mg**
Child (12–24 months)	4 mg	**2.7 mg**

Child (6–14 years) $\left(\dfrac{33}{70}\right)^{0.75} \times 10 = 5.7$

Child (2–5 years) $\left(\dfrac{16}{70}\right)^{0.75} \times 10 = 3.3$

Child (12–25 months) $\left(\dfrac{12}{70}\right)^{0.75} \times 10 = 2.7$

b. **Probably not.** Asthma is a disease of childhood, but occurs at all ages (see Fig. 14-2). Allergic rhinitis can occur at any age, but a 60-year-old patient again probably does not well represent a "typical" patient.

c. **No.** The number (0.21) is simply the ratio of weights. The ratio of weights to the 0.75 power is 0.315, a value closer to the expected relative clearance of the drug.

10. a. **260 mg.**

$$1.5 \times \left(\frac{15}{70}\right)^{0.75} \times 500 \; mg$$

b. **811 mg.**

$$\frac{(140 - 20)}{(140 - 60)} \times \left(\frac{82}{70}\right)^{0.75} \times 500 \; mg$$

c. **277 mg.**

$$\frac{(140 - 92)}{(140 - 60)} \times \left(\frac{63}{70}\right)^{0.75} \times 500 \; mg$$

d. **All three.** The 4-year-old and the 92-year-old patients practically should be given the 250-mg tablet. The 20-month-old patient should be the given the 750-mg tablet.

11. a. **6.7%.** MAC $= 1.32 \times 10^{-0.00303 \times Age}$; $\log_{10}$ MAC $= \log_{10} 1.32 - 0.00303 \times$ Age; Slope $= -0.00303 \; year^{-1}$

In 10 years, the decrease in log MAC is 0.0303, that is, $\Delta(Log_{10}$ MAC$) = 0.0303$. Taking the antilogarithm of both sides of the equation, ΔMAC $= 0.067$ or 6.7%.

b. **Yes, but the apparent change (13% predicted from the equation) is small compared with the variability observed.**

c. **Approximately threefold smaller in the 80-year-old patient.** The anticipated metabolic clearance in the 80-year-old patient is half that in a 20-year-old patient.

$$CL \; (80\text{-}year\text{-}old)\left(\frac{140 - 80}{140 - 20}\right) \cdot CL \; (20\text{-}year\text{-}old)$$

From Fig. 14-24, the MAC is about 0.75 in the 80-year-old patient and 1.2 in the 20-year-old patient (i.e., decreased to 63% of that in the 20-year-old). Thus, the rate of metabolism in the 20-year-old patient at the same anesthetic effect is nearly three times that of the 80-year-old patient.

$$\frac{Rate \; of \; metabolism \; (80\text{-}year\text{-}old)}{Rate \; of \; metabolism \; (20\text{-}year\text{-}old)} = \frac{CL \; (80\text{-}year\text{-}old)}{CL \; (20\text{-}year\text{-}old)} \times \frac{MAC \; (80\text{-}year\text{-}old)}{MAC \; (20\text{-}year\text{-}old)}$$

$$= \quad 0.5 \quad \times \quad 0.63$$
$$= \quad 0.313$$

CHAPTER 15. DISEASE

1. a. **Drugs must be administered cautiously to patients with hepatic and cardiovascular diseases.** Hepatic cirrhosis often requires a reduction in the usual daily dose. Variability in clearance is increased in this condition. Congestive cardiac failure is another disease often requiring adjustment of dosage, particularly for those drugs of high hepatic extraction, because of reduced hepatic blood flow.

b. **Dialysis**—Separation of large from small molecules by the preferential passive movement of small molecules through a semipermeable membrane.
Extracorporeal dialysis—Dialysis of substances outside the body. Substances are delivered from the body to the dializing system by the blood.
Hemodialysis—A form of extracorporeal dialysis in which blood and dialysate fluid each flow past opposite sides of a semipermeable membrane, permitting small molecules to be removed from the body.

Continuous ambulatory peritoneal dialysis—Continuous reinstallation, after a dwell time of 4 to 12 hr, of dialysate fluid into the peritoneal cavity. The peritoneal lining functions as a semipermeable membrane, allowing only small molecules (not large proteins) to move into the peritoneal cavity and be removed from the body.

Dialysis clearance—Rate of removal of a substance in the dialysate relative to its concentration in the plasma entering the dialyzer under steady-state conditions. Blood dialysis clearance and unbound dialysis clearance are the parameters that relate the rate of removal to the drug concentration in blood and plasma water, respectively.

Dialyzer—A general term for the apparatus by which hemodialysis is carried out.

Dialyzer efficiency—Ratio of the rate of removal of a substance to the rate of its presentation to the dialyzer under steady-state conditions.

Clinical dialyzability—A general term for the relative ability of dialysis to remove drug from the body. It is quantified by the ratio of the amount removed during the procedure relative to the amount initially in the body. The value of the ratio is the product of the fraction eliminated by dialysis and the fraction lost by all routes of elimination during the dialysis period.

2. a. **B > D > C > E > A.** Calculated from Eq. 15-8 for a typical 60-year-old, 70-kg patient.

   b. **B and perhaps C and D.** The recommendation depends on how much of a change in systemic exposure one believes is required for it to become clinically important.

3. a. **For both pentazocine and meperidine, the blood clearance in control patients is sufficiently high to expect hepatic bioavailabilities $(1 - CL_b/Q_H)$ of about 8% and 33%, respectively. (Hypothesis: elimination occurs only in the liver and hepatic blood flow is 1.35 L/min).** For both drugs, cirrhosis appears to decrease clearance by about 35% to 37% and to increase bioavailability by 278% and 81%, respectively. Decreased blood flow would explain the decreased clearance but would not explain the extent to which bioavailability is increased. Decreased metabolic activity and shunting of portal blood would explain the effects on both CL and F. Shunting of blood around the liver has been shown to occur in cirrhosis and is probably the major mechanism for the increase in F.

   b. **The bioavailability of pentazocine is more extensively affected by cirrhosis than that of meperidine, because it has the higher hepatic extraction ratio.** The higher the extraction ratio, the lower is the bioavailability and the greater is the effect of a decrease in metabolic activity or shunting on bioavailability.

4. Patients:

	S.W.	B.J.	D.A	B.T.
a. Estimated creatinine clearance (mL/min)*:	134	16	10	27
b. Relative renal function (*RF*):	1.79	0.21	0.13	0.36

5. a. *Patient I:* **42.3 mL/min.**

$$Creatinine\ clearance = \frac{(140 - 29) \times 85}{72 \times 3.1}$$

This is probably an underestimate of the creatinine clearance in the patient. He is likely to be highly muscular and thus to produce creatinine at a rate well above that predicted by his weight. This would give rise to a serum creatinine higher than that which reflects his actual renal function.

Patient II: **28.5 mL/min.**

$$Creatinine\ clearance = \frac{(140 - 84) \times 52}{85 \times 1.2}$$

*See Table 15-3 for equations.

This value is probably an overestimate because her muscle mass is undoubtedly greatly reduced from her having been bedridden for several months, resulting in a lower rate of creatinine production and a lower serum creatinine than that which reflects her actual renal function.

Patient III: **39.4 mL/min, 34.6 to 41.5 mL/min.**

$$Creatinine\ clearance\ =\ \frac{0.48 \times 95}{0.40} \times \left(\frac{17}{70}\right)^{0.75} = 39.4\ mL/min$$

Compare with:

$$Creatinine\ clearance\ (child)\ =\ 120\ mL/min \times \left(\frac{17}{70}\right)^{0.75} = 41.5\ mL/min$$

Patient IV: **74.3 mL/min.**

$$Creatinine\ clearance\ =\ \frac{(140 - 49)}{85 \times 1.8}$$

This value may overestimate her creatinine clearance because this woman is grossly obese. Her creatinine production is not reflected by her additional body weight (fat).

b. **I., 27.8; II., 18.4; IV., 38.6 kg/m².** Calculated from:

$$BMI\ =\ \frac{Wt\ (in\ kg)}{Height\ (in\ meters)^2}$$

6. a. $C_{max,ss}$ = **48 mg/L**; $C_{min,ss}$ = **12 mg/L.**

$$V = 0.4 \times 70 = 28\ L$$

$$C_{max,ss}\ =\ \frac{Dose}{V}\left(\frac{1}{1 - e^{-k\tau}}\right)$$

$$=\ \frac{1000\ mg}{28\ L}\left(\frac{1}{1 - e^{-12 \times 0.693/6}}\right) = 48\ mg/L$$

$$C_{min,ss}\ =\ C_{max,ss} - Dose/V = 12\ mg/L$$

b. **Loading dose = 240 mg [(17/70) × 1000 mg]; Maintenance dose = 120 mg/12 hr.** Creatinine clearance expected in child is

$$\frac{(0.48 \times 108)}{2.7} \times \left(\frac{17}{70}\right)^{0.75} = 6.6\ mL/min$$

Creatinine clearance in a typical patient (60-year-old) is 75 mL/min

$$RF\ (child)\ =\ \frac{7.1\ mL/min}{75\ mL/min} = 0.095;\ fe(n) = 0.95$$

$$R_d =\ RF \cdot fe(t) + [1 - fe(t)]\left[\frac{(140 - Age) \times Wt^{0.75}}{1936}\right] = 0.090 + 0.029;$$

$$R_d = 0.119\ (an\ eightfold\ decrease\ in\ adult\ dosing\ rate).$$

Suggest reducing maintenance dosing rate about eightfold, that is, give 120 mg every 12 hr or 240 mg every 24 hr. For demonstrative purposes, a dosing interval of 12 hr is used.

c. Parameters in child: $CL = 7.1$ mL/min or 0.43 L/hr; $V = 6.8$ L (0.4 L/kg $\times$ 17 kg); $k = 0.063$ hr^{-1}; and $t_{1/2} = 11$ hr.

(1) **Dose: 600 mg every 12 hr, regimen adjusted for age and weight only.**

$$\frac{D_M}{\tau}(child) = \frac{(140 - Age) \times Weight^{0.75}}{1936} \cdot \frac{D_M}{\tau}(reference\ patient)$$

$$= 0.59 \times 1000\ mg/12\ hr$$

$$\approx 600\ mg\ every\ 12\ hr$$

(2) **Dose: 120 mg every 12 hr, adjusted for age, weight, and renal function.**

$$\frac{D_M}{\tau}(child) = R_d \cdot \frac{D_M}{\tau}(reference\ patient)$$

$$= 0.12 \times 1000\ mg/12\ hr$$

$$\approx 120\ mg/12\ hr$$

Note. Table below lists the calculated maximum amounts in the body in the child on approach to steady state on giving the maintenance regimens in (1) and (2). To plot the data, the appropriate scales are

Scale time to 4 to 5 half-lives ~48 hr.

Scale amount in body to $A_{ss,max}$ on regimen of 600 mg every 12 hr.

$$A_{ss,max} = \frac{1}{(1 - e^{-0.063 \times 12})} \approx 1200\ mg$$

TABLE J15-P6	**Maintenance Regimen**							
Time (hr)	0	12	121	24	241	36	361	48
			Amount in body (mg)					
600 mg/12 hr	600	282	882	414	1014	476	1076	505
120 mg/12 hr	120	56	176	83	203	95	215	101

+, just after the dose.

See Fig. J15-P6.

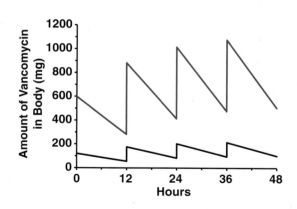

FIGURE J15-P6.

7. a. (1) **Oral bioavailability increased 2.3-fold.**

$$\frac{F_{cirrhotic}}{F_{healthy}} = \frac{\left[\dfrac{AUC_{oral}}{AUC_{i.v.}} \cdot \dfrac{Dose_{i.v.}}{Dose_{oral}}\right]_{cirrhotic}}{\left[\dfrac{AUC_{oral}}{AUC_{i.v.}} \cdot \dfrac{Dose_{i.v.}}{Dose_{oral}}\right]_{healthy}} = \frac{\dfrac{3.36}{1.14} \times \dfrac{100}{400}}{\dfrac{0.52}{0.41} \times \dfrac{100}{400}}$$

(2) **Volume of distribution is virtually unchanged (282 L versus 266 L).**

$$V = \frac{CL \cdot t_{1/2}}{0.693} = \frac{Dose_{i.v.} \cdot t_{1/2}}{AUC_{i.v.} \cdot 0.693}$$

$$V\,(cirrhotic) = \frac{100\ mg}{1.14\ mg\text{-}hr/L} \times \frac{2.1\ hr}{0.693} = 266\ L$$

$$V\,(healthy) = \frac{100\ mg}{0.41\ mg\text{-}hr/L} \times \frac{0.8\ hr}{0.693} = 282\ L$$

The same may not apply to Vu if plasma binding of the drug has changed in cirrhosis.

(3) **Clearance is decreased by a factor of 0.36. Half-life is increased from 0.8 to 2.1 hr.**

	Cirrhotic	*Healthy*
$CL = \dfrac{Dose_{i.v.}}{AUC_{i.v.}}$	$\dfrac{100\ mg}{1.14\ mg\text{-}hr/L}$	$\dfrac{100\ mg}{0.41\ mg\text{-}hr/L}$
	88 L/hr	*244 L/hr*

b. **The plasma clearance in the healthy patients exceeds hepatic blood flow.** No data were given on the ratio of blood and plasma concentrations, but the data suggest a high first-pass metabolism in the liver and, perhaps, even high clearance in extrahepatic tissues. The increased F in cirrhotic patients may be explained by a large fraction of portal blood flow bypassing the functional cells of the liver in cirrhosis. No change in volume of distribution was apparent. Clearance may be decreased because of decreased blood flow to functional liver tissue, although other processes may also be affected.

8. a. **Control: $C_{max,ss} = 50\ \mu g/L$; $C_{min,ss} = 33\ \mu g/L$.**
Tetraplegic: $C_{max,ss} = 68\ \mu g/L$; $C_{min,ss} = 52\ \mu g/L$.

$$C_{max,ss} = \frac{F \cdot Dose}{V} \cdot \frac{1}{(1 - e^{-k\tau})}; \quad C_{min,ss} = C_{max,ss} - \frac{F \cdot Dose}{V}$$

Controls

$$C_{max,ss} = \frac{0.9 \times 2000\ \mu g}{1.5\ L/kg \times 70\ kg} \times \frac{1}{1 - e^{-(0.693/12\ hr) \times 20\ hr}}$$

$$C_{min,ss} = 50\ \mu g/L - \frac{0.9 \times 2000\ \mu g}{1.5\ L/kg \times 70\ kg}$$

Tetraplegics

$$C_{max,ss} = \frac{0.9 \times 2000\ \mu g}{1.6\ L/kg \times 70\ kg} \times \frac{1}{1 - e^{-(0.693312\ hr) \times 31\ hr}}$$

$$C_{min,ss} = 68.3\ \mu g/L = \frac{0.9 \times 2000\ \mu g}{1.6\ L/kg \times 70\ kg}$$

b. (1) **Decreased hepatic blood flow, by itself, seems unlikely to be an explanation.** Clearance is only 78 mL/min/1.8 m^2 in the controls. A change in blood flow should not directly affect CL or $t_{1/2}$ of a low–extraction ratio drug.

(2) **Decreased enzyme activity is a possibility based on the kinetic changes.**

(3) **This is a possibility.** Lorazepam undergoes hepatic recycling through its glucuronide, which is cleaved in the colon. The released drug is reabsorbed. Biliary dyskinesia, more common to these patients, may result in less recycling and an apparent decrease in clearance (increase in half-life).

(4) **Changes in protein binding are unlikely to explain the alterations, as the volume of distribution is unaffected.** An equivalent increase in tissue binding would also have to be involved.

9. **4 mg/L to 8 mg/L.** The unbound concentrations in both the typical and renal failure patients should be the same to obtain the same response. The therapeutic unbound concentration range in the typical patient are 1 to 2 mg/L ($fu \cdot C = 0.1 \times$ 10 to 20 mg/L). In patients with severe renal disease, fu increases to 0.25. The total plasma concentrations equivalent to unbound concentrations of 1 to 2 mg/L are then 4 to 8 mg/L ($C = Cu/fu = (1$ to $2)/0.25$).

10. a. **10.5 mL/min.**

$$\int_0^6 C \cdot dt = C_{av} \cdot 6 = 22 \text{ mg-hr/L}$$

$$CL_D = \frac{Amount\ recovered}{\int_0^6 C \cdot dt} = \frac{14\ mg}{22\ mg\text{-}hr/L} = 10.5\ mL/min$$

b. **3.5%.**

$$Q_b = 0.305\ L/min = 18.3\ L/hr$$

$$Efficiency = \frac{V_D \cdot C_D}{Q_b \cdot \int_0^T C_{B,in} \cdot dt} = \frac{14\ mg}{18.3\ L/hr \times 22\ mg\text{-}hr/L}$$

c. **No. $C_{b,out}/C_{b,in} = 0.965$.**

The ratio of $C_{b,out}$ and $C_{b,in}$ can be calculated from

$$\frac{C_{b,out}}{C_{b,in}} = 1 - Efficiency$$

The concentrations of drug in blood entering and leaving the dialyzer are too close to obtain an accurate estimate of the difference. In addition, only minor differences in flow rates in and out, caused by loss of water into dialysate, can make concentration differences smaller or even negative.

d. **4%.**

$$\frac{Amount\ recovered}{Dose} = \frac{14\ mg}{350\ mg} = 0.04$$

e. **Yes.** 10.5 mL/min measured versus 11.7 mL/min predicted.

$$CL_D = \frac{Dialysis\ clearance}{of\ creatinine} \cdot \sqrt{\frac{113}{252}} \times fu$$

$$CL_D = 83\ min \times 0.67 \times 0.21$$

11. a.

	Unbound Dialysis Clearance* (L/hr)	Dialysis Clearance[†‡] (L/hr)	$\left(\dfrac{t_{1/2}}{t_{1/2,during}}\right)^{\ddagger}$	$t_{1/2}$** (hr)
S-Naproxen M.W. = 230 g/mol	6.3	0.019	1.03	14
Tobramycin M.W. = 4.68 g/mol	4.4	4.1	15	53
Verapamil = 455 g/mol	4.5	0.45	1.0	2.3

$*CLu_D$ = Creatinine dialysis clearance (150 mL/min or 9.0 L/hr) $\cdot \sqrt{\dfrac{113}{MW}}$

$^{\dagger}CLu_D = CLu_D \cdot fu$

$^{\ddagger}\left(\dfrac{t_{1/2}}{t_{1/2,during}}\right) = \dfrac{CL + CL_D}{CL}$

$**t_{1/2} = \dfrac{0.693 \cdot V}{CL}$

b. **Tobramycin is clinically dialyzable. S-Naproxen is poorly dialyzable because of extensive plasma protein binding. Verapamil is poorly dialyzed because of a large V (extensive tissue binding).**

			Clinical Dialyzability
Drug	k_D*	f_D[†]	$f_D(1 - e^{-k_D \cdot t})$[‡]
S-Naproxen	0.0517	0.0194	**0.0036**
Tobramycin	0.196	0.93	**0.51**
Verapamil	0.3	0.0043	**0.003**

$*k_D = \dfrac{CL + CL_D}{V}$

†Eq. 15-29 in text.
‡Eq. 15-30 in text.

12. a. **The manner of calculating dialysis clearance after intraperitoneal (i.p.) administration is the principal cause of the difference in the values.** The amount that entered the body during the first 4-hr dwell time after i.p. administration is unknown. It certainly is not equal to the dose, as was assumed by the authors.
  b. **Clearance, too, is miscalculated, following i.p. administration.** The AUC is less than that after i.v. administration because of the exchange of dialysate at 4 hr. After i.p. administration, $Dose/AUC = CL/F$. It is evident that F is approximately equal to 0.6. This is the same factor by which the peritoneal dialysis clearance after i.p. administration was in error.

13. a. **See Fig. J15-P13.**
  b. **Approximately 7 hr.** Estimate is limited by quality of data during the dialysis treatments. The best estimate is obtained during the dialysis treatment from 66 to 70 hr. Note that less than 1 half-life has elapsed.
  c. **No.** The loss during each treatment appears to be quite small when compared with the amount in the body.

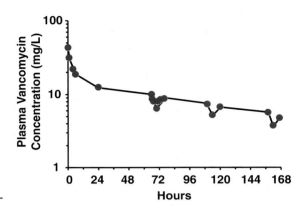

FIGURE J15-P13.

d. **No.** The removal of vancomycin by dialysis is not blood flow limited. Also, because the rate of return to plasma from tissues within the dialysis period is slow, increasing dialysis clearance would not materially increase drug removal from the whole body.

14. a. **Elimination continuously slows from Groups I to V.** Under such changing condition, the peak concentration and the peak time are expected to increase (see Fig.6-5 in Chapter 6, *Kinetics Following an Extravascular Dose*).

b. **4.7 L/hr.**

$$CL_D = \frac{Amount \ in \ dialysate}{AUC(0 - \tau)} = \frac{0.9 \times 30 \ mg}{5.75 \ mg\text{-}hr/L}$$

c. **0.42.**

$$\frac{t_{1/2,during}}{t_{1/2,off}} = \frac{CL}{CL_D + CL}$$

$$\frac{2.05}{5.9} = \frac{CL}{4.7 + CL} \qquad CL = 2.48 \ L/hr$$

$$f_d \cdot (1 - e^{-k_D \cdot t}) = \frac{4.7}{4.7 + 2.48}(1 - e^{-0.693 \times 3/2.05})$$

d. **3.5 L/hr.**

$$CL_D = \frac{Creatinine \ dialysis}{clearance} \cdot \sqrt{\frac{113}{M.W.}} \times fu$$

$$= 158 \ mL/min \times 60 \ min/hr \cdot \sqrt{\frac{113}{407}} \times 0.7$$

e. **4.7 L/hr (measured) versus 3.5 L/hr (predicted).** One explanation for the difference is that the clearance of creatinine begins to approach an upper limit imposed by blood (plasma) flow. Its value is therefore an underestimate of that expected when there is no flow limitation. The dialysis clearance of the drug is smaller than that of creatinine and therefore is not limited by blood flow to the same degree.

CHAPTER 16. NONLINEARITIES

1. a. **5.**
   1. A *more* than proportional increase is expected.
   2. The apparent half-life is *longer* at high concentrations.
   3. The rate increases as the amount in the body increases but approaches a limiting value, *Vm*.

b. **3.**

    1. Induction should produce a concentration *lower* than predicted, because of increased metabolic activity.

    2. A change in *V* should *not affect* the mean steady-state concentration.

c. **1, 2, and 3.**

    4. increased *V* would *not* explain the lack of proportional increase in C_{ss}, unless an increase in *fu* occurred. In this case, *CL* would increase as well.

d. **2 and 4.**

    1. Saturable absorption would lead to a *less* than proportional increase in Ae_∞.

    3. Saturable active tubular secretion would lead to a *less* than proportional increase in the amount excreted unchanged as the dose is increased.

2. a. **Mechanism-based autoinhibition of metabolism refers to a drug that hastens destruction of its own metabolic enzyme(s).** The drug is also called a suicide substrate in that it destroys the enzyme(s) that eliminates it.

  b. **Yes.** The elimination of ticlopidine appears to decrease with time as expected for mechanism-based autoinhibition. The data could also be explained by another mechanism such as the slow accumulation of a long-half metabolite that competitively inhibits the metabolism of tidopidine.

3. a. **I, III, VI.** From the relationship $F \cdot Dose = CL_b \cdot AUC_b$, it is apparent that either *F* is increased or CL_b is decreased.

  b. **I and III.** At steady state, $R_{inf} = CL \cdot C_{ss}$. Clearance must decrease with increasing dosing rate.

  c. **I and III.** From the relationships $Dose = V_b \cdot C_b(0)$ and $Dose = CL_b \cdot AUC_b$ it is evident that volume of distribution is not changed and CL_b is decreased.

4. **Glucose must be actively reabsorbed.** At plasma concentration above 2 g/L, the capacity of the reabsorption system is exceeded, as shown in Fig. J16-P4.

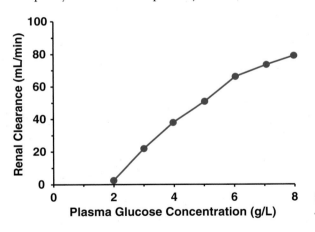

FIGURE J16-P4.

5. Saturable binding to plasma proteins, saturable reabsorption in renal tubules, or autoinduction. The ratio, R_{inf}/C_{ss} is equal to clearance. Calculation of the ratio shows that clearance increases with increasing infusion rate of disopyramide in both patients. The increase in clearance could be a result of saturable binding to plasma proteins (*fu* ↑ with higher infusion rates). This conclusion is supported by its binding to α_1-acid glycoprotein. Drug concentrations in the 2- to 5-mg/L range (6–15 μM) are greater than 20% of the average plasma concentration (15 μM) of this protein. Saturable binding is the explanation: It can be proven by concurrent measurement of protein binding.

    Saturable reabsorption in the renal tubule cannot be substantiated, as no information on reabsorption by a facilitated mechanism in the renal tubule was given. Autoinduction is possible if it occurs within the concentration range in which the observations were made.

6. See Fig. J16-P6.

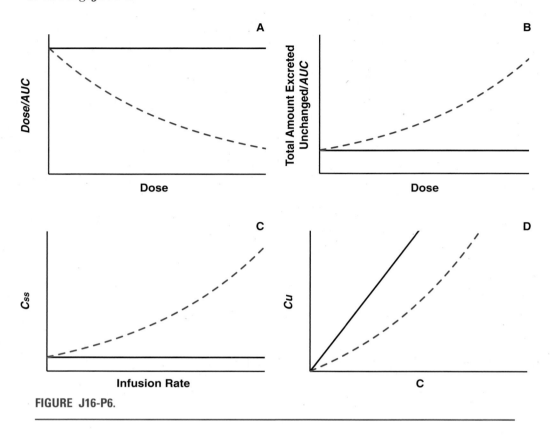

FIGURE J16-P6.

7.

TABLE J16-P7	**Disposition Kinetics and Total and Unbound Steady-State Blood Drug Concentrations are a Function of Dose Dependence in Each of Several Sources Following Oral and Intravenous Administrations**

Source of Dose Dependency	Direction of Change* With Increased Total Daily Dose	Volume of Distribution†	Clearance	Half-life	$\left[\dfrac{\text{Concentration}}{\text{Rate of Administration}}\right]$ Total	Unbound
Oral administration						
Bioavailability	↓	↔	↔	↔	↓	↓
Absorption rate constant	↓	↔	↔	↔**	↔	↔
Intravenous administration						
Fraction unbound in blood						
Low-extraction drug	↑	↑	↑	↔	↓	↔
High-extraction ratio drug	↑	↑	↔	↑	↔	↑

(continued)

TABLE J16-P7	Disposition Kinetics and Total and Unbound Steady-State Blood Drug Concentrations are a Function of Dose Dependence in Each of Several Sources Following Oral and Intravenous Administrations *(Continued)*

Source of Dose Dependency	Direction of Change* With Increased Total Daily Dose	Volume of Distribution†	Clearance	Half-life	Concentration Rate of Administration	
					Total	Unbound
Fraction unbound in tissue	↑	↓	↔	↓	↔	↔
Metabolic clearance	↑	↔	↑	↓	↓	↓
Renal clearance	↓	↔	↓	↑	↑	↑

*Only one example of each direction of change is shown.
†A volume of distribution greater than 50 L.
‡The average steady-state total and unbound blood drug concentrations relative to the rate of administration.
**The terminal half-life increases unless absorption rate-limits elimination of drug.

8. **No.** The peak concentration of dicloxacillin after the 2-g dose is 60 mg/L or 120 μM. This is just the concentration (20% of albumin concentration, 600 μM) expected to produce a 20% increase in *fu* if there is one binding site per molecule. The effect of saturable binding in the *Dose/AUC* value is therefore not expected to be very great at the concentrations observed. Furthermore, if the value of *fu* is increased with time for the 2-g dose relative to the 1-g dose, then renal clearance should be increased, not decreased, as was observed.

9. a. **See Fig. J16-P9.**

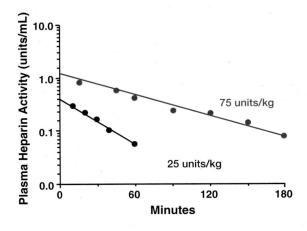

FIGURE J16-P9.

  b. **Yes.** The slop is less (half-life longer) at the higher dose. The intercepts suggest that the volume of distribution may increase slightly with the dose. The *AUC/Dose* increases suggesting a decrease in clearance with dose.
  c. **No.** With Michaelis-Menten kinetics, the slope is the same at a given concentration on a semilogarithmic plot.

$$-\frac{dC}{dt} = \frac{1}{V} \cdot \frac{Vm \cdot C}{Km' + C}$$

$$Slope = \frac{d\ln C}{dt} - \frac{dC/dt}{C} = \frac{1}{V} \cdot \frac{Vm \cdot C}{Km' + C}$$

d. **No.** If all the components measured by the assay behaved linearly, then the curves should superimpose when normalized to dose. The data suggest nonlinear behavior for one or more component.

10. a. **Not accurate.** There is a *more* than proportional increase in $C_{av,ss}$ on increasing the daily dose.

b. **Not accurate.** The renal route is then the only route of elimination ($fe(t) = 1$). At higher plasma drug concentrations, the renal clearance would be higher, leading to a *shorter* half-life.

c. **Not accurate.** It depends on where the target is. For ACE inhibitors, the target is within plasma and clearance increases as the dose is increased. For bosentan, imirestat, and draflazine, which bind to tissue (relative to plasma) components, clearance is not materially changed with dose, but half-life and volume of distribution are.

CHAPTER 17. DRUG INTERACTIONS

1. a. **True.** The patient is often stabilized on one drug and, by adding the second, a change in intensity of response is produced (clarithromycin → cyclosporine). Similarly, a patient may be stabilized on two drugs and withdrawal of one precipitates a clinical problem (carbamazepine → warfarin).

b. **Generally true.** One should realize that "displacer" must bind to the same (or an indirectly affected) site on the same protein as the other drug, and must have a reasonable affinity (association constant) for the site, otherwise even at an equal molar concentration to the binding protein, displacement would be minimal.

c. **True.** The major problem with most displacement reactions is the interpretation of the plasma concentration observed. Seldom is there a therapeutic consequence of this displacement.

d. **True.** Of all the kinds of pharmacokinetic interactions, this mechanism and enzyme induction are generally of greatest therapeutic concern.

e. **True.** The graded nature of the response depends on whether the interaction is *unindirectional, bidirectional,* or *mutual* in nature.

f. **False.** Class 1 compounds are those that have a high aqueous solubility and high cell membrane permeability and, hence, pass through membranes so quickly that transporters tend to have little impact on their pharmacokinetics.

2. a. *fu* **increased. See Fig. J17-P2A.** Colored line is new value.

b. CL_{int} **decreased. See Fig. J17-P2B.** Colored line is new value.

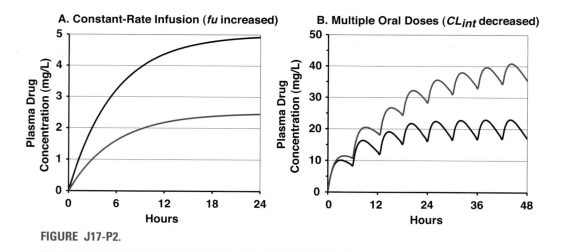

A. Constant-Rate Infusion (*fu* increased)

B. Multiple Oral Doses (CL_{int} decreased)

FIGURE J17-P2.

3. a. (1) See **Fig. J17-P3**. Colored line is new value.

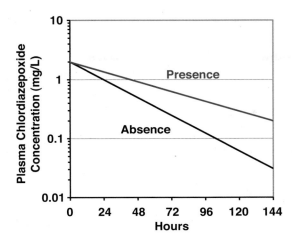

FIGURE J17-P3.

(2)	Without Ketoconazole	With Ketoconazole
V (L)	22.5	22.5
CL (L/hr)	0.65	0.36

b. **CL_{int} decreased.** Low–extraction ratio drug ($CL/Q_H = 1.63 \text{ L/hr}/81 \text{ L/hr}) = 0.02$. Volume of distribution (22.5 L) did not change. Clearance decreased, and the half-life lengthened. A decrease in intrinsic clearance is a logical conclusion. Another possible explanation is an increase in both plasma and tissue binding so that volume of distribution did not change. This would decrease clearance and lengthen half-life. The former has been found to be the mechanism of interaction. *Note:* an increase plasma binding would make little impact on a small volume of distribution drug, but at 22.5 L, chlordiazepoxide is somewhat too large to be classified as such a drug.

4. a. **Drug A is secreted and reabsorbed.** $CL_R/(fu \cdot GFR)$ is 2 in the absence and 0.27 in the presence of Drug B.

b. **Volume of distribution is unchanged.**

$$V = \frac{CL}{k} \qquad CL = \frac{R_{inf}}{C_{ss}} \qquad k = \frac{0.693}{t_{1/2}}$$

Therefore,

$$V = \frac{R_{inf} \times 12 \text{ hr}}{C_{ss} \times 0.693}$$

Absence: $V = \dfrac{2.5 \text{ mg/hr} \times 12 \text{ hr}}{10 \text{ mg/L} \times 0.693} = 43.3 \text{ L}$

Presence: $V = \dfrac{2.5 \text{ mg/hr} \times 25 \text{ hr}}{20.8 \text{ mg/L} \times 0.693} = 43.4 \text{ L}$

c. **Displacement from plasma and tissue binding sites and either inhibition of tubular secretion or enhanced tubular reabsorption (e.g., by a change in urine pH).** The threefold increase in the unbound fraction of Drug A in the presence of Drug

B should have increased the renal clearance threefold; instead the renal clearance decreased from 1.5 to 0.6 L/hr.

The nonrenal clearance increased approximately threefold. For Drug A alone,

$$CL \ (nonrenal) = \frac{25 \ mg/hr}{10 \ mg/L} - 1.5 \ L/hr = 1.0 \ L/hr$$

and in the presence of Drug B,

$$CL \ (nonrenal) = \frac{25 \ mg/hr}{6.7 \ mg/L} - 0.60 \ L/hr = 3.1 \ L/hr$$

By calculation ($V = 1.44 \cdot CL \cdot t_{1/2}$), the volume of distribution of Drug A, 43 L, is seen to not change during coadministration with Drug B. As displacement from plasma proteins occurs, so must displacement occur in tissues to keep the volume of distribution unchanged.

d. The plateau unbound concentration ($fu \cdot C_{ss}$) of Drug A increases from 1 mg/L in the absence to 2 mg/L in the presence of Drug B. This suggests that the response produced by Drug A is increased, perhaps excessively and may require a reduction in the dosing rate. No information is given on A → B.

5. a. $fu \cdot CL_{int} = 289$ L/hr in absence and 27 L/hr in presence of fluoxetine. From the *well-stirred* model.

$$CL_{b,H} = \frac{Q_H \cdot fu_b \cdot CL_{int}}{Q_H \cdot fu_b \cdot CL_{int}}$$

$$F_H = \frac{Q_H}{Q_H \cdot fu_b \cdot CL_{int}}$$

so that $CL_H/F_H = Dose/AUC_b = fu \cdot CL_{int}$, as the plasma-to-blood concentration ratio is close to 1.

b. **Inhibition of desipramine metabolism.** The value of *Dose/AUC* (*CL/F*) is 289 L/hr for desipramine alone. This value greatly exceeds hepatic blood flow (81 L/hr), indicating that *F* may be low due to first-pass metabolism. The drug is extensively metabolized, as supported by *fe* = 0.03. When metabolism primarily occurs in the liver, both a low *F* and a high clearance are expected. The coadministration of fluoxetine then results in diminished metabolism and consequently an increase in *F* and a decrease in *CL*, although the change in the latter may be small as oleanane becomes more sensitive to changes in blood flow than in metabolism.

c. **The change in *CL/F* directly reflects a change in $fu \cdot CL_{int}$ irrespective of whether the drug has a high or low hepatic extraction ratio.** For a high-extraction drug, however, *CL* and half-life are relatively less sensitive to a change in CL_{int} (see first equation in part "a" above). Half-life is increased by a factor of 4.12 (0.693 *V/CL* [fluoxetine present]/0.693 · *V/CL* [fluoxetine absent]). The value of *CL/F* is decreased by a factor of 10.7 (*CL/F* [fluoxetine present]/*CL/F* [fluoxetine absent]).

d. **It would take longer for desipramine to achieve a steady state in the presence of fluoxetine when fluoxetine dosage is initiated in patients already stabilized on desipramine, than when desipramine is added to patients stabilized on fluoxetine.** The reason is that in the later case, desipramine kinetics will be that instantly at that in the presence of a stable fluoxetine plasma concentration, that is 64 hr (Table 17-9), whereas when fluoxetine is added to the regimen of someone stabilized on desipramine, it will take at least 8 days (5 half-lives) for fluoxetine to reach its steady state, and during this time the clearance of desipramine is continually decreasing with the rising concentration of fluoxetine, and only when one has reached a plateau for fluoxetine will desipramine clearance stabilize and then proceed to its new plateau.

e. **Without reducing dosage, there is an increased likelihood of a greater incidence and intensity of adverse effects.** The *AUC* of desipramine after a single dose is increased about 11-fold in the presence of fluoxetine. On chronic administration, the average steady-state concentration should be increased correspondingly. There is a clear case for either choosing another antidepressant that does not interact with fluoxetine, or drastically reducing the dose of desipramine if coadministered with this inhibitor.

6. a. **The design took into account that drug interactions are graded, so it is important that studies are conducted at steady state on a full therapeutic dose, and that the condition is maintained throughout the elimination of the potentially affected drug.** With a half-life of 3 to 5 hr, ritonavir is expected to be at steady state within a day, so waiting to administer digoxin on day 3 (i.e., 48 hr after starting the ritonavir) should ensure steady-state conditions for ritonavir. Administering ritonavir for a further 8 days is to ensure that this steady state condition is maintained throughout the elimination of digoxin, which has a half-life in the order of 1.5 days.

b. **Inhibition of a renal transporter.** Under control conditions, with CL_R (194 *mL/min*) $>$ $fu \cdot GFR$ (0.9 $\times$ 120 *mL/min*), digoxin must be secreted. With ritonavir unlikely to affect *GFR*, the reduction in CL_R of digoxin in the presence of ritonavir, signals inhibition of secretion. The likely mechanism is inhibition of PgP efflux, although involvement of other transporters cannot be excluded.

c. **Yes.** Nonrenal clearance is reduced from 215 (409–194) to 112 (238–126) mL/min. Most nonrenal clearance is hepatic, and being a low extraction ratio, minimally metabolized, compound, the likely mechanism is inhibition by ritonavir of digoxin biliary excretion, although inhibition of hepatic uptake cannot be excluded.

d. **A distinct possibility.** With minimal plasma protein binding, primary events controlling *V* for digoxin are in tissues. Being large and polar, tissue distribution of digoxin is likely to be dependent on transport processes, such as efflux by PgP, which resides in many tissues, which ritonavir inhibits, causing an increase in *V*. Again, involvement of other transporters cannot be excluded. Enhancing tissue digoxin binding by ritonavir is unlikely.

e. **In the presence of ritonavir, both renal and nonrenal clearance are reduced by approximately the same extent, so that *fe* remains unchanged.**

f. **There must be adjustment of the normal digoxin regimen to minimize the risk of excessive toxicity.** With a 50% reduction in clearance, the dosing rate should be halved. However, if contemplated, the initial digitalizing dose may need to be increased, associated with the increase in *V* of digoxin. However, there are several unknowns. One is the impact of ritonavir of the cardiac distribution of digoxin where it acts. Another is the effect of ritonavir on the oral bioavailability of digoxin. If PgP is involved, then an increase in bioavailability is expected, but with an oral bioavailability of digoxin of approximately 0.8, it cannot increase by much.

g. **Both uptake and efflux transporters are likely to be involved in the tissue distribution of digoxin,** given that ritonavir increases, and quinidine decreases, *V*. Both types of transporters may be affected, but clearly, the predominant effect of ritonavir is inhibition of efflux and of quinidine on uptake transport. Finally, notice that by comparison with digoxin pharmacokinetic parameters discussed elsewhere in the book, there is considerable variability in quoted parameter values even among healthy patients, stressing the importance of undertaking, whenever possible, a crossover design when exploring a drug interaction.

7. See Table J17-P7.

TABLE J17-P7	Changes in Pharmacokinetic Parameter Values for Drugs A to G in Various Situations

	Observation				
	Clearance	Volume of Distribution	Half-life	Fraction Excreted Unchanged	Oral Bioavailability
Drug A	↓	↔	↑	↓	↔
Drug B	↑	↔	↓	↔	↔
Drug C	↔	↔	↔	↔	↔
Drug D	↔	↑	↑	↑	↓
Drug E	↔	↓	↓	↔	↔
Drug F	↑	↑	↔	↔	↔
Drug G	↔	↔	↔	↔	↔

8. a. 37.9 mg/L.

$$C_{av,ss} = \frac{F \cdot Dose}{\tau \cdot CL} = \frac{500\ mg}{12\ hr \times 1.1\ L/hr} = 37.9\ mg/L$$

b. (1) 119 mg/L.
For inhibitor

$$Cu_{av,ss,inhibitor} = \frac{fu \cdot F \cdot Dose}{\tau \cdot CL} = \frac{0.04 \times 250\ mg}{12\ hr \times 0.6\ L/hr} = 1.39\ mg/L$$

For tolbutamide

$$CL_{inhibited} = CL \cdot \left[\frac{fm}{(1 + Cu_{av,ss,inhibitor}/K_I)} + (1 - fm) \right]$$

$$= 1.1\ L/hr \times \left[\frac{0.97}{(1 + 1.39\ mg/L/0.6\ mg/L)} + 0.03 \right]$$

$$= 0.35\ L/hr$$

$$C_{av,ss,inhibited} = \frac{F \cdot Dose}{\tau \cdot CL_{inhibited}} = \frac{500\ mg}{12\ hr \times 0.35\ L/hr} = 119\ mg/L$$

(2) Approximately 7 days from initiation of inhibitor administration.
New half-life of tolbutamide

$$t_{1/2,inhibited} = t_{1/2} \cdot CL / CL_{inbibited} = 5.7\ hr \times 1.1L / hr / 0.34\ L/hr = 19.9\ hr$$

For inhibitor

$$t_{1/2} = 0.693 \times V / CL = 0.693 \times 13\ L / 0.6\ L/hr = 15\ hr$$

It takes approximately 2.5 days (4 $t_{1/2}$) for the inhibitor to reach its steady state, and therefore even longer for tolbutamide to reach its new steady state. Being conservative, an additional 4 days (5 $t_{1/2}$) may be required, given that the new half-life of tolbutamide in the presence of a steady state of inhibitor is 19.9 hr.

(3) 250 mg once a day.

Reduced dosing rate of tolbutamide to maintain the same $C_{av,ss}$ is given by

$$\left[\frac{F \cdot Dose}{\tau}\right]_{inhibited} = \left[\frac{F \cdot Dose}{\tau}\right] \cdot \frac{CL_{inhibited}}{CL} = \frac{500\ mg}{12\ hr} \times \frac{0.34\ L/hr}{1.1\ L/hr} = 12.9\ mg/hr$$

Given the increased half-life, tolbutamide can be given once daily in the presence of the inhibitor, corresponding to a total daily dose of 309 mg. It is not practically possible to give this dose. The nearest dose is half a scored 500-mg tablet, that is, 250 mg once daily. This will give a slightly lower (20%) $C_{av,ss}$ than achieved preinhibition, but it should be acceptable. Giving 250 mg twice daily or 500 mg once daily would be (31%) too high.

9. a. **It is probably better not to randomize the study with respect to treatment sequence.** The time course of decline of induction depends on the kinetics of the inducer and that of the enzyme whose synthesis is affected. It may take a long time after stopping the inducer before the effect wears off, and the level of enzyme in the body returns to its control value. This recommendation will not allow separation of treatment and period effects, but generally the period effect is small. The alternative is to randomize the study and leave a long washout phase, but one can never be sure how long this phase should be.

b. **Commensurate with safety, the dosage regimen of the inducer should be as close as possible to the usual recommendation.** Induction, involving an increase in the rate of synthesis of the enzyme, is a graded response; the lower the dosage, the less likely induction will be detected.

c. **The full expression of induction will take time depending on both the kinetics of the inducer and the affected enzyme.** At a minimum, the inducer should be administered for sufficient time to ensure attainment of its steady state, before the drug is given. And, if the half-life of the enzyme (when known) is longer than that of inducer, the inducer should be given even longer to ensure that the new steady-state concentration of enzyme has been achieved. The inducer should then continue to be administered until most of test drug has been eliminated, thereby ensuring the maintenance of the full effects of induction during the elimination of the drug.

d. **Generally, no change in sampling times is recommended, because the shape of the plasma concentration–time profile is not anticipated to change (Fig. J17-P10).** One aspect that may warrant more frequent sampling at earlier times is analytical sensitivity—a sufficient number of precise measurements are needed to allow a good estimate of C_{max}, AUC, and $t_{1/2}$.

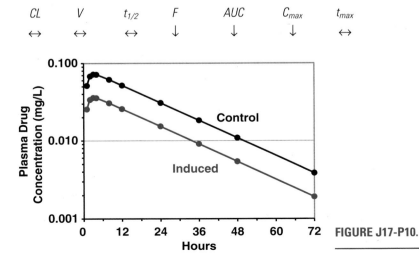

FIGURE J17-P10.

e. **Bioavailability (F).** Because the drug has a high hepatic extraction ratio ($E_H = 0.85$, as $F_H = 0.15$), an increase in enzyme activity results in a decrease in F_H, and only a small change in blood clearance as CL_b approaches hepatic blood flow.

10. Diltiazem is expected to show dose- and time-dependent pharmacokinetics. Being a mechanism-based inhibitor, as it is metabolized, it consumes and inactivates CYP3A4, which then takes time to be resynthesized. Being a substrate of CYP3A4, the intrinsic clearance of diltiazem will decrease in a concentration- and time-dependent manner. The magnitude of effect depends on the control value of *fm* associated with this enzyme; the greater *fm*, the more pronounced the effect. In addition, because it consumes this enzyme, the impact of diltiazem on the clearance and oral first-pass metabolic loss of other substrates of CYP3A4 will be greater than would be anticipated, assuming the mechanism involved was competitive inhibition. In addition, the effect would be evident even after most diltiazem has been eliminated after stopping its administration, because it has a much shorter half-life (4 hr) than that of CYP3A4 (2–4 days), which will slowly return to its prediltiazem level. In practice, the situation is complex, making precise prediction difficult. First, although diltiazem does show dose- and time-dependent pharmacokinetics, the enzymology of its metabolism is incompletely understood. In addition, it forms various metabolites, some active as well as potential inhibitors, many of which are eliminated more slowly than diltiazem, confounding the ability to positively associate time dependencies seen with diltiazem with parent compound.

CHAPTER 18. INITIATING AND MANAGING THERAPY

1. a. In one strategy, the initial dosage regimen for a patient is calculated based on the population pharmacokinetic and pharmacodynamic information, together with the patient-specific data, such as age, body weight, and renal function, which are known to explain some of the interindividual variability in the dose–response relationship. Drug therapy is subsequently managed by monitoring the effects observed; that is, the dose is increased when the desired response is inadequate or decreased when an adverse response is excessive. Digoxin and ganciclovir are examples of drugs administered using this strategy.

   The second strategy is one in which an individual's requirements are determined by starting with a low dose and slowly raising the dosage, until the optimal therapeutic response, without undue adverse effects, is achieved. How quickly the dose is adjusted depends on the kinetics of the drug and its responses. Flecainide, some antiepileptics, and many antidepressants are examples of drugs administered using this second strategy.

   b. Individualizing dosage for infants, children, and frail elderly patients is clearly needed. Individualization before starting therapy may also be prudent when the patient has compromised renal function, hepatic disease, or a genetically related condition in which drug metabolism or drug response is known to be affected. Adjustment to the typical regimen may also be required if concurrently administered drugs interact with the introduced drug. Taking such patient-specific information into account can reduce the occurrence and intensity of harmful events and help to more rapidly establish an individual's optimal dosage requirements.

   c. **The criteria for performing drug concentration monitoring are discussed in the section on Target Concentration Strategy.** Included are good concentration–response relationship, high probability of therapeutic failure, when a problem arises, good population pharmacokinetic information known, and a reliable assay available.

2. a. **Giving a loading dose in several sequential doses allows development of the full beneficial effect of a drug without the occurrence of undue adverse events. The**

use of sequential doses of chloroquine for treating chloroquine-sensitive malaria is an example given in this chapter.

Another example (mentioned in text) of this situation is the loading of digoxin (a drug with a half-life of 1.5–2 days) in the treatment of congestive cardiac failure. Here, the purpose of sequential (often 6 hourly) doses is to titrate the patient to the response desired. The procedure is largely historical in origin. It was established when only crude plant products were available, and the active ingredient and its dose were essentially unknown. Nonetheless, evidence indicates that adopting this approach is safer than giving an anticipated loading dose of digoxin all at one.

b. **The administration of loading doses is driven by the urgency of a need for response, the kinetics of the drug, the kinetics of the response, and tolerance to the adverse effects of the drug.** A loading dose of esmolol, a drug used in treating life-threatening supraventricular tachycardias, is useful even though the drug has a 9-min half-life.

c. Loading doses are sometimes not used for drugs with long half-lives, because the time delay associated with the development of the therapeutic response, as with antidepressants, antihyperlipidemic agents, and drugs used to treat or prevent osteoporosis, is longer than the time required to accumulate the drug. Another reason is that adverse effects associated with rapid loading are not tolerable, as is the case with flecainide acetate, valproic acid, and terazosin.

3. **Plasma drug–concentration monitoring is useful when, for a low therapeutic index drug, much of the *inter*patient variability in response (beneficial or adverse) is accounted for by variability in pharmacokinetics.** This is found with the antiepileptic drug, phenytoin, and the immunosuppressive drug, cyclosporine. The concept of therapeutic concentration monitoring is further enhanced in situations in which the drug is given prophylactically because the desired effect is then the absence of an undesired outcome, such as an epileptic fit or organ transplant rejection. Clearly, plasma concentration monitoring has little to no value when most of the interpatient variability in the dose–response relationship is associated with pharmacodynamics. Recall also that low *intra*patient variability in both pharmacokinetics and pharmacodynamics is required for a low therapeutic index drug; otherwise, a patient could not be well controlled on the drug.

4. **Nitroglycerin—development of tolerance to therapeutic effect; terazosin—tolerance to adverse effect.** These were the two examples given in the text. Tolerance to narcotic analgesics (not mentioned in the text) develops to both therapeutic (analgesic) and adverse (respiratory depression) effects, such that the patient needs and can tolerate more of these drugs when given chronically.

5. **Nonadherence is a deviation, intentional or otherwise, from the prescribed manner of taking a drug product.** Nonadherence occurs in many different ways, which fall into two major categories. The first kind of nonadherence is when there are daily variations in the way the drug is taken. This may involve changes in the time of day when the doses are taken, omitting one or more doses, or taking extra doses, especially to make up for doses not taken. The second kind is when there is a lack of long-term persistence in dosing. For example, doses may be discontinued while on vacation or on a business trip, or patient may decide to stop taking the drug altogether either because they feel better and do not perceive the need to continue with the drug or because the harmful effects experienced override the perceived benefits of the drug.

Adherence is extremely important to therapy, because nonadherence is such a common cause of therapeutic failures, that is, excessive adverse events or ineffective therapy. Adjustment of dosage by the clinician in these situations, based on the belief that the patient has been adherent, is problematic, especially when the dosage is increased because therapy appears to be ineffective. The cause of ineffective therapy may not have been a result of too low a prescribed dose, but rather a lack of systemic drug exposure because of nonadherence (not taking the drug). If the patient now adheres to the regimen of the higher dose, excessive adverse events may ensue.

Clearly, assuring adherence to a drug regimen is essential for therapeutic success, especially in the treatment of AIDS, psychiatric illnesses, and tuberculosis. Patient education, as well as improving behavior of the patient and providing support services, are means to this end.

6. **β-blockers, corticosteroids.** These two examples are given within the text of the chapter. Other examples are those of withdrawing from nicotine abuse (heavy smoking) and withdrawing from narcotic analgesics for those who are highly addicted.

7. See values in table below for the two curves in the figure.

a. **7.5 mg daily. See Fig. J18-P7.**

$$e^{-k\tau} = e^{-\frac{0.693}{20\,hr} \times 24} = 0.435 \qquad F \cdot Dose = 0.9 \times 7.5\ mg = 6.75\ mg$$

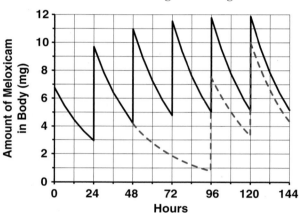

FIGURE J18-P7.

Time (hr)	$A_{max,ss}$ (mg)	Time (hr)	$A_{min,ss}$ (mg)
0+	6.75	24	2.94
24	9.69	48	4.21
48	10.96	72	4.77
72	11.52	96	5.01
96	11.78	120	5.12
120	11.87	144	5.16
144	11.91		

b. **Doses (3rd and 4th doses) missing on days 2 and 3.**

Time (hr)	$A_{max,ss}$ (mg)	Time (hr)	$A_{min,ss}$ (mg)
0+	6.75	24	2.94
24	9.69	48	4.21
48	4.21	72	1.83
72	1.83	96	0.80
96	7.55	120	3.28
120	10.03	144	4.36
144	11.11	—	—

c. $C_{ss,av}$ = **0.811 mg/L.**

$$C_{ss,av} = \frac{F \cdot Dose}{\tau \cdot CL} = \frac{0.9 \times 7.5\ mg}{24\ hr \times 0.3465\ hr^{-1}} = 0.811\ mg/L$$

d. **Extensively reabsorbed:**
   The renal clearance is 0.002 × 347 mL/hr = 6.7 mL/hr or 0.012 mL/min.
   If filtered only, $CL_R = fu \cdot GFR = 0.006 \cdot 100$ mL/min = 0.6 mL/min.
   Therefore, it must be extensively reabsorbed. Only answer 3 is appropriate.

8. a. CL_{cr} = **23 mL/min.**

$$CL_{cr} = \frac{(140 - 85) \times 62}{72 \times 2.1} = 23\ mL/min$$

b. $C_{max,ss}$ = **37 mg/L;** $C_{min,ss}$ = **24 mg/L.**
   From Table 18-7 (Winter method).

$$V = 0.62\ L/kg \times 62\ kg = 38\ L$$

$$CL = CL_{cr} = 23\ mL/min\ or\ 1.38\ L/hr$$

$$k = \frac{CL}{V} = \frac{1.38\ L/hr}{38\ L} = 0.036\ hr^{-1} \qquad t_{1/2} = 0.693/k = 19\ hr$$

Note. Steady state is expected at the time of sampling as the patient has been taking the drug for 3 days (3.8 half-lives).

$$C_{max,ss} = \frac{Dose/V}{(1 - e^{-k\tau})} = \frac{500\ mg/38\ L}{(1 - e^{-0.036 \times 12})} = 37\ mg/L$$

$$C_{min,ss} = C_{max,ss} \cdot e^{-0.036 \times 12} = 24\ mg/L$$

c. **The observed and predicted values are close, so the expected pharmacokinetic parameter values are reasonable estimates.** Because the half-life in this patient is about 19 hr, the dosing interval might be increased to 24 hr (dosing rate halved), a convenient regimen for both the patient and the person administering the drug. On a regimen of 500 mg every 24 hr, the calculated peak and trough values are:

$$C_{max,ss} = \frac{500\ mg/38\ L}{(1 - e^{-0.036 \times 24})} = 23\ mg/L$$

$$C_{min,ss} = C_{max,ss} \cdot e^{-0.036 \times 34} = 9.6\ mg/L$$

This regimen is less likely to produce toxicity, but should be effective.

9. a. **Solid colored curve in Fig. J18-P9.**

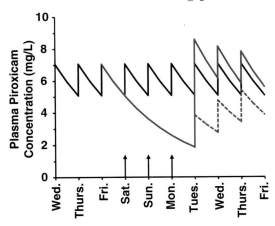

FIGURE J18-P9.

b. **Dashed colored curve in Fig. J18-P9.**

The decease in the plasma piroxicam concentration calculated from $C = C(0)e^{-kt}$, where $k = 0.693/50$ hr. The value of $e^{-k\tau} = \dfrac{5.07}{7.07}$ or $e^{-\frac{0.693 \times 24}{50}} = 0.717$. The

concentration increases by 6 mg/L (3×2 mg/L) on Tuesday morning when three capsules are taken, but only by 2 mg/L when one capsule is taken.

10. a. **93 mL/min or 5.6 L/hr.**

$$CL_{cr}\ (mL/min) = \frac{(140 - 53) \times 82}{85 \times 0.9} = 93\ mL/min$$

$$(5.6\ L/hr\ or\ 0.068\ L/hr/kg)$$

b. **$F = 0.75$; $CL = 6.7$ L/hr; $V = 602$ L, $k = 0.011$ hr^{-1}, $t_{1/2} = 63$ hr.**

Clearance of digoxin is then

$$CL(L/hr/kg) = 0.9 \times 0.068 + 0.02$$

$$(0.0812\ L/hr/kg\ or\ 6.66\ L/hr$$

And volume of distribution is

$$V(L/kg) = 3.8 + 52 \times 0.068\ (7.34\ L/kg\ or\ 602\ L)$$

Elimination rate constant and half-life are then

$$k = CL/V = 0.011\ hr^{-1}$$

$$t_{1/2} = 63\ hr$$

The value of F for digoxin tablets is 0.75.

c. **0.95 to 1.01 mg/L.**

The first question to be addressed is that of the appropriate kinetic model for evaluating this concentration. Presumably, the patient has been taking digoxin for 3 years. The dosing history indicates a single, recently missed dose. Thus, a steady-state model incorporating the missed dose is appropriate. Because the expected half-life is 63 hr and the dosing interval is 24 hr, the fluctuation in concentration should be minor and a constant-rate infusion model should apply. In addition, the blood sample was obtained near the middle of the dosing interval. Alternatively, a steady-state multiple-dose model could be employed. Using the constant-rate infusion model, the concentration expected, $C(t)$, is then $C_{ss} - C(t_1)$, where $C(t_1)$ is the concentration expected 32 hr after administration had only the missed dose been given.

$$C(t) = \underbrace{\frac{F \cdot S \cdot Dose}{CL \cdot \tau}}_{C_{ss}} - \underbrace{\frac{F \cdot S \cdot Dose^{-kt_1} \cdot e^{-kt_1}}{V}}_{C(t_1)}$$

Using a steady-state, multiple-dose model, the concentration expected is that 8 hr (t_2) into the 24-hr dosing interval (τ) minimum $C(t_1)$ as defined above ($t_1 = 32$ hr).

$$C(t) = \frac{F \cdot Dose}{V} \cdot \left[\frac{e^{-kt_2}}{1 - e^{-k\tau}} - e^{kt_1} \right]$$

The values for the two models are 0.95 and 1.01 mg/L, a difference explained by the assumption of *average* steady-state concentration in the first model.

d. **The observed (0.9 μg/L) and expected (0.95 to 1.01 μg/L) values are virtually the same. Revision of parameter values is unnecessary. Furthermore, the clinician** now has some confidence that the patient is handling the drug as expected, and that the concentration observed may be inadequate to control her congestive cardiac failure. A decision must now be made on how much higher a concentration is needed, or if therapy should be augmented with other drugs or changed.

11. **The answers to all the parts of this problem are shown in Fig. J18-P11.** The four parts of the problem are indicated by A, B, C, and D.

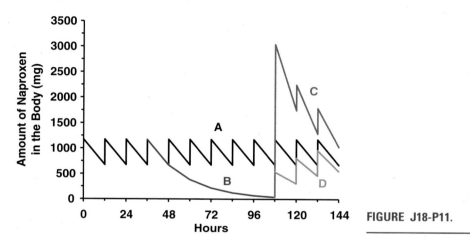

FIGURE J18-P11.

a. The peak and trough amounts in the body (A, black-solid line in Fig. J18-P8) were calculated from the equations.

$$A_{max,ss} = \frac{Dose}{(1 - e^{-k \cdot \tau})} = \frac{500}{(1 - e^{-0.0462hr^{-1} \times 12hr})} = 1175mg$$

$$A_{min,ss} = A_{max,ss} - Dose = 1175\ mg - 500\ mg = 675\ mg$$

b. The amount in the body (B, colored line, 36–108 hr) with time after the first dose was missed (occurred at $t = 36$ hr) was calculated from:

$$A = 675 \cdot e^{-00462 \cdot t} \ (t = \text{time after first dose was missed.})$$

c. (C, colored line, 108 hr onward). The amount in the body at 108 hr, expected just after the six tablets were taken was calculated by the amount remaining in the body plus the dose, 3000 mg. The subsequent minimum amounts were determined by multiplying the initial amount present by the fraction remaining at 12 hr ($e^{-k \cdot \tau}$). A dose of 500 mg was added to the amount remaining at this time to obtain the maximum amount at the beginning of each subsequent dosing interval).

d. The amounts here (D, gray line, 108 hr onward) were calculated as in c., but the dose at 108 hr was 500 mg instead of 3000 mg.

CHAPTER 19. DISTRIBUTION KINETICS

1. *Initial dilution volume (V_1)*—is the volume that a drug appears to occupy initially following an i.v. bolus dose; its value is given by dividing dose by concentration at zero time, a value predicted from an equation that fits the plasma concentration–time data.

Volume of distribution during the terminal phase (V)—is the apparent volume of distribution that a drug occupies after distribution equilibrium between blood and all tissues has been achieved following one or more discrete doses of drug or after stopping drug administration.

Volume of distribution at steady state (V_{ss})—is given by the ratio of the amount of drug in the body at steady state and the corresponding plasma concentration following a constant-rate infusion.

2. a. **True.** The extent of distribution outside blood may be small and the rate of distribution very rapid, in which case frequent sampling at early times after a bolus dose would be needed to observe the kinetics of distribution.

   b. **This is a reasonable representation for most drugs, as the kidneys and the liver are the major organs of elimination, and both organs are highly perfused.** Some drugs are metabolized by many tissues (e.g., nitroglycerin), and for them, the proposition that elimination takes place only in the central compartment is ill founded.

   c. **This statement is true provided that the terminal phase is correctly identified.** If most of the area under the plasma concentration–time curve is associated with the initial phase, then most of the drug is eliminated before distribution equilibrium is achieved and the terminal phase is reached. In this case, the statement is conservative.

3. a. $C_1 = 10,000$ ng/mL; $\lambda_1 = 1.8$ hr^{-1}; $C_2 = 150$ ng/mL; $\lambda_2 = 0.067$ hr^{-1}.

   b. **Clearance = 3.85 L/hr.** Value obtained from:

$$CL = \frac{Dose}{AUC} = \frac{Dose}{\left(\dfrac{C_1}{\lambda_1} + \dfrac{C_2}{\lambda_2}\right)} = \frac{30,000,000\ ng}{\left(\dfrac{10,000\ ng/mL}{1.8\ hr^{-1}} + \dfrac{150\ ng/mL}{0.067\ hr^{-1}}\right)} = 3849\ mL/hr$$

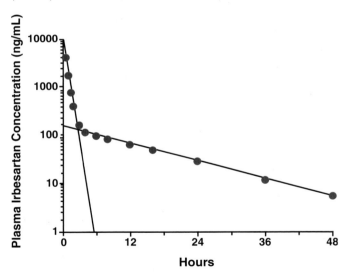

FIGURE J19-P3.

c. $V_1 = 2.96$ L; $V = 57.5$ L. Values obtained from:

$$V_1 = \frac{Dose}{C_1 + C_2} = \frac{30,000,000\ ng}{10,000\ ng/mL + 150\ ng/mL} = 2956\ mL$$

$$V = \frac{CL}{\lambda_2} = \frac{3.85\ L/hr}{0.067\ hr^{-1}} = 57.5\ L$$

d. **2735, 108, 72 ng/mL.** Calculated by substitution into biexponential equation for 45 min, 5, and 11 hr.

e. **168 ng/mL.** The measured concentration is the sum of the contributions from each dose. In this case, at 12 hr after the first dose and 6 hr after the second dose, the values obtained from Table 19-2 are 67 and 101 ng/mL, respectively.

f. **0.71.**

$$\text{Fraction eliminated associated} \atop \text{with first exponent} = \left(\dfrac{C_1/\lambda_1}{C_1/\lambda_1 + C_2/\lambda_2} \right) = \dfrac{10{,}000/1.8}{10{,}000/1.8 + 150/0.067}$$

g. **0.38 hr.** With 71% of irbesartan elimination associated with the first exponential phase, the elimination half-life is associated with this phase, $t_{1/2} = 0.693/1.8 \ hr^{-1}$.

h. **1.3 mg/L.** Calculated from:

$$F \cdot \dfrac{Dose}{\tau} = CL \cdot C_{av,ss}$$

$$C_{av,ss} = \dfrac{F}{CL} \cdot \dfrac{Dose}{\tau} = \dfrac{0.8}{3.85 \ L/hr} \times \dfrac{150 \ mg}{24 \ hr} = 1.3 \ mg/L$$

4. a. **Slow acetylator:** $C_1 = 1.59$ mg/L; $C_2 = 0.65$ mg/L; $\lambda_1 = 5.5 \ hr^{-1}$; $\lambda_2 = 0.11 \ hr^{-1}$.
    Fast acetylator: $C_1 = 1.57$ mg/L; $C_2 = 0.42$ mg/L; $\lambda_1 = 4.2 \ hr^{-1}$; $\lambda_2 = 0.41 \ hr^{-1}$.
    Plots not shown.
   b. **Slow acetylator:** $CL = 12$ L/hr; $V_1 = 33$ L; $V = 110$ L; $MRT = 8.5$ hr; $V_{ss} = 102$ L.

$$MRT = \dfrac{\left(\dfrac{C_1}{\lambda_1^2} + \dfrac{C_2}{\lambda_2^2} \right)}{\left(\dfrac{C_1}{\lambda_1} + \dfrac{C_2}{\lambda_2} \right)} = \dfrac{\left(\dfrac{1.59}{(5.5)^2} + \dfrac{0.65}{(0.11)^2} \right) mg\text{-}hr^2/L}{6.2 \ mg\text{-}hr/L} = 8.5 \ hr$$

$$V_{ss} = MRT \cdot CL = 12 \ L/hr \times 8.5 \ hr = 102 \ L$$

Fast acetylator: $CL = 53$ L/hr; $V_1 = 38$ L; $V = 132$ L; $MRT = 1.85$ hr; $V_{ss} = 98$ L.

$$MRT = \dfrac{\left(\dfrac{C_1}{\lambda_1^2} + \dfrac{C_2}{\lambda_2^2} \right)}{\left(\dfrac{C_1}{\lambda_1} + \dfrac{C_2}{\lambda_2} \right)} = \dfrac{\left(\dfrac{1.57}{(4.2)^2} + \dfrac{0.42}{(0.41)^2} \right) mg\text{-}hr^2/L}{1.4 \ mg\text{-}hr/L} = 1.85 \ hr$$

$$V_{ss} = MRT \cdot CL = 53 \ L/hr \times 1.85 \ hr = 98 \ L$$

The major difference between fast and slow acetylators is in clearance. Although there appears to be some differences in distribution, the difference in values of V is essentially explained by the impact of changes in clearance, as can be seen when comparing V_{ss} values, which are essentially the same.
   c. **Yes.** The initial dilution space (33 and 38 L), well in excess of plasma volume, must include some well-perfused tissues.
   d. **Slow acetylator:** $CL = 12.7$ L/hr; $V = 115$ L. **Fast acetylator:** $CL = 71$ L/hr; $V = 178$ L. In addition to differences in clearance, one might have concluded that differences in distribution (V) also existed, which is not so (see answer to b.).
   e. $f_2 = 0.95$ **(slow acetylator), 0.74 (fast acetylator).**
   f. **Yes.** Since f_2 approaches 1.0 for both patients, the terminal half-life primarily determines the time for the plasma concentration to reach plateau.

5. a. **The fluctuation of halazepam at plateau primarily reflects a balance between the kinetics of absorption and distribution; the 8-hr dosing interval is too short to permit distribution equilibrium to be achieved.**
   b. **Not well, and certainly not within a dosing interval, which is too short relative to the terminal half-life. Theoretically, the terminal half-life could be measured from**

the rising trough concentration on approach to plateau, but in practice, this measurement has too much error to provide a reliable estimate of terminal half-life. The most reliable estimate is gained on stopping drug administration and following the decline in plasma drug concentration.

6. a. $V_1 = 18.2$ L; $CL = 2.8$ L/hr; $V = 295$ L; and $V_{ss} = 70.9$ L.

$$V_1 = \frac{Dose}{C_1 + C_2}, \qquad V = \frac{CL}{\lambda_2}$$

$$CL = \frac{Dose}{\left(\dfrac{C_1}{\lambda_1} + \dfrac{C_2}{\lambda_2}\right)} \cdot V_{ss} = \frac{Dose \cdot \left(\dfrac{C_1}{\lambda_1^2} + \dfrac{C_2}{\lambda_2^2}\right)}{\left(\dfrac{C_1}{\lambda_1} + \dfrac{C_2}{\lambda_2}\right)^2}$$

b. **Only glomerularly filtered.**

$$CLu_R = CL_R/fu = \frac{2.8}{0.37}\ L/hr = 7.6 L/hr\ (\approx GFR)$$

and being polar, the drug is not expected to be reabsorbed. Because the glomerular filtrate comes directly from arterial blood, a model in which elimination occurs from the central compartment only is reasonable.

c. $V > V_{ss}$. Elimination of drug from plasma increases the ratio of drug concentration in slowly equilibrating tissue to that in plasma during the terminal phase. The slower the distribution of drug between plasma and the slowly equilibrating tissues, the greater is the difference between V and V_{ss}.

d. $f_1 = 0.8$; $f_2 = 0.2$. The half-lives of the corresponding exponential coefficients are 3.6 and 73 hr, respectively. The half-lives reflect a composite of distribution and elimination kinetics. In the present case, the majority of drug is eliminated before distribution equilibrium is achieved, and so with respect to elimination, the first half-life is of particular importance. Here, the terminal half-life is only of importance if interest lies in the slowly equilibrating tissues. For most drugs, the majority of drug is eliminated during the terminal phase, that is $f_2 >> f_1$.

e. (1) **5 and 72 hr to reach 50% and 90% of plateau, respectively.** See Table J19-P6. Cannot solve for time explicitly. It is estimated iteratively by successive approximations.

TABLE J19-P6 Fraction of Plateau with Time During a Constant-Rate Infusion

Time (hr)	2	4	5	6	12	24	48	72	96
C/C_{ss}	0.26	0.43	≈0.50	0.55	0.74	0.83	0.87	0.90	0.92

$$\frac{C}{C_{ss}} = f_1(1 - e^{-\lambda_1 t}) + f_2(1 - e^{-\lambda_2 t})$$

$$= 0.8(1 - e^{-0.19t}) + 0.2(1 - e^{-0.0095t})$$

Note that 50% of the plateau value is reached in approximately one initial half-life (3.8 hr; $0.693/\lambda_1$), but that the rise to the 90% value becomes increasingly determined by the long terminal half-life, 73 hr. Under these circumstances, the statement that it takes one half-life to reach 50% of plateau and 3.3 half-lives to reach plateau is misleading.

(2) **A pronounced biexponential curve is observed on stopping the infusion at steady state, because the rate of movement of drug from the slowly equilibrating tissues initially does not match the rapid elimination of drug from plasma.** Eventually, decline of the drug in plasma becomes controlled by movement of drug from the slowly equilibrating tissues to the central compartment.

(3) **Now $f_2 = 0.83$, signifying that distribution equilibrium occurs before much drug is eliminated.** Under this circumstance, although there will still be a biexponential fall on stopping the infusion, the first phase will be very shallow because drug rapidly moves from the tissues as it is eliminated from plasma. Given the general inability to distinguish two concentrations that differ by 10% and have the usual variation in plasma concentrations, it is unlikely that the first phase can be seen; the postinfusion decay would then appear monoexponential, with rate constant λ_2.

7. a. **If all that one wished to describe is the plasma concentration–time profile during and stopping an infusion,** then representing disposition kinetics by the sum of exponentials is adequate. However, if one is also interested in the events occurring in slowly equilibrating tissues, then the use of a compartmental model has an advantage in allowing conceptualization and prediction of the time course of such events, although it is important to keep in mind that the compartments are fictitious and rarely exactly correspond to a physiological space.

   b. **The use of a compartmental model has a definite advantage over the sum of exponentials when attempting to account for variability,** in that one can for example explicitly relate renal clearance solely to renal function, whereas this is not possible when using the sum of exponentials, because clearance enters into each of the parameters defining the exponential model. For this reason, compartmental models are the norm when fitting models to population pharmacokinetic data.

8. **The observation in Fig. 19-29 is explained by differences in the distribution kinetics of these drugs.** For pancuronium, in patients with both normal and impaired renal function, distribution equilibrium is achieved before much drug is eliminated; diminished renal clearance then causes a change in the terminal half-life. For d-tubocurarine, in patients with both normal and impaired renal function, most drug is eliminated from the plasma (and the well-stirred pool) before much drug has distributed; the terminal phase in both cases is then primarily controlled by movement of drug out of the slowly equilibrating tissues. Diminished renal clearance is reflected by a smaller fall in d-tubocurarine concentration before the terminal phase is reached as less drug has been eliminated by that time than in a patient with normal renal function.

9. **It takes time to distribute drug to and from the tissues. With long infusions, the tissues tend to fill up. When the infusion is stopped, the drug slowly returns from the tissues to the vasculature and to the organs of elimination. The greater the amount in the tissues, the less is the tendency for the plasma concentration to drop after the infusion is stopped, and therefore, the plasma concentration stays elevated longer.**
   The two-compartment model may also help in explaining the concept.

10. a. **Alfentanil: $f_1 = 0.072$; $f_2 = 0.206$; $f_3 = 0.722$.**
    Fentanyl: $f_1 = 0.080$; $f_2 = 0.128$; $f_3 = 0.792$.
    Sufentanil: $f_1 = 0.116$; $f_2 = 0.332$; $f_3 = 0.552$.
    b. **For all three drugs, the plasma concentration has fallen by 50% of the value at the end of the 60-min infusion.** Figure J19-P10 shows the decline in plasma concentration for each of the drugs.

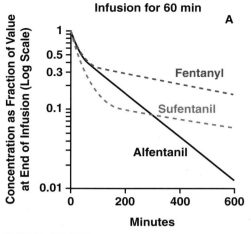

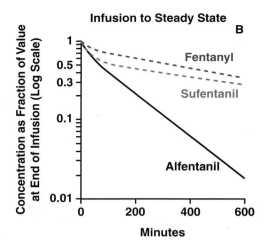

FIGURE J19-P10.

---

   c. **The terminal half-life has no utility in predicting the duration of action on stopping an infusion of drugs such as the i.v. anesthetics, which display pronounced distribution kinetics.** For example, the durations of action of alfentanil, fentanyl, and sufentanil after stopping a 60-min infusion are much shorter at 24.5, 15.6, and 14.8 min, respectively, than, and in the reverse order to the terminal half-lives (111, 462, and 577 min, respectively)

   d. **Yes.** The durations of action (and times for the plasma concentration to fall by 50%) on stopping an infusion at steady state are 62, 307, and 106 min for alfentanil, fentanyl, and sufentanil, respectively.

   e. **The ranking of anticipated duration of action is sensitive to the duration of infusion.** This is readily seen by comparing the times for the plasma concentration of alfentanil, fentanyl, and sufentanil to fall by 50% on stopping an infusion after 1 hr (24.5, 15.6, and 14.8 min, respectively) and at steady state (62, 307, and 106 min, respectively). Collectively, the answers to this question illustrate the need to consider all parameters defining disposition kinetics when predicting temporal events under various input conditions.

11. a. **The increase in duration of action seen after the second, third, and fourth doses of pancuronium is a consequence of distribution kinetics.** The effect of the first dose occurs during the distribution phase of the drug. On successive doses, because of a rising tissue concentration, the tendency of drug to move from plasma into tissues decreases, thereby prolonging the time before the plasma concentration reaches the predetermined value.

   b. **No.** The duration will reach a limiting value when the amount eliminated during the dosing interval equals the dose of drug administered.

12. a. $C_1 = 10.5$ µg/L; $\lambda_1 = 0.18$ min^{-1}; $C_2 = 2.4$ µg/L; $\lambda_2 = 0.019$ min^{-1}.
   Values taken from estimates from the semilogarithmic plot (Fig. J19-P12) using the method of residuals.

   b. λ_2. **Most of the elimination is associated with λ_2 because f_2 is 0.68.**

$$AUC = \frac{10.5}{0.18} + \frac{2.4}{0.019} = 58.3 + 126.3 = 184.6 \, \mu g\text{-}min/L$$

$$f_2 = \frac{126.3}{184.6} = 0.68$$

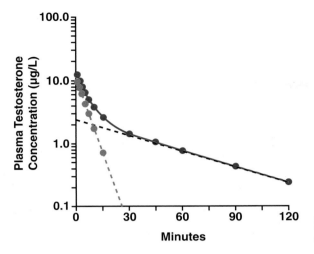

FIGURE J19-P12.

c. $CL = 1.63 \text{ L/min.}$

$$CL = \frac{Dose}{AUC} = \frac{300 \, \mu g}{184.6 \, \mu g - min/L} = 1.63 \, L/min$$

d. **Daily endogenous production of testosterone = 8424 μg or 8.4 mg.**

$$R_t = CL \cdot C_{ss} = 1.63 \, L/min \times 3.6 \, \mu g/L$$

$$= 5.85 \, \mu g/min \times 60 \, min/hr \times 24 \, hr/day$$

$$= 8424 \, \mu g/day \text{ or } 8.4 \, mg/day$$

CHAPTER 20. METABOLITES AND DRUG RESPONSE

1. **Only a.**
   a. Induction leads to an increase in CL_f.

   $$\frac{AUC(m)}{AUC} = \frac{CL_f}{CL(m)}$$

   b. Ratio of areas independent of V or $V(m)$.
   c. Ratio of areas independent of *Dose*.
   d. If alternate pathway is reduced, f_m is increased in proportion to decrease in CL, but CL_f is unaffected.

2. **Elimination of the *trans*-diol metabolite must be rate-limited by its formation from carbamazepine.** The possibility of absorption of carbamazepine being the rate-limiting step is doubtful, even in the absence of any other information; an oral absorption half-life of 30 hr is very uncommon, as very little drug would be absorbed within the usual gastrointestinal transit times of 12 to 48 hr. Independent information (not presented), following oral and i.v. administration, indicates that carbamazepine is absorbed relatively rapidly.

3. **Only the clearance associated with the formation of *N*-acetylprocainamide and the total clearance of *N*-acetylprocainamide.** This follows from the equation $C(m)_{av,ss}/C_{av,ss} = CL_f/CL(m)$. Note that in all patients in whom the ratio is greater than 1.0, the clearance of *N*-acetylprocainamide must be less than the clearance of procainamide.

4. **The rate of renal excretion of salicyluric acid can be taken to be its rate of formation from salicylic acid.** The rate of elimination of salicyluric acid is limited by, and hence essentially equal to, its rate of formation. However, the rate of elimination of salicyluric acid is its rate of renal excretion.

5. a. *fm* **(2-mononitrate) = 0.25.** The amount of metabolite formed after a 5-mg i.v. dose of isosorbide dinitrate is

$$CL(m) \cdot AUC(m) = 23 \ L/hr \times 0.044 \ mg\text{-}hr/L = 1.01 \ mg$$

Hence,

$$f_m = \frac{Amount \ metabolite \ formed}{Dose \ of \ drug} = \frac{1.01 \times \left(\frac{236}{191}\right) \ mg \ drug \ equivalents}{5 \ mg}$$

b. **Assumptions are (i) $CL(m)$ after administration of metabolite equally applies after drug administration, and (ii) all metabolite formed enters the systemic circulation.**

c. **99%.** Percentages of drug converted to the 2- and 5-mononitrates are 25 and 74, respectively.

6. **A major fraction of 4-hydroxypropranolol is formed during the systemic absorption of propranolol, which is subject to extensive first-pass hepatic elimination.** This metabolite has a shorter half-life than propranolol, and so initially the plasma 4-hydroxypropranolol concentration falls faster than that of propranolol; the terminal decline of metabolite is parallel to that of drug because the elimination of metabolite formed from absorbed propranolol is formation rate-limited. The 4-hydroxypropranolol concentration peaks earlier than that of propranolol because it has the shorter half-life. Recall from Chapter 6, *Kinetics Following an Extravascular Dose* the peak is reached when rate of elimination matches the rate of absorption, and it occurs earlier the shorter the half-life of elimination.

7. a. **Counterclockwise.** The metabolite must be formed for the effect to be seen, but the drug must be present first to form metabolite. The requisite drug to metabolite sequence tends to make the drug-to-metabolite ratio decrease with time. This would produce counterclockwise hysteresis.

   b. **Clockwise.** The metabolite would be formed in large amounts during the first pass. The metabolite so formed would disappear quickly compared with the absorbed drug.

8. a. $F_{oral} = 0.19.$

$$F = \frac{\left[\dfrac{AUC}{Dose}\right]_{oral}}{\left[\dfrac{AUC}{Dose}\right]_{i.v.}} = \frac{\left[\dfrac{43 \ nmol - hr/L}{10 \ mg}\right]}{\dfrac{229 \ nmol - hr/L}{10 \ mg}}$$

   b. **Probably.**

$$CL_b = CL \cdot (Plasma\text{-}to\text{-}blood \ concentration \ ratio) = 0.45 \times \frac{101 \ mg \ (or \ 35,000 \ nmol)}{229 \ nmol\text{-}hr/L}$$

$$= 68.7 \ L/hr$$

   If liver is the only site for drug metabolism, the oral bioavailability expected resulting from first-pass hepatic loss is given by

$$F_H = 1 - E_H = 1 - \frac{CL_b \ (1 - fe)}{Q_H}$$

And, as $fe = 0.08$, $Q_H = 81$ L/hr

$$F_H = 1 - \frac{0.92 \times CL_b}{81 \ L/hr} = 0.22$$

c. **Yes.** With very little morphine excreted unchanged ($fe = 0.08$), for the liver to be the sole site of metabolism, the expectation is that the value of $AUC(m)$ should be independent of the route of administration, oral or i.v. Reference to Table 20-8 for both the 3- and 6-glucuronides supports this expectation.

d. **No.** Based on AUC considerations, the systemic bioavailability of morphine is essentially the same whether given orally ($F = 0.19$) or sublingually ($F = 0.21$). Furthermore, the respective AUC values for morphine-3-glucuronide and morphine-6-glucuronide are the same following oral and sublingual administration, suggesting that all sublingually administered morphine is swallowed.

e. **Given that morphine-6-glucuronide has analgesic activity, with comparable C_{max} and AUC values after oral and i.v. administration of morphine, adjustment of the i.v. dose, based on the oral bioavailability of morphine alone tends to overestimate the oral dose of morphine needed to achieve comparable analgesic activity.**

f. **Because the volume of distribution of the more polar acidic glucuronide is likely to be much smaller than that of the more lipophilic and basic parent compound, morphine. Consequently, the value of C_{max} for the glucuronide will be much greater than that for morphine, for a comparable amount in the body.**

g. **Fraction of oral morphine converted to morphine-6-glucuronide is 0.06.**

$$Fraction \ converted = CL(m) \times \frac{AUC \ (m)}{Dose}$$

$$= \frac{5.8 \ L/hr \times 371 \ nmol\text{-}hr/L}{35,000 \ nmol}$$

h. (1) **With a low fe of morphine and a high fe of morphine-6-glucuronide, there will be an increase in the relative exposure of morphine-6-glucuronide to morphine in patients with poor renal function, and as this metabolite is active it may necessitate a reduction in the dosing rate of morphine in such patients or the use of another analgesic agent that is not influenced by reduced renal function.**

(2) **Dosing rate approximately one third of normal dosing rate.** The following calculation is based on observed exposure data. There are several ways of approaching this problem. One approach is adopted here, but whatever one is used the answer should be the same.

Normal renal function. Following i.v. morphine administration, for 6-morphine-glucuronide

$$f(m) = AUC(m) \cdot CL(m)/Dose$$
$$= 313 \ nmol\text{-}hr/L \times 5.8 \ L/hr = 0.052$$

Fraction of morphine converted on single passage though liver $fm_H = \dfrac{fm}{1 - fe} = \dfrac{0.052}{1 - 0.08} = 0.057$

And following oral morphine

Fraction of oral morphine converted to morphine-6-glucuronide $Fm = (1 - F_H) \cdot fm_H + F_H \cdot fm$

$$= 0.81 \times 0.057 + 0.19 \times 0.052 = 0.056$$

Now assuming that the analgesic effect is the sum of the contributions of morphine and morphine-6-glucuronide (which has 10% of activity of morphine), it follows that expressed in activity equivalents at plateau on multiple dosing

$$C_{av,ss} + 0.1 \cdot C(m)_{av,ss} = \frac{Dose}{\tau}\left[\frac{F_H}{CL} + \frac{0.1 \cdot F_m}{CL(m)}\right]$$

$$= \frac{Dose}{\tau}\left[\frac{0.19}{153\ L/hr} + \frac{0.1 \times 0.056}{5.8\ L/hr}\right]$$

$$= \frac{0.0022 Dose}{\tau}$$

Renal impairment. Given that formation of morphine-6-glucuronide all occurs in the liver, which is unaffected by renal impairment, so that F_H and fm_H remain unchanged, and that morphine-6-glucuronide is totally renally excreted unchanged, the expected values are:

$$fm(d) = fm/(1 - fe + RF \cdot fe) = 0.052/(1 - 0.08 + 0.2 \times 0.08) = 0.056$$

Fraction of oral morphine converted to morphine-6-glucuronide $Fm(d) = (1 - F_H) \cdot fm_H + F_H \cdot fm(d)$

$$= 0.81 \times 0.057 + 0.19 \times 0.056 = 0.057$$

That is $Fm(d)$ is only marginally different from Fm because morphine fe is low. Following multiple dosing of morphine

$$C_{av,ss} + 0.1 \cdot C(m)_{av,ss} = \left(\frac{Dose}{\tau}\right)_d\left[\frac{F_H}{CL(d)} + \frac{0.1 \cdot Fm(d)}{CL(m,d)}\right]$$

$$= \left(\frac{Dose}{\tau}\right)_d\left[\frac{F_H}{CL \cdot (1 - fe + RF \cdot fe)} + \frac{0.1 \cdot Fm(d)}{CL(m) \cdot (1 - fe(m) + RF \cdot fe(m))}\right]$$

$$= \left(\frac{Dose}{\tau}\right)_d\left[\frac{0.19}{143\ L/hr} + \frac{0.1 \times 0.057}{1.16\ L/hr}\right]$$

$$= 0.0062\left(\frac{Dose}{\tau}\right)_d$$

Now, as the dosing rate in disease needs to maintain the same degree of analgesia as in a patient with normal renal function, it follows that

$$0.0062\left(\frac{Dose}{\tau}\right)_d = 0.0022\left(\frac{Dose}{\tau}\right)$$

or

$$\left(\frac{Dose}{\tau}\right)_d = 0.035$$

Hence, either the dose must be reduced by threefold, τ increased by threefold, or a combination of changes in both. Finally, it should be noted that although various studies have led to different estimates of *fm*, *Fm*, and relative analgesic activity of morphine-6-glucuronide, which in turn have led to different estimates of the change in dosing rate of morphine, the basis of the calculation remains unchanged.

CHAPTER 21. PROTEIN DRUGS

1. **Protein drugs must generally be given parenterally because they have great difficulty in permeating cell membranes, and they are quickly metabolized (or degraded) before reaching the systemic circulation when administered by any other route.** A few smaller protein drugs can reach the systemic circulation when administered by inhalation, intranasally, or by certain other routes, but there is usually considerable variability and the bioavailability is low.

2. There are several factors that influence the rate and extent of systemic absorption of protein drugs following intramuscular (i.m.) and subcutaneous (s.c.) administration. For example:

   - **Molecular size of the drug molecule.** Larger proteins, especially those greater than 20,000 g/mol in size, are primarily systemically absorbed via the lymphatic system, because of a marked decrease in the permeability of blood capillaries with molecular size.
   - **Degradation.** Metabolism within the interstitial fluid and the lymphatic system often results in reduced bioavailability.
   - **Site of injection is important.** Both rate and extent of absorption can be affected by the location of the injection, even by the same route (e.g., s.c.). Blood flow is one of the components of the site-specific difference in absorption, especially for small molecules. The number of lymph nodes and length of lymphatic vessels traversed before returning to the systemic blood circulation are important for large proteins.
   - **Exercise and rubbing.** Exercise and rubbing influence the rate of systemic absorption as does the volume of fluid injected.

3. **a. Clearance = 0.80 L/hr; Volume of distribution = 7.7 L.**

$$CL = \left[\frac{Dose}{AUC} \right]_{iv} = \frac{\dfrac{40\ units}{kg} \times 60\ kg}{3010\ unit\text{-}hr/L} = 0.80\ L/hr$$

$$V = \frac{CL}{k} = \frac{0.80\ L/hr}{0.693/6.7\ hr} = 7.7\ L$$

   b. Bioavailability = 0.46.

$$F = \frac{(AUC/Dose)_{sc}}{(AUC/Dose)_{iv}} = \frac{1372}{3010}$$

The molecular size of erythropoietin (34,000 g/mol) is such that the majority of a dose probably enters the systemic circulation via the lymphatic, rather than the vascular, system. For loss to occur during the absorption process, the drug must be metabolized (degraded) in the interstitial fluid near the injection site or within the lymphatic system.

c. **Reduced bioavailability, absorption rate-limiting elimination after s.c. administration.** In part, this is caused by the lower bioavailability from the subcutaneous route, but with a bioavailability of 0.46 this alone cannot explain the C_{max} following s.c. administration being 10-fold lower than that after i.v. dosing. The other reason is the slow absorption from the subcutaneous site such that much drug still remains at the absorption site when C_{max} is reached, a characteristic of "flip-flop" kinetics (i.e., when elimination is rate-limited by absorption).

4. a. **Yes, absorption appears to be rate-limiting for s.c. administration into the thigh.** The semilogarithmic plots of the data (Fig. J21-P4) show different terminal slopes. If elimination were always rate-limiting, then the same terminal half-life should be observed. One cannot be sure, however, if absorption is rate-limiting the decline after the injection into the abdomen.

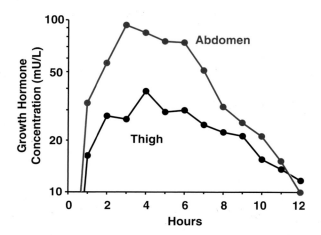

FIGURE J21-P4.

b. **0.54.** The relative bioavailability is not well determined because of the lack of data beyond 12 hr. The value calculated was determined using the trapezoidal rule to 12 hr and C_{last}/k to estimate the area remaining under each curve.

$$F_{rel} = \frac{AUC_{s.c.}\ (thigh)}{AUC_{s.c.}\ (abdomen)} = \frac{0.339\ unit\text{-}hr/L}{0.625\ unit\text{-}hr/L} = 0.54$$

$$k(abdomen) = 0.38\ hr^{-1}\ k(thigh) = 0.17\ hr^{-1}$$

c. $F_{abdomen} = 0.78$

As $F \cdot Dose = CL \cdot AUC$,

$$F_{abdomen} = \frac{CL \cdot AUC}{Dose} = \frac{5.0\ L/hr \times 0.625\ units\text{-}hr/L}{4\ units} = 0.78$$

5. a. **Turnover rate = 5 units/hr.**

$$Turnover\ rate = CL \cdot C_{ss} = \frac{0.5\ L}{hr} \times \frac{10\ units}{L} = 5\ units/hr$$

b. **Turnover time = 8 hr.**

$$Turnover\ time\ (t_t) = \frac{1}{k} = \frac{V}{CL} = \frac{4\ L}{0.5\ L/hr} = 8\ hr$$

c. **Fractional turnover rate = 0.125 hr^{-1}.**

$$Fractional\ turnover\ rate = \frac{CL}{V} = \frac{0.5\ L/hr}{4\ L} = 0.125\ hr^{-1}$$

or

$$= \frac{1}{t_t} = \frac{1}{8\ hr} = 0.125\ hr^{-1}$$

6. a. **Because the drug is also eliminated by renal metabolism.** When renal function goes to zero, as in the case of the two nephrectomized patients, the half-life is virtually more than 100-fold greater than that in healthy patients. Apparently, less than 1% of the elimination normally occurs by nonrenal mechanisms.

b. **There is virtually no other pathway for elimination of hirudin.** The drug is sufficiently small to be glomerularly filtered. Of that filtered, virtually all the dose, the majority undergoes metabolism. This is consistent with the unit nephron hypothesis, which states that chronic renal disease is simply a reduction in the number of functional nephrons.

c. **There is still some renal function remaining in the dialysis group and some renal metabolism as well.** The half-life averages about 33 hr in this group, a value about 20 times that of the healthy group. One can then speculate that, on average, about 5% of renal function remains.

7. a. **No.** The clearance and half-life are virtually unchanged in patients with hepatic disease compared with healthy patients.

b. **~1000 mL/min.** The renal clearance can be crudely estimated by the difference between total clearances for the healthy (1640 mL/min) and renal failure (631 mL/min) groups. Some renal function remains in the latter group, so the renal clearance in the healthy group must be ~1000 mL/min, unless nonrenal clearance is also reduced in renal failure.

c. **Yes.** The renal clearance is greater than $fu \cdot GFR$. No data for fu is given, but its upper limit is 1.0. The ratio $CL_R/(fu \cdot GFR)$ is therefore 10 or more, indicating that the drug undergoes secretion. Very little unchanged drug comes out in the urine, so the high renal clearance is caused by postglomerular metabolism in the tubular cells.

8. a. **28.2 and 11.3 L.**

   Healthy Group

$$V = \frac{\dfrac{Dose}{AUC}}{\dfrac{0.693}{t_{1/2}}} = \frac{\dfrac{70\ mg}{9.5\ mg\text{-}hr/L}}{\dfrac{0.693}{2.64\ hr}} = 28.1\ L$$

   Renal Disease Group

$$V = \frac{\dfrac{Dose}{AUC}}{\dfrac{0.693}{t_{1/2}}} = \frac{\dfrac{70\ mg}{63.7\ mg\text{-}hr/L}}{\dfrac{0.693}{7.15\ hr}} = 11.3\ L$$

b. **The greater drop in the healthy group is a result of rapid elimination of drug from the body, as evidenced by a large percent of the *AUC* being associated with the rapid decline phase.** In the renal disease group, the initial decline in concentration is primarily associated with distribution, not elimination.

c. **The terminal half-life did not change as much as** *AUC* **(and clearance), because the terminal half-life in the healthy patients is not a good estimate of the elimination half-life of the drug.** A good fraction of the area is associated with the more rapid decline. Another view can be expressed using the two-compartment model. In the healthy group, much of the drug is eliminated during the early period leaving only a small fraction of the dose to be distributed to the peripheral compartment. In the renal patients, elimination is slow so that much of the dose distributes to the peripheral compartment before much is lost from the body.

9. **Nonlinear kinetics occurs frequently with protein drugs, because there is a limited capacity for binding of the protein to sites within the body, and the concentrations used in therapy are close to those causing the binding to become nonlinear.** The major binding site is frequently the receptor site for the response. Thus, both the pharmacokinetics and the pharmacodynamics are nonlinear for the same reason, saturable binding to the receptor. Maintenance of a high plasma concentration slows its elimination and maintains a response close to E_{max}, both apparently therapeutically desirable for many protein drugs, especially antibodies.

10. a. **15.9 days and 0.063 day^{-1}.**

$$MRT = \frac{AUMC}{AUC} = \frac{\dfrac{1.5}{1.42^2} + \dfrac{1.2}{0.06^2}}{\dfrac{1.5}{1.42} + \dfrac{1.2}{0.06}} = 15.9 \ days$$

$$k_t = 1/t_t = 1/MRT = 0.063 \ day^{-1}$$

b. **105 and 109 g.**
   Amount in intravascular space

$$V_1 = \frac{Dose^*}{C(0)^*} = \frac{6.7. \ megaBecquerels}{2.7 \ megaBecquerels/L} = 2.5L$$

$$A = V_1 \cdot C(0) = 2.5 \ L \times 42 \ g/L = 105 \ g$$
*Radiolabel

   Total in body

$$V_{ss} = MRT \cdot CL = MRT \cdot Dose/AUC$$
$$= 15.9 \ days \times 6.75 \ megaBequerels/21.06 \ megaBequerels\text{-}hr/L = 5.1 \ L$$
$$A = 5.1 \ L \times 42 \ g/L = 214 \ g$$

   Amount in extravascular space
$$= Total \ in \ body - Amount \ in \ intravascular \ space = 109 \ g$$

c. **13.5 g/day.**
$$R_t = k_t \cdot A_{ss} = k_t \cdot V_{ss} \cdot Css$$
$$= 0.063 \ day^{-1} \times 5.1 \ L \times 42 \ g/L$$

d. **No.** Although the steady-state properties of albumin are defined, these do not allow an insight as to the location(s) for degradation of albumin within the body. Independent data suggest that it occurs in large part within fibroblasts in skin and muscle.

11. a. **Most likely.** Myocardial infarction is known to decrease cardiac output and hepatic blood flow. The high values and similarity in the clearances of t-PA and indocyanine green indicate that the elimination of t-PA is related to hepatic blood flow.
    b. **As both appear to depend on hepatic blood flow, their clearances would be expected to correlate in patients with compromised cardiac output and hepatic**

blood flow. This is one of the unusual examples of a protein drug with a high hepatic extraction ratio. This is in contrast to the large percent of small molecule drugs that have this property.

c. $E_H = 0.80$. Because the two drugs are restricted to plasma, the extraction ratio can be obtained by the ratio of their clearances, 470 mL/min/585 mL/min. The value could also have been obtained by the ratio of their blood clearances that can be determined from the product of their plasma clearances and their plasma/blood concentration ratios ($[470 \times 2]/[585 \times 2]$).

d. **These results suggest that caution might be applied, and adjustments in dosage considered, when t-PA is given to patients with acutely impaired hepatic blood flow or in combination with drugs that may affect hepatic blood flow.**

CHAPTER 22. PREDICTION AND REFINEMENT OF HUMAN KINETICS FROM IN VITRO, PRECLINICAL, AND EARLY CLINICAL DATA

(*No Study Problems*)

APPENDIX A. ASSESSMENT OF *AUC*

1. **Area under the curve to 24 hr = 17.65 mg-hr/L.**

Time (hr)	Plasma Concentration (mg/L)	Time Interval (hr)	Average Concentration* (mg/L)	Area† (mg-hr/L)
0	0	—		
0.5	2.14	0.5	1.070	0.535
1	2.95	0.5	2.545	1.273
1.5	3.25	0.5	3.100	1.550
2	3.27	0.5	3.260	1.630
3	2.68	1	2.975	2.975
4	2.15	1	2.415	2.415
6	1.12	2	1.365	3.270
8	0.611	2	0.865	1.730
10	0.321	2	0.466	0.932
12	0.180	2	0.251	0.502
14	0.101	2	0.141	0.282
24	0.011	10	0.056	0.560
			Total:	17.654

$$* \left[\frac{C(t) + C(t-1)}{2} \right]$$

†Average concentration times time interval.

APPENDIX B. IONIZATION AND THE pH PARTITION HYPOTHESIS

1. a. **61.4%.** Taking the antilog of Eq. B-1 in Appendix B, *Ionization and the pH Partition Hypothesis*, for plasma

$$\frac{Ionized\ Concentration}{Un\text{-}ionized\ Concentration} = 10^{pH - pKa} = 10^{7.4 - 7.2} = 1.58$$

Substituting into Eq. B-4, the percent ionized in blood is

$$\frac{1.58 \times 100}{1.58 + 1} = 61.4\%$$

b. **9.09 %.** Similarly, for the urine,

$$\frac{Ionized\ Concentration}{Un\text{-}ionized\ Concentration} = 10^{pH-pKa} = 10^{6.2-7.2} = 0.1$$

Substituting into Eq. B-4, percent ionized in urine at pH 6.2 is

$$\frac{0.1 \times 100}{0.1 + 1} = 9.09\%$$

2. a. **99%.** Taking the antilog of Eq. B-2, and rearranging, for stomach

$$\frac{Ionized\ Concentration}{Un\text{-}ionized\ Concentration} = 10^{pKa-pH} = 10^{3.8-1.8} = 100$$

Substituting into Eq. B-4, the percent ionized in a pH 1.8 stomach is

$$\frac{100 \times 100}{100 + 1} = 99\%$$

b. **0.025%.** Similarly for the blood.

$$\frac{Ionized\ Concentration}{Un\text{-}ionized\ Concentration} = 10^{pKa-pH} = 10^{3.8-7.4} = 2.5 \times 10^{-4}$$

Substituting into Eq. B-4, the percent ionized in blood is

$$\frac{2.5 \times 10^{-4} \times 100}{2.5 \times 10^{-4} + 1} = 0.025\%$$

APPENDIX C. DISTRIBUTION OF DRUGS EXTENSIVELY BOUND TO PLASMA PROTEINS

1. a.

Percent of Drug in Body* That Is...	Nafcillin	Naproxen	Nitrazepam
In plasma	12	27	2
Unbound	**19**	1	4
In extracellular fluid	34	**67**	6
Outside extracellular fluids	**66**	33	94
Bound to protein	11	27	2
Bound outside the extracellular fluids (in or on tissue cells, Including blood cells)	54	32	**91**

*For a 70-kg person.

b. **Nitrazepam.** See analysis below.

| | $\dfrac{V_R{}^\dagger}{fu_R}$ | V(L)* | | |
		Before	After‡	Percent increase
Nafcillin	147	24.5	41.5	69
Naproxen	1226	11.2	14.9	33
Nitrazepam	958	133	259	94

*70-kg person.

†Estimated from: $V = 7.5 + 7.5 \cdot fu + \dfrac{V_R}{fu_R} \cdot fu$

‡Value after *fu* is doubled.

2. **Unbound volume of distribution (V/fu) is decreased from 2.5 to 1.5 L/kg, whereas unbound clearance shows essentially no change, 300 to 260 mL/hr per kg.** Tolbutamide is unquestionably of low extraction, because CL/Q_H is less than 0.02. The lack of change in unbound clearance indicates no effect of acute viral hepatitis on metabolic activity. The decrease in unbound volume is consistent with the change in fraction unbound for a drug with a small volume of distribution. The half-life shortens because the decrease in binding to plasma proteins decreases the unbound volume.

APPENDIX D. PLASMA-TO-BLOOD CONCENTRATION RATIO

1. a. **40.**

$$Kp_{BC} = \frac{H - 1 + (C_b/C)}{fu \cdot H} = \frac{0.45 - 1 + 1/0.425}{0.1 \times 0.45}$$

b. **0.55.**

$$\frac{C}{C_b} = \frac{1}{1 + H(fu \cdot Kp_{BC} - 1)} = \frac{1}{1 + 0.27(0.1 \times 40 - 1)}$$

The percent change in C/C_b is minor compared to that of the hematocrit. Note that had $fu \cdot Kp_{BC}$ been equal to 1 (drug concentration in blood cells the same as that in plasma); there would have been no change in C/C_b when the hematocrit was altered. Furthermore, if $fu \cdot Kp_{BC}$ is less that 1, then C/C_b increases with a decrease in H. Finally, if $fu \cdot Kp_{BC}$ is greater than 1, then C/C_b decreases with a decrease in H.

$$\frac{C}{C_b} = \frac{1}{1 + H(fu \cdot Kp_{BC} - 1)} = \frac{1}{1 + 0.45(0.32 \times 40 - 1)}$$

The increased value of fu, resulting from the lowered plasma albumin concentration greatly decreases the ratio of C to C_b. Had Kp_{BC} been a small value, the drug would have been largely confined to plasma, and changes in fu would have had a minor effect on the ratio of C to C_b.

APPENDIX E. WELL-STIRRED MODEL OF HEPATIC CLEARANCE

1. a. $E_H = 0.34$

$$E_H = \frac{CL_H \cdot R}{Q_H} = \frac{2.7 L/min \times 0.17}{1.35 L/min}$$

where R is the plasma-to-blood concentration ratio.

b. $CL_{int} = 81.8$ L/min.

$$E_H = \frac{fu_b \cdot CL_{int}}{Q_H + fu_b \cdot CL_{int}} = \frac{fu \cdot R \cdot CL_{int}}{Q_H + fu \cdot R \cdot CL_{int}}$$

Rearranging and collecting terms, yields

$$CL_{int} = \frac{Q_H \cdot E_H}{fu \cdot R \cdot (1 - E_H)} = \frac{1.35 \text{ L/min} \times 0.34}{0.05 \times 0.17 \times (1 - 0.34)} = 81.8 \text{ L/min}$$

c. **Although intrinsic clearance of the drug is much greater than hepatic blood flow, the extraction ratio (0.34) is quite low, because very little of the drug in the perfusing blood is unbound to cross into the hepatocyte as a consequence of its high plasma protein binding and extensive distribution into blood cells.**

2.

$$Cu_{av,ss} = \frac{fu \cdot Dose \cdot F_H}{CL \cdot \tau}$$

When hepatic clearance is uptake permeability rate-limited, then

$$E_H = \frac{fu \cdot R \cdot PS_{influx}}{Q_H + fu \cdot R \cdot PS_{influx}}$$

and

$$F_H = (1 - E_H) = \frac{Q_H}{Q_H + fu \cdot R \cdot PS_{influx}}$$

So that, since $CL = CL_b/R = Q_H \cdot E_H/R$, it follows on substitution that

$$Cu_{av,ss} = \frac{fu \cdot Dose \cdot F_H}{CL \cdot \tau} = \frac{fu \cdot Dose \cdot \left[\dfrac{Q_H}{Q_H + fu \cdot R \cdot PS_{influx}} \right]}{\dfrac{Q_H}{R} \cdot \left[\dfrac{fu \cdot R \cdot PS_{influx}}{Q_H + fu \cdot R \cdot PS_{influx}} \right] \cdot \tau}$$

$$= \frac{Dose}{PS_{influx} \cdot \tau}$$

That is, the unbound concentration at plateau depends only on the dosing rate and PS_{influx}. Clearly, for such a drug, the extraction ratio is low, so therefore is the loss of oral bioavailability caused by hepatic extraction.

APPENDIX F. ABSORPTION KINETICS

1. a. $ka = 1.4$ hr^{-1}; $k = 0.35$ hr^{-1}. **See Fig. JF-P1.**
   b. **Absorption begins immediately because there is no lag time.**
   c. (1) **Clearance = 5.8 L/hr.**
      Assuming $F = 1$, $CL = Dose/AUC = 100$ mg/17.3 mg-hr/L. AUC is obtained using the trapezoidal rule (Appendix A, *Assessment of AUC*).
      (2) $V = CL/k = 17$ **L.**
      If absorption is the rate-limiting step, then $V = 5.8/1.4 = 4.1$ L. This is an unlikely value, so the assignment of values in (a) above is probably correct.

2. **Observations can be explained entirely by a competing reaction.** With a competing reaction, the observed absorption rate constant $ka = ka' + kc$, and $F = ka'/ka$, where ka' is the true rate constant defining the absorption process, and kc is the rate constant of the competing reaction. For both groups calculation indicates that $ka' = ka \cdot F = 0.35$ hr^{-1}. Both the lower bioavailability and the apparent faster absorption of the drug in group A are a result of more extensive degradation in the acidic gastric contents. Lesson: Be careful in interpreting the value of the absorption rate constant when a competing reaction is likely.

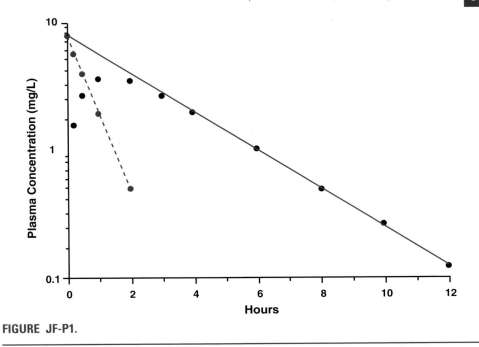

FIGURE JF-P1.

APPENDIX G. WAGNER-NELSON METHOD

1. a. **See table below.**

Estimation of Cumulative Absorption

Time (hr)	Plasma Concentration (mg/L)	Area (mg-hr/L)	Aab/V* (mg/L)	Fraction of Bioavailable Dose Absorbed†
0.0	0.00	0.00	0.00	0.0
0.5	0.76	0.19	0.79	0.055
1	1.42	0.73	1.54	0.11
2	2.48	2.68	2.92	0.20
3	3.24	5.54	4.15	0.29
4	3.75	9.03	5.23	0.36
6	4.27	17.05	7.08	0.49
8	4.31	25.63	8.53	0.59
10	4.09	34.03	9.70	0.67
12	3.72	41.48	10.62	0.73
18	2.46	60.38	12.42	0.86
24	1.45	72.11	13.34	0.93
36	0.43	83.39	14.18	0.98
48	0.11	86.63	14.40	1.00

*$Aab/V = C + k \cdot \int_0^t c \cdot dt$

†Fraction of bioavailability dose absorbed at time t $= \dfrac{\dfrac{Aab}{V}}{\dfrac{(k \cdot AUC(\infty))}{V}} = \dfrac{C + k \cdot \int_0^t Cdt}{k \cdot AUC(\infty)}$

b. **Disposition is described by a (linear) one-compartment model, with no change in disposition kinetics between treatments.**

c. **Approximately 100%**

$$F_{rel} = \frac{\left[\dfrac{AUC}{Dose}\right]_{MR}}{\left[\dfrac{AUC}{Dose}\right]_{solution}} = \frac{\left(\dfrac{86.63}{500}\right)}{\left(\dfrac{86.6}{500}\right)}$$

where MR = modified-release.

d. **First order, the half-life of absorption is 6 hr.** A semilogarithmic plot of fraction of bioavailable dose remaining to be absorbed versus time declines linearly, indicating that absorption is a first-order process. The value of the denominator is 14.4 mg/L. Further, noting that if absorption is first order, then

$$\frac{Aab}{F \cdot Dose} = e^{-ka \cdot t}$$

A semilogarithmic plot of fraction of bioavailable dose remaining to be absorbed $[1 - Aab/F \cdot Dose = 1 - (C + k \cdot \int_0^t C \cdot dt)/(k \cdot AUC(\infty))]$ against time is a straight line with a slope of $-ka$. Such a plot (Fig. JG-P1) shows the decline is linear, with a half-life of 6 hr.

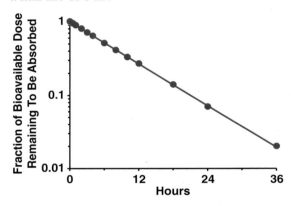

FIGURE JG-P1.

2. a. **Absorption kinetics are listed in table below.**

Time (hr)	Plasma Concentration (µg/L)	AUC (µg-hr/L)	k · AUC* (µg/L)	C + k · AUC (µg/L)	Fraction of Bioavailable Drug Absorbed[†]	Fraction of Drug Absorbed[‡]
0	0	0	0	0	0	0
0.5	0	0	0	0	0	0
2	0.49	0.37	0.13	0.62	0.05	0.025
4	0.99	1.85	0.67	1.70	0.13	0.065
6	1.83	4.67	1.68	3.5	0.28	0.14
8	1.84	8.34	3.00	4.8	0.38	0.19
10	1.93	12.1	4.36	5.9	0.47	0.24
14	1.52	19.0	6.84	8.4	0.67	0.34
18	1.43	24.9	8.96	10.4	0.83	0.42
24	1.63	31.2	11.2	12.9	1.02	0.51
26	0.65	33.5	12.1	12.7	1.01	0.50
28	0.29	34.5	12.4	12.7	1.01	0.50
30	0.10	34.8	12.5	12.6	1.00	0.50

*$k = 0.36 \text{ hr}^{-1}(0.693/1.9 \text{ hr})$.
[†]Fraction = $(C + k \cdot AUC)/k \cdot AUC(0 - \infty)$; $AUC(0-\infty) = 34.83 + 0.1/0.36 = 35.1$ µg-hr/L; $k \cdot AUC(0 - \infty) = 12.6$ µg/L.
[‡]Fraction = $F \times (C + k \cdot AUC)/k \cdot AUC(0 \cdot \infty)$; where $F = 0.50$ (answer from Chapter 10, *Constant-Rate Input*, problem 4.c.).

b. The absorption kinetics approximate, but do not exactly match, the expectation of constant-rate input over a period of 15 hr. A linear plot of the fraction bioavailable with time (not shown) indicates that, after a delay of approximately 1 hr, absorption does proceed at a nearly constant rate for 17 hr, during which time 83% of the bioavailable drug is absorbed. Between 17 and 24 hr, the remaining 17% is absorbed. As such, the device performs reasonable well. A semilogarithmic plot of the fraction absorbed with time shows an increasingly steeper slope, characteristic of a constant-rate process (Fig. JG-P2). Had absorption been a first-order process, the semilogarithmic decline would be linear.

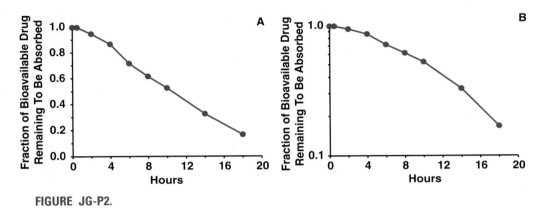

FIGURE JG-P2.

APPENDIX H. MEAN RESIDENCE TIME

1.

$$MRT = \frac{\int_0^\infty C \cdot t \cdot dt}{\int_0^\infty C \cdot dt}$$ (Eq. H-8)

$$C = C(0) \cdot e^{-kt}$$

$$MRT = \frac{C(0) \cdot \int_0^\infty e^{-kt} \cdot t \cdot dt}{C(0) \cdot \int_0^\infty e^{-kt} \cdot dt} = \frac{\int_0^\infty t \cdot e^{-kt} \cdot dt}{\int_0^\infty e^{-kt} \cdot dt}$$

$$= \frac{\left[\dfrac{-e^{-kt}}{k^2}(kt + 1)\right]_0^\infty}{\left[\dfrac{-e^{-kt}}{k}\right]_0^\infty} = \frac{1}{k}$$

2.

$$MRT = \frac{\int_0^{t_{inf}} (Dose - R_{inf} \cdot t)\, dt}{Dose}$$

Since $R_{inf} = Dose/t_{inf}$, then

$$MRT = \frac{Dose \int_0^{t_{inf}} \left(1 - \dfrac{t}{t_{inf}^2}\right) dt}{Dose}$$

$$= \left[t - \frac{t^2}{2t_{inf}}\right]_0 = \frac{2t_{inf}^2 - t_{inf}^2}{2 \cdot t_{inf}} = \frac{t_{inf}}{2}$$

3. a. **4 hr.**

$$\text{Mean infusion time} = 2 \text{ hr } (10\text{--}8) = \frac{t_{inf}}{2}$$

Therefore, $t_{inf} = 4$ hr.

b. **2.77 hr.**

Mean absorption time = 4 hr $(12-8)$.

If absorption is first order and obeys single-compartment kinetics, mean absorption time $= 1/ka$. Therefore, $ka = 0.25 \text{ hr}^{-1}$, and absorption half-life $(0.693/ka)$ = 2.77 hr.

4.

$$\text{Observed MRT} = \frac{\int_0^\infty C \cdot t \cdot dt}{\int_0^\infty C \cdot dt} = \left[\frac{\int_0^\infty (e^{-kt} - e^{-ka \cdot t}) \cdot t \cdot dt}{\int_0^\infty (e^{-kt} - e^{-ka \cdot t}) \cdot dt} \right]$$

$$\text{Observed MRT} = \frac{\left[\dfrac{1}{k^2} - \dfrac{1}{ka^2} \right]}{\left[\dfrac{1}{k} - \dfrac{1}{ka} \right]} = \frac{\left[\dfrac{1}{k} + \dfrac{1}{ka} \right] \cdot \left[\dfrac{1}{k} - \dfrac{1}{ka} \right]}{\left[\dfrac{1}{k} - \dfrac{1}{ka} \right]} = \frac{1}{k} + \frac{1}{ka}$$

Note: Neither *Dose* nor *F* is in the relationship. They cancel on taking the ratio of *AUMC/AUC*.

5. a.   *AUMC/AUC* = **14.7 hr**; *MRT* = **2.7 hr.** The following table lists the calculated values of *AUC* and *AUMC* following both the 24-hr constant-rate i.v. infusion and the administration of the rectal drug delivery device. The values were calculated using the trapezoidal rule (Appendix A, *Assessment of AUC*). From this table, for the i.v. infusion, $AUMC = 1041 \text{ μg-hr}^2/\text{L}$; $AUC = 70.6 \text{ μg-hr/L}$.

$$MRT = \frac{AUMC}{AUC} - \frac{t_{inf}}{2} - 14.7 \text{ hr} - 24 \text{ hr}/2 = 2.7 \text{ hr}$$

Calculation of *AUC* and *AUMC* of Droperidol

	24-hr i.v. Infusion				Rectal Delivery Device			
Time (hr)	C (μg/L)	AUC* (μg-hr/L)	C · t (μg-hr/L)	AUMC* (μg-hr²/L)	C (mg·L)	AUC* (μg-hr/L)	C · t (μg-hr/L)	AUMC* (μg-hr²/L)
0	0	0	0	0	0	0	0	0
0.5	0.9	0.23	0.25	0.06	0	0	0	0
2	1.8	2.3	3.6	3.0	0.49	0.37	0.98	0.25
4	2.6	6.7	9.6	16.2	0.99	1.95	4.0	5.2
6	2.5	11.8	15.0	40.8	1.83	4.7	11.0	20.1
8	2.5	16.8	20.0	75.8	1.84	8.3	14.7	45.8
10	2.7	22.0	27.0	123	1.93	12.1	19.3	79.9
14	2.7	32.8	37.8	252	1.52	19.0	21.3	161
18	2.9	44.0	52.2	432	1.43	24.9	25.3	254
24	3.1	62.0	74.4	812	1.63	31.2	39.1	448

(continued)

Calculation of *AUC* and *AUMC* of Droperidol *(continued)*

	24-hr i.v. Infusion				Rectal Delivery Device			
Time (hr)	C (μg/L)	AUC* (μg-hr/L)	C · t (μg-hr/L)	AUMC* (μg-hr²/L)	C (mg·L)	AUC* (μg-hr/L)	C · t (μg-hr/L)	AUMC* (μg-hr²/L)
26	1.4	66.5	36.4	923	0.65	33.5	16.9	504
28	0.67	67.5	18.8	978	0.29	34.5	8.1	529
30	0.36	69.6	10.8	1008	0.1	34.8	3.0	540
∞	0	70.6†	0	1041‡	0	35.1**	0	549††

*Comulative value to time *t*.

†Extrapolated *AUC* beyond 30 hr = $C(30)/k = 0.36\ \mu g/L/0.36\ hr^{-1} = 1\ \mu g\text{-}hr/L$).

‡Extrapolated *AUMC* beyond 30 hr $= \dfrac{C(30)}{k} \times \left[30 + \dfrac{1}{k} \right] = \dfrac{0.36\ \mu g/L}{0.36\ hr^{-1}} \times (30 + 2.8\ hr) = 32\ \mu g\text{-}hr^2/L.$

**Extrapolated *AUC* beyond 30 hr $= 0.1\ \mu g/L/0.36 hr^{-1} = 0.28\ \mu g\text{-}hr/L.$

††Extrapolated *AUMC* beyond 30 hr $= \dfrac{C(30)}{k} \times \left[30 + \dfrac{1}{k} \right] = \dfrac{0.1\ \mu g/L}{0.36\ hr^{-1}} \times (30 + 2.8) = 9.1\ \mu g\text{-}hr^2/L.$

b. **Yes, reasonably well.** Based on *MRT*, expected $t_{1/2} = 0.693 \times MRT = 0.693 \times 2.7$ hr = 1.87 hr. That estimated from the decline of plasma concentration with time after stopping the infusion is 1.9 hr. The close agreement between the two values of $t_{1/2}$ suggests that the disposition kinetics of droperidol can be approximated by a one-compartment model. Had the disposition kinetics of the drug showed a marked polyexponential character, then the terminal half-life on stopping the infusion would be distinctly greater than $0.693 \times MRT$, which characterizes the body as a single compartment.

c. $(AUMC/AUC)_{\text{rectal device}}$ = **15.6 hr; mean input time = 12.9 hr.** From the table above.

$$\frac{AUMC}{AUC} = \frac{549\ \mu g\text{-}hr^2/L}{35.1\ \mu g\text{-}hr/L} = 15.6\ hr$$

$$Mean\ input\ time = \frac{AUMC}{AUC} - MRT = 15.6\ hr - 2.7\ hr = 12.9\ hr$$

d. **Mean absorption time = 3.9 hr.** For a sequential process:

$$Mean\ input\ time = mean\ release\ time + mean\ absorption\ time$$

Hence,

Mean absorption time = mean input time − mean release time = 12.9 hr − 9 hr = 3.9 hr.

Note: In this calculation the in vitro input time is assumed to apply in vivo. In practice, it may not be so.

APPENDIX I. AMOUNT OF DRUG IN BODY ON ACCUMULATION TO PLATEAU

1. **a. and b. See table that follows.** Note that the sum of the amounts remaining from the first 3 doses plus the last dose, last row, is identical to the sum of the values in column 2. Thus, the accumulation expected after multiple doses can be readily predicted from data following a single dose.

Amount of Diazepam (mg) in the Body Just After Each of Four Successive Daily Doses

Time	First Dose	Second Dose	Third Dose	Fourth Dose
0	10			
τ*	6.07	10		
2τ	3.68	6.07	10	
3τ	2.23	3.68	6.07	10

*τ, 1 day.

c. $A_{max,ss} = 25.4$ mg; $A_{min,ss} = 15.4$ mg.

$$A_{max,ss} = \frac{Dose}{1 - e^{-k\tau}} = \frac{10\ mg}{\left(1 - e^{-0.5day^{-1} \times 1day}\right)} = 25.4\ mg$$

$$A_{min,ss} = A_{max,ss} - Dose = 15.4\ mg$$

or

$$A_{min,ss} = A_{max,ss} \cdot e^{-0.5day^{-1} \times 1day} = 15.4\ mg$$

INDEX

Page numbers in italics refer to figures and tables.

A

Abacavir (Ziagen), inherited variability, 370
Abatacept, protein drugs, *634*
Abciximab (ReoPro), protein drugs, *639, 647*
Absorption
  age factors, 378
  basic models, *25,* 25–28, *26, 27*
  bioavailability, 29
  definition, 29
  disposition rate limitations and, 166–167
  dissolution, *190*
  drug interactions and, 487–489, *488*
  extravascular dose, kinetics, 160–162
    absorption half-life, 160
    absorption rate constant, 160
    first-order process, 160
    kinetics changes, 164–166, *165*
    zero order, 160, 161
  first-pass loss, 29
  intestinal, 29
  kinetic, physiologic concepts, *207,* 207–212
    change in drug disposition, 208–212, *209, 210, 211*
    change in extent, 208
    change in speed, 208, *208*
    impaired renal function, 211
    induction, high extraction ratio, 210
    induction, low extraction ratio, 209–210
    urine pH increase, 211–212, *212*
  peak time and amount, memory aid, *170*
  prediction of, 675–677, *676, 677*
  rate constant, 160
  from solid dosage forms, 198–207, *199,* 200, *200*
    biopharmaceutics classification system, *203,* 203–204
    dissolution, 200, *200*
    gastric emptying and intestinal transit, *201,* 201–203
    modified-release products, 204–207, *205, 206*
    other sites, 207
  from solution, 184–198
    first-pass metabolic loss, 191
    gastrointestinal absorption, 184–189, *185, 187, 188, 189*
    hepatic first-pass loss, gut wall, 192–195, *193, 194, 195*
    hepatic first-pass predictions, 195–196
    intramuscular and subcutaneous sites, 197–198, *198*
    oral bioavailability, 189–192, *190, 191*
    saturable first-pass metabolism, *196,* 196–197
  systemic, 28–29
    bioavailability, 29
Absorption half-life
  effect of changes in, 164, 166 ,*165*
  extravascular dose kinetics, 160
Absorption phase, 163
Accolate. *See* Zafirlukast (Accolate)
Accumulation
  average at plateau, 297–298
  index, 299–300
  maxima, minima to plateau, *296,* 296–297
  in multiple-dose regimens, 313–314
  plasma concentration, *294,* 294–295, *295*
  to plateau, amount of drug in body, *723,* 723–724
    steady state, 724
  rate to plateau, *298,* 298–299
  regimen change, 300

  relative fluctuation, 299
  trough, 297
ACE. *See* Angiotensin-converting enzyme
Acenocoumarol, 223, *225*
  chemical purity, analytic specificity, 20–21
  single dose response, 224–225
Acetaminophen
  BCS, *203*
  biotransformation patterns, *113*
  delayed esophageal transit, 178
  drug absorption, *191*
  gastrointestinal absorption, 185, *185*
  half-life in plasma, *139*
  pharmacokinetic parameters, *327*
  plasma concentration, oral administration, *178*
  rapid dissolution in stomach, 202
Acetazolamide
  half-life in plasma, *139*
  and urine pH, 133, 211, 514
Acetylation, inherited variability, *365,* 365–366
Acetylsalicylic acid. *See* Aspirin
Acidic phospholipids binding of metoprolol, *102*
Active secretion, 131
Active transport systems, 81
Acyclovir
  BCS, *203*
  permeability, 186
  renal extraction, *121*
Adalimumab (Humira)
  bioavailability, *655*
  half-life in plasma, 138, *139*
  protein drugs, 637–638, *639, 642, 647*
  tissue distribution, 103, *104*
Adefovir, drug transport, *82*
Additive, 487
Adherence
  dosage regimen, *11,* 11–12, *12*
  therapy management, 540–543, *541, 542*
  variability in response, 341, *342*
Adinazolam, single and multiple doses, 326
Administration of drugs
  buccal, 23
  extravascular (*See* Extravascular dose)
  in hemodialysis patients, *432,* 432–434, *433*
  intra-arterial, 23, 25, 49
  intradermal, 23
  intramuscular, 23
  intravascular, 23, 49–50
  intravenous, 49–50
  oral (*See* Extravascular dose)
  peritoneal (CAPD patient), 435–436, *436*
  rectal, 23
  regional, 25
  sites of, 23–25, *24*
  subcutaneous
    absorption, 197–198, *198*
    definition, 23
  sublingual, 23
Agalsidase, protein drugs, *634*
Age, 373–395
  absorption changes, 378
  adolescent, 373
  adult, 373
  creatinine clearance, change in, 380–385, *381*
    adults, *383,* 383–385

Age *(continued)*
    children, 383
    elderly, *383,* 383–385
    infants, 380–382, *382*
    neonates, 380–382, *381*
    dosage adjustment and, 390–395, *391*
        adults, *394,* 394–395
        children, 392–394, *393*
        elderly, 395
        infants, 391–392, *392*
        lean body weight, 395
        neonates, 391–392
    elder, 373
    infant, 373
    metabolism, change in, 385–389
        adults, 385, *385*
        children, 385, *385*
        elderly, 385, *385*
        entire lifespan, 385–389, *386, 387, 388, 389*
        infants, 385, *385*
        neonates, 385, *385*
    neonate, 373
    pharmacodynamics, 377–378, *378*
    pharmacokinetics, 378–380
        absorption, 378
        body weight and composition, 378–380, *379, 380*
        disposition, 378–380
        lean body mass, 380
        loading dose, *379,* 379–380
        maintenance dosing rate, 380
    typical patient, *374,* 374–376, *375, 376*
    usual adult dosage regimen, 376–377, *377*
    variability in response, 340
Aggrastat. *See* Tirofiban (Aggrastat)
Agonists, pharmacodynamics, 31
Albendazole, poor dissolution, 202–203
Albumin
    binding decrease to plasma proteins, 414
    binding sites, 464, 489–490, *490*
    glomerular sieving coefficient, 643–644, *644*
    pregnancy and, 390
    turnover, 662
    volume of distribution, 404
Albuterol
    genetic polymorphisms, *360,* 368, *369*
    pharmacodynamic variability, 529
    single-dose therapy, 256
Alcohol
    capacity-limited metabolism, 453–455, *454, 455, 456*
    nonlinear pharmacodynamic relationships, 450
Aldesleukin, protein drugs, *636*
Alefacept
    bioavailability, *655*
    distribution, *642*
Alefacept (Amevive), distribution, *642*
Alemtuzumab (Campath)
    distribution, *642*
    monoclonal antibodies, *639*
    pharmacodynamics, *647*
    target cell destruction, 648
Alendronate sodium (Fosamax)
    adherence, 540, 543
    half-lives, 303
    loading dose, 535, *535*
    permeability, 186, *188*
    pharmacodynamics, 226
    response variability, 342, *530,* 535
Alfentanil
    extraction ratio, 142, *142,* 144
    individual differences, 334, *335*
    kinetic parameters, 601
    pharmacodynamic predictions, *681*
    quantal response, 39, *39*
    variable responses, 334, *335*
Alglucosidase alfa (Myozyme), protein drugs, *634*
Allele, 358
Allometry, disposition kinetics
    application to drugs, 666–670, *667, 668, 669*
    deviation from expectation, *670,* 670–671

    origin, *664,* 664–666, *665, 666*
    protein binding correction, 671, *671*
Allopurinol
    altered turnover, 277
    drug transport, 82
    and mercaptopurine interaction, 213, *214*
All-or-none response, 32–33
Alprazolam, clearance prediction, *674*
Alprenolol
    active metabolites, 255
    hepatic extraction, *611*
    induction, high extraction ratio, 210, *211*
    induction by pentobarbital, 143, *143, 211*
    multiple active species, 255
    saturable first-pass metabolism, *196*
    therapeutic consequences, nonlinearities, 476–477
Alteplase, protein drugs, *636*
Amevive. *See* Alefacept (Amevive)
Amikacin
    permeability, *188*
    in renal dysfunction, 409–410, *410,* 421, *421*
Amiloride, *203*
Aminoglycosides, 321, 470
Aminosalicylic acid
    genetic polymorphisms, *359*
    intestinal reactions, *191*
Amiodarone, in plasma unbound, *98*
Amitriptyline
    active metabolites, 255
    distribution properties, 97, *97*
    volume of distribution, 96
Amoxicillin
    maintenance in therapeutic range, 303–306, *304*
    saturable active transport, *451,* 451–452
Ampicillin
    absorption, 190
    permeability, *127*
    volume of distribution, *94*
Amprenavir (Agenerase)
    Child-Pugh score, *407*
    in cirrhosis, 406
    classification of inhibitors, *499*
Amrinone
    acetylation, 366, *598*
    genetic polymorphisms, *359*
Anakinra (Kineret)
    protein drugs, *634*
    renal disease, 655, *655,* 656, *656,* 661
    volume of distribution, *104*
Analytic specificity, 21–22
Angiomax. *See* Bivalirudin (Angiomax)
Angiotensin-converting enzyme (ACE), 466
Anidulafungin, protein drugs, *635*
Answers to problems, 727–818
Antagonists, pharmacodynamics, 31
Anthelmintic, poor dissolution, 202–203
Antibiotics
    administration, *320,* 320–321, *321*
    clearance, 118
    discontinuation of therapy, 543
    permeability rate limitation, 92
    pharmacodynamics, prediction of, 680
    safety of, 255
    small volume of distribution, 103, *104*
Antihemophilic, protein drugs, *636*
Antipyrine
    lipophilicity, *78*
    perfusion, *123*
Antithrombin III, protein drugs, *637*
Anzemet. *See* Dolasetron mesylate (Anzemet)
Aprepitant (Emend)
    classification of inhibitors, *499*
    mechanism-based inhibition, *509*
Aprotinin, protein drugs, *637*
Aralen. *See* Chloroquine (Aralen)
Arava. *See* Leflunomide (Arava)
Area under concentration–time curve (*AUC*)
    assessment of, 687–688, *688*
        trapezoidal rule, 687, *687*
    systemic exposure–time profile, 20

Aredia. *See* Pamidronate (Aredia)
Aricept. *See* Donepezil (Aricept)
Artificial kidney, 425
Ascorbic acid
    altered clearance, 512
    concentration-dependent renal excretion, 461, *462*
    intestinal reactions, *191*
    nonlinear behavior, 445, 445–446
    saturability, *449,* 464
Asparaginase (Elspar), protein drugs, *636*
Aspirin
    distribution kinetics, *563,* 563–564
    exposure-time profile, 22, *23*
    first-pass loss, 191–192
    intravenous *v.* oral administration, *162*
    response decline, 232–233, *233*
Astemizole, drug interactions, 484
Atenolol
    permeability, 77, *127,* 186, *188*
    pharmacokinetic variability, 249
    plasma protein binding, *98*
    in plasma unbound, *98*
    renal excretion, 63
    renal extraction, *121*
Atorvastatin (Lipitor)
    bioavailability, *193*
    hepatic, renal transporters, *82*
    inhibition, 504
    interconversion, 622
    pharmacokinetic variability, *530*
    and rifampicin interaction, *515,* 515–517
    saturable first-pass metabolism, *196*
    time, therapeutic effect, 316, *317*
AUC. See Area under concentration–time curve
Autoinduction, 465, *471*
Avalide. *See* Irbesartan (Avalide, Avapro)
Avandia. *See* Rosiglitazone (Avandia)
Avapro. *See* Irbesartan (Avalide, Avapro)
Avastin. *See* Bevacizumab (Avastin)
Avodart. *See* Dutasteride (Avodart)
Azathioprine
    genetic polymorphisms, *359*
    S-methylation, 363
Azelastine, drug transport, 84
Azithromycin
    dosage regimens, *302*
    volume of distribution, *94*

B
Bacitracin, protein drugs, *641*
Bacterial resistance, *321*
Barbital, 127
Baseline, response assessment, 33
Basic model, 25, 25–28, *26, 27*
Basiliximab (Simulect), protein drugs, *639, 642*
Baycol. *See* Cerivastatin (Baycol)
Benzodiazepines, receptor affinity, *680*
Benzylpenicillin, hepatic and renal transporters, *82, 121*
Bethanechol chloride, permeability, 79
Bevacizumab (Avastin), protein drugs, *642*
Bexxar. *See* Tositumomab (Bexxar)
Bidirectional interaction, 487
Bile, *128,* 128–129
Biliary secretion, fecal excretion, 30
Bimodal frequency distribution, 338
Binding, and drug distribution
    in blood, 96, *97*
    in plasma, 96–100, *97, 98, 99*
    small volume, of distribution, 103–105, *104, 105*
    in tissues, 100–103, *101, 102*
Binding proteins
    conditions altering plasma concentration, *106*
    in plasma, *94*
Bioavailability
    absorption kinetics
        BCS, *203,* 203–204
        causes of loss, 189–192, *190, 191*
        competing reactions, 190–191, *191*
        hepatic extraction, 195–196

and coefficient of variation, *339*
    definition, 29
    in dialysis patients, 436, *436*
    in multiple-dose regimens, 309–311, 313
    urine, 175–176
Bioequivalence testing, 171–172
Biomarkers
    response classification, 31–32
    safety, 32
    therapy management, 538, *539*
Biopharmaceutics
    classification system, 203–204
    product performance assessment, 170
Biotransformation, 113, *113*
Bivalirudin (Angiomax)
    intravenous infusion, *260*
    protein drugs, *642*
Blood
    clearance, 117–118
    dialysis (*See* Dialysis)
    drug binding, and distribution, 96, *97*
    drug metabolism, 120, *120*
    exposure assessment, 18, *19*
    and plasma, concentration ratio, 118, 703–704
    and plasma water, half-life, 139–140
Blood flow
    altered, kinetic consequences, 145–148, *146, 147*
    and gastrointestinal absorption, 184
    and hepatic extraction ratio, 121–125, *122, 123, 125*
    perfusion rate limitation, 85–91, *87, 88, 89, 90*
    pharmacokinetics in circulatory disorders, 408–409
Blood-brain barrier, 77–78, *78*
Blood-to-plasma concentration ratio, 118, 703–704
Body surface area (BSA). *See* Surface area
Body weight. *See* Weight
Bolus
    AUC assessment, 687, *688*
    distribution kinetics, 563–570
        data presentation, *563,* 563–566, *565, 567*
        elimination, 569–570
        first-order process, 53
        half-life, 54, 58
        and infusion, 269–271, *270, 271, 581,* 581–582
        mathematical aid, 570
        monoexponential equation, 53–54
        MRT, 56
        pharmacodynamic considerations, *589,* 589–590
        pharmacokinetic parameters, 566–569, *568*
        volume of distribution, *51,* 51–52
Bosentan (Tracleer)
    saturability, *451*
    target-mediated drug disposition, 450
    tissue binding, 468, *468,* 491
Brain
    carrier-mediated transport, 82–84, *83*
    perfusion rate-limited distribution, *89*
    protective mechanism, 77–78, *78*
Breast milk, drug disposition, 392
BSA. *See* Surface area
Buccal administration, 23
Budesonide (Pulmicort), first-pass loss, 192
Bufuralol, genetic polymorphisms, *359,* 362
Bumetanide
    drug transport, *82*
    volume of distribution, *104*
Buprenorphine, first-pass loss, 192
Bupropion
    lipophilicity, 392, *392*
    renal disease, *425*
Buspirone
    absorption and grapefruit juice, 208, *209*
    BCS, *203*
    bioavailability, 193, *193*
    hepatic extraction, *611*
    oral AUC, *501*
Busulfan, 32

C

Caffeine, distribution properties, 96, *97*
Calcitonin-salmon (Miacalcin)
    permeability, 77
    protein drugs, *634, 641*
Campath. *See* Alemtuzumab (Campath)
Camptosar. *See* Irinotecan (Camptosar)
Capacity-limited metabolism, 452–459
    alcohol, 453–455, *454, 455, 456*
    Michaelis-Menten kinetics, 452–453
    phenytoin, 455–459, *457, 458, 459*
CAPD. *See* Continuous ambulatory peritoneal dialysis
Capillary permeability, 651, *652*
Capromab pendetide (ProstaScint Kit), *647*
Captopril, *203*
Carbamazepine
    autoinduction, *471*
    circadian variations, 471, *471*
    concentration/dose in children, 393, *393*
    metabolites, 620–621
    in plasma unbound, *98*
    rate-limiting step in metabolism, 628
Carbenicillin
    permeability, *188*
    volume of distribution, *104*
Cardiovascular disease, variability in drug response, 408–409, *409*
Carmustine, lipophilicity, *78*
Carrier-mediated transport, 80–84, *81, 82, 83, 84*
    active transport systems, 81
    concentrating transporter, 81
    efflux transporter, 81
    equilibrating transporter, 81
    influx transporter, 81
    passive facilitated diffusion, 80
    P-glycoprotein, 81
    transport maximum, 81
    transporter, 81
Cefamandole
    permeability, *188*
    and renal function, *438*
    volume of distribution, *104*
Cefazolin
    protein binding, *671*
    renal extraction, *121*
    volume of distribution, *104*
Cefepime, in renal dysfunction, 409, *410*
Cefonicid
    renal clearance, *154*
    saturable binding to plasma, 465, *466*
    volume of distribution, *104*
Ceforanide
    renal function, *438*
    volume of distribution, *104*
Cefotaxime
    drug transport, *82*
    metabolites, *604*
    and renal function, *438*
    volume of distribution, *104*
Cefprozil, hemodialysis, 444, *444*
Cefsulodin, i.p. administration, 434–435, *435*
Ceftazidime
    modality of administration, 320, *320*
    unbound clearance decrease, 411, *411*
Ceftizoxine, half-life, *669*
Ceftriaxone, *398*
Cefuroxime
    half-life, 669, *669*
    and renal function, *438*
Celebrex. *See* Celecoxib (Celebrex)
Celecoxib (Celebrex), genetic polymorphisms, *359*
Celexa. *See* Citalopram (Celexa)
Cell membranes, 74–75, *75*
Cephalexin (Keflex)
    intestinal reactions, 190
    volume of distribution, *104*
Cephalosporin, 409, *410*
Cephalothin
    renal extraction, *121*
    volume of distribution, *104*
Cephradine, volume of distribution, *104*

Cerebrospinal fluid
    drug administration, 25
    permeability, *91*, 91–93
Cerezyme. *See* Imiglucerase (Cerezyme)
Cerivastatin (Baycol), therapeutic drug interaction, 484
Cetirizine, drug transport, 84
Cetuximab (Erbitux)
    monoclonal antibodies, *639*
    volume of distribution, *642*
Charcoal, reversibility of transport, 84–85
Chemical purity, 20–22, *21*
Child-Pugh score, 407, *407*
Children
    creatinine clearance, change in, 383
    dosage adjustment and, 392–394
    metabolism, change in, 385, *385*
    surface area, 385, 392–393
Chlordiazepoxide
    absorption, oral and intramuscular, 206, *206*
    and ketonazole interaction, *521*
    metabolites, *604*
Chloroquine (Aralen)
    and antacids interaction, *485*
    BCS, *203*
    loading dose, 534
    volume of distribution, *94, 139*
Chlorothiazide
    albumin, binding to, *490*
    jejunal permeability, *188*
    volume of distribution, *104*
Chlorpheniramine
    BCS, *203*
    drug transport, 84
Chlorpromazine
    metabolites, *604*
    plasma protein binding, *99*
    volume of distribution, *94*
Chlorthaladone, dosage regimen, 325
Chlorzoxazone
    clearance prediction, *674*
    CYP enzyme substrates, *115, 495*
Cholestyramine
    intestinal reactions, 190
    reversibility of transport, 84–85
Chorionic gonadotropin, protein drugs, *634*
Chronopharmacology
    time-dependent disposition, 468
    variability of response, 344, *344*
Chronotheraphy, *344*
Cidofovir, *180*
Cigarette smoking, and response to drugs, 344
Cilastatin (Primaxin), and Imipenem combination, *486*, 505, *506*
Cimetidine
    classification of inhibitors, *499*
    drug transport, *82*
    metabolism alterations, 458
    permeability, 186, *188*
    plasma concentration monitoring, *544*
    rate control, 204
    renal extraction, *121*
Ciprofibrate, interconversion, 624
Ciprofloxacin, absorption within gastrointestinal tract, 213, *213*
Circulatory disorders, 408–409
Cirrhosis, 404–406, *405, 406*
Cisapride, therapeutic drug interaction, 484
Citalopram (Celexa)
    CYP enzyme substrates, *115, 495*
    mechanism-based inhibition, *509*
Cladribine, intravenous infusion, *260*
Clarithromycin
    classification of inhibitors, *499*
    CYP enzyme substrates, *495*
    mechanism-based inhibition, 471, *506*, 506–508, *509*
    saturability, *449*
    time-dependent disposition, 471, *472*
Classification of drug interactions, *485, 487*
Clearance
    additivity of, 118–119
    concept of (*See* Elimination)

definition, 52
dialysis, 426–429, 434–435, *435*
distribution kinetics, *586*, 586–588, *587*
and drug interactions, 494–512, *495*
   induction, 510–512
   inhibition, 495–496, 496–506
   mechanism-based inhibition, 506–509
   other causes, 512
elimination and, 59, *59*
in general, 115–119, *116*
half-life, in blood and plasma water, 139–140
multiple-dose regimen, 313
organ, process, or site of measurement, 117
plasma *v.* blood, 117–118
plasma-to-blood concentration ratio, 118, 703–704
prediction of, 672–674, *673, 674*
renal, 62–63
in renal dysfunction, 409–411, *410*
total, 55
unbound, 118
volume of distribution and, 51–52, 55–56
Clinical dialyzability, 430
Clinical endpoints, 538
Clinical response, 31
Clobazam, *310*
Clofibric acid
   interconversion, 623–624, *624*
   in nephrotic syndrome, 150
Clonazepam, volume of distribution, *139*
Clonidine
   plasma concentration, 8
   transdermal delivery systems, *262*
Clopidogrel (Plavix)
   maintenance, of level, *302*
   saturability, *449*
Clotting factor IX, *637*
Clotting factor VIIa, *637*
Cloxacillin
   albumin, binding to, *490*
   volume of distribution, *104*
Clozapine, genetic polymorphism, *360*
Cocaine
   hepatic extraction, *121*
   plasma concentration, *70*
Cockcroft-Gault method, *416*
Codeine
   genetic polymorphism, *359, 366–367, 367*
   hepatic extraction, *121, 125, 613*
   metabolites, *604*
   multiple active species, 255
   oxidation, 363
Coefficient of variation, 338, *338, 339*
Collagenase, *635*
Compartments
   absorption and disposition models, 26
   distribution kinetics, 564–566, *565*
Competitive inhibition
   and drug interactions, 496–506
      AUC, *501*
      beneficial interactions, *506*
      classification of inhibitors, *499*
      plasma concentration, *502*
      route of administration, *503*, 503–505
      theophylline and enoxacin, *496*, 496–502, *498*
Computers, pharmacokinetic parameters, 66
Concentrating transporter, 81
Concentration
   blood-to-plasma concentration ratio, 118, 703–704
   plasma
      accumulation, *294*, 294–295, *295*
      renal excretion, *460*, 460–463, *461, 462, 463*
Concentration-dependent renal excretion, 460, *460*,
   460–463, *462, 463*
Concentration–time profile, *473*, 473–475
Conjugation, 113, 363
Constant-rate devices, *261–262*
Constant-rate input
   distribution kinetics, 572–582
      long-term, *573*, 573–582
         bolus plus infusion, *581*, 581–582
         endogenous substances turnover, 577

plateau, 574–577, *575*
   plateau, time to reach, 577–581, *578, 579, 580*
short-term, *572*, 572–573
drug administration, 259–262, *260, 261–262*
exposure–time relationships, 262–271, *263*
   bolus plus infusion, 269–271, *270, 271*
   changing infusion rates, 267–269, *268, 269*
   MRT, 265–266
   plateau, *264*, 264–265
   plateau, time to reach, *266*, 266–267, *267*
   postinfusion, 267
   short-term infusions, 271–272
   steady state, 264
kinetic, physiologic concepts, *284*, 284–286
   drug induction of hepatic metabolism, 285–286
metabolites, 613–617, *614*
   plateau, 615
   postinfusion, 617
   time to plateau, 615–617, *616*
pharmacodynamic considerations, 274–280
   altered turnover, *276*, 276–277
   non–steady-state observations, 279–280, *281*
   onset of response, 274
   response, infusion termination, 274
   response, infusion *v.* single dose, 274, *274*
   steady-state establishment, 277–278, *278, 279, 280*
   turnover, affected systems, 275, *275*
   tolerance, 280–284, *282, 283*
Continuous ambulatory peritoneal dialysis (CAPD), 434–436
Controlled-release
   absorption, solid dosage forms, 204
   extravascular administration, 160
Convolution, 713
Cortisol
   and flesinoxan, 682, *682*
   interconversion, *622, 682*
   non-steady state observations, 280
   plasma binding, *94*
Cosyntropin, *634*
Creatinine clearance
   change in, with age, 380–385, *381*
      adults, *383*, 383–385
      children, 383
      elderly, *383*, 383–385
      infants, 380–382, *382*
      neonates, 380–382, *381*
      premature, change with conceptional age, *382*
   Cockcroft-Gault method, *416*
   estimation of, *416*, 416–419, *417, 418, 419*
   in renal dysfunction, 411, *411*
   Schwartz method, *416*
Crestor. *See* Rosuvastatin (Crestor)
Crixivan. *See* Indinavir (Crixivan)
Crotalidae immune Fab, *639, 647*
Cumulative frequency, 38–39, *39*
Curare, 78
Cyclophosphamide, *666*, 666–667
   allometry and disposition kinetics, *666, 667*
   BCS, *203*
   renal disease, *425*
Cyclosporine
   physicochemical properties, *156*
   therapeutic window, 8, 254
   whole-body physiologic models, 679, *679*
Cytarabine
   drug transport, 81
   intravenous infusion, *260*
Cytarabine (DepoCyt Injection)
   intravenous infusion, *260*
Cytochrome P450 enzymes
   drug oxidation and reduction, 113–115, *114, 115*
   genetic polymorphism, 360–363, *361*
   genetics, 10
   gut wall, and hepatic first-pass loss, 193, *193*
Cytovene. *See* Ganciclovir (Cytovene)

D
Daclizumab (Zenapax)
   antibodies, therapeutic use, *647*
   half-life in plasma, 138, *139*

Dapsone
genetic polymorphism, *367*
interconversion, *622,* 623
pKa values, *692*
Darifenacin, saturable first-pass metabolism, *196*
DDAVP. *See* Desmopressin acetate (DDAVP)
Debrisoquine, genetic polymorphism, 10, 360
Deconvolution, 713
Delavirdine mesylate (Rescriptor), 22
Delayed-release, extravascular dose, 160
Deniluekin diftitox (Ontak), *104*
DepoCyt Injection. *See* Cytarabine (DepoCyt Injection)
Desflurane (Suprane)
MAC, *401*
pharmacodynamics, changes with age, 377, *378*
Desipramine
competitive inhibition, 500, *501*
drug interactions, *495*
drug therapy monitoring, *539*
and fluoxetine, 521, 522, *522*
genetic polymorphism, *367*
metabolites, *604, 611*
Desloratadine, 84
Desmopressin acetate (DDAVP)
absorption, 207
protein drugs, *641*
Detrol. *See* Tolterodine tartrate (Detrol)
Dextrans, sieving coefficient, molecular size and charge, *644*
Dextroamphetamine, 20
Dextromethorphan
drug interactions, *501*
genetic polymorphism, *359*
Dialysis, 425–437
artificial kidney, 425
clinical dialyzability, 430
definition, 425–426
in drug overdose, 436–437
toxic metabolites, 437
extracorporeal, 425
hemodialysis, 425–434, *427*
clearance, 426–429
dialysate, amount recovered, 427–428, *429*
dialysate, rate of recovery, 426–427
drug administration, *432,* 432–434, *433*
drug elimination, 430
in drug overdose, 436–437
effectiveness of procedure, 430–432, *431*
efficiency, 429
extraction coefficient, 429–430
extraction from blood, 426
hemodialyzer, 425
peritoneal, 425
clearance, 434–435, *435*
route of administration, 435–436, *436*
Dialysis clearance, 426–429, *429*
Dialyzability, 430
Diazepam
absorption, 206–207
age and weight factors, 385–388, *386, 387, 388*
BCS, *203*
distribution and elimination, 61
elimination, *115*
half-life in plasma, *139*
hepatic clearance, *121,* 124, *124*
interindividual variability, 333
in plasma unbound, *98*
precipitation, redissolution, 206–207
volume of distribution, *94*
Diclofenac
permeability, 126
volume of distribution, *104*
Dicloxacillin
albumin, binding to, *490*
concentration-dependent renal excretion, 460, *460*
nonlinearities, 481
saturable transport, 464
volume of distribution, *104*
Dicumarol, and phenobarbital interaction, 511, *511*
Didanosine, 202
Diethylcarbamazine, renal clearance, *136*

Diffusion
drug transport, 76–80
blood-brain barrier, 77
membrane characteristics, 79–80
passive, 76
permeability, drug properties and, 76–79, *77, 78*
pH partition hypothesis, 78–79, *79*
equilibrium, 80
Diflunisal, volume of distribution, *104*
Digibind. *See* Digoxin immune Fab (Digibind)
Digitalizing dose, 6
Digitoxin, *218*
Digoxin
absorption, 188–189, *189*
age factors, 376–377, *377*
concentration monitoring, *547–548*
delay in effect, 218, *218*
distribution kinetics, 570–572, *571*
dosage regimen, 4
Fab fragments and detoxification, 648, *648*
half-life, in plasma, *139*
missed dose of, 549, *549*
and rifampin interaction, *189*
and ritonavir interaction, *147*
and quinidine interaction, *514,* 514–515
renal clearance, 140, *147,* 147–148
renal disease and, 423, *423*
reversibility of transport, 84
therapeutic index, 255
Digoxin immune Fab (Digibind)
immunotoxicotherapeutic agents, 648, *648*
protein drugs, *639, 642, 647*
Diltiazem
BCS, *203*
classification of inhibitors, *499*
competitive inhibition, 503, *503*
hepatic extraction, *611*
and lovastatin interaction, *503*
mechanism-based inhibition, *509,* 525
metabolites, *604*
volume of distribution, *94*
Diovan. *See* Valsartan (Diovan)
Diphenhydramine
and alcohol interaction, *485*
BCS, *203*
drug transport, 84
pharmacokinetic data, *397*
Dipyridamole, *94*
Disease states
cardiovascular, 408–409, *409*
hepatic disorders, 404–408, *405, 406, 407, 408*
cirrhosis, *405, 406*
renal dysfunction, 409–425
clearance, 409–411, *410*
creatinine clearance, estimation of, 416–419, *417, 418, 419*
dosage adjustment, 419–422
estimation of, 414–419, *415, 416, 417, 418, 419*
general guidelines and considerations, 422–425, *423, 424, 425*
GFR, estimation of, 415, *415*
loading dose, *421,* 421–422
maintenance rate, *420,* 420–421
plasma protein binding and, 414
unbound clearance, *411,* 411–414, *412, 413*
variability of response and, 341, 403–404
Disopyramide
BCS, *203*
nonlinear binding to ∝, -acid glycoprotein, 480
renal clearance, 461–462, *463*
saturability, *449*
Displacement interactions, 489–491, *490*
acute events, 491–492
conditions favoring, 489–491
kinetics, 492–494
disposition kinetics, 492
plasma concentration–time profile, 494, *494*
plateau, 492, *493*
therapeutic implications, 491–494
Displacer, 489

Disposition. *See also* Distribution; Elimination
  age and body weight, 378–380, *379, 380*
    loading dose, 379–380
    maintenance dosing rate, 380
  basic models, *25,* 25–28, *26, 28*
  changing kinetics, 168, *168, 169*
  definition, 29
  distribution, 29
  elimination, 30
  enterohepatic cycle, 29
  kinetics, 57, *60,* 61
  rate-limitations and absorption, 166, *167*
  rate-limiting step, 164
Dissolution
  absorption from solids, 198, *199,* 200, *200*
  dose dependency, due to, 450, *451*
  of drug, gastrointestinal tract, *190*
  rate-limited, 200
Distribution. *See also* Response
  definition, 29
  and drug interactions, 489–494
    displacement, conditions favoring, 489–491, *490*
  of drugs bound to plasma proteins, *695,* 695–700, *696*
    in body, 698–700, *699*
    of protein, 700
  elimination and, 59–62, *60, 61*
  extent of, 93–103, *94*
    binding, blood, 96, *97*
    plasma protein binding, 96–100, *98, 99*
    tissue distribution, 100–103, *101, 102*
    transporters, 101–103
    volume of distribution, 94–96, *95*
  kinetics
    clearance, *586,* 586–588, *587*
    constant-rate infusion, 572–582
      bolus plus infusion, *581,* 581–582
      endogenous substances turnover, 577
      long-term, *573,* 573–582
      plateau, 574–577, *575*
      plateau, time to reach, 577–581, *578, 579*
      short-term, *572,* 572–573
    drug redistribution, *588,* 588–589
    evidence of, 561–595, *562*–563
    extravascular dose, 570–572, *571*
    intravenous bolus dose, 563–570
      data presentation, *563,* 563–566, *565, 567*
      elimination, 569–570
      mathematical aid, 570
      pharmacokinetic parameters, 566–569, *568*
    multiple dosing, 582–586, *583, 584, 585*
    pharmacodynamic considerations
      multiple dosing, *591,* 591–595, *592, 593, 594*
      single bolus dose, *589,* 589–590
  prediction of, 674–675, *675*
  rate, to tissues, 85–93, *86*
    extravasation, 85
    perfusion, 85
    perfusion limitation, *90,* 90–91
    perfusion-rate limitation, 85–91, *87, 88, 89, 90*
    permeability, 85
    permeability-rate limitation, *91,* 91–93, *93*
    tissue distribution half-life, 89
  small volume of, 103–107
    altered binding, loading dose, 107
    location, in body, 105–107, *106*
    model, 103–105
Distribution phase, 56–57
DNA analysis, genetic polymorphism, 370
Dobutamine, *104*
Dolasetron mesylate (Anzemet), 22
Donepezil (Aricept), *591,* 591–592, *592*
Dornase alfa (Pulmozyme), *641*
Dosage regimen
  adherence, *11,* 11–12, *12*
  adult, 376–377, *377*
  bioavailability and volume, unknown, 310–311
  constant-rate
    altered turnover, *276*
    bolus plus infusion, 269–271, *270, 271*
    drug administration, 259–262, *260, 261–262*

drug induction of hepatic metabolism, 285–286
    exposure–time relationships, 262–271, *263*
    infusion rates, 267–269, *268, 269*
    kinetic, physiologic concepts, *284,* 284–286
    MRT, 265–266
    non–steady-state observations, *280, 281*
    pharmacodynamic considerations, *274,* 274–280
    plateau, time to reach, *266,* 266–267, *267*
    plateau value, *264*
    postinfusion, 267
    short-term infusions, 271–272
    slow tissue distribution, *272,* 272–273, *273*
    steady state, 264, 277–278, *278, 279, 280*
    tolerance, 280–284, *281, 282, 283*
    turnover, of affected systems, 275, *275*
  definition, 3
  design, 307–309, *309*
  empirical approach, *4*
  industrial process, 12–13, *13*
  input–response phases, *4,* 4–8
  multiple-dose regimens
    altered absorption, disposition, 322–324
      extravascular administration, 323
      induction of hepatic metabolism, 324, *324*
      inhibition of hepatic metabolism, 323, *323*
      multiple intravenous dose model, *322,* 322–323
      other situations, 324
    design of regimens using plasma concentration,
        307–311, *309*
      unknown bioavailability and volume, 309–311, *310*
    distribution kinetics, 582–586, *583*
      absorption, 584, *584*
      dosing frequency, 585
      utility of volume terms, *585,* 585–586
    drug accumulation principles, *294,* 294–300, *295*
      accumulation index, 299–300
      accumulation to plateau, 295–297, *296*
      average level, plateau, 297–298
      rate of accumulation to plateau, *298,* 298–299,
          299
      regimen change, 300
    drug maintenance in therapeutic range, 302–306
      half-lives, *302,* 302–303
      reinforcement of principles, 303–306, *304, 305*
    evaluation, 312–315
      accumulation degree, 313–314, *314*
      clearance/bioavailability, 313
      fluctuation degree at plateau, 314–315
      half-life, 313
      other parameters, 315
    extravascular administration, 306–307
    initial, maintenance dosage relationship, 300–302,
        301, 302
    metabolite kinetics, 617, *617*
    modified-release products, 311–312, *312*
    pharmacodynamic considerations, 315–321, *316*
      intermittent administration, 318
      modality of administration, 320–321, *321*
      onset, duration, intensity, 318–319, *319*
      tachyphylaxis, 319
      therapeutic effect, time, *317, 318*
      tolerance, 319–320
    plasma concentration *v.* amount in body, 307
Dose
  initial and maintenance, 300–301, *301*
  loading, 300
  missed, *549,* 549–550
  priming, 300
  starting, 534–535, *535*
  strengths, 539–540
  therapeutic consequences, 450–452
  and time dependencies
    absorption, 450–452, *451*
    capacity-limited metabolism, 452–453, *453*
    capacity-limited metabolism, and alcohol, 453–455,
        454, 455, 456
    capacity-limited metabolism, and phenytoin, 455–459,
        457, 458, 459
    disposition, 468–472, *469, 470, 471, 472*
    nonlinearity, causes, 446

Dose (continued)
  plasma protein and tissue binding, 464–468, 465, 466, 467
  recognition of, nonlinearity, 472–476, 473, 474, 475
  renal excretion, concentration-dependent, 460, 460–463, 461, 462, 463
  saturable first-pass metabolism, 452, 452
  therapeutic consequences, 476–477
  and unequal interval, 552
  titration, 535–536
Dose-dependent metabolic behavior, 445, 446
Dose-independent nonlinear behavior, 446
Dose-response, input-response phases, 4
Dose-time-response relationships, 40, 40–43
  turnover concepts, 41–42, 42
    fractional turnover rate, 41
    pool size, 41
    turnover rate, 41
    turnover time, 41
Doxepin
  BCS, 203
  half-life, in plasma, 139
  hepatic extraction, 611
  oxidation, 362
Doxorubicin
  drug transport, 82
  volume of distribution, 94
Doxycycline
  BCS, 203
  dosage regimen, 301, 301, 302
Draflazine
  saturability, 449
  saturable tissue binding, 468, 469
  time-dependent disposition, 469
Dronabinol (Marinol), 692
Droperidol, 288, 288–289
Drug development, 12–13, 13
Drug idiosyncrasy, 357
Drug interactions. See also specific drugs
  absorption, 487–489, 488
  additive effect, 485, 518
  antagonism, 518
  beneficial interactions, 505, 506
  bidirectional interaction, 487
  classification, 485, 487
  classification of inhibitors, 499
  clearance, 494–512, 495
    competitive inhibition, 496, 496–506, 498, 501, 502
    induction, 510, 510–512, 511
    inhibition, 495–496
    mechanism-based inhibition, 506, 506–509, 507, 509
    noncompetitive inhibition, 495
    other causes, 512
  displacer, 489
  distribution, 489–494
    conditions favoring displacement, 489–491, 490
    therapeutic implications, 491–494, 493, 494
  drug administration sequence, 485–486
  drug transporters, 486
  gradation, 484
  interaction, defined, 487
  isobologram, 518
  mulitfaceted interactions
    atorvastatin-rifampicin, 515, 515–517
    digoxin-quinidine, 514, 514–515
    warfarin-phenylbutazone, 512–513, 513
  multiple-drug therapy, 484
  occurrence of, 484
  pharmacodynamic, 484–485, 516–519
  pharmacokinetic, 485, 486
  route of administration, 502–505, 503, 504, 505
  synergism, 485, 518
  therapeutic, 484
Drug overdose, dialysis, 436–437
Drug transport
  carrier-mediated transport, 80–84, 81, 82, 83, 84
    active transport systems, 81
    concentrating transporter, 81
    efflux transporter, 81
    equilibrating transporter, 81

P-glycoprotein, 81
    influx transporter, 81
    passive facilitated diffusion, 80
    transport maximum, 81
    transporter, 81
  membranes, movement through, 74–75, 75
  permeability-rate limitation, 91, 91–93, 93
  processes, 75–84
    diffusion, 76–80, 77, 78, 79, 80
    paracellular, 75, 76
    protein binding, 75–76
    transcellular, 75, 76
    unbound drug, 75
  reversible nature, of transport, 84–85, 85
  small volume of distribution, 103–107
    altered binding and loading dose, 107
    location, in body, 105–107, 106
    model, 103–105, 104
Drugs
  chemical purity and analytic specificity, 20–22, 21
  generic and brand names, 14–15
  metabolites (See Metabolites)
  pharmacodynamic characteristics and, 39–40
  plasma concentration and, 8
  response, variability, 8–10, 9
Duration, drug therapy, 3
Duration of effect, single dose response, 235–237
Dutasteride (Avodart), 139

E
Efalizumab (Raptiva)
  bioavailability, 655
  cell function alteration, 648
  nonlinearities, 657, 657
  protein drugs, 639
  therapeutic uses, 647
Efavirenz
  clearance, altered, 495
  elimination, 115
  plasma protein binding, 98
  therapeutic exposure, 253
Effect compartment, 227
Effexor. See Venlafaxine (Effexor)
Efflux transporters, 81
Elderly
  creatinine clearance, change in, 383, 383–385
  dosage adjustment and, 395
  metabolism, change in, 385, 385
Electrical resistance, intestinal, 185
Elimination
  active tubular secretion, 147, 147–148
  blood flow, 145–148, 146, 147
  clearance concept, 115–119, 116
    additivity of, 118–119
    blood, 117–118
    organ, process, or site of measurement, 117
    plasma v. blood clearance, 117–118
    plasma-to-blood concentration, 118
    unbound, 118
  definition, 30
  distribution and, 59–62, 60
  excretion, 30
  fraction excreted unchanged, 63
  half-life, 58
  hepatic clearance, 119–129, 120, 121
    acinus, 119
    biliary excretion, enterohepatic cycling, 128, 128–129
    hepatocellular eliminating activity, 125, 125
    intrinsic clearance, 120–121
    intrinsic hepatocellular eliminating activity, 120
    kinetic, physiologic concepts, 140–151
    location of transporters, 127
    memory aid, 125–126
    metabolic interconversion, 30
    metabolism, 30
    perfusion, 121–122, 122, 123
    permeability, 126–127, 127
    plasma protein binding, 122–125, 124

sinusoids, 119
well-stirred model, 125–126
induction of metabolism, *142*, 142–143, *143*
kinetics, and clearance and distribution
half-life, in blood and plasma water, 139–140
half-life, in plasma, 138–139, *139*
metabolic inhibition, 143–145, *144*, *145*
plasma protein binding, *148*, 148–151, *149*, *150*, *151*
primary pharmacokinetic parameters, 140–141
processes, *112*, 112–115, *113*, *114*, *115*
metabolic pathways, 113
microsomal enzymes, 113
microsomes, 113
phase I reactions, 113
phase II reactions, 113
prodrug, 115
renal clearance, 62–63, 129–138
active secretion, 131
glomerular filtration, 130–131
nephron, *129*, 129–137, *130*, *132*, *133*, *134*, *135*, *136*
protein binding, perfusion, 131–132
tubular reabsorption, 132–137
renal metabolism, 137
secondary pharmacokinetic parameters, 141, *141*
Elimination half-life, 58
Elimination phase, 56, 58, 163
Elitek. *See* Rasburicase (Elitek)
Elspar. *See* Asparaginase (Elspar)
Emend. *See* Aprepitant (Emend)
Enalapril
BCS, *203*
genetic polymorphisms, *360*
metabolites, 604, *604*
Enbrel. *See* Etanercept (Enbrel)
Encainide
hepatic extraction, *613*
metabolites, *604*
Endogenous compounds, 33
Enfuvirtide (Fuzeon), *635*
Enoxacin, and theophylline interaction, *496*, 496–498, *498*, 500
Enteric-coated tablets
delayed-release, 160
lag time, 163
rapid dissolution, in intestine, 202
Enterohepatic cycle
definition, 29, *30*
distribution, 29, *30*
Environmental pollutants, 344
Enzymes
autoinduction, 465
cytochrome P448
drug oxidation and reduction, 113–115, *114*, *115*
genetics, 10
gut wall, and hepatic first-pass loss, 193, *193*
and inherited variability, 360–363, *361*
intestinal, 190, 195
in liver disorders, 408, *408*
metabolism, proteins, 647
microsomal, 113
turnover rate, 277
Epinephrine, absorption, 197
Epipodophyllotoxin, *78*
Epoetin alfa (Epogen)
non-steady state observations, 280, *281*
volume of distribution, *104*
Epogen. *See* Epoetin alfa (Epogen)
Eptifibatide (Integrilin)
bolus plus infusion, 269–271, *270*, *271*, *581*, 581–582
infusion rate, 268, *268*
Equilibrating transporter, 81
Equilibrium
diffusion, 80
protein binding, 75–76
renal clearance, *133*, 133–134
volume of distribution, 58
Equivalent time, 671
Erbitux. *See* Cetuximab (Erbitux)
Ergonovine, *203*

Erythromycin
absorption, *191*
elimination, *115*
permeability, 188
and sildenafil interaction, *485*
volume of distribution, *94*
Erythropoietin
bioavailability, *654*
intravenous bolus, *281*
hematocrit and erythrocyte production, *318*
subcutaneous administration, 659
turnover, 660
Esmolol
adherence, 540
dosage regimen, *302*, 303
intravenous infusion, *260*
loading dose, 534
'Essentially similar,' product performance assessment, 171
Estradiol
elimination, 114
transdermal delivery, *262*
Etanercept (Enbrel), *642*
Ethambutol, *203*
Ethchlorvynol, drug overdose kinetics, 476, *476*
Ethinyl estradiol
BCS, *203*
constant-rate devices, *262*
intestinal reactions, *191*
Etonogestrel (NuvaRing), *262*
Excipients, drug formulation, 170
Excretion
definition, 30
MRT, 718, *718*
Exelon. *See* Rivastigmine (Exelon)
Extended-release products, extravascular dose, 160
Extensive metabolizers, inherited variability, 360
Extracorporeal dialysis, 425
Extraction coefficient in dialysis, 429–430
Extraction ratio
hepatic, 121–125, *122*, *123*, *125*
volume of distribution and clearance, 52
Extravasation, 85, 86
Extravascular dose
absorption kinetics, 160–162
absorption half-life, 160
absorption rate constant, 160
first-order process, 160
zero order, 161
changes, dose or absorption kinetics, 164–170
absorption, 164–166, *165*
absorption, disposition rate limitations distinction, 166–167, *167*
disposition, *168*, 168–169, *169*
dose changes, 164
peak changes, 169–170, *170*
definition, 23, *24*
distribution kinetics, 572–574, *573*
intravenous administration comparison, *162*, 162–164, *163*
absorption phase, 163
elimination phase, 163
lag time, 163
in multiple-dose regimens, *306*, 306–307
pharmacokinetic parameters, *172*, 172–176, *173*
plasma and urine data, 176
plasma data alone, 173–175, *175*
urine data alone, 175–176
product performance assessment, 170–172
bioequivalence testing, 171–172, *172*
biopharmaceutics, 170
'essentially similar,' 171
excipients, 170
formulation, 170–171
generic products, 171
routes of administration, 159–160
delayed-release, 160
extended-release, 160
immediate-release products, 160
modified-release dosage forms, 160
Ezetimibe (Zetia), 42

F

Famvir. *See* Felbamate (Famvir)
Fasting, gastric emptying, 201
Fecal excretion, biliary secretion, 30
Felbamate (Famvir), *425*
Felodipine
  absorption, *193*
  inhibition, *501*
  mean demographic data, *399*
  variability in response, 342
Fenoldopam, constant-rate input, 289–290
Fentanyl
  displacement interactions, 492
  disposition kinetic parameters, *601*
  hepatic metabolism, inhibition of, 286
  and itraconazole
    interaction, *144*
  intravenous infusion, *260*
  and naloxone interaction, *485*
  pharmacodynamic predictions, *681*
  and ritonavir
    interaction, *145*
  transdermal delivery, *262*
Fexofenadine (Allegra)
  drug transport, *82,* 84
  intestinal reactions, *191*
  jejunal permeability, 188, *188*
  saturability, *449*
  variability in response, 343, *343*
Fibrinolysin, *635*
Filgrastim (Neupogen)
  drug response, turnover concepts, 42
  protein drugs, *636*
First-order elimination, 52–53
  fractional rate of elimination, 52
  monoexponential equation, 53
  processes, 53
  rate constant, 53
First-order process
  bolus distribution kinetics, 53
  extravascular dose, kinetics of, 160
First-pass loss
  aspirin, 191–192
  definition, 29
  naloxone, 192
  oral bioavailability, 191–192
  orlistat, 191
  pentazocine, 192
  talwin, 192
Flecainide
  dose titration, 535
  drug interactions, *495*
  elimination, *115*
  genetic polymorphisms, *359*
Flesinoxan, 681, *681, 682*
Flip-flop kinetics, 166
Flomax. *See* Tamsulosin (Flomax)
Fluconazole
  classification of inhibitors, *499*
  deviation, from expectation, 670, *670*
  drug interactions, *495,* 503–504, *504*
  renal clearance across mammals, *670*
Fluctuation
  drug accumulation, 295
  in multiple-dose regimen, 314–315
Flumazenil (Romazicon)
  first-pass loss, 192
  intestinal permeability, *188*
Fluorouracil
  molecular size, *653*
  permeability, *78*
  saturable first-pass metabolism, *196*
  therapy management, 538
  variability in response, 344, *344*
Fluoxetine
  BCS, *203*
  classification of inhibitors, *499*
  and desipramine interaction, 521, *522*
  metabolites, *604*
  plasma concentration monitoring, *544*

Flurazepam, 222
Flurbiprofen, in plasma unbound, *98*
Fluvastatin
  distribution properties, *97*
  genetic polymorphisms, *359*
  saturable first-pass metabolism, *196*
Fluvoxamine
  classification of inhibitors, *499*
  drug interactions, *495*
Food
  circadian variations, *470,* 470–471
  variability in response, 342
Forteo. *See* Teriparatide (Forteo)
Fosamax. *See* Alendronate sodium (Fosamax)
Fosamprenavir (Lexiva), 406
Fraction excreted unchanged, 63
Fraction of dose remaining, 54–55
Fraction unbound, 19
Fractional rate of elimination, 52
Fractional turnover rate
  dose-time-response relationships, 41
  one-compartment model, 275–276
  steady state, new constant value, 277–278
Full agonist, 31
Full antagonist, 31
Furosemide
  and phenobarbital interaction, 487
  in plasma unbound, *98*
  protein binding and perfusion, 131, *132*
  response infusion *v.* single dose, 274, *274*
Fuzeon. *See* Enfuvirtide (Fuzeon)

G

Gabapentin, drug transport, 82, 188
Gammagard. *See* Intravenous gamma globulin (Gammagard)
Ganciclovir (Cytovene)
  drug transport, *82*
  renal disfunction, 211, *211, 531*
Gastric emptying
  absorption from solution, 184–185, *185*
  and intestinal transit, *201,* 201–203
    poor dissolution, 202–203
    rapid dissolution, in intestine, 202
    rapid dissolution, in stomach, 202
Gastrointestinal tract
  absorption, 184–189
    gastric emptying, 184–185, *185, 201,* 201–203
    intestinal, 185–189, *187, 188*
  drug metabolism, *190*
Gemcitabine (Gemzar), 81
Gemtuzumab ozogamicin (Mylotarg), *639, 647,* 649
Gemzar. *See* Gemcitabine (Gemzar)
Gender
  pharmacodynamics and, 390
  pharmacokinetics and, 389–390
Generic products, 171
Genetics, 357–359
  allele, 358
  drug idiosyncrasy, 357
  genotype, 357
  metabolic phenotyping, 370
  pharmacodynamic variations, 368–370, *369, 370*
  pharmacogenetics, 357
  pharmacogenomics, 357
  pharmacokinetic variations, 359–368
    acetylation, *365,* 365–366
    conjugation, 363
    extensive metabolizers, 360
    hydrolysis, 366
    S-methylation, 363, *364*
    oxidation, 360–363
    poor metabolizers, 360, *367*
  phenotype, 357
  polymodal frequency distribution, 357
  polymorphism, 358–359, *360,* 366–368, *367*
  therapy management, 534
  unimodal frequency distribution, 357
  variability in response, 339
Genotype, 357

Gentamicin
  antimicrobial effect and dosing interval, *320*
  distribution and elimination, *61*, 61–62
  distribution kinetics, 582–583, *583*, 586, *586*
  in hemodialysis patients, *432*, 432–433, *433*
GFR. *See* Glomerular filtration rate
Gladase, *641*
Glibenclamide, *490*
Glipizide, in plasma unbound, *98*
Glomerular filtration rate (*GFR*), 415, *415*
Glucagon
  altered clearance, 512
  protein drugs, *636*
Glucose
  capacity-limited metabolism, *455*
  nonlinear renal reabsorption, 479
Glyburide
  genetic polymorphisms, *359*
  oxidation, 362
P-glycoprotein
  drug transport, 81
  efflux transporters, 81
Gonadotropin-releasing hormone
  modified-release products, 312
  protein drugs, *634*
  rate limitations, 649, *650*
Goserelin (Zoladex)
  constant-rate devices, *261*
  extravascular administration routes, 160
Graded response
  classification, 32
  exposure and, 36–38, *38*
    steepness factor, 37, *37*
Granulocyte colony-stimulating factor, *657*
Grapefruit juice, buspirone absorption, *209*
Griseofulvin
  bioavailability, 179
  nonlinear absorption, 450, *451*
  nonlinearity, therapeutic consequences, 476–477
  saturability, *449*
  therapeutic consequences, nonlinearities, 476–477
Growth hormone, 208, *208*, 653, *653*
  subcutaneous, 659

H

Halazepam metabolites, 617, *617*
Half-life
  absorption, 160
  in blood and plasma water, 139–140
  bolus distribution kinetics, 54, 58
  in multiple-dose regimens, *302*, 302–303, 313
  phenobarbital, *298*, 298–299
  in plasma, 138–139, *139*
Haloperidol
  constant-rate devices, *261*
  interconversion, *622*
Halothane
  drug interactions, *495*
  elimination, 115
  MAC, *401*
Haplotype, 358
Hematocrit, erythropoietin with time, 317, *318*, 649
Hemodialysis, 425–434, *427*
  clearance, 426–429
  definition, 425
  dialysate, amount recovered, 427–428, *429*
  dialysate, rate of recovery, 426–427
  drug administration, *432*, 432–434, *433*
  drug elimination, 430
  in drug overdose, 436–437
  effectiveness of procedure, 430–432, *431*
  efficiency, 429
  extraction coefficient, 429–430
  extraction from blood, 426
Hemodialyzer, 425
Hemoperfusion, 436
Heparin
  dosage regimens, 246
  intravenous infusion, *260*

nonlinear decline in activity, 482
plasma, serum, whole blood drug concentrations, *19*
protein drugs, *635*
Hepatic clearance
  biliary excretion, enterohepatic cycling, *128*, 128–129
  complexities, 126–128
    location of transporters, 127
    permeability, 126–127, *127*
  kinetic, physiologic concepts, 140–151
  metabolic interconversion, 30
  metabolism, 30
  oral dose, events after, 707
  perfusion, protein binding, and hepatocellular activity,
    119–125, *120*, *121*
    acinus, 119
    hepatocellular eliminating activity, 125, *125*
    intrinsic clearance, 120–121
    intrinsic hepatocellular eliminating activity, 120
    perfusion, 121–122, *122*, *123*
    plasma protein binding, 122–125, *124*
    sinusoids, 119
  rapid equilibration between drug in blood and liver,
    705–706
  well-stirred model
    memory aid, 125–126
    oral dose, events after, 707
    permeability considerations, 706–707
    rapid equilibration, drug in blood and liver, 705–706
Hepatic first-pass
  loss, gut wall and, 192–195, *193*, *194*, *195*
  predictions, 195–196
Hepatitis B immune globulin, *639*
Heptabarbital, *229*
Herceptin. *See* Trastuzumab (Herceptin)
Heterozygous, 358
Hirudin, *642*, *660*
Homozygous, 358
Humira. *See* Adalimumab (Humira)
Hydralazine
  acetylation polymorphism, 366
  genetic polymorphisms, *359*
  saturable first-pass metabolism, *196*
Hydrolysis, 113, 366
Hydrophilic property, 74
Hydrophobic property, 74
Hydroxypropranolol, impact of first-pass metabolism, 630
Hydroxyzine, 84
Hypersensitivity, therapeutic window, 250, *250*
Hysteresis
  concentration–response relationship
    time delay causes, 219–220, 222, *223*, 227, *227*
    time delay detection, 218–219, *219*
  definition, 218, *219*
Hyzaar. *See* Losartan (Hyzaar)

I

Ibandronate, 186–187, *188*
Ibuprofen
  distribution properties, *97*
  plasma protein binding, 99
  in plasma unbound, *98*
  rapid dissolution in stomach, 202
  time delay, 223, *223*
Imiglucerase (Cerezyme), *637*
Imipenem (Primaxin), in renal disease, 423–424, *424*
Imipramine
  BCS, *203*
  genetic polymorphisms, *367*
  half-life, in plasma, *139*
  hepatic extraction, *611*
  metabolites, *604*
Imirestat, saturable tissue binding, 468, *469*
Immediate-release products, extravascular dose, 160
Immunogenic responses, 658
In vitro
  absorption, prediction, 676, *676*
  clearance, prediction, 672–674, *673*
  pharmacodynamic predictions, 680, *680*
  whole-body physiologic models, 678, 679, *679*

Indinavir (Crixivan)
  drug transport, 84, *84*
  hepatic first-pass loss, 195
  plasma protein binding, *98*
Individual variations
  description of, 338–339
  dose strengths, 352–353
  dose-response relationship, 345
  expressions of, 334–339
    coefficient of variation, 338
  kinetic manifestations, 348–352, *349, 350, 351*
  therapeutic exposure, 345–348, *346, 347–348*
Indocyanine green clearance, *409*
Indomethacin, *490*
Industrial process, dosage regimen, 12–13, *13*
Infergen. *See* Interferon alfacon-1 (Infergen)
Infliximab (Remicade)
  half-life, in plasma, 138, *139*
  monoclonal antibodies, *639*
  volume of distribution, *104*
Influx transporter, 81
Infusion. *See* Constant-rate input
Inhalation, 207
Initial dilution space, 57
Insulin
  absorption, *191,* 207
  constant-rate devices, *262*
Insulin glangine, *262*
Integrilin. *See* Eptifibatide (Integrilin)
Interactions. *See* Drug interactions
Interconversion, *622,* 622–624, *623, 624*
Interferon alfacon-1 (Infergen), *635*
Interferon Alpha-2b (Pegintron), *635, 653*
Interferon Beta-1a (Rebif), *635*
Interindividual variability, 333
Interleukin-11 (Neumega), *636, 654*
Intermittent administration, 318
Intestine
  absorption (*See* Absorption)
  competing reactions, 190–191, *191*
  enterohepatic cycling, *128,* 128–129
Intra-arterial administration, 23, 25, 49
Intradermal administration, 23
Intraindividual variability, 333
Intramuscular administration
  absorption, 197–198, *198*
  definition, 23
  protein drugs, 650–655
    absorption, 652–654, *653, 654, 655*
    large proteins, and lymphatic transport, 650–652, *651, 652*
Intranasal route, 207
Intravascular administration, 23, 49–50
Intravenous administration
  overview, 49–50
  protein drugs, 650
Intravenous bolus dose kinetics, 49–68, 563–570
  case study, 56–62, *57*
    clearance and elimination, 59, *59*
    compartment model, 61
    disposition kinetics, 57, *60,* 61
    distribution and elimination, 59–62, *60, 61*
    distribution phase, 56–57
    elimination half-life, 58
    elimination phase, 58
    elimination rate constant, 58
    initial dilution space, 57
    terminal phase, 57–59
    volume of distribution, 58
  data presentation, *563,* 563–566, *565, 567*
    compartment model, 564–566, *565*
    sum, of exponential terms, *563,* 563–564
  distribution kinetics, and elimination, 569–570
  dose adjustment, 67
  elimination pathways, 62–63
    fraction excreted unchanged, 63
    as fraction of total elimination, 63
    renal clearance, 62–63
  kinetic concepts, *50,* 50–56, *51*
    clearance, area and volume of distribution, 55–56

elimination phase, 56
    extraction ratio, 52
    first-order elimination, 52–54, *53*
    first-order elimination rate constant, 53
    first-order process, 53
    fraction of dose remaining, 54–55
    fractional rate of elimination, 52
    half-life, 54
    monoexponential equation, 53–54
    MRT, 56
    total clearance, 55
    volume of distribution and clearance, *51,* 51–52
  mathematical aid, 572
  pharmacokinetic parameters, 63–67, 566–569
    clearance, 566–568, *567*
    computer use, 66
    dose change, 67
    measurement fluid, 66
    plasma and urine data, *64,* 64–66, *65*
    plasma data alone, 63–64, *65*
    precision of, 66
    volume of distribution, *568,* 568–569
Intravenous gamma globulin (Gammagard), *639*
Intravenous infusion, drug examples, *260*
Inulin clearance, *664*
Invirase. *See* Saquinavir (Invirase)
Ionization
  drug transport, 76, 78, *79*
  and pH partition hypothesis, 691–693, *692, 693*
Irbesartan (Avalide, Avapro), *596, 597*
Irinotecan (Camptosar)
  conjugation, 363
  elimination processes, 114
  genetic polymorphisms, *359*
Isobologram, 518, *518*
Isoflurane, *401*
Isoniazid, genetic polymorphism, *359, 365,* 365–366, *401*
Isoproterenol, urinary recover of metabolites, 613
Isosorbide dinitrate
  hepatic extraction, *611*
  metabolite kinetics, 629
  metabolites, *604,* 625, *625*
  saturable first-pass metabolism, *196*
Itraconazole
  classification of inhibitors, *499*
  metabolic inhibition, 144, *144,* 286
  pKa values, *692*

K

Kaletra. *See* Lopinavir (Kaletra)
Keflex. *See* Cephalexin (Keflex)
Ketamine
  maximum effect, of drug, 40
  response, graded, 32, *32,* 36–37
Ketek. *See* Telithromycin (Ketek)
Ketoconazole
  absorption, 189
  classification of inhibitors, *499*
  drug interactions, 509, *509*
  first-pass loss, 192
  and ketonazole pharmacokinetics, *521*
  plasma concentration monitoring, *544*
  saturable first-pass metabolism, *196*
Ketoprofen
  BCS, *203*
  volume of distribution, *94, 104*
Ketorolac, in plasma unbound, *98*
Kidneys
  disorders of, 409–425
    clearance, 409–411, *410*
    creatinine clearance, estimation of, 416–419, *417, 418, 419*
    dosage adjustment, 419–422
    estimation of, 414–419, *415, 416, 417, 418, 419*
    general guidelines and considerations, 422–425, *423, 424, 425*
    GFR, estimation of, 415, *415*
    loading dose, *421,* 421–422

plasma protein binding and, 414
  unbound clearance, *411*, 411–414, *412, 413*
drug disposition, *82, 83*
drug metabolism, 137
elimination, *24*, 25, 112, 117
renal clearance
  active secretion, 131
  concentration-dependent, 460–463, *461, 462, 463*
  elimination pathways, 62–63
  equilibrium, *133*
  glomerular filtration, *130*, 130–131
  nephron anatomy and function, *129*, 129–130
  protein binding and perfusion, 131–132
  tubular reabsorption, 132–137, *133, 134, 135, 136, 137*

L
Labetalol, *203*
Lag time, 163
Lansoprazole
  dissolution, in intestine, 202
  drug interactions, *509*
  genetic polymorphisms, *359*
Laronidase, *634*
Leflunomide (Arava)
  intestinal reactions, 190
  reversibility of transport, *85, 85*
Lepirudin (Refludan), *635*
Leucovorin
  chronopharmacology, 344, *344*
  duration *v.* intensity of exposure, 256
Leukocytes, time delay, pharmacodynamics, *7*, 7–8
Leuprolide acetate
  absorption, 640
  constant-rate devices, *261*
  protein drugs, 641
  rate limitations, 649, *650*
  response, onset, 274
  and testosterone levels, 649, *650*
Levodopa
  absorption, *191*
  BCS, *203*
  drug therapy monitoring, *539*
Levofloxacin, *203*
  dosage with age, 400
Levonorgestrel, 160
Lexiva. *See* Fosamprenavir (Lexiva)
Lidocaine
  absorption, *198*
  clearance, *123*, 147, *147*
  and indocyanine green clearances, *409*
  and metoprolol interaction, *147*
  and propranolol interaction, *147*, 512
Lipitor. *See* Atorvastatin (Lipitor)
Lipophilic property
  drug transport, 91
  membranes and distribution, 74
  permeability, 77
Lipophobic property, 74
Liquids, gastric emptying, 202
Lithium
  dialysis and filtration, *588*, 588–589
  modified-release dosage forms, 312
  in plasma unbound, *98*
  redistribution, *588*
Liver
  clearance (*See* Hepatic clearance)
  disorders of, 404–408, *405, 406, 407, 408*
  drug disposition, *82, 83*
  elimination, *24*, 25, 117
Loading dose
  pharmacokinetic variability, 534–535, *535*
  in renal dysfunction, *421*, 421–422
Local administration, 18
Loglinear decline, 51
Lomefloxacin, *203*
Lomustine, *78*
Loperamide, and quinidine interaction, 509
Lopinavir (Kaletra), *486*

Lorazepam, 441, *441*
Losartan (Hyzaar)
  biotransformation, *113*
  jejunal permeability, *188*
Lovastatin
  and diltiazem interaction, 503, *503*
  inhibition, *501*
  interconversion, 622, *622*
Low therapeutic index, *536*
Lungs
  elimination, 25
  perfusion rate limitation, 86
  pulmonary clearance, 119
Lymphatic transport
  protein drugs, subcutaneous and intramuscular
      administration, 650–652, *651*
    capillary permeability, 651, *652*
    molecular size, 652, *653*
Lymphocyte anti-thymocyte immune globulin, *639, 647*

M
Maintenance dose
  age and weight effects, 380
  in multiple-dose regimens, 302–306
  in renal dysfunction, *420*, 420–421
Maprotiline, distribution properties, *97*
Marinol. *See* Dronabinol (Marinol)
Mavik. *See* Trandolapril (Mavik)
Maximum effect, pharmacodynamic drug characteristics, 40
Mean residence time (*MRT*)
  bolus distribution kinetics, 56
  constant-rate input, 265–266
  excretion data, 718, *718*
  overview, 717–718
  plasma concentration data, *719*, 719–721, *720*
Mechanism-based autoinhibition, 471
Mechanism-based inhibition, *506*, 506–509, *507, 509*
Mefloquine
  drug maintenance, therapeutic range, 303
  half-life, in plasma, *139*
  kinetics of isomers, 328
  loading dose, 534
  renal clearance, 63
Meloxicam, *555, 792*
Memantine, urine pH, 211, *212*
Membranes, movement through. *See* Drug transport
Memory aids
  hepatic clearance, 125–126
  prediction of peak concentration and time, 169, *170*
  secondary pharmacokinetic parameters, 141
Menopur. *See* Menotropin (Menopur)
Menotropin (Menopur), *634*
Meperidine
  BCS, *203*
  hepatic extraction, *121, 613*
  metabolites, *604*
  and pentazocine, *439*
Mercaptopurine
  genetic polymorphisms, *359, 364*
  interaction with alloporinol, 214
  S-methylation, 363
Mesalamine, *449*
Metabolic inhibition, 143–145
Metabolic interconversion, 30, *622*, 622–624, *623, 624*
Metabolic phenotyping, 370
Metabolism
  and age, 385–389
    adults, 385, *385*
    children, 385, *385*
    elderly, 385, *385*
    entire lifespan, 385–389, *386, 387, 388, 389*
    infants, 385, *385*
    neonates, 385, *385*
  definition, 30
  renal, 137
Metabolites
  active, 22, 255
  analytic specificity, 21–22

Metabolites *(continued)*
  constant-rate drug infusion, 613–617, *614*
    plateau, 615
    postinfusion, 617
    time to plateau, 615–617, *616*
  in drug administration, 21–22
  and drug response, 604–605
  formation estimation, 624–625, *625*
  interconversion, *622,* 622–624, *623, 624*
  kinetics of metabolites, 630
  multiple-dose regimen, 617, *617*
  nonlinear formation or elimination, 620–621, *621*
  pharmacokinetic changes, 625–627
  prodrugs and, 22, *23*
  response, 621
  single dose of drug, 605–613
    hepatic extraction, *611,* 611–613, *612*
    plasma concentration, 607–611, *608, 609, 610*
    rate-limiting step, 605–607, *606*
    sequential metabolism, 605
  single-dose data prediction, 618
  systemic exposure-time profile, *23*
  toxic, 437
  variability, 618–620, *619*
Metformin
  drug transport, *82*
  in plasma unbound, *98*
  renal extraction, *121*
Methamphetamine, 134, 134–135, *135*
Method of residuals, 564
Methotrexate
  allometry, and disposition kinetics, 667, *668,* 669
  drug transport, *82*
  duration *v.* intensity of exposure, 256
  permeability, *78*
  renal extraction, *121*
  therapeutic exposure, 254
S-Methylation, inherited variability, 363, *364*
Methyldopa, *188*
Methylphenidate
  chemical purity, analytic specificity, 20, *21*
  saturable first-pass metabolism, 452, *453*
Methylprednisolone
  interconversion, *622*
  plasma concentration, 607–608, *608*
  postinfusion, 617
S-Methyltransferase, genetic polymorphism, *369*
Metoprolol
  BCS, *203*
  distribution properties, *97*
  drug interactions, *501*
  hepatic extraction, 147, *147*
  jejunal permeability, *188*
  poor and extensive metabolizers, *361*
  tissue distribution, *102*
Metronidazole
  BCS, *203*
  permeability, *78*
Miacalcin. *See* Calcitonin-salmon (Miacalcin)
Mibefradil
  distribution properties, 96, *97*
  tissue binding, 100
Michaelis-Menten kinetics, 447, *447,* 452–453
Microdosing, 671–672, *672*
Midazolam
  BCS, *203*
  distribution kinetics, 572
  hepatic first-pass loss, *193*
  individual differences, 334, *335*
  interaction with fluconazole, 504
  intravenous bolus, *57*
  microdosing, 671–672, *672*
  variability, 343, *343*
Minimal inhibitory concentration (MIC), 321, *321*
Minimum alveolar concentration (MAC), 401, *401*
Minocycline, *203*
Minoxidil, *94,* 232, *232,* 234
Misonidazole, *78*
Misoprostol, *203*
Missed dose, monitoring, *549,* 549–550
Modified-release dosage forms, 160

Modified-release products
  absorption from solid dosage forms, 204–207
  in multiple-dose regimens, 311–312, *312*
Monitoring
  data collection, 546
  dosing scenarios, 548–554
    confidence in estimates, 552–554, *553*
    dose and interval unequal, 552, *552*
    missed dose, *549,* 549–550
    9-13-17-21 regimen, *550,* 550–552
  evaluation procedure, 545–548, *546, 547–548*
  target concentration strategy, 543–554
    plasma drug concentrations, 543–546, *544*
Monoexponential equation, 53–54
Montelukast (Singulair), 33, *34*
  dosage in children, 400
Morphine
  metabolites
    hepatic extraction, *611,* 613, *614*
    renal impairment, 619
  modified release, *312*
  therapeutic window, 5–6
Moxalactam, *671*
MRT. See Mean residence time
Multiple active species, 255
Multiple-dose regimens
  altered absorption, disposition, 322–324
    extravascular administration, 323
    induction of hepatic metabolism, 324, *324*
    inhibition of hepatic metabolism, 323, *323*
    multiple intravenous dose model, *322,* 322–323
    other situations, 324
  distribution kinetics, 582–586, *583*
    absorption, 584, *584*
    dosing frequency, 585
    utility of volume terms, *585,* 585–586
  drug accumulation principles, *294,* 294–300, *295*
    accumulation index, 299–300
    accumulation to plateau, 295–297, *296*
    average level, plateau, 297–298
    rate of accumulation to plateau, *298,* 298–299, *299*
    regimen change, 300
    relative fluctuation, 299
  drug maintenance in therapeutic range, 302–306
    half-lives, *302,* 302–303
    reinforcement of principles, 303–306, *304, 305*
  evaluation, 312–315
    accumulation degree, 313–314, *314*
    clearance/bioavailability, 313
    fluctuation degree at plateau, 314–315
    half-life, 313
    other parameters, 315
  extravascular administration, 306–307
  initial, maintenance dosage relationship, 300–302, *301*
    loading dose, 300
    maintenance dose, 300
    priming, 300
  metabolite kinetics, 617, *617*
  modified-release products, 311–312, *312*
  pharmacodynamic considerations, 315–321, *316*
    intermittent administration, 318
    modality of administration, 320–321, *321*
    onset, duration, intensity, 318–319, *319*
    tachyphylaxis, 319
    therapeutic effect, time, *317, 318*
    tolerance, 319–320
  plasma concentration *v.* amount in body, 307
  regimen design, plasma concentration, 307–311, *309*
    unknown bioavailability and volume, 309–311, *310*
Muromomab-CD3, *639*
Mylotarg. *See* Gemtuzumab ozogamicin (Mylotarg)
Myozyme. *See* Alglucosidase alfa (Myozyme)

N
Naloxone
  and fentanyl interaction, *485*
  first-pass loss, 192
  hepatic extraction, *611*
Naphthoxylactic acid, 609, *609,* 612

Naproxen
  delay in pain relief, *219*
  maintenance in therapeutic range, 303–306, *304*
  in plasma unbound, *98*
  saturable binding to plasma proteins, *465*
Nasal cavity, drug permeability, 77, *80*
Nelfinavir mesylate (Viracept)
  absorption, 195
  drug interactions, *501*
  variability in response, 342
Neomycin, *188*
Neonate, 373
Nephron
  active secretion, 131
  anatomy and function, *129,* 129–130
  glomerular filtration, *130,* 130–131
  protein binding and perfusion, 131–132, *132*
  tubular reabsorption, 132–137, *133, 134, 135, 136, 137*
Nesiritide, *260*
Neumega. *See* Interleukin-11 (Neumega)
Neupogen. *See* Filgrastim (Neupogen)
Niacin, *196, 449*
Nicardipine
  distribution kinetics, 577–578, *578*
  intravenous infusion, *260*
  saturability, *449*
  saturable first-pass metabolism, *196, 452, 452*
Nicotine
  hepatic extraction, *121*
  tolerance, 281, *282*
  and urinary pH, *154*
Nifedipine
  absorption, *193,* 193–194
  BCS, *203*
  constant-rate devices, *261*
  kinetics, rectal infusion, *288*
  in plasma unbound, *98*
  tolerance, 281, 281–282, *283*
9-13-17-21 regimen, *550*
Nitrazepam
  distribution parameters, *700, 701*
  hepatic extraction, *121*
  pKa values, *692*
Nitroglycerin
  dosage regimen, *302*
  single-dose therapy, 256
  tolerance, development of, 319–320
Nonadherence
  patterns of, *342,* 540–543
  source of variability, *11*
Noncompetitive inhibition, 495
Nonlinearities
  capacity-limited metabolism, 452–453
    alcohol, 453–455, *454, 455, 456*
    phenytoin, 455–459, *457, 458, 459*
  causes of, 446
  concentration-dependent renal excretion, *460,* 460–463, *461, 462, 463*
  dose-dependent, 445, *446*
  dose-independent, 446
  drug overdose kinetics, 476, *476*
  linear, 446
  metabolite formation or elimination, 620–621, *621*
  nonlinear absorption, 450–452
    saturable active transport, 451–452
    solubility, 450–451, *451*
  nonlinear kinetic behavior, 446
  pharmacodynamics, 449–450, *450*
  principle of superposition, 446
  recognition of, 472–476
    concentration-time profile, *473,* 473–475
    protein-binding data, *474, 475,* 475–476
    urinary recovery, *472,* 472–473
  saturable, 446
  saturable binding to plasma proteins, 448–449, *449,* 464–468, *465, 466, 467*
    autoinduction, 465
    concentration-dependent behavior, 464
  saturable first-pass metabolism, 452, *452, 453*
  saturable metabolism, 446–448, *447, 448*
  saturable transport, 448, 463–464

  therapeutic consequences, 476–477
  time-dependent disposition, 468–472, *469, 470, 471, 472*
  time-dependent kinetics, 446
  tissue binding, 468, *468*
Norelgestromin (Ortho Evra), *262*
Norepinephrine, *127*
Norfloxacin, *499*
Normal immune globulin, *639*
Nortriptyline
  drug interactions, *501, 530*
  and genetic polymorphism, *361*
  half-life, in plasma, *139*
  hepatic extraction, *121, 613*
  metabolites, *604*
  multiple active species, 255
  plasma concentration, *253,* 254, *544*
  studies in twins, *358*
  variable responses, 334, *335, 530*
Norvir. *See* Ritonavir (Norvir)
NuvaRing. *See* Etonogestrel (NuvaRing)

O
Obesity, and dosage, 395
Octreotide
  extravascular administration, 160
  protein drugs, *635*
Olanzapine, and cigarette smoking, 344
Olsalazine, *191*
Omalizumab (Xolair), *639, 642, 655*
Omeprazole
  dissolution, in intestine, 202, 233
  duration, of effect, 237
  pharmacodynamics rate-limits, 233, *234*
  saturable first-pass metabolism, *196*
Ondansetron, *121*
Ontak. *See* Denileukin diftitox (Ontak)
Oral administration, 23
Oral bioavailability
  causes of loss, 189–192, *190, 191*
    first-pass loss, 191–192
    intestinal reactions, 190–191
  in cirrhosis, 405, *405*
Orlistat (Xenical), first-pass loss, 191–192
Ortho Evra. *See* Norelgestromin (Ortho Evra)
Overdose
  dialysis in, 436–437
  kinetics, nonlinearities, 476, *476*
Oxacillin, *127, 139,* 490
Oxaliplatin
  chronopharmacology, 344, *344*
  variability, 345
Oxazepam
  pharmacodynamic prediction, *680*
  in plasma unbound, *98*
  variability, in metabolism, 408
Oxidation
  inherited variability, 360–363
  metabolic reactions, 113–114
Oxycodone
  dosage regimen, maintenance level, *302*
  modified-release dosage forms, 312
Oxytocin
  permeability, 77
  protein drugs, *634*

P
Paclitaxel
  absorption, 195
  drug transport, *82*
  leukocytes in blood, *7*
  permeability, 188
  plasma concentration-time course, 234–235, *235*
  time delay, pharmacodynamics, *7, 7,* 7–8
PAH. *See* Para-aminohippuric acid
Palivizumab (Synagis), *639, 655*
Pamidronate (Aredia), *121*
Pancrelipase, *635, 641*

Pancuronium, *599, 601*
Panitumumab (Vectibix), *639*
Pantoprazole
  dissolution, in intestine, 202
  genetic polymorphisms, *359*
Papain
  immunotoxicotherapeutic agents, 648
  protein drugs, *635*, 637, *638*
  protein drugs, administration, *641*
Para-aminohippuric acid (PAH)
  protein binding, perfusion, 132
  renal clearance, 423
Paracellular, drug transport, 75, *76*
Parenteral administration, 23
Paroxetine
  classification of inhibitors, *499*
  clearance, altered, *495*
  elimination, *115*
  hepatic extraction, *121*
  oxidation, 362
  in plasma unbound, *98*
  saturability, *449*
Partial agonist, 31
Partial antagonist, 31
Partition coefficient, 74
Passive diffusion, 76
Passive facilitated diffusion, 80
Pegintron. *See* Interferon Alpha-2b (Pegintron)
Pegvisomant, *635*
Penciclovir, *121*
Penicillin
  absorption, 166, *167*
  drug maintenance, in therapeutic range, 303
  and probenecid interaction, 505
Penicillin G
  absorption, 166, *167, 191*
  half-life, in plasma, *139*
  permeability-rate limitation, 92
  in plasma unbound, *98*
  saturability, *449*
Pentagastrin, *234, 634*
Pentazocine (Talwin)
  first-pass loss, 192
  and meperidine, *439*
Pentobarbital
  and alprenolol interaction, 143, *143*, 210, *211*
  permeability-rate limitation, 91–92
Pentoxyphylline, in hepatic cirrhosis, 440
Perfusion
  hepatic clearance, 121–122, *122*
  limitation, *90,* 90–91
  rate limitation, 85–91, *87, 88, 89, 90*
  renal clearance, 131–132, *132*
Peritoneal dialysis
  clearance, 434–435, *435*
  definition, 425
  route of administration, 435–436, *436*
Permeability
  absorption and jejunal permeability, *188*
  distribution rate, to tissues, 85
  in drug transport, 76–79, *77, 78*
  hepatic clearance, 126–127, *127*
  rate limitation, *91,* 91–93, *93*
Pertussis immune globulin, *639*
PH
  partition hypothesis, 78–79, 691–693, *692, 693*
  urine, 211–212, *212*
Pharmaceutical formulation, variability, 342, *601*
Pharmacodynamic phase, definition, 4–5
Pharmacodynamics
  agonists, 31
  antagonists, 31
  definition, 5
  drug response assessment, 33–35, *34, 35*
    baseline, 33
    disease progression, 35
    endogenous compounds, 33
    exogenous administration, 33
    placebo effect, 33
  drug therapy applications, *18*

PK/PD modeling, 31
response, exposure relationship, 36–40
  cumulative frequency, 38, *39*
  desirable characteristics, 39–40
  drug potency, 39
  drug specificity, 39
  graded response, 36–38
  maximum effect of drug, 40
  quantal response, 38–39, *39*
  steepness factor, 37
response classification, 31–33, *32*
  all-or-none response, 32
  biomarker, 32
  clinical response, 31
  grade, 32
  quantal response, 32
  safety biomarkers, 32
  surrogate endpoint, 31
time factors, 7
up-or-down regulation, 30
variability, *529*
Pharmacogenetics, 357
Pharmacogenomics, 357
Pharmacokinetic concepts
  absorption and disposition models, *25,* 25–28, *26, 27*
    compartments, 26
  active metabolites and prodrugs, 22
  ADME, *28*
  anatomic, physiologic considerations, 22–25
    drug distribution, 25
    sites of administration, 23–25, *24*
  biliary secretion, 30
  chemical purity, analytic specificity, 20–22, *21*
  definition, 5
  drug therapy applications, *18*
  fecal excretion, 30
  phase, 4–5
  sites of measurement, *19*
  systemic absorption, 28–29, *29*
  systemic exposure, 18
    exposure-time profile, *19,* 19–20
    observation period, 20
    sites of measurement, 18, *19*
    unbound drug concentration, 18–19
Pharmacokinetic parameters
  estimation of, 63–67, *64*
    computer use, 66
    measurement fluid, 66
    plasma and urine data, 64–66, *65*
    plasma data alone, 63–64, *65*
    precision of, 66
  extravascular dose, *172,* 172–176, *173*
    plasma data alone, 173–175, *175*
    urine data alone, 175–176
  fraction excreted unchanged, 63
  multiple-dose regimens, 313–315
    accumulation, 313–314, *314*, 314–315
    clearance/bioavailability, 313
    fluctuation at plateau, 314–315
    half-life, 313
  and physiologic variables, 140–151
    blood flow, 145–147, *146, 147*
    metabolic inhibition, 143–145, *144, 145*
    metabolism induction, *142,* 142–143, *143*
    plasma protein binding, *148,* 148–151, *149, 150, 151*
    primary parameters, 140–141, *141*
    renal tubular secretion, *147,* 147–148
    secondary parameters, 141, *141*
  saturability, of processes and mechanisms, *449*
  variability, 529–534, *532*
Pharmacokinetic-pharmacodynamic (PK/PD) modeling, 31
Phenelzine, *359*
Phenobarbital
  and dicumarol interaction, 511, *511*
  and furosemide interaction, 487
  half-life, *298,* 298–299
  in hemodialysis patients, 431–432, 434
  in plasma unbound, *98*
  reversibility of transport, 84–85
  urine pH and urine flow, *137*

Phenotypes, 357
Phenprocoumon, time delay causes, 224, *225*
Phenylbutazone, and warfarin interaction, 512–513, *513*
Phenytoin
    capacity-limited metabolism, 455–459
    in plasma unbound, *98*
    protein binding in renal disease, *148*, 423
    removal by hemodialysis, 441
    in renal dysfunction, *148*, 148–149
    short-term infusions, 271–272
    therapeutic response, 248–249
    untoward effects, *252*, 253
    variable responses, *9*
Physiologic considerations
    sites of administration
        extravascular, 23, *24*
        intravascular, 23
        parenteral, 23, *24*
        regional, 25
    systemic drug delivery, 25
Physiologic functions, change with age, *383*
Physiologic variables and pharmacokinetic parameters. *See*
        Pharmacokinetic parameters
Pimozide, *509*
Piperacillin, *104*
Piroxicam
    maintenance in therapeutic range, 301–304, *302, 304*
    and nonadherence, 556
Pivampicillin, 190, *191*
PK/PD modeling. *See* Pharmacokinetic-pharmacodynamic
        (PK/PD) modeling
Placebo effect, *33*, 33–35, *35*
Plasma
    and blood, concentration ratio, 118, 703–704
    clearance kinetics, 117–118
    concentration (*See* Plasma concentration)
    disposition of intravenous administration, *50*,
        50–62, *51*
    drug concentrations, 543–545, *544*
    excretion of extravascular dose, 173–174
Plasma concentration
    accumulation, *294*, 294–295, *295*
    concentration-dependent renal excretion, 460, *460*
    data presentation, 50, *50, 51*
    drug accumulation principles, *294*, 294–295, *295*
    drug effects and, 8
    and drug interactions, *502*
    MRT, *719*, 719–721, *720*
    multiple-dose regimens
        and amount in body, 307
        design of regimens, 307–311, *309, 310, 311*
    single dose of drug
        metabolites, 607–611, *608, 609, 610*
    time factors, 7
Plasma-to-blood concentration ratio, 118, 703–704
Plateau
    accumulation
        amount of drug in body, 723–724
    in constant-rate infusion, *264*, 264–265
        events at, 574–577, *575*
        metabolite kinetics, 615–617, *616*
        time to reach, *266*, 266–267, *267*, 577–581, *578, 579,*
        580
        value, *264*, 264–265
    multiple-dose regimens
        accumulation, 295–297, *296*
        average level at, 297–298
        fluctuation degree at, 314–315
        rate of accumulation, *298*, 298–299, *299*
        steady state, 724
Plavix. *See* Clopidogrel (Plavix)
Pleural cavity, drug administration, 25
Polymodal frequency distribution, 357
Polymorphism, genetics. *See* Genetics
Polymyxin B sulfate, *641*
Polypeptide therapeutic agents, *634–637*
Pool size
    constant-rate infusion, 275, *275*
    steady-state establishment, 277–278, *278, 279, 280*
    turnover concepts, 41

Poor metabolizers, 360, *367*
Population pharmacodynamics, 336
Potency, pharmacodynamic drug characteristics, 39
Pravastatin
    drug transport, *82*
    high biliary clearance, 128
    permeability, 127
    therapy management, 538, *539*
Prazepam, *604*
Prediction of human kinetics
    absorption, 675–677, *676, 677*
    allometry and disposition kinetics, 664–672
        application to drugs, 666–670, *667, 668, 669*
        deviation from expectation, 670–671
        origin, *664*, 664–666, *665, 666*
        protein binding correction, *671*
    clearance, 672–674, *673, 674*
    distribution, 674, *675*
    microdosing, 671–672, *672*
    pharmacodynamics, *680*, 680–682, *681, 682*
    virtual patient populations, 682–685, *683, 684, 685*
    whole-body physiologic models, *678*, 678–680, *679*
Prednisolone, metabolites, 622–623, *623*
Prednisone
    drug response, *35*
    interconversion, *622*, 622–623, *623*
    metabolites, *604*
Premature newborn
    creatine clearance, *382*, *382*
    metabolism, 385–386, *386*
Primaquine
    BCS, *203*
    genetic polymorphisms, *9*, 360
Primary parameters, 140–141
Primaxin. *See* Cilastatin (Primaxin); Imipenem (Primaxin)
Primidone, *604*
Priming dose, 300
Principle of superposition, 446
Probenecid
    albumin, binding to, *490*
    and penicillin interaction, 505, 509
    turnover, altered, 277
    volume of distribution, *104*
Procainamide, *177*
Procarbazine, *78*
Prodrugs
    active metabolites and, 22, *23*
    elimination, 115
Progesterone, 262
Proguanil, *367*
Promazine, *203*
Propafenone
    classification of inhibitors, *499*
    saturable first-pass metabolism, *196*
Propofol
    anesthesia, rapid induction, 273
    BCS, *203*
    distribution properties, *98*, 99, *99*, 101, *101*
    duration of anesthesia, *600*
    elimination, *139*, 147, *147*, 149, *149*
    infusion rate, chronic administration, 273
    intravenous infusion, 260
    permeability, *188*
    pharmacodynamics, 355
    saturable first-pass metabolism, *196*
    short-term infusions, 272
    slow tissue distribution, *273*
Propranolol
    in cirrhosis, *405*
    effect of food, 215
    fraction unbound in plasma, 149, *149*
    graded response, *37*, 37–38, *38*
    and lidocaine interaction, 147, *147*, 512
    and pharmacokinetic variability, 529–530, *530*
    plasma protein binding, *99*
    in plasma unbound, *98*
    tissue distribution, 101, *101*, 219
    reduction in exercise tachycardia, 239
    variability in response, 349, *349*, 350, *350*
Propylthiouracil, 359

ProstaScint Kit. *See* Capromab pendetide (ProstaScint Kit)
Protein binding
    altered plasma, *148,* 148–151, *149, 150, 151*
    and drug transport, 75–76
    hepatic clearance, 122–125, *124*
    in plasma, 96–100, *98, 99*
    renal clearance, 131–132, *132*
Protein drugs
    concurrent disease states, 655–656
        hepatic disease, 656
        renal disease, *655,* 655–656, *656*
    and conventional non protein drugs, pharmacokinetics
        absorption, 640
        distribution, 640–643, *641, 642, 643*
        metabolism, 645–646
        renal handling, 643–645, *644, 645*
    immunogenic responses, 658, *658*
    intravenous administration, 650
    nonlinearities, 656–657, *657*
    peptide, polypeptide and protein drugs, 633–639,
        634–637, 638, 639
    pharmacodynamics, 646–650
        of antibody drugs, *647,* 647–649, *648*
        of nonantibody protein drugs, *646,* 646–647
        and pharmacokinetic rate limitations, 649–650, *650*
    subcutaneous and intramuscular administration,
        650–655
        absorption, 652–654, *653, 654, 655*
        large proteins and lymphatic transport, 650–652,
            651, 652
Protein (nonantibody) therapeutic agents, *634–637*
Protein-binding data, nonlinearities, *474, 475,* 475–476
Protriptyline, 301, 320
Pulmicort. *See* Budesonide (Pulmicort)
Pulmonary administration, 23
Pulmozyme. *See* Dornase alfa (Pulmozyme)
Pyridostigmine, low oral bioavailability, 186–187, *188*

Q
Quantal responses
    classification, 32–33
    cumulative frequency, 38–39, *39*
    exposure and, 38–39
Quinacrine, *94*
Quinidine
    and digoxin interaction, *514,* 514–515
    in plasma unbound, *98*

R
Rabies immune globulin, *639*
Ranibizumab (Lucentis), *639*
Ranitidine
    absorption *v.* location in small intestine, 186, *187,* 189
    in plasma unbound, *98*
Rapamune. *See* Sirolimus (Rapamune)
Raptiva. *See* Efalizumab (Raptiva)
Rasburicase (Elitek), *104*
Rate limitation
    extravascular dose
        absorption, disposition, 166–167, *167*
    metabolites, 605–607, *606*
    perfusion, 85–91, *86, 87, 88, 89*
    permeability, *91,* 91–93, *93*
    protein drugs
        pharmacodynamic and pharmacokinetic,
            649–650, *650*
Rebif. *See* Interferon Beta-1a (Rebif)
Reclast. *See* Zoledronic acid (Reclast, Zometa)
Rectal administration, 23
Reduction, 113
Refludan. *See* Lepirudin (Refludan)
Regional administration, 25
Relative fluctuation, 299
Remicade. *See* Infliximab (Remicade)
Remifentanil
    gastric emptying, 185, *185*
    intravenous infusion, *260*
Renal. *See* Kidneys

Renal clearance
    concentration-dependent, *460,* 460–463, *461,
        462, 463*
    elimination pathways, 62–63
    equilibrium, *133,* 133–134
    nephron, 129–137
        active secretion, 131
        anatomy and function, *129,* 129–130
        glomerular filtration, *130,* 130–131
        protein binding and perfusion, 131–132, *132*
        tubular reabsorption, 132–137, *133, 134, 135, 136,
            137*
Renal function (RF), 414–419
    creatinine, estimation of, 416–419, *417, 418, 419*
    GFR, estimation of, *415,* 415–416
Renal metabolism, 137
ReoPro. *See* Abciximab (ReoPro)
Rescriptor. *See* Delavirdine mesylate (Rescriptor)
Residence times, 56
Response
    all-or-none, 32–33
    assessment of, 33–36
        baseline, 33
        disease progression, 36, *36*
        endogenous compounds, 33
        exogenous, 33
        placebo effect, *33,* 33–35, *34*
    biomarker, 31–32
        safety, 32
    classification of, 31–33
    clinical, 31
    to drugs, variability, 8–10, *9*
    and exposure, 36–40
    graded, 32, *32,* 36–38, *38*
        steepness factor, 37, *37*
    metabolite kinetics, 621
    quantal, 32–33, 38–39
        cumulative frequency, 38–39, *39*
    single dose, 217–237
        concentration-response relationship, 226–229, *227,
            228, 229*
        duration of effect, 235–237, *236, 237*
        effect compartment, 227, *227*
        onset of effect, 235
        pharmacodynamic rate-limit decline, 232–235, *233,
            234, 235*
        pharmacodynamics, 220, *220, 221, 222*
        pharmacokinetic rate-limit decline, *230,* 230–232,
            231, 232
        systems in flux, 222–226, *223, 224, 225, 226*
        time delay causes, 219–226
        time delay detection, *218,* 218–219, *219*
    surrogate endpoint, 31
Reversibility of drug transport, 84–85, *85*
RF. *See* Renal function
Rho(D) immune globulin, *639*
Rifampin
    and atorvastatin interaction, *515,* 515–516
    induction, low extraction ratio, 209–210, *210*
    induction of metabolism, 142, *142*
    intestinal absorption, and permeability, 189
    plasma concentration monitoring, *544*
    and warfarin interaction, *485, 495*
Ritonavir (Norvir)
    classification of inhibitors, *499*
    drug interactions, *495,* 509
    hepatic first-pass loss, 195
    high extraction ratio, 144–145, *145*
    interaction with digoxin, 522
    intestinal absorption, permeability, 189
    and lopinavir combination, *486*
    tubular secretion, *147,* 147–148
Rituxan. *See* Rituximab (Rituxan)
Rituximab (Rituxan), *639, 647*
Rivastigmine (Exelon), *196*
Rolipram, 289, *289*
Romazicon. *See* Flumazenil (Romazicon)
Rosiglitazone (Avandia), *203*
Rosuvastatin (Crestor), 127
    interaction with cyclosporine, *505*

Routes of administration
  extravascular, 23, *24*, 159–160
  intravascular, 23, 49–50

S
Safety biomarker, 32
Salicylic acid
  absorption, *191*
  albumin, binding to, *490*
  following aspirin administration, *23*
  biotransformation patterns, *113*
  clearance, altered, 512
  concentration-time profile, *473, 474*
  first-pass loss, 191–192
  hepatic extraction, *121*
  long-term infusion, 576–577
  metabolites, 22, *23, 604*
  nonlinear disposition, *473, 474, 475*
  permeability-rate limitation, *91*, 91–92
  pharmacodynamics, 232
  renal clearance, 136, *136*
  variability in response, *530*
  volume of distribution, *104*
Saquinavir (Invirase)
  absorption, 195
  inhibition, *501*
  intestinal absorption, permeability, 188
  and midazolam interaction, *485*
Saruplase, 670
Saturable, 446
Saturable binding, to plasma proteins, 448–449, *449*, 464–468
Saturable first-pass metabolism
  absorption from solution, *196*
  nonlinearities, 452, *452, 453*
Saturable processes
  pharmacodynamics, 449–450, *450*
  saturable binding to plasma proteins, 448–449
  saturable metabolism, 446–448
    Michaelis-Menten model, 446–447
  saturable transport, 448, *463*, 463–464
Schwartz method of estimation, *416*
Scopolamine, 262
Secondary pharmacokinetic parameters, 141, *141*
Sequential metabolism, 605
Sermorelin, *634*
Sertraline, *499*
Serum creatinine
  age and, *417*
  renal function assessment, 414–419, *415, 416, 418*
Sevoflurane (Ultane), *401*
Sildenafil citrate (Viagra)
  and erythromycin interaction, *485*
  inhibition, *501*
  metabolites, 22
Simulect. *See* Basiliximab (Simulect)
Simvastatin
  biotransformation patterns, *113*
  hepatic first-pass loss, *194,* 194–195, *195*
  turnover, drug response, 42
Single dose response
  concentration-response relationship, 226–229
    effect compartment, 227, *227*
    systems in flux, *228*, 228–229, *229*
  duration of effect, 235–237, *236, 237*
  hysteresis, 218
  onset of effect, 235
  response decline, with time, 229–235
    pharmacodynamics rate-limits decline, 232–235, *233, 234, 235*
    pharmacokinetics rate-limits decline, *230*, 230–232, *231*
  time delay causes
    pharmacodynamic rate-limited response, 222
    pharmacodynamics, *220*, 220–222, *221*
    pharmacokinetic rate-limited response, 222
    systems in flux, 222–226, *223, 224, 225, 226*
    tissue distribution, 219–220
  time delay detection, *218*, 218–219, *219*
Single-dose therapy, 256

Singulair. *See* Montelukast (Singulair)
Sirolimus (Rapamune), 300–301, *302*
Sites of administration, 23–25, *24*
Skin, as a functional membrane, 74, *75*
Solids, absorption of. *See* Absorption
Solubility, nonlinear absorption, 450–451, *451*
Solutions, absorption from. *See* Absorption
Somatropin
  genetic polymorphisms, *634*
  systemic absorption, 653
  volume of distribution, *104*
Sparteine, 370
Specificity, pharmacodynamic drug characteristics, 39
St. John's Wort
  drug interactions, 484
  intestinal absorption, permeability, 189
  variable response, 343, *343*
Starting dose, 534–535, *535*
Steady state
  accumulation to plateau, 724
  constant-rate input, 264, 277–278, *278, 279, 280*
Steepness factor, 37
Stomach. *See also* Gastric emptying
  absorption, 184–185, *187*
Streptomycin, *188*
Subcutaneous administration
  definition, 23
  protein drugs, 650–655
    absorption, 652–654, *653, 654, 655*
    large proteins and lymphatic transport, 650–652, *651, 652*
Sublingual administration, 23
Succinylcholine
  duration of effect, 236–237, *237*
  inherited variability of response, 366
  pharmacokinetics rate-limits, *231*, 231–232
Sucralfate, 200
Sufentanil, *601, 681*
Sulfamethazine, 370
Sulfasalazine, 202
Sulfinpyrazone, *499*
Sulindac
  interconversion, *622*, 622–623
  metabolites, *604*
Sumatriptan, *191*, 207
Suprane. *See* Desflurane (Suprane)
Surface area
  in children, 385, 392–393
  dosage adjustment for age, 390
  and gastrointestinal absorption, 184–186
Surmontil. *See* Trimipramine (Surmontil)
Surrogate endpoint, 31
Surrogates, therapy management, 538
Synagis. *See* Palivizumab (Synagis)
Synergism, 485
Systemic absorption, 28–29, *29*
  bioavailability, 29
  definition, 28–29, 29
  first-pass loss, 29
  intestinal absorption, 29

T
Tachyphylaxis, 319
Tacrolimus
  hepatic first-pass loss, *193,* 193–194
  inhibition, 504
  plasma-to-blood concentration ratio, 153
Talwin. *See* Pentazocine (Talwin)
Talwin, first-pass loss, 192
Tamoxifen
  genetic polymorphism, 367
  pKa values, *692*
Tamsulosin (Flomax), 21
Target concentration. *See* Monitoring
Target-mediated drug disposition, 468
Taxol, *115*, 495
Teicoplanin, 435, *436*
Telithromycin (Ketek), *425, 499*
Tenecteplase (TNKase), *642*

Terazosin, 536, 538
Terbutaline, *188*
Terfenadine, drug interactions, 10, 484
Teriparatide (Forteo), *636*
Testosterone
   after intravenous dose, *602*
   and leuprolide acetate depot formulation, 649, *650*
   in plasma unbound, *98*
Tetanus immune globulin, *639*
Theophylline
   absorption and disposition rate limitations, 166, *167*
   and cigarette smoking, 344
   and enoxacin interaction, *496*, 496–498, *498*, 500
   kinetic manifestations, 349, *349*
   modified-release dosage forms, 312
   plasma concentration-time profile, 70, *70*
   renal clearance and, 462
   therapeutic exposure, 254
   therapeutic index, 303
Therapeutic concentration range, 250
Therapeutic drug interaction, 484
Therapeutic effectiveness, 248
Therapeutic index, 255
Therapeutic relevance
   clinical setting, 3–12
      adherence, *11*, 11–12, *12*
      dosage regimen, 3, *4*
      input-response phases, 4–8
      pharmacodynamic phase, 4, *4*, *7*
      pharmacokinetic phase, 4, *4*
      therapeutic window, *5*, *6*
      variability, drug response, 8–10, *9*
   industrial perspective, 12–13
      drug development, *13*
Therapeutic utility curve, 250
Therapeutic window
   dosage regimen, 5–8, 245–247, *246*
   drug exposure range, *5*
   duration *v.* intensity of exposure, 256
   multiple active species, 255
   plasma drug concentration, *6*
   single-dose therapy, 256
   therapeutic exposure, *247*, 247–255, *249*, *251*, *252*, *253*
      therapeutic concentration range, 250
      therapeutic effectiveness, 248
      therapeutic utility curve, 250
   therapeutic index, 255
   time delays, 256
Therapy
   discontinuation, 543
   dose titration, 535–536
   management
      adherence, 540–543, *541*, *542*
      biomarkers, 538, *539*
      clinical endpoints, 538, *539*
      dose strengths, 539–540
      low therapeutic index, *536*, 536–538, *537*
      surrogates, 538, *539*
      tolerance, 538–539
   pharmacodynamic variability, 529, *529*
   pharmacokinetic variability, 529–534, *530*
      body weight and, 532, *532*
      genetics and, 532, *533*
      measurable characteristics, 530, *531*
   starting dose, 534–535, *535*
   strategies, 527–528, *528*
   target concentration strategy, 543–554
      changes in therapy, 554
      concentration monitoring, 545
      dose and interval unequal, 552
      estimates, 552–554, *553*
      evaluation procedure, 545–548, *546*, *547–548*
      information needed, 545
      missed dose(s), *549*, 549–550
      9-13-17-21 regimen, *550*, 550–552
      plasma drug concentrations, 543–545, *544*
   and variability sources, 528–534
Thioguanine, 363, *364*
Thiopental
   distribution kinetics, 562, *562*, 595, *595*

drug therapy monitoring, *539*
permeability-rate limitation, *91*
pKa values, *692*
rate of distribution to tissues, *86*
Thiopurine methyltransferase (TPMT)
   genetic polymorphism, 363
   pharmacokinetic variability, 533, *533*
Thyroxine, *539*
Ticlid. *See* Ticlopidine (Ticlid)
Ticlopidine (Ticlid), *449*
Time delays, response, 6–8, *7*
Time-dependent disposition, 468–472
   chronopharmacokinetics, 468
   circadian changes, *470*
   time-dependent kinetics, 446, 468, 468–469
Timolol maleate
   genetic polymorphisms, *359*
   variability in response, 342
Tipranavir
   inhibition, *501*
   saturability, *449*
Tirofiban (Aggrastat), *260*
Tissue binding, 468
Tissue-type plasminogen activator (t-PA), 262–263, *263*, *269*, 662
TNKase. *See* Tenecteplase (TNKase)
Tobramycin
   distribution and elimination, *61*
   dosage adjustment, age, 394
Tolbutamide
   albumin, binding to, *490*
   genetic polymorphisms, *359*, 362
   hepatic clearance, 124, *124*
   metabolites, *610*, 610–611
   volume of distribution, *104*
Tolerance
   in constant-rate infusion, 280–284, *281*, *282*, *283*
   in multiple-dose regimens, 319–320
   tachyphylaxis, 319
   therapy management, 538–539
Tolmetin, *104*
Tolterodine tartrate (Detrol), *501*, *674*, *692*
Tositumomab (Bexxar), *639*
Toxicity
   in dosage regimen, 3
   metabolites, 437
   therapeutic window, *249*, 249–250
TPMT. *See* Thiopurine methyltransferase
Tracleer. *See* Bosentan (Tracleer)
Trandolapril (Mavik), 466–468, *467*
Transcellular drug transport, 75, *76*
Transdermal delivery, 207
Transport maximum
   drug transport, 81
   saturable transport, 448
Transport of drugs. *See* Drug transport
Transporter, 81
Trapezoidal rule, 687, *687*
Trastuzumab (Herceptin)
   protein drugs, *639*, *642*
   short-term infusions, 272
   variability in response, 368, *530*
Triazolam
   hepatic first-pass loss, 193, *193*
   inhibition, *501*
   time delay causes, 222
Trimipramine (Surmontil), 532, *533*
Troleandomycin, *142*, 144, *509*
Trough, drug accumulation, 297
Tubocurarine, 590, *590*, *599*
Turnover concepts
   constant-rate input, 275, 275–280
      altered turnover, 275, *276*, 276–277
      non–steady-state, 279–280, *281*
      steady-state, 264, 277–278, *278*, *279*, 280
   creatinine clearance in renal failure, 418–419, *419*
   in drug response, 41–43, *42*
   endogenous substances, 577
Turnover rate, 41, 275, *278*, *279*
Turnover time, 41, 276, *276*, *278*, *279*

Two-compartment model, *565*
Typical patient, *374*, 374–376, *375*

U

Ultane. *See* Sevoflurane (Ultane)
Unbound clearance
  plasma *v.* blood clearance, 118
  renal dysfunction, *411*, 411–414, *412*, *413*
Unbound drug, 75
Unimodal frequency distribution
  inherited variability, 357
  variability in response, 338
Up-or-down regulation, 30
Urine
  bioavailability, 175–176
  nonlinear recovery, *472*, 472–473
  pharmacokinetic parameters, *64*, 64–66, *65*
Urine pH
  drug disposition increase, 211–212, *212*
  and renal clearance, 512
Urokinase, *637*
Usual dosage regimen, 376–377

V

Vaccinia immune globulin, *639*
Valcyte. *See* Valganciclovir (Valcyte)
Valganciclovir (Valcyte)
  intestinal reactions, 191
  renal function, *211*
Valproic acid
  dosage adjustment, for age, *393*
  dose titration, 535
  drug interactions, 489–490, *490*, 492, *493*
  pKa values, *692*
  plasma concentration, *544*
  therapeutic exposures, *253*
Valsartan (Diovan), 127
Vancomycin
  9-13-17-21 regimen, *550*
  dosage in child, 440
  and hemodialysis, *443*
  intestinal absorption, permeability, 187, *188*, 198
  peritoneal dialysis clearance, 442
  target concentration strategy, 545, *547–548*, 551–553
Variability
  dose strengths and, 352–353
  dose-response relationship, 345
  drug response, 8–10, *9*
  individual differences, *334*, 334–339, *335*
    bimodal, 338
    coefficient of variation, 338, *338*, *339*
    describing variability, 338–339
    population pharmacodynamics, 336
    population pharmacokinetics, 336
    quantifying variability, 336–337, *337*
    unimodal, 338
  interindividual, 333
  intraindividual, 333
  kinetic manifestations, 348–352, *349*, *350*, *351*
  in metabolite kinetics, 618–620, *619*
  pharmacodynamic, 529
  reasons for, 339–345, *340*, *341*, *353*
    adherence, 341, *342*
    age and weight and, 340
    chronopharmacology, 344, *344*
    cigarette smoking, 344
    disease and, 341
    environmental pollutants, 344
    food, 342
    genetics and, 339
    herbal preparations, 343, *343*
    persistence, 341
    pharmaceutical formulation, 342
    therapeutic exposure, 345–348, *346*, *347–348*
Varicella-zoster immune globulin (Varivax), *639*
Varivax. *See* Varicella-zoster immune globulin (Varivax)
Vasopressin, *636*
Vectibix. *See* Panitumumab (Vectibix)
Venlafaxine (Effexor), *98*, *509*

Verapamil hydrochloride
  BCS, *203*
  classification of inhibitors, *499*
  and hepatic disease, 406, *406*
  hepatic extraction, *121*
  metabolites, *604*, *611*
  in plasma unbound, *98*
  saturable first-pass metabolism, *196*
  time-dependencies, *471*
  time-dependent disposition, 470, *470*
Viagra. *See* Sildenafil citrate (Viagra)
Vinblastine, 78, *78*
Vincristine, 78
Viomycin, *637*
Viracept. *See* Nelfinavir mesylate (Viracept)
Virtual patient populations, 682–685, *683*, *684*, *685*
Vitamin B_{12}, nonlinear bioavailability and renal excretion,
  463, *463*
Vitamin C, nonlinear bioavailability and renal excretion,
  462, 464
Vitamin K, pharmacodynamic interactions, 516
Volume of distribution
  apparent, 58, *94*, 94–96, *95*
  bolus distribution kinetics, *51*, 51–52
  clearance, area, and, 55–56
  definition, 52
  terminal phase, 57–59
Voriconazole, *196*, 197, *449*, *501*

W

Wagner-Nelson method, 713–715, *714–715*
  convolution, 713
  deconvolution, 713
Warfarin
  absorption, 209–210, *210*
  concentration-response relationship, *228*, 228–229, *229*
  daily dose required, *334*, *389*
  elimination, *113*
  genetics, unbound clearance, and weekly dose, *362*
  individual differences, *335*, 335–336, *336*
  and phenylbutazone interaction, 512–513, *513*
  in plasma unbound, *98*
  response, 6, *7*
  and rifampin interaction, *210*
  therapeutic index, 255
  therapeutic window, *253*
  time-delay, 223–224, *224*
  variability in response, 8, *9*, 10
  volume of distribution, *94*, *104*
Weight
  and aging, 378–380, *379*, *380*
  dosages and, 395–396
  lean body weight, 395
  therapy management, 532
  variability in response, 340
Well-stirred model
  memory aid, 125–126
  oral dose, events after, 707
  permeability considerations, 706–707
  rapid equilibration, drug in blood and liver, 705–706
Whole-body physiologic models, *678*, 678–680

X

Xenical. *See* Orlistat (Xenical)
Xolair. *See* Omalizumab (Xolair)

Z

Zafirlukast (Accolate), 30
Zenapax. *See* Daclizumab (Zenapax)
Zero order, 161
Zetia. *See* Ezetimibe (Zetia)
Ziagen. *See* Abacavir (Ziagen)
Zidovudine, *98*, 114, *203*, *604*
Zileuton (Zyflo), *689*
Zoladex. *See* Goserelin (Zoladex)
Zoledronic acid (Reclast, Zometa), 540
Zyflo. *See* Zileuton (Zyflo)